AACN

PROCEDURE
MANUAL *for*
CRITICAL CARE

AMERICAN
ASSOCIATION
of CRITICAL-CARE
NURSES

AACN
PROCEDURE
MANUAL *for*
CRITICAL CARE

Fifth Edition

Edited by:

Debra J. Lynn-McHale Wiegand
PhD, RN, CCRN, FAAN

Postdoctoral Fellow
Yale University School of Nursing
New Haven, Connecticut
Staff Nurse
Surgical Cardiac Care Unit
Thomas Jefferson University Hospital
Philadelphia, Pennsylvania

Karen K. Carlson
MN, RN, CCNS

Critical Care Clinical Nurse Specialist
The Carlson Consulting Group
Bellevue, Washington
Clinical Faculty
Department of Biobehavioral Nursing
University of Washington
Seattle, Washington

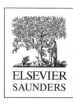

ELSEVIER
SAUNDERS

ELSEVIER
SAUNDERS

11830 Westline Industrial Drive
St. Louis, Missouri 63146

WY
49
A111
2005

AACN Procedure Manual for Critical Care, Fifth Edition
Copyright © 2005, Elsevier Inc. All rights reserved.

NOTICE

Previous editions copyrighted 2001, 1993, 1985, 1980.

ISBN-13: 978-0-7216-0452-7
ISBN-10: 0-7216-0452-8

Executive Publisher: Barbara Nelson Cullen
Developmental Editor: Laura Sieh Chu
Publishing Services Manager: John Rogers
Project Manager: Helen Hudlin
Designer: Kathi Gosche

Printed in United States of America
Last digit is the print number: 9 8 7 6 5 4 3 2

Contributors

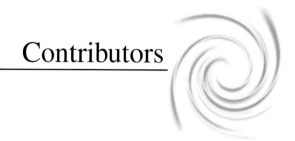

Mary G. Adams, PhD, RN, CNS
Assistant Professor, School of Nursing, The State
University of New York at Buffalo, Buffalo, New York;
Clinical Nurse, Trauma ICU, Eric County Medical Center,
Buffalo, New York
Continuous ST-Segment Monitoring

Nancy M. Albert, PhD(c), MSN, CCNS, CCRN, CNA
Director, Nursing Research and Innovation,
Cleveland Clinic Foundation, Cleveland, Ohio
Cardiac Output Measurement Techniques (Invasive)

Andrei V. Alexandrov, MD
Assistant Professor of Neurology, Director,
Cerebrovascular Ultrasound, University of Texas—Houston
Medical School, Houston, Texas
Transcranial Doppler Monitoring

Richard B. Arbour, MSN, RN, CCRN, CNRN
Staff Nurse, Clinical Researcher, Albert Einstein
Healthcare Network, Philadelphia, Pennsylvania
Bispectral Index Monitoring

Deborah E. Becker, MSN, CRNP, BC
Director, Adult Acute Care Nurse Practitioner Program,
School of Nursing, University of Pennsylvania,
Philadelphia, Pennsylvania
*Pericardiocentesis (Perform); Pericardiocentesis (Assist);
    Temporary Transvenous Pacemaker Insertion (Perform);
    Arterial Catheter Insertion (Perform)*

**Patricia A. Blissitt, PhD, RN, CCRN, CNRN, CCM,
APRN, BC**
Staff Nurse, Neuroscience Intensive Care Unit,
Duke University Hospital, Durham, North Carolina
*Lumbar Subarachnoid Catheter Insertion (Assist) for
    Cerebral Spinal Fluid Pressure Monitoring and Drainage*

Stephanie Bloom, MSN, RN
Research Nurse, Hospital of the University of Pennsylvania,
Philadelphia, Pennsylvania
*Brain Tissue Oxygenation Monitoring: Insertion (Assist),
    Care, and Troubleshooting*

Barbara A. Brown, MS, RN, CCRN, ANP
Nursing Program Manager, SICU and Burn Unit, Ohio
State University Medical Center, Columbus, Ohio
*Calculating Doses, Flow Rates, and Administration of
    Continuous Intravenous Infusions*

Linda Bucher, DNSc, RN
Associate Professor, University of Delaware, Newark,
Delaware; Nursing Research Facilitator, Christiana Care
Health System, Christiana Hospital, Newark, Delaware;
Per Diem Staff Nurse, Emergency Department, Virtua
Health System, Memorial Hospital, Mount Holly,
New Jersey
*Arterial Puncture; Peripheral Intravenous Catheter
    Insertion; Peripherally Inserted Central Catheter;
    Venipuncture*

**Suzanne M. Burns, MSN, RN, RRT, ACNP, CCRN,
FAAN, FCCM**
Professor of Nursing, School of Nursing, University of
Virginia, Charlottesville, Virginia; Advanced Practice
Nurse 2, Medical Intensive Care Unit, University of
Virginia Health System, Charlottesville, Virginia
*Arterial-Venous Oxygen Difference Calculation;
    Auto-PEEP Calculation; Compliance and Resistance
    Measurement; Manual Self-Inflating Resuscitation Bag;
    Indices of Oxygenation; Shunt Calculation; Ventilatory
    Management—Volume and Pressure Modes; Weaning
    Criteria—Negative Inspiratory Pressure, Positive End-
    Expiratory Pressure, Spontaneous Tidal Volume, and
    Vital Capacity Measurement; Weaning Process*

Karen K. Carlson, MN, RN, CCNS
Clinical Faculty, Department of Biobehavioral Nursing,
University of Washington, Seattle, Washington; Critical
Care Clinical Nurse Specialist, The Carlson Consulting
Group, Bellevue, Washington
  *Chest Tube Placement (Assist); Chest Tube Removal
    (Assist); Thoracentesis (Perform); Thoracentesis
    (Assist); Automated External Defibrillation;Nasogastric
    Tube Insertion, Care, and Removal; Paracentesis (Assist);
    Peritoneal Lavage (Assist); Scleral Endoscopic Therapy*

Marianne Chulay, DNSc, RN, FAAN
Consultant, Critical Care Nursing and Clinical Research,
Chapel Hill, North Carolina
  Suctioning: Endotracheal or Tracheostomy Tube

Bonnie L. Curtis, RN, CCRN
Core Charge Nurse, Critical Care, St. Cloud Hospital,
St. Cloud, Minnesota
  *Extubation/Decannulation (Perform);
    Extubation/Decannulation (Assist); Nasopharyngeal
    Airway Insertion; Oropharyngeal Airway Insertion;
    Tracheal Tube Cuff Care; Tracheostomy Tube Care*

Jacqueline M. Davis, RN
Staff Nurse, The Methodist Hospital, Houston, Texas
  Tong and Halo Pin Site Care

Janice Y. Dawson, BSN, RN
Staff Nurse, Department of Cardiology, Lankenau
Hospital, Jefferson Health System, Wynnewood,
Pennsylvania
  Transesophageal Echocardiography (Assist)

Michael W. Day, MSN, RN, CCRN
Adjunct Faculty, Intercollegiate College of Nursing,
Washington State University, Spokane, Washington;
Outreach Educator/Clinical Nurse Specialist, Northwest
MedStar, Spokane, Washington; Staff Nurse, Intensive
Care Unit, Sacred Heart Medical Center, Spokane,
Washington
  *Combitube Insertion and Removal; Laryngeal Mask
    Airway; Esophagogastric Tamponade Tube*

Robyn Dealtry, RN
College of Nursing, The St. George Hospital, Kogarah,
Clinical Nurse Consultant, Multidisciplinary Pain Service,
Westmead Hospital, New South Wales, Australia
  *Epidural Catheters: Assisting With Insertion and Pain
    Management; Peripheral Nerve Blocks (Assist)*

Barbara J. Drew, PhD, RN, FAAN
Professor of Nursing and Clinical Professor of Medicine,
University of California San Francisco, San Francisco,
California
  *Extra Electrocardiographic Leads: Right Precordial and
    Left Posterior Leads*

Phyllis Dubendorf, MSN, CRNP
Lecturer, Adult Acute Care Nurse Practitioner Program,
University of Pennsylvania, Philadelphia, Pennsylvania
  *Cerebrospinal Fluid Drainage Assessment;
    Ice-Water Caloric Testing for Vestibular
    Function (Assist); Lumbar and Cisternal
    Punctures (Assist)*

Margaret M. Ecklund, MS, RN, CCRN, APRN-BC
Clinician V, Advanced Practice Nurse, Rochester General
Hospital, Rochester, New York
  *Percutaneous Endoscopic Gastrostomy (PEG),
    Gastrostomy, or Jejunostomy Tube Care;
    Small-Bore Feeding Tube Insertion and Care*

Eleanor R. Fitzpatrick, MSN, RN, CCRN
Clinical Nurse Specialist, Surgical Critical Care and
Trauma, Thomas Jefferson University Hospital,
Philadelphia, Pennsylvania
  Vacuum-Assisted Closure (V.A.C.) System for Wounds

Desiree A. Fleck, MSN, RN, CCRN, CRNP, ACNP
Adult Nurse Practitioner, Adult Congenital Heart Disease
Center, The Children's Hospital of Philadelphia,
Philadelphia, Pennsylvania
  *Ventricular Assist Devices; Pulmonary Artery Catheter
    Insertion (Perform); Central Venous Catheter Insertion
    (Perform)*

Janet G. Whetstone Foster, PhD, RN, CNS, CCRN
Assistant Professor, Texas Women's University, Houston,
Texas; Director of Clinical Research, Memorial Hermann
Hospital, Houston, Texas; President, Nursing Inquiry and
Intervention, Inc., The Woodlands, Texas
  Peripheral Nerve Stimulators

John J. Gallagher, MSN, RN, CCNS, CCRN, RRT
Clinical Faculty, School of Nursing, Widener University,
Chester, Pennsylvania; Clinical Nurse Specialist, Surgical
Critical Care, Hospital of the University of Pennsylvania,
Philadelphia, Pennsylvania
  *Intraabdominal Pressure Monitoring;
    Intracompartmental Pressure Monitoring*

Karen K. Giuliano, PhD, RN, FAAN
Clinical Research Specialist, Philips Medical Systems,
Andover, Massachusetts
  *Continuous Mixed Venous Oxygen Saturation
    Monitoring*

Margaret T. Goldberg, MSN, RN, CWOCN
Wound Care Consultant, Wound Treatment Center, Delray
Medical Center, Delray Beach, Florida
  *Pressure-Reducing Devices: Lateral Rotation
    Therapy*

Vicki S. Good, MSN, RN, CCRN, CCNS
Director of Acute Care Services, Baylor All Saints Medical Center, Fort Worth, Texas
Continuous End-Tidal Carbon Dioxide Monitoring

Cindy Goodrich, MSN, RN, CCRN
Flight Nurse, Airlift Northwest, Seattle, Washington
Endotracheal Intubation (Perform); Needle Thoracostomy (Perform)

Charlotte A. Green, BSN, CCRN
Staff Nurse, Critical Care Unit, Group Health Cooperative, Eastside Hospital, Redmond, Washington
Automated External Defibrillation

Cynthia Hambach, MSN, RN, CCRN
Staff Nurse, Coronary Intensive Care Unit, Abington Memorial Hospital, Abington, Pennsylvania
Cardioversion; Defibrillation (External)

Joelle Hargraves, MSN, RN, CCRN
Transplant Assist Device Coordinator, Montefiore Medical Center, Bronx, New York
Ventricular Assist Devices

Jan M. Headley, BS, RN
JMH Consulting, Pepperell, Massachusetts
Continuous Mixed Venous Oxygen Saturation Monitoring

M.J. Heffernan, BSN, RN, OCN
Medical Oncology Nurse, Overlake Cancer Center, Overlake Internal Medical Associates, Bellevue, Washington; Procedure Nurse, Seattle Cancer Care Alliance, Seattle, Washington
Bone Marrow Biopsy and Aspiration (Perform); Bone Marrow Biopsy and Aspiration (Assist)

Elizabeth I. Helvig, MS, RN, CWOCN
Burn, Wound, Ostomy Clinical Nurse Specialist, Harborview Medical Center, Seattle, Washington
Donor Site Care; Burn Wound Care

Joanne V. Hickey, PhD, RN, ACNP, BC, FAAN
Professor of Nursing, Health Science Center at Houston, University of Texas, Houston, Texas; Neuroscience Nursing Consultant, The Methodist Hospital, Houston, Texas
External Fixation Device Insertion (Assist); HaloTraction Care; Tong and Halo Pin Site Care; Traction Maintenance

June Hinkle, BSN, MSN, CNP
Director, Bereavement Services, The Ohio State University Hospitals, Columbus, Ohio
Care of the Organ Donor; Identification of Potential Organ Donors; Request for Organ Donation

Linda M. Hoke, PhD, RN, CCRN
Clinical Nurse Specialist, Cardiac Care Unit, Hospital of the University of Pennsylvania, Philadelphia, Pennsylvania
Transesophageal Echocardiography (Assist)

Cindy Hudgens, BSN, CNRN
Manager, Stroke Unit, Methodist Hospital, Houston, Texas
Traction Maintenance

Merrie Jackson, ADN
Staff Nurse, Intensive Care Unit, Creighton University Medical Center, Omaha, Nebraska
Temporary Transvenous and Epicardial Pacing; Left Atrial Catheter: Care and Assisting With Removal

Carol Jacobson, MN, RN
Cardiovascular Clinical Nurse Specialist, Quality Education Service, Seattle, Washington
Atrial Overdrive Pacing (Perform)

Paul R. Jansen, BS, MBA
Director, Product, Technical, and Clinical Advocacy, Cardiodynamics International, San Diego, California
Noninvasive Hemodynamic Monitoring: Impedance Cardiography

Eileen M. Kelly, MSN, RN, CCRN
Clinical Nurse Specialist, Thomas Jefferson University Hospital, Philadelphia, Pennsylvania
Temporary Transcutanous (External) Pacing; External Warming/Cooling Devices

Mary Ellen Kern, MSN, RN, CCRN, APRN, CS
Clinical Nurse Specialist, Medical and Surgical Cardiac Units, Thomas Jefferson University Hospital, Philadelphia, Pennsylvania
Pericardial Catheter Management

Peggy Kirkwood, MSN, RN, ACNP, BC
Cardiovascular Nurse Practitioner, Mission Hospital, Mission Viejo, California; Associate Clinical Faculty, UCLA, Los Angeles, California
Chest Tube Removal (Perform); Chest Tube Removal (Assist); Paracentesis (Perform); Paracentesis (Assist); Peritoneal Lavage (Perform); Peritoneal Lavage (Assist); Wound Closure; Suture Removal

Deborah G. LaMarr, MSN, APRN, ACNP
Surgical Critical Care Nurse Practitioner, Hartford Hospital, Hartford, Connecticut
Emergent Open Sternotomy (Perform); Emergent Open Sternotomy (Assist); Esophageal Doppler Monitoring of Aortic Blood Flow: Probe Insertion; Esophageal Doppler Monitoring of Aortic Blood Flow: Care and Removal

Denise M. Lawrence, MS, RN, ACNP
Critical Care Nurse Practitioner, Hartford Hospital,
Hartford, Connecticut
  *Chest Tube Placement (Perform); Chest Tube Placement
  (Assist); External Counterpressure With Pneumatic
  Antishock Garments*

Jeanne R. Lowe, BA, RN, CCRN, CWCN
Preceptor for the University of Washington Wound
Management Education Program, University of
Washington, Seattle, Washington; Clinical Nurse Educator,
Harborview Medical Center, Seattle, Washington
  Skin Graft Care

Margaret M. Mahon, PhD, RN, FAAN
Senior Fellow, University of Pennsylvania Center for
Bioethics, Philadelphia, Pennsylvania; Advanced Practice
Nurse, Palliative Care and Ethics, Philadelphia,
Pennsylvania
  *Non-Heart-Beating Organ Donation (Donation After
  Cardiac Death); Withholding and Withdrawing
  Life-Sustaining Therapy*

Mary Beth Flynn Makic, MS, RN, CNS, CCRN
Senior Instructor, University of Colorado Health
Science Center, Denver, Colorado; Clinical Nurse
Specialist/Educator, University of Colorado Hospital,
Denver, Colorado
  *Cleaning, Irrigating, Culturing, and Dressing an Open
  Wound; Debridement: Pressure Ulcers, Burns, and
  Wounds; Dressing Wounds With Drains; Drain
  Removal; Pouching a Wound; Vacuum-Assisted Closure
  (V.A.C.) System for Wounds*

Marc Malkoff, MD
Associate Professor of Neurology, University of Texas—
Houston Medical School, Houston, Texas
  Lumbar Puncture (Perform)

**Eileen Maloney-Wilensky, MSN, RN, CRNP,
CCRN, CNRN**
Director, Neurosurgery Clinical Research Division,
Director, In-House CRNP/PA Team, Department of
Neurosurgery, University of Pennsylvania Health System,
Philadelphia, Pennsylvania
  *Brain Tissue Oxygenation Monitoring: Insertion (Assist),
  Care, and Troubleshooting*

Andrea Marshall, BN, RN, IC Cert., MN (Research)
Senior Research Fellow, Critical Care Nursing Professorial
Unit, University of Technology, Sydney, Broadway NSW,
Australia; Royal North Shore Hospital, St. Leonards NSW,
Australia
  *Monitoring Gastrointestinal Perfusion With
  a Gastric Tonometer*

**Rhonda K. Martin, MS, RN, MLT (ASCP), CCRN,
CNS/ANP-C**
Lecturer, School of Medicine, University of California,
San Diego, California; Nurse Practitioner/Clinical Nurse
Specialist, Hepatology and Abdominal Organ Transplant
Programs, San Diego Medical Center, University of
California, San Diego, California
  *Continuous Renal Replacement Therapies; Hemodialysis;
  Peritoneal Dialysis; Apheresis, Plasmapheresis, and
  Plasma Exchange*

Kathy McCloy, MSN, RN, ACNP
Acute Care Nurse Practitioner, Cardiology, UCLA Medical
Center, Los Angeles, California
  Pericardial Catheter Management

Mary G. McKinley, MSN, RN, CCRN
Staff Nurse VI, Ohio Valley Medical Center, Wheeling,
West Virginia
  *Electrophysiologic Monitoring: Hardwire and Telemetry;
  Twelve-Lead Electrocardiogram*

Joanne L. Monroig, BSN, RN, CNRN
Staff Nurse-Mentor, The Methodist Hospital, Houston, Texas
  Halo Traction Care

Patricia Gonce Morton, PhD, RN, ACNP, FAAN
Professor and Assistant Dean for Master's Studies, School
of Nursing, University of Maryland, Baltimore, Maryland,
Acute Care Nurse Practitioner, University of Maryland
Medical Center, Baltimore, Maryland
  Implantable Cardioverter-Defibrillator

Anne C. Muller, BA, MSN, RN, CRNP
Adjunct Faculty, La Salle University, Philadelphia,
Pennsylvania; Clinical Nurse Specialist, Cardiothoracic
Surgery, Hospital of the University of Pennsylvania,
Philadelphia, Pennsylvania
  *Implantable Venous Access Device: Access, Deaccess,
  and Care*

Nancy Munro, MN, RN, CCRN, ACNP
Clinical Instructor, Acute Care Nurse Practitioner Program,
School of Nursing, University of Maryland, Baltimore,
Maryland; Acute Care Nurse Practitioner, Critical Care,
The National Institutes of Health, Bethesda, Maryland
  *Blood Sampling From Central Venous Catheters; Central
  Venous Catheter Removal; Central Venous Catheter Site
  Care; Central Venous/Right Atrial Pressure Monitoring;
  Central Venous Catheter Insertion (Assist)*

Janis Namink, RN, AND
Staff Nurse, Neuroscience Intensive Care Unit, Methodist
Hospital, Houston, Texas
  External Fixation Device Insertion (Assist)

Barbara B. Ott, PhD, RN
Associate Professor, College of Nursing, Villanova
University, Villanova, Pennsylvania
Advance Directives

Michele M. Pelter, PhD, RN
Director of Nursing Research & Outcomes, Washoe Health
System, Reno, Nevada; Assistant Professor, University of
Nevada Reno, Reno, Nevada
Continuous ST-Segment Monitoring

JoAnne K. Phillips, MSN, RN, CCRN, CCNS
Clinical Nurse Specialist, Patient Safety, The Hospital of
the University of Pennsylvania, Philadelphia, Pennsylvania
Gastric Lavage in Hemorrhage and Overdose

Joya D. Pickett, MSN
Clinical Instructor, Department of Behavioral Nursing and
Health Systems, University of Washington, Seattle,
Washington; Critical Care Clinical Nurse Specialist,
Swedish Medical Center, Seattle, Washington
Closed Chest Drainage System

D. Nathan Preuss, MA, RN, CCRN
Clinical Charge Nurse, Neurovascular Intensive Care Unit,
Jefferson Hospital for Neurosciences, Philadelphia,
Pennsylvania
Neurologic Drainage and Pressure Monitoring System

Teresa Preuss, MSN, RN, CCRN
Clinical Charge Nurse, Medical Coronary Care Unit, Thomas
Jefferson University Hospital, Philadelphia, Pennsylvania
*Atrial Electrogram; Blood Sampling From a Pulmonary
Artery Catheter; Pulmonary Artery Catheter Insertion
(Assist) and Presssure Monitoring; Pulmonary Artery
Catheter Removal; Pulmonary Artery Catheter and
Pressure Lines, Troubleshooting; Single- and
Multiple-Pressure Transducer Systems*

Susan Quaal, PhD, RN, APRN
Associate Clinical Professor, University of Utah Health
Science Center, Salt Lake City, Utah; Advanced Practice
Cardiovascular Clinical Specialist, Salt Lake VA
Healthcare System, Salt Lake City, Utah
Intraaortic Balloon Pump Management

Deborah Nolan Reilly, BSN, RN
Electrophysiology Laboratory Supervisor, University of
Maryland Medical Center, Baltimore, Maryland
Implantable Cardioverter-Defibrillator

Christine S. Schulman, MS, RN, CNS, CCRN
ICU Clinical Nurse Specialist, Providence St. Vincent
Medical Center, Portland, Oregon; Adjunct Faculty,
Oregon Health Sciences University, Portland, Oregon
*Continuous Arteriovenous Rewarming; Massive
Infusion Devices*

Sandra L. Schutz, MSN, CCRN
Clinical Nurse Specialist, Swedish Medical Center/Ballard
Campus, Seattle, Washington
Oxygen Saturation Monitoring by Pulse Oximetry

Julianne M. Scott, MA, RN, CCRN
Operations Leader, John Nasseff Heart Hospital, United
Hospital, St. Paul, Minnesota
*Endotracheal Intubation (Assist); Endotracheal Tube and
Oral Care; Autotransfusion*

Liza Severance-Lossin, MSN, RN, CS, CCRN
Lecturer, University of Pennsylvania, Philadelphia,
Pennsylvania; Resource Nurse, Hospital of the University
of Pennsylvania, Philadelphia, Pennsylvania
*Intracranial Bolt Insertion (Assist), Monitoring, Care,
Troubleshooting, and Removal; Intraventricular
Catheter Insertion (Assist), Monitoring, Care,
Troubleshooting, and Removal; Jugular Venous Oxygen
Saturation Monitoring: Insertion (Assist), Care,
Troubleshooting, and Removal; Lumbar Subarachnoid
Catheter Insertion (Assist) for Cerebral Spinal Fluid
Pressure Monitoring and Drainage; Patient-Controlled
Analgesia; Determination of Death*

Rose B. Shaffer, MSN, RN, ACNP-CS, CCRN
Cardiology Nurse Practitioner, Thomas Jefferson
University Hospital, Philadelphia, Pennsylvania
*Arterial Catheter Insertion (Assist), Care and Removal;
Blood Sampling From an Arterial Catheter;
Arterial and Venous Sheath Removal*

Christine Shamloo, MSN, RN, CCRN
Clinical Specialist, Critical Care/Emergency Services,
Washington Hospital Center, Washington, DC
Defibrillation (Internal); Epicardial Pacing Wire Removal

Kirsten N. Skillings, MA, RN, CCNS, CCRN
Critical Care Clinical Nurse Specialist, St. Cloud Hospital,
St. Cloud, Minnesota
*Extubation/Decannulation (Perform);
Extubation/Decannulation (Assist); Nasopharyngeal
Airway Insertion; Oropharyngeal Airway Insertion;
Tracheal Tube Cuff Care; Tracheostomy Tube Care*

Deborah C. Stamps, MS, RN, GNP, CNA, BC
Director of Nursing, Women's and Neonatal Health
Emergency Services and Clinical Bed Coordination,
Rochester General Hospital, Rochester, New York
Enteral Nutrition; Parenteral Nutrition

Jacqueline Sullivan, PhD, RN, CCRN, CNRN
Clinical Assistant Professor, Thomas Jefferson University
Hospital, Philadelphia, Pennsylvania; Clinician Researcher,
Neuroscience and Critical Care Nursing, Thomas Jefferson
University Hospital, Philadelphia, Pennsylvania
*Intracranial Bolt Insertion (Assist), Monitoring, Care,
Troubleshooting, and Removal; Intraventricular Catheter
Insertion (Assist), Monitoring, Care, Troubleshooting,*

and Removal; Jugular Venous Oxygen Saturation Monitoring: Insertion (Assist), Care, Troubleshooting, and Removal; Lumbar Subarachnoid Catheter Insertion (Assist) for Cerebral Spinal Fluid Pressure Monitoring and Drainage; Determination of Death

Nancy L. Tomaselli, MSN, RN, CRNP, CWOCN, CS, CLNC
Distinguished Faculty, College of Nursing and Health Professions, Drexel University, Philadelphia, Pennsylvania
Pressure Reducing Devices: Lateral Rotation Therapy

Maureen Turner, BSN, RN
Director of Clinical Affairs, Deltex Medical, Inc., Severna Park, Maryland
Esophageal Doppler Monitoring of Aortic Blood Flow: Probe Insertion; Esophageal Doppler Monitoring of Aortic Blood Flow: Care and Removal

Karen Vojtko, BSN, CCRN
Senior Partner, University of Maryland Medical Center, Baltimore, Maryland
Implantable Cardioverter-Defibrillator

Kathleen M. Vollman, MSN, RN, CCRN, CCNS, FCCM
Clinical Nurse Specialist/Educator/Consultant, Advanced Nursing, Dearborn, Michigan
Endotracheal Tube and Oral Care; Pronation Therapy

Kathryn T. Von Rueden, MS, RN, FCCM
Faculty Associate, University of Maryland School of Nursing, Baltimore, Maryland; Director, Safety and Quality, Anne Arundel Medical Center, Annapolis, Maryland
Noninvasive Hemodynamic Monitoring: Impedance Cardiography

Kevin B. Wagner, BSBE
Associate Director, Technical Products and Services, Cardiodynamics International, San Diego, California
Noninvasive Hemodynamic Monitoring: Impedance Cardiography

Debra J. Lynn-McHale Wiegand, PhD, RN, CCRN, FAAN
Postdoctoral Fellow, Yale University School of Nursing, New Haven, Connecticut; Staff Nurse, Surgical Cardiac Care Unit, Thomas Jefferson University Hospital, Philadelphia, Pennsylvania

Atrial Electrogram; Blood Sampling From a Pulmonary Artery Catheter; Pulmonary Artery Catheter Insertion (Assist) and Pressure Monitoring; Pulmonary Artery Catheter Removal; Pulmonary Artery Catheter and Pressure Lines, Troubleshooting; Single- and Multiple-Pressure Transducer Systems; Withholding and Withdrawing Life-Sustaining Therapy

Fred Williams, RCIS, RCDS
Pacemaker/ICD Clinical Coordinator, Kaiser Permanente, Silver Spring, Maryland
Permanent Pacemaker (Assessing Function)

Sandi Wind, RN, CWCN, COCN
Stuart, Florida
Pressure-Reducing Devices: Lateral Rotation Therapy

Sue Wingate, DNSc, RN, CS, CRNP
Cardiology Nurse Practitioner, Kaiser Permanente, MidAtlantic States, Silver Spring, Maryland
Permanent Pacemaker (Assessing Function)

Anne W. Wojner-Alexandrov, PhD, RN, CCRN, FAAN
Assistant Professor of Neurology and Neuroscience, Critical Care Medicine, Department of Neurology, University of Texas—Houston Medical School, Houston, Texas; President, Health Outcomes Institute, The Woodlands, Texas
Transcranial Doppler Monitoring; Lumbar Puncture (Perform)

Sandra Schulp Woods, MA, RN, CNS, CCRN
Clinical Nurse Specialist, Critical Care, Creighton University Medical Center, Omaha, Nebraska
Temporary Transvenous and Epicardial Pacing; Left Atrial Catheter: Care and Assisting With Removal

Maribeth Wooldridge-King, BSN, MS, OCN
Clinical Supervisor, Memorial Sloan-Kettering Cancer Center, New York, New York
Blood and Blood Component Administration; Blood Pump Use; Transfusion Reaction Management; Determination of Microhematocrit via Centrifuge

Shu-Fen Wung, PhD, RN, ACNP, BC, FAHA
Associate Professor, College of Nursing, University of Arizona, Tucson, Arizona
Extra Electrocardiographic Leads: Right Precordial and Left Posterior Leads

Reviewers

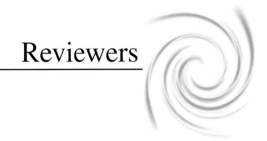

Susan R. Adams, RN, CCRN
Cape Canaveral Hospital
Cocoa Beach, Florida

Mamoona Arif, MSN, RN
Northern Virginia Community Hospital
Arlington, Virginia

Marie Arnone, MA, RN, CCRN
Swedish Medical Center—Providence Campus
Seattle, Washington

Lorraine Avery, BN, MN, RN, CNCC(C)
WRHA Cardiology Sub Program
Winnipeg, Manitoba, Canada

Mona N. Bahouth, MSN, CRNP
University of Maryland Medical Center
Baltimore, Maryland

Nancy Ballard, MSN, RN
WellStar Health System
Marietta, Georgia

Jody Bammann, RN, ADN, CCRN
Mercy Medical Center
Roseburg, Oregon

Mary L. Bessinger, RN
MedCentral Health System
Mansfield, Ohio

Donna Zimmaro Bliss, PhD, RN, FAAN
University of Minnesota School of Nursing
Minneapolis, Minnesota

Patricia A. Blissitt, PhD, RN, CCRN, CNRN, CCM, APRN, BC
Duke University Hospital
Durham, North Carolina

Cathryn D. Boardman, MSN, RN, CCRN
Medical Center East
Birmingham, Alabama

Donna Bond, MSN, RN, BC, CNS, AE-C
Carilion Health System
Roanoke, Virginia

Joann Byler, MSN, RN, CCRN
Parkview Health
Fort Wayne, Indiana

Jim Carlson, PharmD
Group Health Cooperative
Seattle, Washington

Lissa A. Cash, MSN, RN, CCRN, CEN
Sentara Leigh Hospital
Norfolk, Virginia

Sandy Cecil, BS, RN
Legacy Emanuel Hospital
Portland, Oregon

Alice Chan, MN, RN, CS
UCLA Healthcare
Los Angeles, California

Lydia Chan, BSN, RN
Swedish Medical Center
Seattle, Washington

Kathleen Colfer, MSN, RN, LNC
Thomas Jefferson University Hospital
Philadelphia, Pennsylvania

Karen L. Cooper, MSN, RN, CCRN, CS, CNA
Kaiser Permanente Hospital
Sacramento, California

Lisa Covington-Kennedy, MA, RN, CEN, CCRN
Saint Vincent Catholic Medical Centers
New York, New York

Phyllis Daniel, MSN, RN, CHPN, CNS
Carilion Health System
Roanoke, Virginia

Jose Delp, BSN, RN
Upper Chesapeake Health System
Bel Air, Maryland

Sharon P. Dickinson, MSN, RN, CNS, CCRN
University of Michigan Health System
Ann Arbor, Michigan

Lisa Dilorenzo, RN
Evergreen Healthcare
Kirkland, Washington

Susan M. Dirkes, MSA, RN, CCRN
University of Michigan Health System
Ann Arbor, Michigan
NxStage Medical Inc.
Lawrence, Massachusetts

Ross H. Ehrmantraut, BA, RN, CCRN
Harborview Medical Center
Seattle, Washington

Janice R. Ekemo, MN, RN, ARNP
The Polyclinic
Seattle, Washington
Swedish Medical Center
Seattle, Washington
University of Washington
Seattle, Washington

Kathleen L. Emde, MN, RN, CCRN, CEN
Swedish Medical Center
Issaquah, Washington

Debra Ferguson, MSN, RN, CCRN, CNRN
Community Health Network
Indianapolis, Indiana

Susan K. Frazier, PhD, RN
Ohio State University College of Nursing
Columbus, Ohio

Marjorie Funk, PhD, RN, FAHA, FAAN
Yale University School of Nursing
New Haven, Connecticut
Yale–New Haven Hospital
New Haven, Connecticut

Vicki S. Good, RN, MSN, CCRN, CCNS
Baylor All Saints Medical Center
Fort Worth, Texas

Cindy Goodrich, MS, RN, CCRN
Airlift Northwest
Seattle, Washington

Sheryl A. Greco, MN, RN, CCRN
University of Washington Medical Center
Seattle, Washington

Charlotte A. Green, BSN, CCRN
Group Health Cooperative
Redmond, Washington

Peggi Guenter, PhD, RN, CNSN
American Society for Parenteral and Enteral Nutrition
Silver Spring, Maryland

Carl F. Haas, MLS, RRT
University of Michigan Health System
Ann Arbor, Michigan

Karen L. Haight, BSN, CCRN, CNRN
Mission Hospital
Mission Viejo, California
Saddleback College
Mission Viejo, California
Saddleback Memorial Medical Center
Laguna Hills, California

Deborah A. Hanes, MSN, RN, CNS, CRNP
The Cleveland Clinic
Cleveland, Ohio

Linda Harrington, PhD, RN, CNS
JPS Health Network
Fort Worth, Texas
Texas Christian University
Fort Worth, Texas

Karen L. Harvey, RN
Spectrum Health Regional Burn Center
Grand Rapids, Michigan

Kathleen S. Hobson, MS, RN
Virginia Mason Medical Center
Seattle, Washington
Stevens Hospital
Edmonds, Washington

Alan B. Hopkins, PhD, ACNP, CS
Hometown Medical Services
Covington, Tennessee

Melissa L. Hutchinson, RN, MN, CCRN, CWCN
VA Puget Sound Health Care System
Seattle, Washington

Mary Fran Kaminski, RN, CCRN
Sacred Heart Hospital
Allentown, Pennsylvania

Patricia A. Knowles, RN, CCRN
VCU Health System
Richmond, Virginia

Julene B. (Julie) Kruithof, MSN, RN, CCRN
Spectrum Health
Grand Rapids, Michigan

Dana M. Kyles, BSN, RN
Harborview Medical Center
Seattle, Washington

Denise M. Lawrence, MS, RN, APRN, ACNP
Hartford Hospital
Hartford, Connecticut

Janet Leahy, BSN, RN
VA Puget Sound Health Care System
Seattle, Washington

Marykay Livingston, MSN, CRNA, ARNP
Group Health Cooperative
Redmond, Washington

Jeanne R. Lowe, BA, RN, CCRN, CWCN
Harborview Medical Center
Seattle, Washington

Lezli Matthews, BSN, RN
University of Utah Medical Center
Salt Lake City, Utah

Julie A. Marcum, APRN, CCRN, CS
Boise Veterans' Affairs Medical Center
Boise, Idaho

Suzanne A. Meader, RN, MN, ARNP, ACNP, ANP, CCRN
Overlake Hospital Medical Center
Bellevue, Washington

Maureen Merkl, MSN, RN, CEN
Virginia Hospital Center
Arlington, Virginia

Norma A. Metheny, PhD, RN, FAAN
St. Louis University School of Nursing
St. Louis, Missouri

Barbara Miller, MSN, RN, ARNP, CS
Northwest Hospital and Medical Center
Seattle, Washington

Radine A. Mills, BSN, RN, CCRN
Kadlec Medical Center
Richland, Washington

Lynda Minor, MN, RN, ET
Olympic Medical Center
Port Angeles, Washington
University of Washington
Seattle, Washington

June Oliver, MSN, APN/CNS, CCNS
Swedish Covenant Hospital
Chicago, Illinois

Mary O. Palazzo, MS, RN, CCRN
St. Joseph Medical Center
Towson, Maryland

Maria Teresa Palleschi, RN, CCRN, APRN-BC
Harper University Hospital
Detroit, Michigan

Michaelynn Paul, BS, RN, CCRN
Walla Walla College
Portland, Oregon

Kristine J. Peterson, MS, RN, CCNS, CCRN
Park Nicollet Health Services
St. Louis Park, Minnesota

Theresa A. Posani, MS, RN, CCNS, CCRN
Presbyterian Hospital of Dallas
Dallas, Texas

Martha Purrier, MN, RN, AOCN
Virginia Mason Medical Center
Seattle, Washington

Eileen E. Pysznik, BS, RN, CCRN
Baystate Medical Center
Springfield, Massachusetts

Carolyn Reilly, PhD(c), APRN, CCRN, CCNS
Central Maine Medical Center
Lewiston, Maine

Marti Reiser, MSN, RN, NP-C, CDE, CCRN
University Hospitals Health System
Bedford, Ohio

Kelli Rosenthal, MS, RN, BC, CRNI, ANP, APRN
ResourceNurse.com, A Division of Nurses-Station.com, LLC
Oceanside, New York

Robert M. Rothwell, MN, RN, CCRN
VA Puget Sound Health Care System
Seattle, Washington

Sheila Scarbrough, BSN, RN
Medical University of South Carolina
Charleston, South Carolina

Pamela S. Schlicher, RN, CCRN
South Bay Hospital
Sun City Center, Florida

Linda H. Schakenbach, MSN, RN, CNS, CCRN, CWCN, CS
Inova Alexandria Hospital
Alexandria, Virginia

Lynn Schallom, MSN, RN, CCNS, CCRN
Barnes-Jewish Hospital
St. Louis, Missouri

Hildy Schell-Chaple, MS, RN, CCRN, CCNS
UCSF School of Nursing
UCSF Medical Center
San Francisco, California

Maureen A. Seckel, MSN, RN, APRN, BC, CCRN
Christiana Care Health Services
Newark, Deleware

Shirley A. Storch Sherman, BSN, RN, CCRN
Virginia Mason Medical Center
Seattle, Washington

Deborah Sidor, MSN, APRN-BC, CCRN
Harper University Hospital
Detroit, Michigan

Helen Simons, RN, CCRN
University of Washington Medical Center
Seattle, Washington

Joy M. Speciale, MBA, RN, CCRN
Hinsdale Hospital
Hinsdale, Illinois

Valerie Spotts, BSN, RN
University of Michigan Health System
Ann Arbor, Michigan

Barbara Stahl, C-ANP, DNSc, RN
Yale–New Haven Hospital
New Haven, Connecticut

Hilaire J. Thompson, PhD, RN, BC, APRN, CNRN
University of Washington
Seattle, Washington
Harborview Medical Center
Seattle, Washington

Elizabeth Varadi-Ginsberg, BSN, RN, CCRN
University of Michigan Health System
Ann Arbor, Michigan

Kathleen M. Vollman, MSN, RN, CCRN, CCNS, FCCM
Clinical Nurse Specialist/Educator/Consultant
Advanced Nursing
Dearborn, Michigan

Rebecca A. Walsh, MN, RN, CCRN
Virginia Mason Medical Center
Seattle, Washington

Georgita Washington, MSN, RN, CCRN, CCNS
Mountain States Health Alliance
Johnson City, Tennessee

Janice M. Whitman, MSN, RN, CCRN
Overlake Hospital Medical Center
Bellevue, Washington

Michelle Gheen Whitney, MN, CS, ARNP
Overlake Hospital Medical Center
Bellevue, Washington

Patricia J. S. Wilson, MSN, RN, CNS, CS, CCRN
University of Texas M.D. Anderson Cancer Center
Houston, Texas

Catherine Winkler, MPH, RN
Danbury Hospital
Danbury, Connecticut

Janice M. Wojcik, RN, MS, CCRN, APRN, BC
St. Joseph's Regional Medical Center
Paterson, New Jersey

Karen A. Wojcik, BSN, RN
Medtronic Emergency Response Systems
Redmond, Washington

Susan M. Wright, BSN, RN, CCRN
University of Michigan Health System
Ann Arbor, Michigan

Karen Lynn Yarbrough, MN, RN, CRNP
Upper Chesapeake Health System
Bel Air, Maryland

Preface

In this time of dramatic change in health care, it is with great pleasure that we present the fifth edition of the *AACN Procedure Manual for Critical Care*. The changes that our colleagues will find in this edition are a direct reflection of the knowledge and technology explosion that have moved us into the new century. While every attempt was made to capture current clinical practice, we recognize that critical care clinical practice is dynamic and, therefore, any resource to support that practice must be considered a work in progress.

AACN is dedicated to the care of patients experiencing critical illness or injury and their families. AACN's vision is of a health care system driven by the needs of patients and their families in which critical care nurses make their optimal contribution. Toward that vision, it is our hope that this edition of the *AACN Procedure Manual for Critical Care* will be a useful resource for critical care nurses in providing quality patient care.

The fifth edition of the *AACN Procedure Manual for Critical Care* will be an asset for practitioners across the spectrum of acute and critical care practice. The manual includes a comprehensive review of and state of the art information on acute and critical care procedures. Procedures related to new and emerging trends have been added, and all of the procedures have been revised to reflect changes in practice. With the increased presence of advance practice nurses in critical care units, this edition of the *AACN Procedure Manual for Critical Care* contains not only procedures commonly performed by critical care nurses but also includes an even great number of procedures performed by advance practice nurses than the fourth edition. Since we recognize that the procedures included in this manual are only a portion of the repertoire needed by today's critical care practitioners to skillfully care for critically ill patients, we recommend it be used in conjunction with AACN's *Core Curriculum for Critical Care Nursing,* AACN's *Care Review for Critical Care Nursing,* and the upcoming AACN advanced critical nursing reference that is currently in development.

The *AACN Procedure Manual for Critical Care* is designed so that information within each procedure can be found quickly. In an effort to provide high-quality care to seriously ill patients, we need resources that provide us with readily available "need to know" information. This edition, like the fourth, has been organized using the following framework. The manual is organized in units, with most of the units having several sections. All procedures are designed using the same style, starting with a purpose. Following the purpose is the prerequisite nursing knowledge that includes information the nurse needs prior to performing the procedure. The equipment list includes equipment necessary to perform the procedure. Some of the procedures identify additional equipment that may be necessary based on individual situations. A patient and family education section identifies essential information that should be taught to patients and their families. The patient assessment and preparation section includes the specific assessment criteria that should be obtained before the procedure and describes how the patient should be prepared for the procedure. The step-by-step procedure follows and includes the rationale for steps and important special considerations. Associated research and appropriate figures and tables are included to enhance the procedure. Following the procedure is a list of expected and unexpected outcomes. The expected outcomes include the anticipated results of the procedure. The unexpected outcomes include potential complications or untoward outcomes of the procedure. The next section, patient monitoring, includes information related to assessments and interventions that should be completed. The rationale for each item is described and conditions necessitating notification of an advance practice nurse or physician are identified. The documentation section describes what should be documented after the procedure is performed. Lastly, references used within the procedures and additional readings are included.

In the nursing profession, our quest to have our practice driven by research has never been greater. Building on the fourth edition, this edition of the *AACN Procedure Manual for Critical Care* uses a research leveling system. As available, this research-based information is provided to indicate the research-based strength of recommendation for various interventions. While we believe that this is a major step forward in promoting research-based practice, the paucity of research available in many procedures also speaks loudly to the need for further investigation. The research-based leveling system is the same as is used for *AACN Protocols for Practice* and includes:

Level I: Manufacturer's recommendations only.
Level II: Theory based, no research data to support recommendations: recommendations from expert consensus group may exist.
Level III: Laboratory data, no clinical data to support recommendations.
Level IV: Limited clinical studies to support recommendations.
Level V: Clinical studies in more than one or two patient populations and situations to support recommendations.
Level VI: Clinical studies in a variety of patient populations and situations to support recommendations.

Given the nature of critical care, many of the included procedures use electrical equipment. This manual makes the assumption that all equipment is maintained by your institution's bioengineering department according to accepted national and state regulations for the individual piece of equipment.

We hope that you find this book an essential resource for clinical practice. An important complement to the *AACN Procedure Manual for Critical Care* are the *Critical Care Procedure Performance Evaluation Checklists*. The checklists are available on CD-ROM and include checklists for each procedure within this book. These are extremely helpful for use during critical care orientation. This edition of *AACN Procedure Manual for Critical Care* is also available electronically and can be individualized to meet the needs of any given institution.

Acknowledgments

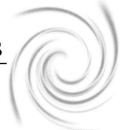

This text could not have been designed or developed without help from numerous people. First, we would like to thank AACN for giving us the opportunity to co-edit this endeavor. Our deep gratitude goes to Ellen French, AACN's Publishing Director, for her continued support of us and her incredible energy that went into making this book a success. We would also like to thank the practice and education team at the AACN National Office and the volunteers who diligently reviewed this work to ensure its quality.

We would also like to thank a number of key people at Elsevier for their support and hard work throughout this entire project. We are extremely grateful to work closely with Barbara Cullen, our editor. Barbara's leadership is instrumental to the procedure manual's success. We would like to thank Laura Sieh Chu and her predecessor, Adrienne Simon, for keeping the progress of the text so organized. We extend a grateful thank you to Helen Hudlin, our production manager; Gina Keckritz, our copyeditor; and Kathi Gosche, our designer. Without the creative and hard-working team at Elsevier, our text would not have been possible.

A simple thank you is inadequate for our critical care colleagues, the experts in our field, who made this book a reality. Their hard work and efforts to produce quality, well-researched procedures will have a long-lasting effect on critical care practice in years to come. As well, we are indebted to our colleagues who served as procedure reviewers. We thank you for taking the time to critically review each procedure and support our efforts to promote excellence. In addition, we would like to thank the AACN volunteers and volunteer groups who provided early reviews of our table of contents.

Lastly, yet very importantly, we would like to thank those close to us who provided personal support. Debra would like to thank her mother and father for their solid foundation and love. She would also like to thank her friends (Rose, Denise, Elly, and Terry) for their support and laughter. Most importantly, Debra would like to thank Jim for his everlasting love and support, and thank Scott and Michael for keeping her grounded in life's priorities. Karen would like to thank her mom, whose years of compassionate bedside nursing helped her to see what being a nurse is really all about, thank her critical care colleagues and friends across the country, especially in the Pacific Northwest, for their continuous support, thank Jim whose love and support makes every day a better day, and Daniel and Katie who help her remember that whatever life brings is a God-given blessing.

Debra J. Lynn-McHale Wiegand

Karen K. Carlson

Contents

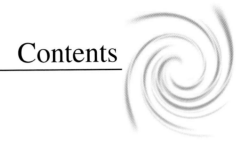

UNIT IX End of Life, 1167

UNIT X Calculating Medication Doses, 1206

AACN

PROCEDURE
MANUAL *for*
CRITICAL CARE

UNIT I
Pulmonary System

SECTION ONE
Airway Management

evolve http://evolve.elsevier.com

P R O C E D U R E

1

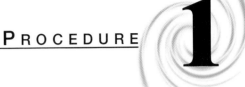

Combitube Insertion and Removal

P U R P O S E : A Combitube may be used to provide an emergency airway while resuscitating a profoundly unconscious patient who requires artificial ventilation and when endotracheal intubation is not readily available or has failed to establish an airway successfully.

Michael W. Day

PREREQUISITE NURSING KNOWLEDGE

- Anatomy and physiology of the upper airway should be understood.
- The Combitube does *not* require direct visualization of the airway for insertion and is inserted in a "blind" fashion, being an adjunct when endotracheal intubation attempts fail or trauma makes visualization of the airway difficult.[2] The Combitube (Fig. 1-1) is available in two sizes, based on patient height.
  - ❖ For patients 48 to 66 inches tall (122 to 168 cm), use the 37 Fr size.
  - ❖ Either size 37 Fr or size 41 Fr is applicable in patients 60 to 66 inches tall (152 to 168 cm).[9]
  - ❖ For patients greater than or equal to 66 inches (168 cm), use the 41 Fr size.
- The Combitube has a unique design:
  - ❖ A double-lumen, semirigid airway
    - ○ Blue lumen opening to the perforations between the cuffs
    - ○ White lumen opening distal to the distal cuff
    - ○ Each lumen fitted with a 15-mm male adapter

- ❖ Two cuffs for occlusion
  - ○ Proximal cuff (85 ml or 100 ml, depending on tube size) to occlude the hypopharynx
  - ○ Distal cuff (12 ml or 15 ml, depending on tube size) to occlude either the esophagus or the trachea
  - ○ Each cuff connected to a pilot balloon and valve—blue for proximal ("No. 1"), white for distal ("No. 2")

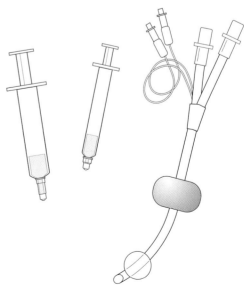

FIGURE 1-1 Components of the Combitube.

- Two black lines indicate the position of the patient's teeth or gumline when first inserted.
- Because of the large inflated cuff in the hypopharynx, the Combitube requires no stabilization or securing after placement.

- The correct placement of a Combitube in the airway is as follows:
  - Esophageal insertion (Figs. 1-2 and 1-3), in which the distal cuff occludes the esophagus and the proximal balloon occludes the hypopharynx, allows ventilation via the blue lumen.
  - Tracheal insertion (see Fig. 1-4), in which the distal cuff occludes the trachea and the proximal balloon occludes the hypopharynx, allows ventilation through the white lumen.
- Before the insertion of a Combitube, adequate ventilation of an unconscious patient with a mouth-to-mask or a bag-valve-mask device is necessary.
- Use of the Combitube is contraindicated for airway management[9] in the following patients:
  - Patients with an intact gag reflex
  - Patients with known esophageal disease
  - Patients who have ingested caustic substances
- The Combitube contains latex and may cause an allergic reaction in patients or personnel handling the device who have a known sensitivity to latex.[9]
- The Combitube is supplied either in a complete kit (with all of the necessary components for insertion), in soft or rigid packaging, or as a single, individual device (without any of the necessary components for insertion). If the single individual device is used, additional components are *required* for insertion.
- Initial and ongoing training is required to maximize insertion success and to minimize complications.[3,9]
- Medications delivered by endotracheal tube *cannot be used* with a Combitube in the esophageal position.[6] Medications may *not* reach the alveolar surfaces of the lung for absorption.

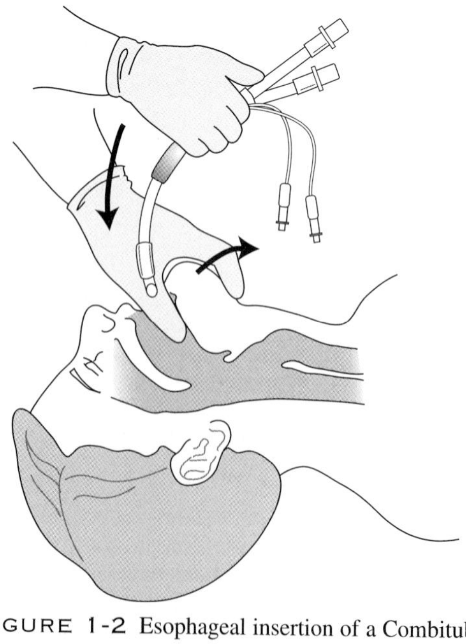

FIGURE 1-2 Esophageal insertion of a Combitube.

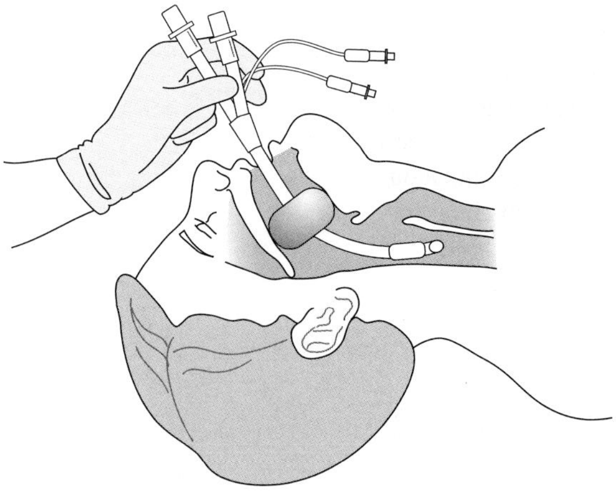

FIGURE 1-3 Combitube in esophageal position.

EQUIPMENT

- Combitube, of the appropriate size for the patient's height
- Large (100 ml) Luer-tip syringe
- Small (20 ml) Luer-tip syringe
- Water-soluble lubricant
- Mouth-to-mask or bag-valve-mask device attached to a high-flow oxygen source
- Gloves, mask, and eye protection
- Suction equipment (suction canister with control head, tracheal suction catheters, Yankauer suction tip)
- Fluid deflector elbow

PATIENT AND FAMILY EDUCATION

- If time allows, provide the family with information about the Combitube and the reason for insertion. ➸*Rationale:* This information assists the family in understanding why the procedure is required and decreases family anxiety.

PATIENT ASSESSMENT AND PREPARATION

Patient Assessment

- Assess level of consciousness and responsiveness. ➸*Rationale:* In an emergency situation, the Combitube should be inserted only into a patient who is profoundly unconscious, unresponsive, and unable to maintain adequate ventilation.[2]
- Assess history and patient information for possibility of esophageal disease or caustic substance ingestion. ➸*Rationale:* A Combitube is contraindicated in patients with these conditions.[2]
- Assess patient's height. ➸*Rationale:* This allows the selection of the appropriate-size Combitube.[2]

Patient Preparation

- Ensure adequate ventilation and oxygenation with either a mouth-to-mask or a bag-valve-mask device. ➤*Rationale:* The patient will be nonresponsive and unable to maintain adequate ventilation without assisted ventilation before the Combitube insertion.

- Ensure that the suction equipment is assembled and in working order. ➤*Rationale:* The patient may regurgitate during the insertion or while the Combitube is in place and require oropharyngeal or tracheal suctioning or both.

Procedure for Combitube Insertion

Steps	Rationale	Special Considerations
1. Wash hands and don protective equipment (goggles, mask, gloves).	Reduces the possible transmission of microorganisms and bodily secretions; minimizes contamination of Combitube.	
2. Open the package and test the integrity of both cuffs. *(Level I: Manufacturer's recommendations only.)*	Ensures that the device is not defective and will work as indicated.	
A. Pull the plunger back on the large syringe to the appropriate volume for the size of the tube and attach it to the proximal (blue) valve, marked "**No. 1.**"	Readies the syringe for inflating the cuff.	Use 85 ml volume for the 37 Fr size and 100 ml volume for the 41 Fr size.[10]
B. Inflate the proximal cuff with the appropriate volume and assess for leaks.	Ensures that the device is not defective and will work as indicated.	If a leak is found, discard the device and secure another.
C. Actively deflate the proximal cuff, leaving the syringe attached to the valve.	Provides for smoother insertion and readies the syringe for inflation after insertion.	
D. Pull the plunger back on the small syringe to the appropriate volume for the size of the tube and attach it to the distal (white) valve, marked "**No. 2.**"	Readies the syringe for inflating the cuff.	Use 12 ml volume for the 37 Fr size and 15 ml volume for the 41 Fr size.[10]
E. Inflate the distal cuff with the appropriate volume and assess for leaks.	Ensures that the device is not defective and will work as indicated.	If a leak is found, discard the device and secure another.
F. Actively deflate the proximal cuff, leaving the syringe attached to the valve.	Provides for smoother insertion and readies the syringe for inflation after insertion.	
3. Lubricate the device with water-soluble lubricant. *(Level I: Manufacturer's recommendations only.)*	Facilitates and eases insertion.	
4. Attach a fluid deflector to the clear lumen marked "**No. 2.**" *(Level I: Manufacturer's recommendations only.)*	Diverts any fluid that may be regurgitated through the tube during insertion away from person inserting the device.	A fluid deflector is included in the kits but *not* in the single, individual devices.

Procedure continues on the following page

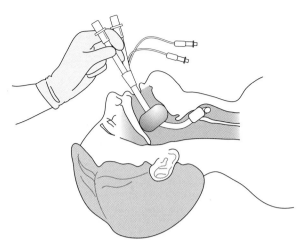

FIGURE 1-4 Combitube in tracheal position.

Procedure for Combitube Insertion—*Continued*

Steps	Rationale	Special Considerations
5. Grasp the patient's jaw with one hand and pull up (or forward if the patient is in a sitting position), maintaining the head in a neutral position (Fig. 1-4).[4] *(Level I: Manufacturer's recommendations only.)*	Pulls the tongue forward and away from the hypopharynx.	With facial trauma, assess for the presence of broken teeth (real or artificial) and remove loose fragments. Maintain cervical spine precautions with suspected or known spine trauma. *Use extreme caution to avoid puncturing the balloons during insertion.*[9]
6. Grasp the Combitube in the other hand so that it curves toward the patient's feet. *(Level I: Manufacturer's recommendations only.)*	Places the Combitube in the appropriate position for insertion.	
7. Insert the tip of the Combitube into the patient's mouth and advance it in a downward curving motion, maintaining a midline position, until the teeth or gumline is between the two black marks on the device. *(Level I: Manufacturer's recommendations only.)*	Allows the Combitube to follow the patient's hypopharynx until it is in the correct position.	*Do not force the Combitube.*[9] If it does not easily advance, attempt to redirect, or remove and reinsert.[9]
8. Inflate the proximal cuff with the appropriate volume, using blue valve, marked "**No. 1.**" *(Level I: Manufacturer's recommendations only.)*	Inflates and seats the proximal cuff into the posterior hypopharynx and seals it.	Use 85 ml volume for the 37 Fr size and 100 ml volume for the 41 Fr size.[10] Significant resistance is felt as the cuff is inflated. Keep the syringe plunger depressed while removing it from the valve to prevent air escaping from the cuff.[4] If an air leak develops, add 10 ml of air at a time until the leak seals. Volumes of 150 ml may be required for some individuals.[4]

Procedure for Combitube Insertion—*Continued*

Steps	Rationale	Special Considerations
9. Inflate the distal cuff with the appropriate volume, using white valve, marked "**No. 2**." *(Level I: Manufacturer's recommendations only.)*	Inflates the distal cuff and seals the esophagus (or trachea) depending on locations. Both locations allow the establishment of an effective airway.	Use 12 ml volume for the 37 Fr size and 15 ml volume for the 41 Fr size.[10]
10. Connect the bag-valve device to the 15-mm adapter on the blue lumen, marked "**No. 1**," and ventilate. *(Level I: Manufacturer's recommendations only.)*	More than 95% of the time, the distal balloon will be in the esophagus.[10] With both cuffs inflated, the only place the ventilation can go is into the trachea.	
11. Assess for tube placement. *(Level I: Manufacturer's recommendations only.)*	Determines placement of the tube and which lumen should be used to ventilate.	
A. Assess for gurgling over the epigastrium, chest rise and fall, and breath sounds in the lung fields with each ventilation.	If the distal cuff is in the esophagus, no gurgling will be heard over the epigastrium, and the ventilation will expand the lungs, causing the chest to rise and fall and breath sounds to be heard over the lung fields. **Go to Step 12.** If the distal cuff is in the trachea, gurgling will be heard over the epigastrium and there will be *no* rise and fall of the chest or breath sounds heard over the lung fields. **Go to Step 11B.** If no gurgling or breath sounds are noted with each ventilation, the Combitube may have been advanced too far into the esophagus, blocking the perforations from the blue lumen. **Go to Step 11C.**	Listening over the epigastrium initially provides rapid determination that the ventilation is going into the esophagus.[1] When assessing for the presence of breath sounds, always consider the possibility of a pneumothorax. This condition can change the breath sounds presentation and lead the inserter to believe that the Combitube is misplaced.
B. Immediately switch the bag-valve device to the clear lumen, marked "**No. 2**," and attempt to ventilate, assessing for gurgling over the epigastrium, chest rise and fall, and breath sounds in the lung fields with each ventilation.	If the distal cuff is in the trachea, no gurgling will be heard over the epigastrium, and the ventilation will expand the lungs, causing the chest to rise and fall and breath sounds to be heard over the lung fields. **Go to Step 12.**	Listening over the epigastrium initially provides rapid determination that the ventilation is going into the esophagus.[1] When assessing for the presence of breath sounds, always consider the possibility of a pneumothorax. This condition can change the breath sounds presentation and lead the inserter to believe that the Combitube is misplaced.
C. Deflate the proximal cuff, using a syringe on blue valve, marked "**No. 1**," withdraw the Combitube approximately 2-3 cm, and reinflate the "**No. 1**" cuff.	Allows for the repositioning of the Combitube so that the blue lumen perforations no longer are occluded by the soft tissue of esophagus. **Return to Step 11.**	If repositioning of the Combitube does *not* establish an effective airway, remove the device and establish an airway with alternative means.

Procedure continues on the following page

Procedure for Combitube Insertion—*Continued*

Steps	Rationale	Special Considerations
12. Further assess device placement with end-tidal carbon dioxide device[4,5] or an esophageal detector device.[1,4,12] (*Level II: Theory based, no research data to support recommendations; recommendations from expert consensus group may exist.*)	Confirms proper placement by two additional methods.[4,5,11]	
13. Continue ventilation through whichever lumen provides the airway (*Level I: Manufacturer's recommendations only.*)	Adequate ventilation can be achieved with the distal cuff of the Combitube in either the esophagus or the trachea.	

Procedure for Combitube Removal

Steps	Rationale	Special Considerations
1. To remove the Combitube:[6,11] (*Level II: Theory based, no research data to support recommendations; recommendations from expert consensus group may exist.*)	Removal is indicated when the patient is breathing spontaneously or there is a need to intubate the patient using endotracheal intubation.	Before removal of the Combitube, ensure that personnel qualified to endotracheal intubate the patient are readily available.[8] The Combitube may be left in place while an endotracheal tube is inserted.[8] A fiberoptic scope may be used to replace a Combitube with an endotracheal tube.[6] If the Combitube has been placed in the trachea, cricoid pressure should be established and maintained until the new airway is established.[6]
A. Decompress the stomach.	Removes any contents from the stomach, making regurgitation less likely with the removal of the device.	If the Combitube is placed in the esophagus, a small suction catheter may be inserted through the white, "No. 2" lumen to decompress the stomach.
B. Attach a 100-ml syringe to the blue valve, marked "**No. 1**," and deflate the cuff.	Deflates the proximal cuff and allows suctioning of the hypopharynx.	
C. Suction the hypopharynx.	Removes secretions that may have accumulated in the hypopharynx.	
D. Attach a 20-ml syringe to the white valve, marked "**No. 2**," and deflate the cuff.	Deflates the distal cuff and allows the Combitube to be withdrawn.	
E. Withdraw the Combitube from the airway, and administer supplemental oxygen.	Allows the patient to breathe on his or her own and supplies supplemental oxygen to counter any hypoxia.	

Expected Outcomes

- Establishment of an effective airway in an emergency situation
- Maintenance of adequate ventilation and oxygenation
- Recovery of spontaneous ventilation

Unexpected Outcomes

- Complications related to the use of the Combitube may be related to insertion technique or excessive cuff pressures
- Sore throat[7]
- Dysphagia[7]
- Bleeding[7]
- Pharyngeal perforation[7]
- Esophageal lacerations[11]
- Esophageal rupture[8]
- Improper placement, resulting in hypoventilation

Patient Monitoring and Care

Steps	Rationale	Reportable Conditions
		These conditions should be reported if they persist despite nursing interventions.
1. Monitor ventilation effectiveness while the Combitube is in place by monitoring:[6] A. Difficulty of ventilation. B. Oxygen saturation (SpO_2). C. End-tidal carbon dioxide ($ETCO_2$).	Determines that the Combitube is functioning correctly and providing adequate ventilation and oxygenation.	• Increased difficulty in ventilation • Unexplained decreases in SpO_2 or $ETCO_2$ levels
2. Monitor for return of spontaneous attempts at breathing.	May indicate need either to remove the device or to use medications (sedatives or nondepolarizing neuromuscular blockade) to prevent the gag reflex.[6]	

Documentation

Documentation should include the following:

- Assessment findings indicating the need for inserting a Combitube
- Confirmation of adequacy of ventilation, with auscultation of gastric area and lung fields
- Any difficulties with placement of the Combitube
- $ETCO_2$ levels
- Need for sedation or neuromuscular blockade or both
- Assessment findings on removal of the Combitube, including work of breathing, breath sounds, SpO_2 levels

- Assessment findings after insertion of Combitube, indicating which lumen ventilates the patient
- Secondary confirmation of adequacy of ventilation, using $ETCO_2$ or an esophageal detection device, in conjunction with SpO_2 levels with ventilation
- Ongoing monitoring of difficulty or ease of ventilation
- SpO_2 levels
- Assessment findings indicating the need to remove the Combitube or replace it with an endotracheal tube

References

1. American Heart Association. (2000). *Guidelines for 2000 for Cardiopulmonary Resuscitation and Emergency Cardiovascular Care for Advanced Cardiac Life Support (ACLS)*. Dallas: Author.
2. Blostein, P.A., Koestner, A.J., and Hoak, S. (1998). Failed rapid sequence intubation in trauma patients: Esophageal tracheal combitube is a useful adjunct. *J Trauma, 44*, 534-7.
3. Calkins, M.D., and Robinson, T.D. (1999). Combat trauma airway management: Endotracheal intubation versus laryngeal mask airway versus combitube used by Navy SEAL and reconnaissance combat corpsmen. *J Trauma, 46*, 927-32.
4. Frass, M. (2001). Combitube. *The Internet Journal of Anesthesiology, 5*(2). Available at: www.ispub.com. Accessed May 10, 2003.
5. Frass, M., et al. (1987). Evaluation of esophageal combitube in cardiopulmonary resuscitation. *Crit Care Med, 15*, 609-11.
6. Hoak, S., and Koestner, A. (1997). Esophageal tracheal Combitube in the emergency department. *J Emerg Nurs, 23*, 347-50.
7. Keller, C., et al. (2002). The influence of cuff volume and anatomic location on pharyngeal, esophageal, and tracheal mucosal pressures with the esophageal tracheal combitube. *Anesthesiology, 96*, 1074-7.
8. Klein, H., et al. (1997). Esophageal rupture associated with the use of the Combitube. *Anesth Analg, 85*, 937-9.
9. Tyco Healthcare. (2000). *Combitube Product Brochure*. Mansfield, MA: Author. Available at: www.kendalhq.com/catalog/brochures/Combitube.pdf. Accessed May 9, 2003.
10. Tyco Healthcare. (2000). *Combitube Product Insert*. Mansfield, MA: Author.

11. Vezina, D., et al. (1999). Esophageal and tracheal distortion by the Esophageal-Tracheal Combitube: A cadaver study. *Can J Anaesth*, 46, 393-7.

12. Wafai, Y., et al. (1995). Effectiveness of the self-inflating bulb in verification of the proper placement of the Esophageal Tracheal Combitube. *Anesth Analg*, 80, 122-6.

Additional Readings

Agro, F., et al. (2002). Current status of the Combitube: A review of the literature. *J Clin Anesth,* 14, 307-14.

Foley, L.J., and Ochroch, E.A. (2000). Bridges to establish an emergency airway and alternate intubating techniques. *Crit Care Clin*, 16, 429-44.

Gaitini, L.A., Vaida, S.J., and Agro, F. (2002). The Esophageal-Tracheal Combitube. *Anesthesiol Clin North Am*, 20, 893-906.

Idris, A.H., and Gabrielli, A. (2002). Advances in airway management. *Emerg Med Clin North Am*, 20, 843-57.

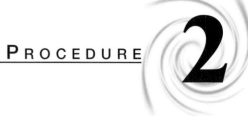

PROCEDURE **2**

AP
Endotracheal Intubation (Perform)

PURPOSE: Endotracheal intubation is performed to establish and maintain a patent airway, facilitate oxygenation and ventilation, reduce the risk of aspiration, and assist with the clearance of secretions.

Cindy Goodrich
Karen K. Carlson

PREREQUISITE NURSING KNOWLEDGE

- Anatomy and physiology of the pulmonary system should be understood.
- Indications for endotracheal intubation include the following:[4]
  - Upper airway obstruction (e.g., secondary to swelling, trauma, tumor, bleeding)
  - Apnea
  - Ineffective clearance of secretions (i.e., inability to maintain airway adequately)
  - High risk of aspiration
  - Respiratory distress
- Pulse oximetry should be used during intubation so that oxygen desaturation can be detected quickly.
- Preoxygenation with 100% oxygen using a bag-valve-mask device with a tight-fitting facemask should be performed for 3 to 5 minutes before intubation.
- Intubation attempts should take no longer than 15 to 30 seconds.
- Applying cricoid pressure (Sellick maneuver) may decrease the incidence of pulmonary aspiration and gastric distention. This procedure is accomplished by applying firm, downward pressure on the cricoid ring, pushing the vocal cords downward so that they are visualized more easily. Once begun, cricoid pressure must be maintained until intubation is completed (Fig. 2-1).

- Two types of laryngoscope blades exist, straight and curved. The straight (Miller) blade is designed so that the tip extends below the epiglottis, lifting and exposing the glottic opening. It is recommended for use in obese patients, pediatric patients, and patients with short necks because their tracheas may be located more anteriorly. When a curved (Macintosh) blade is used, the tip is advanced into the vallecula (the space between the epiglottis and the base of the tongue), exposing the glottic opening.
- Endotracheal tube size reflects the size of the internal diameter of the tube. Tubes range in size from 2.5 mm for neonates to 9 mm for large adults. Endotracheal tubes ranging in size from 7 to 8 mm are used for average-sized women, whereas endotracheal tubes ranging in size from

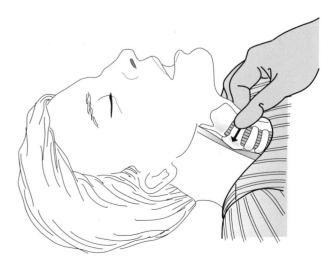

FIGURE 2-1 Cricoid pressure. Firm downward pressure on the cricoid ring pushes the vocal cords downward toward the field of vision while sealing the esophagus against the vertebral column.

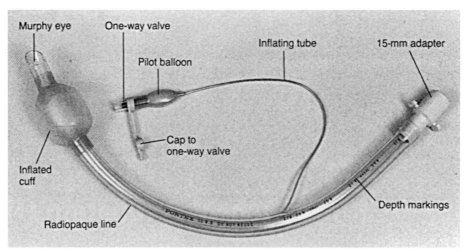

FIGURE 2-2 Parts of the endotracheal tube (soft-cuffed tube by Smiths Industries Medical Systems, Co., Valencia, CA). *(From Kersten, L.D. [1989].* Comprehensive Respiratory Nursing. *Philadelphia: W.B. Saunders, 637.)*

8 to 9 mm are used for average-sized men (Fig. 2-2).[8,9] The tube with the largest clinically acceptable internal diameter should be used to minimize airway resistance and assist in suctioning.[3]

- Endotracheal intubation can be done via nasal or oral routes. The skill of the practitioner performing intubation and the patient's clinical condition determine the route used.
- Nasal intubation is relatively contraindicated in trauma patients with facial fractures or suspected fractures at the base of the skull or postoperatively after cranial surgeries, such as transnasal hypophysectomy.
- In patients with suspected spinal cord injuries, in-line cervical immobilization of the head must be maintained during endotracheal intubation.
- Improper intubation technique may result in trauma to the teeth, soft tissues of the mouth or nose, vocal cords, and posterior pharynx.
- Primary and secondary confirmation of endotracheal intubation should be performed.[3]
  - ❖ Primary confirmation of proper endotracheal tube placement includes visualization of the tube passing through the vocal cords, absence of gurgling over the epigastric area, auscultation of bilateral breath sounds, bilateral chest rise and fall during ventilation, and mist in the tube.
  - ❖ Secondary confirmation of proper endotracheal tube placement is necessary to protect against unrecognized esophageal intubation. Methods include use of disposable end-tidal carbon dioxide (CO_2) detectors, continuous end-tidal CO_2 monitors, and esophageal detection devices.
- End-tidal CO_2 monitoring devices have been shown to be reliable indicators of expired CO_2 in patients with perfusing rhythms.[4,5,11,12,15,17] During cardiac arrest (nonperfusing rhythms), there may not be sufficient expired CO_2 due to low pulmonary blood flow.[16] If CO_2 is detected using an end-tidal CO_2 detector, it is a reliable indicator

of proper tube placement.[6,13] If CO_2 is not detected, use of an esophageal detector device is recommended.[2,5,14,18]

- Disposable end-tidal CO_2 detectors are chemically treated with a nontoxic indicator that changes color in the presence of CO_2, indicating that the endotracheal tube has been placed successfully into the trachea.
- Continuous end-tidal CO_2 monitors may be used to confirm proper endotracheal tube placement after intubation attempts and allows for the detection of future tube dislodgment.
- Esophageal detector devices work by creating suction at the end of the endotracheal tube by compressing a flexible bulb or pulling back on a syringe plunger. When the tube is placed correctly in the trachea, air allows for reexpansion of the bulb or movement of the syringe plunger. If the tube is located in the esophagus, no movement of the syringe plunger or reexpansion of the bulb is seen. These devices may be misleading in patients who are morbidly obese, patients in status asthmaticus, patients late in pregnancy, or patients with large amounts of tracheal secretions.[5]
- Double-lumen endotracheal tubes are used for independent lung ventilation in situations in which there is bleeding of one lung or a large air leak that would impair ventilation of the good lung.
- The endotracheal tube also provides a route for the administration of emergency medication (e.g., lidocaine, epinephrine, atropine, and naloxone).

EQUIPMENT

- Personal protective equipment, including eye protection
- Endotracheal tube with intact cuff and 15-mm connector (women, 7- to 8-mm tube; men, 8- to 9-mm tube)
- Laryngoscope handle with fresh batteries
- Laryngoscope blades (straight and curved)
- Spare bulb for laryngoscope blades
- Flexible stylet

- Self-inflating resuscitation bag with mask connected to supplemental oxygen (greater than or equal to 15 liters/min)
- Oxygen source and connecting tubes
- Swivel adapter (for attachment to resuscitation bag or ventilator)
- Luer-tip 10-ml syringe for cuff inflation
- Water-soluble lubricant
- Rigid pharyngeal suction-tip (Yankauer) catheter
- Suction apparatus (portable or wall)
- Suction catheters
- Bite-block or oropharyngeal airway
- Endotracheal tube–securing apparatus or appropriate tape
  - ❖ Commercially available endotracheal tube holder
  - ❖ Adhesive tape (6 to 8 inches long)
  - ❖ Twill tape (cut into 30-inch lengths)
- Stethoscope
- Monitoring equipment: continuous oxygen saturation and cardiac rhythm
- Secondary confirmation device: disposable end-tidal CO_2 detector, continuous end-tidal CO_2 monitoring device, or esophageal detection device
- Drugs for intubation as indicated (sedation, paralyzing agents, lidocaine, atropine)

  Additional equipment (to have available depending on patient need or practitioner preference) includes the following:
- Anesthetic spray (nasal approach)
- Local anesthetic jelly (nasal approach)
- Magill forceps (to remove foreign bodies obstructing the airway)
- Ventilator

PATIENT AND FAMILY EDUCATION

- Assess level of understanding about condition and rationale for endotracheal intubation. ➟*Rationale:* This assessment identifies the patient's and family's knowledge deficits concerning the patient's condition, the procedure, the expected benefits, and the potential risks; it also allows time for questions to clarify information and voice concerns. Explanations decrease patient anxiety and enhance cooperation.
- Explain the procedure and the reason for intubation. ➟*Rationale:* This enhances patient and family understanding and decreases anxiety.
- If indicated, explain the patient's role in assisting with insertion of endotracheal tube. ➟*Rationale:* This elicits the patient's cooperation, which assists with insertion.
- Explain that patient will be unable to speak while the endotracheal tube is in place, but that other means of communication will be provided. ➟*Rationale:* This enhances patient and family understanding and decreases anxiety.

- Explain that the patient's hands often are immobilized to prevent accidental dislodgment of the tube. ➟*Rationale:* This enhances patient and family understanding and decreases anxiety.

PATIENT ASSESSMENT AND PREPARATION

Patient Assessment

- Assess immediate history of trauma when spinal cord injury is suspected or cranial surgery. ➟*Rationale:* Knowing pertinent patient history allows for selection of the most appropriate method for intubation, helping reduce the risk for secondary injury.
- Assess nothing-by-mouth (NPO) status and signs of gastric distention. ➟*Rationale:* Increased risk of aspiration and vomiting occurs with accumulation of air, food, or secretions. If a patient who has gastric distention or who has eaten recently needs to be intubated, use of cricoid pressure decreases the risk of aspiration.
- Assess level of consciousness, level of anxiety, and respiratory difficulty. ➟*Rationale:* This assessment determines need for sedation or use of paralytic agents and the patient's ability to lie flat and supine for intubation.
- Assess vital signs and for the following:
  - ❖ Tachypnea
  - ❖ Dyspnea
  - ❖ Shallow respirations
  - ❖ Cyanosis
  - ❖ Apnea
  - ❖ Altered level of consciousness
  - ❖ Tachycardia
  - ❖ Cardiac dysrhythmias
  - ❖ Hypertension
  - ❖ Headache

  ➟*Rationale:* Any of these conditions may indicate a problem with oxygenation or ventilation or both.
- Assess patency of nares (for nasal intubation). ➟*Rationale:* Selection of the most appropriate naris facilitates insertion and may improve patient tolerance of tube.
- Assess need for premedication. ➟*Rationale:* Various medications provide sedation or paralysis of the patient as needed.

Patient Preparation

- Ensure that the patient understands preprocedural teaching. Answer questions as they arise, and reinforce information as needed. ➟*Rationale:* Understanding of previously taught information is evaluated and reinforced.
- Before intubation, initiate intravenous access. ➟*Rationale:* Readily available intravenous access may be necessary if the patient needs to be sedated or paralyzed or needs other medications because of a negative response to the intubation procedure.
- Position the patient appropriately.
  - ❖ Positioning of the nontrauma patient is as follows: Place patient supine with head in sniffing position, in

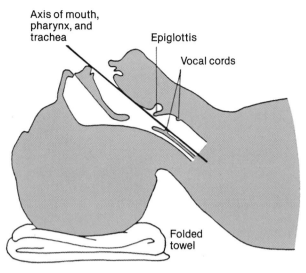

Axis of mouth, pharynx, and trachea

Epiglottis

Vocal cords

Folded towel

FIGURE 2-3 Neck hyperextension in the sniffing position aligns the axis of the mouth, pharynx, and trachea before endotracheal intubation. *(From Kersten, L.D. [1989].* Comprehensive Respiratory Nursing. *Philadelphia: W.B. Saunders, 642.)*

which the head is extended and the neck is flexed. Placement of a small towel under the occiput elevates it several inches, allowing for proper flexion of the neck (Fig. 2-3). ➤*Rationale:* Placing the head in the sniffing position allows for visualization of the larynx and vocal cords by aligning the axes of the mouth, pharynx, and trachea.

❖ Positioning of the trauma patient is as follows: In-line cervical spinal immobilization must be maintained during the entire process of intubation. ➤*Rationale:* Because cervical spinal cord injury must be suspected in all trauma patients until proved otherwise, this position helps prevent secondary injury should a cervical spine injury be present.

• Premedicate as indicated. ➤*Rationale:* Appropriate premedication allows for more controlled intubation, reducing the incidence of insertion trauma, aspiration, laryngospasm, and improper tube placement.

• As appropriate, notify the respiratory therapy department of impending intubation. ➤*Rationale:* Ventilator will be set up before intubation.

Procedure for Performing Endotracheal Intubation

Steps	Rationale	Special Considerations
General Setup 1. Wash hands, and don personal protective equipment, including eye protection.	Reduces transmission of microorganisms and body secretions; standard precautions.	Protective eyewear should be worn to avoid exposure to secretions.
2. Attach patient to pulse oximeter and cardiac monitor.		
3. Set up suction apparatus, and connect rigid suction-tip catheter to tubing.	Prepares for oropharyngeal suctioning as needed.	
4. Check equipment. A. Use 10-ml syringe to inflate cuff on tube, assessing for leaks. Completely deflate cuff.	Verifies that equipment is functional and that tube cuff is patent without leaks; prepares tube for insertion.	
B. Insert the stylet into the endotracheal tube, ensuring that the tip of the stylet does not extend past the end of the endotracheal tube. C. Check the laryngoscope batteries.		Stylet must be recessed by at least ½ inch from the distal end of the tube so that it does not protrude beyond the end of the tube, resulting in damage to the vocal cords and trachea.
5. Position the patient's head by flexing the neck forward and extending the head (sniffing position) (only if neck trauma is not suspected) (see Fig. 2-3).	Allows for visualization of the vocal cords by aligning the mouth, pharynx, and trachea.	Placement of a small towel under the occiput elevates it, allowing for proper neck flexion. Do not flex or extend neck of patient with suspected spinal cord injury; the head must be maintained in a neutral position with in-line cervical spine immobilization.
6. Check the mouth for dentures and remove if present. Suction the mouth and pharynx as needed.	Dentures should be removed before oral intubation is attempted but may remain in place for nasal intubation.	

Procedure for **Performing Endotracheal Intubation**—*Continued*

Steps	Rationale	Special Considerations
7. Insert oropharyngeal airway as indicated (see Procedure 9).	Assists in maintaining upper airway patency.	Use only in unconscious patients.
8. Preoxygenate for 3 to 5 minutes, with 100% oxygen via a nonrebreather mask if ventilations are adequate or via a self-inflating bag-valve-mask device (see Procedure 29) if patient is not adequately ventilating. Provide frequent and gentle breaths.	Helps prevent hypoxemia. Gentle breaths reduce incidence of air entering stomach (leading to gastric distention), decrease airway turbulence, and distribute ventilation more evenly within the lungs.	If patient is breathing, avoid positive-pressure ventilation with a bag-valve-mask due to risk for gastric distention, aspiration, and vomiting.
9. Premedicate patient as indicated. For nasotracheal intubation, proceed to **Step 30**.		
10. Remove oropharyngeal airway if present.		
Orotracheal Intubation		
11. Grasp laryngoscope (with blade in place and illuminated light on) in left hand.	Prepares for efficient blade placement.	Grasp handle as low as possible and keep wrist rigid to prevent using upper teeth as a fulcrum.
12. Use fingers of right hand to open the mouth.	Provides access to oral cavity.	
13. Slowly insert the blade into the right side of the patient's mouth, using it to push the tongue to the left (Fig. 2-4). Advance the blade inward and toward midline past the base of the tongue.	Displaces the tongue to the left, increasing visualization of the glottic opening (Fig. 2-5).	Avoids pressure on the teeth and lips.

Procedure continues on the following page

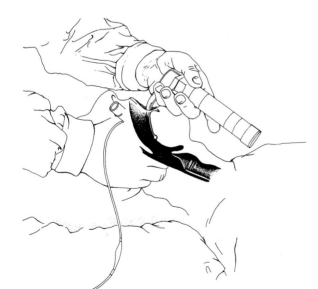

FIGURE 2-4 Technique of orotracheal intubation. The laryngoscope blade is inserted into the oral cavity from the right, pushing the tongue to the left as it is introduced.

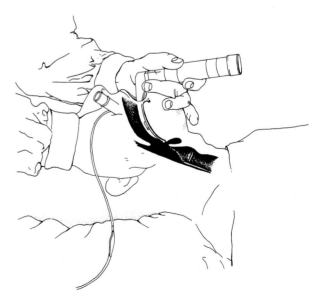

FIGURE 2-5 The blade is advanced into oropharynx, and the laryngoscope is lifted to expose the epiglottis.

Procedure for Performing Endotracheal Intubation—*Continued*

Steps	Rationale	Special Considerations
14. Advance the blade.		
A. Using a curved blade, advance tip into vallecula and exert outward and upward gentle traction at a 45-degree angle to the bed (Fig. 2-6).	Exposes the glottic opening.	Keep left arm and back straight when pulling upward, allowing for use of shoulders when lifting patient's head (decreases use of teeth as a fulcrum).
B. Using a straight blade, advance tip just beneath the epiglottis and exert gentle traction outward and upward at a 45-degree angle to the bed.	Exposes the glottic opening.	Keep left arm and back straight when pulling upward, allowing for use of shoulders when lifting patient's head (decreases use of teeth as a fulcrum).
15. Lift the laryngoscope handle until the vocal cords are visualized.	Allows for correct placement of tube into trachea (Fig. 2-7).	Gentle cricoid pressure (see Fig. 2-1) may assist in visualization of vocal cords and decrease risk of gastric distention and subsequent pulmonary aspiration. When cricoid pressure is begun, it must be continued until the tube is correctly placed.
16. Hold end of tube in right hand with the curved portion downward.	Tube is placed by the right hand.	
17. Under direct vision, gently insert tube from right corner of mouth through the vocal cords (Fig. 2-8) until the cuff is no longer visible and has passed through the vocal cords completely (Fig. 2-9).	Must see tube pass through the vocal cords to ensure proper placement. Advance tube 1.25 to 2.5 cm further into the trachea. When correctly positioned, the tip of the tube should be halfway between the vocal cords and the carina.[3]	The front teeth should be aligned between the 19- and 23-cm depth markings on the tube to ensure the tip of the tube is above the carina.[3] Common tube placement at the teeth is 21 cm for women and 23 cm for men.[9] If intubation is unsuccessful within 30 seconds, remove the tube. Ventilate with 100% oxygen using a bag-valve-mask device before another intubation attempt is made (**repeat Steps 11 through 17**).
18. When tube is correctly placed, continue to hold it securely in place at the lips with right hand while withdrawing the laryngoscope blade and the stylet using left hand.	Firmly holding tube at the lips provides stabilization and prevents inadvertent extubation.	

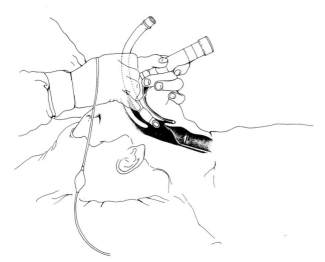

FIGURE 2-6 The tip of the blade is placed in the vallecula, and the laryngoscope is lifted further to expose the glottis. The tube is inserted through the right side of the mouth.

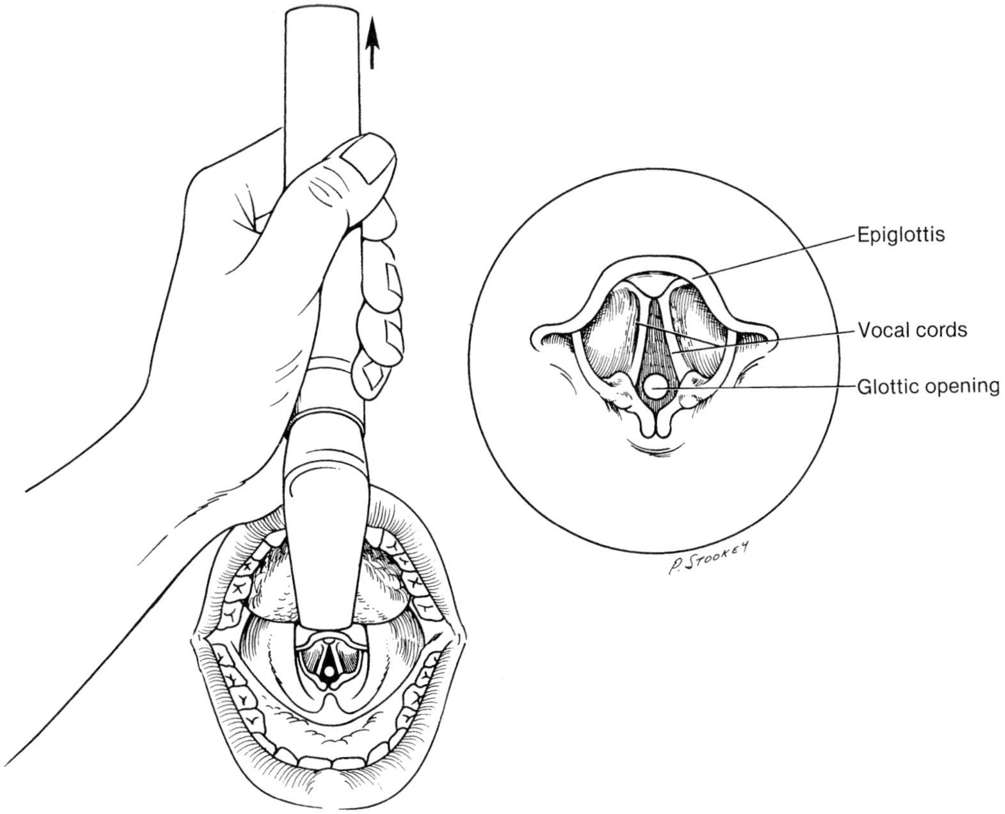

Epiglottis

Vocal cords

Glottic opening

P. STOOKEY

FIGURE 2-7 The endotracheal tube is passed through the vocal cords. *(From Flynn, J.M., and Bruce, N.P. [1993]. Introduction to Critical Care Skills.* St. Louis: Mosby, 56.)

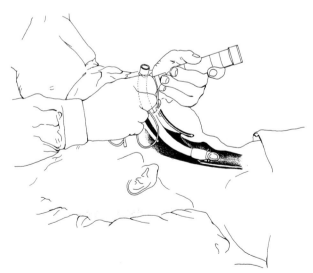

FIGURE 2-8 The tube is advanced through the vocal cords into the trachea.

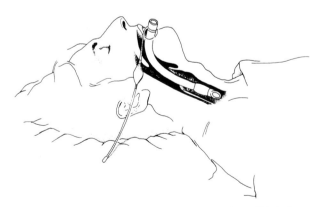

FIGURE 2-9 The tube is positioned so that the cuff is below the vocal cords, and the laryngoscope is removed.

Procedure for Performing Endotracheal Intubation—*Continued*

Steps	Rationale	Special Considerations
19. Inflate cuff with 5 to 10 ml of air depending on the manufacturer's recommendation (see Procedure 11).	Inflation volumes vary depending on manufacturer and size of tube. Keep cuff pressure between 20 and 25 mm Hg to decrease risk of aspiration and prevent ischemia and decreased blood flow.[3,5]	In adults, the minimal intracuff pressure to prevent aspiration is 25 mm Hg. Decreased mucosal capillary blood flow (ischemia) results when pressure is greater than 40 mm Hg.[3]
20. Confirm endotracheal tube placement while manually bagging with 100% oxygen.	Ensures correct placement of endotracheal tube.	
A. Attach disposable end-tidal CO_2 detector. Watch for color change, indicating the presence of CO_2. *(Level VI: Clinical studies in a variety of patient populations and situations.)* *or* Attach continuous end-tidal CO_2 monitor and watch for detection of CO_2.	Disposable CO_2 detectors may be used to assist with identification of proper tube placement.[3,4,6,11-15,17] Detection of CO_2 confirms proper endotracheal tube placement into the trachea.[3] During cardiac arrest (nonperfusing rhythms), there may not be sufficient expired CO_2 due to low pulmonary blood flow.[16]	CO_2 detectors usually are placed between the self-inflating bag and the endotracheal tube. CO_2 detectors should be used in conjunction with physical assessment findings.
Consider use of esophageal detection device in cardiac arrest. *(Level V: Clinical studies in more than one patient population and situation.)*	If CO_2 is detected using an end-tidal CO_2 detector, it is a reliable indicator of proper tube placement. If CO_2 is not detected, use of an esophageal detector device is recommended.[2,7,10,14,18]	
B. Auscultate over epigastrium. *(Level II: Theory based, no research data to support recommendations; recommendations from expert consensus group may exist.)*	Allows for identification of esophageal intubation.[3,5]	If air movement or gurgling is heard, esophageal intubation has occurred. The tube must be pulled and intubation reattempted. Improper insertion may result in hypoxemia, gastric distention, vomiting, and aspiration.
C. Auscultate lung bases and apices for bilateral breath sounds. *(Level II: Theory based, no research data to support recommendations; recommendations from expert consensus group may exist.)*	Assists in verification of correct tube placement into the trachea. A right main stem bronchus intubation results in diminished left-sided breath sounds.[3]	Equal breath sounds indicate proper placement of the endotracheal tube.
D. Observe for symmetric chest wall movement. *(Level II: Theory based, no research data to support recommendations; recommendations from expert consensus group may exist.)*	Assists in verification of correct tube placement.[3]	Absence may indicate right main stem or esophageal intubation.
E. Evaluate SpO_2 by noninvasive pulse oximetry. *(Level II: Theory based, no research data to support recommendations; recommendations from expert consensus group may exist.)*	SpO_2 decreases if the esophagus has been inadvertently intubated. It may or may not change in a right main stem bronchus intubation.[3,5]	SpO_2 findings should be used in conjunction with physical assessment findings.

Procedure for Performing Endotracheal Intubation—*Continued*		
Steps	**Rationale**	**Special Considerations**
21. If CO_2 detection, assessment findings, or SpO_2 reveals that the tube is not correctly positioned, deflate cuff and remove tube immediately. Hyperoxygenate with 100% oxygen for 3 to 5 minutes, then reattempt intubation, beginning with **Step 11**. (*Level II: Theory based, no research data to support recommendations; recommendations from expert consensus group may exist.*)	Esophageal intubation results in gas flow diversion and hypoxemia.[3,5]	
22. If breath sounds are absent on the left, deflate the cuff and withdraw tube 1 to 2 cm. Reevaluate for correct tube placement (**Step 20**).	Absence of breath sounds on the left may indicate right main stem intubation, which is common because of the anatomic position of the right main stem bronchi. When correctly positioned, the tube tip should be halfway between the vocal cords and the carina.[2]	
23. Connect endotracheal tube to oxygen source or mechanical ventilator, using swivel adapter.	Reduces motion on tube and mouth or nares.	
24. Insert a bite-block or oropharyngeal airway (to act as a bite-block) along the endotracheal tube.	Prevents the patient from biting down on the endotracheal tube.	The bite-block should be secured separately from the tube to prevent dislodgment of the tube.
25. Secure the endotracheal tube in place (according to institutional standard). (*Level II: Theory based, no research data to support recommendations; recommendations from expert consensus group may exist.*)	Prevents inadvertent dislodgment of tube.[1,3,8]	Various methods are used for securing endotracheal tubes, including the use of specially manufactured tube holders, twill tape, or adhesive tape.
Use of Commercially Available Endotracheal Tube Holder A. Apply according to manufacturer's directions.	Allows for secure stabilization of the tube, decreasing the likelihood of inadvertent extubation.	These are recommended over the use of other types of endotracheal tube securing methods, such as taping and tying.[2]
Use of Twill Tape A. Double over a 2-foot length of twill tape; tie the tape around the tube, pulling the frayed ends of tape through the looped end; and tie where tube emerges from the lips. B. Pull the tape ends in opposite directions around the patient's neck. C. Tie the two ends of the tape at the side of the patient's neck securely.	Allows for secure stabilization of the tube, decreasing the likelihood of inadvertent extubation. Secures tube and prevents direct pressure on back of neck.	

Procedure continues on the following page

Procedure for Performing Endotracheal Intubation—*Continued*

Steps	Rationale	Special Considerations
Use of Adhesive Tape		
A. Prepare tape as shown in Figure 2-10.	Use of a hydrocolloid membrane (e.g., Duoderm) on the patient's cheeks helps protect the skin.	
B. Secure tube by wrapping double-sided tape around patient's head and torn tape edges around endotracheal tube.		
26. Reconfirm tube placement (**Step 20**).	Verifies that the tube was not inadvertently repositioned during the securing of the tube.	
27. Note position of tube at teeth (use centimeter markings on tube).	Common tube placement at the teeth is 21 cm for women and 23 cm for men.[9]	
28. Hyperoxygenate and suction endotracheal tube and pharynx (see Procedure 10) as needed.	Removes secretions that may obstruct tube or accumulate on the top of the cuff.	
29. Confirmation of correct tube position should be verified by a chest x-ray. (*Level II: Theory based, no research data to support recommendations; recommendations from expert consensus group may exist.*)	Chest x-ray documents actual tube location (distance from the carina). Because chest x-ray is not immediately available, it should not be used as the primary method of tube assessment.[3,5,9]	Endotracheal tubes placed bronchoscopically may not require chest x-ray verification (check institutional standard).
Nasotracheal Intubation		
30. **Follow Steps 1 through 10.**	Steps necessary to initiate nasal intubation. Dentures may be left in place for nasotracheal intubation.	
31. Spray nasal passage with anesthetic and vasoconstrictor, as indicated.	Anesthetizes and vasoconstricts nasal mucosa to decrease incidence of trauma and bleeding.	
32. Lubricate tube with local anesthetic jelly.	Allows for smooth passage of tube.	
33. Slowly insert tube into selected naris, and guide tube up from the nostril, then backward and down into the nasopharynx.	Tube is introduced into airway channel.	
34. Gently advance the tube until maximal sound of moving air is heard through the tube.	Tube is located at opening of trachea.	Breath sounds become maximal just before entering the glottis.

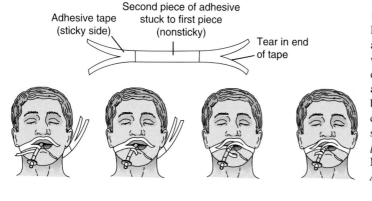

FIGURE 2-10 Methods of securing adhesive tape. Example protocol for securing the endotracheal tube using adhesive tape: (1) Clean the patient's skin with mild soap and water. (2) Remove oil from the skin with alcohol and allow to dry. (3) Apply a skin adhesive product to enhance tape adherence. (When tape is removed, an adhesive remover will be necessary.) (4) Place a hydrocolloid membrane over the cheeks to protect friable skin. (5) Secure with adhesive tape as shown. (*From Henneman, E., Ellstrom, K., and St. John, R.E. [1999].* AACN Protocols for Practice: Care of the Mechanically Ventilated Patient Series. *Aliso Viejo, CA: American Association of Critical-Care Nurses, 56.*)

Procedure for Performing Endotracheal Intubation—*Continued*

Steps	Rationale	Special Considerations
35. While listening, continue to advance tube during inspiration.	Facilitates movement of tube through glottic opening.	Magill forceps may assist with advancement of tube. Cricoid pressure may help align the glottic opening.
36. When endotracheal tube is placed, inflate cuff.		
37. **Follow Steps 20 through 23 and 25 through 29** to evaluate tube placement and secure tube in place.		

Expected Outcomes

- Placement of patent artificial airway
- Properly positioned and secured airway
- Improved oxygenation and ventilation
- Facilitation of secretion clearance

Unexpected Outcomes

- Intubation of esophagus or right main stem bronchus (improper tube placement)
- Accidental extubation
- Cardiac dysrhythmias because of hypoxemia and vagal stimulation
- Broken or dislodged teeth
- Leaking of air from endotracheal tube cuff
- Tracheal injury at tip of tube or at cuff site
- Laryngeal edema
- Vocal cord trauma
- Suctioning of gastric contents or food from endotracheal tube (aspiration)
- Obstruction of endotracheal tube

Patient Monitoring and Care

Steps	Rationale	Reportable Conditions
		These conditions should be reported if they persist despite nursing interventions.
1. Auscultate breath sounds on insertion and every 2 to 4 hours.	Allows for detection of tube movement or dislodgment.	- Absent, decreased, or unequal breath sounds
2. Maintain tube stability, using specially manufactured holder, twill tape, or adhesive tape.	Prevents movement and dislodgment of tube.	- Unplanned extubation
3. Monitor and record position of tube at teeth or nose (in reference to centimeter markings on tube).	Provides for identification of tube migration.	- Tube movement from original position
4. Maintain tube cuff pressure at 20 to 25 mm Hg (see Procedure 11).	Provides adequate inflation to decrease aspiration risk and prevents overinflation of cuff to avoid tracheal damage.[3,5]	- Cuff pressure less than 20 to greater than 25 mm Hg
5. Hyperoxygenate and suction endotracheal tube, as needed (see Procedure 10).	Prevents obstruction of tube and resulting hypoxemia.	- Inability to pass a suction catheter - Copious, frothy, or bloody secretions - Significant change in amount or character of secretions
6. Inspect nares or oral cavity once per shift while patient is intubated.	Allows for the detection of skin breakdown and necrosis.	- Redness, necrosis, skin breakdown

Documentation

Documentation should include the following:

- Patient and family education
- Vital signs before, during, and after intubation, including oxygen saturation
- Type of intubation—oral or nasal
- Number of intubation attempts
- Use of any medications
- Size of endotracheal tube
- Depth of endotracheal tube insertion—centimeters at teeth or nose

- Measurement of cuff pressure
- Assessment of breath sounds
- Confirmation of tube placement including chest radiograph (how placement was confirmed)
- Occurrence of unexpected outcomes
- Nursing interventions
- Secretions
- Patient response to procedure

References

1. Barnason, S., et al. (1998). Comparison of two endotracheal tube securement techniques on unplanned extubation, oral mucosa, and facial skin integrity. *Heart Lung, 27,* 409-17.
2. Bozeman W.P., et al. (1996). Esophageal detector device versus detection of end-tidal carbon dioxide level in emergency intubation. *Ann Emerg Med, 27,* 595-9.
3. Cummins, R.O., ed. (2003). Airway, airway adjuncts, oxygenation, and ventilation. In: *ACLS: Principles and Practice.* Dallas: American Heart Association, 135-80.
4. Goldberg J.S., et al. (1990). Colorimetric end-tidal carbon dioxide monitoring for tracheal intubation. *Anesth Analg, 70,* 191-4.
5. Guidelines 2000 for Cardiopulmonary Resuscitation and Emergency Cardiovascular Care: International Consensus on Science. (2000). Adjuncts for oxygenation, ventilation, and airway control. *Circulation* 102 (Suppl), 95-104.
6. Hayden, S.R., et al. (1995). Colorimetric end-tidal CO_2 detector for verification of endotracheal tube placement in out-of-hospital cardiac arrest. *Acad Emerg Med, 2,* 499-502.
7. Hendey, G. W., et al. (2002). The esophageal detector bulb in the aeromedical setting. *J Emerg Med, 23,* 51-5.
8. Henneman, E., Ellstrom, E., and St. John, R.E. (1999). Airway management. In: *AACN Protocols for Practice: Care of the Mechanically Ventilated Patient Series.* Aliso Viejo, CA: American Association of Critical-Care Nurses.
9. Holleran, R.S. (1996). *Flight Nursing: Principles and Practice.* 2nd ed. St. Louis: Mosby.
10. Kasper, C.L., et al. (1998). The self-inflating bulb to detect esophageal intubation during emergency airway management. *Anesthesiology, 88,* 898-902.
11. MacLeod, B.A., et al. (1991). Verification of endotracheal tube placement with colorimetric end-tidal CO_2 detection. *Ann Emerg Med, 20,* 267-70.
12. Ornato, J.P., et al. (1992). Multicenter study of a portable, hand-size, colorimetric end-tidal carbon dioxide detection device. *Ann Emerg Med, 21,* 518-23.
13. Sanders, K.C., et al. (1994). End-tidal carbon dioxide detection in emergency intubation in four groups of patients. *J Emerg Med, 12,* 771-7.
14. Schaller, R.J., et al. (1997). Comparison of a colorimetric end-tidal CO_2 detector and an esophageal aspiration device for verifying endotracheal tube placement in the prehospital setting: A six-month experience. *Prehospital Disaster Med, 12,* 57-63.
15. Takeda, T., et al. (2003). The assessment of three methods to verify tracheal tube placement in the emergency setting. *Resuscitation, 56,* 153-7.
16. Varon, A.J., et al. (1991). Clinical utility of a colorimetric end-tidal CO_2 detector in cardiopulmonary resuscitation and emergency intubation. *J Clin Monit, 7,* 289-93.
17. Vukmir, R.B., et al. (1991). Confirmation of endotracheal tube placement: A miniaturized infrared qualitative CO_2 detector. *Ann Emerg Med, 20,* 726-9.
18. Zaleski, L., et al. (1993). The esophageal detector device. Does it work? *Anesthesiology, 79,* 244-7.

Additional Reading

Salem, M.R. (2001). Verification of endotracheal tube position. *Anesthesiol Clin North Am, 19,* 813-39.

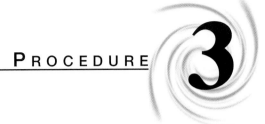
PROCEDURE **3**

Endotracheal Intubation (Assist)

P U R P O S E :   Endotracheal intubation is performed to establish and maintain a patent airway, facilitate oxygenation and ventilation, reduce the risk of aspiration, and assist with the clearance of secretions.

Julianne M. Scott

PREREQUISITE NURSING KNOWLEDGE

- Anatomy and physiology of the pulmonary system should be understood.
- Indications for endotracheal intubation include the following:[4]
    - Upper airway obstruction (e.g., secondary to swelling, trauma, tumor, bleeding)
    - Apnea
    - Ineffective clearance of secretions (i.e., inability to maintain airway adequately)
    - High risk of aspiration
    - Respiratory distress
- Pulse oximetry should be used during intubation so that oxygen desaturation can be detected quickly.
- Preoxygenation with 100% oxygen using a bag-valve-mask device with a tight-fitting facemask should be performed for 3 to 5 minutes before intubation.
- Intubation attempts should take no longer than 15 to 30 seconds.
- Applying cricoid pressure (Sellick maneuver) may decrease the incidence of pulmonary aspiration and gastric distention. This procedure is accomplished by applying firm, downward pressure on the cricoid ring, pushing the vocal cords downward so that they are visualized more easily. Once begun, cricoid pressure must be maintained until intubation is completed (see Fig. 2-1).
- Two types of laryngoscope blades exist, straight and curved. The straight (Miller) blade is designed so that the tip extends below the epiglottis, lifting and exposing the glottic opening. It is recommended for use in obese patients, pediatric patients, and patients with short necks because their tracheas may be located more anteriorly. When a curved (Macintosh) blade is used, the tip is advanced into the vallecula (the space between the epiglottis and the base of the tongue), exposing the glottic opening.
- Endotracheal tube size reflects the size of the internal diameter of the tube. Tubes range in size from 2.5 mm for neonates to 9 mm for large adults. Endotracheal tubes ranging in size from 7 to 8 mm are used for average-sized women, whereas tubes ranging in size from 8 to 9 mm are used for average-sized men (see Fig. 2-2).[4,5] The tube with the largest clinically acceptable internal diameter should be used to minimize airway resistance and assist in suctioning.
- Endotracheal intubation can be done via nasal or oral routes. The skill of the practitioner performing intubation and the patient's clinical condition determine the route used.
- Nasal intubation is relatively contraindicated in trauma patients with facial fractures or suspected fractures at the base of the skull or postoperatively after cranial surgeries, such as transnasal hypophysectomy.
- In patients with suspected spinal cord injuries, in-line cervical immobilization of the head must be maintained during endotracheal intubation.
- Improper intubation technique may result in trauma to the teeth, soft tissues of the mouth or nose, vocal cords, and posterior pharynx.
- Primary and secondary confirmation of endotracheal intubation should be performed.
    - Primary confirmation of proper endotracheal tube placement includes visualization of the tube passing through the vocal cords, absence of gurgling over the epigastric

area, auscultation of bilateral breath sounds, bilateral chest rise and fall during ventilation, and mist in the tube.

  ❖ Secondary confirmation of proper endotracheal tube placement is necessary to protect against unrecognized esophageal intubation. Methods include use of disposable end-tidal carbon dioxide (CO_2) detectors, continuous end-tidal CO_2 monitors, and esophageal detection devices.

- End-tidal CO_2 monitoring devices have been shown to be reliable indicators of expired CO_2 in patients with perfusing rhythms.[3] During cardiac arrest (nonperfusing rhythms), there may not be sufficient expired CO_2 due to low pulmonary blood flow. If CO_2 is detected using an end-tidal CO_2 detector, it is a reliable indicator of proper tube placement. If CO_2 is not detected, use of an esophageal detector device is recommended (see Procedure 2).[3]
- Disposable end-tidal CO_2 detectors are chemically treated with a nontoxic indicator that changes color in the presence of CO_2, indicating that the endotracheal tube has been placed successfully into the trachea.
- Continuous end-tidal CO_2 monitors may be used to confirm proper endotracheal tube placement after intubation attempts and allow for the detection of future tube dislodgment.
- Esophageal detector devices work by creating suction at the end of the endotracheal tube by compressing a flexible bulb or pulling back on a syringe plunger. When the tube is placed correctly in the trachea, air allows for reexpansion of the bulb or movement of the syringe plunger. If the tube is located in the esophagus, no movement of the syringe plunger or reexpansion of the bulb is seen. These devices may be misleading in patients who are morbidly obese, patients in status asthmaticus, patients late in pregnancy, and patients with large amounts of tracheal secretions.[3]
- Double-lumen endotracheal tubes are used for independent lung ventilation in situations in which there is bleeding of one lung or a large air leak that would impair ventilation of the good lung.
- The endotracheal tube also provides a route for the administration of emergency medication (e.g., lidocaine, epinephrine, atropine, and naloxone).

EQUIPMENT

- Personal protective equipment, including eye protection
- Endotracheal tube with intact cuff and 15-mm connector (7- to 8-mm tube, women; 8- to 9-mm tube, men)
- Laryngoscope handle with fresh batteries
- Laryngoscope blades (straight and curved)
- Spare bulb for laryngoscope blades
- Flexible stylet
- Self-inflating resuscitation bag with mask connected to supplemental oxygen (greater than or equal to 15 L/min)
- Oxygen source and connecting tubes
- Swivel adapter (for attachment to resuscitation bag or ventilator)
- Luer-tip 10-ml syringe for cuff inflation

- Water-soluble lubricant
- Rigid pharyngeal suction-tip (Yankauer) catheter
- Suction apparatus (portable or wall)
- Suction catheters
- Bite-block or oropharyngeal airway
- Endotracheal tube–securing apparatus or appropriate tape
  ❖ Commercially available endotracheal tube holder
  ❖ Adhesive tape (6 to 8 inches long)
  ❖ Twill tape (cut into 30-inch lengths)
- Stethoscope
- Monitoring equipment: continuous oxygen saturation and cardiac rhythm
- Secondary confirmation device: disposable end-tidal CO_2 detector, continuous end-tidal CO_2 monitoring device, and esophageal detection device
- Drugs for intubation as indicated (sedation, paralyzing agents, lidocaine, atropine).

Additional equipment (to have available depending on patient need or practitioner preference) includes the following:
- Anesthetic spray (nasal approach)
- Local anesthetic jelly (nasal approach)
- Magill forceps (to remove foreign bodies obstructing the airway)
- Ventilator

PATIENT AND FAMILY EDUCATION

- Assess level of understanding about condition and rationale for endotracheal intubation. ➦*Rationale:* This assessment identifies the patient's and family's knowledge deficits concerning patient condition, procedure, expected benefits, and potential risks and allows time for questions to clarify information and voice concerns. Explanations decrease patient anxiety and enhance cooperation.
- Explain the procedure and the reason for intubation. ➦*Rationale:* This enhances patient and family understanding and decreases anxiety.
- If indicated, explain the patient's role in assisting with insertion of endotracheal tube. ➦*Rationale:* Eliciting the patient's cooperation assists with insertion.
- Explain that the patient will be unable to speak while the endotracheal tube is in place, but that other means of communication will be provided. ➦*Rationale:* This enhances patient and family understanding and decreases anxiety.
- Explain that the patient's hands often are immobilized to prevent accidental dislodgment of the tube. ➦*Rationale:* This enhances patient and family understanding and decreases anxiety.

PATIENT ASSESSMENT AND PREPARATION

Patient Assessment

- Assess immediate history of trauma when spinal cord injury is suspected or cranial surgery. ➦*Rationale:* Knowing pertinent patient history allows for selection of the most appropriate method for intubation, helping reduce the risk for secondary injury.

- Assess nothing-by-mouth (NPO) status and signs of gastric distention. ➤*Rationale:* Increased risk of aspiration and vomiting occurs with accumulation of air, food, or secretions. If a patient who has gastric distention or who has eaten recently needs to be intubated, use of cricoid pressure decreases the risk of aspiration.
- Assess level of consciousness, level of anxiety, and respiratory difficulty. ➤*Rationale:* This determines need for sedation or use of paralytic agents and the patient's ability to lie flat and supine for intubation.
- Assess vital signs, and assess for tachypnea, dyspnea, shallow respirations, cyanosis, apnea, altered level of consciousness, tachycardia, cardiac dysrhythmias, hypertension, and headache. ➤*Rationale:* Any of the aforementioned may indicate a problem with oxygenation or ventilation or both.
- Assess patency of nares (for nasal intubation). ➤*Rationale:* Selection of the most appropriate naris facilitates insertion and may improve patient tolerance of tube.
- Assess need for premedication. ➤*Rationale:* Various medications provide sedation or paralysis of the patient as needed.

Patient Preparation

- Ensure that the patient understands preprocedural teaching. Answer questions as they arise, and reinforce information as needed. ➤*Rationale:* This evaluates and reinforces understanding of previously taught information.

- Before intubation, initiate intravenous access. ➤*Rationale:* Readily available intravenous access may be necessary if the patient needs to be sedated or paralyzed or needs other medications because of a negative response to the intubation procedure.
- Position the patient appropriately.
  - ❖ Positioning of the nontrauma patient is as follows: Place patient supine with head in sniffing position, in which the head is extended and the neck is flexed. Placement of a small towel under the occiput elevates it several inches, allowing for proper flexion of the neck (see Fig. 2-3). ➤*Rationale:* Placing the head in the sniffing position allows for visualization of the larynx and vocal cords by aligning the axes of the mouth, pharynx, and trachea.
  - ❖ Positioning of the trauma patient is as follows: In-line cervical spinal immobilization must be maintained during the entire process of intubation. ➤*Rationale:* Because cervical spinal cord injury must be suspected in all trauma patients until proved otherwise, this position helps prevent secondary injury should a cervical spine injury be present.
- Premedicate as indicated. ➤*Rationale:* Appropriate premedication allows for more controlled intubation, reducing the incidence of insertion trauma, aspiration, laryngospasm, and improper tube placement.
- As appropriate, notify the respiratory therapy department of impending intubation. ➤*Rationale:* Ventilator will be set up before intubation.

Procedure for Assisting With Endotracheal Intubation

Steps	Rationale	Special Considerations
1. Wash hands, and don personal protective equipment.	Reduces transmission of microorganisms and body secretions; standard precautions.	Protective eyewear should be worn to avoid exposure to secretions.
2. Insert oropharyngeal airway (see Procedure 9). Connect patient to pulse oximeter and cardiac monitor.	Assists in maintaining upper airway patency.	Used only in unconscious patients.
3. Set up suction apparatus and connect rigid suction-tip catheter to tubing.	Prepares for oropharyngeal suctioning as needed.	
4. Assist in positioning the patient's head by flexing the neck forward and extending the head (sniffing position).	Allows for visualization of the vocal cords by aligning the three axes of the mouth, pharynx, and trachea.	Placement of a small towel under the occiput elevates it, allowing for proper neck flexion. Do not flex or extend the neck of a patient with suspected spinal cord injury; the head must be maintained in a neutral position with in-line cervical spine immobilization.
5. Check the mouth for dentures, and remove if present. Suction the mouth as needed.	Dentures should be removed before oral intubation is attempted but may remain in place for nasal intubation.	

Procedure continues on the following page

Procedure for Assisting With Endotracheal Intubation—*Continued*

Steps	Rationale	Special Considerations
6. Preoxygenate using a self-inflating bag-valve-mask device (see Procedure 29) attached to 100% oxygen for 3 to 5 minutes. Provide frequent and gentle breaths.	Helps prevent hypoxemia; gentle breaths reduce incidence of air entering stomach (leading to gastric distention), decrease airway turbulence, and distribute ventilation more evenly within the lungs.	
7. Premedicate patient as indicated.		
8. Apply cricoid pressure as requested.	Gentle cricoid pressure (see Fig. 2-1) may assist in visualization of vocal cords and decrease the risk of gastric distention and subsequent pulmonary aspiration. Once cricoid pressure is begun, it must be continued until the tube is correctly placed.	
9. Have manual resuscitation bag connected to 100% oxygen source and facemask ready for hyperoxygenation and manual ventilation.	Intubation attempts should not take longer than 30 seconds. Patients need to be hyperoxygenated and ventilated between intubation attempts.[2]	
10. When the endotracheal tube has been placed, assist to confirm tube placement while bagging with 100% oxygen (see Procedure 2).	Confirms placement of the endotracheal tube. Disposable CO_2 detectors or esophageal detection devices may be used to assist with identification of proper tube placement.[2]	CO_2 detectors or esophageal detection devices usually are placed between the self-inflating bag and the endotracheal tube. CO_2 detectors or esophageal detection devices should be used in conjunction with physical assessment findings.
A. Auscultate over epigastrium. *(Level II: Theory based, no research data to support recommendations; recommendations from expert consensus group may exist.)*	Allows for identification of esophageal intubation.[2]	If air movement or gurgling is heard, esophageal intubation has occurred; the tube must be pulled and intubation reattempted. Improper insertion may result in hypoxemia, gastric distention, vomiting, and aspiration.
B. Auscultate lung bases and apices for bilateral breath sounds. *(Level II: Theory based, no research data to support recommendations; recommendations from expert consensus group may exist.)*	Assists in verification of correct tube placement into the trachea. A right main stem bronchus intubation results in diminished left-sided breath sounds.[2]	Equal breath sounds indicate proper placement of the endotracheal tube.
C. Observe for symmetric chest wall movement. *(Level II: Theory based, no research data to support recommendations; recommendations from expert consensus group may exist.)*	Assists in verification of correct tube placements.[2]	Absence may indicate right main stem or esophageal intubation.
D. Evaluate oxygen saturation (Spo₂) by noninvasive pulse oximetry. *(Level II: Theory based, no research data to support recommendations; recommendations from expert consensus group may exist.)*	Spo₂ decreases if the esophagus has been inadvertently intubated; it may or may not change in a right main stem bronchus intubation.[2,3]	Spo₂ findings should be used in conjunction with physical assessment findings.

Procedure for Assisting With Endotracheal Intubation—*Continued*

Steps	Rationale	Special Considerations
11. If CO_2 detection, assessment findings, or SpO_2 level reveals that the tube has not been positioned correctly, assist with reintubation. Hyperoxygenate with 100% oxygen for 3 to 5 minutes, and reattempt intubation, beginning with **Step 1**. (*Level II: Theory based, no research data to support recommendations; recommendations from expert consensus group may exist.*)	Esophageal intubation results in gas flow diversion and hypoxemia.[2,3]	
12. If breath sounds are absent on the left, the cuff should be deflated and the tube pulled 1 to 2 cm. Reevaluate for correct tube placement (**Step 10**).	Absence of breath sounds on the left may indicate right main stem intubation, which is common as a result of the anatomic position of the right main stem bronchi. When correctly positioned, the tip of the tube should be halfway between the vocal cords and the carina.[2]	
13. Connect endotracheal tube to oxygen source or mechanical ventilator, using swivel adapter.	Reduces motion on tube and mouth or nares.	
14. Insert a bite-block or oropharyngeal airway (to act as a bite-block) along the endotracheal tube.	Prevents the patient from biting down on the endotracheal tube.	The bite-block should be secured separately from the tube to prevent dislodgment of the tube.
15. Secure the endotracheal tube in place (according to institutional standard). (*Level II: Theory based, no research data to support recommendations; recommendations from expert consensus group may exist.*)	To prevent inadvertent dislodgment of tube.[1,2,4]	Various methods are used for securing endotracheal tubes, including use of specially manufactured tube holders, twill tape, and adhesive tape.
Use of Twill Tape A. Double over a 2-foot length of twill tape; tie the tape around the tube, pulling frayed ends of tape through the looped end; and tie where tube emerges from the lips. B. Pull the tape ends in opposite directions around the patient's neck.	Allows for secure stabilization of the tube, decreasing the likelihood of inadvertent extubation.	
C. Tie the two ends of the tape at the side of the patient's neck securely.	Secures tube and prevents direct pressure on back of neck.	
Use of Adhesive Tape A. Prepare tape as shown in Figure 2-10.	Use of a hydrocolloid membrane (e.g., Duoderm) on the patient's cheeks helps protect the skin.	
B. Secure tube by wrapping double-sided tape around patient's head and torn tape edges around endotracheal tube.		
16. Reconfirm tube placement (**Step 10**).	Verifies that the tube was not inadvertently repositioned during the securing of the tube.	

Procedure continues on the following page

Procedure for Assisting With Endotracheal Intubation—*Continued*

Steps	Rationale	Special Considerations
17. Note position of tube at teeth (use centimeter markings on tube).	Common tube placement at the teeth is 21 cm for women and 23 cm for men.[5]	
18. Hyperoxygenate and suction endotracheal tube and pharynx (see Procedure 10) as needed.	Remove secretions that may obstruct tube or accumulate on top of cuff.	
19. Confirmation of correct tube position should be verified by a chest x-ray. (*Level II: Theory based, no research data to support recommendations; recommendations from expert consensus group may exist.*)	Chest x-ray documents actual tube location (distance from the carina). Because chest x-ray is not immediately available, it should not be used as the primary method of tube assessment.[2-4]	Endotracheal tubes placed bronchoscopically may not require chest x-ray verification (check institutional standard).

Expected Outcomes

- Placement of patent artificial airway
- Properly positioned and secured airway
- Improved oxygenation and ventilation
- Facilitation of secretion clearance

Unexpected Outcomes

- Intubation of esophagus or right main stem bronchus (improper tube placement)
- Accidental extubation
- Cardiac dysrhythmias as a result of hypoxemia and vagal stimulation
- Broken or dislodged teeth
- Leaking of air from endotracheal tube cuff
- Tracheal injury at tip of tube or at cuff site
- Laryngeal edema
- Vocal cord trauma
- Suctioning of gastric contents or food from endotracheal tube (aspiration)
- Obstruction of endotracheal tube

Patient Monitoring and Care

Steps	Rationale	Reportable Conditions
		These conditions should be reported if they persist despite nursing interventions.
1. Auscultate breath sounds on insertion and every 2 to 4 hours.	Allows for detection of tube movement or dislodgment.	• Absent or unequal breath sounds
2. Maintain tube stability, using specially manufactured holder, twill tape, or adhesive tape.	Prevents movement and dislodgment of tube.	• Unplanned extubation
3. Monitor and record position of tube at teeth or nose (in reference to centimeter markings on tube).	Provides for identification of tube migration.	• Tube movement from origingal position
4. Maintain tube cuff pressure at 20 to 25 mm Hg (see Procedure 11).	Provides adequate inflation, decreases aspiration risk, and prevents overinflation of cuff to avoid tracheal damage.[2,3]	• Cuff pressure less than 20 or greater than 25 mm Hg
5. Hyperoxygenate and suction endotracheal tube as needed.	Prevents obstruction of tube and resulting hypoxemia.	• Inability to pass a suction catheter • Copious, frothy, or bloody secretions • Significant change in amount or character of secretions
6. Inspect nares or oral cavity once per shift while patient is intubated.	Allows for the detection of skin breakdown and necrosis.	• Redness, necrosis, skin breakdown

Documentation

Documentation should include the following:

- Patient and family education
- Vital signs before, during, and after intubation, including oxygen saturation
- Type of intubation—oral or nasal
- Use of any medications
- Size of endotracheal tube
- Depth of endotracheal tube insertion (centimeters at teeth or nose)
- Measurement of cuff pressure
- Assessment of breath sounds
- Confirmation of tube placement, including chest radiograph (how placement was confirmed)
- Occurrence of unexpected outcomes
- Nursing interventions
- Secretions
- Patient response to procedure

References

1. Barnason, S., et al. (1998). Comparison of two endotracheal tube securement techniques on unplanned extubation, oral mucosa, and facial skin integrity. *Heart Lung,* 27, 409-17.
2. Cummins, R.O., ed. (2003). Airway, airway adjuncts, oxygenation, and ventilation. In: *ACLS: Principles and Practice.* Dallas: American Heart Association, 135-80.
3. Guidelines 2000 for Cardiopulmonary Resuscitation and Emergency Cardiovascular Care: International Consensus on Science. (2000). Adjuncts for oxygenation, ventilation, and airway control. *Circulation,* 102(Suppl), 95-104.
4. Henneman, E., Ellstrom, K., and St. John, R.E. (1999). Airway management. In: *AACN Protocols for Practice: Care of the Mechanically Ventilated Patient Series.* Aliso Viejo, CA: American Association of Critical-Care Nurses.
5. Holleran, R.S. (1996). *Flight Nursing: Principles and Practice.* 2nd ed. St. Louis: Mosby.

Additional Readings

American College of Emergency Physicians. (2002). Policy statement on verification of endotracheal tube placement. *Ann Emerg Med,* 40, 551-2.
Committee on Trauma. (1997). *American College of Surgeons: Advanced Trauma Life Support Manual.* Chicago: American College of Surgeons.
Holleran, R.S. (2003). *Air and Surface Patient Transport: Principles and Practice.* St. Louis: Mosby.
Huggins, R.M., et al. (2003). Cardiac arrest from succinylcholine-induced hyperkalemia. *Am J Health-Syst Pharm,* 60, 693-7.
National Association of Emergency Technicians. (2003). *PHTLS: Basic and Advanced Prehospital Trauma Life Support.* 5th ed. St. Louis: Mosby.
Roberts, J.R., and Hedges, J.R., eds. (2004). *Clinical Procedures in Emergency Medicine.* 4th ed. Philadelphia: W.B. Saunders.
Society of Critical Care Medicine. (2001). *Fundamental Critical Care Support Course Text.* 3rd ed. Des Plaines, IL: Society of Critical Care Medicine.

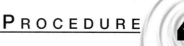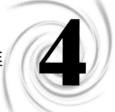
PROCEDURE **4**

Endotracheal Tube and Oral Care

P U R P O S E : Endotracheal tube and oral care is performed to prevent buccal, oropharyngeal, and tracheal trauma from the tube and cuff; to provide oral hygiene; to promote ventilation; and to decrease the risk of ventilator-associated pneumonia (VAP).

Julianne M. Scott
Kathleen M. Vollman

PREREQUISITE NURSING KNOWLEDGE

- Anatomy and physiology of the pulmonary system should be understood.
- Anatomy and physiology of the oral cavity should be understood.
- Endotracheal tubes are used to maintain a patent airway or to facilitate mechanical ventilation. Presence of these artificial airways, especially endotracheal tubes, prevents effective coughing and secretion removal, requiring periodic removal of pulmonary secretions with suctioning. In acute care situations, suctioning always is performed as a sterile procedure to prevent nosocomial pneumonia.
- Suctioning of airways should be performed only for a clinical indication and not as a routine, fixed-schedule treatment (see Procedure 10).
- Adequate systemic hydration and supplemental humidification of inspired gases assist in thinning secretions for easier aspiration from airways.
- Appropriate cuff care (see Procedure 11) helps prevent major pulmonary aspirations, prepares for tracheal extubation, decreases the risk of inadvertent extubation, provides a patent airway for ventilation and removal of secretions, and decreases the risk of iatrogenic infections.
- Constant pressure from the endotracheal tube on the mouth or nose can cause skin breakdown.
- If the patient is anxious or uncooperative, using two caregivers when retaping or repositioning the endotracheal tube helps prevent accidental dislodgment of the tube.
- The incidence of ventilator-associated pneumonia is increased in patients intubated for longer than 24 hours.

Ventilator-associated pneumonia is thought to be related to aspiration of gastric or oral secretions (or both) and the colonization of the mouth related to dental plaque.[2,10,12,23,29] Ventilator-associated pneumonia not only increases ventilator days, but also the overall length of stay in the critical care unit and hospital and overall morbidity and mortality.[2,16,19,24]

EQUIPMENT

- Goggles or glasses and mask
- Bite-block or oral airway if needed
- Adhesive or twill tape; commercial endotracheal tube holder (design ensures ability to provide oral care and suctioning)
- Normal saline solution
- Soft pediatric/adult toothbrush or suction toothbrush
- Toothettes/oral swab/oral suction swab
- Oral cleansing solution (e.g., 1.5% H_2O_2, chlorhexidine, toothpaste[4,9,11,14,18])

Additional equipment (have available depending on patient need) includes the following:
- Closed-suction setup with a catheter of appropriate size (see Table 10-1)
- Sterile saline lavage containers (5 to 10 ml)
- Suction catheter for oral and nasal suctioning (single use, Yankauer, covered Yankauer, oral saliva ejector)
- Two sources of suction or a connection device (wall mounted or portable)
- Connecting tube (4 to 6 feet)
- Nonsterile gloves
- Stethoscope

PATIENT AND FAMILY EDUCATION

- Explain procedure to patient and family, including purpose of endotracheal tube care and importance of effective oral care in preventing infection. ➤*Rationale:* This identifies patient and family knowledge deficits concerning patient condition, procedure, expected benefits, and potential risks and allows time for questions to clarify information and voice concerns. Explanations decrease patient anxiety and enhance cooperation.
- If indicated, explain patient's role in assisting with endotracheal tube care. ➤*Rationale:* Eliciting the patient's cooperation assists with care.
- Explain that the patient will be unable to speak while the endotracheal tube is in place, but that other means of communication will be provided. ➤*Rationale:* This enhances patient and family understanding and decreases anxiety.
- Explain that the patient's hands often are immobilized to prevent accidental dislodgment of the tube. ➤*Rationale:* This enhances patient and family understanding and decreases anxiety.

PATIENT ASSESSMENT AND PREPARATION

Patient Assessment

- Assess for signs and symptoms indicating that oral cavity and endotracheal tube care is required.
  - ❖ Excessive secretions (oral or tracheal)
  - ❖ Plaque buildup on teeth
  - ❖ Soiled tape or ties
  - ❖ Patient biting or kinking tube
  - ❖ Pressure areas on naris, corner of mouth, or tongue
  - ❖ Tube moving in and out of mouth
  - ❖ Patient able to verbalize
  - ➤*Rationale:* Assessment provides for early recognition that endotracheal tube care is needed.
- Assess level of consciousness and level of anxiety. ➤*Rationale:* This assessment determines need for sedation during endotracheal tube care.

Patient Preparation

- Ensure that the patient understands preprocedural teaching. Answer questions as they arise, and reinforce information as needed. ➤*Rationale:* This evaluates and reinforces understanding of previously taught information.
- Assist the patient to a position that is comfortable for the patient and the nurse, generally semi-Fowler or Fowler (greater than 30°). ➤*Rationale:* This promotes comfort and reduces physical strain and the risk of aspiration.

Procedure for Endotracheal Tube and Oral Care

Steps	Rationale	Special Considerations
1. Wash hands, and don personal protective equipment.	Decreases transmission of microorganisms and body secretions; standard precautions.	
2. Ensure that endotracheal tube is connected to the ventilator using a swivel adapter.	Decreases pressure exerted by ventilator tubing on the endotracheal tube, minimizing risk of pressure ulceration.	
3. Support the endotracheal tube and tubing as needed.		
4. If suctioning is clinically indicated, hyperoxygenate and suction endotracheal tube (see Procedure 10).	Suctioning of airways should be performed only for a clinical indication and not as a routine, fixed-schedule treatment. Removes secretions that may obstruct tube.	
5. Loosen and remove old tape and ties.		If the method to secure the endotracheal tube obstructs the ability to provide effective oral care, consider changing the method of securing.

Procedure continues on the following page

Procedure | for Endotracheal Tube and Oral Care—*Continued*

Steps	Rationale	Special Considerations
6. If patient is nasally intubated, clean around endotracheal tube using saline-soaked gauze or cotton swabs. **Proceed to Step 8.**	Removes secretions that could cause pressure and subsequent skin breakdown.	The Centers for Disease Control and Prevention (CDC) recommends that patients intubated nasally be reintubated orally as soon as possible to reduce the risk of VAP.[2]
7. If patient is intubated orally, remove bite-block or oropharyngeal airway (acting as bite-block) **Proceed to Step 8.**	The bite-block or oropharyngeal airway prevents the patient from biting down on the endotracheal tube and occluding airflow.	The bite-block should be secured separately from the tube to prevent dislodgment of the endotracheal tube. The bite-block may be a barrier to providing good oral care.
8. Perform oral hygiene, using pediatric or adult (soft) toothbrush, at least twice a day. Gently brush patient's teeth to clean and remove plaque from teeth. *(Level IV: Limited clinical studies to support recommendations.)*	Good oral hygiene reduces oropharyngeal colonization, which is associated with ventilator-associated pneumonia.[5,6,10-12]	Pediatric or soft bristle toothbrushes may be easier to use in adult intubated patients.[11,20]
9. In addition to brushing twice daily, use oral swabs with a 1.5% hydrogen peroxide solution to clean mouth every 2 to 4 hours. With each cleansing, apply a mouth moisturizer to the oral mucosa and lips to keep tissue moist. *(Level IV: Limited clinical studies to support recommendations.)*	Oral care given every 2 to 4 hours seems to show a greater improvement in oral health. If oral care is not provided for 4 to 6 hours, previous benefits are thought to be lost.[5,7,13,20,24] Most studies support the safety and efficacy of greater than 1% or less than 3% H_2O_2 as a cleanser for plaque removal and maintaining overall gingival health.[18,24,25,32] Saliva serves a protective function. Mechanical ventilation causes drying of the oral mucosa, affecting salivary flow and contributing to mucositis and gram-negative bacteria colonization.[19]	Foam swabs are effective in stimulating mucosal tissue but less effective in plaque removal.[5,8,21] Implementation of a comprehensive oral care program is recommended by the CDC to reduce VAP.[2] Use of mouthwash as a cleansing agent is not recommended.[11] Postoperative cardiac surgery patients are the only population in which 2% chlorhexidine gluconate is being recommend for twice-daily application to the oral cavity after brushing.[2,4] The CDC has not reached a consensus for recommendation of 2% chlorhexidine gluconate in other critically ill populations.[2,9,14,17,22]
10. Suction oral cavity/pharynx frequently. *(Continuous suctioning: Level II: Theory based, no research data to support recommendations; recommendations from expert consensus group may exist.) (Intermittent suctioning: Level IV: Limited clinical studies to support recommendations.)*	Removes secretions that may accumulate on top of the cuff and cause microaspiration.[2,27,28] Continuous subglottic suctioning using a specially designed endotracheal tube has been shown to reduce ventilator-associated pneumonia.[26,31,32] Intermittent deep oral cleansing as a part of a comprehensive oral care program has been shown to reduce ventilator-associated pneumonia in a quality improvement project.[24]	Oral suction equipment and suction tubing should be changed every 24 hours. Non-disposable oral suction apparatus should be rinsed with sterile isotonic sodium chloride solution after each use and placed on a paper towel if not disposable or covered.[2,24,27,28] Placement of tonsil suction back into the package is associated withgreater colonization.[2,27] Disconnection of a closed suction system to provide oral suctioning may contribute to increased bacterial colonization at the point of the disconnection.[19,27]

Procedure for Endotracheal Tube and Oral Care—*Continued*

Steps	Rationale	Special Considerations
11. Move oral tube to the other side of the mouth. Replace bite-block or oropharyngeal airway (to act as bite-block) along the endotracheal tube if necessary to prevent biting.	Prevents or minimizes pressure areas on lips, tongue, and oral cavity.	
12. Ensure proper cuff inflation (see Procedure 11) using minimal leak volume or minimal occlusion volume.	Decreases risk of aspiration; ensures airflow to lungs rather than to stomach.	
13. Reconfirm tube placement (see Procedure 2), and note position of tube at teeth or naris.	Common tube placement at the teeth is 21 cm for women and 23 cm for men.	
14. Secure the endotracheal tube in place (according to institutional standard) (see Procedure 2). *(Level IV: Limited clinical studies to support recommendations.)*	Prevents inadvertent dislodgment of the tube.[1,2,8,14]	Various methods are used for securing endotracheal tubes, including use of specially manufactured tube holder, twill tape, or adhesive tape. The method for securing the endotracheal tube should not interfere with caregivers' ability to provide frequent, comprehensive oral care.

Expected Outcomes

- Patent airway
- Secured endotracheal tube
- Removal of oral secretions
- Intact oral and nasal mucous membranes
- Reduced oral colonization
- Moist, pink oral cavity

Unexpected Outcomes

- Dislodged endotracheal tube
- Occluded endotracheal tube
- Cuff leak
- Pressure sores in mouth, lip, or naris
- Ventilator-associated pneumonia

Patient Monitoring and Care

Steps	Rationale	Reportable Conditions
		These conditions should be reported if they persist despite nursing interventions.
1. Keep head of bed elevated at least 30 degrees, unless contraindicated.[2,6,30] *(Level IV: Limited clinical studies to support recommendations.)*	Contraindications include hemodynamic instability, decreased cerebral perfusion pressure, or patient in the prone position.	
2. Suction endotracheal tube if clinically indicated.	Maintains patent airway.	• Inability to pass suction catheter
3. Monitor amount, type, and color of secretions (see Procedure 10).		• Change in quantity or characteristics of secretions
4. If patient is nasally intubated, monitor for nasal drainage.		• Purulent drainage
5. Assess oral cavity and lips every 8 hours, and perform oral care (as outlined in **Steps 8 and 9**) every 2 to 4 hours and as needed. *(Level IV: Limited clinical studies to support recommendations.)*	If oral care is omitted for 4 to 6 hours, previous benefits are lost.[5,7,8,20,24,32] Early recognition of pressure or drainage allows for prompt intervention.	• Breakdown of lip, tongue, or oral cavity • Presence of mouth sores

Procedure continues on the following page

Patient Monitoring and Care—*Continued*

Steps	Rationale	Reportable Conditions
6. With oral care, assess for buildup of plaque on teeth or potential infection related to oral abscess.	Assessment and removal of plaque decreases bacteria in the mouth.	• Continued plaque buildup on teeth
7. Reconfirm tube placement (see Procedure 2), and note position of tube at teeth or naris. Retape or secure endotracheal tube every 24 hours and as needed for soiled or loose securing devices.	Ensures secured tube.	• Tube moving in and out of mouth

Documentation

Documentation should include the following:

- Patient and family education
- Patient tolerance to suctioning
- Aspirate amount, type, and color
- Presence of nasal drainage
- Repositioning of endotracheal tube
- Retaping of endotracheal tube

- Oral care, moisturization, and oral suctioning
- Condition of lips, mouth, and tongue
- Presence of cuff leak
- Amount of air used to inflate cuff
- Centimeter mark on endotracheal tube
- Which naris endotracheal tube is in

References

1. Barnason, S., et al. (1998). Comparison of two endotracheal tube securement techniques on unplanned extubation, oral mucosa, and facial skin integrity. *Heart Lung,* 27, 409-17.
2. Centers for Disease Control and Prevention. (2004). Guidelines for preventing health-care associated pneumonia, 2003: Recommendations of CDC and the Healthcare Infection Control Practices Advisory Committee. *MMWR Morb Mortal Wkly Rep,* 53(No. RR-3), 1-40.
3. Cummins, R.O., ed. (2003). Adjuncts for airway control, oxygenation, and ventilation. In: *ACLS: Principles and Practice.* Dallas: American Heart Association, 167.
4. DeRiso, A.J., 2nd, et al. (1996). Chlorhexidine gluconate 0.12% oral rinse reduces the incidence of total nosocomial respiratory infection and nonprophylactic systemic antibiotic use in patients undergoing heart surgery. *Chest,* 109, 1556-61.
5. DeWalt, E.M. (1975). Effect of timed hygienic measures on oral mucosa in a group of elderly subjects. *Nurs Res,* 24, 104-8.
6. Drakulovic, M.B., et al. (1999). Supine body position as a risk factor for nosocomial pneumonia in mechanically ventilated patients: A randomized trial. *Lancet,* 354, 1851-8.
7. Ginsberg, M.K. (1961). A study of oral hygiene nursing care. *AJN,* 61, 67-9.
8. Fitch, J.A., et al. (1999). Oral care in the adult intensive care unit. *Am J Crit Care,* 8, 314-8.
9. Ferretti, G.A., et al. (1987). Chlorhexidine for prophylaxis against oral infections and associated complications in patients receiving bone marrow transplants. *J Am Dent Assoc,* 114, 461-7.
10. Fourrier, F., et al. (1998). Colonization of dental plaque, a source of nosocomial infections in intensive care unit patients. *Crit Care Med,* 26, 301-8.
11. Gagari, E., and Kabani, S. (1995). Adverse effects of mouthwash use: A review. *Oral Surg Oral Med Oral Pathol Oral Radiol Endod,* 80, 432-9.
12. Garrouste-Orgeas, M., et al. (1997). Oropharyngeal or gastric colonization and nosocomial pneumonia in adult intensive care unit patients: A prospective study based on genomic DNA analysis. *Am J Respir Crit Care Med,* 156, 1647-55.
13. Grap, M.J., et al. (2003). Oral care interventions in critical care: Frequency and documentation. *Am J Crit Care,* 12, 113-9.
14. Grap, M.J., et al. (2004). Duration of action of a single, early oral application of chlorhexidine on oral microbial flora in mechanically ventilated patients: A pilot study. *Heart Lung,* 33, 83-91.
15. Henneman, E., Ellstrom, K., and St. John, R.E. (1999). In: *AACN Protocols for Practice: Care of the Mechanically Ventilated Patient Series.* Aliso Viejo, Ca: American Association of Critical-Care Nurses.
16. Hixson, S., Sole, M.L., and King, T. (1998). Nursing strategies to prevent ventilator-associated pneumonia. *AACN Clin Issues,* 9, 76-90.
17. Houston, S., et al. (2002). Effectiveness of 0.12% chlorhexidine gluconate oral rinse in reducing prevalence of nosocomial pneumonia in patients undergoing heart surgery. *Am J Crit Care,* 11, 567-70.
18. Marshall, M.V., Cancro, L.P., and Fischman, S.L. (1995). Hydrogen peroxide: A review of its use in dentistry. *J Periodontol,* 66, 786-96.
19. Munro, C.L., and Grap, M.J. (2004). Oral health and care in the intensive care unit: State of the science. *Am J Crit Care,* 13, 25-33.
20. O'Reilly, M. (2003). Oral care of the critically ill: A review of the literature and guidelines of practice. *Aust Crit Care,* 16, 101-10.
21. Pearson, L.S., and Hutton, J.L. (2002). A controlled trial to compare the ability of foam swabs and toothbrushes to remove dental plaque. *J Adv Nurs,* 39, 480-9.
22. Rutkauskas, J.S., and Davis, J.W. (1993). Effects of chlorhexidine during immunosuppressive chemotherapy: A preliminary report. *Oral Surg Oral Med Oral Pathol Oral Radiol Endod,* 76, 441-7.
23. Scannapieco, F.A., Stewart, E., and Mylotte, J. (1992). Colonization of dental plaque by respiratory pathogens in medical intensive care patients. *Crit Care Med,* 20, 740-5.
24. Schleder, B., Stott, K., and Lloyd, R.C. (2002). The effect of a comprehensive oral care protocol on patients at risk for ventilator-associated pneumonia. *J Advocate Health Care,* 4, 27-30.

25. Shibly, O., et al. (1997). Clinical evaluation of a hydrogen peroxide mouth rinse, sodium chlorhexidine, for prophylaxis against oral infections and associated bicarbonate dentifrice, and mouth moisturizer on oral health. *J Clin Dent,* 8, 145-9.

26. Shorri, A., and O'Malley, P. (2001). Continuous subglottic suctioning for the prevention of VAP: Potential economic impact. *Chest,* 119, 228-38.

27. Sole, M.L., et al. (2002). Suctioning techniques and airway management practices: Pilot study and instrument evaluation. *Am J Crit Care,* 11, 141-9.

28. Sole, M.L., et al. (2003). A multisite survey of suctioning techniques and airway management practices. *Am J Crit Care,* 12, 220-32.

29. Sumi, Y., Nakamura, Y., and Michiulaki, Y. (2002). Colonization of denture plaque by respiratory pathogens in dependent elderly. *Gerontology,* 19, 25-9.

30. Torres, A., et al. (1992). Pulmonary aspiration of gastric contents in patients receiving mechanical ventilation: The effect of body position. *Ann Intern Med,* 116, 540-3.

31. Vallés, J., and Rello, J. (1997). Nonpharmacologic strategies for preventing nosocomial pneumonia. *Clin Pulm Med,* 4, 141-7.

32. Van Drimmelen, J., and Rollins, H.F. (1969). Evaluation of a commonly used oral hygiene agent. *Nurs Res,* 18, 327-32.

33. Wilson, D.J., and Shepherd, K.E. (1994). Modern airway appliances and their long-term complications. In: Robert, J.T., ed. *Clinical Management of the Airway.* Philadelphia: W.B. Saunders, 461.

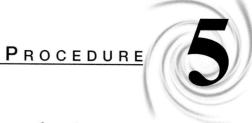

PROCEDURE **5**

AP
Extubation/Decannulation (Perform)

PURPOSE: The purpose of extubation and decannulation is to remove the artificial airway to allow the patient to breathe independently.

Kirsten N. Skillings
Bonnie L. Curtis

PREREQUISITE NURSING KNOWLEDGE

- *Extubation* refers to removal of an endotracheal tube, whereas *decannulation* refers to removal of a tracheostomy tube.
- Indications for extubation and decannulation include the following:[1,3]
  - Underlying condition that led to the need for an artificial airway is reversed or improved.
  - Hemodynamic stability is achieved, with no new reasons for continued artificial airway support.
  - Patient is able to clear pulmonary secretions.
  - Airway problems have resolved; there is minimal risk for aspiration.
  - Mechanical ventilatory support no longer is needed.
- Most extubations or decannulations are planned. Planning allows for preparation of the patient physically and emotionally and decreases the likelihood of reintubation and hypoxic sequelae. Unintentional or unplanned extubation complicates a patient's overall recovery.[2]
- Extubation usually occurs within 24 hours of successful weaning from mechanical ventilatory support, whereas decannulation occurs much later. The patient with a tracheostomy tube is weaned gradually from the tracheostomy tube using a combination of techniques, including downsizing the tube diameter, using fenestration, and capping the tracheostomy. The tracheostomy tube is removed when the patient is able to breathe comfortably, maintain adequate ventilation and oxygenation, and manage secretions.

EQUIPMENT

- Suctioning equipment
- Personal protective equipment
- Sterile suction catheter or suction kit
- Self-inflating resuscitation bag connected to 100% oxygen source
- Scissors
- Supplemental oxygen with aerosol
- 10-ml syringe
- Rigid pharyngeal suction-tip (Yankauer) catheter
- Sterile dressing for tracheal stoma
  Additional equipment (to have available depending on patient need) includes the following:
- Endotracheal intubation supplies
- Emergency cart

PATIENT AND FAMILY EDUCATION

- Explain the procedure and the reason the endotracheal tube or tracheostomy tube is no longer needed. →*Rationale:* This identifies the patient's and family's knowledge deficits concerning the patient's condition, the procedure, and the expected benefits and allows time for questions to clarify information and voice concerns. Explanations decrease patient anxiety and enhance cooperation.
- Explain the purpose and necessity of extubation. →*Rationale:* Communication and explanation of therapy encourage cooperation and minimize anxiety.
- Discuss the suctioning process and the importance of coughing and deep breathing. →*Rationale:* Understanding therapy encourages cooperation with the follow-up procedures necessary to maintain a patent airway.
- Explain that the patient's voice may be hoarse after extubation or decannulation. For patients who have a tracheostomy tube removed, occlusion of the stoma may be necessary to facilitate normal speech and coughing.

➨*Rationale:* Knowledge minimizes the patient's and family's fear and anxiety.

- Explain that the patient may need continued oxygen or humidification support. ➨*Rationale:* Many patients continue to require oxygen support for some time after extubation. Continued humidification often helps decrease hoarseness and liquefy secretions.

PATIENT ASSESSMENT AND PREPARATION

Patient Assessment

- Desired level of consciousness has been achieved (for most patients, patient is awake and able to follow commands).[4]
- Assess signs and symptoms associated with independent breathing.[1,3,4]
  - ❖ Stable respiratory rate of less than 25 breaths/min
  - ❖ Absence of dyspnea
  - ❖ Absence of accessory muscle use
  - ❖ Negative inspiratory pressure less than or equal to −20 cm H_2O
  - ❖ Positive expiratory pressure greater than or equal to +30 cm H_2O

- ❖ Spontaneous tidal volume greater than or equal to 5 ml/kg
- ❖ Vital capacity greater than or equal to 10 to 15 ml/kg
- ❖ Minute ventilation less than or equal to 10 liters/min
- ❖ Fraction of inspired oxygen (FIO_2) less than or equal to 50%
- ❖ Stable pulse and blood pressure and absence of serious cardiac dysrhythmias

  ➨*Rationale:* Evaluation of the patient's respiratory status identifies that intubation is no longer necessary.
- Assess patient's ability to cough. ➨*Rationale:* The ability to cough and clear secretions is important for successful airway management after extubation.

Patient Preparation

- Ensure that patient understands preprocedural teaching. Answer questions as they arise, and reinforce information as needed. ➨*Rationale:* This evaluates and reinforces understanding of previously taught information.
- Place patient in semi-Fowler position. ➨*Rationale:* Respiratory muscles are more effective in an upright position versus a prone position. This position facilitates coughing and minimizes the risk of vomiting and consequent aspiration.

Procedure for Performing Extubation and Decannulation

Steps	Rationale	Special Considerations
1. Wash hands, and don personal protective equipment.	Reduces the transmission of microorganisms and body secretions; standard precautions.	
2. Hyperoxygenate and suction endotracheal tube and pharynx (see Procedure 10).		
3. Cut twill tape or remove tape to free tube.		
4. Insert syringe into one-way valve in pilot balloon.	Prepares for cuff deflation.	
5. Instruct patient to deep breathe.	Promotes hyperinflation.	A manual resuscitation bag can assist in hyperinflation.
6. At the peak of a deep inspiration, deflate the cuff and remove the tube in one motion on inspiration.	Assists in a smooth, quick, less traumatic removal. Vocal cords are maximally abducted at peak inspiration. Additionally, initial cough response expected following extubation should be more forceful if started from maximal inspiration versus expiration.[1]	Alternative methods to facilitate removal of secretions while tube is removed include application of positive pressure while the cuff is deflated; insertion of suction catheter 1 to 2 inches (5 cm) below distal end of tube; and application of suction while cuff is deflated and tube removed.[4]
7. Encourage the patient to deep breathe and cough.	Promotes hyperinflation; helps remove secretions.	
8. Suction the pharynx.	Removes secretions.	

Procedure continues on the following page

Procedure for Performing Extubation and Decannulation—*Continued*

Steps	Rationale	Special Considerations
9. Apply supplemental oxygen and aerosol, as appropriate.	Promotes warmth and moisture and prevents oxygen desaturation. Cool humidification is usually preferred after extubation to help minimize upper airway swelling.[1]	
10. Place a dry, sterile, 4 × 4 dressing over stoma when tracheostomy tube is removed.	Contains secretions that leak out of stoma.	Tracheostomy stoma closure usually occurs within a few days.

Expected Outcomes	Unexpected Outcomes
• Smooth, atraumatic extubation or decannulation • Stable respiratory status	• Fatigue and respiratory failure • Persistent hoarseness • Tracheal stoma narrowing • Aspiration • Laryngospasm • Trauma to soft tissue

Patient Monitoring and Care

Steps	Rationale	Reportable Conditions
		These conditions should be reported if they persist despite nursing interventions.
1. Monitor vital signs, respiratory status, and oxygenation immediately after extubation, within 1 hour, and per institutional standard.	Change in vital signs and oxygenation after extubation or decannulation may indicate respiratory compromise, necessitating reintubation.	• Tachycardia • Tachypnea • Blood pressure greater than 110% baseline • Oxygen saturation (SpO_2) less than or equal to 90% • Stridor • Breathing difficulty • Chest-abdominal asynchrony
2. Promote optimal oxygenation by providing supplemental oxygen as needed.	Decreases incidence of oxygen desaturation immediately after extubation.	• SpO_2 less than or equal to 90%
3. Monitor for aspiration related to pooled secretions.	Failure to suction or ineffective suctioning of the pharynx allows accumulated secretions to advance further into the trachea on cuff deflation.	• Patient unable to handle secretions
4. Encourage coughing and deep breathing.	Prevents atelectasis and secretion accumulation.	• Ineffective cough
5. Assess swallowing ability.	Presence of tube over extended periods may result in impaired swallow.	• Inability to handle secretions • Inability to swallow without coughing

Documentation

Documentation should include the following:

• Patient and family education
• Respiratory and vital signs assessment before and after procedure
• Date and time when procedure is performed.

• Patient response
• Unexpected outcomes
• Nursing interventions taken

References

1. Henneman, E., Ellstrom, K., and St. John, R. (1999). Airway management. In: *AACN Protocols for Practice: Care of the Mechanically Ventilated Patient Series.* Aliso Viejo, CA: American Association of Critical-Care Nurses.
2. O'Meade, M., Guyatt, G., and Cook, D. (2001). Weaning from mechanical ventilation: The evidence from clinical research. *Respir Care,* 12, 78-83.
3. Twibel, R., Siela, D., and Mahmoodi, M. (2003). Subjective perceptions in physiological variables during weaning from mechanical ventilation. *Am J Crit Care,* 12, 101-12.
4. Wojahn, A. (2002). *Adult Ventilation Management.* Corexcel. Available at: http://www.corexcel.com/online-courses.html.

Additional Readings

Bach, J.R., and Saporito, L.R. (1996). Criteria for extubation and tracheostomy tube removal for patients with ventilatory failure. *Chest,* 110, 1566-71.
Boulain, T., Association des Reanimateurs du Centre-Quest. (1998). Unplanned extubations in the adult intensive care unit. *Am J Respir Care Med,* 157(4 Pt 1), 1131-7.
Durbin, C.G., Campbell, R.S., and Branson, R.D. (1999). AARC clinical practice guideline: Removal of the endotracheal tube. *Respir Care,* 44, 85-90.
Henneman, E. (2001). Liberating patients from mechanical ventilation: A team approach. *Crit Care Nurse,* 21, 25-33.

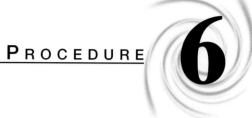
PROCEDURE **6**

Extubation/Decannulation (Assist)

P U R P O S E : The purpose of extubation and decannulation is to remove the artificial airway to allow the patient to breathe independently.

Kirsten N. Skillings
Bonnie L. Curtis

PREREQUISITE NURSING KNOWLEDGE

- *Extubation* refers to removal of an endotracheal tube, and *decannulation* refers to removal of a tracheostomy tube.
- Indications for extubation and decannulation include the following:[1,3]
  - ❖ The underlying condition that led to the need for an artificial airway is reversed or improved.
  - ❖ Hemodynamic stability is achieved, with no new reasons for continued artificial airway support.
  - ❖ The patient is able to clear pulmonary secretions.
  - ❖ Airway problems have resolved; there is minimal risk for aspiration.
  - ❖ Mechanical ventilatory support is no longer needed.
- Most extubations or decannulations are planned. Planning allows for preparation of the patient physically and emotionally and decreases the likelihood of reintubation and hypoxic sequelae. Unintentional or unplanned extubation complicates a patient's overall recovery.[2]
- Extubation usually occurs within 24 hours of successful weaning from mechanical ventilatory support, whereas decannulation occurs much later. A patient with a tracheostomy tube is weaned gradually from the tracheostomy tube using a combination of techniques, including downsizing the tube diameter, using fenestration, and capping the tracheostomy. The tracheostomy tube is removed when the patient is able to breathe comfortably, maintain adequate ventilation and oxygenation, and manage secretions.

EQUIPMENT

- Suctioning equipment
- Personal protective equipment
- Sterile suction catheter or suction kit
- Self-inflating resuscitation bag connected to 100% oxygen source
- Scissors
- Supplemental oxygen with aerosol
- 10-ml syringe
- Rigid pharyngeal suction-tip (Yankauer) catheter
- Sterile dressing for tracheal stoma

  Additional equipment (to have available depending on patient need) includes the following:
- Endotracheal intubation supplies
- Emergency cart

PATIENT AND FAMILY EDUCATION

- Explain the procedure and the reason the endotracheal tube or tracheostomy tube is no longer needed. ➤*Rationale:* This identifies patient and family knowledge deficits concerning the patient's condition, procedure, and expected benefits and allows time for questions to clarify information and voice concerns. Explanations decrease patient anxiety and enhance cooperation.
- Explain the purpose and necessity of extubation. ➤*Rationale:* Communication and explanation for therapy encourage cooperation and minimize anxiety.
- Discuss the suctioning process and the importance of coughing and deep breathing. ➤*Rationale:* Understanding therapy encourages cooperation with the follow-up procedures necessary to maintain a patent airway.
- Explain that the patient's voice may be hoarse after extubation or decannulation. For patients who have a tracheostomy tube removed, occlusion of the stoma may be necessary to facilitate normal speech and coughing. ➤*Rationale:* Knowledge minimizes patient and family fear and anxiety.
- Explain that the patient may need continued oxygen or humidification support. ➤*Rationale:* Many patients

continue to require oxygen support for some time after extubation. Continued humidification often helps to decrease hoarseness and liquefies secretions.

PATIENT ASSESSMENT AND PREPARATION

Patient Assessment

- Desired level of consciousness has been achieved (for most patients, patient is awake and able to follow commands).[4]
- Assess the patient's respiratory status.
  - ❖ Stable respiratory rate of less than 25 breaths/min
  - ❖ Absence of dyspnea
  - ❖ Absence of accessory muscle use
  - ❖ Negative inspiratory pressure less than or equal to -20 cm H_2O
  - ❖ Positive expiratory pressure greater than or equal to $+30$ cm H_2O
  - ❖ Spontaneous tidal volume greater than or equal to 5 ml/kg
  - ❖ Vital capacity greater than or equal to 10 to 15 ml/kg
  - ❖ Minute ventilation less than or equal to 10 liters/min
  - ❖ Fraction of inspired oxygen less than or equal to 50%
  - ❖ Stable pulse and blood pressure and absence of serious cardiac dysrhythmias

    ➤*Rationale:* Evaluation of the patient's respiratory status identifies that intubation is no longer necessary. Signs and symptoms associated with independent breathing are as follows:[1,3,4]

- Assess the patient's ability to cough. ➤*Rationale:* The ability to cough and clear secretions is important for successful airway management after extubation.

Patient Preparation

- Ensure that the patient understands preprocedural teaching. Answer questions as they arise, and reinforce information as needed. ➤*Rationale:* This evaluates and reinforces understanding of previously taught information.
- Place the patient in a semi-Fowler position. ➤*Rationale:* Respiratory muscles are more effective in an upright position versus a supine position. This position facilitates coughing and minimizes the risk of vomiting and consequent aspiration.

Procedure | for Assisting With Extubation and Decannulation

Steps	Rationale	Special Considerations
1. Wash hands, and don personal protective equipment.	Reduces transmission of microorganisms and body secretions; standard precautions.	
2. Hyperoxygenate and suction endotracheal tube and pharynx (see Procedure 10).	Removes secretions, including those above the cuff.	
3. Cut twill tape, or remove tape to free tube.	Removes means for securing above the cuff.	
4. Instruct patient to deep breathe.	Promotes hyperinflation.	A manual resuscitation bag can assist in hyperinflation. (see Procedure 29).
5. While the tube is being removed, at the peak of inspiration, monitor and support the patient.	Provides reassurance and possibly distraction as patient experiences removal of the tube.	
6. Encourage the patient to deep breathe and cough.	Promotes hyperinflation; helps remove secretions.	Alternative methods to facilitate removal of secretions while tube is removed include application of positive pressure while the cuff is deflated; insertion of suction catheter 1 to 2 inches (5 cm) below distal end of tube, and application of suction while cuff is deflated and tube removed.[4]
7. Suction the pharynx.	Removes secretions.	
8. Apply supplemental oxygen and aerosol, as appropriate.	Promotes warmth and moisture and prevents oxygen desaturation. Cool humidification usually is preferred after extubation to help minimize upper airway swelling.[1]	

Procedure continues on the following page

Procedure for Assisting With Extubation and Decannulation—*Continued*

Steps	Rationale	Special Considerations
9. Place a dry, sterile, 4 × 4 dressing over stoma when tracheostomy tube is removed.	Contains secretions that leak out of stoma.	Tracheostomy stoma closure usually occurs within a few days.
10. Document in patient's record.		

Expected Outcomes

- Smooth, atraumatic extubation or decannulation
- Stable respiratory status

Unexpected Outcomes

- Fatigue and respiratory failure
- Persistent hoarseness
- Tracheal stoma narrowing
- Aspiration
- Laryngospasm
- Trauma to soft tissue

Patient Monitoring and Care

Steps	Rationale	Reportable Conditions
		These conditions should be reported if they persist despite nursing interventions.
1. Monitor vital signs, respiratory status, and oxygenation immediately after extubation, within 1 hour, and per institutional standard.	Change in vital signs and oxygenation after extubation or decannulation may indicate respiratory compromise, necessitating reintubation.	• Tachycardia • Tachypnea • Blood pressure greater than 110% baseline • Oxygen saturation (SpO_2) less than or equal to 90% • Stridor • Breathing difficulty • Chest-abdominal asynchrony
2. Promote optimal oxygenation by providing supplemental oxygen as needed.	Decreases incidence of oxygen desaturation immediately after extubation.	• SpO_2 less than or equal to 90%
3. Monitor for aspiration related to pooled secretions.	Failure to suction or ineffective suctioning of the pharynx allows accumulated secretions to advance further into the trachea on cuff deflation.	• Patient unable to handle secretions
4. Encourage coughing and deep breathing.	Prevents atelectasis and secretion accumulation.	• Ineffective cough
5. Assess swallowing ability	Presence of tube over extended periods may result in impaired swallow.	• Inability to handle secretions • Inability to swallow without coughing

Documentation

Documentation should include the following:

- Patient and family education
- Respiratory and vital signs assessment before and after procedure
- Date and time when procedure is performed

- Patient response
- Unexpected outcomes
- Nursing interventions taken

References

1. Henneman, E., Ellstrom, K., and St. John, R. (1999). Airway management. In: *AACN Protocols for Practice: Care of the Mechanically Ventilated Patient Series*. Aliso Viejo, CA: American Association of Critical-Care Nurses.

2. O'Meade, M., Guyatt, G., and Cook, D. (2001). Weaning from mechanical ventilation: The evidence from clinical research. *Respir Care,* 12, 78-83.

3. Twibel, R., Siela, D., and Mahmoodi, M. (2003). Subjective perceptions in physiological variables during weaning from mechanical ventilation. *Am J Crit Care,* 12, 101-12.

4. Wojahn, A. (2002). *Adult Ventilation Management.* Corexcel, Inc. Available at: http://www.corexcel.com/online-courses.html.

Additional Readings

Bach, J.R., and Saporito, L.R. (1996). Criteria for extubation and tracheostomy tube removal for patients with ventilatory failure. *Chest,* 110, 1566-71.

Boulain, T., and Association des Reanimateurs du Centre-Quest. (1998). Unplanned extubations in the adult intensive care unit. *Am J Respir Care Med,* 157(4 Pt 1), 1131-7.

Durbin, C.G., Campbell, R.S., and Branson, R.D. (1999). AARC clinical practice guideline: Removal of the endotracheal tube. *Respir Care,* 44, 85-90.

Henneman, E. (2001). Liberating patients from mechanical ventilation: A team approach. *Crit Care Nurse,* 21, 25-33.

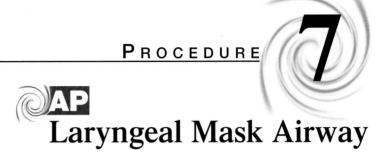
PROCEDURE 7

Laryngeal Mask Airway

P U R P O S E :   A laryngeal mask airway (LMA) may be used to provide an emergency airway while resuscitating a profoundly unconscious patient who requires artificial ventilation and when endotracheal intubation is not readily available or has failed to establish an airway successfully.

Michael W. Day

PREREQUISITE NURSING KNOWLEDGE

- The requirement for rapid airway management in an unconscious patient should be understood.
- The anatomy and physiology of the upper airway should be understood.
- The design of the LMA should be understood (Fig. 7-1):
  - ❖ An airway tube connects the mask and the 15-mm male adapter.
  - ❖ The mask's cuff, when inflated, conforms to the contours of the hypopharynx, positioning the opening of the air tube directly over the laryngeal opening. Two aperture bars cross the opening where the tube exits into the mask.
  - ❖ An inflation line is fitted with a valve and pilot balloon that leads to the mask's cuff.
- The final placement of an LMA in the airway should be understood (Fig. 7-2).
- The ability to ventilate an unconscious patient adequately with a mouth-to-mask or bag-valve-mask device is necessary.
- An understanding of the limitations of the LMA is needed. Limitations are as follows:
  - ❖ The LMA does *not* protect the airway from aspiration of stomach contents, and the risks of insertion and aspiration must be weighted against the need to establish an airway.[10,11]
  - ❖ The presence of a nasogastric tube may make regurgitation more likely because of its effect on the esophageal sphincter tone.[10,11]
  - ❖ The LMA should not be used on patients requiring high ventilator pressures (e.g., pulmonary fibrosis) because the LMA provides a low-pressure seal.[10,11]
  - ❖ The LMA should not be used in an emergency situation in which the patient is *not* profoundly unconscious and may resist insertion of the device.[10,11]
  - ❖ The LMA should be used with caution in patients with oropharyngeal trauma, only when all other means of

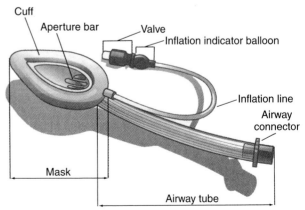

FIGURE 7-1 Components of the laryngeal mask airway. *(From The Laryngeal Mask Company Limited. [2000]. Instruction Manual: LMA-Classic. San Diego: Author, 1.)*

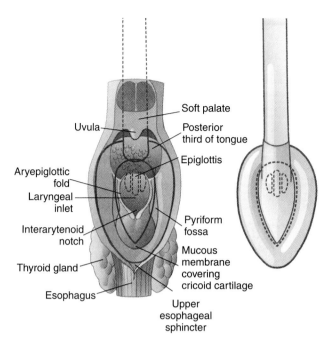

FIGURE 7-2 Dorsal view of the laryngeal mask airway showing position in relation to pharyngeal anatomy. *(From The Laryngeal Mask Company Limited. [2000]. Instruction Manual: LMA-Classic. San Diego: Author, 2.)*

establishing an airway fail[1] and when the risks of insertion are weighed against the need to establish an airway.

- "There are no absolute contraindications to the LMA if the alternative is loss of the airway with its associated complications (p. 851)."[6]
- The LMA may provide a more viable means of ventilation than a bag-valve-mask device in patients with a beard or without teeth.[9]
- Initial and ongoing training is required to maximize insertion success and minimize complications.[9]
- This procedure refers specifically to the LMA-Unique, a disposable model of the nondisposable LMA-Classic. Other types of LMA devices are available that provide additional features, such as endotracheal intubation through the LMA or gastric suctioning.
- The LMA-Unique is latex-free.[11]

EQUIPMENT

- Two LMA-Unique of the appropriate size for patient weight[2]
Weight ranges listed for LMA-Unique sizes are only approximations. Emerging clinical data suggest that using a larger size provides an effective seal without associated higher pharyngeal pressures.[2]
  - ❖ Size 3—30 to 50 kg
  - ❖ Size 4—50 to 70 kg
  - ❖ Size 5—70 to 100 kg
  - ❖ Size 6—greater than 100 kg
- 60-ml Luer-tip syringe
- Water-soluble lubricant
- Gloves, mask, and eye protection
- Suction equipment (suction canister with control head, tracheal suction catheters, Yankauer suction tip)
- Mouth-to-mask or bag-valve-mask device, with peak pressure manometer, attached to a high-flow oxygen source
- Bite-block, at least 3 cm thick
- Tape or commercially available tube securing device

PATIENT AND FAMILY EDUCATION

- If time allows, provide family information regarding the LMA and the reason for insertion ➤➤*Rationale:* This information assists the family in understanding why the procedure is required and decreases family anxiety.

PATIENT ASSESSMENT AND PREPARATION

Patient Assessment

- Assess level of consciousness and responsiveness. ➤➤*Rationale:* In an emergency situation, the LMA should be inserted only into a patient who is profoundly unconscious and unresponsive.[10,11]
- Assess history or patient information for possibility of delayed gastric emptying (e.g., hiatal hernia, recent food ingestion, poorly controlled diabetes). ➤➤*Rationale:* In a patient with delayed gastric emptying, the benefits of inserting the LMA must be weighed against the possibility of regurgitation.[10,11]
- Assess history and patient information for possibility of decreased pulmonary compliance (i.e., pulmonary fibrosis). ➤➤*Rationale:* The high pressures required to ventilate a patient with decreased pulmonary compliance may override the occlusive pressure of the LMA.[10,11]

Patient Preparation

- Ensure adequate ventilation and oxygenation with either a mouth-to-mask or bag-valve-mask device. ➤➤*Rationale:* The patient would be nonresponsive and apneic without assisted ventilation before the LMA insertion.
- Ensure that the suction equipment is assembled and in working order. ➤➤*Rationale:* The patient may regurgitate during the insertion or while the LMA is in place and require oropharyngeal or tracheal suctioning.

Procedure for Laryngeal Mask Airway (LMA-Unique) Insertion

Steps	Rationale	Special Considerations
1. Wash hands, and don protective equipment, including protective eyewear.	Reduces the possible transmission of microorganisms and bodily secretions; minimizes contamination of LMA.	
2. Ensure that a spare LMA of the same size is immediately available. *(Level I: Manufacturer's recommendations only.)*	Provides for a "backup" device should the initial device fail.	
3. Remove the LMA from the package and inspect. *(Level I: Manufacturer's recommendations only.)*	Ensures that the device is not defective and will work as indicated.	
A. Inspect the exterior of the mask for any cuts, tears, or scratches.	Ensures that the exterior surface of the device has not been damaged in any way.	Discard the device if any evidence of damage is found, and open the backup device.
B. Inspect the interior of the airway tube for any particles.	Particles in the airway tube may be inhaled when the device is used.	Discard the device if any particles cannot be removed from the tube, and open the backup device.
C. Examine the airway opening in the mask, ensuring that the aperture bars are intact.	Broken aperture bars may allow the epiglottis to obstruct the airway.	Discard the device if the aperture bars are broken or otherwise damaged, and open the backup device.
D. Examine the 15-mm male connector at the end of the airway tube and ensure that it fits tightly into the tube.	The 15-mm male connector is essential for ventilation with a bag-valve device or ventilator.	*Do not twist the connector because this breaks the seal.*[10,11] Discard the device if the connector does not fit tightly into the airway tube, and open the backup device.
4. Perform the deflation and inflation tests. *(Level I: Manufacturer's recommendations only.)*	Ensures that the device is not defective and will work as indicated.	
A. Expel the air from the 60-ml syringe, and connect it to the pilot balloon valve.	The appropriate-size syringe is needed to inflate the cuff to the proper test level.	
B. Pull back the syringe plunger to deflate the cuff fully, then examine the cuff to ensure that it remains fully deflated (Fig. 7-3).	Full deflation of the cuff helps ensure its patency.	Discard the device if the cuff does not remain fully deflated, and open the backup device.

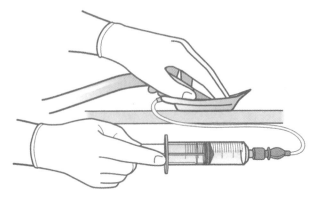

FIGURE 7-3 Method for deflating the laryngeal mask airway cuff. *(From The Laryngeal Mask Company Limited. [2000]. Instruction Manual: LMA-Classic. San Diego: Author, 19.)*

Procedure for Laryngeal Mask Airway (LMA-Unique) Insertion—*Continued*

Steps	Rationale	Special Considerations
C. Remove the syringe from the valve, pull back on the syringe to volume required for the each LMA size, reattach to the valve, and inflate the cuff (Table 7-1).	Ensures that the device is not defective and will work as indicated.	
D. Examine the inflated cuff to ensure that it is symmetrical without bulges.	Ensures that the device is not defective and will work as indicated.	Discard the device if the cuff bulges asymmetrically, and open the backup device.
E. Examine the pilot balloon to ensure that its inflated shape is elliptical.	Ensures that the device is not defective and will work as indicated.	Discard the device if the pilot balloon is spherical or bulges, and open the backup device.
5. Deflate the cuff by placing it, aperture side down, on a hard, flat surface, smoothing out any wrinkles as air is withdrawn from the cuff with the syringe. Leave the syringe attached to the valve (see Fig. 7-3). *(Level I: Manufacturer's recommendations only.)*	Facilitates smooth insertion and avoids deflection of the epiglottis.	Before insertion, the cuff should appear smooth, without wrinkles (Fig. 7-4).
6. Lubricate the posterior tip of the cuff with water-soluble lubricant. *(Level I: Manufacturer's recommendations only.)*	Facilitates smooth insertion	Ensure that the lubricant does *not* spread to the anterior portion of the cuff because it may be aspirated.[10] Do *not* use lidocaine lubricants because they may delay the return of protective reflexes and may cause an allergic reaction.[10]
7. Place the patient's head in a "sniffing" position. *(Level II: Theory based, no research data to support recommendations: recommendations from expert consensus group may exist.)*	Facilitates smooth insertion.	The patient's head may be left in a neutral position if there is a possibility of cervical spine injury.[4,5]
8. Use index finger method of insertion. *(Level II: Theory based, no research data to support recommendations: recommendations from expert consensus group may exist.)*	Ensures proper placement of the LMA.[10]	This method provides for better final placement of the LMA compared with other methods.[2]

Procedure continues on the following page

TABLE 7-1	Test Cuff Inflation Volumes
Laryngeal Mask Airway Size	**Air Volume for Testing *Only***
3	30 ml
4	45 ml
5	60 ml
6	75 ml

From The Laryngeal Mask Company Limited. (2000). *Instruction Manual: LMA-Classic*. San Diego: Author.

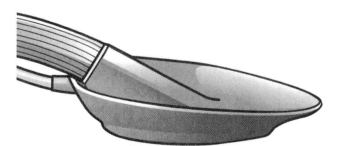

FIGURE 7-4 Laryngeal mask airway cuff properly deflated for insertion. *(From The Laryngeal Mask Company Limited. [2000]. Instruction Manual: LMA-Classic. San Diego: Author, 4.)*

Procedure for Laryngeal Mask Airway (LMA-Unique) Insertion—*Continued*		
Steps	**Rationale**	**Special Considerations**
A. Assume a position at the patient's head, and slightly lift the patient's head with the nondominant hand, maintaining upward pressure during the insertion.	Facilitates proper body position for the person inserting the device and the patient's head during insertion.	
B. Hold the LMA so that the dominant hand's index finger and thumb grasp the airway tube just behind the cuff (Fig. 7-5A).	Facilitates proper device position for insertion.	The mask aperture must face toward the patient's feet, and the black line on the airway tube must face toward the patient's nose.
C. Insert the LMA into the patient's mouth, directing it upward toward the hard palate (Fig. 7-5B).	Assists in maneuvering the LMA into the proper position.	
D. Using the middle finger, open the patient's jaw and look into the mouth to ensure that the cuff is flattened against the hard palate (Fig. 7-5C).	Assists in maneuvering the LMA into the proper position.	If the LMA does not flatten against the hard palate, remove and reinsert.

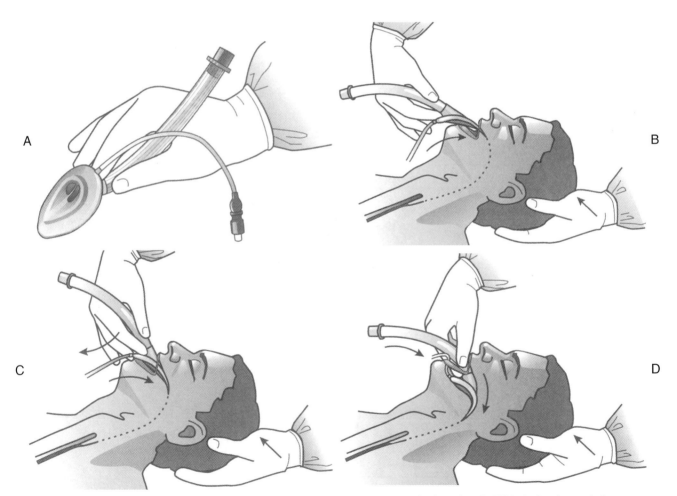

FIGURE 7-5 **A,** Method for holding the laryngeal mask airway (LMA) for insertion. **B,** With the head extended and the neck flexed, the caregiver carefully flattens the LMA tip against the hard palate. **C,** To facilitate LMA introduction into the oral cavity, the caregiver gently presses the middle finger down on the jaw. **D,** The index finger pushes the LMA in the cranial direction following the contours of the hard and soft palates.

Continued

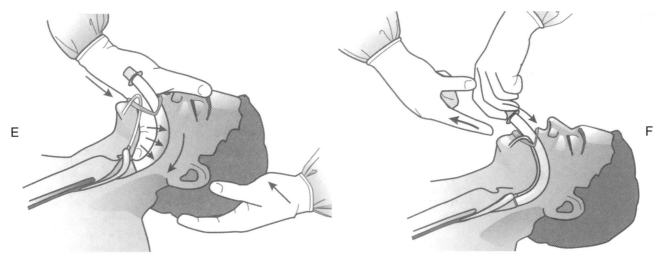

E

F

FIGURE 7-5 CONT'D, **E,** Maintaining pressure with the finger in the tube in the cranial direction, the caregiver advances the LMA until definite resistance is felt at the base of the hypopharynx. Note the flexion of the wrist. **F,** The caregiver gently maintains cranial pressure with the nondominant hand while removing the index finger. *(From The Laryngeal Mask Company Limited. [2000].* Instruction Manual: LMA-Classic. *San Diego: Author, 23-26.)*

Procedure **for Laryngeal Mask Airway (LMA-Unique) Insertion**—*Continued*

Steps	Rationale	Special Considerations
E. Using the index finger, advance the LMA into hypopharynx, in one smooth movement (Fig. 7-5D).	Moves the device into the proper position in the back of the mouth.	*Do not use force.* If the LMA does not advance, remove, reventilate, and reinsert.
F. Continue advancing the LMA until resistance is felt (Fig. 7-5E).	Continues moving the LMA into the proper final position.	*Do not* hold the jaw open during this maneuver because it may cause the epiglottis or tongue to prevent advancement of the LMA.
		Depending on the size of the person's hand inserting the LMA and the size of the patient, the final resistance may not be met.
G. Remove the nondominant hand from behind the patient's head, and use it to stabilize the airway tube. Remove the dominant hand index finger from the patient's mouth (Fig. 7-5F).	Maintains position of the LMA before the removal of the index finger.	The mask *must* be pressed up against the hard palate to be inserted correctly.[10,11] If the cuff curls or fails to flatten against the hard palate, remove, reventilate, and reinsert.[10,11] If the cuff becomes obstructed by the tonsils, a diagonal maneuver is often successful.[10,11]
9. Use thumb method of insertion. *(Level II: Theory based, no research data to support recommendations: recommendations from expert consensus group may exist.)*	May be used when accessing the patient from behind or above the head.[10]	

Procedure continues on the following page

Procedure **for Laryngeal Mask Airway (LMA-Unique) Insertion**—*Continued*

Steps	Rationale	Special Considerations
A. Approach the patient from the front.	Facilitates proper body position for the person inserting the device.	
B. Hold the LMA with dominant hand, with the thumb at the angle of the mask and airway tube (Fig. 7-6A).	Facilitates proper device position for insertion.	
C. As the LMA is advanced into the patient's mouth, the dominant hand fingers are spread up over the patient's face, and the thumb pushes the LMA into the hypopharynx (Fig. 7-6B).	Facilitates proper device position for insertion.	The mask *must* be pressed up against the hard palate to be inserted correctly.[10,11] If the cuff curls or fails to flatten against the hard palate, remove, reventilate, and reinsert.[10,11]

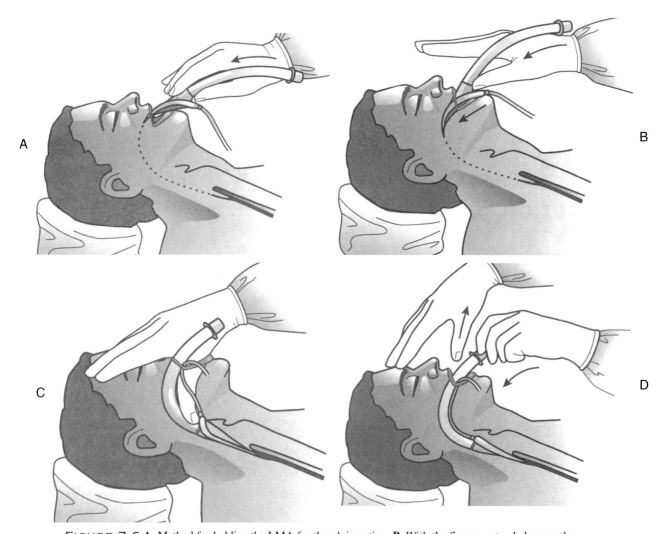

FIGURE 7-6 **A,** Method for holding the LMA for thumb insertion. **B,** With the fingers extended, press the thumb along the posterior pharynx. **C,** Advance the thumb to its fullest extent. **D,** Press LMA gently into place with the nondominant hand while removing the thumb. *(From The Laryngeal Mask Company Limited. [2000]. Instruction Manual: LMA-Classic. San Diego: Author, 29-30.)*

Procedure for Laryngeal Mask Airway (LMA-Unique) Insertion—*Continued*

Steps	Rationale	Special Considerations
		If the cuff becomes obstructed by the tonsils, a diagonal maneuver is often successful.[10,11]
D. Continue advancing the device until the thumb is fully extended into the patient's mouth (Fig. 7-6C).	Moves the LMA into proper position.	Neck flexion may be maintained by either a head support or the nondominant hand.
E. Using the nondominant hand, grasp the airway tube, and gently advance the mask, until resistance is met, before removing the thumb (Fig. 7-6D).	Stabilizes the LMA while removing the thumb.	
10. Release the airway tube,[10,11] and inflate the cuff to create a seal, with intracuff pressure approximately 60 cm H$_2$O (Fig. 7-7).[13] (*Level I: Manufacturer's recommendations only.*)	Releasing the airway tube during inflation allows the cuff to "seat" into the proper position during inflation.	Only one half of maximum inflation volume is necessary to create a seal (Table 7-2).[10,11] *Avoid overinflation of the cuff.*
11. Observe for one or more signs indicating correct placement and inflation: slight outward movement of the airway tube, slight bulging of the neck around the cricothyroid area, or no cuff visible in the mouth. (*Level I: Manufacturer's recommendations only.*)	Ensures correct placement and inflation of the cuff.	If *none* of these signs is observed, consider deflation of the cuff and removal of the LMA. Reventilate, and insert the backup LMA.
12. Connect 15-mm male adapter to bag-valve device and *gently* ventilate, using peak airway pressures of less than 20 cm H$_2$O, with tidal volumes less than or equal to 8 ml/kg of body weight.[10]	Maintaining low ventilatory pressures prevents overriding the pressure in the cuff, creating a leak or forcing air into the stomach.	The cuff may leak with the first few breaths, as it settles into position. If the leak continues, ensure that the ventilator pressures are low.[10,11]

Procedure continues on the following page

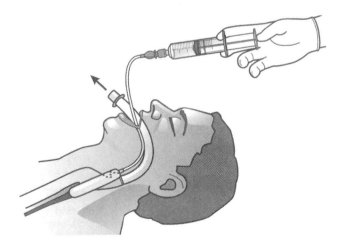

FIGURE 7-7 Inflation without holding the tube allows the mask to seat itself optimally. (*From The Laryngeal Mask Company Limited. [2000]. Instruction Manual: LMA-Classic. San Diego: Author, 27.*)

TABLE 7-2	Maximal Cuff Inflation Volumes
Laryngeal Mask Airway Size	**Cuff Inflation Volume**
3	20 ml
4	30 ml
5	40 ml
6	50 ml

From The Laryngeal Mask Company Limited. (2000). *Instruction Manual: LMA-Classic.* San Diego: Author.

AP This procedure should be performed only by physicians, advanced practice nurses, and other health care professionals (including critical care nurses) with additional knowledge, skills, and demonstrated competence per professional licensure or institutional standard.

Procedure for Laryngeal Mask Airway (LMA-Unique) Insertion—*Continued*

Steps	Rationale	Special Considerations
13. Further assess device placement with end-tidal carbon dioxide device or an esophageal detector device. *(Level I: Manufacturer's recommendations only.)*	Confirms proper placement by two additional methods.[1]	
14. Secure the LMA. *(Level II: Theory based, no research data to support recommendations; recommendations from expert consensus group may exist.)*	Prevents disturbing the correct placement.	
A. Insert a bite-block.	Prevents the patient from biting down on the airway tube, causing displacement of the cuff or occlusion of the airway tube.	Maintain the bite-block in place until the LMA is removed.[10,11]
B. Press the airway tube up toward the palate.	Secures the airway tube in position.	
C. Apply tape or commercially prepared device to hold the airway tube in place (Fig. 7-8).	Prevents movement of the airway tube and cuff.	
15. Remove the LMA as follows:	Removal, when appropriate, may prevent agitation, regurgitation, and laryngeal spasm.	
A. Gently assist with ventilations when the patient begins spontaneously breathing.	Prevents excess ventilatory pressures.	
B. Observe for signs of swallowing.	Indicates a return of some protective reflexes.	Tape or tube-securing device may be removed at this time. Leave the bite-block in place. Avoid suctioning because it may cause laryngeal spasm. The cuff should prevent aspiration.[10]
C. When the patient can open mouth to command, deflate the cuff. The LMA and bite-block are removed together.[10]	If LMA is removed before effective swallowing and coughing, secretions may enter the larynx, causing bronchospasm.	
D. Continue to assess for airway and breathing effectiveness.	Maintains monitoring of the airway and patient's ability to breathe on his or her own.	

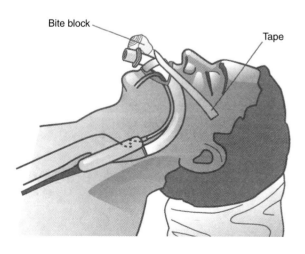

Bite block

Tape

FIGURE 7-8 The bite-block and airway tube are taped together with the tube taped downward against the chin. *(From The Laryngeal Mask Company Limited. [2000]. Instruction Manual: LMA-Classic. San Diego: Author, 31.)*

Expected Outcomes

- Establishment of an effective airway in an emergency situation
- Maintenance of adequate ventilation
- Recovery of spontaneous ventilation

Unexpected Outcomes

- Complications related to the use of the LMA that may be related to poor insertion technique or excessive cuff pressures:
  - Regurgitation
  - Aspiration
  - Bronchospasm
  - Gagging
  - Retching
  - Trauma to tissues
  - Damage to various nerves
  - Sore or dry mouth
  - Hoarseness, stridor
  - Dysphagia, dysarthria, dysphonia
  - Cuff separation from airway tube[9]

Patient Monitoring and Care

Steps	Rationale	Reportable Conditions
		These conditions should be reported if they persist despite nursing interventions.
1. Monitor the patient and LMA during ventilation for potential problems. *(Level II: Theory based, no research data to support recommendations; recommendations from expert consensus group may exist.)*	Ensures proper ventilation and airway management. Pressure-controlled and volume-controlled ventilation may be used, although pressure-controlled ventilation may require lower peak airway pressures.[7] If mechanically ventilated, tidal volume, respiratory rate, and inspiratory-to-expiratory ratios need to be adjusted to prevent high peak airway pressures.[8]	• Inability to ventilate patient
A. Attach a pulse oximeter and monitor for trends.	Monitors adequate oxygenation.	• Decreased oxygen levels despite adequate oxygen delivery.
B. Watch for air leaks around the cuff that may be caused by malposition. If suspected, assess for normal smooth, oval swelling around cricothyroid membrane. If absent, in conjunction with prolonged expiratory phase, remove the LMA, reventilate, and reinsert.[10]	May indicate problems with the LMA position. *Do not add more air to the cuff* because it may force the soft cuff off of the larynx.[10]	• Indications of an air leak, especially with a prolonged expiratory phase or lack of normal smooth, oval swelling around the cricothyroid membrane.
C. If regurgitation occurs, as indicated by fluid in the airway tube, immediately tilt the patient head down and turn body to one side, remove bag-valve device, and suction through airway tube (see Procedure 10).	Allows drainage and clearance of fluid from airway tube. If airway problems, difficulty with ventilation, or regurgitation continues, remove the LMA and establish an airway by other means.[10]	• Airway problems, difficulty with ventilation, or regurgitation.

Documentation

Documentation should include the following:

- Initial patient assessment indicating a need for LMA insertion
- Performance of visual inspection, inflation and deflation tests
- After insertion, assessment of end-tidal carbon dioxide and chest rise and fall
- Before removal, presence of swallowing and ability to open mouth
- Any complications while the LMA is in place (e.g., regurgitation or air leaks)

- Preoxygenation and ventilation before LMA insertion
- Insertion technique (index finger or thumb)
- Initial cuff inflation pressure
- Signs of correct placement and cuff inflation
- Placement of bite-block and securing of the LMA
- After removal, patency of airway, effectiveness of breathing, pulse oximetery and vital sign readings, patient complaints, or signs of complications

References

1. American Heart Association. (2000). *Guidelines for 2000 for Cardiopulmonary Resuscitation and Emergency Cardiovascular Care for Advanced Cardiac Life Support (ACLS)*. Dallas: Author.
2. Brimacombe, J., and Berry, A. (1993). Insertion of the laryngeal mask airway: A prospective study of four techniques. *Anaesth Intensive Care, 21,* 89-92.
3. Burgard, G., Möllhoff, T., and Prien, T. (1996). The effect of laryngeal mask cuff pressure on postoperative sore throat incidence. *J Clin Anesth, 8,* 198-201.
4. Drain, C.B. (2002). *Perianesthesia Nursing: A Critical Care Approach.* Philadelphia: W.B. Saunders.
5. Hand, H. (2002). Cardiopulmonary resuscitation: The laryngeal mask airway. *Emerg Nurse, 10,* 31-37.
6. Idris, A.H., and Gabrielli, A. (2002). Advances in airway management. *Emerg Med Clin N Am, 20,* 843-857.
7. Natalini, G., et al. (2001). Pressure controlled versus volume controlled ventilation with laryngeal mask airway. *J Clin Anesth, 13,* 436-439.
8. Ovassapian, A., and Meyer, R.M. (1998). Airway management. In: Longnecker, D.E., Tinker, J.H., and Morgan, G.E., Jr., editors. *Principles and Practice of Anesthesiology.* 2nd ed. St. Louis: Mosby.

9. Shuster, M., Nolan, J., and Barnes, T.A. (2002). Airway and ventilation management. *Emerg Cardiovasc Care, 20,* 23-35.
10. The Laryngeal Mask Company Limited. (2000). *Instruction Manual: LMA-Classic.* San Diego: Author.
11. The Laryngeal Mask Company Limited. (2001). *Instruction Manual: LMA-Unique.* San Diego: Author.

Additional Readings

Bogetz, M.S. (2002). Using the laryngeal mask airway to manage the difficult airway. *Anesthesiol Clin North Am, 20,* 863-870.
Burns, S.M. (2001). Safely caring for patients with a laryngeal mask airway. *Crit Care Nurse, 21,* 72-74.
Gabrielli, A., et al. (2002). Alternative ventilation strategies in cardiopulmonary resuscitation. *Curr Opin Crit Care, 8,* 199-211.
Maltby, J.R., Loken, R.G., and Watson, N.C. (1990). The laryngeal mask airway: Clinical appraisal in 250 patients. *Can J Anesth, 37,* 509-513.
Nolan, J.D. (2001). Prehospital and resuscitative airway care: Should the gold standard be reassessed? *Curr Opin Crit Care, 7,* 413-421.

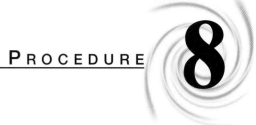

PROCEDURE **8**

Nasopharyngeal Airway Insertion

P U R P O S E :   Nasopharyngeal airways are used to maintain a patent airway to the hypopharynx and to facilitate the removal of tracheobronchial secretions by directing the catheter and by averting tissue trauma that is associated with repeated suction attempts.[2,3]

Kirsten N. Skillings
Bonnie L. Curtis

PREREQUISITE NURSING KNOWLEDGE

- The nasopharyngeal airway is a flexible piece of rubber. It is passed through the nose and follows the posterior nasal and oropharyngeal walls to the base of the tongue (Fig. 8-1).
- The nasopharyngeal airway has three parts: flange, cannula, and bevel or tip. The flange is the wide, trumpet-like end that prevents further slippage into the airway. The hollow shaft of the cannula permits airflow into the hypopharynx. The bevel or tip is the opening at the distal end of the tube. When properly inserted, the tip can be seen resting posterior to the base of the tongue.
- The external diameter of the nasopharyngeal airway should be slightly smaller than the patient's external naris opening. The length of the nasopharyngeal airway is determined by measuring the distance between the naris and the tragus of the ear (Fig. 8-2).[1] Improperly sized nasopharyngeal airways may result in increased airway resistance, limited airflow (if the airway is too small), kinking and mucosal trauma, gagging, vomiting, and gastric distention (if the airway is too large). Some manufacturers provide nasopharyngeal airways shaped specifically for the right and left nares.
- The advantages of the nasopharyngeal airway include increased comfort and tolerance in a conscious patient, stable airway positioning for long periods, decreased incidence of gag reflex stimulation, and minimal incidence of mucosal trauma during frequent suctioning.
- Nasopharyngeal airways are especially useful for relieving airway obstruction associated with mandibular-type injuries that result in jaw immobility or soft tissue obstruction. Examples of these injuries include jaw wiring,

trismus, pain, edema, jaw spasms, and mechanical impairment such as temporomandibular joint fractures and zygomatic fractures. In selected patient situations, a nasopharyngeal airway may be used to facilitate the passage of a fiberoptic bronchoscope and to tamponade small, bleeding blood vessels in the nasal mucosa.
- Insertion of the nasopharyngeal airway in an alert patient may stimulate the gag reflex, causing retching and vomiting.
- The nasopharyngeal airway is used most commonly in the postanesthesia recovery period to facilitate pulmonary toilets and in situations in which the patient is semiconscious.

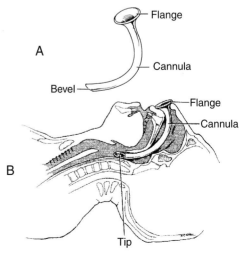

FIGURE 8-1 Nasopharyngeal airway. **A,** Airway parts. **B,** Proper placement. *(From Eubanks, D.H., and Bone, R.C. [1990].* Comprehensive Respiratory Care: A Learning System. *St. Louis: C.V. Mosby, 518.)*

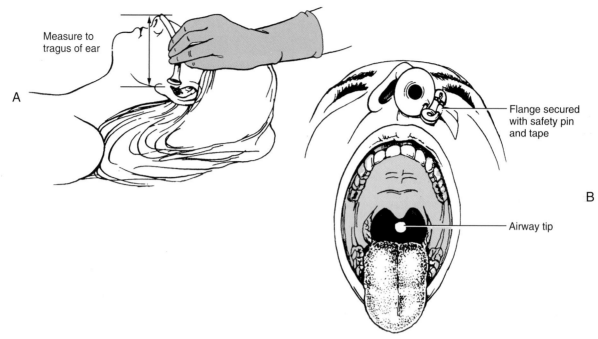

FIGURE 8-2 **A,** Estimating nasopharyngeal airway size. **B,** Nasopharyngeal position after insertion. *(From Eubanks, D.H., and Bone, R.C. [1990].* Comprehensive Respiratory Care: A Learning System. *St. Louis: C.V. Mosby, 552.)*

- Contraindications to use of a nasopharyngeal airway are as follows:
  - ❖ Patients receiving anticoagulation therapy
  - ❖ Patients prone to epistaxis
  - ❖ Patients with obstructed nasal passageways
  - ❖ Patients with facial or head trauma when basilar skull fracture or cranial vault communication is suspected

EQUIPMENT

- Appropriately sized nasal airway (Table 8-1)
- Nonsterile gloves
- Water-soluble lubricant
- Tape
- Suction equipment
- Flashlight
- Tongue depressor
  Additional equipment (to have available depending on patient need) includes the following:
- Cotton swabs
- Topical anesthetic

TABLE 8-1	Nasopharyngeal Airway Sizing
Approximate Body Weight	**Size (mm)**
Small adult	6-7
Medium adult	7-8
Large adult	8-9

From Cummins, R.O., editor. (2003). Airway, airway adjuncts, oxygenation, and ventilation. In: *ACLS: Principles and Practice.* Dallas: American Heart Association, 145-6.

PATIENT AND FAMILY EDUCATION

- Explain the purpose of the airway and the necessity of the procedure to conscious patients or to the family of an unconscious patient. ➤*Rationale:* Communication and explanation regarding therapy are cited as an important need of patients and families; they relieve anxiety and encourage communication.
- Explain the patient's role in assisting with insertion of the airway. ➤*Rationale:* Patient cooperation is elicited, and tube insertion is facilitated.
- Discuss the sensory experiences associated with nasal airway insertion, including the presence of a rubber airway in the nose and possible gagging. ➤*Rationale:* Knowledge of anticipated sensory experiences reduces anxiety and distress.

PATIENT ASSESSMENT AND PREPARATION

Patient Assessment

- Assess cardiopulmonary status. ➤*Rationale:* Evaluation of the patient's cardiopulmonary status assists in determining the need for an artificial airway.
- Assess patent nasal passageway. With finger pressure, occlude one nostril; feel for air movement under the open nostril. Patency also can be assessed by inspection of each naris with a flashlight. ➤*Rationale:* Assessment of patency promotes smooth, quick, unobstructed airway insertion.

Patient Preparation

- Ensure that the patient understands preprocedural teaching. Answer questions as they arise, and reinforce information as needed. ➧*Rationale:* This evaluates and reinforces understanding of previously taught information.

- Position patient. Unless contraindicated, a supine or high Fowler position is acceptable. ➧*Rationale:* This positioning promotes patient and nurse comfort and provides easy access to the external nares.

Procedure for Nasopharyngeal Airway Insertion

Steps	Rationale	Special Considerations
1. Wash hands; don personal protective equipment.	Reduces transmission of microorganisms and body secretions; standard precautions.	For copious secretions, don protective eyewear, facemask, or both.
2. Prepare the nasopharyngeal airway. A. Inspect for smooth edges. B. Generously lubricate the tip and outer cannula with water-soluble lubricant.	Decreases chances of mucosal trauma during insertion. Decreases incidence of trauma by preventing friction against dry mucosal membrane.[3]	
3. Remove excess secretions from naris.	Allows for visual inspection of naris; removes possible source of obstruction; removes medium for organism growth.	Nasopharyngeal and nasotracheal suction are contraindicated in patients with actual or suspected maxillofacial and skull injuries.
4. When difficult insertion is anticipated (e.g., with nasal polyps, septal deviation), apply topical anesthetic to cotton swabs, insert as far as possible, and coat the nasal passageway.	Topical anesthetics with a vasoconstrictor help shrink nasal mucosa and decrease the incidence of trauma and bleeding. Vasoconstrictor property acts on capillaries to decrease bleeding.	Check with physician, advanced practice nurse, or institutional standards for topical anesthetic usage and indications.
5. Gently slide airway into nostril. Guide it medially and downward along the nasal passage.	Following the natural contour of the nasal passage decreases the incidence of trauma.	If resistance is encountered, rotate the tube and continue gentle forward pressure. Do not force the tube. If resistance continues, withdraw the tube and try the other nostril. While inserting the tube, if the patient experiences increasing dyspnea or respiratory distress, consider removing the tube.
6. Ask patient to open his or her mouth, or hold the patient's mouth open. Control the tongue with a tongue depressor. Illuminate the oral cavity, and visualize the tip of the nasopharyngeal airway behind the uvula (see Fig. 8-2).	Verifying the location of the airway in the pharynx verifies proper airway positioning and allows for inspection of posterior pharynx for excessive bleeding or mucus.	
7. Verify patency of airway. Feel for air movement over the flange. Auscultate breath sounds bilaterally.	Optimal airway positioning allows for forward gas flow, removal of secretions, and possible prevention of airway occlusion.	
8. Secure airway by taping it in place.	Minimizes dislodgment, removal, and deeper penetration into the nasopharynx.	
9. Suction secretions as needed.	Maintains patent airway.	Recheck flange for proper position.
10. Reassess patient's respiratory status.	Indicates effectiveness of the nasal airway.	

Expected Outcomes

- Improvement of respiratory status
- Long-term patent airway
- Diminished mucosal edema and trauma related to frequent suction passes

Unexpected Outcomes

- Inability to pass nasopharyngeal airway
- Airway obstruction
- Head or ear pain
- Epistaxis
- Naris and nasal mucosal ulceration

Patient Monitoring and Care

Steps	Rationale	Reportable Conditions
		These conditions should be reported if they persist despite nursing interventions. • Redness • Swelling • Drainage • Bleeding • Skin breakdown
1. Assess skin in contact with nasal airway.		
2. Facilitate removal of secretions. Hyperoxygenate and suction as needed (see Procedure 10).	Retained secretions increase the potential for airway obstruction and pulmonary infections. Aging results in diminishing mucociliary clearance.	• Change in character or amount of secretions
3. Monitor respiratory status every 2 to 4 hours.	Change in respiratory status may indicate displacement of oral airway or worsening respiratory condition.	• Change in respiratory status not corrected with repositioning of airway or suctioning
4. Provide meticulous mouth care every 4 to 8 hours and as needed (see Procedure 4).	Prevents secretions, encrustations, mouth infections, and airway port occlusions.	• Lacerations • Ulcerations • Areas of necrosis

Documentation

Documentation should include the following:

- Patient and family education
- Insertion of nasopharyngeal airway
- Size of nasopharyngeal airway
- Any difficulties with insertion
- Patient tolerance, including respiratory and vital signs assessment before and after procedure
- Verification of proper placement
- Appearance and thickness of tracheal secretions, if present
- Skin integrity around tube
- Unexpected outcomes
- Nursing interventions

References

1. Cummins, R.O., editor. (2003). Airway, airway adjuncts, oxygenation, and ventilation. In: *ACLS: Principles and Practice.* Dallas: American Heart Association, 145-6.
2. Eubanks, D.H., and Bone, R.C. (1990). *Comprehensive Respiratory Care: A Learning System.* St. Louis: C.V. Mosby, 491-5.
3. Pierce, L. (1995). *Guide to Mechanical Ventilation and Intensive Respiratory Care.* Philadelphia: W.B. Saunders.

Additional Reading

St. John, R. (1999). Protocols for practice: Applying research at the bedside; airway management. *Crit Care Nurse,* 19, 79-83.

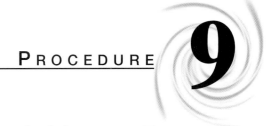

http://evolve.elsevier.com

PROCEDURE **9**

Oropharyngeal Airway Insertion

P U R P O S E : Oropharyngeal airways are inserted to relieve airway obstruction, provide short-term maintenance of an airway, and facilitate removal of tracheobronchial secretions.

Kirsten N. Skillings
Bonnie L. Curtis

PREREQUISITE NURSING KNOWLEDGE

- Oropharyngeal airways are usually disposable and made of hard, curved plastic.
- Oral airways are inserted through the open mouth with the posterior tip resting in the patient's pharynx. The oral airway is placed over the tongue. The curvature or body of the airway displaces the tongue forward from the posterior pharyngeal wall, a common site of airway obstruction.
- An oral airway has four parts: flange, body, tip, and channel (Fig. 9-1). The flange, or flat surface, protruding from the mouth rests against the lips. This design protects against aspiration into the airway. The body of the airway curves over the tongue. The tip is the distal-most part of the airway toward the base of the tongue. The channel enables passage of a suction catheter.

- The Guedel airway is tubular with a flattened-oval inner diameter. A suction catheter passes through the central lumen or channel.
- The Berman airway has a channel on either side that guides the catheter along the edge of the airway into the pharyngeal space.
- Oral airways are manufactured in a variety of lengths and widths for adults, children, and infants. Sizing depends on the age and size of the patient (Table 9-1). An alternative method used to select the size of an oral airway is to measure the airway by placing the flange alongside the

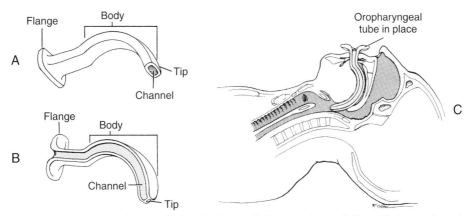

FIGURE 9-1 Oropharyngeal airways. **A,** Guedel airway. **B,** Berman airway. **C,** Properly inserted oropharyngeal tube. *(From Eubanks, D.H., and Bone, R.C. [1990]. Comprehensive Respiratory Care: A Learning System. St. Louis: C.V. Mosby, 518.)*

TABLE 9-1	Oral Airway Sizes	
Size of Patient	Diameter of Oral Airway (mm)	Size of Oral Airway (Guedel)
Large adult	100	5
Medium adult	90	4
Small adult	80	3

From Cummins, R.O., editor. (2003). Airway, airway adjuncts, oxygenation, and ventilation. In: *ACLS: Principles and Practice.* Dallas: American Heart Association, 145.

patient's lips and the oral airway tip alongside the angle of the jaw (Fig. 9-2). Improperly sized airways can cause airway obstruction (if they are too small) and tongue displacement against the oropharynx (if they are too large).

- Oropharyngeal airways are used most commonly in unconscious patients because they may stimulate vomiting in a conscious or semiconscious patient.
- Oral airways facilitate suctioning of the pharynx and prevent patients from biting their tongues, grinding their teeth, or occluding their endotracheal or oral gastric tubes. Additionally, an oropharyngeal airway may be used in conjunction with an oral endotracheal tube to facilitate artificial ventilation, to act as a bite-block, and to prevent damage to the tongue and soft tissues of the mouth.
- Improper or rough insertion techniques can result in tooth damage or loss and lacerations to the roof of the mouth. Improper lip, mouth, and tube care can result in pressure sores, cracked lips, and stomatitis.
- Oropharyngeal airway placement should never be attempted in a patient who is actively seizing. If the patient has an aura preceding the seizure, an airway may be placed prophylactically.

EQUIPMENT

- Appropriately sized oral airway
- Nonsterile gloves

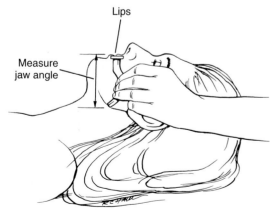

FIGURE 9-2 Alternative method for selecting size of an oropharyngeal airway. (*From Eubanks, D.H., and Bone, R.C. [1990].* Comprehensive Respiratory Care: A Learning System. *St. Louis: C.V. Mosby, 552.*)

- Tongue depressor
- Tape
  Additional equipment (to have available based on patient needs) includes the following:
- Suction equipment
- Goggles, glasses, or facemask

PATIENT AND FAMILY EDUCATION

- Explain the procedure (if the patient's condition and time allow) and the reason for the airway insertion. ➤*Rationale:* This identifies patient and family knowledge deficits about the patient's condition, the procedure, its expected benefits, and its potential risks and allows time for questions to clarify information and voice concerns. Explanations decrease patient anxiety and enhance cooperation.
- Explain the patient's role in assisting with insertion of the airway. ➤*Rationale:* Patient cooperation is elicited, and tube insertion is facilitated.
- Discuss the sensory experiences associated with oral airway insertion, including the inability to clench teeth together, the presence of a hard plastic airway in the mouth, the inability to move tongue freely, and the possibility of gagging. ➤*Rationale:* Knowledge of anticipated sensory experiences reduces anxiety and distress.

PATIENT ASSESSMENT AND PREPARATION

Patient Assessment

- Assess the patient's need for long-term airway maintenance. ➤*Rationale:* Oropharyngeal airways are generally used for temporary airway maintenance.[1-3]
- Assess condition of oral mucosa, dentition, and gums. ➤*Rationale:* Preprocedural assessment provides baseline information for later comparison.
- Remove loose-fitting dentures and any foreign objects (including partial plates and tongue studs) from the mouth. ➤*Rationale:* Removal ensures that objects will not be advanced further into the airway during insertion.

Patient Preparation

- Ensure that patient understands preprocedural teaching. Answer questions as they arise, and reinforce information as needed. ➤*Rationale:* This evaluates and reinforces understanding of previously taught information.
- Position patient. A semi-Fowler or supine position is preferred for a conscious patient. ➤*Rationale:* This positioning promotes patient and nurse comfort and provides easy access to the oral cavity.
- Hyperextend the patient's neck using the head-tilt, chin-lift technique; use the jaw-thrust technique for the unconscious patient. ➤*Rationale:* Airway obstructions can result from posterior displacement of the tongue and epiglottis (not in the trauma patient).

Procedure for Oropharyngeal Airway Insertion

Steps	Rationale	Special Considerations
1. Wash hands, and don personal protective equipment.	Reduces transmission of microorganisms and body secretions; standard precautions.	Protective eyewear or facemasks should be worn in the presence of copious secretions.
2. Suction the mouth and pharynx using a rigid pharyngeal suction tip (Yankauer) catheter.	Clears airway of secretions, blood, and vomit so that they do not enter into the airway with airway insertion.	
3. Open the mouth using the crossed-finger technique (Fig. 9-3). Remove dentures, if present.	Provides access to oral cavity and leverage to open a tightly closed mouth.	
4. Insert oral airway.		
A. Hold oral airway with curved end up (Fig. 9-4).	Provides patent upper airway and prevents posterior tongue displacement.	
B. Advance oral airway over the base of the tongue until the flange is parallel with the patient's nose.	Positions airway appropriately.	Remove the airway immediately if the patient gags, gasps for air, or begins breathing irregularly.
C. Rotate the tip 180 degrees to point down (see Fig. 9-4).	Provides for open pathway from the mouth to the pharynx.	A tongue depressor may assist in tongue control during insertion.
5. Recheck the size and position of the oral airway. Verify airway patency.	Proper placement and size are essential for securing and maintaining a patent airway.	When the oral airway is properly sized, the flange should rest against the patient's lips (see Fig. 9-2). Gagging may indicate that the airway is too long. Ensure the lips and tongue are not between the teeth and airway.[3]
6. Consider securing the airway.	Taping is indicated to prevent expulsion of the airway. Leaving the airway untaped is indicated in patients who need to be able to cough out the airway if gagging should occur because gagging may stimulate vomiting and aspiration (i.e., in a postanesthesia or semiconscious patient).	Follow institutional standards. Use care not to tape over air channel.

Procedure continues on the following page

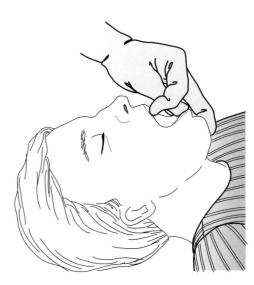

FIGURE 9-3 Crossed-finger technique for opening the mouth. *(From Eubanks, D.H., and Bone, R.C. [1990]. Comprehensive Respiratory Care: A Learning System. St. Louis: C.V. Mosby, 631.)*

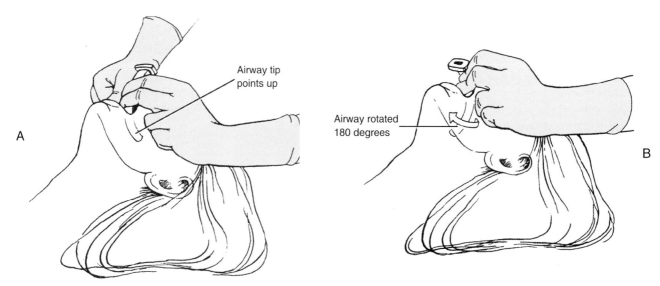

Airway tip
points up

A

Airway rotated
180 degrees

B

FIGURE 9-4 Insertion of an oropharyngeal airway. **A,** Advance airway with curved end up. **B,** Rotate airway 180 degrees. *(From Eubanks, D.H., and Bone, R.C. [1990]. Comprehensive Respiratory Care: A Learning System. St. Louis: C.V. Mosby, 551.)*

Procedure for Oropharyngeal Airway Insertion

Steps	Rationale	Special Considerations
7. Hyperoxygenate and suction pharynx as needed (see Procedure 10).	Maintains patent airway; pooled secretions provide a medium for bacterial growth.	
8. Reassess patient's respiratory status.	Validates the effectiveness of the oral airway.	

Expected Outcomes

- Improvement of respiratory status
- Short-term patent airway

Unexpected Outcomes

- Airway obstruction
- Pulmonary aspiration
- Trauma to the lips and oral cavity
- Inability to insert oral airway because patient is combative or seizing or patient's mouth cannot be opened

Patient Monitoring and Care

Steps	Rationale	Reportable Conditions
		These conditions should be reported if they persist despite nursing interventions.
1. Reposition the oral airway every 1 to 2 hours, assessing the lips, tongue, and mouth with each position change.	Pressure of the flange on the lips may produce ulcers and necrosis.	• Lacerations • Ulcerations • Areas of necrosis
2. Apply water-soluble jelly, petrolatum, or lip balm to the lips.	Prevents mucosal drying and cracking.	• Cracked and bleeding lips

Patient Monitoring and Care—*Continued*

Steps	Rationale	Reportable Conditions
3. Provide meticulous oral care every 4 to 8 hours and as needed. (see Procedure 4)	Decreases secretions, encrustations, oral infections, and airway port occlusions.	• Lacerations • Ulcerations • Areas of necrosis • Drainage
4. Remove the oral airway every 24 hours or as needed. Clean airway and reinsert, as needed.	Allows for more complete inspection of the lips and oral cavity; enables complete oral hygiene.	
5. Monitor respiratory status every 2 to 4 hours.	Change in respiratory status may indicate displacement of oral airway or worsening respiratory condition.	• Stridor • Crowing • Gasping respirations • Snoring

Documentation

Documentation should include the following:

- Patient and family education
- Insertion of oropharyngeal airway
- Type and size of oral airway
- Any difficulties in insertion
- Patient tolerance, including respiratory and vital signs assessments before and after procedure
- Verification of proper placement
- Appearance and thickness of tracheal or oral secretions, if present
- Oral care
- Skin integrity around tube
- Unexpected outcomes
- Nursing interventions

References

1. Cummins, R.O., editor. (2003). Airway, airway adjuncts, oxygenation, and ventilation. In: *ACLS: Principles and Practice.* Dallas: American Heart Association, 145-6.
2. Eubanks, D.H., and Bone, R.C. (1990). *Comprehensive Respiratory Care: A Learning System.* St. Louis: C.V. Mosby, 491-5.
3. Pierce, L. (1995). *Guide to Mechanical Ventilation and Intensive Respiratory Care.* Philadelphia: W.B. Saunders.

Additional Reading

St. John, R. (1999). Protocols for practice: Applying research at the bedside; airway management. *Crit Care Nurse,* 19, 79-83.

PROCEDURE **10**

Suctioning: Endotracheal or Tracheostomy Tube

P U R P O S E :   Endotracheal or tracheostomy tube suctioning is performed to maintain the patency of the artificial airway and to improve gas exchange, decrease airway resistance, and reduce infection risk by removing secretions from the trachea and main stem bronchi. Suctioning also may be performed to obtain samples of tracheal secretions for laboratory analysis.

Marianne Chulay

PREREQUISITE NURSING KNOWLEDGE

- Endotracheal and tracheostomy tubes are used to maintain a patent airway and to facilitate mechanical ventilation. Presence of these artificial airways, especially endotracheal tubes, prevents effective coughing and secretion removal, requiring periodic removal of pulmonary secretions with suctioning. In acute care situations, suctioning is always performed as a sterile procedure to prevent nosocomial pneumonia.
- Suctioning is performed using one of two basic methods. In the open-suction technique, after disconnection of the endotracheal or tracheostomy tube from any ventilatory tubing or oxygen sources, a single-use suction catheter is inserted into the open end of the tube. In the closed-suction technique, also referred to as *in-line suctioning,* a multiple-use suction catheter inside a sterile plastic sleeve is inserted through a special diaphragm attached to the end of the endotracheal or tracheostomy tube (Fig. 10-1). The closed-suction technique allows for the maintenance of oxygenation and ventilation support, which may be beneficial when high levels of inspired oxygen or positive end-expiratory pressure (PEEP) are required during mechanical ventilation. In addition, the closed-suction technique decreases the risk for aerosolization of tracheal secretions during suction-induced coughing. Use of the closed-suction technique should be considered in patients who develop cardiopulmonary

instability during suctioning with the open technique, who have high levels of PEEP (greater than 10 cm H_2O) or inspired oxygen (greater than 80%) or both, who have grossly bloody pulmonary secretions, or in whom active tuberculosis is suspected.
- Indications for suctioning include the following:
  - ❖ Secretions in the artificial airway
  - ❖ Suspected aspiration of gastric or upper airway secretions
  - ❖ Auscultation of adventitious lung sounds over the trachea or main stem bronchi or both
  - ❖ Increase in peak airway pressures when patient is on mechanical ventilation
  - ❖ Increase in respiratory rate or frequent coughing or both
  - ❖ Gradual or sudden decrease in arterial blood oxygen (PaO_2), arterial blood oxygen saturation (SaO_2), or arterial saturation levels via pulse oximetry (SpO_2) levels
  - ❖ Sudden onset of respiratory distress, when airway patency is questioned
- Suctioning of airways should be performed only for a clinical indication and not as a routine, fixed-schedule treatment.
- Hyperoxygenation always should be provided before and after each pass of the suction catheter into the endotracheal tube, whether done with the open or closed suctioning method.
- Suctioning is a necessary procedure for patients with artificial airways. When clinical indicators of the need for

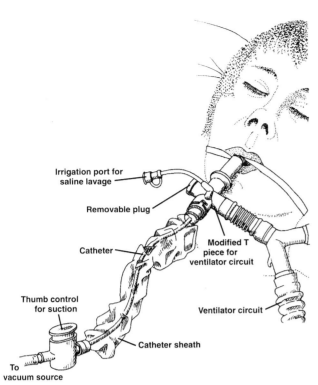

FIGURE 10-1 Closed-suction technique. *(From Sills, J.R. [1991]. Respiratory Certification Guide. St. Louis: C.V. Mosby.)*

Labels on figure:
- Irrigation port for saline lavage
- Removable plug
- Catheter
- Modified T piece for ventilator circuit
- Thumb control for suction
- Ventilator circuit
- Catheter sheath
- To vacuum source

suctioning exist, there is no absolute contraindication to suctioning. In situations in which the development of a suctioning complication would be poorly tolerated by the patient, strong evidence of a clinical need for suctioning should exist.

- Complications associated with suctioning of artificial airways include the following:
  ❖ Respiratory arrest
  ❖ Cardiac arrest
  ❖ Cardiac dysrhythmias
  ❖ Hypertension or hypotension
  ❖ Decreases in mixed venous oxygen saturation (Svo_2)
  ❖ Increased intracranial pressure
  ❖ Bronchospasm
  ❖ Pulmonary hemorrhage or bleeding
- Tracheal mucosal damage (epithelial denudement, hyperemia, loss of cilia, edema) occurs during suctioning when tissue is pulled into the catheter tip holes. These areas of damage increase the risk of infection and bleeding. Use of special-tipped catheters, low levels of suction pressure,

or intermittent suction pressure has not been shown to decrease tracheal mucosal damage with suctioning.

- Postural drainage and percussion may improve secretion mobilization from small to large airways in diseases with large mucus production (e.g., cystic fibrosis, bronchitis).
- Adequate systemic hydration and supplemental humidification of inspired gases assist in thinning secretions for easier aspiration from airways. Instillation of a bolus of normal saline (5 to 10 ml) does not thin secretions, may cause decreases in arterial and mixed venous oxygenation, and may contribute to lower airway contamination secondary to the mechanical dislodgment of bacteria within the artificial airway or from contamination of saline during instillation.
- The suction catheter should not be any larger than half of the internal diameter of the endotracheal or tracheostomy tube.

EQUIPMENT

Open Technique

- Suction catheter of appropriate size (Table 10-1)
- Sterile water-soluble lubricant or sterile saline solution
- Sterile gloves
- Sterile solution container or sterile basin
- Source of suction (wall mounted or portable)
- Connecting tube, 4 to 6 ft
- Self-inflating manual resuscitation bag (MRB) connected to an oxygen flowmeter, set at 15 liters/min (not required if using the ventilator to deliver hyperoxygenation breaths)
- Goggles or glasses and mask
  Additional equipment (to have available depending on patient need) includes the following:
- PEEP valve (for patients on greater than 5 cm H_2O PEEP)

Closed Technique

- Closed-suction setup with a catheter of appropriate size (see Table 10-1)
- Sterile saline lavage containers (5 to 10 ml)
- Suction catheter (individually packaged) for oral and nasal suctioning
- Source of suction (wall mounted or portable)
- Connecting tube (4 to 6 feet)
- Nonsterile gloves
- Goggles or glasses and mask

TABLE 10-1	Guideline for Catheter Size for Endotracheal and Tracheostomy Tube Suctioning*		
Patient Age	**Endotracheal Tube Size (mm)**	**Tracheostomy Tube Size (mm, inner diameter)**	**Suction Catheter Size (Fr)**
Small child (2-5 years)	4.0-5.0	3.5-4.5	6-8
School-age child (6-12 years)	5.0-6.0	4.5-5.0	8-10
Adolescent to adult	7.0-9.0	5.0-9.0	10-16

*This guide should be used as an estimate only. Actual sizes depend on the size and individual needs of the patient.
From Henneman, E., Ellstrom, K., and St. John, R.E. (1999). Airway management. In: *AACN Protocols for Practice: Care of the Mechanically Ventilated Patient Series.* Aliso Viejo, CA: American Association of Critical-Care Nurses.

PATIENT AND FAMILY EDUCATION

- Explain the procedure for endotracheal or tracheostomy tube suctioning. ➤*Rationale:* The explanation reduces anxiety.
- Explain that suctioning may be uncomfortable, causing the patient to experience shortness of breath. ➤*Rationale:* This reduces anxiety and elicits patient cooperation.
- Explain the patient's role in assisting with secretion removal by coughing during the procedure. ➤*Rationale:* This encourages cooperation and facilitates removal of secretions.

PATIENT ASSESSMENT AND PREPARATION

Patient Assessment

- Assess for signs and symptoms of airway obstruction:
  - ❖ Secretions in the airway
  - ❖ Inspiratory wheezes
  - ❖ Expiratory crackles
  - ❖ Restlessness
  - ❖ Ineffective coughing
  - ❖ Decreased level of consciousness
  - ❖ Decreased breath sounds
  - ❖ Tachypnea
  - ❖ Tachycardia or bradycardia
  - ❖ Cyanosis
  - ❖ Hypertension or hypotension
  - ❖ Shallow respirations

➤*Rationale:* Physical signs and symptoms result from inadequate gas exchange associated with airway obstruction.
- Note peak airway pressures on the ventilator. ➤*Rationale:* These indicate potential secretions in the airway, increasing resistance to gas flow.
- Evaluate SaO_2 and SpO_2 levels. ➤*Rationale:* These indicate potential secretions in the airway, decreasing gas exchange.
- Assess signs and symptoms of inadequate breathing patterns.
  - ❖ Dyspnea
  - ❖ Shallow respirations
  - ❖ Intercostal and suprasternal retractions
  - ❖ Frequent triggering of ventilator alarms
  - ❖ Increased respiratory rate

➤*Rationale:* Respiratory distress is a late sign of lower airway obstruction.

Patient Preparation

- Ensure that the patient understands preprocedural teaching. Answer questions as they arise, and reinforce information as needed. ➤*Rationale:* This communication evaluates and reinforces understanding of previously taught information.
- Assist the patient in achieving a position that is comfortable for the patient and nurse, generally semi-Fowler or Fowler. ➤*Rationale:* This positioning promotes comfort, oxygenation, and ventilation and reduces strain.
- Secure additional personnel to assist with the MRB to provide hyperoxygenation (open-suction technique only). ➤*Rationale:* Two hands are necessary to inflate the MRB for adult tidal volume levels (greater than 600 ml).

Procedure | for Endotracheal or Tracheostomy Tube Suctioning

Steps	Rationale	Special Considerations
1. Wash hands, and don personal protective equipment.	Reduces transmission of microorganisms and body secretions; standard precautions.	
2. Turn on suction apparatus, and set vacuum regulator to 100 to 120 mm Hg. (*Level II: Theory based, no research data to support recommendations; recommendations from expert consensus group may exist.*) Follow manufacturer's directions for suction pressure levels when using closed-suction catheter systems. (*Level I: Manufacturer's recommendation only.*)	The amount of suction applied should be only enough to remove secretions effectively. High negative-pressure settings may increase tracheal mucosal damage.[1,19,22]	
3. Secure one end of the connecting tube to the suction machine, and place the other end in a convenient location within reach.	Prepares suction apparatus.	
4. Monitor patient's cardiopulmonary status before, during, and after the	Observes for signs and symptoms of complications: decreased arterial	Development of cardiopulmonary instability, particularly cardiac

Procedure for Endotracheal or Tracheostomy Tube Suctioning—*Continued*

Steps	Rationale	Special Considerations
suctioning period. *(Level II: Theory based, no research data to support recommendations; recommendations from expert consensus group may exist.)*	and mixed venous oxygen saturation, cardiac dysrhythmias, bronchospasm, respiratory distress, cyanosis, increased blood pressure or intracranial pressure, anxiety, agitation, or changes in mental status.[1,7-9,13-15,19,20,23,28,30,32,34,35]	dysrhythmias or arterial desaturation, requires immediate termination of the suctioning procedure.
5a. Open-Suction Technique Only		
A. Open sterile catheter package on a clean surface, using the inside of the wrapping as a sterile field.	Prepares catheter and prevents transmission of microorganisms.	
B. Set up the sterile solution container or sterile field. Be careful not to touch the inside of the container. Fill with approximately 100 ml of sterile normal saline solution or water.	Prepares catheter flush solution.	
C. Don sterile gloves.	Maintains sterility and standard precautions.	In the event that one sterile glove and one nonsterile glove are used, apply the nonsterile glove to the nondominant hand and the sterile glove to the dominant hand. Handle all nonsterile items with the nondominant hand.
D. Pick up suction catheter, being careful to avoid touching nonsterile surfaces. With the nondominant hand, pick up the connecting tubing. Secure the suction catheter to the connecting tubing.	Maintains catheter sterility. Connects the suction catheter and the connecting tubing.	The dominant hand should not come in contact with the connecting tubing. Wrapping the suction catheter around the sterile dominant hand helps prevent inadvertent contamination of the catheter.
E. Check equipment for proper functioning by suctioning a small amount of sterile saline solution from the container. **Proceed to Step 6**.	Ensures equipment function.	
5b. Closed-Suction Technique Only		
A. Connect the suction tubing to the closed system suction port, according to manufacturer's guidelines.		
6. Hyperoxygenate the patient for at least 30 seconds by one of the following three methods *(Level VI: Clinical studies in a variety of patient populations and situations.)*	Hyperoxygenation with 100% oxygen is used to prevent a decrease in arterial oxygen levels during the suctioning procedure.[1,4,10,12,13,19,28-30,32,39,40]	Limited data indicate that use of a ventilator to deliver the hyperoxygenation may be more effective in increasing arterial oxygen levels.[4,17]
A. Press the suction hyperoxygenation button on the ventilator with the nondominant hand. *or*		
B. Increase the baseline fraction of inspired oxygen (FIO_2) level on the mechanical ventilator.		When using this method, caution must be used to return the FIO_2 to baseline levels after completion of suctioning.

Procedure continues on the following page

Procedure **for Endotracheal or Tracheostomy Tube Suctioning**—*Continued*

Steps	Rationale	Special Considerations
C. Disconnect the ventilator or gas delivery tubing from the end of the endotracheal or tracheostomy tube, attach the MRB to the tube with the nondominant hand, and administer five to six breaths over 30 seconds.	Attach a PEEP valve to the MRB for patients on greater than 5 cm H_2O PEEP. Verify 100% oxygen delivery capabilities of MRB by checking manufacturer's guidelines or with direct measurement with an in-line oxygen analyzer when baseline ventilator oxygen delivery to the patient is greater than 60%. Some models of MRB entrain room air and deliver less than 100% oxygen.	Use of a second person to deliver hyperoxygenation breaths with the MRB significantly increases tidal volume delivery. One-handed "bagging" rarely achieves adult tidal volume breaths (greater than 500 ml).[15-17,21]
7. With the suction off, gently but quickly insert the catheter with the dominant hand into the artificial airway until resistance is met, then pull back 1 cm.[1,19] *(Level II: Theory based, no research data to support recommendations; recommendations from expert consensus group may exist.)*	Suction should be applied only as needed to remove secretions and for as short a time as possible to minimize decreases in arterial oxygen levels.	Directional or coudé catheters are available for selective right or left main stem bronchus placement. Straight catheters usually enter the right main stem bronchus.[24,26] Saline should not be instilled routinely into the artificial airway before suctioning. *(Level VI: Clinical studies in a variety of populations and situations.)*[1-3,5,6,11,18,33,36,37]
8. Place the nondominant thumb over the control vent of the suction catheter and apply continuous or intermittent suction. *(Level III: Laboratory data; no clinical data to support recommendations.)* Rotate the catheter between the dominant thumb and forefinger as you withdraw the catheter for less than or equal to 10 seconds into the sterile catheter sleeve (closed-suction technique) or out of the open airway (open-suction technique). *(Level II: Theory based, no research data to support recommendations; recommendations from expert consensus group may exist.)*	Tracheal damage from suctioning is similar with intermittent or continuous suction.[14,25,27,31] Decreases in arterial oxygen levels during suctioning can be kept to a minimum with brief suction periods.[1,19,38]	
9. Hyperoxygenate for 30 seconds as described in **Step 6**. *(Level VI: Clinical studies in a variety of patient populations and situations.)*		
10. One or two more passes of the suction catheter, as delineated in **Steps 7 and 8,** may be performed if secretions remain in the airway and the patient is tolerating the procedure. *(Level II: Theory based, no research data to support recommendations; recommendations from expert consensus group may exist.)*	Arterial oxygen desaturation and cardiopulmonary complications increase with each successive pass.[2,19,22]	If secretions remain in the airways after two or three suction catheter passes, allow the patient to rest before additional suctioning passes.

Procedure for Endotracheal or Tracheostomy Tube Suctioning—*Continued*

Steps	Rationale	Special Considerations
Provide 30 seconds of hyperoxygenation before and after each pass of the suction catheter. *(Level VI: Clinical studies in a variety of patient populations and situations.)* See **Step 6.**		
11. If the patient does not tolerate suctioning despite hyperoxygenation, try the following steps. *(Level II: Theory based, no research data to support recommendations; recommendations from expert consensus group may exist.)* A. Ensure that 100% oxygen is being delivered. B. Maintain PEEP during suctioning. Check that the PEEP valve is attached properly to the MRB if using that method for hyperoxygenation. C. Switch to another method of suctioning (e.g., closed-suctioning technique). D. Allow longer recovery intervals between suction passes. E. Hyperventilation may be used in situations in which the patient does not tolerate suctioning with hyperoxygenation alone, using either the MRB or the ventilator.	Use of a different suctioning technique may be physiologically less demanding.[39]	
12. Rinse the catheter and connecting tubing with sterile saline solution until clear.	Removes buildup of secretions in the connecting tubing and, when using the closed-suction catheter system, in the in-line suction catheter.	
13. When the lower airway has been cleared adequately of secretions, perform nasal or oral pharyngeal suctioning. *(Level II: Theory based, no research data to support recommendations; recommendations from expert consensus group may exist.)* A separate suction catheter must be opened for this step when using the closed-suction technique.	Prevents contamination of the lower airways with upper airway organisms, particularly gram-negative bacilli.[8a]	Care should be taken to avoid nasal or oral pharyngeal tissue trauma and gagging during suctioning.
14. *Open-suction technique only:* On completion of upper airway suctioning, wrap the catheter around the dominant hand. Pull glove off inside out. Catheter remains in glove. Pull off other glove in same fashion, and discard. Turn off suction device.	Reduces transmission of microorganisms.	
15. Reposition patient.		
16. Wash hands.		

Procedure continues on the following page

Procedure for Endotracheal or Tracheostomy Tube Suctioning—*Continued*

Steps	Rationale	Special Considerations
17. Discard remaining normal saline solution and solution container. If basin is nondisposable, place in soiled utility room. Suction collection tubing and canisters may remain in use for multiple suctioning episodes. *(Level II: Theory based, no research data to support recommendations; recommendations from expert consensus group may exist.)*	Solutions and catheters that come in direct contact with the lower airways during suctioning must be sterile to decrease the risks for nosocomial pneumonia. Devices that are not in direct contact have not been shown to increase infection risk.[8a]	Check institutional standards for equipment removal.

Expected Outcomes

- Removal of secretions from the large airways
- Improved gas exchange
- Airway patency
- Amelioration of clinical signs or symptoms of need for suctioning (e.g., adventitious breath sounds, coughing, high airway pressures)
- Sample for laboratory analysis

Unexpected Outcomes

- Cardiac dysrhythmias (premature contractions, tachycardias, bradycardias, heart blocks, asystole)
- Hypoxemia
- Bronchospasm
- Excessive increases in arterial blood pressure or intracranial pressure
- Nosocomial infections
- Cardiopulmonary distress
- Decreased level of consciousness
- Airway obstruction

Patient Monitoring and Care

Steps	Rationale	Reportable Conditions
		These conditions should be reported if they persist despite nursing interventions.
1. Monitor patient's cardiopulmonary status before, during, and after the suctioning period. *(Level II: Theory based, no research data to support recommendations; recommendations from expert consensus group may exist.)*	Observes for signs and symptoms of complications.[1,7-9,13,15,19,20,23,28,30,32,34,35]	• Decreased arterial or mixed venous oxygen saturation • Cardiac dysrhythmias • Bronchospasm • Respiratory distress • Cyanosis • Increased blood pressure or intracranial pressure • Anxiety, agitation, or changes in mental status
2. Reassess patient for signs of suctioning effectiveness. *(Level II: Theory based, no research data to support recommendations; recommendations from expert consensus group may exist.)*		• Diminished breath sounds • Decreased oxygenation • Increased peak airway pressures • Coughing • Increased work of breathing

Documentation

Documentation should include the following:

- Patient and family education
- Presuctioning assessment, including clinical indication for suctioning
- Suctioning of endotracheal or tracheostomy tube
- Size of suction catheter
- Type of hyperoxygenation method used
- Number of passes of the suction catheter
- Volume, color, consistency, and odor of secretions obtained
- Any difficulties during catheter insertion or hyperoxygenation
- Tolerance of suctioning procedure, including development of any unexpected outcomes during or after the procedure
- Nursing interventions
- Postsuctioning assessment

References

1. AARC Clinical Practice Guideline. (1993). Endotracheal suctioning of mechanically ventilated adults and children with artificial airways. *Respir Care,* 38, 500-04.
2. Ackerman, M. (1993). The effect of saline lavage prior to suctioning. *Am J Crit Care,* 2, 326-30.
3. Ackerman, M., and Mick, D. (1998). Instillation of normal saline before suctioning in patients with pulmonary infections: A prospective randomized controlled trial. *Am J Crit Care,* 7, 261-6.
4. Anderson, K. (1989). Effects of manual bagging vs mechanical ventilatory sighing on oxygenation during the suctioning procedure. *Heart Lung,* 18, 301-2.
5. Blackwood, B. (1999). Normal saline instillation with endotracheal suctioning: *Primum non nocere* (first do no harm). *J Adv Nurs,* 29, 928-34.
6. Bostick, J., and Wendelgass, S. (1986). Normal saline instillation as part of the suctioning procedure: Effects on PaO_2 and amount of secretions. *Heart Lung,* 16, 532-7.
7. Brown, B., and Peeples, D. (1991). The effects of hyperventilation and lidocaine on intracranial pressure. *Heart Lung,* 21, 286.
8. Campbell, V. (1991). Effects of controlled hyperoxygenation and endotracheal suctioning on intracranial pressure in head-injured adults. *Appl Nurs Res,* 4, 138-40.
8a. Centers for Disease Control and Prevention. (2004). Guidelines for prevention of health-care-associated pneumonia, 2003: Recommendations of CDC and the Healthcare Infection Control Practices Advisory Committee. *MMWR,* 53, (No. RR-3), 1-35.
9. Chase, D., et al. (1989). Hemodynamic changes associated with endotracheal suctioning. *Heart Lung,* 18, 292-3.
10. Chulay, M. (1988). Arterial blood gas changes with a hyperinflation and hyperoxygenation suctioning intervention in critically ill patients. *Heart Lung,* 17, 654-61.
11. Chulay, M. (1994). Why do we keep putting saline down endotracheal tubes? It's time for a change in the way we suction! *Capsules Comments,* 2, 7-11.
12. Chulay, M., and Graeber, G. (1988). Efficacy of a hyperinflation and hyperoxygenation suctioning intervention. *Heart Lung,* 17, 15-22.
13. Clark, A., et al. (1990). Effects of endotracheal suctioning on mixed venous oxygen saturation and heart rate in critically ill adults. *Heart Lung,* 19, 552-7.
14. Czarnik, R., et al. (1991). Differential effects of continuous versus intermittent suction on tracheal tissue. *Heart Lung,* 20, 144-51.
15. Glass, C., et al. (1991). Nurse performance of hyperoxygenation. *Heart Lung,* 20, 299.
16. Glass, C., et al. (1993). Nurses' ability to achieve hyperinflation and hyperoxygenation with a manual resuscitation bag during endotracheal suctioning. *Heart Lung,* 22, 158-65.
17. Grap, M.J., et al. (1996). Endotracheal suctioning: Ventilator versus manual delivery of hyperoxygenation breaths. *Am J Crit Care,* 5, 192-7.
18. Hanley, M., Rudd, T., and Butler, J. (1978). What happens to intratracheal instillations? (Abstract). *Am Rev Respir Dis,* 177(Suppl), 124.
19. Henneman, E., Ellstrom, K., and St. John, R. (1999). Airway management. In: *AACN Protocols for Practice: Care of the Mechanically Ventilated Patient Series.* Aliso Viejo, CA: American Association of Critical-Care Nurses.
20. Hepburn, D., et al. (1990). Electrocardiographic changes associated with endotracheal suctioning (Abstract). *Circulation,* 82(Suppl 4), 210.
21. Hess, D., and Goff, G. (1987). The effects of two-hand versus one-hand ventilation on volumes delivered during bag-valve ventilation at various resistances and compliances. *Respir Care,* 32, 1025-8.
22. Kersten, L. (1989). *Comprehensive Respiratory Nursing: A Decision-Making Approach.* Philadelphia: W.B. Saunders.
23. Kinloch, D. (1999). Instillation of normal saline during endotracheal suctioning: Effects on mixed venous oxygen saturation. *Am J Crit Care,* 8, 231-42.
24. Kirimili, B., King, J., and Pfaeffle, H. (1970). Evaluation of tracheal bronchial suction techniques. *J Cardiovasc Surg,* 59, 340-4.
25. Kleiber, C., Krutzfield, N., and Rose, E. (1988). Acute histologic changes in the tracheobronchial tree associated with different suction catheter insertion techniques. *Heart Lung,* 17, 10-4.
26. Kubota, Y., et al. (1986). Is a straight catheter necessary for selective bronchial suctioning in the adult? *Crit Care Med,* 14, 755-6.
27. Kuzenski, B. (1978). Effect of negative pressure on tracheobronchial trauma. *Nurs Res,* 27, 260-3.
28. Lookinkind, S., and Appel, P.L. (1991). Hemodynamic and oxygen transport changes following endotracheal suctioning in trauma patients. *Nurs Res,* 40, 133-9.
29. Mancinelli-Van Atta, J., and Beck, S. (1991). Preventing hypoxemia and hemodynamic compromise related to endotracheal suctioning. *Am J Crit Care,* 1, 62-79.
30. McCauley, C., and Boller, L. (1986). Bradycardiac responses to endotracheal suctioning. *Crit Care Med,* 16, 1165-6.
31. Ogburn-Russell, L. (1987). The effect of continuous and intermittent suctioning on the tracheal mucosa of dogs. *Heart Lung,* 16, 297.
32. Preusser, B., et al. (1987). The effect of two methods of preoxygenation (manual versus ventilator) on mean arterial pressure, peak airway pressure and postsuctioning hypoxemia. *Heart Lung,* 16, 317-22.
33. Raymond, S. (1995). Normal saline instillation before suctioning: helpful or harmful? A review of the literature. *Am J Crit Care,* 4, 267-71.
34. Rudy, E., et al. (1986). The relationship between endotracheal suctioning and changes in intracranial pressure: a review of the literature. *Heart Lung,* 15, 488-93.

35. Rudy, E., et al. (1991). Endotracheal suctioning in adults with head injury. *Heart Lung,* 20, 667-74.
36. Rutula, W., Stiegel, M., and Sarubbi, F. (1984). A potential infection hazard associated with the use of disposable saline vials. *Infect Control,* 5, 170-2.
37. St. John, R.E. (1999). Airway management. *Crit Care Nurs,* 19, 79-83.
38. St. John, R.E. (1998). The pulmonary system. In: Alspach J, editor. *Core Curriculum for Critical Care Nursing.* 5th ed. Philadelphia: W.B. Saunders, 1-136.
39. Stone, K., et al. (1988). Effect of lung hyperinflation on cardiopulmonary hemodynamics and post suctioning hypoxemia. *Heart Lung,* 17, 309.
40. Walsh, J., et al. (1989). Unsuspected hemodynamic alterations during endotracheal suctioning. *Chest,* 95, 162-5.

Additional Readings

Akgul, S., and Akyolcu, N. (2002). Effects of normal saline on endotracheal suctioning. *J Clin Nurs,* 11, 826-30.
Birdsall, C. (1986). How do you use a closed suction adapter? *Am J Nurs,* 86, 1222-3.
Gunderson, L., Stone, K., and Hamlin, R. (1991). Endotracheal suctioning-induced heart rate alterations. *Nurs Res,* 40, 139-43.
Kerr, M., et al. (1999). Effect of endotracheal suctioning on cerebral oxygenation in traumatic brain-injured patients. *Crit Care Med,* 27, 2776-81.
Labarca, J., et al. (1999). A multistate outbreak of *Ralstonia pickettii* colonization associated with an intrinsically contaminated respiratory care solution. *Clin Infect Dis,* 29, 1281-6.
Paul-Allen, J., and Ostrow, C. (2000). Survey of nursing practices with closed-system suctioning. *Am J Crit Care,* 9, 9-19.
Redick, E. (1993). Closed-system, in-line endotracheal suctioning. *Crit Care Nurse,* 13, 47-51.
Schwenker, D., Ferrin, M., and Gift, A. (1998). A survey of endotracheal suctioning with instillation of normal saline. *Am J Crit Care,* 7, 255-60.
Stone, K.S., Bell, S.D., and Preusser, B.A. (1991). The effect of repeated endotracheal suctioning on arterial blood pressure. *Appl Nurs Res,* 4, 152-8.

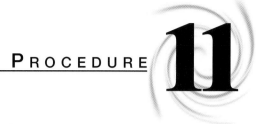

PROCEDURE 11

Tracheal Tube Cuff Care

PURPOSE: The tracheal tube cuff helps stabilize the tracheal tube and maintain an adequate airway seal so that air moves through the tube into the lungs. The cuff also may decrease the risk of aspiration of large food particles, but it does not protect against aspiration of liquid.

Kirsten N. Skillings
Bonnie L. Curtis

PREREQUISITE NURSING KNOWLEDGE

- The tracheal tube cuff is an inflatable "balloon" that surrounds the shaft of the tracheal tube near its distal end. When inflated, the cuff presses against the tracheal wall to prevent air leakage and pressure loss from the lungs.
- Appropriate cuff care helps prevent major pulmonary aspirations, prepares for tracheal extubation, decreases the risk of inadvertent extubation, provides a patent airway for ventilation and removal of secretions, and decreases the risk of iatrogenic infections.
- Although a variety of cuffs exists, the most desirable cuff provides a maximal airway seal with minimal tracheal wall pressure. The most widely used cuff is the high-volume, low-pressure cuff (Fig. 11-1). This cuff has a relatively large inflation volume requiring lower filling pressure to obtain a seal (less than 25 mm Hg or 34 cm H_2O).
- High-volume, low-pressure cuffs allow a large surface area to come into contact with the tracheal wall, distributing the pressure over a much greater area. The older cuff design (low volume, high pressure) may require 40 mm Hg (54.4 cm H_2O) to obtain an effective seal and is undesirable.
- The amount of pressure and volume necessary to obtain a seal and prevent mucosal damage depends on tube size and design, cuff configuration, mode of ventilation, and the patient's arterial blood pressure.
- A variety of devices are available to measure cuff pressures, including bedside sphygmomanometers, special aneroid cuff manometers, and electronic cuff pressure devices. Ideally the cuff pressures should be between 20 and 25 mm Hg, while still meeting the goals of cuff use. Tracheal capillary perfusion pressure is 25 to 35 mm Hg for normotensive patients. Lower cuff pressures are associated with less mucosal damage, but also are associated with silent aspiration, which has been shown to be more prevalent at cuff pressures less than 20 mm Hg.[3,4,6]
- Two techniques, minimal leak technique (MLT) and minimal occlusion volume (MOV), are employed to inflate and monitor air in the cuff.
  - ❖ MLT involves air inflation of the tube cuff until any leak stops, then a small amount of air is removed slowly until a small leak is heard on inspiration.[3-6]
  - ❖ MOV consists of injecting air into the cuff until no leak is heard, then withdrawing the air until a small leak is heard on inspiration, then adding more air until no leak is heard on inspiration.[3-6]
- Each technique has distinct advantages. MLT decreases mucosal injury and assists in mobilizing secretions forward into the pharynx. MOV decreases the incidence of aspiration and is most effective for patients who are changing position frequently and are at increased risk for tube movement.[4]
- Although rare since the use of high-volume, low-pressure devices became common, the adverse effects of tracheal tube cuff inflation include tracheal stenosis, necrosis, tracheoesophageal fistulas, and tracheomalacia. These complications may be more likely to occur in conditions that adversely affect tissue response to mucosal injury, such as hypotension. Two major mechanisms are mainly responsible for airway damage: tube movement and pressure. Duration of intubation also plays a significant role.[4]

SOFT CUFF
■ High volume
■ Exerts low and equal lateral tracheal wall pressure (TWP) *(arrows)*
■ Minimizes tracheal injury

HARD CUFF
■ Low volume
■ Exerts high and unequal lateral TWP *(arrows)*
■ Causes tracheal injury

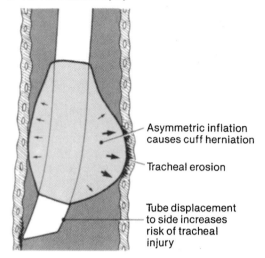

Cuff conforms to trachea

Centrally positioned tube

Asymmetric inflation causes cuff herniation

Tracheal erosion

Tube displacement to side increases risk of tracheal injury

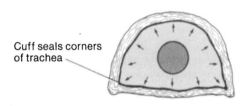

Cuff seals corners of trachea

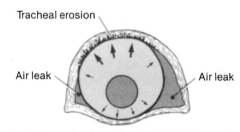

Tracheal erosion

Air leak   Air leak

FIGURE 11-1 Cross-sectional view in D-shaped trachea. Effects of soft and hard cuff inflation on the tracheal wall. *(From Kersten, L.D. [1989].* Comprehensive Respiratory Nursing. *Philadelphia: W.B. Saunders, 648.)*

- Routine cuff deflation is unnecessary but may be indicated to evaluate cuff leak, to clear upper airway secretions, after cardiopulmonary resuscitation, and after surgery to reevaluate the number of milliliters of air in the cuff.[1,4]
- Unintentional extubation and tube manipulation can occur with ineffective patient restraint, inadequate securing of the tube, inadequate sedation, incorrect tube size and length, improper support or respiratory underinflation of endotracheal cuff, and prolonged intubation.[4]

EQUIPMENT

- 10-ml syringe
- Pressure manometer with extension line
- Three-way stopcock
- Stethoscope
- Manual resuscitation bag connected to oxygen
  Additional equipment (for cuff inflation with faulty inflating device) includes the following:
- Scissors
- Padded hemostats
- Short, 18-gauge or 23-gauge blunt needle
- Tongue depressor
- Tape (1 inch wide)
- Reintubation equipment, in case of accidental extubation
- Suction supplies (see Procedure 10)

PATIENT AND FAMILY EDUCATION

- Explain the procedure (if patient condition and time allow) and the reason for tracheal tube cuff care. ➤*Rationale:* This communication identifies patient and family knowledge deficits concerning the patient's condition, procedure, expected benefits, and potential risks and allows time for questions to clarify information and voice concerns. Explanations decrease patient anxiety and enhance cooperation.
- Explain the patient's role in assisting with cuff care. ➤*Rationale:* This elicits patient cooperation.
- Explain that the procedure can be uncomfortable and cause the patient to cough. ➤*Rationale:* This explanation elicits patient cooperation.

PATIENT ASSESSMENT AND PREPARATION

Patient Assessment

- Assess presence of bilateral breath sounds. ➤*Rationale:* This assessment assists in verifying tube placement.
- Assess signs and symptoms of cuff leakage, as follows.
  ❖ Audible or auscultated inspiratory leak over larynx
  ❖ Patient able to vocalize audibly

❖ Pilot balloon deflation
❖ Loss of inspiratory and expiratory volume on mechanically ventilated patient

➤➤*Rationale:* An adequate seal of cuff to tracheal wall does not permit air to flow past the cuff.

- Assess signs and symptoms of inadequate ventilation, as follows.
  ❖ Rising arterial carbon dioxide tension
  ❖ Chest-abdominal dyssynchrony
  ❖ Patient-ventilator dyssynchrony
  ❖ Dyspnea
  ❖ Headache
  ❖ Restlessness
  ❖ Confusion
  ❖ Lethargy
  ❖ Increasing (early sign) or decreasing (late sign) arterial blood pressure
  ❖ Activation of expiratory or inspiratory volume alarms on mechanical ventilator

  ➤➤*Rationale:* Inadequate ventilation results when cuff seal is improper or cuff leak is extensive.

- Assess amount of air or pressure previously used to inflate the cuff. ➤➤*Rationale:* The amount of air previously used to inflate the cuff can be used as a guideline to determine changes in volume or pressure or both.
- Assess size of tracheal tube and size of patient. ➤➤*Rationale:* Volume and pressure of air needed to seal the airway depend on the relationship of tube and trachea diameters.

Patient Preparation

- Ensure that the patient understands preprocedural teaching. Answer questions as they arise, and reinforce information as needed. ➤➤*Rationale:* This communication evaluates and reinforces understanding of previously taught information.
- Place patient in semi-Fowler position. ➤➤*Rationale:* This positioning promotes general relaxation, oxygenation, and ventilation. It also reduces stimulation of the gag reflex and risk of aspiration.

Procedure | **for Tracheal Tube Cuff Care**

Steps	Rationale	Special Considerations
Deflation and Inflation		
1. Wash hands, and don personal protective equipment.	Reduces transmission of microorganisms and body secretions; standard precautions.	
2. Remove oxygen tubing attached to the endotracheal or tracheostomy tube.	Accesses tube opening.	
3. Hyperoxygenate and suction tracheobronchial tree (see Procedure 10) and pharynx before cuff deflation.	Clears secretions in the lower airway and decreases incidence of aspiration.	A fresh sterile catheter is necessary.
MOV Technique		
4. Deflate cuff while applying positive pressure.	Prepares for measurement of cuff pressure and prevents aspiration of pharyngeal secretions.	Instruct the alert, cooperative patient to cough.
5. Insert air-filled, 10-ml syringe tip into inflating tube valve.	Provides a pathway between air source and cuff.	Most cuffs are sufficiently inflated with less than 10 ml of air.
6. Slowly inject air on inhalation until sounds cease over larynx.	The trachea dilates during inhalation. The cuff needs to seal the airway during inhalation so that air is directed toward the lung. Cessation of air movement on auscultation indicates that the cuff is sealed against the tracheal mucosal wall.	Hazards of cuff inflation include cuff overinflation, distention, and rupture.

Procedure continues on the following page

Procedure for Tracheal Tube Cuff Care—*Continued*

Steps	Rationale	Special Considerations
7. Apply positive pressure with manual resuscitation bag.	The cuff is inflated when an audible leak is not heard.	The alert, cooperative patient may be asked to speak. If the trachea is sealed, vocalization is not possible.
8. **Proceed to Step 11**.		
MLT Technique		
9. Place a stethoscope over larynx.	Indirectly assesses inflation of cuff.	
10. Slowly withdraw air (in 0.1-ml increments) from the cuff until a small leak is heard by auscultation on inspiration.	Auscultation of air movement indicates air escaping through the larynx.	Intracuff pressure measurement provides an approximation of cuff-to-tracheal wall pressure.[4]
11. Remove syringe tip.	Keeping a syringe on the inflation valve can cause it to become stuck in the open position allowing air to escape.[4]	
12. Replace any oxygen or humidity tubing. Check and secure ventilator connections, as needed.	Allows for oxygen flow and prevents oxygen desaturation.	
13. Reassess patient's airway and respiratory status.	Identifies effects of tracheal cuff care.	
Cuff Pressure Measurement		
14. Wash hands, and don personal protective equipment.	Reduces transmission of microorganisms; standard precautions.	
15. Connect the manometer line to the patient inflation system with a three-way stopcock (turned "off" to the patient) (Fig. 11-2).	Develops an intracuff pressure-monitoring device.	This device is made easily using parts of a blood pressure cuff (e.g., aneroid manometer device).

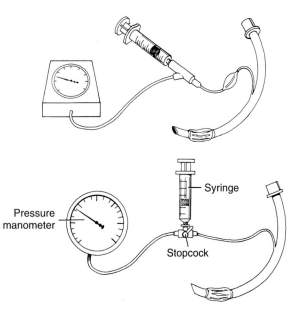

FIGURE 11-2 Measuring cuff pressure by way of a homemade pressure monitor. (*From Eubanks, D.H., and Bone, R.C. [1990]. Comprehensive Respiratory Care. 2nd ed. St. Louis: C.V. Mosby.*)

Procedure for Tracheal Tube Cuff Care—*Continued*

Steps	Rationale	Special Considerations
16. With the thumb, occlude the open port, and with an air-filled syringe, inject air into the tubing leading to the manometer until the needle of the manometer reads between 20 and 25 mm Hg.	Measures the pressure of the air applied from the system.	Pressure should be kept at a level to maintain a seal between cuff and tracheal wall. The volume necessary to create the seal depends on tube size and cuff configuration. Contributing factors to airway damage are excessive head movement, tube size, duration of intubation, and cuff pressure.[4]
17. Turn the stopcock off to the open port (syringe). Read the cuff pressure now shown on the aneroid face.	The connecting channel is now between the manometer and the patient's inflation line, allowing evaluation of pressure in the patient's cuff.	
18. Turn the stopcock off to the inflating tube, and disconnect the manometer line from the patient's inflation line.	The connecting channel to the inflating tube is now closed, maintaining air in the cuff.	
19. Detach the manometer line with three-way stopcock from the patient's inflation system.	Removes apparatus to monitor cuff pressure.	
Troubleshooting Tracheal Cuff Problems *Faulty Inflating Valve*		
20. Identify faulty inflating valve.	Determines need for repair.	When inflating line becomes faulty and reintubation is undesirable, consider instituting an emergency cuff-inflation technique (Fig. 11-3).
Cuff Pressure Measurement		
21. Insert three-way stopcock into the distal opening of the inflating balloon.	Provides access to cuff.	
22. Inflate the cuff using MOV **(Steps 6-8, 11)** or MLT **(Steps 9-11)** technique.	Allows for cuff inflation; restores tracheal wall and cuff seal.	
23. Clamp the inflating tube by applying a padded hemostat distal to the pilot balloon.	Maintains air in cuff; provides a quick occlusion of the inflating tube.	

Procedure continues on the following page

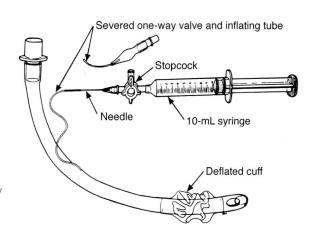

FIGURE 11-3 Attachments for emergency cuff inflation for faulty inflating line. *(From Sills, J. [1986]. An emergency cuff inflation technique.* Respir Care, *31, 200.)*

Procedure for **Tracheal Tube Cuff Care**—*Continued*

Steps	Rationale	Special Considerations
24. Turn the stopcock off to the inflating tube; remove clamp.	Provides for temporary use of the tracheal tube, while maintaining cuff pressure.	
Faulty Inflating Line		
25. Identify malfunctioning of inflating line.	Determines need for and method of repair.	
26. Cut off faulty end of inflation line with scissors (see Fig. 11-3).	Prepares inflation line for repair.	
27. Insert short 18-gauge to 23-gauge blunt needle into inflation line.	Provides inflation access.	Maintain care to avoid puncture or severing of inflation line or skin.
28. Attach three-way stopcock to a blunt needle.	Provides control of airflow in and out of inflating line.	
29. Using a 10-ml syringe, inflate the cuff with air using MOV (**Steps 6-8, 11**) or MLT (**Steps 9-11**) technique.	Allows cuff inflation; restores tracheal wall and cuff seal.	
30. Turn stopcock off to the inflating tube.	Provides for temporary use of the tracheal tube, while maintaining cuff pressure.	
31. Secure assembled device with tape to a tongue depressor.	Provides for stabilization and protection.	
32. Assemble equipment for trach replacement.		

Expected Outcomes

- Tracheal tube remains in correct position
- Cuff pressure is kept at a level to maintain a seal between cuff and tracheal wall (usually between 20 and 25 mm Hg)
- Cuff remains intact

Unexpected Outcomes

- Extubation or tube dislodgment
- Mucosal ischemia
- Faulty cuff and inflating line
- Cuff overinflation and distention over the end of the tube
- Cuff rupture

Patient Monitoring and Care

Steps	Rationale	Reportable Conditions
1. Assess respiratory status for optimal ventilation.	Inadequate interface between tracheal cuff and tracheobronchial mucosa decreases inspiratory flow.	*These conditions should be reported if they persist despite nursing interventions.* • Rising arterial carbon dioxide tension • Chest-abdominal dyssynchrony • Patient-ventilator dyssynchrony • Dyspnea • Headache • Restlessness • Confusion • Lethargy • Increasing (early sign) or decreasing (late sign) arterial blood pressure • Activation of expiratory or inspiratory volume alarms on the mechanical ventilator

Patient Monitoring and Care—*Continued*

Steps	Rationale	Reportable Conditions
2. Measure cuff pressure every 8 hours, maintaining cuff pressure between 20 and 25 mm Hg.[1,5] *(Level II: Theory based, no research data to support recommendations: recommendations from expert consensus group may exist.)*	Prevents tracheal injury and aspiration. Excessive cuff pressure is cited as the most frequent problem of tracheal intubation and the best predictor of tracheolaryngeal injury.[3,4]	• Cuff pressure less than 20 mm Hg or greater than 25 mm Hg.
3. Maintain tracheal tube cuff integrity.	Manipulation of the tracheal tube increases the likelihood of cuff disruption. Cuff leak or rupture is evident when the pressure on the manometer continues to decrease.	• Inability to maintain cuff inflation • Audible air through the patient's nose or mouth • Low-pressure or low-volume alarm sounds on the mechanical ventilator • Audible or auscultated inspiratory leak over larynx • Patient able to vocalize audibly • Pilot balloon deflation • Loss of inspiratory and expiratory volume on mechanically ventilated patients
4. Hyperoxygenate and suction patient based on assessment (see Procedure 10).	Removal of secretions reduces chance for partial or complete airway obstruction.	
5. Reinflate cuff using MOV or MLT whenever deflation is necessary. *(Level II: Theory based, no research data to support recommendations: recommendations from expert consensus group may exist.)*	Cuff should be deflated only when problems arise[1] or every 48 to 72 hours.[2] If the number of milliliters needed to seal the airway increases, evaluate patient for tracheal dilation using chest radiography of cuff diameter-to-tracheal diameter ratio. Increasing number of milliliters also may indicate leak in cuff or pilot balloon valve. Hypoxemia, overinflation of the cuff on reinflation, and pulmonary aspiration occur with periodic cuff deflation.[4]	
6. Compare patient's cardiopulmonary status before and after tracheal tube cuff care.	Identifies the effects of tracheal tube cuff care on the cardiovascular system.	• Decreased arterial oxygen saturation • Cardiac dysrhythmias • Bronchospasm • Respiratory distress • Cyanosis • Increased blood pressure or intracranial pressure • Anxiety, agitation, or changes in level of consciousness
7. Reassess cuff pressure and volume when transporting patient from one altitude to another (i.e., air transport) or during hyperbaric therapy without environmental pressurization.	Changes in altitude change the volume of gas in the cuff; volume and pressure need to be reevaluated during and after transport.	

Documentation

Documentation should include the following:

- Patient and family education
- Cardiopulmonary and vital sign assessment before and after procedure
- Method of cuff inflation
- Cuff inflation volume and cuff pressure
- Patient's tolerance

- Appearance and characteristics of tracheal secretions, if present
- Unexpected outcomes
- Use of medications
- Use of restraints
- Date, time, and frequency with which procedure is performed
- Nursing interventions

References

1. Guyton, D., Banner, M.J., and Kirgby, R.R. (1991). High-volume, low-pressure cuffs: are they always low pressure? *Chest,* 100, 1076-81.
2. Henneman, E., Ellstrom, K., and St. John, R. (1999). Airway management. In: *AACN Protocols for Practice: Care of the Mechanically Ventilated Patient Series.* Aliso Viejo, CA: American Association of Critical Care Nurses.
3. MacIntyre, N., and Branson, R. (2001). The patient-ventilation interface: Ventilator circuits airway care and suctioning. In: *Mechanical Ventilation.* Philadelphia: W.B. Saunders, 92-4.
4. Pierce, L. (1995). Airway maintenance. In: *Guide to Mechanical Ventilation and Intensive Respiratory Care.* Philadelphia: W.B. Saunders, 81-91.
5. Plambeck, A. (2004). *Adult Ventilation Management.* Corexcel, Inc. Available at: http://www.corexcel.com/courses/vent.htm. Accessed April 22, 2004.
6. St. John, R. (1999). Protocols for practice: Applying research at the bedside; airway management. *Crit Care Nurse,* 19, 79-83.

Additional Reading

Swartz, C. (2001). Nursing protocol: Artificial airway management. *Int J Trauma Nurs,* 7, 101-3.

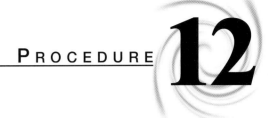

PROCEDURE **12**

Tracheostomy Tube Care

PURPOSE: Tracheostomy tube care is performed to maintain airway patency and to decrease infection risk by removing secretions accumulating within the inner cannula.

Kirsten N. Skillings
Bonnie L. Curtis

PREREQUISITE NURSING KNOWLEDGE

- *Tracheotomy* refers to the surgical procedure in which an incision is made below the cricoid cartilage through the second to fourth tracheal rings (Fig. 12-1). *Tracheostomy* refers to the opening, or stoma, made by the incision. The tracheostomy tube is the artificial airway inserted into the trachea during tracheotomy (Fig. 12-2).
- Tracheostomy tubes have a variety of parts (Fig. 12-3) and are available in various types. A tracheostomy tube is shorter than but similar in diameter to an endotracheal tube and has a squared-off distal tip for maximizing airflow. The outer cannula forms the body of a tracheostomy tube with a cuff. The neck flange, attached to the outer cannula, assists in stabilizing the tube in the trachea and provides the small holes necessary for proper securing of the tube. Some tracheostomy setups have an inner cannula inserted into the outer cannula. The inner cannula is removable for easy cleaning without compromising the airway. The cuff is a balloon inflated with air to maintain a seal around the tube. As the air flows through the one-way inflation valve, the pilot balloon inflates, indicating the volume of air present in the cuff.
- A cuffed tube is appropriate for use in patients who require mechanical ventilation or when aspiration is a problem. The cuff limits aspiration of oral and gastric secretions. Uncuffed tubes are commonly used in children, in adults with laryngectomies, and during decannulization of the tracheostomy.
- A tracheostomy is performed as either an elective procedure or an emergency procedure for a variety of reasons

(Table 12-1). Most often, the procedure is elective and performed in the operating room under sterile conditions. An emergency tracheotomy is performed at the bedside under aseptic technique or before arrival in the critical care unit when swelling, injury, or other upper airway obstruction prevents intubation with an endotracheal tube. Percutaneous tracheostomies also are performed at the bedside. This procedure consists of passing a needle into the trachea, placing a J-tipped guidewire, progressively

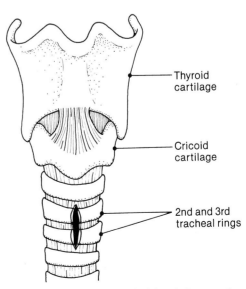

FIGURE 12-1 Vertical tracheal incision during a tracheotomy procedure. *(From Kersten, L.D. [1989].* Comprehensive Respiratory Nursing. *Philadelphia: W.B. Saunders, 654.)*

79

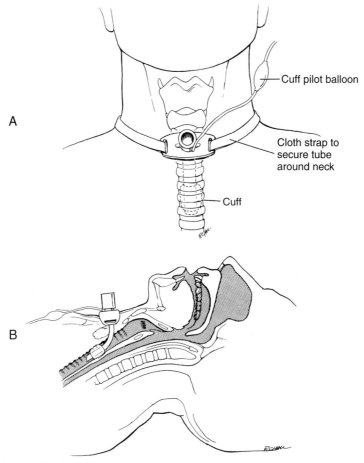

FIGURE 12-2 **A,** Anterior view of tracheostomy tube after insertion. **B,** Lateral view of tracheostomy tube after insertion. *(From Eubanks, D.H., and Bone, R.C. [1990]. Comprehensive Respiratory Care. 2nd ed. St. Louis: C.V. Mosby, 554.)*

dilating the trachea, and placing the tracheostomy tube. The percutaneous procedure has achieved outcomes comparable to outcomes with the surgical technique.[4]

- Protocols for emergency tracheotomy vary among institutions. Often, nurses at the bedside take an active role in assisting with tracheotomy and insertion of a tracheostomy tube; however, some institutions have surgical personnel at the bedside to assist with the procedure.

- During insertion, the obturator replaces the inner cannula. Its smooth surface protrudes from the outer cannula, minimizing tracheal trauma. When the tracheostomy tube is inserted, the obturator is removed and replaced with the inner cannula, which locks in place. The obturator should be placed in a plastic bag and kept at the bedside in case the tube must be reinserted emergently.

- The decision for a tracheostomy in long-term mechanically ventilated patients is made on the basis of the team's projection regarding length of time that mechanical ventilation or an artificial airway will be required. A tracheostomy tube is the preferred method of airway maintenance in a patient requiring intubation for more than 14 to 21 days. Each case must be reviewed individually.[1,4]

- When compared with an endotracheal tube, tracheostomy tubes provide added benefits to patients, including the following:
  - ❖ Prevention of further laryngeal injury from the translaryngeal tube
  - ❖ Improved patient comfort, acceptance, and toleration
  - ❖ Decreased work of breathing owing to less airflow resistance
  - ❖ Provision of a speech mechanism
  - ❖ Increased patient mobility
  - ❖ Easier secretion removal
  - ❖ Reduced risk of unintentional decannulation

- A fenestrated tracheostomy tube has an opening in the curvature of the posterior wall of the outer cannula. Fenestration allows for speech with cuff deflation, removal of inner cannula, and occlusion of outer cannula because air is permitted to flow through the upper airway and tracheostomy opening.

- A tracheostomy is viewed by the body as foreign material. The body responds by increasing mucus production. Also, ciliary movement is impaired, limiting the forward movement of the mucociliary escalator. Because the

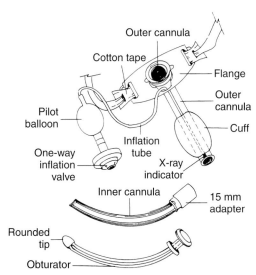

FIGURE 12-3 Parts of a tracheostomy tube. *(From Eubanks, D.H., and Bone, R.C. [1990]. Comprehensive Respiratory Care. 2nd ed. St. Louis: C.V. Mosby, 570.)*

TABLE 12-1	Indications for Tracheostomy

Bypass acute upper airway obstruction
Prolonged need for artificial airway
Prophylaxis for anticipated airway problems
Reduction of anatomic dead space
Prevention of pulmonary aspiration
Retained tracheobronchial secretions
Chronic upper airway obstruction

tracheostomy bypasses the upper airway and its protective and hydrating mechanisms, patients are at increased risk of infection. Lack of hydration by the upper airway can lead to thick mucus, increasing the risk of airway obstruction.[5,6]
- The tracheostomy creates a more stable airway, making it feasible for the patient to transfer out of the critical care unit when his or her overall condition warrants. Also, care of the patient, such as suctioning, mouth care, and ability to meet nutritional needs, is simplified.
- A stoma less than 48 hours old has not fully formed a tracheostomy tract. If the tracheostomy tube is accidentally dislodged, the tracheostomy may close, compromising the patient's airway.
- A small amount of bleeding is expected for the first few days after a tracheotomy. Bright, frank bleeding or constant oozing is not expected and should be brought to the attention of the physician or advanced practice nurse
- Consideration should be given to obtaining assistance with tracheostomy care, especially when changing tracheal ties or with an agitated patient. An extra pair of hands can minimize the risk for accidental dislodgment.

EQUIPMENT

Some institutions may use tracheostomy care kits, which include some or all of the following items:
- Personal protective equipment
- Hydrogen peroxide (H_2O_2)
- Sterile normal saline (NS) or water
- Twill tape or tracheal ties
- Sterile cotton swabs
- Sterile basin

- Sterile 4 × 4 gauze pad (three)
- Sterile precut tracheostomy dressing
- Small, sterile brush
- Scissors
- Sterile, disposable inner cannula (if disposable setup is used)
- Suction supplies
- Two sterile gloves
- Self-inflating manual resuscitation bag and mask
  Additional equipment (to have available based on patient need) includes the following:
- Second practitioner (if changing tracheal ties)
- Extra obturator at bedside

PATIENT AND FAMILY EDUCATION

- Explain the purpose and the necessity of tracheotomy or tracheostomy care. ➟*Rationale:* Communication and explanation regarding therapy encourage cooperation, minimize anxiety, and are a continual patient and family need.

PATIENT ASSESSMENT AND PREPARATION

Patient Assessment
- Assess increased production of secretions. ➟*Rationale:* Tube irritation to mucosa results in increased production of secretions.
- Assess cardiopulmonary status.
  - ❖ Decreased arterial oxygen saturation
  - ❖ Cardiac dysrhythmias
  - ❖ Bronchospasm
  - ❖ Respiratory distress
  - ❖ Cyanosis
  - ❖ Increased blood pressure or intracranial pressure
  - ❖ Anxiety, agitation, or changes in level of consciousness
  ➟*Rationale:* Evaluation of the patient's cardiopulmonary status provides valuable information about need for and tolerance of tracheostomy tube care.

Patient Preparation
- Ensure that the patient understands preprocedural teaching. Answer questions as they arise, and reinforce information as needed. ➟*Rationale:* This communication evaluates and reinforces understanding of previously taught information.

Procedure for Tracheostomy Tube Care

Steps	Rationale	Special Considerations
1. Wash hands, and don personal protective equipment.	Reduces the transmission of microorganisms and body secretions; standard precautions.	Protective eyewear or facemask should be worn when secretions are copious.
2. To make new ties, cut twill tape at a length that wraps around the patient's neck two times.	Provides length for circumferential wrapping around the patient's neck.	Premade Velcro tracheal ties also may be used. The tracheostomy tube may be sutured in place and no ties used (e.g., for patients with new laryngectomy and flap).
3. Hyperoxygenate and suction trachea and pharynx as needed (see Procedure 10).	Reduces risk of hypoxemia; removes secretions and diminishes patient's need to cough during the procedure.	
4. Remove soiled dressing.		
5. Remove soiled gloves, and set up sterile saline solution container on sterile field. Be careful not to touch the inside of the container. Fill with equal parts sterile NS or water and H_2O_2, totaling approximately 100 ml.		
6. Don sterile gloves.	Reduces transmission of microorganisms; standard precautions.	
7. Remove oxygen source and inner cannula, placing it in the 1:1 solution of H_2O_2 and NS or water.	Removes inner cannula for cleaning. Hydrogen peroxide loosens debris from inner cannula.	This is not required when patient has a disposable inner cannula. Cleaning a disposable inner cannula with H_2O_2 disrupts the integrity of the structural material, causing pitting of a metal inner cannula. Only sterile NS should be used for cleaning a metal tracheostomy tube. Reusable inner cannulas made of plastic may be cleaned with H_2O_2 followed by NS.
8. Apply tracheostomy collar oxygen source over outer cannula, or, if ventilator assistance is needed, attach outer cannula to connector on ventilator.	Maintains oxygen supply. Maintains mechanical ventilation, as appropriate.	
9. Clean inner cannula with a small brush.	Assists in the removal of debris and thick secretions.	There is not agreement in the literature as to the frequency of tracheostomy care.[2]
10. Rinse inner cannula by pouring NS over the cannula.	Removes hydrogen peroxide and debris.	
11. Remove oxygen source from over outer cannula.	Allow access to opening of outer cannula.	
12. Insert inner cannula and lock into place.	Secures inner cannula.	
13. Reapply oxygen or ventilator oxygen source.	Reestablishes oxygen supply.	

Procedure for Tracheostomy Tube Care—*Continued*

Steps	Rationale	Special Considerations
14. Moisten swabs and 4 × 4 gauze pads with H_2O_2. Clean stoma site and outer cannula surface by wiping with cotton-tipped swabs and 4 × 4 gauze pads.	Removes debris and secretions from the stoma area.	Some institutions may use only NS for cleaning. While there have not been studies done that demonstrate that H_2O_2 is superior to NS, cleaning often appears to be easier if H_2O_2 is used.
15. Rinse stoma site and outer cannula with NS-soaked, cotton-tipped swabs and 4 × 4 gauze pads.	Rinses H_2O_2 and removes additional debris. Hydrogen peroxide can be irritating to the skin and must be rinsed thoroughly from the skin.	
16. Pat dry the skin area surrounding the stoma site.	Dry surface decreases likelihood of microorganism growth and skin breakdown.	
17. Have assistant hold neckplate securely.	Decreases the incidence of tracheal tube decannulation.	
18. Cut and remove current twill tape.	Prepares for new twill tape.	Assistant must maintain hold while ties are not secure.
19. Insert one new tie end through the faceplate and pull until one half of the tape is through the eyelet. (Tape will not be "doubled.") Slide the doubled tie around the back of neck, insert through the second eyelet, bring one tie around neck, pull snug, and tie in double square knot on the side of the neck (Fig. 12-4).	Reestablishes secure tracheal faceplate. Knot should be visible on side of neck to be able to observe that it remains tied.	Allow one finger space between twill tape and neck to allow for venous outflow.
20. Apply clean, precut tracheostomy dressing under faceplate.	Promotes drainage absorption.	Never cut a 4 × 4 gauze pad because cut edges fray and provide a potential source for infection.
21. Provide appropriate oral care (see Procedure 4).		
22. Document in patient record.		

Expected Outcomes

- Airway patency
- Infection prevention
- Healing promotion

Unexpected Outcomes

- Prolonged apnea, increasing hypoxemia, or cardiopulmonary arrest
- Hemorrhage
- Interstitial air: subcutaneous emphysema, pneumothorax, pneumopericardium, and pneumoperitoneum
- Thyroid gland injury
- Cardiac dysrhythmias
- Tube-tip erosion into the tracheal innominate artery
- Stoma infection
- Bronchopulmonary infection
- Displacement or dislodgment out of trachea
- Excessive cuff pressure
- Leaking airway cuff
- Airway obstruction from misalignment, cuff overinflation, and dried or excessive secretions
- Agitation
- Tracheal stenosis, malacia, or tracheoesophageal fistula
- Tracheal ischemia, necrosis, or dilation
- Laryngeal disorders
- Dysphasia

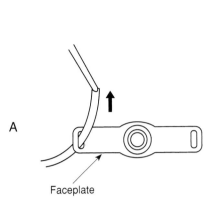

A

Faceplate

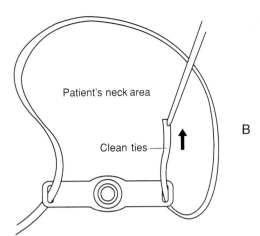

Patient's neck area

Clean ties

B

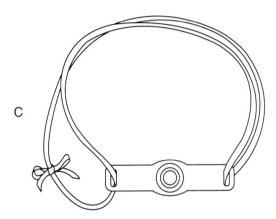

C

FIGURE 12-4 Placement of tracheostomy twill tape.
A, Faceplate with threading of twill tape (to prevent decannulation, an additional person needs to stabilize faceplate). **B,** Advancing of the twill tape around the back of the neck and looping through the other side if faceplate. **C,** Doubling of the twill tape and securing in a knot.

Patient Monitoring and Care

Steps	Rationale	Reportable Conditions
		These conditions should be reported if they persist despite nursing interventions.
1. Provide continuous humidified air or oxygen. Warm or cool delivered gas as appropriate. *(Level III: Laboratory data, no clinical data to support recommendations.)*	Artificial airways bypass the nose and mouth, preventing normal warming, humidification, and filtering.[3,5,6]	
2. Check proper placement by auscultation every shift. *(Level II: Theory based, no research data to support recommendations: recommendations from expert consensus group may exist.)*	Displacement into the bronchus or at the carina is rare with tracheostomy tube because of the short length. Because of the variety of tracheal tube lengths and patient sizes, however, the potential for displacement exists. Improper placement may lead to inadequate ventilation and complications.	• Decreased or delayed chest motion • Unilateral breath sounds • Excessive coughing • Localized expiratory wheeze • Bilateral decreased breath sounds
3. Inspect and palpate for air under skin every shift.	Air may escape into the incision, causing subcutaneous emphysema. *Special Note: Subcutaneous emphysema usually does not harm patients*	• Subcutaneous emphysema

Patient Monitoring and Care—*Continued*

Steps	Rationale	Reportable Conditions
	with an airway already in place. Puffiness of the soft tissue may result, however, and, if significant, can change the patient's appearance, alarming the patient and the family.	
4. Assess for frank bleeding or constant oozing of blood every shift.	Surgical procedures increase the risk of potential injury to adjacent tissues and structures. Stoma placement below the second and third cartilaginous rings incidence results in an increased of innominate artery erosion.	• Frank bleeding or constant oozing of blood
5. Palpate the tube for pulsation every shift.	If pulsations are felt in the tracheal tube, it is suggestive of impending erosion of major blood vessels.	• Pulsation of the tracheal tube
6. Assess for presence of pain every shift.	Pain and discomfort increase the incidence of anxiety and disorientation.	• Uncontrolled pain
7. Maintain mucosal tissue integrity using appropriate cuff care procedures (see Procedure 11).	Constant pressure and irritation of the mucosal tissue can result in blood vessel and cellular damage.	• Need for increasing pressure or volume to maintain tracheal cuff seal
8. Tracheostomy care should be performed at least every shift. *(Level II: Theory based, no research data to support recommendations: recommendations from expert consensus group may exist.)*	Keeps tube free of mucus or encrustations that may impede airway patency; decreases risk of infection. There is not agreement in the literature as to the frequency of tracheostomy care.[2,3]	
9. Assess skin for signs of infection or inflammation.	Moisture promotes maceration and skin breakdown at stomal opening.	• Redness • Swelling • Purulent drainage
10. Maintain dry, clean dressing.	Decreases risk of skin breakdown. Moisture promotes maceration of the tracheal opening.	• Copious drainage • Change in characteristics of drainage
11. Monitor secretions (color, amount, and consistency). Hyperoxygenate and suction (see Procedure 10) based on assessment.	Suctioning should be based on patient need rather than on a standard frequency. Change in secretion characteristics may indicate infection or inadequate hydration.	• Excessively thick secretions • Copious or purulent secretions
12. Maintain head of bed at 30 degrees for approximately 24 hours and during enteral feedings.	An elevated head of bed promotes oropharyngeal and nasopharyngeal drainage and minimizes the risk of aspiration. Withholding enteral feeding when gastric residual volumes are high is also important in the prevention of regurgitation and pulmonary aspiration.	

Procedure continues on the following page

Patient Monitoring and Care—*Continued*

Steps	Rationale	Reportable Conditions
13. Ensure that tube is securely in place (using twill tape or tracheal Velcro tie).	During the initial 48 hours after tracheostomy tube insertion, the tube should not be removed. If removed too early, the newly created stoma may collapse, making reintubation difficult.	
14. Perform oral hygiene every 2 to 4 hours (see Procedure 4).	Prevents bacterial overgrowth and promotes patient comfort.	
15. Promote effective patient-provider communication (paper and pencil, letter or word boards, one-way speaking valves, if appropriate).	The patient cannot talk, which may result in fear and anxiety. Patients need an established communication mechanism.	

Documentation

Documentation should include the following:

- Patient and family education
- Respiratory and vital signs assessment before and after procedure
- Type and size of tube
- Nursing interventions taken
- Use of medications for sedation or pain
- Placement of inner cannula
- Expected and Unexpected outcomes

- Patient response to procedure
- Date, time, and frequency with which procedure is performed
- Type and amount of secretions
- General condition of stoma and surrounding skin
- Nursing interventions
- Retaping of endotracheal tube
- Mouth care

References

1. Brook, A.D., et al. (2000). Early versus late tracheostomy in patients who require prolonged mechanical ventilation. *Am J Crit Care,* 9, 352-9.
2. Burns, S.M., et al. (1998). Are frequent inner cannula changes necessary? A pilot study. *Heart Lung,* 27, 58-62.
3. Henneman, E., Ellstrom, K., and St. John, R.E. (1999). Airway management. In: *AACN Protocols for Practice: Care of the Mechanically Ventilated Patient Series.* Aliso Viejo, CA: American Association of Critical-Care Nurses.
4. Mittendorf, E.A., et al. (2002). Early and late outcome of bedside percutaneous tracheostomy in the intensive care unit. *Am Surg,* 68, 342-6.
5. Rankin, N. (1998). What is optimum humidity? *Respir Care Clin North Am,* 4, 321-8.
6. Williams, R., et al. (1996). Relationship between the humidity and temperature of inspired gas and the function of the airway mucosa. *Crit Care Med,* 24, 1920-9.

Additional Readings

Plambeck, A. (2004). *Adult Ventilation Management.* Corexcel, Inc. Available at: http://www.corexcel.com/courses/vent.htm.
Tamburri, L.M. (2000). Care of the patient with a tracheostomy. *Orthop Nurs,* 19, 49-58.

SECTION TWO

Special Pulmonary Procedures

PROCEDURE **13**

Continuous End-Tidal Carbon Dioxide Monitoring

PURPOSE: End-tidal carbon dioxide (CO_2) monitoring is used to monitor a patient's ventilatory status and pulmonary blood flow, allowing the practitioner to detect changes in the ventilation-perfusion ratio (V/Q) of the lung.[1] The partial pressure of end-tidal CO_2 ($PETCO_2$) is assumed to represent alveolar gas, which under normal V/Q matching in the lungs closely parallels arterial levels of CO_2.

Vicki S. Good

PREREQUISITE NURSING KNOWLEDGE

- The principles of ventilation should be understood. CO_2 is a by-product of oxygen used by the cells after aerobic metabolism. When the CO_2 reaches the lungs, the CO_2 of venous blood ($PVCO_2$) diffuses from the capillaries to the alveoli ($PACO_2$). The normal $PVCO_2$ is 45 mm Hg, and the normal $PACO_2$ is 40 mm Hg. This pressure difference of 5 mm Hg causes the CO_2 to diffuse out of the capillaries into the alveoli for elimination. As the blood passes through the pulmonary capillaries, the $PVCO_2$ equals the $PACO_2$ of 40 mm Hg.[4] In patients with normal V/Q relationships, $PACO_2$, partial pressure of CO_2 in arterial blood ($PaCO_2$), $PVCO_2$ and $PETCO_2$ closely resemble one another. $PETCO_2$ can be used as an estimate of $PaCO_2$, with $PETCO_2$ generally 1 to 5 mm Hg lower than $PaCO_2$.[11]
- The principles of arterial blood gas sampling (see Procedure 79) and interpretation should be understood.
- Indications for continuous end-tidal CO_2 monitoring include the following:
  - ❖ Determine a baseline CO_2 waveform and $PETCO_2$.
  - ❖ Continuously monitor the patency of the airway and the presence of breathing.
  - ❖ Provide mechanism for early detection of changes in waveform pattern or $PETCO_2$ value that may accompany a sudden or gradual change in CO_2 production or

elimination (permissive hypercapnia, hyperthermia, hyperventilation therapy) or reduction in circulation (pulmonary blood flow).[1,11]

- Basic principles of $PETCO_2$ monitoring should be understood. The end-tidal CO_2 monitor may be a stand-alone system or a module incorporated into the patient's bedside hemodynamic monitor. An infrared capnograph passes light through an expiratory gas sample and, using a photodetector, measures absorption of that light by the gas. The capnograph determines the amount of CO_2 in the gas sample based on the absorption properties of CO_2. The capnograph also visually graphs the pattern in which CO_2 is exhaled and provides a display called a *capnogram* or *$PETCO_2$ waveform*.[8]
- The capnograph samples exhaled CO_2 by one of two methods: aspiration (sidestream) or nonaspiration (mainstream) sampling. In the sidestream method, a sample of gas is transported via small-bore tubing to the bedside monitor for analysis. In the mainstream system, analysis occurs directly at the patient-ventilator circuit.[3]
- The normal capnographic waveform has the following characteristics (Fig. 13-1).
  - ❖ A zero baseline represents the completion of inspiration and the beginning of exhalation of CO_2-free gas from anatomic dead space. This gas comes from the large airways, oropharynx, and nasopharynx (A-B).

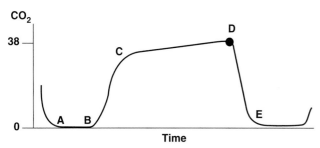

FIGURE 13-1 Essentials of the normal capnographic waveform. *(Reprinted by permission of Nellcor Puritan Bennett Incorporated, Pleasanton, CA.)*

- ❖ A rapid, sharp upstroke occurs as the gas from the intermediate airways, containing a mixture of fresh gas and CO_2, begins to be exhaled from the lungs (B-C).
- ❖ A nearly flat alveolar plateau occurs as exhaled flow velocity slows, and mixed gas is displaced by alveolar gas (C-D). Alveolar exhalation of CO_2 is nearing completion.
- ❖ A distance end-tidal point most closely reflects the maximal concentration of exhaled CO_2 and the end of exhalation (D).
- ❖ A rapid downstroke occurs as the patient begins the inspiration of gas that is essentially devoid of CO_2 (D-E).
- ❖ The positively deflected limb occurs with exhalation, whereas the negatively deflected limb occurs with inhalation. This is opposite from other respiratory waveforms, including the respirogram, spirograms, and flow-volume loop. The capnogram deviates from normal whenever there is a physiologic or mechanical disruption of the breath.
- The common physiologic basis for $PaCO_2$ and $PETCO_2$ abnormalities is incomplete alveolar emptying and increased alveolar dead space; this results in $PETCO_2$ values more than 5 mm Hg below $PaCO_2$.
- The ideal gas exchanging unit has a V/Q ratio of 1. Practically speaking, V/Q ratio in the normal human lung is something other than 1 because areas of high V/Q and low V/Q exist within the normal physiologic realm. Under normal V/Q conditions, $PaCO_2$ and $PETCO_2$ values are equal or nearly equal to the $PETCO_2$ values, an average of 2 to 5 mm Hg less than the $PaCO_2$. This difference is known as the a-$ADCO_2$ gradient. It is determined by subtracting the $PETCO_2$ value from the $PaCO_2$ value.
- In conditions in which abnormally large numbers of alveolar-capillary units are underperfused in relation to their ventilation (high V/Q units) or in which lung units are ventilated but totally nonperfused (dead space units), transfer of CO_2 gas from blood to lung is impaired. When

employing $PETCO_2$ monitoring, a lower exhaled CO_2 concentration than that measured in arterial blood (widened a-$ADCO_2$) is observed. This lower concentration occurs because the CO_2-free gas exhaled from nonperfused units mixes with CO_2-rich gas from perfused units, diluting the overall concentration of CO_2 exhaled. At the opposite end of the V/Q spectrum are low V/Q units and shunt units. In these situations, perfusion exceeds ventilation. Although low V/Q and shunt units are known contributors to the development of hypoxemia, they do not result in abnormal widening of the a-$ADCO_2$.

- Caution should be observed when interpreting $PETCO_2$ in the presence of decreased pulmonary blood flow because the $PETCO_2$ may not reflect $PaCO_2$ accurately.[6]

EQUIPMENT

- Capnograph
- Airway adapter

PATIENT AND FAMILY EDUCATION

- Discuss the rationale for implementing capnography. ➥*Rationale:* Discussion reduces anxiety for the patient and family associated with an additional monitor, related interventions, and unfamiliar procedures.
- If the patient is alert, explain the procedure to the patient. ➥*Rationale:* This communication informs the patient of the purpose of monitoring, improves cooperation with interventions, and reduces anxiety.

PATIENT ASSESSMENT AND PREPARATION

Patient Assessment

- Assess indications for $PETCO_2$ monitoring.
  - ❖ Acute airway obstruction or apnea (or potential for)
  - ❖ Dead space ventilation (or potential for)
  - ❖ Incomplete alveolar emptying (or potential for)
  - ➥*Rationale:* Assessment for initiation of $PETCO_2$ monitoring ensures that patients at risk for inadequate ventilation and gas exchange receive monitoring for such occurrences, allowing for early institution of appropriate interventions.

Patient Preparation

- Ensure that the patient understands preprocedural teaching. Answer questions as they arise, and reinforce information as needed. ➥*Rationale:* Understanding of previously taught information is evaluated and reinforced.

Procedure for Continuous End-Tidal Carbon Dioxide Monitoring

Steps	Rationale	Special Considerations
1. Obtain order for continuous $PETCO_2$ monitoring by capnography.	Order provides guideline for duration of monitoring, acceptable parameters for results, and appropriate interventions for abnormal results.	
2. Assess for proper functioning of capnograph, including airway adapter, sensor, and display monitor; check electrical grounding and accurate setup; and secure connections.	Ensures reliability of $PETCO_2$ values and waveforms obtained.	
3. Wash hands, and don personal protective equipment.	Reduces transmission of microorganisms; standard precautions.	
4. Connect capnograph into grounded wall outlet, and connect appropriate patient cable into display monitor; turn instrument on.	Decreases incidence of electrical interference.	Check capnograph's battery capacity and charging time, if applicable.
5. Perform calibration routine. Calibration procedure should occur daily or more often when instrument is in clinical use. *(Level I: Manufacturer's recommendations only.)*	Accurate measurement depends on proper calibration. Improper calibration may lead to erroneous $PETCO_2$ values.	All monitors have some type of calibration procedure; see operator's manual for exact steps.
6. Assemble airway adapter, sensor, and display monitor, and connect to patient circuit as close as possible to the patient's ventilation connection. *(Level I: Manufacturer's recommendations only.)*	Decreases incidence of improper gas sampling.	Sampling errors and gas leaks in system are major causes of inaccurate readings. Place adapter or sampling port as close as possible to the patient's airway to decrease response time to detect a change in CO_2.
7. Ensure that the sampling port is placed at the right angle to the endotracheal tube or ventilator circuit (applicable in sidestream sampling). *(Level I: Manufacturer's recommendations only.)*	Decreases secretion accumulation on CO_2 port where gas is drawn for sampling.	
8. Set appropriate alarms; alarm limits should include respiratory rate, apnea default, high and low $PETCO_2$, and minimal levels of inspiratory CO_2. *(Level VI: Clinical studies in a variety of patient populations and situations.)*	Alerts the nurse to potentially life-threatening problems.[3,6,11]	The $PETCO_2$ alarm is set 5% above and below acceptable parameter or per institutional standard. If monitor is interfaced with other equipment (electrocardiogram monitor, mechanical ventilator, pulse oximeter), ensure alarms are set consistently among all monitors.
9. Wash hands.	Reduces transmission of microorganisms.	

Expected Outcomes

- Significant changes in ventilatory status are detected
- Alterations in the a-ADCO$_2$ gradient are identified

Unexpected Outcomes

- Inaccurate measurements of $PETCO_2$ are displayed
- Inaccurate measurements resulting from calibration drift or contamination of optics with moisture or secretions are displayed
- Equipment malfunction occurs
- Inadvertent extubation due to weight of sensor

Patient Monitoring and Care

Steps	Rationale	Reportable Conditions
		These conditions should be reported if they persist despite nursing interventions.
1. Observe artificial airway for patency.	The airway adapter often adds weight to the airway and increases the risk of dislodgment or kinking. If kinking occurs, support the airway with an artificial support or towel.[3]	• Endotracheal or tracheal tube dislodgment
2. Observe waveform for quality.	If waveform is of poor quality, the numerical PETCO$_2$ value should not be accepted. If the PETCO$_2$ waveform is acceptable and the PETCO$_2$ numerical reading is questionable, obtain arterial blood gas measurement to confirm changes in PETCO$_2$.[3,6]	• Poor-quality waveform • Questionable PETCO$_2$ reading
3. Observe waveform for gradually increasing PETCO$_2$ (Fig. 13-2).	Increasing PETCO$_2$ occurs from absorption of CO$_2$ from exogenous sources and increased CO$_2$ production.[3,4] Clinical conditions in which increasing PETCO$_2$ is found include increased metabolism, hyperthermia (usually indicated by a rapid rise in PETCO$_2$), sepsis, hypoventilation or inadequate minute ventilation, neuromuscular blockade, decreased alveolar ventilation, partial obstruction of the airway, use of respiratory depressant drugs, and conditions that cause metabolic alkalosis.[7]	• PETCO$_2$ increase of greater than 10% of baseline
4. Observe for a gradual increase in baseline and PETCO$_2$ value (Fig. 13-3).	Reflects rebreathing of previously exhaled gas. Clinical conditions in which a gradual increase in baseline and PETCO$_2$ levels is found include defective exhalation valve on mechanical ventilator and excessive mechanical dead space in ventilator circuit.[9]	• Malfunction of the ventilator

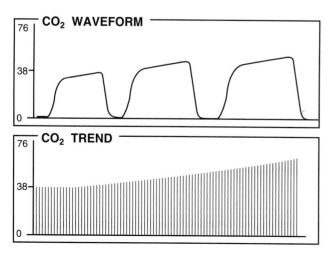

FIGURE 13-2 Gradually increasing PETCO$_2$. *(Reprinted by permission of Nellcor Puritan Bennett Incorporated, Pleasanton, CA.)*

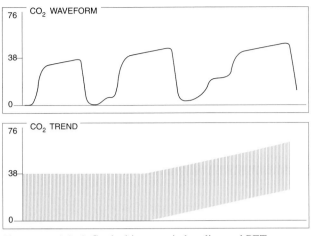

FIGURE 13-3 Gradual increase in baseline and PETCO$_2$ value. *(Reprinted by permission of Nellcor Puritan Bennett Incorporated, Pleasanton, CA.)*

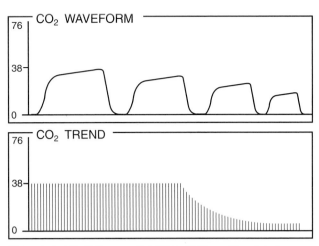

FIGURE 13-4 Exponential fall in PETCO$_2$. *(Reprinted by permission of Nellcor Puritan Bennett Incorporated, Pleasanton, CA.)*

Patient Monitoring and Care—*Continued*

Steps	Rationale	Reportable Conditions
5. Observe for an exponential fall in PETCO$_2$ (Fig. 13-4).	Indicates a widening of the a-ADCO$_2$ gradient from a sudden increase in dead space ventilation. a-ADCO$_2$ gradient widening is seen in clinical conditions such as cardiopulmonary bypass, cardiopulmonary arrest, pulmonary embolism, and severe pulmonary hypoperfusion.[2,4,9,11,12]	• Cardiopulmonary arrest • Fall greater than 10% in baseline
6. Observe for decreased PETCO$_2$ (with a normal waveform) (Fig. 13-5).	Gradual decreases indicate a decrease in perfusion or a decrease in production of CO$_2$ and may be seen in patients with high minute volumes, hypothermia, metabolic acidosis, decreased cardiac output, and hypovolemia.[12]	• PETCO$_2$ decreased greater than 10% of baseline
7. Observe for a sudden decrease in PETCO$_2$ to low values (Fig. 13-6).	Incomplete sampling or full exhalation is not detected in the system. This may be seen in patients with leak in airway system, partial airway obstruction,	• PETCO$_2$ decreased greater than 10% of baseline

Procedure continues on the following page

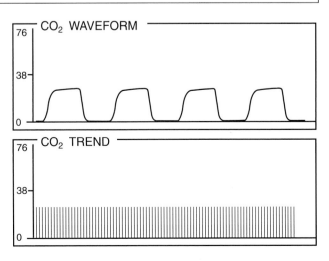

FIGURE 13-5 Decreased PETCO$_2$. *(Reprinted by permission of Nellcor Puritan Bennett Incorporated, Pleasanton, CA.)*

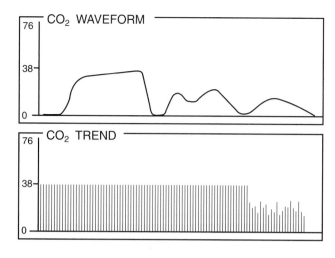

FIGURE 13-6 Sudden decrease in PETCO₂ values. *(Reprinted by permission of Nellcor Puritan Bennett Incorporated, Pleasanton, CA.)*

Patient Monitoring and Care—*Continued*

Steps	Rationale	Reportable Conditions
	mechanical ventilator malfunction, or partial disconnection of ventilator circuit.[3,4,6,11]	
8. Observe for a sudden decrease in PETCO₂ to near zero (Fig. 13-7).	Drop in waveform to baseline or near baseline (baseline equals zero) implies that no respirations are present.[11]	• Dislodged endotracheal tube • Complete airway obstruction • Mechanical ventilator malfunction • Airway disconnection • Esophageal intubation
9. Observe for a sustained low PETCO₂ without alveolar plateau (Fig. 13-8).	Sustained low PETCO₂ values indicate incomplete alveolar emptying, such as in partially kinked endotracheal tube, bronchospasm, mucous plugging, improper exhaled gas sampling, or insufficient expiratory time on the ventilator.[11]	• Complete airway obstruction requiring reintubation • PETCO₂ decreased greater than 10% of baseline
10. Routinely monitor the airway adapter or sampling port for signs of obstruction.	If the adapter or the port becomes obstructed, the quality of the capnographic waveform is poor and PETCO₂ is not reliable.[11]	• Obstruction in the airway adapter or sampling port
11. Evaluate the patient's response to activities that may positively or negatively affect ventilation (e.g., suctioning, repositioning, change in mechanical support, nutritional supplementation, cardiopulmonary resuscitation,[5] neuromuscular blockade,[11] verification of endotracheal tube placement[10]).		

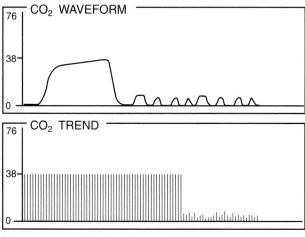

FIGURE 13-7 Sudden decrease in PETCO$_2$ to near zero. *(Reprinted by permission of Nellcor Puritan Bennett Incorporated, Pleasanton, CA.)*

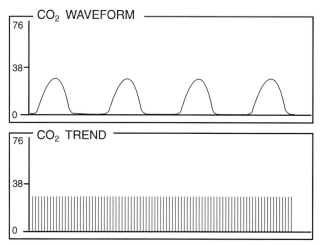

FIGURE 13-8 Low PETCO$_2$ without alveolar plateau. *(Reprinted by permission of Nellcor Puritan Bennett Incorporated, Pleasanton, CA.)*

Documentation

Documentation should include the following:

- Patient and family education
- Mechanical ventilator settings
- PETCO$_2$ value and capnogram
- PaCO$_2$-PETCO$_2$ gradient
- Arterial blood gases
- Times of calibration
- Respiratory therapies

- Medications that may affect respiratory system (e.g., neuromuscular blockers, sedatives, or bronchodilators)
- Respiratory assessment (e.g., respiratory rate, breathing patterns, adventitious sounds)
- Unexpected outcomes
- Nursing interventions

References

1. AARC. (2003). AARC clinical practice guideline: Capnography/capnometry during mechanical ventilation—2003 revision and update. *Respir Care, 48,* 534-8.
2. Ahrens, T., et al. (2001). End-tidal carbon dioxide measurements as a prognostic indicator of outcome in cardiac arrest. *Am J Crit Care, 10,* 391-8.
3. Frakes, M.A. (2001). Measuring end-tidal carbon dioxide: Clinical applications and usefulness. *Crit Care Nurse, 21,* 23-6.
4. La-Valle, T.L., and Perry, A.G. (1995). Capnography: Assessing end-tidal CO$_2$ levels. *Dimensions Crit Care Nurs, 14,* 70-7.
5. Levine, P.D., and Pizov, R. (1997). End-tidal carbon dioxide and outcome of out-of-hospital cardiac arrest. *N Engl J Med, 337,* 301-6.
6. Martin, S., and Wilson, M. (2002). Monitoring gaseous exchange: Implications for nursing care. *Aust Crit Care, 15,* 8-13.
7. Miner, J.R., Heegaard, W., and Plummer, D. (2002). End-tidal carbon dioxide monitoring during procedural sedation. *Acad Emerg Med, 9,* 275-80.
8. Petterson, M.T. (1990). Questions and answers on capnography. *Crit Care Choices, 1,* 12-7.
9. Rhoades, C., and Thomas, F. (2002). Capnography: Beyond the numbers. *Air Med J, 21,* 43-8.
10. Sitzwohl, C., et al. (1998). The arterial to end-tidal carbon dioxide gradient increases with uncorrected but not with temperature-corrected PaCO$_2$ determination during mild to moderate hypothermia. *Anesth Analg, 85,* 1131-6.
11. St. John, R.E. (1996). End tidal CO$_2$ monitoring. In Burns S: *American Association of Critical-Care Nurses Technology Series.* Aliso Viejo, CA: American Association of Critical-Care Nurses, 1-31.
12. Tyburski, J.G., et al. (2002). End-tidal CO$_2$-derived values during emergency trauma surgery correlated with outcome: A prospective study. *J Trauma Inj Infect Crit Care, 53,* 738-43.

Additional Reading

Pierce, L.N.B. (1995). *Mechanical Ventilation and Intensive Respiratory Care.* Philadelphia: W.B. Saunders.

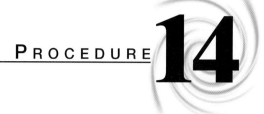
PROCEDURE 14

Continuous Mixed Venous Oxygen Saturation Monitoring

P U R P O S E : Mixed venous oxygen saturation (Svo_2) monitoring is performed to measure the oxygen saturation of the venous blood in the pulmonary artery (PA). Continuous assessment of the balance between a patient's oxygen delivery and oxygen consumption can be monitored using a specialized fiberoptic PA catheter and a computer.

Karen K. Giuliano
Jan M. Headley

PREREQUISITE NURSING KNOWLEDGE

- Anatomy and physiology of the cardiopulmonary system should be understood.
- Physiologic principles related to invasive hemodynamic monitoring should be understood.
- Technical aspects of PA pressure monitoring should be understood.
- Physiologic concepts of oxygen delivery, oxygen demand, and tissue oxygen consumption should be understood.
- Svo_2 is the percent of venous oxygen saturation. Because the blood in the PA is a mixture of all venous blood, it is represents a measurement of overall venous oxygen saturation.
- Clinically, Svo_2 provides an index of overall oxygen balance because it is a reflection of the dynamic relationship between the patient's oxygen delivery and oxygen consumption (VO_2). Whenever there is a threat to the oxygen balance, the body's primary compensatory mechanisms are to increase delivery by increasing cardiac output or to increase extraction at the tissue level.
- In a critically ill patient, if cardiac output is limited, increased extraction occurs to meet the demand for oxygen at the tissue level. The result is a decreased level of oxygen returning to the heart, and a lower Svo_2 measurement. Many factors can affect the requirements for oxygen and subsequently Svo_2 (Table 14-1).[4,6,7,10]

- Svo_2 does not correlate directly with any of the determinants of oxygen delivery or oxygen consumption. Because a critically ill patient is in a dynamic state with rapidly changing oxygen demand and oxygen consumption, Svo_2 must be viewed in the light of these changing determinants and considered an index of oxygen balance.[1-4]
- A normal Svo_2 generally is considered to be 60% to 80%,[8] and a clinically significant change in Svo_2 ($\pm$5-10%) can be an early indicator of physiologic instability.[2,8] Svo_2 values of less than 60% may result from either inadequate oxygen delivery or excess oxygen consumption. Svo_2 monitoring is used in critically ill patients for earlier detection of oxygenation instability than that obtained through traditional PA monitoring.
- The proper setup and maintenance of the bedside computer or module is necessary for accurate monitoring. Additionally, proper blood sampling techniques from the distal port of the PA catheter are necessary for ensuring accurate values for calibration. There are two separate calibrations that must be done to ensure accurate Svo_2 monitoring. The light source must be electronically calibrated before catheter insertion (in vitro calibration). The second calibration is done by comparing Svo_2 values from a laboratory-analyzed sample with the Svo_2 monitor samples to ensure accuracy of continuous monitoring samples (in vivo calibration). This second calibration should be performed daily.[1,5]

TABLE 14-1	Common Conditions and Activities Affecting Mixed Venous Oxygen Saturation Values

Decreased Mixed Venous Oxygen Saturation

Decreased Oxygen Delivery
Decreased cardiac output
Decreased hemoglobin
Decreased arterial oxygen saturation
Decreased arterial partial pressure of oxygen

Increased Oxygen Consumption
Fever
Pain
Shivering
Seizures
Increased work of breathing
Agitation
Infection and sepsis
Vasoactive and β-agonist medications
Multiple organ failure
Burns
Head injury
Increased musculoskeletal activities
Numerous nursing procedures (e.g., dressing changes, suctioning, turning, and chest physiotherapy)

Increased Mixed Venous Oxygen Saturation

Increased Oxygen Delivery
Increased cardiac output
Increased hemoglobin
Increased arterial oxygen saturation
Increased arterial partial pressure of oxygen

Decreased Oxygen Consumption
Hypothermia
Hypothyroidism
Pharmacologic paralysis and sedation
Anesthesia
Cellular dysfunction
Decreased work of breathing
Decreased musculoskeletal activities

- Continuous monitoring is performed with a three-component system (Fig. 14-1):[1,4,5,7]
  - ❖ A fiberoptic PA catheter contains two fiberoptic filaments, exiting at the distal port. One filament serves as a sending fiber for the emission of light; the other serves as a receiving fiber for the light reflected back from the blood in the PA.
  - ❖ The optic module houses the light-emitting diodes (LEDs), which transmit various wavelengths of light, and a photodetector, which receives light back. Various wavelengths of lights are shone through a blood sample. Desaturated hemoglobins, saturated hemoglobins (oxyhemoglobin), and dyshemoglobins (carboxyhemoglobin, methemoglobin) have different light absorption characteristics. The ratio of hemoglobin to oxyhemoglobin is determined and reported as a percentage value.[10] All previous patient data, including calibration of SvO_2 values and patient identification information, are stored in this component. This module should not be disconnected. If the module must be disconnected, refer to the manufacturer's instructions for a disconnection procedure that does not result in memory loss.
  - ❖ An oximeter computer, which can be a stand-alone unit or module for a bedside monitor, has a microprocessor

that converts the light information from the optic module into an electrical display, updated every few seconds for continuous monitoring. This information is displayed as a continuous graphic trend, a numeric display, or both, depending on the manufacturer.

EQUIPMENT

- Fiberoptic PA catheter (7.5 Fr or 8 Fr)
- Optic module
- Oximeter computer or bedside monitor module
- Equipment required for PA catheterization and pressure monitoring (see Procedure 71)

Additional equipment (to have available depending on patient need) includes the following:

- Printer

PATIENT AND FAMILY EDUCATION

- Assess patient and family understanding of the clinical benefits of SvO_2 monitoring. ➥*Rationale:* To provide the most appropriate information, it is important to assess the level of patient and family understanding of need for SvO_2 monitoring.
- Explain the continuous nature of this monitoring system and the significance of the alarms. ➥*Rationale:* Explanation of the procedure to the patient and family helps to alleviate fears and concerns. Additional monitors may produce increased anxiety in the patient and family.

PATIENT ASSESSMENT AND PREPARATION

Patient Assessment

- Indications for use of SvO_2 monitoring include the following.[4,8,9]
  - ❖ High-risk cardiovascular surgery
  - ❖ Heart failure
  - ❖ Myocardial infarction
  - ❖ Respiratory failure
  - ❖ Severe burns
  - ❖ Sepsis
  - ❖ Anemia and hemorrhage
  - ❖ Multisystem organ dysfunction
  - ❖ Trauma
  - ❖ Acute respiratory distress syndrome
  - ❖ Use of positive end-expiratory pressure

  ➥*Rationale:* SvO_2 monitoring is useful in the early detection of oxygenation imbalance, which can facilitate the use of early and more appropriate interventions.

Patient Preparation

- Answer patient questions as they arise, and reinforce information as needed. ➥*Rationale:* This communication evaluates and reinforces understanding of previously taught information.

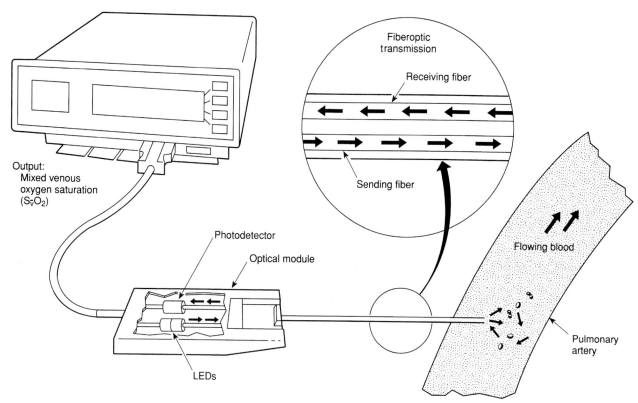

FIGURE 14-1 A mixed venous oxygen saturation system using reflection spectophotometry. *(From American Edwards Laboratories. [1987].* Understanding Continuous Mixed Venous Oxygen Saturation (SvO$_2$) Monitoring With the Swan Ganz Oximetry TD System. *Irvine, CA: Author.)*

Procedure for Continuous Mixed Venous Oxygen Saturation Monitoring

Steps	Rationale	Special Considerations
1. Assemble necessary equipment and supplies for continuous monitoring. *(Level II: Theory based, no research data to support recommendations; recommendations from expert consensus group may exist.)*	Ensures equipment is ready and available for the procedure.[3,4]	
2. Connect alternating current (AC) power cord to computer, turn on, and observe system check on the computer screen. *(Level I: Manufacturer's recommendation only.)*	Allows electronics to warm up; confirms component function.[1,5]	Warm-up times may vary by manufacturer
3. Connect optics module to computer. *(Level I: Manufacturer's recommendation only.)*	LEDs are housed in optics module. Approximately 20 minutes is required to warm light source sufficiently.[1,5]	
4. Remove outer wrap of catheter package and aseptically peel back the inner wrap portion covering the optic connector of the catheter. *(Level I: Manufacturer's recommendation only.)*	Provides access to inner package.[2,8] Isolates connector from catheter tip to maintain sterility during in vitro calibration.[1,5]	
5. Firmly connect the optic connector to the optic module. *(Level I: Manufacturer's recommendation only.)*	Ensures connections are tight and properly aligned for light transmission.[1,5]	

Procedure for Continuous Mixed Venous Oxygen Saturation Monitoring—*Continued*

Steps	Rationale	Special Considerations
6. Perform in vitro calibration or standardization. *(Level I: Manufacturer's recommendation only.)*	Standardizes or calibrates the light source to the catheter. Calibration is performed before catheter insertion. Catheter tip should be left in the calibration cup or container in the package during in vitro calibration.[1,5]	Catheter lumens must be dry. Do not flush catheter before performing this step or in vitro calibration is invalid.
7. Pull back remaining wrap covering catheter package using aseptic technique. *(Level I: Manufacturer's recommendation only.)*	Prepares catheter for insertion.[1,5]	
8. Carefully remove catheter from tray using sterile technique. Pull catheter tip up and out of the calibration cup. *(Level I: Manufacturer's recommendation only.)*	Prevents the transmission of microorganisms; prevents damage to the balloon.[1,5]	Fiberoptics in catheter and balloon are fragile and may be damaged if not handled properly.
9. Attach pressure tubing, and prime lumens with flush solution (see Procedure 72).	Enables monitoring of chamber pressures during insertion; maintains patency of lumens. Refer to institutional standards for use of heparinized flush solution.[8]	
10. Assist physician or advanced practice nurse with PA catheter insertion (see Procedure 71).		
11. Observe waveforms during insertion (see Procedure 71).	Central PA catheter tip placement is necessary for optimal light reflection.[1,5]	A light intensity or signal indicator verifies adequate reflection of the light signals after the catheter tip is placed correctly.
12. Note amount of air required to inflate balloon.	Inflation volume of 1.25 to 1.5 ml is recommended for proper catheter tip placement.[1,5]	Less than optimal inflation volume to obtain a wedge tracing may indicate distal catheter migration. A change in the intensity or signal indicator also may alert the clinician to this condition.
13. Set high and low alarm limits and activate alarms. *(Level II: Theory based, no research data to support recommendations; recommendations from expert consensus group may exist.)*	Individualizes alarm settings according to patient baseline. Audible alarms notify the clinician of significant changes in Svo_2 values and trends.[3,4]	
14. Input patient height and weight data as per institutional standard.	Allows for calculation of derived parameters.[4,5]	
15. Apply a sterile dressing to insertion site.	Reduces transmission of microorganisms.	Use institutional standard for central venous catheter dressings.
16. Firmly secure the optic module near the patient.	Excessive tension on catheter or optic module may cause breakage of optic fibers.[1,5]	
17. After calibration and insertion of catheter, obtain baseline set of hemodynamic and oxygenation indices (see Procedure 72).	Provides baseline information for comparison with patient's response to interventions.[1,5]	

Procedure continues on the following page

Procedure for Continuous Mixed Venous Oxygen Saturation Monitoring—*Continued*

Steps	Rationale	Special Considerations
18. Continuously monitor PA pressure tracings and $S\bar{v}O_2$ values. *(Level II: Theory based, no research data to support recommendations: recommendations from expert consensus group may exist.)*	Spontaneous catheter migration may occur after insertion. As a reflection of post–capillary arterialized blood and the vessel wall, the $S\bar{v}O_2$ value may increase.[7,8]	
Mixed Venous Blood Sampling Skill/In Vivo Calibration		
19. Draw mixed venous blood sample (see Procedure 62).	In vivo calibration is required to verify the accuracy of the computer and value displayed after insertion of the fiberoptic PA catheter. Follow specific recommendations from the manufacturer about the frequency of calibration and specific steps to implement the process. Ideally the patient's hemodynamic and oxygenation status should be stable for optimal calibration.[3,5,8]	Mixed venous samples should be drawn only from the PA.[10]
20. Perform a verification or in vivo calibration per institutional standard.	Typically, this is done every 24 hours or whenever the displayed value is in question. In vivo calibration verifies the accuracy of the $S\bar{v}O_2$ being displayed.[1,5]	
21. Ensure measurement is performed with a cooximeter. *(Level II: Theory based, no research data to support recommendations: recommendations from expert consensus group may exist.)*	Cooximetry measures saturation; blood gas analyzers calculate saturation from measured partial pressure values. A calculated saturation value from a gas analyzer may not correlate with the actual patient value and, if used for calibration, may produce erroneous results.[8]	
22. Observe bedside oscilloscope for PA tracing and resume $S\bar{v}O_2$ monitoring	Reconfirms catheter tip placement in the PA.	

Expected Outcomes

- $S\bar{v}O_2$ values and trends within normal range (60% to 80%)[1,3,8]
- $S\bar{v}O_2$ trends not fluctuating greater than 10% of baseline value
- Hemodynamic and oxygenation parameters optimal for patient condition

Unexpected Outcomes

- $S\bar{v}O_2$ values less than 60% or greater than 80%
- $S\bar{v}O_2$ value trends greater than 10% from baseline
- Infection from presence of an indwelling PA catheter
- PA infarction or rupture

Patient Monitoring and Care

Steps	Rationale	Reportable Conditions
		These conditions should be reported if they persist despite nursing interventions.
1. Ensure that there are no kinks or bends in the catheter.	Fiberoptics are fragile and can break if not handled carefully. Overtightening of the introducer connector can cause crimping and breakage of the fiberoptics.[6,7]	- Change in PA waveform or $S\bar{v}O_2$ value that does not correlate to patient condition

Patient Monitoring and Care—*Continued*

Steps	Rationale	Reportable Conditions
	Subclavian or internal jugular approaches for insertion may cause kinking in the vessel if the vessel is tortuous. Sending and receiving wavelengths may show either a change in light signal or values that do not reflect the patient's status.	
2. Monitor PA waveforms continuously. *(Level II: Theory based, no research data to support recommendations: recommendations from expert consensus group may exist.)*	Migration of the catheter tip may reflect post–capillary arterialized blood causing an elevation in the SvO_2 value. Uncorrected catheter migration places the patient at risk for PA infarction or rupture	• Permanent wedge waveform
3. Observe SvO_2 value and trends.	Normal SvO_2 values range from 60% to 80%[3,4,8]; values outside this range may indicate an imbalance between oxygen delivery and consumption. A value greater than 10% may signify a clinically significant change. If the patient's clinical presentation differs from the observed SvO_2 value or trends, recheck the accuracy of the monitoring system.	• SvO_2 values greater than 80% or less than 60%

Documentation

Documentation should include the following:

- Patient and family education
- SvO_2 whenever the hemodynamic profile is recorded
- Additional oxygenation indices as indicated
- Specific nursing activities (e.g., suctioning, turning the patient, or titrating a vasoactive drug) and the relationship of the event with the SvO_2, especially if the event produces a marked change in the value
- Hard copy printout (as available)
- Unexpected outcomes
- Nursing interventions

References

1. Abbott Laboratories. (2003). *Oximetrix 3 System SO₂/CO Computer (Operator's Manual)*. North Chicago, IL: Author.
2. Bishop, M.H., et al. (1995). Prospective, randomized trial of survivor values of cardiac index, oxygen delivery, and oxygen consumption as resuscitation endpoints in severe trauma. *J Trauma, 38,* 780-7.
3. Daily, E.K. (1991). Hemodynamic monitoring. In: Dolan J, editor. *Critical Care Nursing: Clinical Management Through the Nursing Process*. Philadelphia: F.A. Davis, 828-54.
4. Darovic, G.O. (2002). *Hemodynamic Monitoring: Invasive and Non-Invasive Clinical Application*. 3rd ed. Philadelphia: W.B. Saunders.
5. Edwards Lifesciences. (2003). Vigilance: Continuous cardiac output and SvO₂ monitoring system. In: *Operations Manual*. Irvine, CA: Baxter Healthcare Corp.
6. Gawlinski, A. (1998). Can measurement of mixed venous oxygen saturation replace measurement of cardiac output in patient with advanced heart failure? *Am J Crit Care, 7,* 374-80.
7. Headley, J.M. (1995). Strategies to optimize the cardiorespiratory status of the critically ill. *AACN Clin Issues Crit Care Nurs, 6,* 121-34.
8. Jesurum, J.T. (1998). SvO₂ monitoring. In: *AACN Protocols for Practice: Hemodynamic Monitoring*. Aliso Viejo, CA: American Association of Critical-Care Nurses.
9. Vedrinne, C., et al. (1997). Predictive factors for usefulness of fiberoptic pulmonary artery catheter for continuous oxygen saturation in mixed venous blood monitoring in cardiac surgery. *Anesth Analg, 85,* 2-10.
10. White, K.M. (1993). Using continuous SvO₂ to assess oxygen supply/demand balance in the critically ill patient. *AACN Clin Issues Crit Care Nurs, 4,* 134-47.

Additional Readings

Edwards, J.D., and Mayall, R.M. (1998). Importance of the sampling site for measurement of mixed venous oxygen saturation in shock. *Crit Care Med,* 26, 1356-60.

Keckeisen, M. (1998). Pulmonary artery pressure monitoring. In: *AACN Protocols for Practice: Hemodynamic Monitoring.* Aliso Viejo, CA: American Association of Critical-Care Nurses.

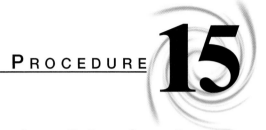

PROCEDURE **15**

Oxygen Saturation Monitoring by Pulse Oximetry

P U R P O S E : Pulse oximetry is a noninvasive monitoring technique used to estimate the measurement of arterial oxygen saturation (Sao$_2$) of hemoglobin.

Sandra L. Schutz

PREREQUISITE NURSING KNOWLEDGE

- Oxygen saturation is an indicator of the percentage of hemoglobin saturated with oxygen at the time of the measurement. The reading, obtained through pulse oximetry, uses a light sensor containing two sources of light (red and infrared) that are absorbed by hemoglobin and transmitted through tissues to a photodetector. The infrared light is absorbed by the oxyhemoglobin, and the red light is absorbed by the reduced hemoglobin. The amount and type of light transmitted through the tissue is converted to a digital value representing the percentage of hemoglobin saturated with oxygen (Fig. 15-1).
- Oxygen saturation values obtained from pulse oximetry (Spo$_2$) represent one part of a complete assessment of a patient's oxygenation status and are not a substitute for measurement of arterial partial pressure of oxygen (Pao$_2$) or of ventilation (as measured by arterial partial pressure of carbon dioxide [Paco$_2$]).
- The accuracy of Spo$_2$ measurements requires consideration of many physiologic variables. Patient variables include the following:
  - ❖ Hemoglobin level
  - ❖ Arterial blood flow to the vascular bed
  - ❖ Temperature of the digit or the area where the oximetry sensor is located
  - ❖ Patient's oxygenation ability
  - ❖ Fraction of inspired oxygen (percentage of inspired oxygen)
  - ❖ Evidence of ventilation-perfusion mismatch
  - ❖ Amount of ambient light seen by the sensor
  - ❖ Venous return at the sensor location

- A complete assessment of oxygenation includes evaluation of oxygen content and delivery, which includes the following parameters: Pao$_2$, Sao$_2$, hemoglobin, cardiac output, and, when available, mixed venous oxygen saturation.
- Normal oxygen saturation values are 97% to 99% in a healthy individual on room air. An oxygen saturation value of 95% is clinically accepted in a patient with a normal hemoglobin level. Using the oxyhemoglobin dissociation curve, an oxygen saturation value of 90% is generally equated with a Pao$_2$ of 60 mm Hg.
- Tissue oxygenation is not reflected by arterial or oxygen saturation obtained by pulse oximetry. The affinity of

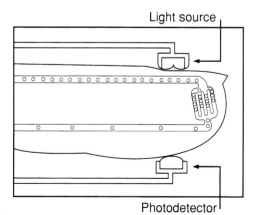

Light source

Photodetector

FIGURE 15-1 A sensor device that contains a light source and a photodetector is placed around a pulsating arteriolar bed, such as the finger, great toe, nose, or earlobe. Red and infrared wavelengths of light are used to determine arterial saturation. *(Reprinted by permission of Nellcor Puritan Bennett Incorporated, Pleasanton, CA.)*

hemoglobin to oxygen may impair or enhance oxygen release at the tissue level.

- ❖ Oxygen is more readily released to the tissues when pH is decreased (acidosis), body temperature is increased, $PaCO_2$ is increased, and 2,3-diphosphoglycerate levels (a by-product of glucose metabolism also found in stored blood products) are increased (*decreased oxygen affinity*).
- ❖ When hemoglobin has greater affinity for oxygen, less is available to the tissues (*increased oxygen affinity*). Conditions such as increased pH (alkalosis), decreased temperature, decreased $PaCO_2$, and decreased 2,3-diphosphoglycerate increase oxygen binding to the hemoglobin and limit its release to the tissue.
- Oxygen saturation values may vary with the amount of oxygen usage by the tissues. In some patients, there is a difference in SpO_2 values at rest compared with values during activity, such as ambulation or positioning.
- Oxygen saturation does not reflect the patient's ability to ventilate. The true measure of ventilation is determination of the $PaCO_2$ in arterial blood. Use of SpO_2 in a patient with obstructive pulmonary disease may result in erroneous clinical assessments of condition. As the degree of lung disease increases, the patient's drive to breathe may shift from an increased carbon dioxide stimulus to a hypoxic stimulus. Enhancing the patient's SpO_2 may limit his or her ability to ventilate. The normal baseline SpO_2 for a patient with known severe restrictive disease and more definitive methods of determining the effectiveness of ventilation must be known before considering interventions that enhance oxygenation.
- Any discoloration of the nail bed can affect the transmission of light through the digit. Dark nail polish, such as blue, green, brown, or black colors,[1,12] and bruising under the nail can limit the transmission of light and result in an artificially decreased SpO_2 value. If the nail polish cannot be removed, the sensor can be placed in a lateral side-to-side position on the finger to obtain readings if no other method of sampling the arterial bed is available.[1]
- Pulse oximetry has not been shown to be affected by the presence of an elevated bilirubin.[2]
- Pulse oximeters are unable to differentiate between oxygen and carbon monoxide bound to hemoglobin. Readings in the presence of carbon monoxide are falsely elevated. Pulse oximetry should never be used in suspected cases of carbon monoxide exposure. An arterial blood gas reading always should be obtained to determine the accurate oxygen saturation.
- It has been suggested that dark skin may affect the ability of the pulse oximeter to detect arterial pulsations. One study found a more frequent difference between the SpO_2 and SaO_2 with black patients compared with lighter skinned patient[6]; another study did not find a significant difference.[7]
- A pulse oximeter should not be used as a predictive indicator of the actual arterial blood gas saturation.
- A pulse oximeter should never be used during a cardiac arrest situation because of the extreme limitations of

blood flow during cardiopulmonary resuscitation and the pharmacologic action of vasoactive agents administered during the resuscitation effort.

EQUIPMENT

- Oxygen saturation meter and monitor
- Oxygen saturation cable and sensor
- Manufacturer's recommended germicidal agent for cleaning the nondisposable sensor (used for cleaning between patients)

PATIENT AND FAMILY EDUCATION

- Explain the need for determination of oxygen saturation with a pulse oximeter. ➥*Rationale:* This explanation informs the patient of the purpose of monitoring, enhances patient cooperation, and decreases patient anxiety.
- Explain that the values displayed may vary by patient movement, amount of environmental light, patient level of consciousness (awake or asleep), and position of the sensor. ➥*Rationale:* This explanation decreases patient and family anxiety over the constant variability of the values.
- Explain that the use of pulse oximetry is part of a much larger assessment of oxygenation status. ➥*Rationale:* This prepares the patient and family for other possible diagnostic tests of oxygenation (e.g., arterial blood gas).
- Explain the equipment to the patient. ➥*Rationale:* This facilitates patient cooperation in maintaining sensor placement.
- Explain the need for an audible alarm system for determination of oxygen saturation values below a set acceptable limit. Demonstrate the alarm system, alerting the patient and family to the possibility of alarms, including causes of false alarms. ➥*Rationale:* Providing an understanding of the use of an alarm system and its importance in the overall management of the patient and of circumstances in which a false alarm may occur assists in patient understanding of the values seen while at the bedside.
- Explain the need to move or remove the sensor on a routine basis to prevent complications related to the type of sensor used or the degree of tightness in which the sensor is secured around the finger. ➥*Rationale:* Providing an understanding of the need to move the sensor routinely assists in patient understanding of the frequency of sensor movement.

PATIENT ASSESSMENT AND PREPARATION

Patient Assessment

- Signs and symptoms of decreased ability to oxygenate include the following.
  - ❖ Cyanosis
  - ❖ Dyspnea
  - ❖ Tachypnea
  - ❖ Decreased level of consciousness
  - ❖ Increased work of breathing

❖ Loss of protective airway (patients undergoing conscious sedation)
❖ Agitation
❖ Confusion
❖ Disorientation
❖ Tachycardia/bradycardia

➤*Rationale:* Patient assessment determines the need for continuous pulse oximetry monitoring. Anticipation of conditions in which hypoxia could be present allows earlier intervention before unfavorable outcomes occur.

• Assess the extremity (digit) or area where the sensor will be placed including the following.
  ❖ Decreased peripheral pulses
  ❖ Peripheral cyanosis
  ❖ Decreased body temperature
  ❖ Decreased blood pressure

❖ Exposure to excessive environmental light sources (e.g., examination lights)
❖ Excessive movement or tremor in the digit
❖ Presence of dark nail polish or bruising under the nail
❖ Presence of artificial nails
❖ Clubbing of the digit tips

➤*Rationale:* Assessment of factors that may inhibit accuracy of the measurement of oxygenation before attempting to obtain the SpO_2 reading enhances the validity of the measurement and allows for correction of factors as possible.

Patient Preparation

• Ensure that patient understands preprocedural teaching. Answer questions as they arise, and reinforce information as needed. ➤*Rationale:* This communication evaluates and reinforces understanding of previously taught information.

Procedure for Oxygen Saturation Monitoring by Pulse Oximetry

Steps	Rationale	Special Considerations
1. Wash hands, and use personal protective equipment.	Reduces the transmission of microorganisms and body secretions; standard precautions.	
2. Select the appropriate pulse oximeter sensor for the area with the best pulsatile vascular bed to be sampled (Fig. 15-2). Use of finger sensors has been found to produce the best results over other sites.[3] *(Level IV: Limited clinical studies to support recommendations.)*	The correct sensor optimizes signal capture and minimizes artifact-related difficulties.[3,4,8,10]	Several different types of sensors are available, including disposable and nondisposable sensors that may be applied over a variety of vascular beds. Do not use one manufacturer's sensors with another manufacturer's pulse oximeter unless compatibility has been verified.
3. Select desired sensor site. If using the digits, assess for warmth and capillary refill. Confirm the presence of an arterial blood flow to the area monitored.	Adequate arterial pulse strength is necessary for obtaining accurate SpO_2 measurements.	Avoid sites distal to indwelling arterial catheters, blood pressure cuffs, military antishock trousers (MAST), or venous engorgement (e.g., arteriovenous fistulas, blood transfusions).
4. Plug oximeter into grounded wall outlet if the unit is not portable. If the unit is portable, ensure sufficient battery charge by turning it on before using. Plug patient cable into monitor.	When using electrical outlets, grounded outlets decrease the occurrence of electrical interference.	Portable systems have rechargeable batteries and depend on sufficient time plugged into an electrical outlet to maintain the proper level of battery charge. When system is used in the portable mode, always check battery capacity.
5. Apply the sensor in a manner that allows the light source (light-emitting diodes) to be: A. Directly opposite the light detector (photodetector). *(Level IV: Limited clinical studies to support recommendations.)*	To determine a pulse oximetry value properly, the light sensors must be in opposing positions directly over the area of the sample.[3,5,11,14]	

Procedure continues on the following page

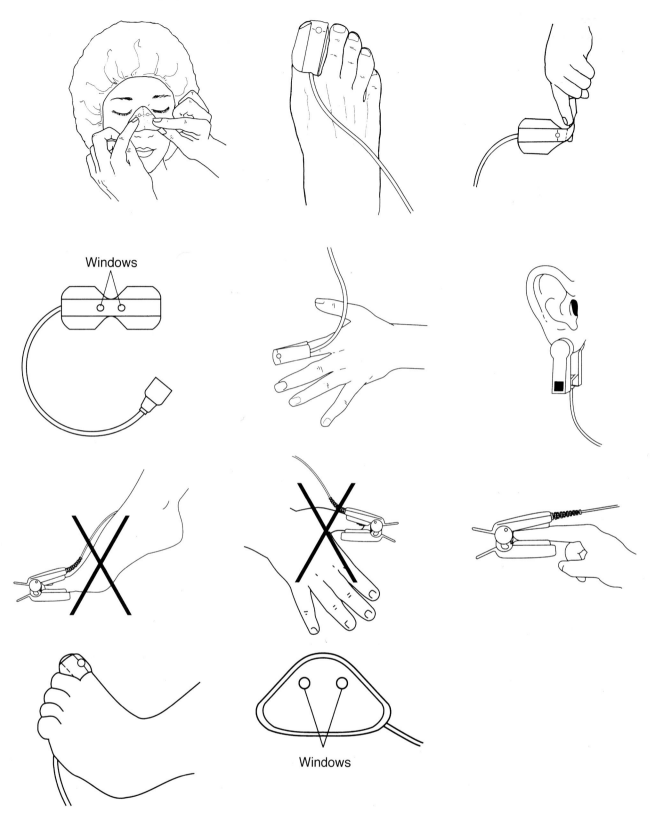

FIGURE 15-2 Sensor types and sensor sites for pulse oximetry monitoring. Use "wrap" or "clip" style sensors on the fingers (including thumb), great toe, and nose. The windows for the light source and photodetector must be placed directly opposite each other on each side of the arteriolar bed to ensure accuracy of SpO_2 measurements. Choosing the correct size of the sensor helps decrease the incidence of excess ambient light interference and optical shunting. "Clip" style sensors are appropriate for fingers (except the thumb) and the earlobe. Ensuring that the arteriolar bed is well within the clip with the windows directly opposite each other decreases the possibility of excess ambient light interference and optical shunting. *(Reprinted by permission of Nellcor Puritan Bennett Incorporated, Pleasanton, CA.)*

Procedure for Oxygen Saturation Monitoring by Pulse Oximetry—*Continued*

Steps	Rationale	Special Considerations
B. Shielded from excessive environmental light. *(Level V: Clinical studies in more than one patient population and situation.)*	Light from sources such as examination lights or overhead lights can cause elevated oximetry values.[5,11,14]	If the oximeter sensor fails to detect a pulse when perfusion seems adequate, excessive environmental light (overhead examination lights, phototherapy lights, infrared warmers) may be blinding the light sensor. Troubleshoot by reapplying the sensor or shielding the sensor with a towel or blanket.
C. Positioned so that all sensor-emitted light comes in contact with perfused tissue beds and is not seen by the other side of the sensor or without coming in contact with the area to be read.	If the light is seen directly from the sensor without coming in contact with the vascular bed, too much light can be seen by the sensor, resulting in either a falsely high reading or no reading.	Known as *optical shunting,* the light bypasses the vascular bed; shielding the sensor does not eliminate this if the sensor is too large or not properly positioned.
6. Gently position the sensor so that it does not cause restriction to arterial flow or venous return. *(Level IV: Limited clinical studies to support recommendations.)*	The pulse oximeter is unable to distinguish between true arterial pulsations and fluid waves (e.g., venous engorgement or fluid accumulation).[3,4,9,13]	Restriction of arterial blood flow can cause a falsely low value and lead to vascular compromise, causing potential loss of viable tissues. Edema from restriction of venous return can cause venous pulsation. Elevating the site above the level of the heart reduces the possibility of venous pulsation. Moving the sensor to another site on a routine schedule also reduces tissue compromise. Never place the sensor on an extremity that has decreased or absent sensation because the patient may not be able to identify discomfort or the signs and symptoms of loss of circulation or tissue compromise.
7. Plug sensor into oximeter patient cable.	Connects the sensor to the oximeter, allowing SpO$_2$ measurement and analysis of waveforms.	
8. Turn instrument on with the power switch.		Allow 30 seconds for self-testing procedures and for detection and analysis of waveforms before values are displayed.
9. Determine accuracy of detected waveform by comparing the numeric heart rate value with that of a monitored heart rate or an apical heart rate or both.	If there is insufficient arterial blood flow through the sensor, the heart rate values vary significantly. If the pulse rate detected by oximeter does not correlate with the patient's heart rate, the oximeter is not detecting sufficient arterial blood flow for accurate values.	Consider moving the sensor to another site, such as the earlobe or the nose. This problem occurs particularly with the use of the fingers and the toes in conditions of low blood flow.
10. Set appropriate alarm limits.	Alarm limits should be set appropriate to the patient's condition.	Oxygen saturation limits should be 5% less than patient acceptable baseline. Heart rate alarms should be consistent with the cardiac monitoring limits (if monitored).

Procedure continues on the following page

Procedure for Oxygen Saturation Monitoring by Pulse Oximetry—*Continued*

Steps	Rationale	Special Considerations
11. Wash hands.	Reduces transmission of microorganisms to other patients.	
12. Cleanse nondisposable sensor, if used, between patients with manufacturer's recommended germicidal agent.	Reduces transmission of microorganisms to other patients.	

Expected Outcomes

- All changes in oxygen saturation are detected
- The number of oxygen desaturation events is reduced
- The need for invasive techniques for monitoring oxygenation is reduced
- False-positive pulse oximeter alarms are reduced

Unexpected Outcomes

- Accurate pulse oximetry is not obtainable because of movement artifact
- Low perfusion states or excessive edema prevents accurate pulse oximetry measurements
- Disagreements occur in SaO_2 and oximeter SpO_2

Patient Monitoring and Care

Steps	Rationale	Reportable Conditions
		These conditions should be reported if they persist despite nursing interventions.
1. Evaluate laboratory data along with the patient for evidence of poor oxygenation.	SpO_2 values are one segment of a complete evaluation of oxygenation and supplemental oxygen therapy. Data should be integrated into a complete assessment to determine the overall status of the patient. If SpO_2 is used as an indicator of SaO_2, an arterial blood gas should be done to determine if the values correlate consistently.	- Inability to maintain oxygen saturation levels as desired
2. Evaluate sensor site every 2 to 4 hours (if a disposable sensor is used) or every 2 hours (if a rigid encased nondisposable sensor is used). Rotate the site of a reusable sensor every 4 hours; replace a disposable sensor every 24 hours[8] or more frequently if the securing mechanism is compromised or soiled.	Assessment of the skin and tissues under the sensor identifies skin breakdown or loss of vascular flow, allowing appropriate interventions to be initiated.	- Change in skin color - Loss of warmth of tissue unrelated to vasoconstriction - Loss of blood flow to the digit - Evidence of skin breakdown due to the sensor - Change in color of the nail bed indicating compromised circulation to the nail
3. Monitor the site for excessive movement.	Excessive movement of the sampled site may result in unreliable saturation values. Moving the sensor to a less physically active site reduces motion artifact; using a lightweight sensor also helps. If the digits are used, ask the patient to rest the hand on a flat or secure surface.	
4. Compare and monitor the actual heart rate with the pulse rate value from the oximeter to determine accuracy of values.	The two numeric heart rate values should correlate closely. A difference in heart rate values may indicate excessive movement or a loss of pulsatile flow detection.	- Inability to correlate actual heart rate and pulse rate from oximeter

Documentation

Documentation should include the following:

- Patient and family education
- Indications for use of pulse oximetry
- Patient's pulse with SpO_2 measurements
- Fraction of inspired oxygen delivered (if patient is receiving oxygen)
- Patient clinical assessment at the time of the saturation measurement
- Sensor site
- Simultaneous arterial blood gases (if available)
- Recent hemoglobin measurement (if available)
- Skin assessment at sensor site
- Oximeter alarm settings
- Events precipitating acute desaturation
- Unexpected outcomes
- Nursing interventions

References

1. Chan, M.M. (2003). What is the effect of fingernail polish on pulse oximetry? *Chest,* 123, 2163-4.
2. Chelluri, L., Snyder, J.V., and Bird, J.R. (1991). Accuracy of pulse oximetry in patients with hyperbilirubinemia. *Respir Care,* 36, 1383-6.
3. Grap, M.J. (In press). Pulse oximetry. In: *AACN Protocols for Practice: Technology Series.* Aliso Viejo, CA: American Association of Critical-Care Nurses.
4. Grap, M.J. (1998). Pulse oximetry. *Crit Care Nurse,* 18:94-9.
5. Hanowell, L., Eisele, J.H., and Downs, D. (1987). Ambient light affects pulse oximeters. *Anesthesiology,* 67, 864-5.
6. Jubran, A. (1990). Reliability of pulse oximetry in titrating supplemental oxygen therapy in ventilator-dependent patients. *Chest,* 97, 1420-5.
7. Kelleher, J.F. (1989). Pulse oximetry. *J Clin Monit,* 5, 37-62.
8. McConnell, E.A. (1999). Performing pulse oximetry. *Nursing 99,* 11, 17.
9. Robertson, R.E., and Kaplan, R.F. (1991). Another site for the pulse oximeter probe. *Anesthesiology,* 74, 198.
10. Rutherford, K.A. (1989). Principles and application of pulse oximetry. *Crit Care Nurs Clin Am,* 1, 649-57.
11. Siegel, M.N., and Garvenstein, N. (1987). Preventing ambient light from affecting pulse oximetry. *Anesthesiology,* 67, 280.
12. Soubani, A.O. (2001). Noninvasive monitoring of oxygen and carbon dioxide. *Am J Emerg Med,* 19, 141-6.
13. Szarlarski, N.L., and Cohen, N.H. (1989). Use of pulse oximetry in critically ill adults. *Heart Lung,* 18, 444-53.
14. Zablocki, A.D., and Rasch, D.K. (1987). A simple method to prevent interference with pulse oximetry by infrared heating lamps. *Anesth Analg,* 66, 915.

Additional Readings

Attin, M., et al. (2002). An educational project to improve knowledge related to pulse oximetry. *Am J Crit Care,* 11, 529-34.

Clark, A.P. (2002). Legal lessons: "But his O_2 sat was normal!" *Clin Nurse Specialist,* 16, 162-3.

Seguin, P., et al. (2000). Evidence for the need of bedside accuracy of pulse oximetry in an intensive care unit. *Crit Care Med,* 28, 703-6.

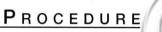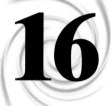

PROCEDURE **16**

Pronation Therapy

P U R P O S E : The prone position may be used in conjunction with other supportive strategies in an attempt to improve oxygenation in patients with acute lung injury or acute respiratory distress syndrome (ARDS). The position also may be used for mobilization of secretions as a postural drainage technique, posterior wound management that allows excellent visualization and management of the site, relief of pressure in the sacral region, positioning for operative or diagnostic procedures, and therapeutic sleep for critically ill patients who normally sleep on their abdomen at home.

Kathleen M. Vollman

PREREQUISITE NURSING KNOWLEDGE

- Prone positioning is used as an adjunct short-term, supportive therapy in an attempt to improve gas exchange in a critically ill patient with severely compromised lungs. Based on more recent studies and a systematic review of the literature, greater than 70% of all acute respiratory distress syndrome patients studied responded to prone positioning with a 20% increase in partial pressure of arterial oxygen (Pao_2) or an increase in Pao_2-to-fraction of inspired oxygen (Fio_2) ratio greater than 20% within 2 hours of the turn.[3-5,7,8,12,17-19,23] To enhance an understanding of how prone positioning may affect gas exchange, it is important to understand the factors that influence the distribution of ventilation and perfusion within the lung.

- *Distribution of ventilation:* Regional pleural pressures and local lung compliance jointly determine the volume of air distributed regionally throughout the lungs. Three major factors—gravity and weight of the lung, compliance, and heterogeneously diseased lungs—influence regional distribution. In an upright individual, the pleural pressure next to the diaphragm is less negative than at the pleural apices. The weight of the lung and the effect of gravity on the lung and its supporting structures in the upright position create this difference in regional pleural pressures. This relationship results in a higher functional residual capacity (FRC) in the nondependent zone or the

apices, redirecting ventilation to the dependent zone.[14,24] When body position changes, there are changes in regional pleural pressures, compliance, and volume distribution. In the supine position, distribution becomes more uniform from apex to base. The ventilation of dependent lung units exceeds that of nondependent lung units, however, and a reduction in FRC is seen.[14,24] The two factors contributing to the reduction in FRC seen when going from the upright to supine position include (1) the pressure of the abdominal contents on the diaphragm[9] and (2) the position of the heart and the relationship of the supporting structures to the lung and its influence on pleural pressure gradients.[16]

- ❖ The first factor to influence pleural pressure, regional volumes, and FRC is the impact of the abdominal contents on the function of the diaphragm. In spontaneously breathing individuals in the supine position, the diaphragm acts as a shield against the pressure exerted by the abdominal contents, preventing the contents from interfering with dependent lung volume distribution. When patients are mechanically ventilated with positive-pressure breaths, sedated, or paralyzed, the active muscle tension in the diaphragm is lost, resulting in a cephalad displacement of the diaphragm and allowing abdominal pressures to decrease dependent lung volume inflation and FRC.[9] The only way to modify this influence is to change the posture to a prone position with the abdomen unsupported.[7,9,19]

- The second factor to influence pleural pressure, regional volumes, and FRC and compliance is the position of the heart and supporting structures. The heart and the diaphragm extend farther dorsally and rest against a rigid spine in the supine position, squeezing the lungs beneath them. This pressure on the lungs generates more positive pleural pressures, resulting in a greater propensity to collapse of the alveoli at end expiration. In the prone position, the heart and upper abdomen rest against the sternum, exerting less weight on the lung tissue. There is less effect on pleural pressure; this leaves the pleural pressures less positive, maintaining open alveoli.[16,19]

- A third factor that contributes to the distribution of volume is heterogeneously or unevenly distributed diseased lung. The acute respiratory distress syndrome lung weight is increased twofold to threefold from normal. The increased weight is due to edema and the resulting hydrostatic forces. A progressive squeezing of gas along a vertical-dorsal axis results. This decrease of regional inflation along the vertical axis results in dependent/dorsal lung collapse. In the prone position, these densities shift. The pattern almost completely reverts toward normal. The inflation gradient is less steep, and the difference results in a more homogeneous regional inflation. This inflation may be related to a redistribution of gas because of the change in hydrostatic forces caused by differences in pleural pressure, as described earlier.[10,11,19]

- *Distribution of perfusion:* Similar to ventilation, regional distribution of perfusion is influenced by three factors— cardiac output, pulmonary vascular resistance, and gravity or body position.

- In an upright individual, blood flow decreases as it moves from base to apex with virtually no flow at the apex. This decrease is caused by the influence of gravity on pulmonary vascular pressures within the lung (Fig. 16-1). In zone 1, near the apex, alveolar pressure exceeds arterial pressure, creating little or no flow. In zone 2, the pulmonary artery pressure exceeds alveolar pressure, which exceeds the venous pressure. Blood flow in this area occurs based on the differences in pressure between the arterial and alveolar. In zone 3, the arterial pressure is greater than the venous pressure, which is greater than the alveolar pressure. In this zone, the influence of the alveolar pressure on blood flow is reduced, resulting in freedom of flow in this region.[24,25] In supine and lateral positions, apical region blood flow changes. There is no real change in basilar units, but a greater dependent versus nondependent blood flow occurs. In the prone position, there is a marked reduction, however, in the gravitational perfusion gradient, suggesting no gravity-dependent benefit to flow in the prone position.[16]

- Based on the current available data as outlined here, it seems that changes in oxygenation may be related to differences in the regional inflation/ventilation of the lung while prone and are not related to a redistribution of blood flow.[9,16,18,19]

- Suggested criteria for use of the prone position include:
  - PaO_2/FIO_2 ratio less than 200 on a FIO_2 greater than 50% with sufficient positive end-expiratory pressure used to recruit alveoli.

- Contraindications and precautions to pronation therapy include the following:[20]
  - Patient unable to tolerate a head-down position
  - Increased intracranial pressure

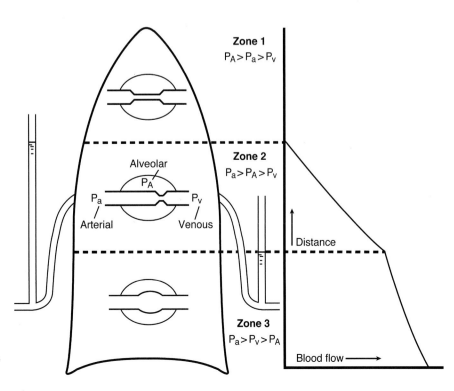

FIGURE 16-1 Zone model of the lung. Three-zone model of the lung is used to explain distribution of blood flow based on pressure variations. *(From West, J.B., Dollery, C.T., and Naimark, A. [1964]. Distribution of blood flow in isolated lung; relation to vascular and alveolar pressures.* J Appl Physiol, *19, 713-24.)*

❖ Unstable spine (unless Stryker Frame® used)
❖ Hemodynamically unstable patient (as defined by a systolic blood pressure less than 90 mm Hg with fluid and vasoactive support in place)
❖ If using a support frame, patient weight greater than 135 kg
❖ Weight 160 kg or greater
❖ Extracoporeal membrane oxygenator cannula placement problems
❖ Open chest/unstable chest wall
❖ Unstable pelvis
❖ Pregnant patient
❖ Bifurcated endotracheal tube

EQUIPMENT

• Pillows or foam blocks
• Four or five staff members
• Lift sheets
or
• Vollman Prone Positioner® (VPP) (Hill-Rom, Inc.) (Fig. 16-2)
• Three staff members (with VPP)
• Resuscitation bag and mask available
Additional equipment (to have available depending on patient need) includes the following:
• Lateral rotation therapy bed with or without prone accessory kit
• Stryker Frame® for use in patients with unstable spines
• Capnography monitor

PATIENT AND FAMILY EDUCATION

• Explain to the patient and family the patient's lung/oxygenation problem and the reason for the use of the prone position. ➤*Rationale:* This explanation decreases patient and family anxiety by providing information and clarification.
• Explain the standard of care to the patient and family, including positioning procedure, perceived benefit,

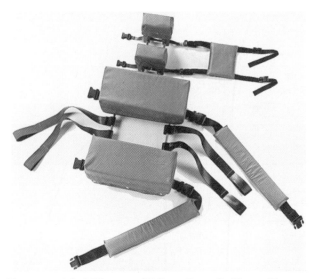

FIGURE 16-2 Diagram of Vollman Prone Positioner. (*From Hill-Rom, Inc.*)

frequency of assessments, expected response, and parameters for discontinuation of the positioning technique and equipment (if special bed or frame is initiated). ➤*Rationale:* This communication provides an opportunity for the patient and family to verbalize concerns or ask questions about the procedure.

PATIENT ASSESSMENT AND PREPARATION

Patient Assessment

• Assess time interval from injury to position change. ➤*Rationale:* A trial of prone positioning should be performed within 48 hours in the course of acute lung injury to assess the patient's level of response. A response is defined by a PaO_2/FIO_2 ratio greater than 20% or a PaO_2 greater than 10 mm Hg.[19] If initial positioning does not elicit a positive response, however, this should not rule out periodic attempts to assess the patient's responsiveness throughout the course of lung injury. Response to severe position change has been noted at all stages of acute lung injury.
• Assess hemodynamic status of the patient to identify ability to tolerate a position change. ➤*Rationale:* Imbalances between oxygen supply and demand must be addressed before the pronation procedure to offset any increases in oxygen demand that may be created by the physical turning. The final decision to place a hemodynamically unstable patient prone rests with the physician or advanced practice nurse, who must weigh the risks against the potential benefits of using the prone position.
• Assess mental status before use of the prone position. ➤*Rationale:* Agitation—whether caused by delirium, anxiety, or pain—can have a negative effect when using the prone position. Nevertheless, agitation is not a contraindication for use of the prone position. The health care team should strive to manage the agitation effectively to provide a safe environment for the use of the prone position.
• Assess size and weight load, to determine the ability to turn within the narrow critical care bed frame and to weigh the potential risk of injury to the health care worker. ➤*Rationale:* When turning a patient prone in a hospital bed, with or without a frame, one must determine whether a 180-degree turn can be accomplished within the confines of the space available. Critical care bed frames are narrow, making it difficult to complete the turn on patients who weigh more than 160 kg. The team must consider the potential for injury to the health care workers when making the decision to turn morbidly obese patients prone.

Patient Preparation

• Ensure that the patient understands preprocedural teaching. Answer questions as they arise and reinforce information as needed. ➤*Rationale:* This communication evaluates and reinforces understanding of previously taught information.
• Assessment of agitation with a reliable scale and appropriate management before, during, and after the turn are key to accomplishing a safe procedure.

- Turn off the tube feeding 1 hour before the prone position turn. ➤*Rationale:* This assists with gastric emptying and reduces the risk of aspiration during the turning procedure.[22]
- Before positioning the patient prone, the following care activities should be performed. ➤*Rationale:* These activities prevent areas of pressure and potential breakdown; avoid complications related to injury or accidental extubation; and promote the delivery of comprehensive care before, during, and after the pronation therapy.
  - ❖ Remove electrocardiogram leads from the anterior chest wall.
  - ❖ Perform eye care including lubrication and taping of the eyelids closed in a horizontal fashion.
  - ❖ Ensure the tongue is inside the patient's mouth. If the tongue is swollen or protruding, insert a bite-block.
  - ❖ Ensure the tape/ties of the endotracheal tube or tracheotomy tube are secure. Changing of the ties may be required on return to the supine position if not secure. If adhesive tape is used to secure the endotracheal tube, double taping or wrapping completely around the head is recommended because increased salivary drainage occurs in the prone position and may loosen the adhesive.[1,6]
  - ❖ If a wound dressing on the anterior body is due to be changed during the prone position sequence, perform the dressing change before the turn. If saturated on return from the prone position, the dressing needs to be changed.
  - ❖ Empty ileostomy/colostomy bags before positioning.
  - ❖ Capnography monitoring is suggested to help ensure proper positioning of the tube during the turning procedure and while in the prone position.

Procedure for Manual Pronation Therapy

Steps	Rationale	Special Considerations
1. Wash hands, and don personal protective equipment.	Reduces risk of transmission of microorganisms and body secretions; standard precautions.	If using the frame, ensure it has been cleaned with an appropriate hospital-approved disinfectant.
2. Ensure that emergency equipment is available.	In the event of an emergency (i.e., accidental extubation or hemodynamic instability), having equipment available allows for rapid patient stabilization.	
3. Place a lift sheet under the patient to assist with turning.	A lift sheet allows for the use of correct body alignment during the turning procedure.	A lift sheet is unnecessary if the patient is on a low air-loss surface and a support frame is being used.
4. Without a frame: Two staff members are positioned on each side of the bed, with another staff member positioned at the head of the bed. **Proceed to Step 6.**	Four to five individuals are required to position a patient safely prone without a frame. Additional personnel may be required, based on the size of the patient.[1,6]	The individual at the head of the bed is responsible for monitoring the stability and position of the endotracheal tube (ETT), ventilator tubing, and monitoring/intravenous lines located by the patient's head. For increased airway security, the individual at the head of the bed should hold the ETT during the turn.
5. With a frame: One staff member is positioned on either side of the bed, with another staff member positioned at the head of the bed. (*Level IV: Limited clinical studies to support recommendations.*)	Three staff members are required for the turn; two perform the actual lifting and turning, and the third is positioned at the head of the bed.[20,23]	
6. Correctly position all tubes and invasive lines.	All intravenous tubing and invasive lines are adjusted to prevent kinking, disconnection, or contact with the body during the turning procedure and while the patient remains in the prone position.	If the patient is in skeletal traction, one individual needs to apply traction to the leg while the lines and weights are removed for the turn. If a skeletal pin comes in contact with the bed, a pillow needs to be placed in the correct position to alleviate pressure points.

Procedure continues on the following page

Procedure **for Manual Pronation Therapy**—*Continued*

Steps	Rationale	Special Considerations
A. Lines inserted in the upper torso are aligned with either shoulder, and the excess tubing is placed at the head of the bed. The only exception to this rule is for chest tubes.	Disconnecting lines before the turn may help to prevent dislodgment, but places the patient at an increased risk for infection.	
B. Chest tubes and lines or tubes placed in the lower torso are aligned with either leg and extend off the end of the bed.	Consider adding an extension tube to lines that are too short to be placed at the head of bed or the end of the bed.	
C. If the patient has an open abdomen, cover with a synthetic material before positioning, and identify a positioning strategy that allows the abdomen to be free of restriction.	Open abdomens are not a contraindication for use of the prone position. A cover employing a synthetic material and a support such as an abdominal binder may be used effectively to secure the abdomen.[15]	
7. If on a low air-loss surface, maximally inflate.	Maximally inflating the air surface firms up the mattress, making it easier to perform the turn.	
8. Always turn the patient in the direction of the mechanical ventilator.	These maneuvers are performed to prevent disconnection of the ventilator tubing or kinking of the ETT during the turning procedure.[20,23]	
A. Turn the patient's head so that it is facing away from the ventilator. Without disconnecting the ventilator tubing from the endotracheal tube, place the portion of the tubing extending out from the endotracheal tube on the side of the patient's face that is turned away from the ventilator.		
B. Loop the remaining ventilator tubing above the patient's head (Fig. 16-3). (*Level IV: Limited clinical studies to support recommendations.*)		
9. If a frame is used, the straps, which secure the positioner to the body, are placed under the patient's head, chest (axillary area), and pelvic region at this time.		
Placing Chest/Pelvic Support or the Vollman Prone Positioner®		
1. When turning prone without a frame and using the abdomen-unrestricted position, gather pillows at this time for manual placement under the head, upper chest, and pelvic region at a later phase in the procedure.	For lateral rotation beds with a prone position accessory kit, follow manufacturer's instructions for preparing air cushions for the prone position.	

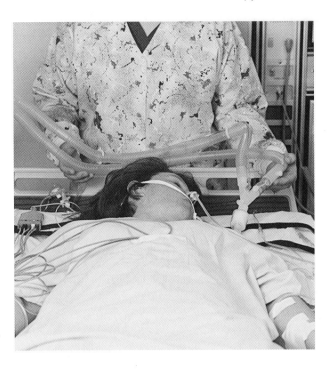

FIGURE 16-3 Positioning of ventilator tubing.
(From Hill-Rom, Inc.)

Procedure **for Manual Pronation Therapy**—*Continued*		
Steps	**Rationale**	**Special Considerations**
2. If using the VPP: Attach the frame to the patient while in the supine position. Lay the frame gently on top of the patient. Align the chest piece to rest between the clavicle and sixth rib. *(Level IV: Limited clinical studies to support recommendations.)*	The chest piece is the only nonmovable part and serves as the marker piece for proper placement and alignment of the device.[20,23]	
3. Adjust the pelvic piece to rest 1/2 inch above the iliac crest. *(Level IV: Limited clinical studies to support recommendations.)*	This prevents direct pressure over bony prominences and provides sufficient distance between the chest and pelvis to allow the abdomen to be free of restriction, while preventing bowing of the back.[20,23]	
4. Adjust the forehead and chin pieces to provide full facial support in a face-down or a side-lying position without interfering with the endotracheal tube.		If the patient has limited neck range of motion or a short neck, the face-down position is optimal. Because it is difficult to readjust the head to relieve pressure points, it is recommended to move both headpieces up to the top of the frame. Only the head cushion supports the forehead, and the chin is suspended to reduce the risk of skin breakdown from pressure.
5. Fasten the positioner to the patient using the soft adjustable straps. As the straps are tightened, the cushions compress. When fastened, lift the positioner to assess whether a secure fit has been obtained. Readjust as	If the device is not secured tightly before the turn, the patient may develop shear/friction injuries on the chest and pelvic area during the turning process.	When the device is secured correctly, it appears uncomfortable and possibly painful. As a result, the practitioner has a tendency not to fasten the device as tightly as is needed to prevent injury.

Procedure continues on the following page

Procedure	for Manual Pronation Therapy—*Continued*	
Steps	**Rationale**	**Special Considerations**
necessary. (*Level I: Manufacturer's recommendation only.*)		When secured correctly, the device creates a feeling of pressure and a sense of security for the patient during the turning process.
Turning Prone Using the Half-Step Technique 1. Using a draw sheet, move the patient to the edge of the bed farthest away from the ventilator in preparation for the prone turn. The individual closest to the patient maintains body contact with the bed at all times, serving as a side rail to ensure a safe environment. (*Level IV: Limited clinical studies to support recommendations.*)	Provides sufficient room to rotate the body safely 180 degrees within the confines of a narrow critical care bed.[20,23]	
2. Turning without a frame: Ensure there is a bottom sheet under the patient. Tuck arms slightly under the buttock. Place a sheet over the patient.[1] A. Nurses on both sides of the bed take the top and bottom sheets and roll them together tightly toward the patient. B. Slide the patient over to the edge of the mattress away from the ventilator (Fig. 16-4). C. Tilt the patient fully onto his or her side. The patient can be placed in the abdomen-unrestricted position at this time by inserting pillows under the head, chest, and pelvic region (see Fig. 16-4).	It is important to use a wide base of support to improve balance and prevent self-injury during the turning procedure.	

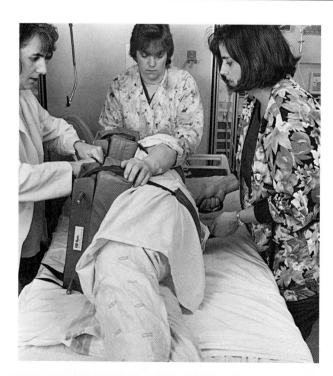

FIGURE 16-4 Turning patient prone on Vollman Prone Positioner.

Procedure for Manual Pronation Therapy—*Continued*		
Steps	**Rationale**	**Special Considerations**
D. Using a three count, the patient is rolled using the sheets into a prone position. The staff member at the head of the bed supports the head during the turn, while ensuring that all tubes and lines are secure (see Fig. 16-4).		
3. Gently rotate the arms parallel to the body, then flex them into a position of comfort so that they are lying adjacent to the head. Minor adjustments of the patient's body may be necessary to obtain correct alignment when in the prone position, whether using a frame or not.		Many patients have range-of-motion limitations to the shoulder area that may make it difficult to keep the arms in a flexed position. There are many ways to position the arms for comfort. The arms can be left in a side-lying position, aligned with the body, or one up and one down, similar to a swimmer position.
4. Turning with the VPP: A. Tuck the straps on the bar located between the chest and pelvic piece underneath the patient. B. Tuck the patient's arm and hand that now rest in the center of the bed under the buttocks, after position alignment with the edge of the mattress is achieved. C. Cross the leg closest to the edge of the bed over the opposite leg at the ankle. *(Level IV: Limited clinical studies to support recommendations.)*	Helps with forward motion when the turning process begins.[20,23]	
5. Turn the patient to a 45-degree angle toward the ventilator. A. The staff member on the ventilator side of the bed grips the upper steel bar. B. The staff member on the opposite side of the bed grasps the straps attached to the lower steel bar. C. Using a three count, lift the patient by the frame into a prone position. D. During the turning procedure, the staff member at the head of the bed ensures that all tubes and lines are secure and patent (see Fig. 16-4). *(Level IV: Limited clinical studies to support recommendations.)*	It is extremely important to use a wide base of support to improve balance and prevent self-injury during the turning procedure.[20,23]	
6. With the VPP: Loosen the straps at this time. If the patient is unstable, it is recommended to keep the straps fastened securely to facilitate a safe, quick return to the supine position in the event of an emergency (see Fig. 16-5).	The procedure for returning to the supine position takes less than 1 minute if the straps are fastened and a support frame is used.	

Procedure continues on the following page

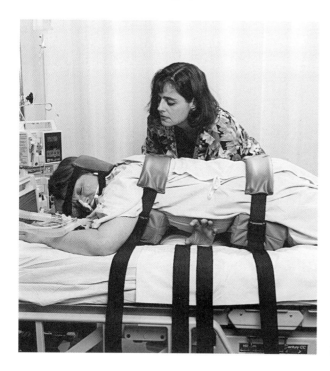

FIGURE 16-5 Patient lying prone on Vollman Prone Positioner. *(From Hill-Rom, Inc.)*

Procedure | for Manual Pronation Therapy—*Continued*

Steps	Rationale	Special Considerations
7. If on a low air-loss surface, release the maximal inflation.	A return to normal pressures on the surface helps to alleviate pressure at various bony prominences while in the prone position.	If on a standard hospital mattress, the thigh-knee-calf area must be supported to minimize the risk of pressure injury and prevent discomfort.
8. Place a support or other pillow under the ankle area.	A support in this area allows for correct body alignment and prevents tension on the tendons in the foot and ankle region.	If the patient is tall enough, dangling the feet over the edge of the mattress may be a sufficient alternative to support the ankles and feet in correct alignment.
Returning to the Supine Position 9. Align the patient with the edge of the mattress closest to the ventilator.		The patient would be turning toward the center of the mattress, away from the ventilator.
10. Arrange the ventilator tubing to provide sufficient mobility and length to prevent pulling during the turning procedure.	The staff member at the head of the bed is responsible for monitoring placement of the ventilator tubing, monitoring wires, and invasive lines.	
11. Straighten the patient's arms from a flexed position and bring them to rest on either side of the head. Remove leg and ankle pillow supports. If on a low air-loss surface, maximally inflate.		
12. Cross the leg closest to the edge of the bed over the opposite leg at the ankle.		

Procedure for Manual Pronation Therapy—*Continued*

Steps	Rationale	Special Considerations
13. Without a frame: Turn the patient to a 45-degree angle using the lift sheet and the patient's body, then roll the patient onto his or her back.	Lifting and realignment in the center of the bed may be necessary when returning to the supine position if a support frame is not used.	
14. Stretch the arms parallel to the body and bring them into a downward position.		
15. With the VPP: Fasten the straps tightly before repositioning.		
16. Turn the patient to a 45-degree angle using the steel bars, then roll the patient onto his or her back (Fig. 16-6).	The steel bars on the positioning frame allow lifting as the patient is realigned into the center of the bed.	
17. Unfasten the positioner, and remove from the patient. The straps may be left under the patient in preparation for the next turn.		

Expected Outcomes

- Increased oxygenation
- Improved secretion clearance
- Improved compliance of the lungs and alveolar recruitment

Unexpected Outcomes

- Agitation
- Disconnection or dislodgment of tubes and lines
- Peripheral arm nerve injury
- Periorbital and conjunctival edema
- Skin injuries or pressure ulcers
- Eye pressure

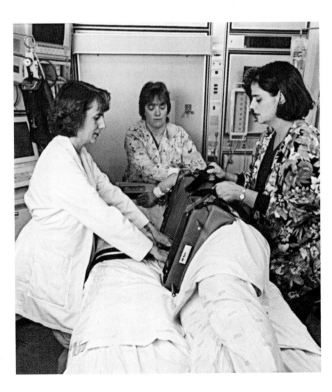

FIGURE 16-6 Patient returning to supine position. *(From Hill-Rom, Inc.)*

Patient Monitoring and Care

Steps	Rationale	Reportable Conditions
		These conditions should be reported if they persist despite nursing interventions.
1. Assess patient's tolerance to the turning procedure: • Respiratory rate and effort • Heart rate and blood pressure	Oxygen saturation is not used as a measure of intolerance to the turning procedure because patients often experience desaturation with a deep lateral turn; however, if the patient responds to the prone position, he or she stabilizes quickly when settled into the prone position. The lateral-turn decrease in oxygen saturation may deter the health care team from trying the prone position. If respiratory rate and effort, heart rate, and blood pressure do not return to normal within 10 minutes of the turn, the patient may be displaying initial signs of intolerance.[21,26]	• Failure of the respiratory rate, respiratory effort, heart rate, and blood pressure to return to normal 5 to 10 minutes after the turn
2. Assess the patient's response to the prone position: • Pulse oximetry (SpO_2) • Mixed venous oxygenation saturation (SvO_2) and hemodynamics • Arterial blood gases 30 minutes after position change • PaO_2/FIO_2 ratio	Of all acute lung injury patients turned prone, greater than 70% improved their oxygenation.[3-5,7,8,12,17,18,23] A response is defined by a PaO_2/FIO_2 ratio of greater than 20% or a PaO_2 greater than 10 mm Hg.[19] The time response varies among patients. Some patients immediately respond, whereas others may take 6 hours to show maximal response to the position change. Hemodynamic measurements are accurate in the prone position compared with supine as long as the zero reference point is calibrated at the phlebostatic axis.[22]	• Decrease from baseline in the SpO_2 or failure of the SvO_2 to return to baseline after 5 to 10 minutes.
3. Reposition the patient's head on an hourly basis while in the prone position to prevent facial breakdown. While one staff member lifts the patient's head, a second staff member moves the headpieces to provide support for the head in a different position.	The face and ears have minimal structural padding to reduce the risk of skin breakdown. Patients with short necks or limited neck range of motion have difficulty assuming a head side-lying position. These patients are more likely to develop facial breakdown, making it necessary to turn the patient more frequently to prevent breakdown or to use the technique described in procedure **Step 4, Special Considerations.**	• Skin breakdown
4. Assess skin frequently for areas of nonblanchable redness or breakdown. Place a hydrocolloid dressing over areas where shearing and friction injuries are likely to occur (i.e., chest, pelvis, elbows, and knees). *(Level I: Manufacturer's recommendation only.)*	Greater than 2 hours on a standard surface without changing position increases a patient's risk for breakdown. If on a pressure-reduction surface, the time remaining in a stationary position can be lengthened. The use of a hydrocolloid may serve as a protective barrier, reducing the risk of shearing and friction injuries.[6,13] If using the VPP and a skin injury occurs on the chest or pelvis, reassess tightness of the device before the	• Nonblanchable redness • Shearing and friction injuries

Patient Monitoring and Care—*Continued*

Steps	Rationale	Reportable Conditions
	prone position turn. The injury is most likely related to a loose-fitting apparatus.	
5. Provide frequent oral care and suctioning of the airway as needed.	The prone position promotes postural drainage through the natural use of gravity. Drainage from the nares may be a clinical sign of an undetected sinus infection.	• Drainage from the nares • Change in amount or character of secretions
6. Maintain tube feeding as tolerated.	The risk for aspiration is minimal in the prone position because the patient is already in a head-down, side-lying position that maximizes the use of gravity to move vomited matter safely. A reverse Trendelenburg position changes that relationship and increases the risk of aspiration.[22]	• Evidence of tube feeding material when suctioning
7. Scheduling frequency: The positioning schedule is based on whether the patient is able to sustain improvements in PaO_2 made while in the prone position. A schedule of every 6 hours in the prone position is suggested.[18] Time spent in the supine position is based on the length of time the patient is able to sustain or maintain the improvement in gas exchange that occurred while prone. • If the patient maintains the improvement in PaO_2 when repositioned supine, the patient can remain in the supine to lateral position for a maximum of 4 to 6 hours or return to the prone position when or if a decrease in PaO_2 is seen. *(Level V: Clinical studies in more than one patient population and situation.)* • If the patient is unable to maintain the improvement in gas exchange seen with the prone position when returned to a supine position, the patient should remain in the supine/lateral position for only 1 hour before being repositioned prone. • The use of the prone position is discontinued when the patient no longer shows a positive response to the position change.	Without a clear direction from the literature on frequency of position change, the health care team must weigh other physiologic factors when a patient remains in a stationary position for an extended period. Following the principles of pressure relief used when positioning patients laterally or supine can minimize the potential for skin injury and edema formation. Longer time spent in a single position requires that the support surface provide greater pressure reduction or relief than a standard hospital mattress. Combining the literature on the prone position and surface interface pressure, a safe suggestion for frequency of repositioning is between 4 and 6 hours.[3-5,7,8,12,13,17,18,21,23] It is suggested to use lateral rotation therapy in conjunction with prone positioning so that when the patient is returned to a supine position, he or she is laterally rotated. The use of continuous lateral rotation therapy has been associated with a reduction in pulmonary complications.[2,21] The literature has not clearly identified when the use of prone positioning should be discontinued. One suggestion for discontinuation is when the patient's PaO_2/FIO_2 ratio is greater than 200 on less than 50% FIO_2 and less than or equal to 10 cm of H_2O of positive end-expiratory pressure.	• Clinically significant decreases in oxygenation (greater than 10 mm Hg) or oxygen saturation (less than 88%)

Documentation

Documentation should include the following:

- Patient and family education
- Ability to tolerate the turning procedure
- Length of time in the prone position
- Maximal oxygenation response while in the prone position
- Oxygenation response when returned to the supine position
- Positioning schedule used

- Complications noted during or after the procedure
- Use of continuous lateral rotation therapy
- Amount and type of secretions
- Unexpected outcomes
- Nursing interventions

References

1. Balas, M.C. (2000). Prone positioning of patients with acute respiratory distress syndrome: Applying research to practice. *Crit Care Nurse, 20*, 24-36.
2. Basham, K.R., Vollman, K.M., and Miller, A. (1997). To everything turn turn turn: An overview of continuous lateral rotation therapy. *Respir Care Clin North Am, 3*, 109-34.
3. Brussel, T., et al. (1993). Mechanical ventilation in the prone position for acute respiratory failure after cardiac surgery. *J Cardiothorac Vasc Anesth, 7*, 541-6.
4. Chatte, G., et al. (1997). Prone position in mechanically ventilated patients with severe acute respiratory failure. *Am J Respir Crit Care Med, 155*, 473-8.
5. Curley, M.A.Q. (1999). Prone positioning of patients with acute respiratory distress syndrome: A systematic review. *Am J of Crit Care, 8*, 397-405.
6. Dirkes, S.M., and Dickinson, S.P. (1998). Common questions about prone positioning for ARDS. *AJN, 98*, 16-JJ-NN.
7. Douglas, W.W., et al. (1977). Improved oxygenation in patients with acute respiratory failure: The prone position. *Am Rev Respir Dis, 115*, 559-66.
8. Fridrich, P., et al. (1996). The effects of long-term prone positioning in patients with trauma induced adult respiratory distress syndrome. *Anesth Analg, 83*, 1206-11.
9. Froese, A.B., and Bryan, A.C. (1974). Effects of anesthesia and paralysis on diaphragmatic mechanics in man. *Anesthesiology, 41*, 242-55.
10. Gattinoni, L., et al. (1988). Relationships between lung computed tomographic density, gas exchange and PEEP in acute respiratory failure. *Anesthesiology, 69*, 824-32.
11. Gattinoni, L., et al. (1991). Body position changes redistribute lung computed tomographic density in patients with acute respiratory failure. *Anesthesiology, 74*, 15-23.
12. Gattinoni, L., et al. (2001). Effect of prone positioning on the survival of patients with acute respiratory failure. *N Engl J Med, 345*, 568-73.
13. Glavis, C., and Barbara, S. (1990). Pressure ulcer prevention in critical care: State of the art. *AACN Clin Issues, 1*, 602-13.
14. Kaneko, K., et al. (1966). Regional distribution of ventilation and perfusion as a function of body position. *J Appl Physiol, 21*, 767-77.
15. Murray, T.A., and Patterson, L.A. (2002). Prone positioning of trauma patients with acute respiratory distress syndrome and open abdominal incisions. *Crit Care Nurse, 22*, 52-6.
16. Mutoh, T., et al. (1992). Prone position alters the effect of volume overload on regional pleural pressures and improves hypoxemia in pigs in vivo. *Am Rev Respir Dis, 146*, 300-6.
17. Pappert, D., et al. (1994). Influence of positioning on ventilation-perfusion relationships in severe adult respiratory distress syndrome. *Chest, 106*, 1511-6.
18. Pelosi, P., et al. (1998). Effects of the prone position on respiratory mechanics and gas exchange during acute lung injury. *Am J Respir Crit Care Med, 157*, 387-93.
19. Pelosi, P., Brazzi, L., and Gattinoni, L. (2002). Prone position in ARDS. *Eur Respir J, 20*, 1017-28.
20. Vollman, K.M. (1989). *The effect of suspended prone positioning on PaO_2 and A-a gradients in adult patients with acute respiratory failure.* Masters Thesis, California State University, Long Beach.
21. Vollman, K.M. (1997). Prone positioning for the ARDS patients. *Dimen Crit Care Nurs, 16*, 184-93.
22. Vollman, K.M. (2001). What are the practice guidelines for prone positioning of acutely ill patients? Specifically, what are the recommendations related to hemodynamic monitoring and tube feeding? *Crit Care Nurse, 21*, 84-6.
23. Vollman, K.M., and Bander, J.J. (1996). Improved oxygenation utilizing a prone positioner in patients with acute respiratory distress syndrome. *Intensive Care Med, 22*, 1105-11.
24. West, J.B. (1985). *Respiratory Physiology: The Essentials.* 3rd ed. Baltimore: Williams & Wilkins, 11-66.
25. West, J.B., Dollery, C.T., and Naimark, A. (1964). Distribution of blood flow in isolated lung: Relation to vascular and alveolar pressures. *J Appl Physiol, 19*, 713-24.
26. Winslow, E.H., et al. (1990). Effects of a lateral turn on mixed venous oxygen saturation and heart rate in critically ill adults. *Heart Lung, 19*, 555-61.

Additional Readings

Albert, R.E., et al. (1987). The prone position improves arterial oxygenation and reduces shunt in oleic acid induced acute lung injury. *Am Rev Respir Dis, 135*, 628-33.

Ball, C. (1999). Use of prone positioning in the management of acute respiratory distress syndrome. *Clin Effectiveness Nurs, 3*, 36-46.

Breiburg, A.N., et al. (2000). Efficacy and safety of prone positioning for patients with acute respiratory distress syndrome. *J Adv Nurs, 32*, 922-9.

Bryan, A.C., et al. (1964). Factors affecting regional distribution of ventilation and perfusion in the lung. *J Appl Physiol, 19*, 395-402.

Goettler, C.E., Pryor, J.P., and Reilly, P.M. (2002). Brachial plexopathy after prone positioning. *Crit Care Forum, 6*, 1-6.

Johannigman, J.A., et al. (2000). Prone positioning for acute respiratory distress syndrome in the surgical intensive care unit: Who, when and how long? *Surgery, 128*, 708-16.

Langer, M., et al. (1988). The prone position in ARDS patients: A clinical study. *Chest, 91*, 103-7.

Vollman, K.M., and Aulbach, R.K. (1998). Acute respiratory distress syndrome. In: Kinney, M.G., et al., editors. *AACN Clinical Reference for Critical Care Nursing.* 4th ed. St. Louis: Mosby, 529-64.

Wiener, C.M., Kir, W., and Albert, R.K. (1990). Prone position reverses gravitational distribution of perfusion in dog lungs with oleic acid induced injury. *J Appl Physiol, 68*, 1386-92.

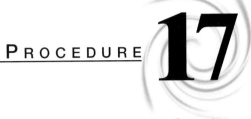
SECTION THREE

Thoracic Cavity
Management

Autotransfusion

P U R P O S E : Autotransfusion is the collection and filtration of blood from an active bleeding site and reinfusion of that blood into the same patient for the maintenance of blood volume.

Julianne M. Scott

PREREQUISITE NURSING KNOWLEDGE

- Understanding of transfusion and intravenous therapy and fluid balance is necessary.
- Autotransfusion is commonly used for trauma victims and for patients undergoing cardiovascular and orthopedic procedures, reducing the need for banked blood transfusions and the risk of transfusion reactions and disease transmission.
- A variety of autotransfusion devices are available. An autotransfusion system may be a standard water-seal chest drainage system (see Fig. 22-1A), a separate autotransfusion setup, or a modified chest drainage autotransfusion system. In addition, continuous and intermittent systems are available. A continuous system has an intravenous line connected directly from the drainage unit collection chamber to the patient. An intermittent system uses a blood collection bag in-line between the chest tube and the collection chamber.
- Many disposable systems available today have the ability to act as a reservoir for autotransfusion if the need arises. To initiate autotransfusion, the autotransfusion bag is disconnected from the disposable system and connected to the saline-filled blood administration tubing. Nurses should gain familiarity with their institution's autotransfusion system.
- Indications for autotransfusion in the appropriate patient populations include active bleeding (greater than 100 ml/hr) and the accumulation of greater than 300 ml of drainage in the collection chamber.
- Contraindications to autotransfusion include the following:
  - ❖ Active infection or contamination of shed blood
  - ❖ Malignant cells in shed blood
  - ❖ Renal or hepatic insufficiency

- ❖ Established coagulopathies
- ❖ Blood that has been in the autotransfusion system for longer than institutional standards allow
- Any contraindications to autotransfusion are overruled in the presence of exsanguinating hemorrhage in the absence of an adequate supply of banked blood.
- As with banked blood, patients may refuse to receive blood based on their religious beliefs.
- Informed consent should be obtained in nonemergency situations.

EQUIPMENT

- Personal protective equipment
- Autotransfusion collection system
- Autotransfusion system replacement bag
- Blood administration set
- 40-mcg microemboli filter
- Normal saline (NS)

PATIENT AND FAMILY EDUCATION

- Explain procedure to the patient, if appropriate, and the family, including the risks and benefits of using the patient's own blood. ➥*Rationale:* Information enhances patient and family understanding and decreases anxiety.

PATIENT ASSESSMENT AND PREPARATION

Patient Assessment
- Signs and symptoms of hypovolemia and associated hypoperfusion include the following:
  - ❖ Pale, clammy skin
  - ❖ Hypotension

❖ Tachycardia

❖ Dyspnea

❖ Decreased central venous pressure, pulmonary artery pressure, or pulmonary artery wedge pressure

❖ Decreased cardiac output or index

❖ Oliguria

❖ Decreased hemoglobin or hematocrit

➺*Rationale:* Significant blood loss, related systemic hypoperfusion, and the associated decrease in oxygen-carrying capacity, with its impact on hypoxemia, often require the replacement of blood with whole blood or packed cells. In appropriate patient populations (trauma, cardiovascular, or orthopedic surgical patients), autotransfusion should be considered as the need to replace blood becomes apparent.

Patient Preparation

• Ensure that the patient understands preprocedural teaching. Answer questions as they arise, and reinforce information as needed. ➺*Rationale:* This communication evaluates and reinforces understanding of previously taught information.

Procedure for Autotransfusion		
Steps	**Rationale**	**Special Considerations**
1. Wash hands, and don personal protective equipment.	Decreases the transmission of microorganisms; standard precautions.	
2. Assemble equipment.		
3. Set up autotransfusion unit. (See manufacturer's instructions.)	Suction is required to drain blood into drainage unit.	
4. If instructed by manufacturer's recommendations, inject anticoagulant into the autotransfusion bag before collecting blood from the patient. (*Level II: Theory based, no research data to support recommendations: recommendations from expert consensus group may exist.*)	Several different anticoagulants may be used. Citrate phosphate dextrose is commonly used (1 ml per 7 ml blood).[1,2]	Use of anticoagulants is controversial.
5. Connect the patient's drainage or chest tube to the collection bag directly or via a water-seal setup.	Allows for collection of shed blood in preparation for autotransfusion.	Although autotransfusion is often performed with blood drained from the thoracic cavity, it also can be done after orthopedic procedures.
6. Before disconnecting the filled collection bag for patient infusion, a new collection system should be prepared.	Allows for the collection of additional blood and keeping the system closed and sterile.	
7. Clamp the tubes (attached to the tubing by the manufacturer) on the new collection bag.	Clamping eliminates the risk of air entering the system.	
8. Close the clamp on the patient drainage tubing.	Stops further drainage into the bag.	
9. If the collection bag is part of the water-seal system (see Fig. 22-1), close the clamps on the tubing connected to the water-seal drainage unit.	Prepares the system for disconnection.	
10. Disconnect the filled bag from the patient system, maintaining sterility at all times.		
11. Take the previously prepared new collection bag; attach it to the water-seal unit or to the patient's chest tube or drainage tube.	Allows for continued collection of blood.	

Procedure for Autotransfusion—*Continued*

Steps	Rationale	Special Considerations
12. Ensure that all connections are secure; open clamps on autotransfusion bag and patient drainage tubing.	Connections must be secured to create suction for drainage.	
13. Prime the blood administration tubing with NS. Connect filled collection bag to blood administration set with microfilter. *(Level II: Theory based, no research data to support recommendations: recommendations from expert consensus group may exist.)*	Filters should be used to reduce the danger of microembolization.[1,2] Do not apply pressure or use with pressure device when transfusing.	A 40-mcg filter is commonly used for autotransfusion.
14. Initiate infusion as prescribed (see Procedure 121).	Restores blood volume.	Reinfuse blood within 6 hours (if stored at room temperature) of collection.[1]
15. Repeat procedure as needed.		
16. Discard disposable supplies with blood in infectious waste.	Prevent exposure to blood; standard precautions.	

Expected Outcomes

- Patient infused with own blood in a timely manner
- Improved hemoglobin and hematocrit
- Improved oxygenation through increased oxygen-carrying capacity of blood
- Hemodynamic stability

Unexpected Outcomes

- Blood transfusion reaction
- Fluid overload

Patient Monitoring and Care

Steps	Rationale	Reportable Conditions
		These conditions should be reported if they persist despite nursing interventions.
1. Assess cardiopulmonary status and vital signs in 15 minutes, then hourly until 1 hour after the transfusion is completed (see Procedure 121).	Provides baseline and ongoing assessment of patient's condition.	• Tachypnea • Decreased or absent breath sounds • Hypoxemia • Tracheal deviation • Subcutaneous emphysema • Neck vein distention • Muffled heart tones • Tachycardia • Hypotension • Dysrhythmias • Fever
2. Evaluate and maintain drainage tube patency every 2 to 4 hours.	In chest tubes, obstruction of drainage interferes with lung reexpansion.	• Inability to establish patency
3. Monitor amount and type of drainage from collection system hourly for 8 hours, then every 2 hours.	Volume loss can cause patients to become hypovolemic. Decreased or absent drainage associated with respiratory distress	• Bloody drainage greater than 200 ml/hr • New onset of clots • Sudden decrease or absence of drainage

Procedure continues on the following page

Patient Monitoring and Care—*Continued*

Steps	Rationale	Reportable Conditions
	may indicate obstruction; decreased or absent drainage without respiratory distress may indicate lung reexpansion.	
4. Mark the drainage level on the outside of the drainage-collection chamber in hourly or shift increments, and document in patient record.	Provides reference point for future measurements and assists in monitoring how quickly blood is accumulating for possible autotransfusion. Sudden flow of dark, bloody drainage occurring with position change is often old blood that finds its way into the chest tube.	• Drainage greater than 200 ml/hr • Sudden decrease or absence of drainage • Change in characteristics of drainage
5. Monitor for blood transfusion reaction (see Procedure 125).	A patient receiving autotransfusion is unlikely to experience a blood transfusion reaction.	• Temperature spike • Chills • Tachycardia • Abdominal pain or back pain • Hypotension • Hematuria

Documentation

Documentation should include the following:

- Patient and family education
- Amount of drainage system loss
- Amount of blood autotransfused
- Date and time when collection of blood started

- Patient tolerance
- Unexpected outcomes
- Nursing interventions

References

1. American Association of Blood Banks. (1997). *Guidelines for Blood Recovery and Reinfusion in Surgery and Trauma.* Bethesda, MD: American Association of Blood Banks.
2. Purcell, T.B. (2004). Autotransfusion. In: Roberts, J.R., and Hedges, J.R., editors. *Clinical Procedures in Emergency Medicine.* 4th ed. Philadelphia: W.B. Saunders, 410-26.

Additional Readings

American Association of Blood Banks. (2002). *Guidance for Standards for Perioperative Autologous Blood Collection and Administration.* Bethesda, MD: American Association of Blood Banks.

Brown, M., and Whalen, P.K. (2000). Red blood cell transfusion in critically ill patients: Emerging risks and alternatives. *Crit Care Nurse,* Dec(Suppl), 1-14.
Cross, M.H. (2001). Autotransfusion in cardiac surgery. *Perfusion,* 16, 391-400.
Ley, S.J. (1996). Intraoperative and postoperative blood salvage. *AACN Clin Issues,* 7, 238-48.
Oeltjen, A.M., and Santrach, P.J. (1997). Autologous transfusion techniques. *J Intraven Nurs,* 20, 305-10.

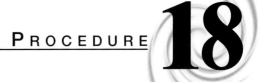

PROCEDURE **18**

@AP
Chest Tube Placement (Perform)

P U R P O S E :   Chest tubes are placed for the removal or drainage of air, blood, or fluid from the intrapleural or mediastinal space. They also are used to introduce sclerosing agents into the pleural space, preventing a reaccumulation of fluid.

Denise M. Lawrence

PREREQUISITE NURSING KNOWLEDGE

- The thoracic cavity, under normal conditions, is a closed airspace. Any disruption results in the loss of negative pressure within the intrapleural space. Air or fluid entering the space competes with the lung, resulting in collapse of the lung. Associated conditions are the result of disease, injury, surgery, or iatrogenic causes.
- Chest tubes are sterile, flexible vinyl, silicone nonthrombogenic catheters approximately 20 inches (51 cm) long, varying in size from 12 Fr to 40 Fr. The size of the tube placed is determined by the condition. Chest tubes inserted for traumatic hemopneumothorax or hemothorax (blood) should be large (36 Fr to 40 Fr). Medium tubes (26 Fr to 36 Fr) should be used for fluid accumulation (pleural effusions). Tubes inserted for pneumothorax (air) should be small (12 Fr to 26 Fr).
- Indications for chest tube insertion include the following:
  - ❖ Pneumothorax (collection of air in the pleural space)
  - ❖ Hemothorax (collection of blood)
  - ❖ Hemopneumothorax (accumulation of air and blood in the pleural space)
  - ❖ Tension pneumothorax
  - ❖ Thoracostomy (e.g., open heart surgery, pneumonectomy)
  - ❖ Pyothorax or empyema (collection of pus)
  - ❖ Chylothorax (collection of chyle from the thoracic duct)
  - ❖ Cholothorax (collection of fluid containing bile)
  - ❖ Hydrothorax (collection of noninflammatory serous fluid)
  - ❖ Pleural effusion
- A pneumothorax may be classified as an open, closed, or tension pneumothorax.
  - ❖ *Open pneumothorax:* The chest wall and the pleural space are penetrated, allowing air to enter the pleural space, as in penetrating injury or trauma; surgical incision in the thoracic cavity (i.e., thoracotomy); or iatrogenically, occurring as complication of surgical treatment (e.g., unintentional puncture during invasive procedures, such as thoracentesis or central venous catheter insertion).
  - ❖ *Closed pneumothorax:* The pleural space is penetrated, but the chest wall is intact, allowing air to enter the pleural space from within the lung, as in spontaneous pneumothorax. A closed pneumothorax occurs without apparent injury and often is seen in individuals with chronic lung disorders (e.g., emphysema, cystic fibrosis, tuberculosis, necrotizing pneumonia) and in young, tall men who have a greater than normal height-to-width chest ratio; after blunt traumatic injury; or iatrogenically, occurring as a complication of medical treatment (e.g., intermittent positive-pressure breathing, mechanical ventilation with positive end-expiratory pressure).
  - ❖ *Tension pneumothorax:* Air leaks into the pleural space through a tear in the lung and has no means to escape from the pleural cavity, creating a one-way valve effect. With each breath the patient takes, air accumulates, pressure within the pleural space increases, and the lung collapses. This causes the mediastinal structures (i.e., heart, great vessels, and trachea) to shift to the

opposite or unaffected side of the chest. Venous return and cardiac output are impeded, along with the possibility of collapse of the unaffected lung. This is a life-threatening emergency that requires prompt recognition and intervention.

❖ *Special applications:* Chest tubes can be used to instill anesthetic solutions and sclerosing agents.

• There are no absolute contraindications to chest tube therapy. Use of chest tubes in patients with multiple adhesions, giant blebs, or coagulopathies is carefully considered; however, these relative contraindications are superseded by the need to reinflate the lung.

• The site selected for chest tube insertion is determined by the indication. If draining air, the tube is placed near the apex of the lung (second intercostal space); if draining fluid, the tube is placed near the base of the lung (fifth or sixth intercostal space) (Fig. 18-1).

• Mediastinal tubes generally are placed in the operating room by a surgeon after cardiac surgery.

EQUIPMENT

• Antiseptic solution
• Sterile gloves, caps, gowns, masks, drapes
• Protective eyewear (goggles)
• Local anesthetic: 1% lidocaine solution
• Tube thoracotomy tray
  ❖ Sterile towels, 4 × 4 sterile gauze
  ❖ Scalpel with No. 11 blade
  ❖ Two Kelly clamps, curved clamps
  ❖ Needle holder
  ❖ 2-0, 3-0 silk suture with cutting needle
  ❖ Suture scissors
  ❖ Two hemostats
  ❖ 10-ml syringe with 20-gauge, 1½-inch needle

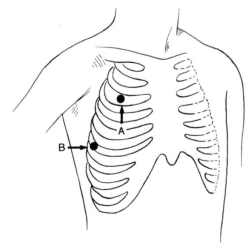

FIGURE 18-1 Standard sites for tube thoracostomy. **A,** The second intercostal space, midclavicular line. **B,** The fourth or fifth intercostal space, midaxillary line. Most clinicians prefer midaxillary line placement for all chest tubes, regardless of pathology. Placing the tube too far posteriorly does not allow the patient to lie down comfortably. *(From Roberts, J.R., and Hedges, J.R., editors. [2004]. Clinical Procedures in Emergency Medicine. 4th ed. Philadelphia: W.B. Saunders.)*

• 5-ml syringe with 25-gauge, 1-inch needle
• Thoracostomy tube (choose size appropriate to condition)
• Closed chest drainage system
• Suction source
• Suction connector and connecting tubing (usually 6 feet for each tube)
• Y connector
• 1-inch adhesive tape or Parham bands
• Dressing materials (4 × 4 gauze pads, slit drain sponges, petroleum gauze, tape)

PATIENT AND FAMILY EDUCATION

• Explain the procedure (if patient condition and time allows) and the reason for the chest tube insertion. ➥*Rationale:* This communication identifies patient and family knowledge deficits concerning the patient's condition, procedure, expected benefits, and potential risks and allows time for questions to clarify information and to voice concerns. Explanations decrease patient anxiety and enhance cooperation.

• Explain that the patient's participation during the procedure is to remain as immobile as possible and do relaxed breathing. ➥*Rationale:* This facilitates insertion of the chest tube and prevents complications during insertion.

• After the procedure, instruct the patient to sit in a semi-Fowler position (unless contraindicated). ➥*Rationale:* This position facilitates drainage from the lung by allowing air to rise and fluid to settle to be removed via the chest tube. This position also makes breathing easier.

• Instruct the patient to turn and change position every 2 hours. The patient may lie on the side with the chest tube but should keep the tubing free of kinks. ➥*Rationale:* Turning and changing position prevent complications related to immobility and retained pulmonary secretions. Keeping the tube free of kinks maintains patency of the tube, facilitates drainage, and prevents the accumulation of pressure within the pleural space that interferes with lung reexpansion.

• Instruct the patient to cough and deep breathe, splinting the affected side. ➥*Rationale:* Coughing and deep breathing increase pressure within the pleural space, facilitating drainage, promoting lung reexpansion, and preventing respiratory complications associated with retained secretions. The application of firm pressure over the chest tube insertion site (i.e., splinting) decreases pain and discomfort.

• Encourage active or passive range-of-motion exercises of the arm on the affected side. ➥*Rationale:* The patient may limit movement of the arm on the affected side to decrease the discomfort at the insertion site, resulting in joint discomfort and potential joint contractures.

• Instruct the patient and family about activity as prescribed while maintaining the drainage system below the level of the chest. ➥*Rationale:* This facilitates gravity drainage and prevents backflow and potential infectious contamination into the pleural space.

• Instruct the patient about the availability of prescribed analgesic medication and other pain relief strategies. ➤*Rationale:* Pain relief ensures comfort, and facilitates coughing, deep breathing, positioning, range of motion, and recuperation.

PATIENT ASSESSMENT AND PREPARATION

Patient Assessment

• Assess significant medical history or injury, including chronic lung disease, spontaneous pneumothorax, hemothorax, pulmonary disease, therapeutic procedures, and mechanism of injury. ➤*Rationale:* Medical history or injury may provide the etiologic basis for the occurrence of pneumothorax, empyema, pleural effusion, or chylothorax.

• Assess baseline cardiopulmonary status for signs and symptoms requiring chest tube insertion.
  ❖ Tachypnea
  ❖ Decreased or absent breath sounds on affected side
  ❖ Crackles adjacent to the affected area
  ❖ Shortness of breath, dyspnea
  ❖ Asymmetrical chest excursion with respirations
  ❖ Cyanosis
  ❖ Decreased oxygen saturation
  ❖ Hyperresonance in the affected side (pneumothorax)
  ❖ Subcutaneous emphysema (pneumothorax)
  ❖ Dullness or flatness in the affected side (hemothorax, pleural effusion, empyema, chylothorax)
  ❖ Sudden, sharp chest pain
  ❖ Anxiety, restlessness, apprehension
  ❖ Tachycardia
  ❖ Hypotension
  ❖ Dysrhythmias
  ❖ Tracheal deviation to the unaffected side (tension pneumothorax)
  ❖ Neck vein distention (tension pneumothorax)
  ❖ Muffled heart sounds (tension pneumothorax)
  ➤*Rationale:* Accurate assessment of signs and symptoms allows for prompt recognition and treatment. Baseline assessment provides comparison data for evaluating changes and outcomes of treatment.

• Diagnostic tests (if patient's condition does not necessitate immediate intervention) include chest x-ray and arterial blood gases. ➤*Rationale:* Diagnostic testing confirms the presence of air or fluid in the pleural space, a collapsed lung, hypoxemia, and respiratory compromise.

Patient Preparation

• Ensure that the patient understands preprocedural teaching. Answer questions as they arise, and reinforce information as needed. ➤*Rationale:* This communication evaluates and reinforces understanding of previously taught information.

• Obtain informed consent if circumstances allow. ➤*Rationale:* Invasive procedures, unless performed under implied consent in a life-threatening situation, require written consent of the patient or significant other.

• Determine insertion site. ➤*Rationale:* The insertion site is determined by the indication for the chest tube. For air, use the second intercostal space; for fluid, use the fifth or sixth intercostal space.

• Assist the patient to the lateral, supine (for pneumothorax), or semi-Fowler position (for hemothorax). ➤*Rationale:* This positioning enhances accessibility to the insertion site for positioning of the chest tube.

• Administer prescribed analgesics or sedatives as needed. ➤*Rationale:* Analgesics and sedatives reduce the discomfort and anxiety experienced, facilitating patient cooperation.

Procedure for Performing Chest Tube Placement		
Steps	**Rationale**	**Special Considerations**
1. Wash hands, and don sterile personal protective equipment.	Reduces the transmission of microorganisms and body secretions; standard precautions.	Chest tube insertion is a sterile procedure and requires full attire, unless performed in a life-threatening situation.
2. Open the chest tube insertion tray using sterile technique.	Reduces transmission of microorganisms.	

3. Prepare equipment.
  A. Check that all equipment is present.
  B. Pour antiseptic solution into basin using aseptic technique.
	Facilitates insertion of the tube.	

Procedure continues on the following page

Procedure for Performing Chest Tube Placement—*Continued*

Steps	Rationale	Special Considerations
C. Attach needle holder to suture. D. Apply a large Kelly clamp to proximal end of tube. E. Prepare syringe with lidocaine solution.		
4. Identify insertion site and have assistant position the patient. *(Level II: Theory based, no research data to support recommendations: recommendations from expert consensus group may exist.)*	Assists in preparing area for insertion and proper placement of tube.[1,5]	*Air:* right or left second intercostal space. *Fluid:* right or left fifth or sixth intercostal space, midaxillary line. Incision site is one rib below insertion site (see Fig. 18-1).
5. Surgically prepare the skin with antiseptic solution, and drape the area surrounding the insertion site. *(Level II: Theory based, no research data to support recommendations: recommendations from expert consensus group may exist.)*	Inhibits growth of bacteria at insertion site; maintains sterility.[3,4,7]	Prepare the area from the clavicle to umbilicus; mid chest to anterior axillary line.
6. Anesthetize the skin, subcutaneous tissue, muscle, and periosteum with 1% lidocaine solution. A. Using a 5-ml syringe (25-gauge needle), inject a subcutaneous wheal of lidocaine at the insertion site. B. Using a 10-ml syringe (20-gauge, 1½-inch needle), advance the needle/syringe, aspirating as you go, until air or pleural fluid is confirmed. Inject the lidocaine deeper, and slowly withdraw the syringe, generously anesthetizing rib periosteum, subcutaneous tissue, and pleura (Fig. 18-2). *(Level II: Theory based, no research data to support recommendations: recommendations from expert consensus group may exist.)*	Results in loss of sensation and decreased pain during insertion.[1,2,5]	When infiltrating with lidocaine, aspirate as you go to confirm the presence of air or fluid; 30 to 40 ml of lidocaine may be required for anesthesia.
7. Using a No. 11 blade, make a 3-cm transverse skin incision directly over the inferior aspect of the anesthetized rib below the insertion site (Fig. 18-3).	Allows for the diameter of the chest tube.[1,2,5]	When making the incision, incise down through the subcutaneous tissue; the space should be large enough to admit a finger.

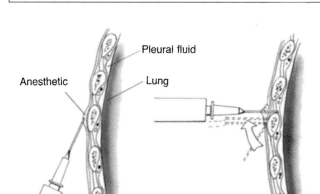

Pleural fluid

Anesthetic

Lung

FIGURE 18-2 Insertion of a chest tube can be relatively painless with proper infiltration of the skin and pleura with local anesthetic. The liberal use of *buffered* 1% lidocaine without epinephrine (maximum lidocaine dose 5 mg/kg) is recommended. *(From Roberts, J.R., and Hedges, J.R., editors. [2004]. Clinical Procedures in Emergency Medicine. 4th ed. Philadelphia: W.B. Saunders.)*

Procedure for Performing Chest Tube Placement—*Continued*

Steps	Rationale	Special Considerations
(Level II: Theory based, no research data to support recommendations: recommendations from expert consensus group may exist.)		
8. Introduce the curved clamp through the incision, with the tips down, creating a tunnel through the subcutaneous tissue and muscle; use an opening and spreading maneuver; aim toward the superior aspect of the rib until the pleural space is reached (Fig. 18-4). *(Level II: Theory based, no research data to support recommendations: recommendations from expert consensus group may exist.)*	Facilitates insertion of the tube. Blunt dissection minimizes trauma to the neurovascular bundle.[1,5,7]	Additional lidocaine is infiltrated as needed. The direction of the tunnel created through the subcutaneous tissue and muscle determines the direction the chest tube takes after insertion. Make sure the clamp stays close to the ribs to avoid injury to the neurovascular bundle.
9. When the clamp is just over the superior portion of the rib, close the clamp and push it with steady pressure through the parietal pleura and into the pleural space. Widen the hole in the pleural space by spreading the clamp (Fig. 18-5).	Ensures opening is large enough for the chest tube. Steady, even, controlled pressure provides control of the clamp once the pleura is perforated.[1,5,7]	This maneuver requires more pressure than might be anticipated; a lunging motion or use of the trocar may cause a hole in lung or injury to the liver or spleen.

Procedure continues on the following page

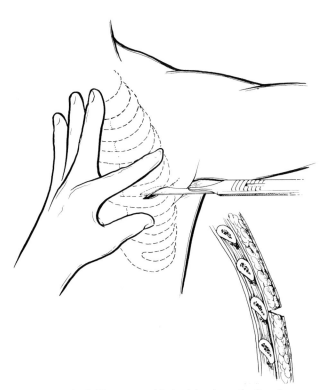

FIGURE 18-3 Transverse skin incision is made directly over the inferior aspect of the anesthetized rib down to the subcutaneous tissue. *(From Dumire, S.M., and Paris, P.M. [1994]. Atlas of Emergency Procedures. Philadelphia: W.B. Saunders.)*

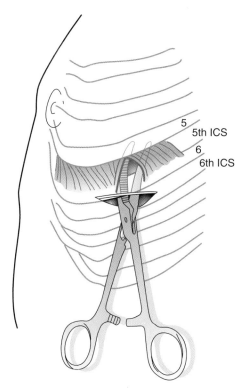

FIGURE 18-4 Blunt dissection is accomplished by forcing a closed clamp through the incision and by using an opening-and-spreading maneuver, creating a tunnel to the pleura. *ICS*, intercostal space.

Procedure for Performing Chest Tube Placement—*Continued*

Steps	Rationale	Special Considerations
(Level II: Theory based, no research data to support recommendations: recommendations from expert consensus group may exist.)		
10. Insert the index finger to dilate the tract and hole in the pleura. *(Level II: Theory based, no research data to support recommendations: recommendations from expert consensus group may exist.)*	Relieves air or fluid when penetration of the space is made. Ensures entry into the pleural space and not into a space inadvertently created between the parietal pleura and chest wall.[1,6,7]	Feel for lung tissue (lung should expand and meet finger on inspiration), diaphragm, or adhesions. Break up clot, if found.
11. Insert the chest tube into the chest cavity using a curved Kelly clamp, holding the proximal end to guide the tip into the pleural space (Fig. 18-6). Remove the clamp and guide the tube, in a rotating motion, through the tract and into the space. The tube is advanced until the last hole is in the pleural space. Condensation of air or fluid in the tube should be noted.	Confirms placement of the tube.	To drain air, aim the tube posteriorly and superiorly toward the apex of the lung; to drain fluid, aim the tube inferiorly and posteriorly. Do not allow any side holes of the tube to remain outside the thoracic cavity.
12. Connect the chest tube to the closed chest drainage system (see Procedure 22) and check for respiratory variation of the H_2O column. Have assistant apply ordered amount of suction.	Ensures the tube is properly positioned.	
13. Suture the tube to the chest wall. Wrap the free ends of the suture around the tube (similar to lacing a shoe). Tie the ends of the suture snugly around the top of the tube (Fig. 18-7).	Secures the position of the tube.[4,6,7] Secures the tube snugly to prevent subcutaneous air/emphysema.	Type of stitch used depends on the individual; the goal is to prevent displacement of the chest tube.

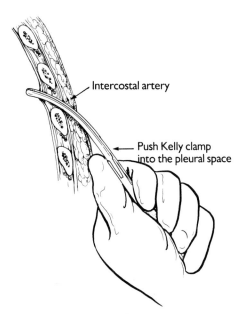

FIGURE 18-5 Just over the superior portion of the rib, close the clamp, and push with steady pressure into the pleura. *(From Dumire, S.M., and Paris, P.M. [1994]. Atlas of Emergency Procedures. Philadelphia: W.B. Saunders.)*

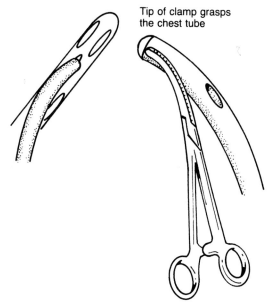

FIGURE 18-6 The tube is grasped with the curved clamp, with the tube tip protruding from the jaws. *(From Roberts, J.R., and Hedges, J.R., editors. [2004]. Clinical Procedures in Emergency Medicine. 4th ed. Philadelphia: W.B. Saunders.)*

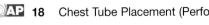

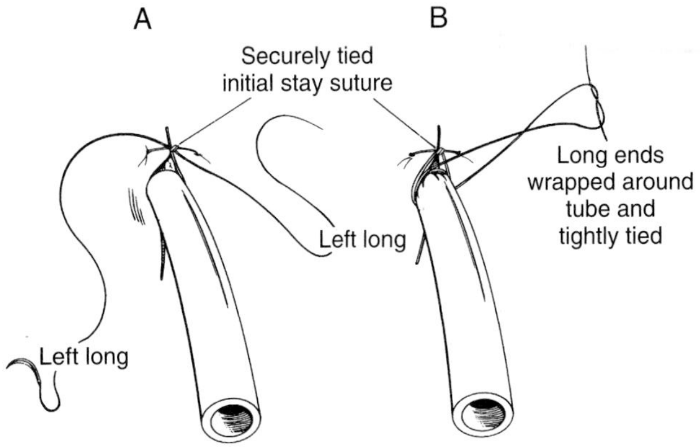

A   B

Securely tied
initial stay suture

Long ends
wrapped around
tube and
tightly tied

Left long

FIGURE 18-7 A "stay" suture is placed first next to the tube to close the skin incision. **A,** The knot is tied securely, and the ends, which subsequently are wrapped around the chest tube, are left long. **B,** The ends of the suture are wound twice about the tube tightly enough to indent the tube slightly and are tied securely. *(From Roberts, J.R., and Hedges, J.R., editors. [2004]. Clinical procedures in Emergency Medicine, 4th ed. Philadelphia: W.B. Saunders.)*

Left long

Procedure for Performing Chest Tube Placement—*Continued*

Steps	Rationale	Special Considerations

14. Apply occlusive dressing.
  A. Petrolatum gauze is used around the chest tube, or follow institutional standard.
  B. Split drain sponges are placed around the chest tube, one from top, one underneath.
  C. Cover with 4 × 4 gauze.
  D. Tape dressing.
	Provides airtight seal around the chest tube.[3,6]	

15. Tape all connection points to the drainage system. *(Level II: Theory based, no research data to support recommendations: recommendations from expert consensus group may exist.)*	Creates an airtight system. Airtight connections prevent air leaks into the pleural space.[3,6]	Check that all holes are in the pleural space.
16. Obtain a chest x-ray. *(Level II: Theory based, no research data to support recommendations: recommendations from expert consensus group may exist.)*	Confirms placement of tube and expansion of lung and removal of fluid.[2-5]	Document location, tube size, complications, and result of chest x-ray in the chart.
17. Dispose of equipment in receptacle. Document procedure in patient record.	Standard precautions.	

Expected Outcomes

- Removal of air, fluid, or blood from the pleural space
- Relief of respiratory distress
- Reexpansion of the lung (validated by chest x-ray)
- Restoration of negative pressure within the pleural space

Unexpected Outcomes

- Hemorrhage/shock
- Increasing respiratory distress
- Infection
- Damage to intercostal nerve resulting in neuropathy or neuritis
- Incorrect tube placement
- Chest tube kinking, clogging, or dislodgment from chest wall
- Subcutaneous emphysema

Patient Monitoring and Care

Steps	Rationale	Reportable Conditions
1. Assess cardiopulmonary and vital signs every 2 hours and as needed.	Provides baseline and ongoing assessment of patient's condition. Abnormalities can indicate recurrence of the condition that required chest tube insertion.	*These conditions should be reported if they persist despite nursing interventions.* • Tachypnea • Decreased or absent breath • Hypoxemia • Tracheal deviation • Subcutaneous emphysema • Neck vein distention • Muffled heart tones • Tachycardia • Hypotension • Dysrhythmias • Fever
2. Monitor output every 2 hours, and record amount and color.	Provides data for diagnosis.	• Bloody drainage greater than or equal to 200 ml/hr • Sudden cessation of drainage • Change in character of drainage
3. Assess for pain at the insertion site or for chest discomfort.	Interferes with adequate deep breathing. Pain at insertion site, particularly with inspiration, may indicate improper tube placement.	• Pain at insertion site
4. Evaluate the chest drainage system for fluctuation in water-seal chamber (see Procedure 22). Check connections.	Water level normally rises and falls with respiration until lung is expanded. Bubbling immediately after insertion and with exhalation and coughing is normal; persistent bubbling indicates an air leak and should be corrected.	• Absence of fluctuation in water-seal chamber • Persistent bubbling
5. Assess insertion site and surrounding skin for presence of subcutaneous air and signs of infection or inflammation with each dressing change or every day.	Skin integrity is altered during insertion and can lead to infection.	• Fever • Redness around insertion site • Purulent drainage • Subcutaneous emphysema

Documentation

Documentation should include the following:

- Patient and family education
- Reason for chest tube insertion
- Respiratory and vital sign assessment before and after insertion
- Description of procedure, including tube size, date and time of insertion, insertion site, and any complications associated with procedure
- Results of procedure, type and amount of drainage
- Presence of fluctuation and bubbling
- Amount of suction
- Patient's tolerance to procedure
- Postinsertion chest x-ray results
- Unexpected outcomes
- Nursing interventions

References

1. Chen, H., Sola, J.E., and Lillemae, K.D. (1996). *Manual of Common Bedside Surgical Procedures.* Baltimore: Williams & Wilkins, 100-8.
2. Dunmire, S.M., and Paris, P.M. (1991). *Atlas of Emergency Procedures.* Philadelphia: W.B. Saunders, 50-70.
3. Iberti, T.J., and Stern, P.M. (1998). Chest tube thoracostomy. *Crit Care Clin,* 14, 879-92.
4. Kravis, T.C., Warner, C.G., and Jacobs, L.M. (1994). *Emergency Medicine Procedures Manual.* New York: Raven Press, 51-5.
5. Lewinter, J.R. (1992). Tube thoracostomy. In: Jastremski, M.S., Dumas, M., and Penalver, L., editors. *Emergency Procedures.* Philadelphia: W.B. Saunders, 391-97.
6. Wilson, R.F. (1996). Thoracic trauma. In: Tininalli, J.E., Ruiz, E., and Krome, R.L., editors. *Emergency Medicine: A Comprehensive Guide.* 4th ed. New York: McGraw Hill, 1156-82.

7. Wright, S.W. (2004). Tube thoracostomy. In: Roberts, J.R., and Hedges, J.R., editors. *Clinical Procedures in Emergency Medicine.* 4th ed. Philadelphia: W.B. Saunders, 148-71.

Additional Readings

Altman, B., et al. (2001). Modified Seldinger technique for the insertion of chest tubes. *Am J Surg,* 181, 354-5.

Bailey, R.C. (2000). Complications of tube thoracostomy in trauma. *J Accidental Emerg Med,* 17, 111-4.

Cerfolio, R.J. (2002). Advances in tube thoracostomy. *Surg Clin North Am,* 82(4), 833-48.

Singh, S. (2003). Abandon the trocar. *Intens Care Med,* 29, 142-43.

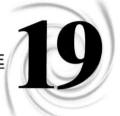

PROCEDURE **19**

Chest Tube Placement (Assist)

P U R P O S E : Chest tubes are placed for the removal or drainage of air, blood, or fluid from the intrapleural or mediastinal space. They also are used to introduce sclerosing agents into the pleural space, preventing a reaccumulation of fluid.

Denise M. Lawrence
Karen K. Carlson

PREREQUISITE NURSING KNOWLEDGE

- The thoracic cavity, under normal conditions, is a closed airspace. Any disruption results in the loss of negative pressure within the intrapleural space. Air or fluid entering the space competes with the lung, resulting in collapse of the lung. Associated conditions are the result of disease, injury, surgery, or iatrogenic causes.
- Chest tubes are sterile, flexible vinyl, silicone nonthrombogenic catheters approximately 20 inches (51 cm) long, varying in size from 12 Fr to 40 Fr. The size of the tube placed is determined by the condition. Chest tubes inserted for traumatic hemopneumothorax or hemothorax (blood) should be large (36 Fr to 40 Fr). Medium tubes (26 Fr to 36 Fr) should be used for fluid accumulation (pleural effusions). Tubes inserted for pneumothorax (air) should be small (12 Fr to 26 Fr).
- Indications for chest tube insertion include the following:
  - ❖ Pneumothorax (collection of air in the pleural space)
  - ❖ Hemothorax (collection of blood)
  - ❖ Hemopneumothorax (accumulation of air and blood in the pleural space)
  - ❖ Tension pneumothorax
  - ❖ Thoracostomy (e.g., open heart surgery, pneumonectomy)
  - ❖ Pyothorax or empyema (collection of pus)
  - ❖ Chylothorax (collection of chyle from the thoracic duct)
  - ❖ Cholothorax (collection of fluid containing bile)
  - ❖ Hydrothorax (collection of noninflammatory serous fluid)
  - ❖ Pleural effusion

- A pneumothorax may be classified as an open, closed, or tension pneumothorax.
  - ❖ *Open pneumothorax:* The chest wall and the pleural space are penetrated, allowing air to enter the pleural space, as in penetrating injury or trauma; surgical incision in the thoracic cavity (i.e., thoracotomy); or iatrogenically, occurring as complication of surgical treatment (e.g., unintentional puncture during invasive procedures, such as thoracentesis or central venous catheter insertion).
  - ❖ *Closed pneumothorax:* The pleural space is penetrated, but the chest wall is intact, allowing air to enter the pleural space from within the lung, as in spontaneous pneumothorax. A closed pneumothorax occurs without apparent injury and often is seen in individuals with chronic lung disorders (e.g., emphysema, cystic fibrosis, tuberculosis, necrotizing pneumonia) and in young, tall men who have a greater than normal height-to-width chest ratio; after blunt traumatic injury; or iatrogenically, occurring as a complication of medical treatment (e.g., intermittent positive-pressure breathing, mechanical ventilation with positive end-expiratory pressure).
  - ❖ *Tension pneumothorax:* Air leaks into the pleural space through a tear in the lung and has no means to escape from the pleural cavity, creating a one-way valve effect. With each breath the patient takes, air accumulates, pressure within the pleural space increases, and the lung collapses. This causes the mediastinal structures (i.e., heart, great vessels, and trachea) to shift to the opposite or unaffected side of the chest. Venous return and cardiac output are impeded, along with the

possibility of collapse of the unaffected lung. This is a life-threatening emergency that requires prompt recognition and intervention.

❖ *Special applications:* Chest tubes can be used to instill anesthetic solutions and sclerosing agents.

- There are no absolute contraindications to chest tube therapy. Use of chest tubes in patients with multiple adhesions, giant blebs, or coagulopathies is carefully considered; however, these relative contraindications are superseded by the need to reinflate the lung.

- The insertion site selected for chest tube insertion is determined by the indication. If draining air, the tube is placed near the apex of the lung (second intercostal space); if draining fluid, the tube is placed near the base of the lung (fifth or sixth intercostal space) (see Fig. 18-1).

- When the tube is in place, the tube is sutured to the skin to prevent displacement, and an occlusive dressing is applied (Fig. 19-1). The chest tube also is connected to a chest drainage system (see Procedure 22) to remove air and fluid from the pleural space; this facilitates reexpansion of the collapsed lung. All connection points are secured with tape or Parham bands to ensure that the system remains airtight (Fig. 19-2).

- Mediastinal tubes generally are placed in the operating room by a surgeon after cardiac surgery.

EQUIPMENT

- Antiseptic solution
- Sterile gloves, caps, gowns, masks, drapes
- Protective eyewear (goggles)
- Local anesthetic: 1% lidocaine solution
- Tube thoracotomy tray
  ❖ Sterile towels, 4 × 4 sterile gauze
  ❖ Scalpel with No. 11 blade
  ❖ Two Kelly clamps, curved clamps
  ❖ Needle holder
  ❖ 2-0, 3-0 silk suture with cutting needle
  ❖ Suture scissors
  ❖ Two hemostats
  ❖ 10-ml syringe with 20-gauge, 1½-inch needle
  ❖ 5-ml syringe with 25-gauge, 1-inch needle
  ❖ Thoracostomy tube (choose size appropriate to condition)

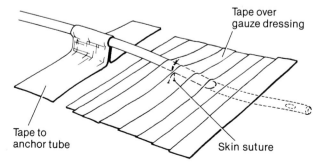

FIGURE 19-1 Occlusive chest tube dressing. *(From Kersten, L.D. [1989]. Comprehensive Respiratory Nursing. Philadelphia: W.B. Saunders.)*

Tape over gauze dressing

Tape to anchor tube

Skin suture

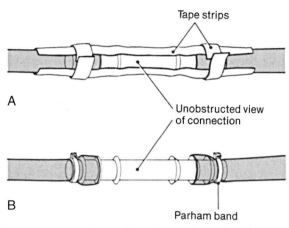

Tape strips

Unobstructed view of connection

Parham band

FIGURE 19-2 The securing of connection points. **A,** Tape. **B,** Parham bands. *(From Kersten, L.D. [1989]. Comprehensive Respiratory Nursing. Philadelphia: W.B. Saunders.)*

- Closed chest drainage system
- Suction source
- Suction connector and connecting tubing (usually 6 feet for each tube)
- Y connector
- 1-inch adhesive tape or Parham bands
- Dressing materials (4 × 4 gauze pads, slit drain sponges, petroleum gauze, tape)

PATIENT AND FAMILY EDUCATION

- Explain the procedure (if patient condition and time allows) and the reason for the chest tube insertion. ➥*Rationale:* This communication identifies patient and family knowledge deficits concerning the patient's condition, procedure, expected benefits, and potential risks and allows time for questions to clarify information and to voice concerns. Explanations decrease patient anxiety and enhance cooperation.

- Explain that the patient's participation during the procedure is to remain as immobile as possible and do relaxed breathing. ➥*Rationale:* This facilitates insertion of the chest tube and prevents complications during insertion.

- After the procedure, instruct the patient to sit in a semi-Fowler position (unless contraindicated). ➥*Rationale:* This position facilitates drainage from the lung by allowing air to rise and fluid to settle to be removed via the chest tube. This position also makes breathing easier.

- Instruct the patient to turn and change position every 2 hours. The patient may lie on the side with the chest tube but should keep the tubing free of kinks. ➥*Rationale:* Turning and changing position prevent complications related to immobility and retained pulmonary secretions. Keeping the tube free of kinks maintains patency of the tube, facilitates drainage, and prevents the accumulation of pressure within the pleural space that interferes with lung reexpansion.

- Instruct the patient to cough and deep breathe, splinting the affected side. ➤**Rationale:** Coughing and deep breathing increase pressure within the pleural space, facilitating drainage, promoting lung reexpansion, and preventing respiratory complications associated with retained secretions. The application of firm pressure over the chest tube insertion site (i.e., splinting) decreases pain and discomfort.
- Encourage active or passive range-of-motion exercises of the arm on the affected side. ➤**Rationale:** The patient may limit movement of the arm on the affected side to decrease the discomfort at the insertion site, resulting in joint discomfort and potential joint contractures.
- Instruct the patient and family about activity as prescribed while maintaining the drainage system below the level of the chest. ➤**Rationale:** This facilitates chest gravity drainage and prevents backflow and potential infectious contamination into the pleural space.
- Instruct the patient about the availability of prescribed analgesic medication and other pain relief strategies. ➤**Rationale:** Pain relief ensures comfort, and facilitates coughing, deep breathing, positioning, range of motion, and recuperation.

PATIENT ASSESSMENT AND PREPARATION

Patient Assessment

- Assess significant medical history or injury, including chronic lung disease, spontaneous pneumothorax, hemothorax, pulmonary disease, therapeutic procedures, and mechanism of injury. ➤**Rationale:** Medical history or injury may provide the etiologic basis for the occurrence of pneumothorax, empyema, pleural effusion, or chylothorax.
- Assess baseline cardiopulmonary status for signs and symptoms requiring chest tube insertion.
  - ❖ Tachypnea
  - ❖ Decreased or absent breath sounds on affected side
  - ❖ Crackles adjacent to the affected area
  - ❖ Shortness of breath, dyspnea
  - ❖ Asymmetrical chest excursion with respirations
  - ❖ Cyanosis
  - ❖ Decreased oxygen saturation
  - ❖ Hyperresonance in the affected side (pneumothorax)

- ❖ Subcutaneous emphysema (pneumothorax)
- ❖ Dullness or flatness in the affected side (hemothorax, pleural effusion, empyema, chylothorax)
- ❖ Sudden, sharp chest pain
- ❖ Anxiety, restlessness, apprehension
- ❖ Tachycardia
- ❖ Hypotension
- ❖ Dysrhythmias
- ❖ Tracheal deviation to the unaffected side (tension pneumothorax)
- ❖ Neck vein distention (tension pneumothorax)
- ❖ Muffled heart sounds (tension pneumothorax)
  ➤**Rationale:** Accurate assessment of signs and symptoms allows for prompt recognition and treatment. Baseline assessment provides comparison data for evaluating changes and outcomes of treatment.
- Diagnostic tests (if patient's condition does not necessitate immediate intervention) include chest x-ray and arterial blood gases. ➤**Rationale:** Diagnostic testing confirms the presence of air or fluid in the pleural space, a collapsed lung, hypoxemia, and respiratory compromise.

Patient Preparation

- Ensure that the patient understands preprocedural teaching. Answer questions as they arise, and reinforce information as needed. ➤**Rationale:** This communication evaluates and reinforces understanding of previously taught information.
- Obtain consent if circumstances allow. ➤**Rationale:** Invasive procedures, unless performed under implied consent in a life-threatening situation, require written consent of the patient or significant other.
- Determine insertion site. ➤**Rationale:** The insertion site is determined by the indication for the chest tube. For air, use the second intercostal space; for fluid, use the fifth or sixth intercostal space.
- Assist the patient to the lateral, supine (for pneumothorax), or semi-Fowler position (for hemothorax). ➤**Rationale:** This positioning enhances accessibility to the insertion site for positioning of the chest tube.
- Administer prescribed analgesics or sedatives as needed. ➤**Rationale:** Analgesics and sedatives reduce the discomfort and anxiety experienced, facilitating patient cooperation.

Procedure   for Assisting With Chest Tube Placement

Steps	Rationale	Special Considerations
1. Wash hands, and don sterile personal protective equipment.	Reduces the transmission of microorganisms and body secretions; standard precautions.	Chest tube insertion is a sterile procedure and requires full attire, unless performed in a life-threatening situation.

Procedure for Assisting With Chest Tube Placement—*Continued*		
Steps	**Rationale**	**Special Considerations**
2. Open the chest tube insertion tray using sterile technique.	Reduces transmission of microorganisms.	
3. Assist with preparation of the equipment. A. Check that all equipment is present. B. Pour antiseptic solution into basin using aseptic technique. C. Apply a large Kelly clamp to proximal end of tube. D. Assist to prepare a syringe with lidocaine.	Facilitates insertion of the tube.	
4. Assist the patient to the lateral, supine (for pneumothorax), or semi-Fowler position (for hemothorax).		
5. Assist the physician or advanced practice nurse with preparation of the insertion site.	Assists in preparing area for insertion and proper placement of tube.[1,5]	*Air:* right or left second intercostal space. *Fluid:* right or left fifth or sixth intercostal space, midaxillary line. Incision site is one rib below insertion site (see Fig. 18-1).
6. Connect the chest tube to the closed chest drainage system (see Procedure 22), and check for respiratory variation of the H_2O column. Apply ordered amount of suction.	Ensures the tube is properly positioned.	
7. Assist with suturing of the tube to the chest wall.	Secures the position of the tube.[4,6,7] Secures the tube snugly to prevent subcutaneous air/emphysema.	Type of stitch used depends on the individual; the goal is to prevent displacement of the chest tube.
8. Apply occlusive dressing (see Fig. 19-1). A. Petrolatum gauze is used around the chest tube, or follow institutional standard. B. Split drain sponges are placed around the chest tube, one from top, one underneath. C. Cover with 4 × 4 gauze. D. Tape dressing.	Provides airtight seal around the chest tube.[3,6]	
9. Tape all connection points to the drainage system. (*Level II: Theory based, no research data to support recommendations: recommendations from expert consensus group may exist.*)	Creates an airtight system. Airtight connections prevent air leaks into the pleural space.[3,6]	Check that all holes are in the pleural space.
10. Obtain a chest x-ray. (*Level II: Theory based, no research data to support recommendations: recommendations from expert consensus group may exist.*)	Confirms placement of tube and expansion of lung and removal of fluid.[2-5]	Document location, tube size, complications, and result of chest x-ray in the chart.
11. Dispose of equipment in receptacle.	Standard precautions.	
12. Document in patient record.		

Expected Outcomes

- Removal of air, fluid, or blood from the pleural space
- Relief of respiratory distress
- Reexpansion of the lung (validated by chest x-ray)
- Restoration of negative pressure within the pleural space

Unexpected Outcomes

- Hemorrhage/shock
- Increasing respiratory distress
- Infection
- Damage to intercostal nerve resulting in neuropathy or neuritis
- Incorrect tube placement
- Chest tube kinking, clogging, or dislodgment from chest wall
- Subcutaneous emphysema

Patient Monitoring and Care

Steps	Rationale	Reportable Conditions
		These conditions should be reported if they persist despite nursing interventions.
1. Assess cardiopulmonary and vital signs every 2 hours and as needed.	Provides baseline and ongoing assessment of patient's condition. Abnormalities can indicate reoccurrence of the condition that required chest tube insertion.	• Tachypnea • Decreased or absent breath sounds • Hypoxemia • Tracheal deviation • Subcutaneous emphysema • Neck vein distention • Muffled heart tones • Tachycardia • Hypotension • Dysrhythmias • Fever
2. Monitor output every 2 hours, and record amount and color (see Procedure 22).	Provides data for diagnosis.	• Bloody drainage greater than or equal to 200 ml/hr • Sudden cessation of drainage • Change in character of drainage
3. Assess for pain at the insertion site or for chest discomfort.	Interferes with adequate deep breathing. Pain at insertion site, particularly with inspiration, may indicate improper tube placement.	• Pain at insertion site
4. Evaluate the chest drainage system for fluctuation in water-seal chamber (see Procedure 22). Check connections.	Water level normally rises and falls with respiration until lung is expanded. Bubbling immediately after insertion and with exhalation and coughing is normal; persistent bubbling indicates an air leak and should be corrected.	• Absence of fluctuation in water-seal chamber • Persistent bubbling
5. Assess insertion site and surrounding skin for presence of subcutaneous air and signs of infection or inflammation with each dressing change or every day.	Skin integrity is altered during insertion and can lead to infection.	• Fever • Redness around insertion site • Purulent drainage • Subcutaneous emphysema

Documentation

Documentation should include the following:

- Patient and family education
- Reason for chest tube insertion
- Respiratory and vital sign assessment before and after insertion
- Description of procedure, including tube size, date and time of insertion, insertion site, and any complications associated with the procedure
- Results of procedure, type and amount of drainage
- Presence of fluctuation and bubbling
- Amount of suction
- Patient's tolerance to procedure
- Postinsertion chest x-ray results
- Unexpected outcomes
- Nursing interventions

References

1. Chen, H., Sola, J.E., and Lillemae, K.D. (1996). *Manual of Common Bedside Surgical Procedures.* Baltimore: Williams & Wilkins, 100-8.
2. Dunmire, S.M., and Paris, P.M. (1991). *Atlas of Emergency Procedures.* Philadelphia: W.B. Saunders, 50-70.
3. Iberti, T.J., and Stern, P.M. (1998). Chest tube thoracostomy. *Crit Care Clin,* 14, 879-92.
4. Kravis, T.C., Warner, C.G., and Jacobs, L.M. (1994). *Emergency Medicine Procedures Manual.* New York: Raven Press, 51-5.
5. Lewinter, J.R. (1992). Tube thoracostomy. In: Jastremski, M.S., Dumas, M., and Penalver, L., editors. *Emergency Procedures.* Philadelphia: W.B. Saunders, 391-97.
6. Wilson, R.F. (1996). Thoracic trauma. In: Tininalli, J.E., Ruiz, E., and Krome, R.L., editors. *Emergency Medicine: A Comprehensive Guide.* 4th ed. New York: McGraw Hill, 1156-82.
7. Wright, S.W. (2004). Tube thoracostomy. In: Roberts, J.R., and Hedges, J.R., editors. *Clinical Procedures in Emergency Medicine.* 4th ed. Philadelphia: W.B. Saunders, 148-71.

Additional Readings

Altman, B., et al. (2001). Modified Seldinger technique for the insertion of chest tubes. *Am J Surg,* 181, 354-5.
Bailey, R.C. (2000). Complications of tube thoracostomy in trauma. *J Accidental Emerg Med,* 17, 111-4.
Cerfolio, R.J. (2002). Advances in tube thoracostomy. *Surg Clin North Am,* 82, 833-48.
Singh, S. (2003). Abandon the trocar. *Inten Care Med,* 29, 142-43.

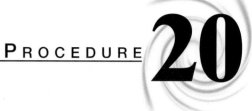
PROCEDURE **20**

⦿AP
Chest Tube Removal (Perform)

P U R P O S E :   Chest tube removal is performed to discontinue a chest tube when it is no longer needed for the removal or drainage of air, blood, or fluid from the intrapleural or mediastinal space.

Peggy Kirkwood

PREREQUISITE NURSING KNOWLEDGE

- Chest tubes are placed in the pleural or the mediastinal space to evacuate an abnormal collection of air or fluid or both.
- Indications for removal are based on the reason for insertion and include the following:
  - Drainage has decreased to 50 to 100 ml in 24 hours if tube was placed for hemothorax, empyema, or pleural effusion.
  - Drainage has changed from bloody to serosanguineous, no air leak is present, and amount is less than 100 ml in the past 8 hours (if tube was placed after cardiac surgery).
  - Lungs are reexpanded (as shown on chest x-ray).
  - Respiratory status has improved (i.e., nonlabored respirations, equal bilateral breath sounds, absence of shortness of breath, decreased use of accessory muscles, symmetrical respiratory excursion, and respiratory rate less than 24 breaths/min).
  - Fluctuations are absent in the water-seal chamber of the collection device, and the level of solution rises in the chamber.
  - Air leaks have resolved for at least 24 hours (assessed by the air-leak chamber or the absence of continuous bubbling in the water-seal chamber), and lung is fully reinflated on x-ray.
- The water-seal chamber should bubble gently immediately on insertion of the chest tube during expiration and

with coughing. Continuous bubbling in this chamber indicates a leak in the system. Fluctuations in the water level in the water-seal chamber of 5 to 10 cm, rising during inhalation and falling during expiration, should be observed with spontaneous respirations. If the patient is on mechanical ventilation, the pattern of fluctuation is just the opposite. If suction is being applied, this must be disconnected temporarily to assess correctly for fluctuations in the water-seal chamber.
- Pleural tubes are placed after cardiac surgery if the pleural cavity has been entered. They typically are removed singly and within 24 to 48 hours after surgery.
- Mediastinal chest tubes most often are removed 24 to 36 hours after cardiac surgery.
- Pleural tubes placed for reasons other than post–cardiac surgery necessity remain until the patient no longer needs them (i.e., no persistent air leak, ongoing fluid leak or bleeding has stopped, or lung is reexpanded on chest x-ray).
- Chest tubes that remain in place for more than 7 days increase the risk of infection along the chest tube tract.
- Chest x-rays are done periodically to determine whether the lung has reexpanded. Reexpanded lungs, along with respiratory assessments that show improvement in the patient's respiratory status, are the basis for the decision to remove the chest tube.
- While the tubes are in place, patients may experience related discomfort. Prompt removal of chest tubes encourages patients to increase ambulation and respiratory measures to improve lung expansion after surgery (e.g., coughing, deep breathing). Additionally, removal of the chest tube is a painful procedure for the patient.[5,9,10]
- The types of sutures used to secure chest tubes vary according to the preference of the physician, the physician assistant, or the advanced practice nurse. One common type is the horizontal mattress or purse-string suture, which

is threaded around and through the wound edges in a U shape with the ends left unknotted until the chest tube is removed. Usually there are one or two anchor stitches accompanying the purse-string suture (Fig. 20-1).

- A primary goal of chest tube removal is to remove tubes without introducing air or contaminants into the pleural space.

EQUIPMENT

- Suture removal set
- Povidone-iodine swabs
- Petrolatum gauze
- Kelly clamps (two per chest tube) or disposable umbilical clamps
- Wide, occlusive tape (2 inch)
- Dry 4 × 4 gauze sponges (two to four)
- Towel or Chux pad
- Personal protective equipment (goggles, sterile and non-sterile gloves, mask, gown)

Additional equipment (to have available depending on patient need) includes the following:

- Specimen collection cup (if catheter tip is to be sent to the laboratory for analysis)
- Scissors

PATIENT AND FAMILY EDUCATION

- Assess patient and family understanding of the procedure. ➤➤*Rationale:* This assessment identifies patient and family knowledge deficits concerning patient condition,

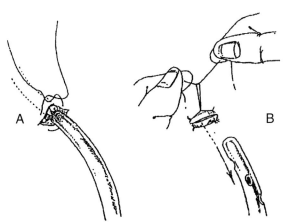

FIGURE 20-1 Purse-string suture. Removing the chest tube. **A,** First throw of a knot in the mattress suture. **B,** Removal of the chest tube and tying of purse-string suture. *(From Leonar, S., and Nikaidoh, H. [1990]. Thoracentesis and chest tube insertion. In: Levin, D., and Morriss, F., editors.* Essentials of Pediatric Intensive Care. *St. Louis: Quality Medical Publishing.)*

procedure, expected benefits, and potential risks and allows time for questions to clarify information.

- Explain the procedure, reason for removal, and sensations to be expected.[4,9-12] ➤➤*Rationale:* This explanation decreases patient anxiety and enhances cooperation.
- Explain the patient's role in assisting with removal. Explain that when prompted, the patient should perform the Valsalva maneuver. ➤➤*Rationale:* This explanation elicits patient cooperation and facilitates removal.
- Instruct the patient to turn and reposition every 2 hours after the chest tube has been removed. ➤➤*Rationale:* This prevents complications related to immobility and retained secretions.
- Instruct the patient to cough and deep breathe after the chest tube has been removed, splinting the affected side or sternum (with mediastinal tubes). ➤➤*Rationale:* This prevents respiratory complications associated with retained secretions. The application of firm pressure over the insertion site (i.e., splinting) decreases pain and discomfort.
- Instruct the patient regarding the availability of prescribed analgesic medication. ➤➤*Rationale:* Analgesics alleviate pain and facilitate coughing, deep breathing, and repositioning.[10-12]
- Instruct the patient and family to report signs and symptoms of respiratory distress or infection immediately. ➤➤*Rationale:* Immediate reporting facilitates prompt intervention to relieve a recurrent pneumothorax or to treat an infection.

PATIENT ASSESSMENT AND PREPARATION

Patient Assessment

- Assess respiratory status.
  - ❖ Oxygen saturation within normal limits
  - ❖ Nonlabored respirations
  - ❖ Absence of shortness of breath
  - ❖ Decreased use of accessory muscles
  - ❖ Respiratory rate of less than 24 breaths/min
  - ❖ Equal bilateral breath sounds

  ➤➤*Rationale:* Assessment of respiratory status ensures the patient's readiness for chest tube removal.
- Assess chest tube drainage (less than 50 to 100 ml in 24 hours or less than 100 ml in 8 hours after cardiac surgery). ➤➤*Rationale:* Assessment of drainage verifies patient readiness for chest tube removal.
- Assess absence of fluctuation in water-seal chamber and air leak indicator. ➤➤*Rationale:* This indicates if lung is reexpanded and air leak is not present.
- Assess chest x-ray. ➤➤*Rationale:* Lung reexpansion indicates that need for chest tube is resolved.
- Assess vital signs and (optional) arterial blood gases. ➤➤*Rationale:* Vital signs indicate if patient can tolerate chest tube removal.

Patient Preparation

- Ensure that the patient understands preprocedural teaching. Answer questions as they arise, and reinforce information as needed. ➤➤*Rationale:* This communication evaluates and reinforces understanding of previously taught information. Anticipatory preparation may prepare patients for a better experience.[9-12]

- Premedicate the patient with adequate analgesics at least 15 minutes before procedure. Intravenous morphine may be used, or, in conjunction with the cardiac surgeon, subfascial lidocaine may be injected into the chest tube tract.

➤➤**Rationale:** Pain medication reduces the discomfort and anxiety experienced, facilitating patient cooperation.[9-12]

- Place the patient in the semi-Fowler position. Alternatively place the patient on the unaffected side with the bed protector (towel or Chux pad) underneath. ➤➤**Rationale:** This position enhances accessibility to the insertion site of the chest tube and protects the bed from drainage.

Procedure for Performing Chest Tube Removal

Steps	Rationale	Special Considerations
1. Wash hands, and don personal protective equipment.	Reduces transmission of microorganisms and body secretions; standard precautions.	
2. Open the sterile suture removal set and prepare petrolatum gauze dressing and two to four 4 × 4 gauze sponges.	Aseptic technique is maintained to prevent contamination of the wound. Removal of pleural chest tubes must be accomplished rapidly with the simultaneous application of an occlusive dressing to prevent air from entering the pleural space.	
3. Discontinue suction from chest drainage system and check for air leakage in water-seal chamber. Observe the water-seal chamber while the patient coughs. A. If tube was placed for a pneumothorax, protocol may require 6 to 24 hours of water-seal and another x-ray before removal. *(Level IV: Limited clinical studies to support recommendations.)*	Bubbling in this chamber is associated with an air leak. When an air leak is present, removal of the chest tube can cause development of a pneumothorax. Ensures a recurrent pneumothorax has not occurred.[2]	If an air leak is present, the tube should not be removed. Consult with the physician or advanced practice nurse to determine appropriate action.
4. Remove existing tape, clean area around tubes with povidone-iodine, and determine type of suture that secures each chest tube. Clip appropriately. If a purse-string suture is present, leave the long suture ends intact.	Allows access to the chest tube at the skin level and prepares the sutures for removal.	
5. Confirm that the tube is free from the suture and the tape.		
6. Clamp each tube to be removed with two Kelly clamps or umbilical clamps.	Prevents air from being introduced into the pleural space.	
7. According to protocol, tube is removed while patient is performing Valsalva maneuver at either end inspiration or end expiration. *(Level IV: Limited clinical studies to support recommendations.)*	Valsalva maneuver is needed to provide positive pressure in the pleural cavity and decreases the incidence of an involuntary gasp by the patient when the tube is removed.[1]	

Procedure for Performing Chest Tube Removal—*Continued*

Steps	Rationale	Special Considerations
A. *End inspiration:* Instruct patient to take a deep breath and hold it while performing the Valsalva maneuver for each tube removed. If the patient is receiving ventilator support, pause the ventilator. If the patient is receiving ventilator support and is unable to follow instructions, the tube during peak inspiration remove phase. B. *End expiration:* Instruct patient to perform the Valsalva maneuver at end expiration. C. According to protocol, patients may need to hold their breath until sutures are tied.		
8. Remove chest tubes rapidly, smoothly, and individually while patient is performing Valsalva maneuver. A. Hold sutures in hand closest to head of patient, and apply mild pressure over exit site with folded 4 × 4 gauze pad. B. If tube was "Y" connected to another tube, cut the removed tube below the clamp to allow for easier manipulation when removing the remaining chest tubes.	Prevents accidental entrance of air into the pleural space.	Some resistance is expected; however, if strong resistance is encountered and rapid removal of the tube is not possible, stop the procedure and consult with the physician immediately. Resistance may indicate that the tube was inadvertently sutured during surgery or sternal closure.
9. Tie purse-string suture using a square knot, if available (see Fig. 20-1).	Creates a firm closure of the chest tube site.	Avoid pulling the suture too tight to prevent tissue necrosis at the site and to facilitate easier removal later.
10. Cover pleural insertion sites with petrolatum gauze dressing and mediastinal insertion site with 4 × 4 gauze pads. Secure with tape.	Avoids the influx of air.	Sterile petrolatum gauze should be applied over the skin site immediately after removal if tube was in pleural space or if no purse-string suture was present.
11. Examine each chest tube to verify that all of the tube has been removed.	If portion of tube is not removed, resternotomy is necessary to remove it.	Consult with physician or advanced practice nurse immediately.
12. Assess the patient after the procedure, and compare the results with previous assessment.	Ensures stable respiratory status after the procedure.	Increased work of breathing, decreased oxygen saturation, increased restlessness, complaints of chest discomfort, and diminished breath sounds on the affected side are warning signs to be observed.

Procedure continues on the following page

Procedure for Performing Chest Tube Removal—*Continued*

Steps	Rationale	Special Considerations
13. Obtain a portable chest x-ray per order or protocol (generally 1 to 24 hours after removal) or as clinically indicated. *(Level V: Clinical studies in more than one patient population and situation.)*	Assesses that the lung has remained expanded.[3,6-8]	
14. Dispose of equipment in appropriate receptacle.	Standard precautions.	
15. Wash hands.	Decreases transmission of microorganisms.	
16. Document in patient record.		

Expected Outcomes

- Patient is comfortable and experiences no respiratory distress
- Lung remains expanded after chest tube removal
- Site remains free of infection

Unexpected Outcomes

- Pneumothorax
- Bleeding
- Skin necrosis
- Retained chest tube
- Infected chest tube insertion site

Patient Monitoring and Care

Steps	Rationale	Reportable Conditions
		These conditions should be reported if they persist despite nursing interventions.
1. Ensure adequate respiratory status. Obtain chest x-ray if difficulties arise.	Diminished respiratory status could indicate a pneumothorax. Pneumothorax could be from removal of the chest tube before all the air, fluid, or blood in the pleural space had been drained, or it may recur after removal of the chest tube if air is introduced accidentally into the pleural space through the chest tube tract.	• Decreased oxygen saturation on pulse oximetry • Increased work of breathing • Diminished breath sounds on affected side • Increased restlessness and complaints of chest discomfort
2. Monitor insertion site for bleeding. Apply pressure at site. Place a tight occlusive dressing over site.	Persistent bleeding from insertion site could mean chest tube was against a vein or artery of chest wall before removal.	• Persistent bleeding
3. Monitor purse-string suture site for signs of skin necrosis. If seen, remove the suture and cleanse wound.	If purse-string suture was pulled too tightly closed when chest tube was removed, skin necrosis may be seen.	• Dark or inflamed skin with necrotic areas visible
4. Monitor site for signs of infection. If seen, prepare for wound cultures.	Prolonged insertion of a chest tube increases the risk that the tract created by the chest tube may become infected, or infection may occur after removal of the chest tube if the opening created by the removal becomes contaminated.	• Purulent drainage • Increased body temperature • Inflammation • Tenderness • Warmth at site
5. Monitor insertion area for development of subcutaneous emphysema.	Air may leak into the surrounding tissues causing crepitus.	• Crepitus

Patient Monitoring and Care—*Continued*

Steps	Rationale	Reportable Conditions
6. Monitor for signs and symptoms of pericardial effusion or cardiac tamponade.	Removal of chest tubes may cause increased bleeding into pericardium. Pericardial bleeding may continue after chest tubes removed.	• Distant heart tones • Decreased blood pressure, tachycardia • Pulsus paradoxus • Narrowed pulse pressure • Equalized pulmonary artery pressures

Documentation

Documentation should include the following:

- Patient and family education
- Respiratory and vital signs assessments before and after procedure
- Date, time, and by whom procedure was performed
- Amount, color, and consistency of any drainage
- Application of a sterile, occlusive dressing
- Type of suture in place and what was done to it (cut or tied)
- Patient's tolerance of the procedure
- Completion and results of chest x-ray
- Specimens sent to laboratory (if applicable)
- Unexpected outcomes
- Nursing interventions

References

1. Bell, R.L., et al. (2001). Chest tube removal: End-inspiration or end-expiration? *J Trauma,* 50, 674-7.
2. Martino, K., et al. (1999). Prospective randomized trial of thoracostomy removal algorithms. *J Trauma,* 46, 369-71.
3. McCormick, J.T., et al. (2002). The use of routine chest x-ray films after chest tube removal in postoperative cardiac patients. *Ann Thorac Surg,* 74, 2161-4.
4. Mimnaugh, L., et al. (1999). Sensations experienced during removal of tubes in acute postoperative patients. *Appl Nurs Res,* 12, 78-85.
5. Mueller, X.M., Tinguely, F., and Tavaearai, H.T. (2000). Impact of duration of chest tube drainage on pain after cardiac surgery. *Eur J Cardiothorac Surg,* 18, 570-4.
6. Pacanowski, J.P., et al. (2000). Is routine roentgenography needed after closed tube thoracostomy removal? *J Trauma,* 48, 684-8.
7. Palesty, J.A., McKelvey, A.A., and Dudrick, S.J. (2000). The efficacy of x-rays after chest tube removal. *Am J Surg,* 179, 13-6.
8. Pizano, L.R., Houghton, D.E., and Cohn, S.M. (2002). When should a chest radiograph be obtained after chest tube removal in mechanically ventilated patient? A prospective study. *J Trauma,* 53, 1073-7.
9. Puntillo, K., et al. (2001). Patients' perceptions and responses to procedural pain: Results from Thunder Project II. *Am J Crit Care,* 10, 238-51.
10. Puntillo, K., et al. (2002). Practices and predictors of analgesic intervention for adults undergoing painful procedures. *Am J Crit Care,* 11, 415-29.
11. Summer, G.H., and Puntillo, K. (2001). Management of surgical and procedural pain in a critical care setting. *Crit Care Nurs Clin North Am,* 13, 233-42.
12. Thompson, C.L., et al. (2001). Translating research into practice: Implications of the thunder project II. *Crit Care Nurs Clin North Am,* 13, 541-6.

Additional Readings

Charnock, Y., and Evans, D. (2001). Nursing management of chest drains: A systematic review. *Aust Crit Care,* 14, 156-60.

Christensen, M. (2002). Nurse-led chest drain removal in a cardiac high dependency unit. *Nurs Crit Care,* 7, 67-72.

Davis, J.W., et al. (1994). Randomized study of algorithms for discontinuing tube thoracostomy drainage. *J Am Coll Surg,* 179, 553-7.

Kirkwood, P. (2000). What is the current consensus or standard of practice for nurses removing chest tubes in a postoperative setting? *Crit Care Nurse,* 20, 97-8.

Tang, A.T.M., Velissaris, R.J., and Weeden, D.F. (2002). An evidence-based approach to drainage of the pleural cavity: Evaluation of best practice. *J Eval Clin Pract,* 8, 333-40.

Thomson, S.C., Wells, S., and Maxwell, M. (1997). Chest tube removal after cardiac surgery. *Crit Care Nurse,* 17, 34-8.

Younes, R.N., et al. (2002). When to remove a chest tube? A randomized study with subsequent prospective consecutive validation. *J Am Coll Surg,* 195, 658-62.

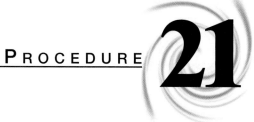
PROCEDURE **21**

Chest Tube Removal (Assist)

PURPOSE: Chest tube removal is performed to discontinue a chest tube when it is no longer needed for the removal or drainage of air, blood, or fluid from the intrapleural or mediastinal space.

Peggy Kirkwood
Karen K. Carlson

PREREQUISITE NURSING KNOWLEDGE

- Chest tubes are placed in the pleural or the mediastinal space to evacuate an abnormal collection of air or fluid or both.
- Indications for removal are based on the reason for insertion and include the following:
  - Drainage has decreased to 50 to 100 ml in 24 hours if tube was placed for hemothorax, empyema, or pleural effusion.
  - Drainage has changed from bloody to serosanguineous, no air leak is present, and amount is less than 100 ml in the past 8 hours (if tube was placed after cardiac surgery).
  - Lungs are reexpanded (as shown on chest x-ray).
  - Respiratory status has improved (i.e., nonlabored respirations, equal bilateral breath sounds, absence of shortness of breath, decreased use of accessory muscles, symmetrical respiratory excursion, and respiratory rate less than 24 breaths/min).
  - Fluctuations are absent in the water-seal chamber of the collection device, and the level of solution rises in the chamber.
  - Air leaks have resolved for at least 24 hours (assessed by the air-leak chamber or the absence of continuous bubbling in the water-seal chamber), and lung is fully reinflated on x-ray.
- The water-seal chamber should bubble gently immediately on insertion of the chest tube during expiration and with coughing. Continuous bubbling in this chamber indicates a leak in the system. Fluctuations in the water level in the water-seal chamber of 5 to 10 cm, rising during inhalation and falling during expiration, should be observed with

spontaneous respirations. If the patient is on mechanical ventilation, the pattern of fluctuation is just the opposite. If suction is being applied, this must be disconnected temporarily to assess correctly for fluctuations in the water-seal chamber.
- Pleural tubes are placed after cardiac surgery if the pleural cavity has been entered. They typically are removed singly and within 24 to 48 hours after surgery.
- Mediastinal chest tubes most often are removed 24 to 36 hours after cardiac surgery.
- Pleural tubes placed for reasons other than post–cardiac surgery necessity remain until the patient no longer needs them (i.e., no persistent air leak, ongoing fluid leak or bleeding has stopped, or lung is reexpanded on chest x-ray).
- Chest tubes that remain in place for more than 7 days increase the risk of infection along the chest tube tract.
- Chest x-rays are done periodically to determine whether the lung has reexpanded. Reexpanded lungs, along with respiratory assessments that show improvement in the patient's respiratory status, are the basis for the decision to remove the chest tube.
- While the tubes are in place, patients may experience related discomfort. Prompt removal of chest tubes encourages patients to increase ambulation and respiratory measures to improve lung expansion after surgery (e.g., coughing, deep breathing). Additionally, removal of the chest tube is a painful procedure for the patient.[5,9,10]
- The types of sutures used to secure chest tubes vary according to the preference of the physician, the physician assistant, or the advanced practice nurse. One common type is the horizontal mattress or purse-string suture, which is threaded around and through the wound

edges in a U shape with the ends left unknotted until the chest tube is removed. Usually there are one or two anchor stitches accompanying the purse-string suture (see Fig. 20-1).
- A primary goal of chest tube removal is to remove tubes without introducing air or contaminants into the pleural space.

EQUIPMENT

- Suture removal set
- Povidone-iodine swabs
- Petrolatum gauze
- Kelly clamps (two per chest tube) or disposable umbilical clamps
- Wide, occlusive tape (2 inch)
- Dry 4 × 4 gauze sponges (two to four)
- Towel or Chux pad
- Personal protective equipment (goggles, sterile and nonsterile gloves, mask, gown)
  Additional equipment (to have available depending on patient need) includes the following:
- Specimen collection cup (if catheter tip is to be sent to the laboratory for analysis)
- Scissors

PATIENT AND FAMILY EDUCATION

- Assess patient and family understanding of the procedure. ➻*Rationale:* This assessment identifies patient and family knowledge deficits concerning patient condition, procedure, expected benefits, and potential risks and allows time for questions to clarify information.
- Explain the procedure, reason for removal, and sensations to be expected.[4,9-12] ➻*Rationale:* This explanation decreases patient anxiety and enhances cooperation.
- Explain the patient's role in assisting with removal. Explain that when prompted, the patient should perform the Valsalva maneuver. ➻*Rationale:* This explanation elicits patient cooperation and facilitates removal.
- Instruct the patient to turn and reposition every 2 hours after the chest tube has been removed. ➻*Rationale:* This prevents complications related to immobility and retained secretions.
- Instruct the patient to cough and deep breathe after the chest tube has been removed, splinting the affected side or sternum (with mediastinal tubes). ➻*Rationale:* This prevents respiratory complications associated with retained secretions. The application of firm pressure over the insertion site (i.e., splinting) decreases pain and discomfort.
- Instruct the patient regarding the availability of prescribed analgesic medication. ➻*Rationale:* Analgesics

alleviate pain and facilitate coughing, deep breathing, and repositioning.[10-12]
- Instruct the patient and family to report signs and symptoms of respiratory distress or infection immediately. ➻*Rationale:* Immediate reporting facilitates prompt intervention to relieve a recurrent pneumothorax or to treat an infection.

PATIENT ASSESSMENT AND PREPARATION

Patient Assessment

- Assess respiratory status.
  - ❖ Oxygen saturation within normal limits
  - ❖ Nonlabored respirations
  - ❖ Absence of shortness of breath
  - ❖ Decreased use of accessory muscles
  - ❖ Respiratory rate of less than 24 breaths/min
  - ❖ Equal bilateral breath sounds
  ➻*Rationale:* Assessment of respiratory status ensures the patient's readiness for chest tube removal.
- Assess chest tube drainage (less than 50 to 100 ml in 24 hours or less than 100 ml in 8 hours after cardiac surgery). ➻*Rationale:* Assessment of drainage verifies patient readiness for chest tube removal.
- Assess absence of fluctuation in water-seal chamber and air leak indicator. ➻*Rationale:* This indicates if lung is reexpanded and air leak is not present.
- Assess chest x-ray. ➻*Rationale:* Lung reexpansion indicates that need for chest tube is resolved.
- Assess vital signs and (optional) arterial blood gases. ➻*Rationale:* Vital signs indicate if patient can tolerate chest tube removal.

Patient Preparation

- Ensure that the patient understands preprocedural teaching. Answer questions as they arise, and reinforce information as needed. ➻*Rationale:* This communication evaluates and reinforces understanding of previously taught information. Anticipatory preparation may prepare patients for a better experience.[9-12]
- Premedicate the patient with adequate analgesics at least 15 minutes before procedure. Intravenous morphine may be used, or, in conjunction with the cardiac surgeon, subfascial lidocaine may be injected into the chest tube tract. ➻*Rationale:* Pain medication reduces the discomfort and anxiety experienced, facilitating patient cooperation.[9-12]
- Place the patient in the semi-Fowler position. Alternatively, place the patient on the unaffected side with the bed protector (towel or chux pad) underneath. ➻*Rationale:* This position enhances accessibility to the insertion site of the chest tube and protects the bed from drainage.

Procedure for Assisting With Chest Tube Removal

Steps	Rationale	Special Considerations
1. Wash hands, and don personal protective equipment.	Reduces the transmission of microorganisms and body secretions; standard precautions.	
2. Open the sterile suture removal set, and prepare petrolatum gauze dressing and two to four 4 × 4 gauze sponges.	Aseptic technique is maintained to prevent contamination of the wound. Removal of pleural chest tubes must be accomplished rapidly with the simultaneous application of an occlusive dressing to prevent air from entering the pleural space.	
3. Discontinue suction from chest drainage system, and check for air leakage in water-seal chamber. Observe the water-seal chamber while the patient coughs. A. If tube was placed for a pneumothorax, protocol may require 6 to 24 hours of water-seal and another x-ray before removal. *(Level IV: Limited clinical studies to support recommendations.)*	Bubbling in this chamber is associated with an air leak. When an air leak is present, removal of the chest tube can cause development of a pneumothorax. Ensures a recurrent pneumothorax has not occurred.[2]	If an air leak is present, the tube should not be removed. Consult with the physician or advanced practice nurse to determine appropriate action.
4. Remove existing tape, clean area around tubes with povidone-iodine, and determine type of suture that secures each chest tube. Clip appropriately. If a purse-string suture is present, leave the long suture ends intact.	Allows access to the chest tube at the skin level and prepares the sutures for removal.	
5. Confirm that the tube is free from the suture and the tape.		
6. Clamp each tube to be removed with two Kelly clamps or umbilical clamps.	Prevents air from being introduced into the pleural space.	
7. According to protocol, tube is removed while patient is performing Valsalva maneuver at either end inspiration or end expiration. *(Level IV: Limited clinical studies to support recommendations.)* A. *End inspiration:* instruct patient to take a deep breath and hold it while performing the Valsalva maneuver for each tube removed. If the patient is receiving ventilator support, pause the ventilator. If the patient is receiving ventilator support and is unable to follow instructions, remove the tube during peak inspiration phase. B. *End expiration:* Instruct patient to perform the Valsalva maneuver at end expiration. C. According to protocol, patients may need to hold their breath until sutures are tied.	Valsalva maneuver is needed to provide positive pressure in the pleural cavity and decreases the incidence of an involuntary gasp by the patient when the tube is removed.[1]	

Procedure for Assisting With Chest Tube Removal—*Continued*

Steps	Rationale	Special Considerations
8. Cover pleural insertion sites with petrolatum gauze dressing and mediastinal insertion site with 4 × 4 gauze pads. Secure with tape.	Avoids the influx of air.	Sterile petrolatum gauze should be applied over the skin site immediately after removal if tube was in pleural space or if no purse-string suture was present.
9. Obtain a portable chest x-ray per order or protocol (generally 1 to 24 hours after removal) or as clinically indicated. (*Level IV: Limited clinical studies to support recommendations.*)	Assesses that the lung has remained expanded.[3,6-8]	
10. Dispose of equipment in appropriate receptacle.	Standard precautions.	
11. Wash hands.	Decreases transmission of microorganisms.	

Expected Outcomes

- Patient is comfortable and experiences no respiratory distress
- Lung remains expanded after chest tube removal
- Site remains free of infection

Unexpected Outcomes

- Pneumothorax
- Bleeding
- Skin necrosis
- Retained chest tube
- Infected chest tube insertion site

Patient Monitoring and Care

Steps	Rationale	Reportable Conditions
		These conditions should be reported if they persist despite nursing interventions.
1. Ensure adequate respiratory status. Obtain chest x-ray if difficulties arise.	Diminished respiratory status could indicate a pneumothorax. Pneumothorax could be from removal of the chest tube before all the air, fluid, or blood in the pleural space had been drained, or it may recur after removal of the chest tube if air is introduced accidentally into the pleural space through the chest tube tract.	• Decreased oxygen saturation on pulse oximetry • Increased work of breathing • Diminished breath sounds on affected side • Increased restlessness and complaints of chest discomfort
2. Monitor insertion site for bleeding. Apply pressure at site. Place a tight occlusive dressing over site.	Persistent bleeding from insertion site could mean chest tube was against a vein or artery of chest wall before removal.	• Persistent bleeding
3. Monitor purse-string suture site for signs of skin necrosis. If seen, remove the suture and cleanse wound.	If purse-string suture was pulled too tightly closed when chest tube was removed, skin necrosis may be seen.	• Dark or inflamed skin with necrotic areas visible
4. Monitor site for signs of infection. If seen, prepare for wound cultures.	Prolonged insertion of a chest tube increases the risk that the tract created by the chest tube may become infected, or infection may occur after removal of the chest tube if the opening created by the removal becomes contaminated.	• Purulent drainage • Increased body temperature • Inflammation • Tenderness • Warmth at site

Procedure continues on the following page

Patient Monitoring and Care—*Continued*

Steps	Rationale	Reportable Conditions
5. Monitor insertion area for development of subcutaneous emphysema.	Air may leak into the surrounding tissues causing crepitus.	• Crepitus
6. Monitor for signs and symptoms of pericardial effusion or cardiac tamponade.	Removal of chest tubes may cause increased bleeding into pericardium. Pericardial bleeding may continue after chest tubes removed.	• Distant heart tones • Decreased blood pressure, tachycardia • Pulsus paradoxus • Narrowed pulse pressure • Equalized pulmonary artery pressures

Documentation

Documentation should include the following:

- Patient and family education
- Respiratory and vital signs assessments before and after the procedure
- Date, time, and by whom procedure was performed
- Amount, color, and consistency of any drainage
- Application of a sterile, occlusive dressing

- Type of suture in place and what was done to it (cut or tied)
- Patient's tolerance of the procedure
- Completion and results of chest x-ray
- Specimens sent to laboratory (if applicable)
- Unexpected outcomes
- Nursing interventions

References

1. Bell, R.L., et al. (2001). Chest tube removal: End-inspiration or end-expiration? *J Trauma,* 50, 674-7.
2. Martino, K., et al. (1999). Prospective randomized trial of thoracostomy removal algorithms. *J Trauma,* 46, 369-71.
3. McCormick, J.T., et al. (2002). The use of routine chest x-ray films after chest tube removal in postoperative cardiac patients. *Ann Thorac Surg,* 74, 2161-4.
4. Mimnaugh, L., et al. (1999). Sensations experienced during removal of tubes in acute postoperative patients. *Appl Nurs Res,* 12, 78-85.
5. Mueller, X.M., Tinguely, F., and Tavaearai, H.T. (2000). Impact of duration of chest tube drainage on pain after cardiac surgery. *Eur J Cardiothorac Surg,* 18, 570-4.
6. Pacanowski, J.P., et al. (2000). Is routine roentgenography needed after closed tube thoracostomy removal? *J Trauma,* 48, 684-8.
7. Palesty, J.A., McKelvey, A.A., and Dudrick, S.J. (2000). The efficacy of x-rays after chest tube removal. *Am J Surg,* 179, 13-6.
8. Pizano, L.R., Houghton, D.E., and Cohn, S.M. (2002). When should a chest radiograph be obtained after chest tube removal in mechanically ventilated patient? A prospective study. *J Trauma,* 53, 1073-7.
9. Puntillo, K., et al. (2001). Patients' perceptions and responses to procedural pain: Results from Thunder Project II. *Am J Crit Care,* 10, 238-51.
10. Puntillo, K., et al. (2002). Practices and predictors of analgesic intervention for adults undergoing painful procedures. *Am J Crit Care,* 11, 415-29.
11. Summer, G.H., and Puntillo, K.A. (2001). Management of surgical and procedural pain in a critical care setting. *Crit Care Nurs Clin North Am,* 13, 233-42.
12. Thompson, C.L., et al. (2001). Translating research into practice: Implications of the Thunder Project II. *Crit Care Nurs Clin North Am,* 13, 541-6.

Additional Readings

Charnock, Y., and Evans, D. (2001). Nursing management of chest drains: A systematic review. *Aust Crit Care,* 14, 156-60.

Christensen, M. (2002). Nurse-led chest drain removal in a cardiac high dependency unit. *Nurs Crit Care,* 7, 67-72.

Davis, J.W., et al. (1994). Randomized study of algorithms for discontinuing tube thoracostomy drainage. *J Am Coll Surg,* 179, 553-7.

Kirkwood, P. (2000). What is the current consensus or standard of practice for nurses removing chest tubes in a postoperative setting? *Crit Care Nurse,* 20, 97-8.

Tang, A.T.M., Velissaris, R.J., and Weeden, D.F. (2002). An evidence-based approach to drainage of the pleural cavity: Evaluation of best practice. *J Eval Clin Pract,* 8, 333-40.

Thomson, S.C., Wells, S., and Maxwell, M. (1997). Chest tube removal after cardiac surgery. *Crit Care Nurse,* 17, 34-8.

Younes, R.N., et al. (2002). When to remove a chest tube? A randomized study with subsequent prospective consecutive validation. *J Am Coll Surg,* 195, 658-62.

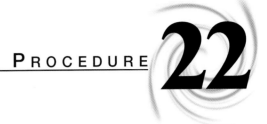

PROCEDURE **22**

Closed Chest Drainage System

P U R P O S E :   Closed chest drainage systems are used to facilitate the evacuation of fluid, blood, and air from the pleural space or the mediastinum or both; restore negative pressure to the pleural space; and promote reexpansion of a collapsed lung.

Joya D. Pickett

PREREQUISITE NURSING KNOWLEDGE

- Closed chest drainage systems include wet suction with a traditional water-seal; dry suction with a traditional water-seal; dry suction with a one-way valve; and one-, two-, three-, and four-bottle setups.
- Closed chest drainage systems use gravity, suction, or both to restore negative pressure and remove air, fluid, and blood from the pleural space or the mediastinum.
- Closed chest drainage systems use a one-way mechanism created by a water-seal, permitting air and fluid to be removed while preventing backflow into the chest.
- Closed chest drainage systems require that the pressure within the chest be greater than the pressure within the system. This is accomplished by keeping the drainage unit at least 1 foot below the chest tube insertion site and the tubing free of dependent loops and obstructions.
- Normal intrapleural pressures measure approximately -4 cm H_2O. At end inhalation, pressure decreases to -8 cm H_2O.
- The addition of a suction source can enhance drainage when large volumes of air or fluid must be evacuated.
    - Some disposable systems and suction devices (i.e., Emerson pump) contain an exit vent from the water-seal chamber so that the drainage unit remains vented when the suction device is off.
    - When using chest drainage systems without an exit vent and wall-mounted suction devices, from a pipeline vacuum system or Venturi suction, drainage systems should be disconnected from these suction devices before they are turned off.[12]
    - Some wall-mounted suction devices need control and pressure gauges to regulate and monitor for potential surges in suction levels.[12]
- Some disposable wet suction with traditional water-seal drainage systems can provide suction levels greater than -25 cm H_2O. The suction chamber vent holes can be occluded by using a nonporous tape or replaced with the manufacturer's special pronged vent plug and connecting it directly to a wall regulator suction. Suction levels must be converted from prescribed levels of cm H_2O suction to mm Hg of wall suction (Table 22-1).
- Disposable chest drainage units are an alternative to traditional glass bottle chest drainage systems and correlate to the three-bottle drainage system, with collection, water-seal, and suction control chambers positioned side by side in a molded plastic disposable unit (Fig. 22-1).
- Disadvantages of a bottle system include the risk for error during assembly because of multiple parts and connections, increased risk for contamination because of the multiple parts, difficulty in transportation because of the weight and awkwardness of the system, and increased risk of breakage.
- Some disposable drainage systems have a positive-pressure relief valve used to prevent a tension pneumothorax if the suction tubing becomes accidentally occluded or the suction source fails. Additionally, automatic and

TABLE 22-1	Pressure Conversion Chart*	
cm H_2O	**mm Hg**
20	15
25	18
30	22
35	26
40	30
45	33
50	37
60	44

*Approximate values.
Reprinted with permission of Atrium Medical Corporation, Hudson, NH.

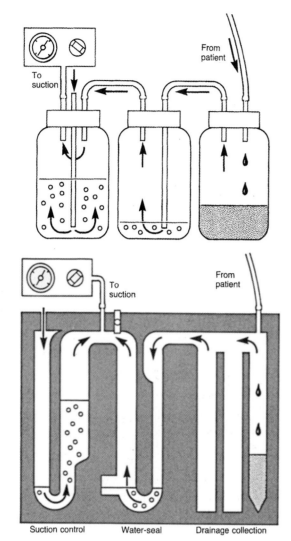

FIGURE 22-1 Disposable system correlates with three-bottle system. *(From Luce, J.M., Tyler, M.L., and Pierson, D.J. [1984]. Intensive Respiratory Care. Philadelphia: W.B. Saunders.)*

manual pressure relief valves vent excessive negative pressure, such as may occur during deep inspiration or milking of the chest tube.

- Tension pneumothorax is a critical condition in which increasing pressure from air trapped in the chest may displace vital organs, leading to shock and circulatory collapse.[11]
- Some disposable chest drainage systems use dry suction with a traditional water-seal and either a regulator or a restricted orifice mechanism. Although water is added to the water-seal chamber, it is not necessary to add water to the suction chamber. Instead, the suction source (usually a wall regulator) is increased until an indicator appears.
- Some disposable chest drainage systems are waterless, referred to as *dry-dry drains,* and have a one-way valve, eliminating the need to fill any chambers (except an air-leak indicator zone, as needed). A valve opens on expiration allowing patient air to exit, then closes to prevent atmospheric air from entering during inspiration. This one-way valve feature allows the system to be used in the vertical or horizontal position without loss of the seal; these systems are safe if accidentally tipped. The amount of suction delivered is regulated by an adjustable dial.

- Advantages of dry suction are ease of setup; higher, more precise levels of suction; and a quiet system.
- Disposable systems have self-sealing ports or collection tubes for aspiration of drainage samples and removal of excess chamber fluid levels.
- Some disposable chest drainage units have replaceable collection chambers, which can be removed when filled and replaced with a new one without changing the entire unit. Latex-free tubing is used in many disposable drainage units.
- Some disposable chest drainage systems have accessories to convert them to an autotransfusion unit. Normal saline (NS) is recommended when preparing these units.
- Some clinicians suggest using the Emerson pump (Fig. 22-2) for patients with large bronchopleural air leaks because they are high-volume, low-resistance, portable suction devices capable of handling high air flow rates.[6]
- Tidaling, fluctuations that occur with inspiration/expiration, provides a continuous manometer of the pressure changes in the pleural space and indicates overall respiratory effort. Absence of oscillations suggests obstruction of the drainage system due to clots, contact with lung tissue, kinks, loss of subatmospheric pressure due to fluid-filled dependent loops, or complete reexpansion of the lung.[1,2]
- The most common amount of suction pressure is -20 cm H_2O.[1,8,11] Suction levels higher than -40 cm H_2O suction are not recommended to prevent complications, such as persistent pleural air leaks, lung tissue entrapment, and reexpansion pulmonary edema.[5,9]
- Except for the exit vent, an airtight system is required to assist in maintaining negative pressure in the pleura and to prevent air entrapment in the pleural space.[11]
- In general, clamping of chest tubes is contraindicated. Clamping a chest tube in a patient with a pleural air leak may cause a tension pneumothorax. There are a few situations in which chest tubes may be clamped briefly (i.e., less than 1 minute): to locate the source of an air leak, to replace the chest drainage system, and to determine if a patient is ready to have the chest tube removed.[1,2,5,6]
- No references were found in the literature to support the routine practice of medication instillation into chest tubes.

EQUIPMENT

Disposable Setup (Wet and Dry Systems)
- Disposable chest drainage unit
- Gloves
- Suction source
- Connecting tubing
- Tape (1 inch), one roll, or Parham bands

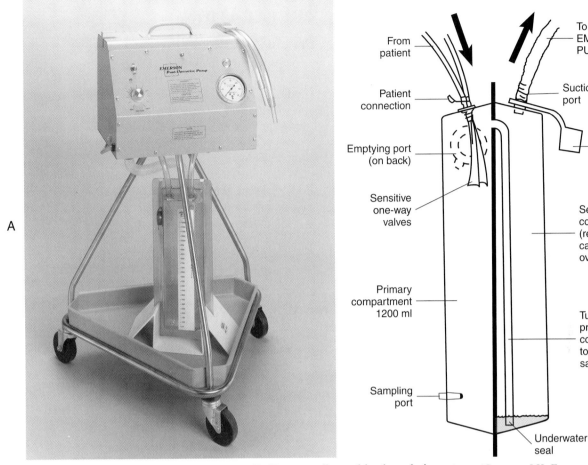

FIGURE 22-2 **A,** Emerson pump. **B,** Emerson disposable chest drain system. *(Courtesy J.H. Emerson, Cambridge, MA.)*

- 1-liter bottle of sterile water or normal saline (NS) (for systems that use water)
- 50-ml irrigation syringe (if not supplied with unit) for systems that use water

Emerson Pump (Disposable Setup)
- Disposable chest drainage unit
- Gloves
- Emerson pump
- 1-liter bottle of sterile water or NS
- Flexible corrugated tubing
- Drainage tubes
- Bottle stand

All Bottle Systems
- Gloves
- Sterile water or NS
- Rack or holder for the bottles
- Tape (1 inch), one roll
- Parham bands

One-Bottle System
- Sterile 2-liter bottle
- One short straw

- One long straw
- Sterile rubber stopper with two holes

Two-Bottle System
- Two sterile 2-liter bottles
- Three short straws
- One long straw
- Two sterile rubber stoppers, one with two holes and the other with either two or three holes (depending on which type of double-bottle system is used)
- Sterile connecting tubing (6 feet)
- One short sterile connecting tubing
- Suction source, if prescribed

Three-Bottle System
- Three sterile 2-liter bottles
- Five short straws
- Two long straws
- Two sterile rubber stoppers with two holes
- One sterile rubber stopper with three holes
- Suction source
- Sterile connecting tubing (6 feet)
- Two short sterile connecting tubings
- Suction source

Four-Bottle System

- Four sterile 2-liter bottles
- Seven short straws
- Three long straws
- Two sterile rubber stoppers with two holes
- Two sterile rubber stoppers with three holes
- Sterile connecting tubing (6 feet)
- Three short sterile connecting tubings
- Suction source

PATIENT AND FAMILY EDUCATION

- Explain the procedure and how the closed chest drainage system works. ➤*Rationale:* This communication identifies patient and family knowledge deficits about the patient's condition, procedure, expected benefits, and potential risks and allows time for questions to clarify information and to voice concerns. Explanations decrease patient anxiety and enhance cooperation.
- After chest tube insertion, instruct the patient to sit in a semi-Fowler position (unless contraindicated). ➤*Rationale:* This position facilitates drainage from the lung, by allowing air to rise and fluid to settle, enhancing removal via the chest tube. This position also makes breathing easier.
- Instruct the patient to turn and reposition every 2 hours. The patient may lie on the side with the chest tube but should keep the tubing free of kinks. ➤*Rationale:* Turning and positioning prevents complications related to immobility and retained secretions. Keeping the tubing free of kinks maintains patency of the tube, facilitates drainage, and prevents the accumulation of pressure within the pleural space, which interferes with lung reexpansion.
- Instruct the patient to cough and deep breathe, splinting the affected side or sternum (if mediastinal tube is in place). ➤*Rationale:* Coughing and deep breathing increase pressure within the pleural space, facilitating drainage, promoting lung reexpansion, and preventing respiratory complications associated with retained secretions. Applying firm pressure over the chest tube insertion site (i.e., splinting) decreases pain and discomfort.
- Encourage active or passive range-of-motion exercises of the arm on the affected side. ➤*Rationale:* The patient may limit the movement of the arm on the affected side to decrease the discomfort at the insertion site, resulting in joint discomfort and potential joint complications.
- Instruct the patient and family about activity as prescribed while maintaining the drainage system below the level of the chest. ➤*Rationale:* The drainage system is maintained below the level of the chest to facilitate gravity drainage and to prevent backflow into the pleural space and potential infectious contamination into the pleural space.
- Instruct the patient and family about the availability of prescribed analgesic medication and other pain relief strategies. ➤*Rationale:* Pain relief ensures comfort and facilitates coughing, deep breathing, positioning, range-of-motion exercises, and recuperation.

PATIENT ASSESSMENT AND PREPARATION

Patient Assessment

- Assess significant medical history or injury, including chronic lung disease, spontaneous pneumothorax, pulmonary disease, therapeutic procedures, and mechanism of injury. ➤*Rationale:* Medical history or injury may provide the etiologic basis for the occurrence of pneumothorax, hemothorax, empyema, pleural effusion, or chylothorax.
- Assess baseline cardiopulmonary status, as follows.
  - ❖ Vital signs (blood pressure, heart rate, respiratory rate): hypotension, tachycardia, dysrhythmias, tachypnea
  - ❖ Shortness of breath or dyspnea
  - ❖ Anxiety, restlessness, or apprehension
  - ❖ Cyanosis
  - ❖ Decreased oxygen saturation (SpO_2, SaO_2)
  - ❖ Decreased or absent breath sounds on the affected side
  - ❖ Crackles adjacent to the affected area
  - ❖ Asymmetrical chest excursion with respirations
  - ❖ Hyperresonance in the affected side (pneumothorax)
  - ❖ Dullness or flatness in the affected side (hemothorax, pleural effusion, empyema, or chylothorax)
  - ❖ Subcutaneous emphysema/crepitus (pneumothorax)
  - ❖ Sudden sharp focal chest pain
  - ❖ Tracheal deviation to the unaffected side (tension pneumothorax)
  - ❖ Neck vein distention (tension pneumothorax)
  - ❖ Muffled heart sounds (tension pneumothorax)
  ➤*Rationale:* Accurate assessment of signs and symptoms allows for prompt recognition and treatment. Baseline assessment provides comparison data for evaluating changes and outcomes of treatment.
- Assess diagnostic tests (if patient's condition does not necessitate immediate intervention).
  - ❖ Chest x-ray
  - ❖ Arterial blood gases
  ➤*Rationale:* Diagnostic testing confirms the presence of air or fluid in the pleural space, a collapsed lung, hypoxemia, and respiratory compromise.

Patient Preparation

- Ensure that the patient understands preprocedural teaching. Answer questions as they arise, and reinforce information as needed. ➤*Rationale:* This communication evaluates and reinforces understanding of previously taught information.
- Assist the patient to the lateral, supine (for pneumothorax), or semi-Fowler position (for hemothorax). ➤*Rationale:* These positions enhance accessibility to the insertion site for positioning of the chest tube.
- Administer prescribed analgesics or sedatives as needed. ➤*Rationale:* Analgesics and sedatives reduce the discomfort and anxiety experienced, facilitating patient cooperation.

Procedure for Using Closed Chest Drainage Systems

Steps	Rationale	Special Considerations

These Steps Should Be Followed for Wet and Dry Disposable Units, Emerson Pump, and Bottle Units

Steps	Rationale	Special Considerations
1. Wash hands, and don personal protective equipment.	Reduces transmission of microorganisms and body secretions; standard precautions.	
2. Open sterile packages.	Maintains aseptic technique whenever making changes to the system.	

Disposable Wet Suction System
Proceed to Step 3.

Disposable Dry Suction System
Proceed to Step 10.

Emerson Pump Disposable Suction
Proceed to Step 16.

One-Bottle System
Proceed to Step 23.

Two-Bottle System
Proceed to Step 30.

Three-Bottle System
Proceed to Step 55.

Four-Bottle System
Proceed to Step 72.

Disposable Wet Suction Chest Drainage System

Steps	Rationale	Special Considerations
3. Stabilize unit. Some systems have a floor stand. For systems with an in-line connector, move the patient tube clamp down next to the in-line connector.	Keeping the clamp visible helps prevent inadvertent clamping.	Clamping of chest tubes can cause air trapped in the pleural space to accumulate and may cause tension pneumothorax.
4. Remove the connector cap from the short tubing of the water-seal chamber, and use the funnel provided or a 50 ml syringe to add sterile water or NS to the 2 cm level.	Depth of solution required to establish a water-seal; the water-seal permits air and fluid to be removed from the chest while preventing backflow of air.	Water-seal levels greater than 2 cm increase the work of breathing; levels less than 2 cm can expose the water-seal to air and increase the risk for pneumothorax.
5. For gravity drainage, leave the short tubing from the suction control chamber open to air.	Creates the exit vent for the escape of air.	Clamping or occlusion of the exit vent can cause air to remain trapped in the pleural space, which may cause tension pneumothorax.
6. For suction drainage, fill the suction control chamber with sterile water or NS to the prescribed level (usually –20 cm H_2O suction). Connect the short tubing from the suction control chamber to the suction source.	Suction is regulated by the height of the solution level in this chamber.	Refill the solution level as necessary to the prescribed amount to replace solution lost through evaporation. Remove excess fluid as necessary via self-sealing grommet.
7. Hang chest drainage unit from bed frame, or set it on a floor stand. (*Level IV: Limited clinical studies to support recommendations.*)	Drainage unit must be kept below the level of the chest to promote gravity drainage and to prevent backflow of drainage into the pleural space, which interferes with lung expansion.[5,10]	

Procedure continues on the following page

Procedure for **Using Closed Chest Drainage Systems**—*Continued*

Steps	Rationale	Special Considerations
8. Connect the long tubing from the drainage collection chamber to the chest tube.	Creates the drainage collection system; avoid dependent or fluid-filled loops.	Dependent or fluid-filled loops may create back-pressure and decrease the effectiveness of suction.
9. Turn on the suction source if prescribed, to elicit gentle, constant bubbling.	Activates suction.	Some systems have a suction control feature to maintain the desired suction level automatically despite fluctuations in the suction source.

Proceed to Step 94.

Disposable Dry Suction Chest Drainage System

Steps	Rationale	Special Considerations
10. Stabilize unit. Some systems have a floor stand. For systems with an in-line connector, move the patient tube clamp down next to the in-line connector.	Keeping the clamp visible helps prevent inadvertent clamping.	Clamping of chest tubes can cause air trapped in the pleural space to accumulate and may cause tension pneumothorax.
11. *Dry suction with a traditional water-seal:* Remove the connector cap from the short tubing of the water-seal chamber, and use the funnel provided or a 50-ml syringe to add sterile water or NS to the 2 cm level. Some systems provide prefilled sterile water containers. *Dry suction with a one-way valve:* Fill air-leak monitor zone.	Depth of solution required to establish a water-seal; the water-seal permits air and fluid to be removed from the patient, while preventing the backflow of air into the chest.	Water-seal levels greater than 2 cm increase the work of breathing; levels less than 2 cm can expose the water-seal to air and increase the risk for pneumothorax.
12. Hang drainage unit from bed frame or set it on a floor stand. *(Level IV: Limited clinical studies to support recommendations.)*	Drainage unit must be kept below the level of the chest to promote gravity drainage and to prevent backflow of drainage into the pleural space, which interferes with lung expansion.[5,10]	
13. Connect the long tubing from the drainage collection chamber to the chest tube.	Creates the closed chest drainage system; avoid dependent or fluid-filled loops.	Dependent or fluid-filled loops may create back-pressure and decrease the effectiveness of suction.
14. For gravity drainage, leave the suction control chamber open to air.	Creates the exit vent for the escape of air.	Clamping of chest tubes can cause air trapped in the pleural space to accumulate and may cause tension pneumothorax.
15. To initiate suction, dial in the prescribed amount of suction (usually –20 cm H_2O), then increase suction source until indicator mark appears according to manufacturer's guidelines.	Activates suction.	Apply suction as per manufacturer's guidelines: to apply –20 cm H_2O suction, use a minimum vacuum pressure of –80 mm Hg. Suction source vacuum should be greater than –80 mm Hg when multiple chest drains are used. For a suction level less than –20 cm H_2O, any observed bellows expansion across the monitor window confirms adequate suction operation. To decrease suction, set the dial, confirm patient on suction, then depress the high-negativity vent, venting to the newer lower amount.

Proceed to Step 94.

Procedure for Using Closed Chest Drainage Systems—*Continued*

Steps	Rationale	Special Considerations
Emerson Disposable Suction System Setup (see Fig. 22-2)		
16. Add sterile water or NS through the suction port into the secondary compartment (overflow compartment) up to the water-seal line.	Depth of solution required to establish a water-seal; the water-seal permits air and fluid to be removed from the chest, while preventing the backflow of air.	Water-seal levels greater than 2 cm increase the work of breathing; levels less than 2 cm can expose the water-seal to air and increase the risk for pneumothorax.
17. Secure the drainage system in the Emerson pump stand using the strings supplied, or with the accessory metal hangers suspend the drainage set from the patient's bed.	Drainage unit must be kept below the level of the chest to promote gravity drainage and to prevent backflow of drainage into the pleural space, which interferes with lung expansion.	
18. Connect the patient tube(s) to the patient connection fittings. If the patient has only one chest tube, leave the second unused port fitting capped.	This helps to maintain a closed drainage system.	
19. Connect the patient's chest tube(s) to the patient connection tubing.	Creates the closed drainage system; avoid dependent loops.	Dependent or fluid-filled loops may create back-pressure and decrease the effectiveness of suction.
20. For gravity drainage, leave the flexible corrugated tubing off of the suction port on the secondary compartment (overflow compartment).	Creates the exit vent for the escape of air.	Clamping of chest tubes can cause air trapped in the pleural space to accumulate and may cause tension pneumothorax.
21. For suction drainage, connect the flexible corrugated tube to the suction port and to the corresponding fitting in the bottom of the Emerson pump cabinet.	Creates the suction drainage system.	
22. Dial in the amount of prescribed continuous suction on the Emerson pump dial. **Proceed to Step 94**.	Activates suction.	
One-Bottle Setup (Fig. 22-3)		
23. Fill the water-seal bottle with sterile water or NS so that the bottom of the long straw is immersed approximately 2 cm.	Immersing the long straw in normal saline is required to establish a water-seal. The water-seal permits air and fluid to be removed from the chest, while preventing the backflow of air.[1]	Water-seal levels greater than 2 cm increase the work of breathing; levels less than 2 cm expose the water-seal to air and increase the risk for pneumothorax. If a large amount of drainage is anticipated, a two-bottle system is preferred, or empty the bottle whenever it is one quarter or more filled with fluid or according to institutional policy.[12]
24. Seal the bottle with the rubber stopper.	Except for the exit vent, an airtight system is required to maintain pleural negative pressure and to prevent air entrapment in the pleural space.	

Procedure continues on the following page

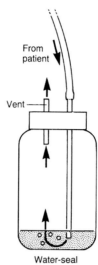

From
patient

Vent —

Water-seal

FIGURE 22-3 One-bottle chest drainage system. *(From
Luce, J.M., Tyler, M.L., and Pierson, D.J. [1984].* Intensive
Respiratory Care. *Philadelphia: W.B. Saunders.)*

Procedure for Using Closed Chest Drainage Systems—*Continued*

Steps	Rationale	Special Considerations
25. Insert the short straw through one of the openings in the stopper and leave open to air.	The exit vent permits pleural air to escape from the system; otherwise, pressure can build up in the system, preventing further removal of pleural air and fluids.	Clamping or occlusion of the exit vent can cause air to remain trapped in the pleural space and may cause tension pneumothorax.
26. Insert the long straw through the second opening, immersing it 2 cm (less than 1 inch) beneath the surface of the solution.	Creates the water-seal.	Immersing the straw deeper than 2 cm increases the work of breathing.
27. Stabilize the drainage bottle on the floor or in a special holder.	The bottle must be kept below the level of the chest to provide gravity drainage and prevent backflow of drainage into the pleural space, which interferes with lung expansion.	Disruption of the system may permit the entrance of atmospheric air into the pleural space, which may collapse the lung.
28. Connect the patient drainage tubing to the long straw of the water-seal bottle.	This creates the water-seal drainage collection bottle.	
29. Connect the patient drainage tubing to the chest tube. **Proceed to Step 94.**	Creates the closed chest drainage system.	
Two-Bottle Setup With a Drainage Collection Bottle and a Water-Seal Bottle (Fig. 22-4A)		
30. Seal one bottle with a rubber stopper with two openings.	Except for the exit vent, an airtight system is required to maintain pleural negative pressure and to prevent air entrapment in the pleural space.	
31. Insert two short straws into the rubber stopper.	Creates the drainage collection bottle.	
32. Fill the water-seal bottle with sterile water or NS so that the bottom of the long straw is immersed approximately 2 cm.	Depth of solution required to establish a water-seal; the water-seal permits air and fluid to be removed from the chest, while preventing the backflow of air.[1]	Water-seal levels greater than 2 cm increase the work of breathing; levels less than 2 cm expose the water-seal to air and increase the risk for pneumothorax.

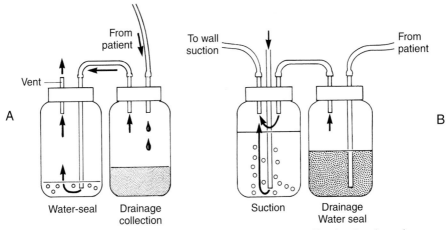

FIGURE 22-4 Two-bottle chest drainage system. **A,** Drainage collection bottle and a water-seal bottle. **B,** Water-seal/drainage collection bottle and a suction control bottle. *(From Luce, J.M., Tyler, M.L., and Pierson, D.J. [1984]. Intensive Respiratory Care. Philadelphia: W.B. Saunders.)*

Procedure for Using Closed Chest Drainage Systems—*Continued*

Steps	Rationale	Special Considerations
33. Seal the other bottle with a rubber stopper with two openings.	Except for the exit vent, an airtight system is required to maintain pleural negative pressure and to prevent air entrapment in the pleural space.	
34. Insert the short straw through one of the openings in the stopper.	Creates the exit vent for the escape of air or for connection to the suction source.	
35. Insert the long straw through the second opening, immersing it 2 cm beneath the surface of the solution.	Creates the water-seal and protects the patient from air leaks or loss of water-seal.	Immersing the straw deeper than 2 cm increases the work of breathing.
36. Use the sterile tubing to connect one of the short straws of the drainage collection bottle to the long straw of the water-seal bottle.	Connects the drainage collection bottle to the water-seal bottle.	
37. Stabilize the bottles on the floor or in a special holder.	The bottles must be kept below the level of the chest, to prevent backflow of drainage into the pleural space, which interferes with lung expansion.	Disruption of the system may permit the entrance of atmospheric air into the pleural space, which may cause tension pneumothorax.
38. Connect the patient drainage tubing to the second short straw of the drainage collection bottle.	Creates a drainage avenue.	
39. Connect the patient drainage tubing to the chest tube.		
40. For gravity drainage, leave the exit vent of the water-seal bottle open to air. To apply suction, connect the suction source (i.e., Emerson pump) to the exit vent, and adjust to the prescribed level (usually –20 cm H_2O suction level). **Proceed to Step 94.**	Suction increases pressure differences between the pleural space and the drainage system, which facilitates drainage from the pleural space.	Some systems have a suction control feature to maintain the desired suction level automatically despite fluctuations in the suction source. When connected to a suction system that has no exit vent, there is no in-flow of air to equilibrate

Procedure continues on the following page

Procedure for Using Closed Chest Drainage Systems—*Continued*

Steps	Rationale	Special Considerations
		the pressure in the chamber, causing potential surges in suction.
		If a wall-mounted suction device is used, the exit vent of the drainage system should be disconnected if the device is turned off.[12]

Two-Bottle Setup With a Water-Seal/Drainage Collection Bottle and a Suction Control Bottle (Fig. 22-4B)

Steps	Rationale	Special Considerations
41. Fill the water-seal/drainage collection bottle with sterile water or NS so that the bottom of the long straw is immersed approximately 2 cm.	Depth of solution required to establish a water-seal; the water-seal permits air and fluid to be removed from the patient, while preventing the backflow of air.[1]	
42. Seal the bottle with a rubber stopper with two openings.	Except for the exit vent, an airtight system is required to maintain pleural negative pressure and to prevent air entrapment in the pleural space.	
43. Insert the short straw through one of the openings in the stopper.	Initial step for connecting the drainage bottle to the water-seal bottle.	
44. Insert the long straw through the second opening, immersing it 2 cm beneath the surface of the solution.	Creates the water-seal and protects the patient from air leaks or loss of water-seal.	Immersing the straw deeper than 2 cm increases the work of breathing.
45. Add prescribed amount of sterile water or NS to the suction bottle (usually −20 cm H_2O suction level).	Creates at least −20 cm H_2O of suction.	The depth the straw is immersed in the solution determines the amount of suction delivered to the chest tube.
46. Seal the suction bottle with the rubber stopper with three openings.	Except for the exit vent, an airtight system is required to maintain pleural negative pressure and to prevent air entrapment in the pleural space.	
47. Insert the long straw through the middle opening (leaving one end immersed in the solution and the other end open to the atmosphere).	Creates an air vent.	
48. Insert the two short straws into the remaining openings of the stopper.	Creates the setup for attachment to suction and to the overflow drainage bottle.	
49. Use the sterile tubing to connect the short straw from the water-seal/drainage collection bottle to one of the short straws of the suction bottle.	Connects the water-seal bottle to the suction source.	
50. Attach one end of the 6-foot connecting tubing to the second short straw of the suction bottle and the other end to the suction source.	Connects the suction bottle to the suction source.	
51. Stabilize the drainage bottles on the floor or in a special holder. (*Level IV: Limited clinical studies to support recommendations.*)	The bottles must be kept below the level of the chest to prevent backflow of drainage into the pleural space, which interferes with lung expansion.[5,10]	Disruption of the system may permit the entrance of atmospheric air into the pleural space, which may collapse the lung.
52. Connect the patient drainage tube to the long straw of the water-seal/drainage collection bottle.	Creates the water-seal/drainage collection bottle.	

Procedure **for Using Closed Chest Drainage Systems**—*Continued*

Steps	Rationale	Special Considerations
53. Connect the patient drainage tube to the chest tube.	Creates the chest drainage system.	The chest tube drainage system should be connected to the chest tube before suction is turned on.
54. Turn on the suction source to elicit gentle, constant bubbling in the suction. **Proceed to Step 94.**	Activates suction.	
Three-Bottle Setup (Fig. 22-5) 55. Seal one of the bottles with the rubber stopper with two openings.	Except for the exit vent, an airtight system is required to maintain pleural negative pressure and to prevent air entrapment in the pleural space.	
56. Insert two short straws into the rubber stopper.	This creates the drainage collection bottle.	This bottle can be calibrated if it is not already by placing a piece of tape on the side so that drainage can be measured and recorded.
57. Fill the water-seal bottle with sterile water or NS so that the bottom of the long straw is immersed approximately 2 cm.	Depth of solution required to establish a water-seal; the water-seal permits air and fluid to be removed from the patient, while preventing the backflow of air into the chest.[1]	Water-seal levels greater than 2 cm increase the work of breathing; levels less than 2 cm expose the water-seal to air and increase the risk for pneumothorax.
58. Seal the water-seal bottle with a rubber stopper with two openings.	Except for the exit vent, an airtight system is required to maintain pleural negative pressure and to prevent air entrapment in the pleural space.	
59. Insert the short straw through one of the openings in the stopper.	Creates the exit vent for the escape of air or for connection to the suction source.	
60. Insert the long straw through the second opening, immersing it 2 cm beneath the surface of the solution.	Creates the water-seal and protects the patient from air leaks or loss of water seal.	Immersing the straw deeper than 2 cm increases the work of breathing.
61. Add prescribed amount of sterile water or NS to the suction bottle (usually −20 cm H_2O suction level).	Creates at least −20 cm H_2O of suction.	The depth the straw is immersed in the solution determines the amount of suction delivered to the chest tube.

Procedure continues on the following page

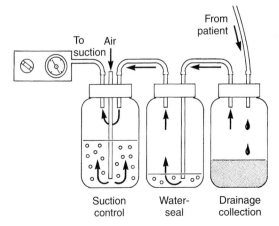

FIGURE 22-5 Three-bottle chest drainage system. *(From Luce, J.M., Tyler, M.L., and Pierson, D.J. [1984]. Intensive Respiratory Care. Philadelphia: W.B. Saunders.)*

Procedure **for Using Closed Chest Drainage Systems**—*Continued*

Steps	Rationale	Special Considerations
62. Seal the suction bottle with the rubber stopper with three openings.	Except for the exit vent, an airtight system is required to maintain pleural negative pressure and to prevent air entrapment in the pleural space.	
63. Insert the long straw through the middle opening (leaving one end immersed in the solution and the other end open to the atmosphere).	Creates the suction bottle.	
64. Insert the two short straws into the remaining openings of the stopper.	Creates the setup for attachment to suction and to the overflow drainage bottle.	
65. Use the sterile tubing to connect the short straw of the drainage collection bottle to the long straw of the water-seal bottle.	Connects the water seal bottle to the suction bottle.	
66. Use the sterile tubing to connect the short straw from the water-seal bottle to one of the short straws of the suction bottle.	Connects the water-seal bottle to the suction bottle.	
67. Attach one end of the 6-foot connecting tubing to the second short straw of the suction bottle and the other end to the suction source.	Connects the suction bottle to the suction source.	
68. Stabilize the drainage bottles on the floor or in a special holder. (*Level IV: Limited clinical studies to support recommendations.*)	The bottles must be kept below the level of the chest to prevent backflow of drainage into the pleural space, which interferes with lung expansion.[5,10]	Disruption of the system may permit the entrance of atmospheric air into the pleural space, which may collapse the lung.
69. Connect the patient drainage tube to the short straw of the drainage collection bottle.	Provides a route for drainage to flow from the patient to the collection bottle.	
70. Connect the patient drainage tube to the chest tube.		The chest tube drainage system should be connected to the chest tube before suction is turned on.
71. Turn the suction source on to elicit gentle, constant bubbling in the suction.	Activates suction.	

Proceed to Step 94.

Four-Bottle Setup (Three-Bottle Setup With Vented Water-Seal Bottle) (Fig. 22-6)

72. Fill the vented water-seal bottle with sterile water or NS so that the bottom of the long straw is immersed approximately 2 cm.	Depth of solution required to establish a water-seal; the water-seal permits air and fluid to be removed from the patient, while preventing the backflow of air into the chest.[1]	
73. Seal the bottle with a rubber stopper with two openings.	Except for the exit vent, an airtight system is required to maintain pleural negative pressure and to prevent air entrapment in the pleural space.	
74. Insert the long straw through one of the openings, immersing it 2 cm beneath the surface of the solution.	Creates the water-seal and protects the patient from air leaks or loss of water-seal.	Immersing the straw deeper than 2 cm increases the work of breathing.

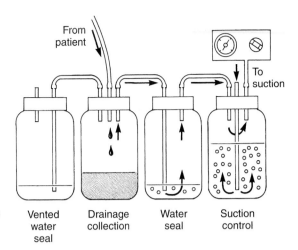

From patient

To suction

FIGURE 22-6 Four-bottle chest drainage system. *(From Luce, J.M., Tyler, M.L., and Pierson, D.J. [1984].* Intensive Respiratory Care. *Philadelphia: W.B. Saunders.)*

Vented water seal   Drainage collection   Water seal   Suction control

Procedure for Using Closed Chest Drainage Systems—*Continued*

Steps	Rationale	Special Considerations
75. Insert a short straw through the second opening in the stopper and leave open to air.	Creates the vented water-seal that acts as a safety feature to allow the escape of positive pressure in case of problems with the suction source.	
76. Seal the drainage collection bottle with a rubber stopper with three openings.	Except for the exit vent, an airtight system is required to maintain pleural negative pressure and to prevent air entrapment in the pleural space.	
77. Insert three short straws into the rubber stopper.	This creates the drainage collection bottle.	This bottle can be calibrated if it is not already by placing a piece of tape on the side so that drainage can be measured and recorded.
78. Fill the water-seal bottle with sterile water or NS so that the bottom of the long straw is immersed approximately 2 cm.	Depth of solution required to establish a water-seal and to protect the patient from air leak or loss of water-seal.	
79. Seal the bottle with a rubber stopper with two openings.	Except for the exit vent, an airtight system is required to maintain pleural negative pressure and to prevent air entrapment in the pleural space.	
80. Insert the short straw through one of the openings in the stopper.	Creates the exit vent for the escape of air for connection to the suction source.	
81. Insert the long straw through the second opening, immersing it 2 cm beneath the surface of the solution.	Creates the water-seal and protects the patient from air leaks or loss of water-seal.	Immersing the straw deeper than 2 cm increases the work of breathing.
82. Add prescribed amount of sterile water or NS to the suction bottle (usually −20 cm H_2O suction level).	Creates at least −20 cm H_2O of suction.	The depth the straw is immersed in the solution determines the amount of suction delivered to the chest tube.

Procedure continues on the following page

Procedure for Using Closed Chest Drainage Systems—*Continued*

Steps	Rationale	Special Considerations
83. Seal the suction bottle with the rubber stopper with three openings.	Except for the exit vent, an airtight system is required to maintain pleural negative pressure and to prevent air entrapment in the pleural space.	
84. Insert the long straw through the middle opening (leaving one end immersed in the solution and the other end open to the atmosphere).	Creates the manometer tube or air vent.	
85. Insert the two short straws into the remaining openings.	Creates the setup for attachment to suction and to the overflow-drainage bottle.	
86. Use the sterile tubing to connect the long straw of the vented water seal bottle to one of the short straws of the drainage collection bottle.	Provides for communication between the drainage system bottle and the vented water-seal bottle.	
87. Use the sterile tubing to connect the second straw of the drainage collection bottle to the long straw of the water-seal bottle.	Connects the drainage collection bottle to the water-seal bottle.	
88. Use the sterile tubing to connect the short straw from the water-seal bottle to one of the short straws of the suction bottle.	Connects the water-seal bottle to the suction bottle.	
89. Attach one end of the 6-foot connecting tubing to the second short straw of the suction bottle and the other end to the suction source.	Connects the suction bottle to the suction source.	
90. Stabilize the drainage bottles on the floor or in a special holder. (*Level IV: Limited clinical studies to support recommendations.*)	The bottles must be kept below the level of the chest to prevent backflow of drainage into the pleural space, which interferes with lung expansion.[5,10]	Disruption of the system may permit the entrance of atmospheric air into the pleural space, which may collapse the lung.
91. Connect the patient drainage tube to the middle short straw of the drainage collection bottle.	Provides a route for drainage to flow from the patient to the collection bottle.	
92. Connect the patient drainage tube to the chest tube.		The chest tube drainage system should be connected to the chest tube before suction is turned on.
93. Turn the suction source on to elicit gentle, constant bubbling in the suction bottle.	Activates suction.	
94. Tape all connection points in the chest drainage system (see Fig. 19-2).	Except for the exit vent, a secure and airtight system is required to avoid inadvertent disconnection causing potential air entrapment in the pleural space and decreased pleural negative pressure.	Parham bands may be used to secure connections instead of tape.
A. 1-inch tape is placed horizontally extending over the connections (a portion of the connector may be left unobstructed by the tape).	This technique secures the connections, but allows visualization of drainage in the connector.	

Procedure for Using Closed Chest Drainage Systems—*Continued*

Steps	Rationale	Special Considerations
B. Reinforce the horizontal tape with tape placed vertically so that it encircles both ends of the connector.		
95. Dispose of equipment in appropriate receptacle.	Standard precautions.	
96. Wash hands.	Reduces transmission of microorganisms.	

Expected Outcomes

- Removal of air, fluid, or blood
- Fluctuation or tidaling noted in the water-seal chamber (until lung reexpanded)
- Relief of respiratory distress
- Reexpansion of the collapsed lung validated by chest x-ray

Unexpected Outcomes

- Tension pneumothorax
- Hemorrhagic shock
- Absence of drainage and fluctuation or tidaling, or continuous bubbling in the water-seal chamber with continued respiratory distress
- Lung not showing evidence of reexpansion
- Fever, purulent drainage, and redness around the insertion site or purulent drainage in the chest tube

Patient Monitoring and Care

Steps	Rationale	Reportable Conditions
		These conditions should be reported if they persist despite nursing interventions.
1. Assess cardiopulmonary and vital signs (including SpO_2) every 2 hours and as needed.	Provides baseline and ongoing assessment of patient's condition.	• Tachypnea • Decreased or absent breath sounds • Hypoxemia • Tachycardia • Dysrhythmias • Hypotension • Muffled heart tones • Tracheal deviation • Subcutaneous emphysema (crepitus) • Neck vein distention • Fever • Absence of fluctuations in water-seal chamber with respiratory distress
2. Mark the drainage level on the outside of the drainage collection chamber in hourly or shift increments and document.	Provides reference point for future measurements. Drainage should decrease gradually and change from bloody to pink to straw colored.[2] Sudden flow of dark bloody drainage that occurs with position change is often old blood.	• Drainage greater than 100 ml/hr • Sudden decrease or absence of drainage • Change in characteristics of drainage
3. Monitor amount and type of drainage from chest tube.	Volume loss can cause patients to become hypovolemic.	• Bloody drainage greater than 100 ml/hr • New onset of clots

Procedure continues on the following page

Patient Monitoring and Care—*Continued*

Steps	Rationale	Reportable Conditions
	Decreased or absent drainage associated with respiratory distress may indicate obstruction; decreased or absent drainage without respiratory distress may indicate lung reexpansion.	• Sudden decrease or absence of drainage
4. Maintain and check tube patency every 2 to 4 hours. Milk the tubing when a visible clot or other obstructing drainage is present in the tubing.[4] (*Level IV: Limited clinical studies to support recommendations.*)	Obstruction of drainage from the chest tube interferes with lung reexpansion. If drainage is bloody or thick, small segments of the tubing may need to be milked to keep it patent. Milking is done by manually squeezing and releasing the chest tubing between the fingers. Stripping the entire length of the chest tube is contraindicated because it results in transient high negative pressures in the pleural space and lung entrapment.[3] No significant differences are reported between the amount of drainage when the tubing is milked as opposed to stripped.[6]	• Inability to establish patency • Excessive drainage
5. Keep the drainage tubing free of dependent loops (i.e., placing the tube horizontally on the bed and down into the collection chamber, coiling the tubing on the bed). If a dependent loop cannot be avoided, lift and drain the tubing every 15 minutes. (*Level IV: Limited clinical studies to support recommendations.*)	Drainage accumulating in dependent loops obstructs chest drainage into the collecting system and increases pressure within the lung[5-7,10]; allow enough length for patient movement.	• Loops or kinks that cannot be removed
6. Refill the solution level as necessary (usually every 8 hours for suction chamber and every 24 hours for water-seal) to the prescribed amount to replace solution lost through evaporation.	To maintain prescribed water-seal and suction levels and to prevent complications.	• Inability to maintain a water-seal or to keep suction at prescribed level
7. Assess for air leaks in the system, as indicated by constant bubbling in the water-seal bottle or chamber. (Some disposable chest drainage systems have an air-leak assessment chamber.) To assess location of a leak, intermittently occlude for a moment (i.e., less than 1 minute) the chest tube or drainage tubing, beginning at the insertion site and progressing to the chest drainage unit.	An airtight system is required to help reestablish negative pressure in the pleural space. Chest tube drainage from a mediastinal tube should not cause bubbling in the water-seal chamber (if noted, it indicates communication with the pleural space—notify physician). Intermittent bubbling when suction is initially turned on occurs when air is displaced by fluid drainage in the collection chamber, patient has a small leak in the pleural space, or patient exhales or coughs.[2]	• New or increasing air leak in the chest or around the chest tube insertion site

Patient Monitoring and Care—*Continued*

Steps	Rationale	Reportable Conditions
	If the bubbling in the water-seal chamber stops when the chest tube is occluded at the dressing site, the air leak is inside the patient's chest or under the dressing. If a new-onset air leak, reinforce the dressing and notify the physician. If the bubbling stops when the drainage tubing is occluded along its length, the air leak is between the occlusion and the patient's chest; check to ensure all connections are airtight.[2] If the bubbling does not stop with occlusion, replace the chest drainage unit.	
8. Assess for patent system: Note fluctuations or tidaling of fluid level in the water-seal chamber (disposable chest drainage system) or the long straw of the water-seal bottle (bottle chest drainage system) with respirations.[1]	Indicates effective communication between the pleural space and drainage system and provides an indication of lung expansion. Fluctuations or tidaling stops when the lung is reexpanded or when the tubing is obstructed by a kink, a fluid-filled loop, the patient lying on the tubing, or a clot or tissue at the distal end.[2] (If a suction source has been added, it must be disconnected momentarily to assess accurately for fluctuations or tidaling.)	• Absence of fluctuations or tidaling
9. Assess drainage systems equipped with a float valve, for increases in the patient's negative intrathoracic pressure, noted in the water-seal level (e.g., after milking of chest tubes or when decreasing the level of suction). First, ensure the chest drainage system is operating on suction. Second, temporarily depress the filtered manual vent, until the float valve releases and the water column lowers.	Changes in the patient's intrathoracic pressure are reflected by the height of the water in the water-seal column. Do not lower water-seal column when suction is not operating or when patient is on gravity drainage. Resume patient to suction operation while performing this procedure.	• Sustained increases in negative pressures
10. Assess insertion site and surrounding skin for presence of subcutaneous air and signs of infection or inflammation with each dressing change or every day. Dressings should be changed when soiled, every 2 to 3 days, or when ordered by physician or advanced practice nurse.	Crepitus may indicate chest tube obstruction or improper tube position. Skin integrity is altered during insertion and can lead to infection.	• Subcutaneous emphysema (crepitus) • Fever • Redness around insertion site • Purulent drainage
11. Monitor collection chamber for total amount of fluid. Change chest drainage system when approaching full or if system	When the patient has an air leak or pneumothorax, clamping of the chest tube may precipitate a tension pneumothorax because the air has	• Respiratory distress noted during or after procedure • Changes in breath sounds postprocedure • Nonfunctioning chest drainage system

Procedure continues on the following page

Patient Monitoring and Care—*Continued*

Steps	Rationale	Reportable Conditions
integrity is interrupted (i.e., cracked). Assess patient, and auscultate breath sounds before and after procedure. Prepare new chest drainage system. Then briefly (i.e., less than 1 minute) cross clamp the chest tube close to the patient's chest. Attach the new system, unclamp the chest tube, check connections, and assess function of drainage system.	no escape route and may accumulate in the pleural space.[2,12] Clamping of the chest tube should be as brief as possible.	
12. Monitor patient's pain and intervene appropriately.	Pain relief ensures comfort and facilitates coughing, deep breathing, positioning, range-of-motion exercises, and improved outcomes.	• Pain unrelieved by nursing interventions
13. Obtaining a drainage specimen with disposable chest drainage systems: Use a syringe with a 20-gauge needle to withdraw the specimen from the self-sealing diaphragm.	Provides a specimen for analysis.	• Inability to obtain specimen

Documentation

Documentation should include the following:

- Patient and family education
- Cardiopulmonary and vital sign assessment
- Type of drainage system used
- Amount of suction, fluctuation or tidaling, type and amount of drainage
- Air leak—absence, presence, resolution, and severity
- Patient's tolerance of the therapy

- Respiratory, thoracic, and vital sign assessment with changes in therapy
- Completion and results of the postinsertion chest x-ray and any other ordered diagnostic tests
- Unexpected outcomes
- Nursing interventions (i.e., measures used to control pain)

References

1. Allibone, L. (2003). Nursing management of chest drains. *Nurs Stand,* 17, 45-56.
2. Carroll, P. (2000). Exploring chest drain options. *RN,* 63, 50-8.
3. Duncan, C., and Erickson, R. (1982). Pressures associated with chest tube stripping. *Heart Lung,* 11, 166-71.
4. Golden, P. (1999). Follow-up chest radiographs after traumatic pneumothorax or hemothorax in the outpatient setting: A retrospective review. *Int J Trauma Nurs,* 5, 88-94.
5. Gordon, P.A., et al. (1997). Positioning of chest tubes: Effects on pressure and drainage. *Am J Crit Care,* 6, 33-8.
6. Gordon, P.A., Norton, J.M., and Merrell, R. (1995). Redefining chest tube management: Analysis of the state of practice. *Dimens Crit Care Nurs,* 14, 6-13.
7. Gross, S.B. (1993). Current challenges, concepts and controversies in chest tube management. *AACN Clin Issues Crit Care Nurs,* 4, 260-75.
8. Jung, I. (2002). Chest tube management: What controls the amount of suction applied to a chest tube drainage system? *Nurs Netw,* 8, 2.
9. Kam, A.C., O'Brien, M., and Kam, P.C.A. (1993). Pleural drainage systems. *Anaesthesia,* 48, 154-61.
10. Schmelz, J.O., et al. (1999). Effects of position of chest drainage tube on volume drained and pressure. *Am J Crit Care,* 8, 319-23.
11. Tang, A.T., and Ragheb, H. (1999). A regional survey of chest drains: Evidence-based practice? *Postgrad Med J,* 75, 471.
12. Tang, A.T., Velissaris, T.J., and Weeden, D.F. (2002). An evidence-based approach to drainage of the pleural cavity: Evaluation of best practice. *J Eval Clin Pract,* 8, 333-40.

Additional Readings

Atrium. (1999). Managing chest drainage. *Atrium Medical Corporation,* 1-38.
Atrium. (1999). Managing dry suction chest drainage. *Atrium Medical Corporation,* 1-38.
Carroll, P. (2000). Exploring chest drain options. *RN,* 10, 2-11.
Carroll, P.F. (2003). Ask the experts: Atrium dry suction chest drainage system. *Crit Care Nurse,* 23, 73-4.
Charnock, Y., and Evans, D. (2001). Nursing management of chest drains: A systematic review. *Aust Crit Care,* 14, 156-60.
Deshpande, K.S., Tortolani, A.J., and Kvetan, V. (2003). Troubleshooting chest tube complications: How to prevent—or quickly correct—the major problems. *J Crit Illness,* 18, 275-80.

Kirkwood, P. (2002). Are chest tubes routinely milked, stripped, or suctioned to maintain patency? *Crit Care Nurse,* 22, 70-2.

Lim-Levy, F., et al. (1986). Is milking and stripping chest tubes really necessary? *Ann Thorac Surg,* 42, 77-80.

McCarthy, K. (2003). *Understanding Chest Drainage.* Available at: http://www.nursingceu.com/NCEU/courses/chestdrainagekm.

O'Hanlon-Nichols, T. (1996). Commonly asked questions about chest tubes. *Am J Nurs,* 5, 60-4.

Pfister, S., and Bullas, J.B. (1985). Caring for a patient with a chest tube connected to the Emerson pump. *Crit Care Nurse,* 5, 26-32.

Schrader, K. (2001). Instilling medication into chest tubes. *Crit Care Nurse,* 21, 77-8.

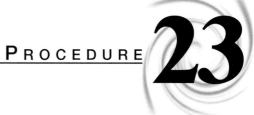

P R O C E D U R E **23**

Needle Thoracostomy (Perform)

P U R P O S E : Needle thoracostomy is performed to reduce a tension pneumothorax to a simple pneumothorax in a rapidly deteriorating patient. This is a temporary measure and is followed quickly by the insertion of a chest tube for more definitive management.

Cindy Goodrich

PREREQUISITE NURSING KNOWLEDGE

- Anatomy and physiology of the pulmonary system should be understood.
- The thoracic cavity, under normal conditions, is a closed airspace. Any disruption results in the loss of negative pressure within the intrapleural space. Air or fluid entering the space competes with the lung, resulting in collapse of the lung. Associated conditions are the result of disease, injury, surgery, or iatrogenic causes.
- A pneumothorax is classified as open, closed, or tension pneumothorax. In patients with tension pneumothorax, air leaks into the pleural space through a tear in the lung and, having no means to escape from the pleural cavity, creates a one-way valve effect. With each breath the patient takes, air accumulates, pressure within the pleural space increases, and the lung collapses. As a result, the mediastinal structures (i.e., heart, great vessels, and trachea) shift to the opposite or unaffected side of the chest. Venous return and cardiac output are impeded, and the possibility of collapse of the unaffected lung exists.
- Tension pneumothorax is a medical emergency, requiring immediate intervention. Accurate assessment of signs and symptoms allows for prompt recognition and treatment:
  - ❖ Tracheal deviation to the unaffected side
  - ❖ Neck vein distention
  - ❖ Muffled heart sounds
  - ❖ Tachypnea
  - ❖ Decreased or absent breath sounds on the affected side
  - ❖ Shortness of breath, dyspnea
  - ❖ Asymmetrical chest excursion with respirations
- Needle thoracostomy is performed by placing a needle into the pleural space to remove air and reestablish negative pressure in unstable patients with tension pneumothorax (Fig. 23-1).

EQUIPMENT

- Personal protective equipment
- 14-gauge to 16-gauge hollow needle or catheter with one-way valve attached or commercially available (Heimlich) flutter valve
- Povidone-iodine solution
- 4 × 4 gauze dressing
- Tape
  Additional equipment (to have available depending on patient need) includes the following:
- Scissors
- Sterile glove (powder-free)
- Small rubber band
  The above-listed equipment can be used to create a one-way valve. Cut a finger off the glove and attach it to the needle using the rubber band. Sterilize before use.
- Oxygen
- Manual resuscitation bag with mask

PATIENT AND FAMILY EDUCATION

- Explain the procedure and reason for needle thoracostomy. ➡*Rationale:* This communication identifies patient and family knowledge deficits concerning the patient's condition, procedure, expected benefits, and potential risks and allows time for questions to clarify information and to voice concerns. Explanations decrease patient anxiety and enhance cooperation.

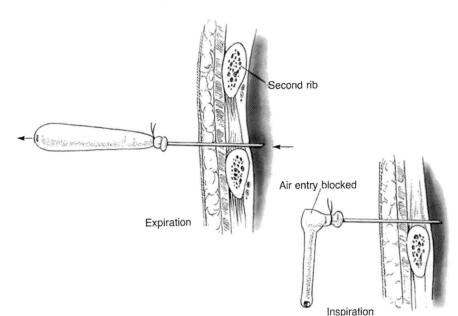

FIGURE 23-1 Use of a needle and a sterile finger cot or a finger from a sterile glove to fashion a one-way (flutter) valve for emergency evacuation of a tension pneumothorax. A small opening is made in the free end of the glove finger to allow air to escape during expiration. *(From Cosgniff, J.H. [1978]. An Atlas of Diagnostic and Therapeutic Procedures for Emergency Personnel. Philadelphia: J.B. Lippincott.)*

- If indicated, explain the patient's role in assisting with needle thoracostomy. ➧*Rationale:* Eliciting the patient's cooperation assists with insertion of flutter valve.

PATIENT ASSESSMENT AND PREPARATION

Patient Assessment

- Signs and symptoms consistent with tension pneumothorax include the following.
  - ❖ Tracheal deviation to the unaffected side
  - ❖ Neck vein distention
  - ❖ Muffled heart sounds
  - ❖ Tachypnea
  - ❖ Decreased or absent breath sounds on the affected side
  - ❖ Shortness of breath, dyspnea
  - ❖ Asymmetrical chest excursion with respirations
  - ❖ Cyanosis
  - ❖ Decreased oxygen saturation
  - ❖ Subcutaneous emphysema

- ❖ Sudden, sharp chest pain
- ❖ Anxiety, restlessness, apprehension
- ❖ Tachycardia
- ❖ Hypotension
- ❖ Dysrhythmias

➧*Rationale:* Accurate assessment of signs and symptoms allows for prompt recognition and treatment. Baseline assessment provides comparison data for evaluating changes and outcomes of treatment. Tension pneumothorax is a medical emergency, requiring immediate intervention.

Patient Preparation

- Ensure that the patient understands preprocedural teaching. Answer questions as they arise, and reinforce information as needed. ➧*Rationale:* This communication evaluates and reinforces understanding of previously taught information.
- Position patient in supine position with the head of the bed flat. ➧*Rationale:* This positioning allows for identification of landmarks for proper placement of needle and flutter valve.

Procedure	**for Performing Needle Thoracostomy**	
Steps	**Rationale**	**Special Considerations**
1. Wash hands, and don personal protective equipment.	Reduces the transmission of microorganisms and body secretions; standard precautions.	

Procedure continues on the following page

Procedure for Performing Needle Thoracostomy—*Continued*

Steps	Rationale	Special Considerations
2. Administer high-flow oxygen and ventilate as needed.	Allows for oxygenation and ventilation before needle insertion.	
3. Locate the second intercostal space at the midclavicular line on the side of the suspected tension pneumothorax (see Fig. 18-1).	Identification of landmarks for needle thoracostomy.	
4. Cleanse area with providone-iodine solution, using a circular motion.	Cleanses area before needle insertion.	
5. Locate the upper margin of the third rib with several fingers. Insert flutter valve into the second intercostal space at the midclavicular line, pointing the needle posterior but slightly upward and sliding it over the top of the third rib.	Allows the proper placement of the flutter valve into the pleural space. Insert flutter valve above third rib to avoid damaging the nerve, artery, and vein that lie just beneath each rib.	Flutter valve acts as a one-way valve, preventing reentry of air into pleural space during inspiration, but allowing for escape of air during expiration (see Fig. 23-1).
6. Puncture the parietal pleural space. Listen for an audible escape of air as the needle enters the parietal pleural space.	Although an audible rush of air indicates that needle decompression has been successful, a dramatic improvement in the patient's clinical condition is the best indicator of successful intervention.	
7. Apply a small dressing around the flutter valve or suture the valve in place.	Allows for temporary stabilization of flutter valve until a chest tube can be inserted.	
8. Prepare for immediate chest tube insertion (see Procedure 18).	Definitive treatment of tension pneumothrax.	

Expected Outcomes

- Removal of air from pleural space
- Reestablishment of negative intrapleural pressure
- Tension pneumothorax conversion to simple pneumothorax
- Improved oxygenation and ventilation

Unexpected Outcomes

- Resultant pneumothorax in patient without tension pneumothorax
- Damage to nerves, veins, or arteries because of improper flutter valve placement
- Local hematoma or cellulitis
- Pleural infection

Patient Monitoring and Care

Steps	Rationale	Reportable Conditions
		These conditions should be reported if they persist despite nursing interventions.
1. Stabilize flutter valve with dressing until chest tube is inserted.	Prevents movement and dislodgment of flutter valve.	• Dislodged flutter valve
2. Constantly monitor for signs and symptoms of tension pneumothorax.	Determines if chest decompression has been successful and allows for early identification of new pneumothorax until chest tube has been placed.	• Tracheal deviation to the unaffected side • Neck vein distention • Muffled heart sounds • Tachypnea • Decreased or absent breath sounds on the affected side • Shortness of breath, dyspnea

Patient Monitoring and Care—*Continued*

Steps	Rationale	Reportable Conditions
		• Asymmetric chest excursion with respirations • Cyanosis • Decreased oxygen saturation • Subcutaneous emphysema • Sudden sharp chest pain • Anxiety, restlessness, apprehension • Tachycardia • Hypotension • Dysrhythmias

Documentation

Documentation should include the following:

- Patient and family education
- Vital signs before and after insertion of flutter valve
- Location of flutter valve
- Size of flutter valve used
- Response after flutter valve placement
- Unexpected outcomes
- Nursing interventions
- Occurrence of unexpected outcomes

Additional Readings

American College of Surgeons Committee on Trauma. (1997). *Advanced Trauma Life Support Manual*. Chicago: American College of Surgeons.

Holleran, R.S. (2003). *Air and Surface Patient Transport: Principles and Practice*. 3rd ed. St. Louis: Mosby.

Prehospital Trauma Life Support Committee of the National Association of Emergency Technicians in cooperation with the Committee on Trauma of the American College of Surgeons. (1999). *PHTLS: Basic and Advanced Prehospital Trauma Life Support*. 4th ed. St. Louis: Mosby.

Roberts, J.R., and Hedges, J.R., editors. (2004). *Clinical Procedures in Emergency Medicine*. 4th ed. Philadelphia: W.B. Saunders.

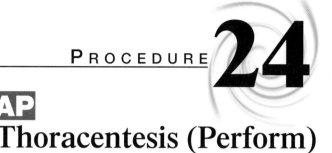
PROCEDURE **24**

AP

Thoracentesis (Perform)

PURPOSE: Thoracentesis is performed to assist in the diagnosis and management of patients with pleural effusions.

Karen K. Carlson

PREREQUISITE NURSING KNOWLEDGE

- Thoracentesis is not used to verify the presence of pleural effusion. Pleural effusions are verified by chest x-ray, ultrasound, or computed tomography scan.
- Diagnostic thoracentesis is indicated for differential diagnosis for patients with pleural effusion of unknown etiology. A diagnostic thoracentesis may be repeated if initial results fail to yield a diagnosis.
- Therapeutic thoracentesis is indicated to relieve the symptoms (e.g., dyspnea) caused by a pleural effusion.
- Thoracentesis is performed by inserting a needle or a catheter into the pleural space, allowing for removal of pleural fluid.
- Samples of pleural fluid are analyzed and assist in distinguishing between exudative and transudative etiologies of effusion. Pleural fluid laboratory results alone do not establish a diagnosis; instead the laboratory results must be correlated with the clinical findings and serum laboratory results.
- Exudative pleural effusions meet one of the following criteria:[7]
  - Pleural fluid lactate dehydrogenase (LDH)-to-serum LDH ratio is greater than 0.6 international unit/ml.
  - Pleural fluid LDH is more than two thirds of the upper limit of normal for serum LDH.
  - Pleural fluid protein-to-serum protein ratio is greater than 0.5 g/dl.
- A transudative pleural effusion is considered when none of the exudative criteria are met.

- Transudative effusions usually are associated with systemic etiologies (e.g., heart failure), whereas exudative effusions indicate a local etiology (e.g., pulmonary embolus, infection).
- Relative contraindications for performing a thoracentesis include the following:
  - Patient anatomy that hinders the practitioner from clearly identifying the appropriate landmarks
  - Patients receiving anticoagulants or having an uncorrectable coagulation disorder
  - Patients receiving positive end-expiratory pressure therapy
  - Patients with splenomegaly, elevated left hemidiaphragm, and left-sided pleural effusion
  - Patients with only one lung as a result of a previous pneumonectomy
  - Patients with known lung disease
- Ultrasound-guided thoracentesis is thought to reduce complications, especially when used in the last four patient groups listed in the relative contraindications list.[3-5]
- Pneumothorax is the most common postthoracentesis complication; however, it is infrequently necessary to place a chest tube.[1]

EQUIPMENT

For Diagnostic Thoracentesis
- Sterile gloves
- Sterile drapes
- Sterile towels
- Adhesive bandage or adhesive strip
- Antiseptic solution
- Sterile 4 × 4 gauze pads
- Local anesthetic (1% or 2% lidocaine)
- One small needle (25-gauge, ⅝ inch long)
- 5-ml syringe for local anesthetic
- Three large needles (20-gauge to 22-gauge, 1½ to 2 inches long)

- Three-way stopcock
- Sterile 20-ml syringe
- Sterile 50-ml syringe
- Two chemistry blood tubes
- Aqueous heparin (1:1000)
- Hemostat or Kelly clamp
- Pulse oximetry equipment

For Therapeutic Thoracentesis

The following equipment is needed in addition to equipment for diagnostic thoracentesis:
- 14-gauge needle
- 16-gauge catheter
- Sterile 50-ml syringe
- VACUTAINERS® or evacuated bottles (1- to 2-liter) with pressure tubing

Additional equipment (to have available depending on patient need) includes the following:
- Two complete blood count tubes
- One anaerobic and one aerobic media bottle for culture and sensitivity
- Sterile tubes for fungal and tuberculosis cultures

PATIENT AND FAMILY EDUCATION

- Explain the procedure and purpose for thoracentesis, including potential complications, such as pneumothorax, pain at insertion site, cough, infection, hypoxemia, and hypovolemia. Also, include an explanation of amount of fluid expected to be withdrawn, duration of time procedure may last, and expectation of and reason for coughing during or after thoracentesis. ➤➤*Rationale:* This communication identifies patient and family knowledge deficits concerning patient condition, procedure, expected benefits, and potential risks and allows time for questions to clarify information and voice concerns. Explanations decrease patient anxiety and enhance cooperation.
- Explain the patient's role in thoracentesis. ➤➤*Rationale:* This explanation increases patient compliance, facilitates needle and catheter insertion, and enhances fluid removal.

PATIENT ASSESSMENT AND PREPARATION

Patient Assessment

- Signs and symptoms of pleural effusion include the following:
  - ❖ Trachea deviated away from the affected side
  - ❖ Affected side dull to flat by percussion
  - ❖ Absent or decreased breath sounds
  - ❖ Tactile fremitus

➤➤*Rationale:* Although physical findings may suggest a pleural effusion, radiography confirms the presence of a pleural effusion.
- Assess chest x-ray findings. ➤➤*Rationale:* If at least half the hemidiaphragm is obliterated on anterior-posterior x-ray, there is sufficient fluid in the pleural space to perform a thoracentesis. If there is a small amount of loculated fluid, however, a decubitus x-ray should be obtained. If the pleural effusion is greater than 10 mm on decubitus x-ray, a diagnostic thoracentesis can be performed. If the pleural effusion is less than 10 mm in diameter or loculated, ultrasonography is required to distinguish between pleural effusion and pleural lesion. Ultrasound-guided thoracentesis may be necessary if a pleural effusion has been confirmed.
- Assess past medical history of pleuritic chest pain, cough, dyspnea, malignancy, or heart failure. ➤➤*Rationale:* Past medical history may provide valuable clues to the cause of a patient's pleural effusion.
- Assess baseline vital signs, including pulse oximetry. ➤➤*Rationale:* Having baseline assessment data provides information about patient status and allows for comparison during and after the procedure.
- Assess recent serum laboratory results, including the following.
  - ❖ Complete blood count
  - ❖ Platelet count
  - ❖ Prothrombin time
  - ❖ Partial thromboplastin time

  ➤➤*Rationale:* These studies help determine if the patient is at increased risk for bleeding.

Patient Preparation

- Ensure that the patient understands preprocedural teaching. Answer questions as they arise and reinforce information. ➤➤*Rationale:* This communication evaluates and reinforces understanding of previously taught information.
- Ensure that written informed consent for the procedure has been obtained. ➤➤*Rationale:* Invasive procedures, unless performed under implied consent in a life-threatening situation, require written consent of the patient or significant other.
- Position the patient. Several alternative positions may be used, as follows. ➤➤*Rationale:* Positioning enhances ease of withdrawal of pleural fluid.
  - ❖ If the patient is alert and able, position him or her on the edge of the bed with legs supported and arms resting on a pillow on the elevated bedside table (Fig. 24-1).
  - ❖ The patient may sit on a chair backward and rest arms on a pillow on the back of the chair.
  - ❖ If the patient is unable to sit, position him or her on the unaffected side, with the back near the edge of the bed and the arm on the affected side above the head. Elevate the head of the bed to 30 or 45 degrees, as tolerated.
- Have an additional member of the health care team positioned in front of the patient. ➤➤*Rationale:* This

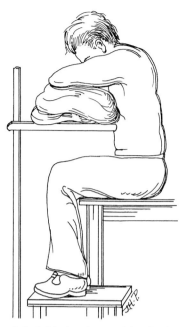

FIGURE 24-1 Ideal patient position for thoracentesis.

reassures or comforts the patient and provides additional assistance.

- Select appropriate site by percussing until dullness is heard. Dullness indicates the highest point of the pleural effusion. Mark this site with a pen. The insertion site is one intercostal space below this point. ➤*Rationale:* This provides the practitioner with an identified site.
- Consider sedation or paralysis. ➤*Rationale:* Sedation or paralysis may be necessary to maximize positioning.
- Have atropine available. ➤*Rationale:* Bradycardia, from a vasovagal reflex, is a common occurrence during thoracentesis.
- Initiate pulse oximetry monitoring. ➤*Rationale:* Pulse oximetry provides a noninvasive means for monitoring oxygenation at the bedside, allowing for prompt recognition of problems.

Procedure for Diagnostic and Therapeutic Thoracentesis

Steps	Rationale	Special Considerations
1. Wash hands, and don personal protective equipment.	Reduces the transmission of microorganisms and body secretions; standard precautions.	
2. Percuss the affected side posteriorly to determine the highest point of the pleural effusion. Identify the intercostal space below this point.	This identifies the superior border of the pleural effusion and identifies and validates the planned site for thoracentesis.	Use the posterior axillary line as the insertion point to avoid the spinal cord. If the space identified for insertion is below the eighth intercostal space, ultrasonography should be done to mark the fluid level and its relationship to the diaphragm. This helps identify a safe point of entry to avoid solid-organ damage.
3. Heparinize the 50-ml syringe.	Prepares syringe for use in accessing pleural fluid.	
4. Prepare site with antiseptic. Don sterile gloves, and drape area with sterile drape.	Reduces skin contaminants, reducing the risk of infection.	
5. Anesthetize the skin with lidocaine (25-gauge, $^5/_8$-inch needle) in the typical wheal fashion around the insertion site.	Increases comfort for patient by anesthetizing the periosteum of the rib and pleura.	
6. Using 2% lidocaine and a 20-gauge to 22-gauge, $1^1/_2$-inch to 2-inch needle, insert the needle through the wheal. Inject the lidocaine into the deep tissue and periosteum of the underlying rib superiorly and laterally.	To anesthetize the work area for optimal patient comfort.	Always aspirate before injecting to prevent lidocaine from entering a blood vessel or the pleural space.

Procedure **for Diagnostic and Therapeutic Thoracentesis**—*Continued*

Steps	Rationale	Special Considerations
7. After anesthetizing the periosteum of the underlying rib, gently advance the needle and alternately aspirate and inject lidocaine until pleural fluid is obtained in the syringe.	Anesthetizes the parietal pleura. The pleural space is identified by pleural fluid aspirate in the syringe.	
8. When pleural fluid is obtained, place a sterile gloved finger on the needle at the point where the needle exits the skin. Withdraw the needle and syringe.	This approximates the length of insertion for the thoracentesis needle or catheter.	
For Therapeutic Thoracentesis, Proceed to Step 13		
9. Attach a three-way stopcock and heparinized 50-ml syringe to a 20-gauge to 22-gauge, $1^1/_2$-inch or 2-inch needle. Open the stopcock valve between the syringe and the needle.	The open stopcock valve allows for aspiration of pleural fluid during needle insertion. The aqueous heparin ensures accurate pH and blood cell counts.	
10. Insert the selected needle via the anesthetized tract and continually aspirate until pleural fluid is obtained, filling the 50-ml syringe.	The pleural fluid is used for laboratory testing for the differential diagnosis. A change in patient position can be attempted to facilitate fluid drainage.	It is possible that no fluid will be accessed (dry tap). A larger gauge needle may be needed for thick or loculated fluid, or the needle may have been inserted above or below the pleural fluid. When pleural fluid is aspirated, the needle may be stabilized by placing a hemostat or clamp on the needle at the skin site to keep the needle from advancing further into the pleural space, preventing lung puncture.
11. Fill the specimen tubes from the pleural fluid–filled syringe. Send the specimen tubes to the laboratory for appropriate analysis.	Analysis may aid in determining an etiology of the pleural effusion.	To interpret pleural fluid laboratory values, serum chemistry laboratory values must be obtained (e.g., pH, total protein, glucose, and LDH). When collecting pleural fluid for cytology or estrogen receptor analysis, add 10,000 units of heparin to the specimen sample. Contrary to common practice, at least one study showed that there is no need for immediate pH evaluation or placement of the sample on ice if this measurement is delayed.[8]
12. On completion of diagnostic thoracentesis, withdraw the needle. Apply pressure to the puncture site for a few minutes, then apply an adhesive strip or adhesive bandage over the puncture site.		Without concrete clinical indications, chest x-ray is not necessary after a routine thoracentesis.[2,3,5,6]

Procedure continues on the following page

Procedure for Diagnostic and Therapeutic Thoracentesis—*Continued*		
Steps	**Rationale**	**Special Considerations**

For Therapeutic Thoracentesis

Steps	Rationale	Special Considerations
13. Insert a 14-gauge needle attached to a 20-ml syringe, bevel down, into the anesthetized tract until pleural fluid is returned.	The 14-gauge needle is selected because it allows for insertion and passage of a 16-gauge catheter; a smaller sized catheter may be unstable and fold or kink on itself.	
14. When pleural fluid is obtained, remove the syringe from the needle, occluding the needle with an index finger.	Occluding the needle helps prevent the possible occurrence of a pneumothorax.	
15. Insert the 16-gauge catheter through the 14-gauge needle. Advance the catheter slowly through the needle, angling the catheter in a downward fashion toward the costodiaphragm until the catheter moves freely in the pleural space.	Advancing the catheter toward the costodiaphragm allows for optimal drainage of pleural fluid.	In therapeutic thoracentesis, a catheter is preferred over a needle because the lung is expected to reexpand. A needle could puncture the lung during reexpansion, causing a pneumothorax.
16. While advancing the catheter beyond the needle tip, remove the needle and leave the catheter in the pleural space. Attach a three-way stopcock with a 50-ml heparinized syringe to the end of the catheter.	Never pull the catheter back through the needle because the catheter may be cut or sheared by the needle tip.	
17. Fill the 50-ml heparinized syringe with pleural fluid. Fill the specimen tubes from the pleural fluid–filled syringe. Send the specimen tubes to the laboratory for appropriate analysis.	When changing syringes, be certain the stopcock is positioned such that air does not enter the pleural space. Analysis may aid in determining an etiology of the pleural effusion.	To interpret pleural fluid chemistry laboratory values, serum chemistry laboratory values also must be obtained (e.g., pH, total protein, glucose, LDH). When collecting pleural fluid for cytology or estrogen receptor analysis, add 10,000 units of heparin to the specimen sample. Contrary to common practice, at least one study showed that there is no need for immediate pH evaluation or placement of the sample on ice if this measurement is delayed.[8]
18. Attach the VACUTAINER® or evacuated bottles with tubing to the three-way stopcock. Open the valve to the VACUTAINER®, and fill the VACUTAINER®.	The VACUTAINER® or evacuated bottles use negative pressure to withdraw pleural fluid from the pleural space, providing therapeutic relief. Reposition catheter or patient or both if drainage stops to determine if fluid is still present.	Do not remove greater than 1000 to 1500 ml of pleural fluid at one time; removing more than this can cause hypovolemia, hypoxemia, or even reexpansion pulmonary edema. The patient may feel the need to cough as the lung reexpands.
19. On completion of thoracentesis, remove the catheter. Apply pressure to the puncture site for a few minutes, then apply an adhesive strip or adhesive bandage over the puncture site.		Without concrete clinical indications, chest x-ray is not necessary after a routine thoracentesis.[2,3,5,6]
20. Document in patient record.		

Expected Outcomes

- Patient will be comfortable and will experience decreased respiratory distress.
- Lung reexpansion will occur.
- Site will remain infection-free.
- Procedure will aid in diagnosing etiology of pleural effusion.

Unexpected Outcomes

- Pneumothorax
- Vasovagal response
- Dyspnea
- Hypovolemia
- Hematoma
- Hemothorax
- Liver or splenic laceration
- Reexpansion pulmonary edema

Patient Monitoring and Care

Steps	Rationale	Reportable Conditions
		These conditions should be reported if they persist despite nursing interventions.
1. Monitor vital signs and cardiopulmonary status before and after thoracentesis and as needed.	Any change in vital signs may alert the practitioner of possible unexpected outcomes. Use of supplemental oxygen may be necessary in certain patient populations.	• Tachypnea • Decreased or absent breath sounds on the affected side • Shortness of breath, dyspnea • Asymmetric chest excursion with respirations • Decreased oxygen saturation • Subcutaneous emphysema • Sudden sharp chest pain • Anxiety, restlessness, apprehension • Tachycardia • Hypotension • Dysrhythmias • Tracheal deviation to the unaffected side • Neck vein distention • Muffled heart sounds
2. If indicated, obtain a postthoracentesis expiratory chest x-ray. *(Level V: Clinical studies in more than one patient population and situation.)*	A chest x-ray is used to evaluate for lung reexpansion and evidence of a possible pneumothorax or hemothorax. If a pneumothorax or hemothorax is present, a chest tube may be necessary. Without concrete clinical indications, chest x-ray is not necessary after a routine thoracentesis.[2,3,5,6]	• Pneumothorax • Expanding pleural effusion • Catheter migration

Documentation

Documentation should include the following:

- Patient and family teaching
- Insertion of catheter or needle
- Catheter or needle size used
- Any difficulties in insertion
- Patient tolerance
- Pleural fluid aspirate characteristics
- Total amount of pleural fluid aspirated
- Site assessment
- Occurrence of unexpected outcomes
- Postthoracentesis x-ray results
- Laboratory test ordered and results as available
- Interpretation of laboratory results
- Nursing interventions

References

1. Colt, H.G., Brewer, N., and Barbur, E.B. (1999). Evaluation of patient-related and procedure-related factors contributing to pneumothorax following thoracentesis. *Chest,* 116, 134-8.
2. Doyle, J.J., et al. (1996). Necessity of routine chest roentgenography after thoracentesis. *Ann Intern Med,* 124, 816-20.
3. Gervais, D.A., et al. (1997). US-guided thoracentesis: Requirement for post procedure chest radiography in patients who receive mechanical ventilation versus patients who breathe spontaneously. *Radiology,* 204, 503-6.
4. Jones, P.W., et al. (2003). Ultrasound-guided thoracentesis: Is it a safer method? *Chest,* 123, 418-23.
5. Lichtenstein, D., et al. (1999). Feasibility and safety of ultrasound-aided thoracentesis in mechanically ventilated patients. *Intensive Care Med,* 25, 955-8.
6. Peterson, W.G., and Zimmerman, R. (2000). Limited utility of chest radiograph after thoracentesis. *Chest,* 117, 1038-42.
7. Qureshi, N., Momin, Z.A., and Brandstetter, R.D. (1994). Thoracentesis in clinical practice. *Heart Lung,* 23, 376-83.
8. Sarodia, B.D., et al. (2000). Does pleural fluid pH change significantly at room temperature during the first hour following thoracentesis? *Chest,* 117, 1043-8.

Additional Readings

Heffner, J.E., Brown, L.K., and Barbieri, C.A. (1997). Diagnostic value of tests that discriminate between exudative and transudative pleural effusions. *Chest,* 111, 970-80.

Klima, L.D., and Benditt, J.O. (1997). Pulmonary procedures. In: Goldstein, R.H., O'Connell, J.J., and Karlinsky, J.B., editors. *A Practical Approach to Pulmonary Medicine.* Philadelphia: Lippincott-Raven, 39-54.

Light, R.W., et al. (1992). Pleural effusion: The diagnostic separation of transudates and exudates. *Ann Intern Med,* 77, 507-13.

Quigley, R.L. (1995). Thoracentesis and chest tube drainage. *Crit Care Clin,* 11, 111-26.

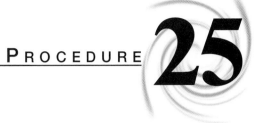
PROCEDURE **25**

Thoracentesis (Assist)

PURPOSE: Thoracentesis is performed to assist in the diagnosis and management of patients with pleural effusions.

Karen K. Carlson

PREREQUISITE NURSING KNOWLEDGE

- Thoracentesis is not used to verify the presence of pleural effusion. Pleural effusions are verified by chest x-ray, ultrasound, or computed tomography scan.
- Diagnostic thoracentesis is indicated for differential diagnosis for patients with pleural effusion of unknown etiology. A diagnostic thoracentesis may be repeated if initial results fail to yield a diagnosis.
- Therapeutic thoracentesis is indicated to relieve the symptoms (e.g., dyspnea) caused by a pleural effusion.
- Thoracentesis is performed by inserting a needle or a catheter into the pleural space, allowing for removal of pleural fluid.
- Samples of pleural fluid are analyzed and assist in distinguishing between exudative and transudative etiologies of effusion. Pleural fluid laboratory results alone do not establish a diagnosis; instead the laboratory results must be correlated with the clinical findings and serum laboratory results.
- Exudative pleural effusions meet one of the following criteria:[7]
  - ❖ Pleural fluid lactate dehydrogenase (LDH)-to-serum LDH ratio is greater than 0.6 international unit/ml.
  - ❖ Pleural fluid LDH is more than two thirds of the upper limit of normal for serum LDH.
  - ❖ Pleural fluid protein-to-serum protein ratio is greater than 0.5 g/dl.
- A transudative pleural effusion is considered when none of the exudative criteria are met.
- Transudative effusions usually are associated with systemic etiologies (e.g., heart failure), whereas exudative effusions indicate a local etiology (e.g., pulmonary embolus, infection).
- Relative contraindications for performing a thoracentesis include the following:
  - ❖ Patient anatomy that hinders the practitioner from clearly identifying the appropriate landmarks
  - ❖ Patients receiving anticoagulants or having an uncorrectable coagulation disorder
  - ❖ Patients receiving positive end-expiratory pressure therapy
  - ❖ Patients with splenomegaly, elevated left hemidiaphragm, and left-sided pleural effusion
  - ❖ Patients with only one lung as a result of a previous pneumonectomy
  - ❖ Patients with known lung disease
- Ultrasound-guided thoracentesis is thought to reduce complications, especially when used in the last four patient groups listed in the relative contraindications list.[3-5]
- Pneumothorax is the most common postthoracentesis complication; however, it is infrequently necessary to place a chest tube.[1]

EQUIPMENT

For Diagnostic Thoracentesis

- Sterile gloves
- Sterile drapes
- Sterile towels
- Adhesive bandage or adhesive strip
- Antiseptic solution
- Sterile 4 × 4 gauze pads
- Local anesthetic (1% or 2% lidocaine)
- One small needle (25-gauge, ⅝ inch long)

181

- 5-ml syringe for local anesthetic
- Three large needles (20-gauge to 22-gauge, 1½ to 2 inches long)
- Three-way stopcock
- Sterile 20-ml syringe
- Sterile 50-ml syringe
- Two chemistry blood tubes
- Aqueous heparin (1:1000)
- Hemostat or Kelly clamp
- Pulse oximetry equipment

For Therapeutic Thoracentesis

The following equipment is needed in addition to equipment for diagnostic thoracentesis:
- 14-gauge needle
- 16-gauge catheter
- Sterile 50-ml syringe
- VACUTAINERS® or evacuated bottles (1- to 2-liter) with pressure tubing

Additional equipment (to have available depending on patient need) includes the following:
- Two complete blood count tubes
- One anaerobic and one aerobic media bottle for culture and sensitivity
- Sterile tubes for fungal and tuberculosis cultures

PATIENT AND FAMILY EDUCATION

- Explain the procedure and purpose for thoracentesis, including potential complications, such as pneumothorax, pain at insertion site, cough, infection, hypoxemia, and hypovolemia. Also, include an explanation of amount of fluid expected to be withdrawn, duration of time procedure may last, and expectation of and reason for coughing during or after thoracentesis. ➥*Rationale:* This communication identifies patient and family knowledge deficits concerning patient condition, procedure, expected benefits, and potential risks and allows time for questions to clarify information and voice concerns. Explanations decrease patient anxiety and enhance cooperation.
- Explain the patient's role in thoracentesis. ➥*Rationale:* This explanation increases patient compliance, facilitates needle and catheter insertion, and enhances fluid removal.

PATIENT ASSESSMENT AND PREPARATION

Patient Assessment

- Signs and symptoms of pleural effusion include the following.
  - ❖ Trachea deviated away from the affected side
  - ❖ Affected side dull to flat by percussion
  - ❖ Absent or decreased breath sounds
  - ❖ Tactile fremitus

➥*Rationale:* Although physical findings may suggest a pleural effusion, radiography confirms the presence of a pleural effusion.
- Assess chest x-ray findings. ➥*Rationale:* If at least half the hemidiaphragm is obliterated on anterior-posterior x-ray, there is sufficient fluid in the pleural space to perform a thoracentesis. If there is a small amount of loculated fluid, however, a decubitus x-ray should be obtained. If the pleural effusion is greater than 10 mm on decubitus x-ray, a diagnostic thoracentesis can be performed. If the pleural effusion is less than 10 mm in diameter or loculated, ultrasonography is required to distinguish between pleural effusion and pleural lesion. Ultrasound-guided thoracentesis may be necessary if a pleural effusion has been confirmed.
- Assess past medical history of pleuritic chest pain, cough, dyspnea, malignancy, or heart failure. ➥*Rationale:* Past medical history may provide valuable clues to the cause of a patient's pleural effusion.
- Assess baseline vital signs, including pulse oximetry. ➥*Rationale:* Having baseline assessment data provides information about patient status and allows for comparison during and after the procedure.
- Assess recent serum laboratory results, including the following.
  - ❖ Complete blood count
  - ❖ Platelet count
  - ❖ Prothrombin time
  - ❖ Partial thromboplastin time

  ➥*Rationale:* These studies help determine if the patient is at increased risk for bleeding.

Patient Preparation

- Ensure that the patient understands preprocedural teaching. Answer questions as they arise and reinforce information. ➥*Rationale:* This communication evaluates and reinforces understanding of previously taught information.
- Ensure that written informed consent for the procedure has been obtained. ➥*Rationale:* Invasive procedures, unless performed under implied consent in a life-threatening situation, require written consent of the patient or significant other.
- Position the patient. Several alternative positions may be used, as follows. ➥*Rationale:* Positioning enhances ease of withdrawal of pleural fluid.
  - ❖ If the patient is alert and able, position him or her on the edge of the bed with legs supported and arms resting on a pillow on the elevated bedside table (see Fig. 24-1).
  - ❖ The patient may sit on a chair backward and rest arms on a pillow on the back of the chair.
  - ❖ If the patient is unable to sit, position him or her on the unaffected side, with the back near the edge of the bed and the arm on the affected side above the head. Elevate the head of the bed to 30 or 45 degrees, as tolerated.
- Have an additional member of the health care team positioned in front of the patient. ➥*Rationale:* This reassures or comforts the patient and provides additional assistance.

- Select appropriate site by percussing until dullness is heard. Dullness indicates the highest point of the pleural effusion. Mark this site with a pen. The insertion site is one intercostal space below this point. ➤*Rationale:* This provides the practitioner with an identified site.
- Consider sedation or paralysis. ➤*Rationale:* Sedation or paralysis may be necessary to maximize positioning.

- Have atropine available. ➤*Rationale:* Bradycardia, from a vasovagal reflex, is a common occurrence during thoracentesis.
- Initiate pulse oximetry monitoring. ➤*Rationale:* Pulse oximetry provides a noninvasive means for monitoring oxygenation at the bedside, allowing for prompt recognition of problems.

Procedure for Assisting With Diagnostic and Therapeutic Thoracentesis

Steps	Rationale	Special Considerations
1. Wash hands, and don personal protective equipment.	Reduces the transmission of microorganisms and body secretions; standard precautions.	
2. Heparinize the 50-ml syringe.	Prepares syringe for use in accessing pleural fluid.	
3. Assist in site preparation with antiseptic. Drape area with sterile drape.	Reduces skin contaminants, reducing the risk of infection.	
4. Assist physician or advanced practice nurse practitioner to draw up lidocaine for anesthetizing the site.	Increases comfort for patient by anesthetizing the periosteum of the rib and pleura.	
For Therapeutic Thoracentesis, Proceed to Step 8		
5. Attach a three-way stopcock and heparinized 50-ml syringe to a 20-gauge to 22-gauge, 1½-inch or 2-inch needle. Open the stopcock valve between the syringe and the needle.	The open stopcock valve allows for aspiration of pleural fluid during needle insertion. The aqueous heparin ensures accurate pH and blood cell counts.	
6. Fill the specimen tubes from the pleural fluid–filled syringe. Send the specimen tubes to the laboratory for appropriate analysis.	Analysis may aid in determining an etiology of the pleural effusion.	To interpret pleural fluid laboratory values, serum chemistry laboratory values must be obtained (e.g., pH, total protein, glucose, and LDH). When collecting pleural fluid for cytology or estrogen receptor analysis, add 10,000 units of heparin to the specimen sample. Contrary to common practice, at least one study showed that there is no need for immediate pH evaluation or placement of the sample on ice if this measurement is delayed.[8]
7. On completion of diagnostic thoracentesis, apply pressure to the puncture site for a few minutes, then apply an adhesive strip or adhesive bandage over the puncture site.		Without concrete clinical indications, chest x-ray is not necessary after a routine thoracentesis.[2,3,5,6]
8. After catheter has been inserted, fill the 50-ml heparinized syringe with pleural fluid. Fill the specimen tubes from the pleural fluid–filled syringe. Send the specimen tubes to the laboratory for appropriate analysis.	When changing syringes, be certain the stopcock is positioned such that air does not enter the pleural space. Analysis may aid in determining an etiology of the pleural effusion.	To interpret pleural fluid chemistry laboratory values, serum chemistry laboratory values also must be obtained (e.g., pH, total protein, glucose, LDH).

Procedure continues on the following page

Procedure for Assisting With Diagnostic and Therapeutic Thoracentesis—*Continued*

Steps	Rationale	Special Considerations
		When collecting pleural fluid for cytology or estrogen receptor analysis, add 10,000 units of heparin to the specimen sample. Contrary to common practice, at least one study showed that there is no need for immediate pH evaluation or placement of the sample on ice if this measurement is delayed.[8]
9. Attach the VACUTAINER® or evacuated bottles with tubing to the three-way stopcock. Open the valve to the VACUTAINER®, and fill the VACUTAINER®.	The VACUTAINER® or evacuated bottles use negative pressure to withdraw pleural fluid from the pleural space, providing therapeutic relief. Reposition catheter or patient or both if drainage stops to determine if fluid is still present.	Do not remove greater than 1000 to 1500 ml of pleural fluid at one time. Removing more than this can cause hypovolemia, hypoxemia, or reexpansion pulmonary edema. The patient may feel the need to cough as the lung reexpands.
10. On completion of thoracentesis, apply pressure to the puncture site for a few minutes, then apply an adhesive strip or adhesive bandage over the puncture site.		Without concrete clinical indications, chest x-ray is not necessary after a routine thoracentesis.[2,3,5,6]

Expected Outcomes

- Patient will be comfortable and will experience decreased respiratory distress.
- Lung reexpansion will occur.
- Site will remain infection-free.
- Procedure will aid in diagnosing etiology of pleural effusion.

Unexpected Outcomes

- Pneumothorax
- Vasovagal response
- Dyspnea
- Hypovolemia
- Hematoma
- Hemothorax
- Liver or splenic laceration
- Reexpansion pulmonary edema

Patient Monitoring and Care

Steps	Rationale	Reportable Conditions
1. Monitor vital signs and cardiopulmonary status before and after thoracentesis and as needed.	Any change in vital signs may alert the practitioner of possible unexpected outcomes. Use of supplemental oxygen may be necessary in certain patient populations.	*These conditions should be reported if they persist despite nursing interventions.* • Tachypnea • Decreased or absent breath sounds on the affected side • Shortness of breath, dyspnea • Asymmetric chest excursion with respirations • Decreased oxygen saturation • Subcutaneous emphysema • Sudden sharp chest pain • Anxiety, restlessness, apprehension • Tachycardia • Hypotension

Patient Monitoring and Care—*Continued*

Steps	Rationale	Reportable Conditions
		• Dysrhythmias • Tracheal deviation to the unaffected side • Neck vein distention • Muffled heart sounds
2. If indicated, obtain a postthoracentesis expiratory chest x-ray. *(Level V: Clinical studies in more than one patient population and situation.)*	A chest x-ray is used to evaluate for lung reexpansion and evidence of a possible pneumothorax or hemothorax. If a pneumothorax or hemothorax is present, a chest tube may be necessary. Without concrete clinical indications, chest x-ray is not necessary after a routine thoracentesis.[2,3,5,6]	• Pneumothorax • Expanding pleural effusion • Catheter migration

Documentation

Documentation should include the following:

- Patient and family teaching
- Insertion of catheter or needle
- Catheter or needle size used
- Any difficulties in insertion
- Patient tolerance
- Pleural fluid aspirate characteristics
- Total amount of pleural fluid aspirated

- Site assessment
- Occurrence of unexpected outcomes
- Postthoracentesis x-ray results
- Laboratory test ordered and results as available
- Interpretation of laboratory results
- Nursing interventions

References

1. Colt, H.G., Brewer, N., and Barbur, E.B. (1999). Evaluation of patient-related and procedure-related factors contributing to pneumothorax following thoracentesis. *Chest,* 116, 134-8.
2. Doyle, J.J., et al. (1996). Necessity of routine chest roentgenography after thoracentesis. *Ann Intern Med,* 124, 816-20.
3. Gervais, D.A., et al. (1997). US-guided thoracentesis: Requirement for post procedure chest radiography in patients who receive mechanical ventilation versus patients who breathe spontaneously. *Radiology,* 204, 503-6.
4. Jones, P.W., et al. (2003). Ultrasound-guided thoracentesis: Is it a safer method? *Chest,* 123, 418-23.
5. Lichtenstein, D., et al. (1999). Feasibility and safety of ultrasound-aided thoracentesis in mechanically ventilated patients. *Intensive Care Med,* 25, 955-8.
6. Peterson, W.G., and Zimmerman, R. (2000). Limited utility of chest radiograph after thoracentesis. *Chest,* 117, 1038-42.
7. Qureshi, N., Momin, Z.A., and Brandstetter, R.D. (1994). Thoracentesis in clinical practice. *Heart Lung,* 23, 376-83.
8. Sarodia, B.D., et al. (2000). Does pleural fluid pH change significantly at room temperature during the first hour following thoracentesis? *Chest,* 117, 1043-8.

Additional Readings

Heffner, J.E., Brown, L.K., and Barbieri, C.A. (1997). Diagnostic value of tests that discriminate between exudative and transudative pleural effusions. *Chest,* 111, 970-80.
Klima, L.D., and Benditt, J.O. (1997). Pulmonary procedures. In: Goldstein, R.H., O'Connell, J.J., and Karlinsky, J.B., editors. *A Practical Approach to Pulmonary Medicine.* Philadelphia: Lippincott-Raven, 39-54.
Light, R.W., et al. (1992). Pleural effusion: The diagnostic separation of transudates and exudates. *Ann Intern Med,* 77, 507-13.
Quigley, R.L. (1995). Thoracentesis and chest tube drainage. *Crit Care Clin,* 11, 111-26.

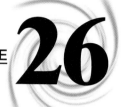

PROCEDURE **26**

Arterial-Venous Oxygen Difference Calculation

PURPOSE: The arterial-venous oxygen difference (a-vDo$_2$) is calculated in a mechanically ventilated patient to provide an indication of oxygen delivery, oxygen consumption, and adequacy of tissue oxygenation.

Suzanne M. Burns

PREREQUISITE NURSING KNOWLEDGE

- Most oxygen carried in the blood is bound to hemoglobin and is referred to as *oxygen saturation*. A small percentage also is dissolved in the plasma. The total blood *oxygen content* is determined by adding the amount of oxygen bound to hemoglobin to that dissolved in the plasma. Oxygen content can be calculated for the arterial blood (Cao$_2$) and the venous blood (Cvo$_2$). By calculating the oxygen contents for arterial and venous blood and subtracting them, a rough estimate of oxygen use can be made. A normal a-vDo$_2$ is 5 vol% (range is 4 to 6 vol%). In general, because the contribution of dissolved oxygen is slight, it is not used clinically to calculate Cao$_2$.
- Mixed venous oxygen pressure (Pvo$_2$) and mixed venous oxygen saturation (Svo$_2$) reflect tissue oxygenation under most conditions. When blood flow does not increase to meet higher tissue oxygen demands (as in hypotension), more oxygen is extracted from the arterial blood, and the Pvo$_2$ and Svo$_2$ decrease. The gradient between Cao$_2$ and Cvo$_2$ widens. Conversely, when blood flow is increased (e.g., hyperdynamic flow, as in sepsis), less oxygen is extracted from the arterial blood; Pvo$_2$ and Svo$_2$ increase, and a-vDo$_2$ decreases.
- A major clinical goal of positive-pressure ventilation (PPV) and positive end-expiratory pressure (PEEP) is improved oxygenation. One potential complication of these therapies is hypotension secondary to the effect of increased intrathoracic pressures on venous return.
- Calculation of a-vDo$_2$ may reflect tissue oxygenation in some cases; however, it is not a direct measurement and can be used only for approximation. The measurement of

lactic acid is thought to be a more accurate assessment of tissue hypoxia; however, the formation of lactic acid occurs late in the clinical course and is often irreversible.[1,2]
- One of the most important variables affecting oxygen use is cardiac output. When cardiac output is low, more oxygen is extracted from the arterial blood, lowering the Cvo$_2$. A decline in Pvo$_2$ may reflect decreased perfusion.
- The product of cardiac output and Cao$_2$ is oxygen delivery. Oxygen consumption may be calculated by determining the product of cardiac output and a-vDo$_2$.
- Measurement of cardiac output is necessary for oxygen delivery and oxygen consumption calculations (see Procedure 63).
- Confirmation of pulmonary artery catheter placement is necessary (see Procedure 72).
- Sampling of arterial blood from an indwelling catheter or arterial puncture should be done (see Procedure 60 or 79).
- Sampling of mixed venous blood from the pulmonary artery catheter should be done (see Procedure 62).
- Interpretation of arterial blood gases is necessary.

EQUIPMENT

- Calculator and mathematical equations
- Arterial blood gas and saturation*
- Mixed venous blood gas and saturation*
- Hemoglobin level
- Hemodynamic profile (if calculating of oxygen delivery/consumption, cardiac output is required)

---

*Note: To obtain accurate arterial and venous saturations, a heparinized blood sample needs to be sent for analysis by cooximeter. The saturation calculated from a blood gas is less accurate.

PATIENT AND FAMILY EDUCATION

- Inform the patient and the family of the patient's perfusion status and changes in therapy, and interpret the changes. If the patient or another family member requests specific information about arterial venous oxygen content differences, explain the general relationship between $a\text{-}vDo_2$ and perfusion. ➤*Rationale:* Most patients and families are less concerned with the diagnostic and therapeutic details and more concerned with how the patient is progressing overall or in relation to a specific physiologic function.

PATIENT ASSESSMENT AND PREPARATION

Patient Assessment

- Assess signs and symptoms of inadequate tissue oxygenation.
  - ❖ Thirst
  - ❖ Nausea
  - ❖ Anxiety
  - ❖ Apprehension
  - ❖ Skin temperature
  - ❖ Bounding pulse
  - ❖ Tachycardia
  - ❖ High cardiac output with low systemic vascular resistance
  - ❖ Cool skin
  - ❖ Weak pulse
  - ❖ Low cardiac output
  - ❖ Hypotension
  - ❖ Decreased mentation
  - ❖ Metabolic acidosis
  - ❖ Decreased pulse pressure
  - ❖ Increased systemic vascular resistance
  - ❖ Tachypnea
  - ❖ Decreased urine output
  - ➤*Rationale:* Calculation of $a\text{-}vDo_2$ is indicated to provide a rough quantitative estimate of tissue perfusion and oxygenation.

Patient Preparation

- Ensure that the patient understands preprocedural teaching. Answer questions as they arise, and reinforce information as needed. ➤*Rationale:* This communication evaluates and reinforces understanding of previously taught information.

Procedure	for Arterial-Venous Oxygen Difference Calculation	
Steps	**Rationale**	**Special Considerations**
1. After obtaining arterial blood gas and mixed venous blood gas results (including saturation), determine and record the value to be used for oxygen-carrying capacity (either 1.39 or 1.34). *(Level II: Theory based, no research data to support recommendations; recommendations from expert consensus group may exist.)*	Use the same oxygen-carrying capacity value consistently for all $a\text{-}vDo_2$ calculations per patient. This prevents erroneous results.[1,2]	
2. Calculate Cao_2 using the modified Fick equation: $Cao_2 = 1.39$ (or 1.34) $\times$ Hgb $\times$ %Sao_2 (use decimal)	Only approximation is needed for clinical purposes.[1,2]	If using dissolved oxygen, add $(0.003 \times Pao_2)$; this is generally not necessary because it adds little to content.
3. Calculate Cvo_2 using the modified Fick equation: $Cvo_2 = 1.39$ (or 1.34) $\times$ Hgb $\times$ %Svo_2 (use decimal)	Only approximation is needed for clinical purposes.[1,2]	If using dissolved oxygen in the equation, add $(0.003 \times Pvo_2)$; this is not usually necessary.
4. Subtract Cvo_2 from Cao_2.	Results in $a\text{-}vDo_2$ value.	
5. Consult with physician or advance practice nurse if needed changes in therapy exceed therapeutic guidelines.	Large changes in $a\text{-}vDo_2$ value may indicate need for revising the therapeutic guidelines. Provides integrated trend data to evaluate tissue oxygenation in light of pulmonary function and ventilator parameters and shows appropriate use of diagnostic and monitoring tests to evaluate therapy and alter therapy if needed.	

Expected Outcome

- Titration of PPV parameters (e.g., tidal volume, PEEP, inspiratory-expiratory ratio) to maintain adequate perfusion and tissue oxygenation

Unexpected Outcome

- Hemodynamic instability

Patient Monitoring and Care

Steps	Rationale	Reportable Conditions
1. Observe trend in a-vDo$_2$.	PPV, particularly with a large tidal volume and PEEP, can compromise hemodynamics from increased intrathoracic pressure. A narrowing difference may indicate hyperdynamic perfusion as seen with sepsis. A widening difference may indicate hypodynamic perfusion, such as with cardiogenic shock. The effect of PPV therapy on perfusion needs to be explored. (Unless a therapeutic plan has been predetermined, decisions related to interventions need to be made with each measurement. For example, although an increase in PEEP may be thought to have resulted in hypotension and a widened a-vDo$_2$, the intervention may be to give fluid instead of lowering PEEP.)	*These conditions should be reported if they persist despite nursing interventions.* • Acute changes in a-vDo$_2$

Documentation

Documentation should include the following:

- Patient and family education
- The a-vDo$_2$ and arterial blood gas and hemoglobin results with which it was calculated
- The time, date, and position of the patient (e.g., supine, prone, semiprone)

- Ventilator parameters at the time the blood gas samples were drawn
- Changes in therapy based on a-vDo$_2$ value
- Patient response to interventions
- Unexpected outcomes

References

1. Barone, J.E. (1994). Maximization of oxygen delivery: A plea for moderation. II. *J Trauma,* 37, 337-8.
2. Silance, P.G., Simon, C., and Vincent, J.L. (1994). The relationship between cardiac index and oxygen extraction in acutely ill patients. *Chest,* 105, 1190-7.

Additional Readings

Ahrens, T.S., and Powers, C.C. (1998). Pulmonary clinical physiology. In: Kinney, M.R., et al., editors. *AACN's Clinical Reference for Critical Care Nursing.* 4th ed. St. Louis: Mosby, 491-516.

Ahrens, T.S., and Rutherford, K.A. (1993). *Essentials of Oxygenation.* Boston: Jones & Bartlett.

West, J.B. (1999). *Respiratory Physiology: The Essentials.* 6th ed. Baltimore: Williams & Wilkins.

West, J.B. (2000). *Pulmonary Physiology and Pathophysiology: An Integrated Case-Based Approach.* Baltimore: Williams & Wilkins.

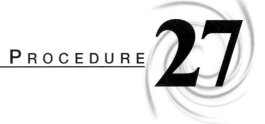

PROCEDURE **27**

Auto-PEEP Calculation

PURPOSE: Auto positive end-expiratory pressure (Auto-PEEP) is measured in a mechanically ventilated patient to identify the presence of auto-PEEP, to quantify the level to assess patient risk and the need for changes in ventilator therapy, and to quantify the level to calculate static compliance accurately.

Suzanne M. Burns

PREREQUISITE NURSING KNOWLEDGE

- Auto-PEEP is often called *occult* because it is not set on the ventilator; instead, it is a result of inadequate exhalation time (Fig. 27-1).
- Auto-PEEP is associated with high minute ventilation requirements, small-diameter endotracheal tubes, bronchospasm, long inspiratory times, high respiratory rates, and mechanical factors such as water accumulation in the ventilator tubing.
- Auto-PEEP may result in increased work of breathing. The set sensitivity of the ventilator does not reflect the pressure required to initiate a breath; the patient has to generate a pressure equal to the set sensitivity plus auto-PEEP.
- Auto-PEEP elevates static pressure (i.e., plateau pressure). High plateau pressures can result in barotrauma and hemodynamic compromise.[1,4,5]
- Auto-PEEP may be a desirable outcome of select ventilator settings (e.g., pressure-controlled inverse ratio ventilation). In these cases, auto-PEEP restores functional residual capacity and reduces shunt.
- Interventions to offset auto-PEEP include the use of sedatives and narcotics, large-diameter endotracheal tubes, bronchodilators, short inspiratory times, slower respiratory rates, and frequent emptying of ventilator circuit water accumulation (heated circuits may eliminate this complication). Occasionally the addition of set-PEEP is used to offset auto-PEEP. An example is in the case of a patient with chronic obstructive pulmonary disease, in whom early airway closure during exhalation results in gas trapping. The addition of set-PEEP serves as a splint by keeping the airway open throughout exhalation, decreasing auto-PEEP.[1,3-5]

EQUIPMENT

Generally, no additional equipment is necessary because most ventilators have an end-expiratory hold button to use for determining auto-PEEP. If the ventilator is an old one, auto-PEEP can be measured manually.

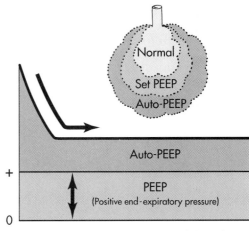

FIGURE 27-1 Auto-PEEP is PEEP over and above the set PEEP. It can be measured by performing an end-expiratory hold maneuver and observing the airway pressure manometer. Auto-PEEP is caused by insufficient expiratory time (e.g., high rates, inverse ratios, obstructions). Too much PEEP can increase pulmonary pressures, decrease systematic blood pressure, and risk diverting blood flow to poorly ventilated alveoli, thus increasing hypoxemia. *PEEP*, positive end-expiratory pressure. *(From Kinney, M., et al. [1998].* AACN Clinical Reference for Critical Care Nursing. *4th ed. St. Louis: Mosby.)*

PATIENT AND FAMILY EDUCATION

- Inform the patient and family about the patient's respiratory status, changes in therapy, and how to interpret the changes. If the patient or family requests specific information about auto-PEEP measurements, explain the general relationship between auto-PEEP, the work of breathing, and complication risks. ➥*Rationale:* Most patients and families are less concerned with the diagnostic and therapeutic details and more concerned with how the patient is progressing overall or in relation to a specific physiologic function.

PATIENT ASSESSMENT AND PREPARATION

Patient Assessment

- Assess for the presence of auto-PEEP; have a high index of suspicion if any of the following is noted:
  - Minute ventilation requirements are greater than 10 L/min.
  - The patient has chronic obstructive pulmonary disease.
  - The patient has bronchospasm.
  - The respiratory rate is rapid (i.e., greater than or equal to 20/min).
  - The inspiratory time is long (i.e., greater than 1 second).
  - Any of the above is present in conjunction with bronchospasm.
  - Dyssynchrony exists between patient and ventilator, especially when the ventilator does not cycle with patient inspiration.[1,3-5] ➥*Rationale:* Auto-PEEP increases the work of breathing by increasing the threshold load

to trigger inspiration. The increased work of breathing may cause fatigue.

- The presence of auto-PEEP (when any of the above-listed criteria are present) and whether the patient is hypotensive or shows signs of barotrauma.
- Patients in status asthmaticus (*high risk*). Consider the presence of auto-PEEP secondary to vigorous bagging, high ventilator rates, or large tidal volumes, especially if hypotension is present.[5] ➥*Rationale:* Auto-PEEP, similar to intentional PEEP, puts the patients at risk for barotrauma secondary to increased intraalveolar pressures. In patients with asthma, lung compliance is good, but airway resistance is high, encouraging dynamic hyperinflation (alveolar overdistention) and potential barotrauma. Hemodynamic compromise occurs when the increased alevolar pressure collapses or squeezes the capillaries; decreased venous return and hypotension result.

- Auto-PEEP may not be detected in some patients with severe asthma despite its presence. This situation may occur if the end-expiratory hold maneuver is too short to allow complete equilibration of pressures and with airway obstruction. In cases in which the presence of auto-PEEP is not detected but is likely (status asthmaticus), monitoring plateau pressure may provide useful information as an alternative to the auto-PEEP maneuver (see Procedure 28).[2]

Patient Preparation

- Ensure that the patient understands preprocedural teaching. Answer questions as they arise, and reinforce information as needed. ➥*Rationale:* This communication evaluates and reinforces understanding of previously taught information.

Procedure for Auto-PEEP Calculation

Steps	Rationale	Special Considerations
1. Identify the end-expiratory hold button on the ventilator. *(Level V: Clinical studies in more than one patient population or situation.)* If no end-expiratory hold button is available, proceed to **Step 3**.	Normally the pressure in the ventilator is exposed to atmospheric pressure during exhalation, and the airway pressure needle will fall to 0 or the set PEEP level. End-expiratory hold buttons close the ventilator systems to atmospheric pressure at end exhalation. The presence and degree of auto-PEEP can be measured because the maneuver allows for the equalization of pressure within the system.[4,5]	
2. A. Push the end-expiratory hold button at the end of exhalation (right before the next inspiration).[2-4] *(Level V: Clinical studies in more than one patient population or situation.)*	Auto-PEEP is the level of PEEP between set PEEP and the highest level noted during this maneuver. Hold until the airway pressure manometer rests on the final auto-PEEP level.	

Procedure for Auto-PEEP Calculation—*Continued*

Steps	Rationale	Special Considerations
B. Observe the baseline pressure level on the airway pressure manometer or on the digital readout. C. If auto-PEEP is present, the baseline (0 or set PEEP level) increases to the level of auto-PEEP. *(Level V: Clinical studies in more than one patient population or situation.)* D. Record the total PEEP over the set PEEP level.	In patients with rapid respiratory rates and in agitated patients, auto-PEEP is difficult to measure accurately. Using sedatives, muscle relaxants, or both may be necessary. In patients with asthma, an end-expiratory hold may not exhibit auto-PEEP despite the presence of significant dynamic hyperinflation. Plateau pressure may be a better measure to assess the results of therapeutic interventions in these cases.[2-4]	
3. Occlude the expiratory port of the ventilator with a gloved hand at the end of expiration, just before initiation of the subsequent mechanical breath. While watching the airway pressure manometer during this maneuver, note where the needle rests. Immediately release the expiratory port.		
4. Document the presence and amount of auto-PEEP and total PEEP.		
5. Consult physician or advance practice nurse as needed for changes in therapy.		

Expected Outcomes

- Auto-PEEP will be identified, monitored, and eliminated (if undesirable).
- Therapy will be titrated, if possible, to minimize or eliminate auto-PEEP.

Unexpected Outcomes

- Pulmonary barotrauma
- Cardiovascular depression

Patient Monitoring and Care

Steps	Rationale	Reportable Conditions
		These conditions should be reported if they persist despite nursing interventions. • Presence of auto-PEEP
1. Evaluate the presence of auto-PEEP in the conditions noted in patient assessment.	Prevent complications by determining the presence of auto-PEEP and intervening appropriately; this is especially important in patients with profound hyperinflation (i.e., status asthmaticus). Interventions may need to be aggressive; the patient may require paralytics and sedatives so that ventilatory support can be reduced to allow for more complete exhalation.	

Patient Monitoring and Care—*Continued*

Steps	Rationale	Reportable Conditions
	Hypercarbia is expected and is called *permissive hypercarbia.* The clinical goal is to reduce dynamic hyperinflation and potential lung injury.	
2. Assess for signs and symptoms of barotraumas, hemodynamic compromise, or both.	Barotrauma is a potential complication of auto-PEEP.	• Decreased breath sounds or absent breath sounds on one side • Respiratory distress • Unexplained vital sign changes

Documentation

Documentation should include the following:

- Patient and family education
- Presence and degree of auto-PEEP
- Any changes in ventilator parameters
- Unexpected outcomes
- Nursing interventions taken

References

1. Georgopoulos, D., Giannouli, E., and Patakas, D. (1993). Effects of extrinsic positive end-expiratory pressure on mechanically ventilated patients with chronic obstructive pulmonary disease and dynamic hyperinflation. *Intensive Care Med,* 19, 197-203.
2. Leatherman, J.W., and Ravenscraft, S.A. (1996). Low-measured auto-positive end-expiratory pressure during mechanical ventilation of patients with severe asthma: Hidden auto-positive end expiratory pressure. *Crit Care Med,* 24, 541-6.
3. MacIntyre, N.R., Cheng, K.C., and McConnell, R. (1997). Applied PEEP during pressure support reduces inspiratory threshold of intrinsic PEEP. *Chest,* 111, 188-93.
4. Pepe, P.E., and Marini, J.J. (1994). Occult positive end-expiratory pressure in mechanically ventilated patients with airflow obstruction. *Am Rev Respir Dis,* 126, 166-73.
5. Smith, T.C., and Marini, J.J. (1988). Impact of PEEP on lung mechanics and work of breathing in severe airflow obstruction. *J Appl Physiol,* 65, 1488-99.

Additional Readings

MacIntyre, N.R. (1995). Complications of positive pressure ventilation. In: Dantzker, D.R., MacIntyre, N.R., and Bakow, E.D., editors. *Comprehensive Respiratory Care.* Philadelphia: W.B. Saunders, 447-50.
Rossei, A., and Ranieri, M.V. (1994). Positive end-expiratory pressure. In: Tobin, M.J., editor. *Principles and Practice of Mechanical Ventilation.* New York: McGraw-Hill, 288-9.

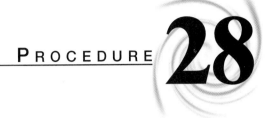
PROCEDURE **28**

Compliance and Resistance Measurement

PURPOSE: Clinical measurements of compliance and resistance are performed to assess trends in respiratory status, to determine the effectiveness of therapy, and to titrate therapy.

Suzanne M. Burns

PREREQUISITE NURSING KNOWLEDGE

- *Compliance* is a measure of lung (and chest wall) distensibility. Conditions that decrease compliance include acute respiratory distress syndrome (ARDS), pulmonary edema, atelectasis, pneumonia, obesity, pulmonary fibrosis, and kyphoscoliosis. Compliance increases with emphysema.
- *Resistance* is a measure of how easy it is to move gases down the airways. Examples of conditions that adversely affect resistance include bronchospasm, secretions, and endotracheal tube size.
- Compliance and resistance are reflected in a mechanically ventilated patient by changes in peak inspiratory and plateau pressures (i.e., volume modes) or by changes in volume (i.e., pressure modes) or both. By monitoring changes in volume per unit change in pressure (ml/cm H_2O), trends can be measured and therapies adjusted.
- Although spirometry or plethysmography or both are required for the exact measurement of airways flow resistance and lung compliance, two clinical measurements frequently are employed to estimate the contributions of each in a mechanically ventilated patient: *dynamic compliance* (C_{dyn}), which is more accurately called *dynamic characteristic*, and *static compliance* (C_{stat}).
  - ❖ The measurements of C_{dyn} and C_{stat} are obtained on volume modes of ventilation. C_{dyn} requires that the delivered volume be divided by the peak inspiratory pressure (PIP) minus positive end-expiratory pressure (PEEP). Because gases are actively moving down the airways during volume breath delivery, PIP reflects the

contribution of airways resistance and lung compliance. *Dynamic characteristic* is a more accurate term than *dynamic compliance.*
  - ❖ C_{stat} is measured during a breath-hold maneuver (i.e., end inspiration). By stopping gas flow, the pressure in the system equilibrates, and the resultant pressure reflects the pressure required to distend the lungs separate from the pressure needed to move gases down the airways. The pressure measured during the breath hold is called *static pressure* (also called *plateau, alveolar,* or *distending pressure*). By also subtracting PEEP, this number becomes the denominator for the calculation of C_{stat} (i.e., tidal volume ÷ [plateau pressure–PEEP]). The normal gradient between PIP and static pressure is 10 to 15 cm H_2O. By comparing the difference between the two, the contribution of airways resistance is easily noted. Although using PIP and static pressure is helpful for monitoring trends clinically, calculating C_{dyn} and C_{stat} is most useful for quantifying the degree of improvement or compromise over time.
- Static pressure is especially helpful to monitor when the lung is stiff (e.g., ARDS) and when there is great potential for barotrauma (e.g., in air leak phenomena) and volutrauma (e.g., in alveolar injury).[1,4] In a randomized controlled trial by the ARDS Network, patients ventilated with low-volume ventilation (i.e., 6 ml/kg) had a lower mortality rate than patients ventilated at larger "traditional" volumes (i.e., 12 ml/kg).[3] The plateau pressures associated with the low-volume ventilation were less than 30 cm H_2O. The clinical goal for patients with ARDS may be to ensure that the plateau

pressure is maintained at a level of 30 cm H_2O or less regardless of the mode of ventilation[3] (see Procedure 32).

- Although the risk is low, measuring static pressure may increase the risk of barotrauma or cardiovascular compromise.

EQUIPMENT

- Calculator
- Values to be collected: tidal volume, PIP, static pressure, PEEP, and auto-PEEP, if present (see Procedure 27)

PATIENT AND FAMILY EDUCATION

- Inform the patent and family about the patient's respiratory status, changes in therapy, and how to interpret the changes. If the patient or a family member requests specific information about C_{dyn} or C_{stat}, explain the relationship between the measurements and how easy it is to get air into the lungs and down the airway. ➤➤*Rationale:* Most patients and families are less concerned with diagnostic and therapeutic details and more concerned with how the patient is progressing overall.

PATIENT ASSESSMENT AND PREPARATION

Patient Assessment

- Determine PIP to assess gradual or acute changes. ➤➤*Rationale:* Given a constant tidal volume, a change in PIP indicates a change in airway resistance or lung compliance.
- Assess changes in ease or difficulty of compression of the manual self-inflating resuscitation bag. ➤➤*Rationale:* Compliance is change in volume for a change in pressure. If more pressure is required to inflate the lungs, ventilation is affected.

Patient Preparation

- Ensure that the patient understands preprocedural teaching. Answer questions as they arise, and reinforce information as needed. ➤➤*Rationale:* This communication evaluates and reinforces understanding of previously taught information.
- Premedicate as needed. ➤➤*Rationale:* This measurement may be extremely difficult in a patient who is breathing rapidly or is agitated. Sedation and paralytics are sometimes necessary.

Procedure for Compliance and Resistance Measurement

Steps	Rationale	Special Considerations
Dynamic Characteristic (C_{dyn}) *(Level VI: Clinical studies in a variety of patient populations and situations.)*	C_{dyn} and C_{stat} have been extensively tested at bedside in many patient populations.[2-4]	
1. Identify the PIP.	PIP is used as a rough estimate of the mechanical properties of the lung and chest wall and airways resistance.	
2. Identify the delivered exhaled tidal volume.	Data collection for calculation.	Air leaks around the artificial airway or through chest tubes prevent an accurate measurement of C_{dyn}. Ensure the cuff leak is minimal. Exhaled tidal volume differs from inspired tidal volume with large leaks.
3. Identify the amount of PEEP and auto-PEEP.	Data collection for calculation.	If auto-PEEP is present, add to PEEP as total PEEP to ensure accurate calculation (see Procedure 27).
4. Record PIP, tidal volume, and total PEEP (i.e., PEEP plus auto-PEEP).	Data collection for calculation.	
5. Subtract total PEEP from PIP.	Reflects PIP without PEEP.	
6. Divide tidal volume by the number obtained in **Step 5**. The result equals the C_{dyn}.	Compliance is defined as the unit change in volume per unit change in pressure.	
7. Record C_{dyn} in ml/cm H_2O.	Communicates data.	
8. Document in patient record.		

Procedure for Compliance and Resistance Measurement—*Continued*

Steps	Rationale	Special Considerations
Static Compliance (C_{stat})		
9. Observe several ventilator respiratory cycles.	Determines timing of the end of inspiration.	
10. Identify initiation of the ventilator inspiratory cycle.	Determines timing of the beginning of inspiration.	
11. At the end of inspiration, activate the inspiratory pause (inflation hold), while watching the pressure gauge. Note the drop and plateau of the PIP needle (plateau pressure), and immediately deactivate the inspiratory pause, allowing exhalation.	At this point, the flow of gas through the airway stops, causing the inspiratory pressure level to drop. The resultant pressure is the static (also called *plateau, alveolar,* and *distending*) pressure.	This maneuver requires hand-eye coordination to ensure a short inspiratory pause (i.e., less than 2 seconds). This measurement may be extremely difficult in a patient who is breathing rapidly or agitated. Administering sedation and paralytics is sometimes necessary.
12. Record the static pressure.	Data collection for calculation.	
13. Subtract total PEEP (PEEP plus auto-PEEP) from plateau pressure.	Reflects pressure plateau without PEEP.	
14. Divide tidal volume by the number obtained in **Step 13.**	C_{stat} is the relationship of the tidal volume to the plateau (static) pressure.	Air leaks around the artificial airway or through chest tubes prevent an accurate measurement of static compliance. Ensure an intact cuff.
15. Document in patient record.		

Expected Outcome

- Therapy titrated to patient response

Unexpected Outcomes

- Pulmonary barotrauma
- Cardiovascular depression

Patient Monitoring and Care

Steps	Rationale	Reportable Conditions
1. Observe trends in C_{dyn} and C_{stat}.	Increasing values with a constant tidal volume indicate improvement in underlying disease process and effectiveness of interventions. Decreasing values with constant tidal volume indicate increased airway resistance (C_{dyn}) or progression of underlying disease process and ineffective interventions (C_{dyn} and C_{stat}).	*These conditions should be reported if they persist despite nursing interventions.* • Bradycardia • Tachycardia • Decrease in saturation to less than or equal to 90% • Changes or trends

Documentation

Documentation should include the following:

- Patient and family education
- C_{dyn} and C_{stat} calculations
- Patient tolerance

- Unexpected outcomes
- Nursing interventions

References

1. Dreyfuss, D., et al. (1988). High inflation pressure pulmonary edema: Respective effects of high airway pressure, high tidal volume, and positive end-expiratory pressure. *Am Rev Respir Dis,* 137, 1159-64.
2. Pepe, P.E., and Marini, J.J. (1982). Occult positive end-expiratory pressure in mechanically ventilated patients with airflow obstruction. *Am Rev Respir Dis,* 126, 166-70.
3. The Acute Respiratory Distress Syndrome Network. (2000). Ventilation with lower tidal volumes as compared with traditional tidal volumes for acute lung injury and the acute respiratory distress syndrome. *N Engl J Med,* 342, 1301-7.
4. Truwit, J.D. (1997). Lung mechanics. In: Dantzker, D.R., MacIntyre, N.R., and Bakow, E.D., editors. *Comprehensive Respiratory Care.* Philadelphia: W.B. Saunders, 20-6.

Additional Readings

Ahrens, T.S., and Powers, C.C. (1998). Pulmonary clinical physiology. In: Kinney, M.R., et al., editors. *AACN's Clinical Reference for Critical Care Nursing.* 4th ed. St. Louis: Mosby-Year Book, 494-5.
Tobin, M.J., and Van De Graaff, W.B. (1994). Monitoring of lung mechanics and work of breathing. In: Tobin, M.J., editor. *Principles and Practice of Mechanical Ventilation.* New York: McGraw-Hill, 978-84.

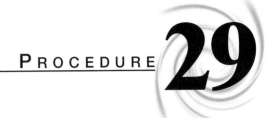

PROCEDURE **29**

Manual Self-Inflating Resuscitation Bag

P U R P O S E : The manual self-inflating resuscitation bag is used to provide ventilation and oxygenation with or without an artificial airway in place and is called *bagging*.

Suzanne M. Burns

PREREQUISITE NURSING KNOWLEDGE

- Bagging is an essential skill used in emergency situations, such as cardiopulmonary arrest. Bagging also is indicated for the following:
    - To provide oxygenation and ventilation before and after suctioning airway procedures and during patient transports
    - To assess airway patency and placement
    - To evaluate the interaction of patient and ventilator
    - To alter the ventilatory pattern
- Bagging should result in chest movement and auscultatory evidence of bilateral air entry.
- In patients without an artificial airway in place, effective bagging requires an unobstructed airway, slight head and neck hyperextension (i.e., the same technique used for mouth-to-mouth ventilation), and firm placement of the facemask over the nose and mouth (Fig. 29-1). Effective bagging is best accomplished with two people: one to secure the mask and ensure head and neck placement and one to bag. An exception to this technique is known cervical spine injury.
- In patients with artificial airways, such as endotracheal or nasotracheal tubes or tracheostomies, the nurse must understand the components of artificial airways and the relationship of the airways to the upper airway anatomy (see Procedures 1, 2, 7, 8, 9, 11, or 12).
- When signs and symptoms of respiratory distress are noted in a mechanically ventilated patient, the patient should be bagged if troubleshooting does not elucidate the problem immediately.
- Large breaths and rapid rates provided during bagging may result in dynamic hyperinflation and resultant hypotension.[4,5] Dynamic hyperinflation most commonly

is associated with bronchospasm and chronic obstructive pulmonary disease.[4] Hyperinflation occurs when exhalation time is inadequate, which results in auto–positive end-expiratory pressure (PEEP) and decreased venous return (see Procedure 27). A high index of suspicion is necessary if hypotension occurs with bagging. A brief disconnection from the bag or the provision of longer exhalation times or both result in a rapid increase in blood pressure. Bagging is resumed at a slower rate and with longer expiratory times.

EQUIPMENT

- Manual self-inflating resuscitation bag (of appropriate size) and mask (Fig. 29-2)
- Oxygen source (flowmeter or needle valve) and tubing
- PEEP valve or PEEP attachment (if patient on greater than 5 cm H_2O of PEEP)

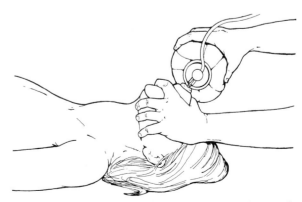

FIGURE 29-1 Proper technique of ventilation with manual self-inflating resuscitation bag and facemask. *(From Wilkins, R.L., and Stoller, J.K. [2003]. Egan's Fundamentals of Respiratory Care. 8th ed. St. Louis: Mosby.)*

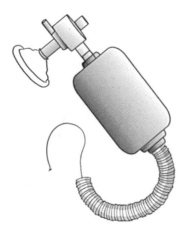

Bag-valve assembly with rear bag reservoir

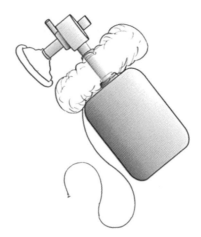

Bag-valve assembly with collar reservoir

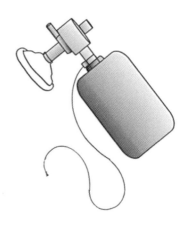

Bag-valve assembly without reservoir

FIGURE 29-2 Manual self-inflating bags: bag-valve assembly with and without reservoir.

Additional equipment (to have available depending on patient need) includes the following:
- Oxygen analyzer when specific fraction of inspired oxygen (F_{IO_2}) is desired
- Portable respirometer if accurate tidal volume delivery on a breath-to-breath basis is required (e.g., during patient transports)

PATIENT AND FAMILY EDUCATION

- Inform the patient and family that disconnection from the ventilator will occur and that bagging will be performed, and describe the reason (e.g., suctioning, transporting, making patient more comfortable). Explain that if the patient is dyspneic or otherwise distressed, it is important that bagging be done immediately. ➤*Rationale:* Information about the patient's therapy is an important need of patients and family members. Dyspnea is uncomfortable and frightening. It leads to anxiety, fear, and distrust. Failure to diagnose promptly and alleviate the cause of respiratory distress puts the patient at risk for further decompensation.
- Inform the patient and family that the patient may be in different positions during bagging (i.e., side-lying, prone, supine, Trendelenburg, reverse Trendelenburg, semi-Fowler). Bagging may be more difficult, however, if the diaphragm and abdominal contents are in positions that resist lung inflation. ➤*Rationale:* Positioning is not an impediment to bagging as long as an intact airway is in place. Bagging may be more difficult in some positions.
- Discuss the sensory experience associated with bagging. ➤*Rationale:* Knowledge of anticipated sensory experiences decreases anxiety and distress.
- Instruct the patient to communicate discomfort with breathing during bagging. ➤*Rationale:* The bagging technique can be altered to produce a comfortable breathing pattern.
- Offer the opportunity for the patient and family to ask questions about bagging. ➤*Rationale:* Being able to ask questions and to have questions answered honestly are cited consistently as the most important needs of patients and families.

PATIENT ASSESSMENT AND PREPARATION

Patient Assessment
- Determine oxygenation and ventilation status and observe for the following signs.
  - ❖ Sudden decrease in arterial oxygen saturation (SaO_2)
  - ❖ Sudden change in mental status
  - ❖ Tachycardia
  - ❖ Tachypnea
  - ❖ Respiratory distress
  ➤*Rationale:* Any acute change in patient status may indicate that bagging is indicated. Rapid response with 100% F_{IO_2} protects the patient and allows for rapid evaluation of airways resistance, placement and function of artificial airway, and interaction of patient and ventilator.
- Determine airways resistance (how easy it is to move air down the airways) and lung compliance (how easy it is to distend the lungs and chest wall). ➤*Rationale:* Airways resistance and lung compliance can be assessed by bagging the patient with breaths that are similar in volume and rate to the breaths provided by the ventilator. Focus on the degree of ease (or difficulty) with which the bag is compressed during inspiration. If it is difficult to bag the patient, look for causes of high airway resistance (e.g., obstructed airway, bronchospasm) or low lung compliance (e.g., pulmonary edema, pneumonia, acute respiratory distress syndrome, pneumothorax). Compare findings with findings after interventions, such as suctioning and bronchodilator use. Changes in resistance and compliance can be confirmed by evaluating dynamic characteristic and static compliance when the patient is placed back on the ventilator (see Procedure 28).
- Ensure proper placement and function of the artificial airway (see Procedures 1, 2, 7, 8, 9, 11, or 12). ➤*Rationale:* This ensures the positioning and patency of the airway.
- Evaluate interaction of patient and ventilator, and specifically note dyssynchrony of patient and ventilator, by observing for the following.

- Breathing pattern not in synchrony with ventilator breaths
- Wheezing
- Restlessness
- Dyspnea
- Altered level of consciousness
- Agitation
- Decreased or unequal breath sounds
- Tachycardia or bradycardia
- Dysrhythmias
- Cyanosis
- Hypertension or hypotension

➤**Rationale:** Bagging may aid in the return of a synchronous breathing pattern and recognition of the cause (e.g., obstruction). If signs and symptoms persist despite bagging, other causes (e.g., pulmonary embolus) should be considered. Therapeutic interventions to ensure synchrony and effective oxygenation and ventilation may be necessary and may include administering medications such as sedatives, narcotics, and bronchodilators. Additional diagnostic evaluations also may be required (e.g., bronchoscopy, ventilation-perfusion scans).

Patient Preparation

- Ensure that the patient understands preprocedural teaching. Answer questions as they arise, and reinforce information as needed. ➤**Rationale:** This communication evaluates and reinforces understanding of previously taught information.

Procedure for Manual Self-Inflating Resuscitation Bag		
Steps	**Rationale**	**Special Considerations**
Using the Manual Self-Inflating Bag for Respiratory Distress or Evaluation of Pulmonary Status (*Level IV: Limited clinical studies to support recommendations.*)[2]		
1. Check that bag is attached to oxygen source, which is turned on.	Safety precaution. Allows oxygen to flow to the bag.	
2. If the patient is mechanically ventilated, disconnect patient from the ventilator. Activate alarm silence. Connect bag to artificial airway.	Allows for manual ventilation.	
3. Observe patient's breathing pattern and rate. Attempt to synchronize manual breaths with the patient's spontaneous effort. Because it is difficult to provide larger breaths with manual ventilation compared with breaths provided by the ventilator, a higher manual rate may be required initially.[3]	Helps patient gain control over breathing by ensuring ventilation and adequate oxygenation.[1]	
4. Encourage patient to relax as manual breaths are provided.	Provides synchrony between patient breaths and manual breaths.	
5. Gradually slow the rate of manual breaths to approximate the ventilator frequency or to a rate that meets the patient's demand.	Reestablishes synchrony. When respiratory distress is relieved with a rate and volume comparable with that delivered by the ventilator, the patient can be reconnected. If the patient is on a low rate (e.g., intermittent mandatory ventilation of 4) or low-pressure support level, common during weaning, the distress may be the result of fatigue. A return to higher ventilator support settings is required after bagging.	

Procedure continues on the following page

Procedure for Manual Self-Inflating Resuscitation Bag—*Continued*

Steps	Rationale	Special Considerations
6. Ascertain whether the patient is comfortable with the manual breaths. Assess the ease or difficulty with which the bag is deflated.	Promotes comfort.	
A. If signs and symptoms of distress are absent, the patient can be reconnected to the ventilator.	Indicates that respiratory distress is relieved.	If the patient becomes distressed after reconnection, consider further assessment to determine etiology and potential interventions. Additional steps are as follows: Call for assistance while bagging, and look for additional confirmatory physical assessment findings, such as tympanic percussion (i.e., pneumothorax), diminished breath sounds with consolidation (i.e., atelectasis, pneumonia), or crackles (i.e. pulmonary edema) to determine etiology of acute distress.
B. If distress is not eliminated with bagging, consider the following steps: Provide higher level of ventilator support if distress is evident on lower levels as in weaning trials; hyperoxygenate and suction (see Procedure 10); assess for the presence of bilateral breath sounds and symmetrical chest expansion; assess the ease (or difficulty) with which the bag can be inflated; evaluate ventilator functioning. Obtain assistance (respiratory care or experienced nurse) to determine adequacy of ventilator function; consider anxiety and discomfort as potential causes of dyspnea.	Indicates respiratory distress cannot be relieved with bagging. Further assessment is required. Distress may be a result of fatigue. Suction will provide information related to the presence of secretions or airway obstruction. By auscultating the lungs during bagging, essential information related to tube placement (e.g., migration to right main stem) or patient status (e.g., bronchospasm, pulmonary edema) can be obtained. Asymmetrical chest expansion may be the result of a displaced artificial airway, pneumothorax, or obstruction. A change in ease of bagging provides gross data about increasing (improved) or decreasing (deteriorating) lung compliance. Alarms should deactivate automatically, unless the problem has not been adequately addressed. A leak or other malfunction results in patient distress and inadequate oxygenation and ventilation. Although psychological reasons for respiratory distress are possible, rule out physiologic causes first.	These data should correlate with changes in positive inspiratory pressure (volume ventilation) or tidal volume (pressure ventilation) on the ventilator. In some situations, such as pulmonary embolus, no distinct physical assessment findings may be immediately evident. Whether or not distress is alleviated with bagging and returns with reconnection, the ventilator may be malfunctioning or the settings may be inadequate for the patient's acute change in physical status. Support the patient until appropriate interventions are accomplished. The use of anxiolytics or analgesics or both is appropriate to decrease anxiety and pain, regardless of the etiology. It is essential, however, that a thorough evaluation of the cause of distress be undertaken after their administration.
7. Return patient to ventilator when respiratory distress is relieved. Reactivate and check ventilator alarms and settings. Observe breathing pattern, patient ventilator synchrony, positive inspiratory pressure (volume ventilation), and tidal volume and frequency (pressure ventilation). Check that call bell is within patient reach, if appropriate.	Safety precautions. Ensures nurse is alerted to actual or potential life-threatening problems.	

Procedure	for Manual Self-Inflating Resuscitation Bag—*Continued*	
Steps	**Rationale**	**Special Considerations**

8. Document event in patient record.

Maintenance Ventilation
(It is highly recommended that portable ventilators be used during transport instead of manual bagging. Regardless, it is possible that bagging will be required for long intervals. The following procedure is designed to provide a ventilatory pattern similar to that provided by the ventilator. Procedures may vary depending on institutional standards.)

Steps	Rationale	Special Considerations
1. Check that bag is attached to oxygen source, which is turned on.	Safety precaution. Provides direct route for oxygen to flow into the bag.	
2. Disconnect patient from ventilator. Silence ventilator alarms.	Because the nurse is at the bedside and there is no problem with the patient or ventilator, there is no reason for the alarms to summon help or disturb other patients.	
3. Insert portable respirometer between bag and artificial airway.	Ensures that tidal volume delivery approximates that provided by ventilator.	
4. Bag patient at approximate rate depth and pattern as ventilator breaths.	Maintains ventilation pattern similar to that provided by ventilator.	
5. Analyze average tidal volume delivered manually. Adjust bag compressions as necessary to produce tidal volume that approximates ventilator tidal volume. Repeat until approximate tidal volume is reproducible.	Achieves reproducible manual breaths.	
6. Remove portable respirometer, and insert portable oxygen analyzer between bag and artificial airway or use 1.0 FIO_2.	Allows FIO_2 to be analyzed.	Policies vary among institutions. Generally, 1.0 FIO_2 is used during patient transports, and analysis of oxygen level is not necessary.
7. Analyze FIO_2 delivered. Adjust liter flow of oxygen to produce same FIO_2 as ventilator breaths or to maintain SaO_2 at desired level.	Prevents hypoxia and maintains prescribed FIO_2.	FIO_2 delivered with bag depends on delivered oxygen liter flow and the type of manual resuscitation bag used. Reservoir tubing may be needed to ensure desired oxygen in some cases.
8. Remove oxygen analyzer and manually ventilate patient at tidal volume, ventilator frequency, and FIO_2 that approximate ventilator settings.	Approximates baseline ventilation and oxygenation.	
9. Periodically ascertain that the patient is comfortable with the bagging technique. Adjustments may be needed to maintain patient comfort with manual ventilation.	Promotes patient comfort.	The patient who is being ambulated may require larger minute ventilation than usual to match increased carbon dioxide production and oxygen consumption during activity.
10. Reconnect patient to ventilator. Reactivate ventilator alarms. Ensure that call bell is within patient reach.	Safety precautions. Ensures that the nurse will be alerted to actual or potential life-threatening problems.	
11. Record in patient record.		

Expected Outcomes

- Maintenance of adequate oxygenation and ventilation
- Resolution of acute respiratory distress

Unexpected Outcomes

- Hemodynamic instability secondary to dynamic hyperinflation
- Pulmonary barotrauma (e.g., pneumothorax)
- Inability to restore adequate ventilation and oxygenation with bagging
- Inadvertent extubation during bagging
- Equipment failure and inability to bag

Patient Monitoring and Care

Steps	Rationale	Reportable Conditions
		These conditions should be reported if they persist despite nursing interventions.
1. Evaluate trends or sudden changes in lung compliance or airways resistance.	Improvement or deterioration in lung function can be approximated by evaluation of patient's response to bagging.	• Difficulty bagging (stiff) • No observable chest movement • Agitation • Diaphoresis • Hypertension or hypotension • Tachycardia or bradycardia
2. Observe for signs and symptoms of patent upper and lower airways, including comfortable appearance; stable or improved level of consciousness; synchrony of patient and ventilator; symmetrical breath sounds; stable heart rate, rhythm, and blood pressure; and absence of rhonchi, wheezes, and dyspnea.	Proper technique results in a comfortable, synchronous breathing pattern.	• Dyssynchronous breathing
3. Observe the patient during bagging. The patient should look comfortable. The chest should rise and fall evenly with bagging deflations and inflations.	Proper technique results in a comfortable, synchronous breathing pattern.	• Dyssynchronous breathing
4. Monitor SaO_2 for maintenance of adequate oxygenation during bagging. End-tidal carbon dioxide tension ($PETCO_2$) may be used to monitor adequacy of ventilation (e.g., carbon dioxide with acceptable limits).	If adequate oxygen is being delivered and ventilation is adequate, SaO_2 and $PETCO_2$ should be unchanged or improve with bagging.	• Decrease in SaO_2 greater than 10% • Increase of $PETCO_2$ greater than 10%

Documentation

Documentation should include the following:

- Patient and family education
- Reason for bagging (e.g., to suction during transport)
- Frequency

- Response of the procedure
- Unexpected outcomes
- Nursing interventions

References

1. Chulay, M. (1997). Airway and ventilatory management. In: Chulay, M., Guzetta, C., and Dossey, B., editors. *AACN Handbook of Critical Care Nursing.* Stamford, CT: Appleton & Lange, 119-53.
2. Grap, M.J., et al. (1996). Endotracheal suctioning: Ventilator vs manual delivery of hyperoxygenation breaths. *Am J Crit Care,* 5, 192-7.
3. Henneman, E., Ellstrom, K., and St. John, R. (1999). Airway management. In: *AACN Protocols for Practice: Care of the Mechanically Ventilated Patient Series.* Aliso Viejo, CA: American Association of Critical-Care Nurses.
4. Pepe, P.E., and Marini, J.J. (1982). Occult positive end-expiratory pressure in mechanically ventilated patients with airflow obstruction. *Am Rev Respir Dis,* 126, 166-70.
5. Wilmoth, D.F., and Carpenter, R.M. (1996). Preventing complications of mechanical ventilation: Permissive hypercapnia. *AACN Clin Issues,* 7, 473-81.

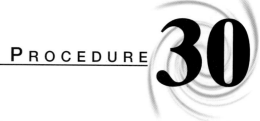
PROCEDURE **30**

Indices of Oxygenation

PURPOSE: Alveolar-arterial oxygen difference (A-aDo$_2$), arterial partial pressure of oxygen-to-fraction of inspired oxygen (Pao$_2$:Fio$_2$) ratio (P:F ratio), and arterial partial pressure of oxygen-to-alveolar partial pressure of oxygen (Pao$_2$:Pao$_2$) ratio (a:A ratio) are calculated to identify shunt as the primary mechanism of hypoxemia, to assess trends in oxygenation, and to determine effectiveness and titration of therapies.

Suzanne M. Burns

PREREQUISITE NURSING KNOWLEDGE

- Pao$_2$ is primarily determined by the concentration of inspired oxygen and the amount of carbon dioxide in the alveolus.
- In normal lungs, alveolar oxygen diffuses rapidly into the pulmonary capillaries, and arterial oxygenation approximates that of the alveolus. The normal A-aDo$_2$ in a patient breathing 21% oxygen is 10 to 30 mm Hg (i.e., Pao$_2$ [100]–Pao$_2$ [80]). When 100% oxygen is inspired, the normal gradient is 50 to 70 mm Hg.
- Trends in alveolar-arterial (A-a) gradient are evaluated most accurately when the Pao$_2$ and Pao$_2$ are measured after inspiration of 100% oxygen for 15 minutes.
- Other clinical indices of oxygenation that are commonly used include a:A ratio and P:F ratio. These indices all are relatively easy to use and are helpful to estimate trends in shunt. The advantage of the a:A ratio and P:F ratio is that a more constant value, despite changes in Fio$_2$, can be calculated. A normal a:A ratio is 0.8 to 1. The smaller the number, the higher the degree of shunt. The normal value for P:F ratio is greater than 300. A smaller P:F ratio reflects a higher degree of shunt. A P:F ratio of 200 to 300 is used to define acute lung injury, whereas a P:F ratio of less than 200 is associated with acute respiratory distress syndrome.
- In patients with shunt (perfusion to unventilated lung units), venous blood is shunted past the closed alveoli without becoming oxygenated. Even though Pao$_2$ may be normal because of an increase in Fio$_2$, a shunt exists. The A-a gradient increases. A-a gradient is considered a useful,

albeit crude, clinical estimate of shunt. It is helpful to trend changes in oxygenation status and the effect of therapies and other interventions.
- Concepts related to shunt and the refractory nature of shunt to increasing Fio$_2$ are inherent in all the indices (i.e., shunt is not responsive to oxygen).
- The gold standard for quantifying shunt is calculation of shunted blood flow-to-total blood flow ratio (Qs:Qt). Calculation of Qs:Qt requires analysis of a mixed venous sample (from a pulmonary artery catheter or venous oxygen saturation [Svo$_2$] catheter); A-a gradient, Pao$_2$:Fio$_2$, and Pao$_2$:Pao$_2$ do not.
- Accurate interpretation of arterial and mixed venous blood gas analysis is necessary.

EQUIPMENT

- Arterial blood gas (ABG) results (after 15 minutes of 100% Fio$_2$) for calculation of A-aDo$_2$. If other indices are used (i.e., a:A ratio, P:F ratio), record the Fio$_2$ level when the ABG is drawn.
- Calculator

PATIENT AND FAMILY EDUCATION

- Inform the patient and family about the patient's oxygenation status and the rationale and implications for changes in therapy. If the patient or a family member requests specific information about A-a oxygen differences, explain the general relationship between A-aDo$_2$ and hypoxemia.

➤➤*Rationale:* Most patients and families are less concerned with the diagnostic and therapeutic details and more concerned with how the patient is progressing overall.

PATIENT ASSESSMENT AND PREPARATION

Patient Assessment

- Assess for signs and symptoms of inadequate oxygenation.
  - ❖ Decreasing arterial oxygen tension
  - ❖ Tachypnea
  - ❖ Dyspnea
  - ❖ Central cyanosis
  - ❖ Restlessness
  - ❖ Confusion
  - ❖ Agitation
  - ❖ Tachycardia
  - ❖ Bradycardia
  - ❖ Dysrhythmias
  - ❖ Intercostal and suprasternal retractions
  - ❖ Increasing or decreasing arterial blood pressure
  - ❖ Adventitious breath sounds
  - ❖ Decreasing urine output
  - ❖ Metabolic acidosis
  - ➤➤*Rationale:* Clinical findings may indicate problems with oxygenation.
- Determine arterial oxygen tension or saturation.
  ➤➤*Rationale:* Hypoxemia is confirmed by a decreasing Pao_2 or Sao_2, or an absolute Pao_2 of less than 60 mm Hg or an absolute Sao_2 of less than 90% confirms oxygenation problems.
- Determine trend of indices and therapies. ➤➤*Rationale:* Improvement or deterioration can be quantified by monitoring indices over time.

Procedure for Oxygenation Indices

Steps	Rationale	Special Considerations
Calculation of Oxygenation Indices *When calculating A-aDo$_2$, adjust the FIO$_2$ to 1.0 for 15 minutes before drawing the ABG. For calculation of the a:A ratio and P:F ratio, ABGs may be drawn without adjustment to the FIO$_2$.*		
1. Use the equation in Table 30-1 for calculation of A-aDo$_2$.		
2. Use the equation in Table 30-2 for calculation of a:A ratio.		
3. Use the equation in Table 30-3 for calculation of P:F ratio.		
4. Document indices in patient record with the following data: A. ABG results. B. Ventilator parameters, including FIO$_2$ at the time ABG were drawn. C. Position of patient at the time the blood was drawn. D. Date and time ABG were drawn. E. Changes in therapy, if any, based on indices.	All the data viewed together are needed for decision making regarding changes in therapy. Positioning (e.g., placing patient in prone position) may be used as a means to improve shunt.	

TABLE 30-1	Calculation of A-aDo$_2$

$$P_{AO_2} = F_{IO_2}(P_{Bar} - PH_2O) - \frac{PaCO_2}{RQ}$$
$$P_{AO_2} - Pao_2 = A\text{-}aDo_2$$

P_{Bar}, barometric pressure (713 mm Hg); PH_2O, pressure of water (vapor) (47 mm Hg); RQ, respiratory quotient (0.8).

TABLE 30-2	Equation for Calculation of Arterial:Alveolar Ratio

Pao$_2$ (obtained from arterial blood gas) ÷ P$_{AO_2}$ (see Table 30-1)

TABLE 30-3	Equation for Calculation of Pao$_2$:Fio$_2$ (P:F) Ratio

Pao$_2$ (obtained from arterial blood gas) ÷ FIO$_2$ (expressed as a decimal)

Expected Outcomes

- Maintenance of adequate oxygenation (i.e., SaO_2, PaO_2)
- Timely decrease in FIO_2 and titration of positive end-expiratory pressure

Unexpected Outcomes

- Hemodynamic instability
- Pulmonary barotrauma
- Oxygen toxicity

Patient Monitoring and Care

Steps	Rationale	Reportable Conditions
		These conditions should be reported if they persist despite nursing interventions.
1. Observe trends in oxygenation indices.	Oxygenation indices reflect the approximate degree of shunting as a mechanism of hypoxemia. Changes may reflect either worsening of disease process or ineffective therapy or an improving disease process or effective therapy.	• Significant change in indices
2. Observe for increasing PaO_2 or SaO_2. When PaO_2 is greater than 60 mm Hg or SaO_2 is greater than 90% on an FIO_2 of less than 0.40, monitoring of the indices is rarely helpful.	Shunting, as a mechanism of hypoxemia, requires high oxygen concentrations to maintain marginal oxygenation. Shunting is not contributing significantly to hypoxemia if the patient has an adequate arterial oxygen tension on an FIO_2 of less than 0.40.	• Acceptable PaO_2 or SaO_2 with FIO_2 less than 0.40

Documentation

Documentation should include the following:

- Patient and family education
- Oxygenation index value, ABG results, FIO_2, and ventilator parameters at time blood was drawn
- Time, date, and position of patient (e.g., supine or left lateral)
- Changes in therapy based on the $A\text{-}aDO_2$
- Patient response to interventions
- Unexpected outcomes
- Nursing interventions

Additional Readings

Ahrens, T.S., and Powers, C.C. (1998). Pulmonary clinical physiology. In: Kinney, M.R., et al., editors. *AACN's Clinical Reference for Critical Care Nursing.* 4th ed. St. Louis: Mosby, 496-503.

Ahrens, T.S., and Rutherford, K.A. (1993). *Essentials of Oxygenation.* Boston, Jones & Bartlett.

Dantzker, D.R. (1995). Pulmonary gas exchange. In: Dantzker, D.R., MacIntyre, N.R., and Bakow, E.D., editors. *Comprehensive Respiratory Care.* Philadelphia: W.B. Saunders, pp 98-118.

West, J.B. (1999). *Respiratory Physiology: The Essentials.* 6th ed. Baltimore: Williams & Wilkins.

West, J.B. (2000). *Pulmonary Physiology and Pathophysiology: An Integrated Case-Based Approach.* Baltimore, Williams & Wilkins.

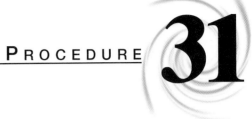

PROCEDURE **31**

Shunt Calculation

P U R P O S E : Shunt calculation is performed to differentiate shunting from other mechanisms of hypoxemia, to quantify the shunt, to assess trends in progression or improvement of shunt, and to determine the effectiveness and duration of therapy.

Suzanne M. Burns

PREREQUISITE NURSING KNOWLEDGE

- *Right-to-left intrapulmonary shunting* (variously called *physiologic shunting, wasted blood flow,* and *venous admixture*) is the pathologic phenomenon whereby venous blood is shunted past the alveoli without taking up oxygen. This blood then returns to the left side of the heart as venous blood with a low oxygen tension.
- Right-to-left intrapulmonary shunting is expressed as a fraction or percentage of shunted blood flow to total blood flow (Q_S/Q_T). The normal physiologic shunt is less than 5% and is caused by venous blood from the bronchial and coronary veins returning to the left side of the heart as desaturated blood.
- Shunting of blood past the alveoli means that a certain percentage of the blood flows through an area of lung that receives no ventilation. Examples of conditions in which shunt is present include acute respiratory distress syndrome, atelectasis, pneumonia, and pulmonary edema with fluid-filled alveoli.
- As the percentage of the shunted cardiac output increases, the mixture of venous shunted blood with arterial blood increases with a concomitant decrease in the arterial oxygen tension. The extent of the hypoxemia depends on the amount of the lung parenchyma that is not ventilated.
- The hallmark of right-to-left intrapulmonary shunting is persistent hypoxemia despite high concentrations of inspired oxygen (called *refractory* hypoxemia).

- For evaluation of shunt, heparinized arterial and mixed venous blood samples are analyzed by cooximeter to determine saturation. Use of the calculated saturation obtained in conjunction with blood gas analysis is not as accurate.

EQUIPMENT

- Calculator
- Q_S/Q_T equation
- Mixed venous and arterial blood gases and saturations
- Pulmonary artery catheter, for drawing mixed venous blood samples, or venous oxygen saturation (S_{vO_2}) catheter. If an S_{vO_2} catheter is used, the mixed venous saturation recorded on the monitor can be used for the calculation (as long as in vitro and in vivo calibrations have been done according to manufacturer's recommendations).

PATIENT AND FAMILY EDUCATION

- Keep the patient and family informed about the patient's oxygenation status. Inform them of changes in therapy and how to interpret the changes. If the patient or a family member requests specific information about intrapulmonary shunting, explain the general relationship between Q_S/Q_T and hypoxemia. ➤➤*Rationale:* Most patients and families are less concerned with the diagnostic and therapeutic details and more concerned with how the patient is progressing overall or in relation to a specific physiologic function.

PATIENT ASSESSMENT AND PREPARATION

Patient Assessment

- Signs and symptoms of inadequate oxygenation include the following.
  - ❖ Decreasing arterial oxygen tension and saturation
  - ❖ Tachypnea
  - ❖ Dyspnea
  - ❖ Central cyanosis
  - ❖ Restlessness
  - ❖ Confusion
  - ❖ Agitation
  - ❖ Tachycardia
  - ❖ Bradycardia
  - ❖ Dysrhythmias
  - ❖ Intercostal and suprasternal retractions
  - ❖ Increasing or decreasing arterial blood pressure
  - ❖ Adventitious breath sounds
  - ❖ Decreasing urine output

- ❖ End-organe failure or metabolic acidosis or both
- ➤*Rationale:* Calculation of Qs/Qt is indicated to help differentiate between the mechanisms of hypoxemia.

Patient Preparation

- Determine arterial oxygen tension or saturation.
  ➤*Rationale:* Hypoxemia is confirmed by a decreasing arterial partial pressure of oxygen (Pao_2), decreasing arterial oxygen saturation (Sao_2), an absolute Pao_2 of less than 60 mm Hg, or an absolute Sao_2 of less than 90%. A low Pao_2 and low Sao_2 with increasing supplemental oxygen confirm hypoxemia caused by right-to-left intrapulmonary shunting.
- Determine Qs/Qt trends with therapies and interventions.
  ➤*Rationale:* Calculation of Qs/Qt is indicated to help differentiate mechanisms of hypoxemia and to provide appropriate interventions. The effect of therapies such as positive end-expiratory pressure (PEEP), selected ventilator modes (e.g., pressure release ventilation, inverse ratio), and prone positioning on shunting and oxygenation can be quantified.

Procedure for Shunt Calculation

Steps	Rationale	Special Considerations
1. Draw heparinized blood sample slowly from distal port of the pulmonary artery catheter or obtain the Svo_2 from the Svo_2 monitor. Be sure to discard the first 3 ml because it will contain flush solution.	If sample is drawn rapidly, it is possible to aspirate arterialized blood from the capillary bed; calculation of Qs/Qt would be inaccurate. The calculation of Qs/Qt has been used as the gold standard for clinical shunt measurement.[1-3]	
2. Draw arterial blood sample simultaneously or within a few minutes of drawing mixed venous sample.	Ensures accuracy.	
3. Send the samples to be analyzed. Analysis of saturation is best done by cooximeter.	Use of calculated saturation obtained via blood gas analysis is less accurate.	
4. Obtain Qs/Qt by using the equation in Table 31-1.		
5. Document in patient record.		

TABLE 31-1 Q_S/Q_T Calculation

$$Q_S/Q_T = \frac{C\bar{c}co_2 - Cao_2}{C\bar{c}co_2 - C\bar{v}o_2}$$

Where Q_S = intrapulmonary shunted blood flow
Q_T = total lung blood flow
$C\bar{c}co_2$ = end capillary O_2
$C\bar{c}co_2$ = (Hgb × 1.34* × Sat[†] [1.0]) + (Pao_2[‡] × 0.003)
Cao_2 = arterial oxygen content in ml/100 ml of blood
(Hgb × 1.34* × Sao_2) + (Pao_2 × 0.003)
$C\bar{v}o_2$ = mixed venous oxygen content in ml/100 ml of blood
(Hgb × 1.34* × $S\bar{v}o_2$) + ($P\bar{v}o_2$ × 0.003)

For ease of calculation, the portion of the equation that determines the O_2 dissolved in plasma may be eliminated because the contribution of the dissolved portion of O_2 to O_2 content is extremely small. For continuity purposes, this should be determined by unit policy.
*Depending on institutional policy, standards between 1.34 and 1.39 are used.
[†]In this equation, saturation is assumed to be 100% as in an "ideal" capillary with no shunt.
[‡]$Pao_2 = Fio_2 (713) - \frac{Paco_2}{0.8}$ (see Table 30-1 for calculation of Pao_2).

Expected Outcomes

- Maintenance of adequate Pao_2
- Timely titration of PEEP and fraction of inspired oxygen (Fio_2) and the application of other therapies, such as prone positioning, as appropriate

Unexpected Outcomes

- Severe hypoxemia
- Hemodynamic instability

Patient Monitoring and Care

Steps	Rationale	Reportable Conditions
		These conditions should be reported if they persist despite nursing interventions.
1. Observe trend in Q_S/Q_T.	An increasing shunt indicates worsening of the disease process or ineffective therapy. A decreasing shunt indicates improving disease process or effective therapy. The greater the blood flow past unoxygenated alveoli, the greater the shunt and the greater the hypoxemia.	• A change in Q_S/Q_T of greater than 5%
2. Observe for increasing Pao_2 or Sao_2 in conjunction with Fio_2 and PEEP levels.	Shunt, as a mechanism of hypoxemia, requires high oxygen concentrations to maintain marginal oxygenation. Shunting is not contributing significantly to hypoxemia if the patient has adequate arterial oxygen tension on an Fio_2 of less than or equal to 0.40. When Pao_2 is greater than 60 mm Hg or Sao_2 is greater than 90% on an Fio_2 of less than or equal to 0.45, monitoring of Q_S/Q_T is no longer necessary.	• Pao_2 less than 60 mm Hg

• Sao_2 less than 90% |

Documentation

Documentation should include the following:

- Patient and family education
- Q_S/Q_T percent
- Date and time Q_S/Q_T was performed
- Arterial and mixed venous blood gas results calculated
- Time, date, position of patient (e.g., supine or left lateral)
- Fio_2 and ventilator parameters at the time blood gases were drawn
- Changes in therapy based on the calculated Q_S/Q_T
- Patient response to interventions
- Unexpected outcomes
- Nursing interventions

References

1. Ahrens, T.S., and Powers, C.C. (1998). Pulmonary clinical physiology. In: Kinney, M.R., et al., editors. *AACN's Clinical Reference for Critical Care Nursing.* 4th ed. St. Louis: Mosby-Year Book, 491-516.
2. Ahrens, T.S., and Rutherford, K.A. (1993). *Essentials of Oxygenation.* Boston: Jones & Bartlett Publishers.
3. West, J.B. (2004). *Respiratory Physiology: The Essentials.* 7th ed. Baltimore: Williams & Wilkins.

Additional Reading

West, J.B. (2000). *Pulmonary Physiology and Pathophysiology: An Integrated Case-Based Approach.* Baltimore: Williams & Wilkins.

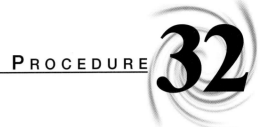
PROCEDURE **32**

Ventilatory Management—Volume and Pressure Modes

PURPOSE: Initiation and maintenance of positive-pressure ventilation (PPV) maintains or improves oxygenation, maintains or improves ventilation, and provides respiratory muscle rest.

Suzanne M. Burns

PREREQUISITE NURSING KNOWLEDGE

- Indications for the initiation of mechanical ventilation include the following:
  - Apnea (e.g., neuromuscular or cardiopulmonary collapse)
  - Acute ventilatory failure, which is generally defined as a pH of less than or equal to 7.25 with an arterial partial pressure of carbon dioxide ($PaCO_2$) greater than or equal to 50 mm Hg
  - Impending ventilatory failure
  - Severe hypoxemia. An arterial partial pressure of oxygen (PaO_2) of less than or equal to 50 mm Hg on room air indicates a critical level of oxygen in the blood. Although oxygen delivery devices may be employed before intubation, the refractory nature of shunt (perfusion without ventilation) may require that positive pressure be applied to reexpand closed alveoli. Restoration of functional residual capacity (FRC) (lung volume that remains at the end of a passive exhalation) is the goal.
  - Respiratory muscle fatigue. The muscles of respiration can become fatigued if they are made to contract repetitively at high workloads. Fatigue occurs when muscles' energy stores become depleted. Weakness, hypermetabolic states, and chronic lung disease are examples of conditions in which patients are especially prone to fatigue. When fatigue occurs, the muscles no longer contract optimally, hypercarbia results,[4,9] and 12 to 24 hours of rest typically are required to rest the muscles. Respiratory muscle rest requires that the

workload of the muscles (or muscle *loading*) be offset so that mitochondrial energy stores can be repleted.[4,9] In general, when hypercarbia is present, mechanical ventilation is necessary to relieve the work of breathing.[43] Muscle *unloading* is accomplished differently, depending on whether the mode is a volume or pressure mode.[7,8,25,30]

- Ventilators are categorized as either negative or positive pressure. Although negative-pressure ventilation (e.g., the iron lung) was used extensively in the 1940s, introduction of the cuffed endotracheal tube resulted in the dominance of positive-pressure ventilation (PPV) in clinical practice during the second half of the 20th century. Although there continues to be sporadic interest in negative-pressure ventilation, the cumbersome nature of the ventilators and the lack of airway protection associated with this form of ventilation preclude a serious resurgence of negative-pressure ventilation.

- Positive-pressure ventilators are categorized into volume and pressure ventilators.
  - With *volume ventilation,* a predetermined tidal volume (Vt) is delivered with each breath regardless of resistance and compliance. Vt is stable from breath to breath, but airway pressure may vary. To rest the respiratory muscles with volume ventilation, the ventilator rate must be increased until spontaneous respiratory effort ceases. When spontaneous effort is present, such as when initiating an assist control (AC) breath, respiratory muscle work continues throughout the breath.[30]
  - With *pressure ventilation,* the clinician selects the desired pressure level, and the Vt is determined by the selected pressure level, resistance, and compliance.

This is an important characteristic to note when caring for an unstable patient on a pressure mode of ventilation. Careful attention to Vt is necessary to prevent inadvertent hyperventilation or hypoventilation. To ensure respiratory muscle rest on pressure-support ventilation (PSV), workload must be offset with the appropriate adjustment of the pressure-support (PS) level. To accomplish this, the PS level is increased to lower the spontaneous respiratory rate to less than or equal to 20/min and to attain a Vt of 8 to 12 mm/kg.[7,8,25]

- For a description of volume and pressure ventilation modes, see Table 32-1.

- Volume ventilation traditionally has been the most popular form of PPV, largely because Vt and minute ventilation (MV) are ensured; this is an essential goal in the acutely ill patient. In contrast, with pressure ventilation, Vt can change drastically with changes in compliance or resistance. Initially, pressure ventilation was described for use only in stable weaning patients; however, pressure ventilation became extremely popular in the 1990s for use in acutely ill patients as well. This change has occurred for several reasons.

  ❖ A decelerating flow pattern is associated with pressure ventilation. Pressure ventilation provides for an augmented inspiration (pressure is maintained throughout inspiration). The flow pattern (speed of the gas) is described as decelerating. That is, gas flow delivery is high at the beginning of the breath and tapers off toward the end of the breath. This is in contrast to volume ventilation, in which the flow rate is typically the same at the beginning of the breath as at the end of the breath. The decelerating flow pattern associated with pressure ventilation is thought to provide better gas distribution and more efficient ventilation.[8,25]

  ❖ The concept of volu-pressure trauma has evolved. Investigators have shown that large volumes, traditionally used to ventilate the noncompliant lung (e.g., in acute respiratory distress syndrome [ARDS]), result in high plateau pressures and lung injury. Plateau pressures of greater than or equal to 30 cm H_2O for greater than 48 to 72 hours have been associated with acute lung injury. Volu-pressure trauma results in the loss of alveolar integrity (i.e., alveolar fractures) and movement of fluids and proteins into the alveolar space (sometimes called *non-ARDS*).[13,18,35,45]

  ❖ The ARDS Network showed in a randomized controlled trial that smaller volumes (6 ml/kg) compared with more "traditional" volumes (i.e., 12 ml/kg) resulted in a lower mortality.[42] As a result, current recommendations are to limit volumes (and lower pressures) in patients with stiff lungs. With pressure ventilation, pressure is limited by definition, ensuring this clinical goal. Until additional evidence emerges on the efficacy of controlling pressures versus volumes in ARDS, a goal should be to ensure a Vt in the 6 ml/kg range.

  ❖ Increasingly sophisticated ventilator technology has developed with volume-assured pressure modes of ventilation. Ventilator manufacturers have responded rapidly to the request of clinicians that pressure modes of ventilation be designed in such a way that volume be guaranteed on a breath-to-breath basis. The potential value of such modes is obvious. The more desirable decelerating flow pattern may be provided and plateau pressures controlled, while ensuring Vt and MV.

  ❖ Additional modes of ventilation have been promoted for use in patients with ARDS, including high-frequency oscillation, pressure-release ventilation, and other ventilator specific modes such as biphasic ventilation.[11,27,28,41] Although some data exist that suggest the modes may be beneficial in ARDS patients, to date no change in mortality has been noted, although trends in variables of interest do appear positive.[11]

TABLE 32-1	**Common Modes of Mechanical Ventilation**

Volume Modes

Control Ventilation (CV) or Controlled Mandatory Ventilation (CMV)
Description: With this mode, the ventilator provides all of the patient's minute ventilation. The clinician sets the rate, Vt, inspiratory time, and PEEP. Generally, this term is used to describe situations in which the patient is chemically relaxed or is paralyzed from a spinal cord or neuromuscular disease and is unable to initiate spontaneous breaths. The ventilator mode setting may be set on CMV, assist/control (A/C), or synchronized intermittent mandatory ventilation (SIMV) because all these options provide volume breaths at the clinician-selected rate.

Assist/Control (A/C) or Assisted Mandatory Ventilation (AMV)
Description: This option requires that a rate, Vt, inspiratory time, and PEEP be set for the patient. The ventilator sensitivity also is set, and when the patient initiates a spontaneous breath, a full-volume breath is delivered.

Intermittent Mandatory Ventilation (IMV) and Synchronized Intermittent Mandatory Ventilation (SIMV)
Description: This mode requires that rate, Vt, inspiratory time, sensitivity, and PEEP are set by the clinician. In between "mandatory breaths," patients can spontaneously breathe at their own rates and Vt. With SIMV, the ventilator synchronizes the mandatory breaths with the patient's own inspirations.

Pressure Modes

Pressure Support Ventilation (PSV)
Description: This mode provides an augmented inspiration to a spontaneously breathing patient. With PS, the clinician selects an inspiratory pressure level, PEEP, and sensitivity. When the patient initiates a breath, a high flow of gas is delivered to the preselected pressure level, and pressure is maintained throughout inspiration. The patient determines the parameters of Vt, rate, and inspiratory time.

Pressure-Controlled/Inverse Ratio Ventilation (PC/IRV)
Description: This mode combines pressure-limited ventilation with an inverse ratio of inspiration to expiration. The clinician selects the pressure level, rate, inspiratory time (1:1, 2:1, 3:1, 4:1), and PEEP level. With prolonged inspiratory times, auto-PEEP may result. The auto-PEEP may be a desirable outcome of the inverse ratios. Some clinicians use PC without IRV. Conventional inspiratory times are used, and rate, pressure level, and PEEP are selected.

Positive End-Expiratory Pressure (PEEP) and Continuous Positive Airway Pressure (CPAP)
Description: This ventilatory option creates positive pressure at end exhalation. PEEP restores FRC. The term *PEEP* is used when end-expiratory pressure is provided during ventilator positive pressure breaths.

Continuous Positive Airway Pressure (CPAP)
Description: Similar to PEEP, CPAP restores FRC. This pressure is continuous during spontaneous breathing; no positive-pressure breaths are present.

- Complications of PPV include hemodynamic changes, pulmonary barotrauma, and volu-pressure trauma.
  - ❖ The extent of hemodynamic changes depends on the level of positive pressure applied, the duration of positive pressure during different phases of the breathing cycle, the amount of pressure transmitted to the vascular structures, the patient's intravascular volume, and the adequacy of hemodynamic compensatory mechanisms. PPV can reduce venous return, shift the intraventricular septum to the left, and increase right ventricular afterload as a result of increased pulmonary vascular resistance. The hemodynamic effects of PPV may be prevented or corrected by optimizing filling pressures to accommodate the PPV-induced changes in intrathoracic pressures; by minimizing the peak pressure, plateau pressure, and positive end-expiratory pressure (PEEP); and by optimizing the inspiratory-to-expiratory (I:E) ratio.
  - ❖ Pulmonary barotrauma is damage to the lung from extrapulmonary air that may result from changes in intrathoracic pressures during PPV. Barotrauma is manifested by pneumothorax, pneumomediastinum, pneumopericardium, pneumoperitoneum, or subcutaneous emphysema. The risk of barotrauma in a patient receiving PPV is increased with preexisting lung lesions (e.g., localized infections, blebs), high inflation pressure (i.e., large Vt, PEEP, main stem bronchus intubation, patient-ventilator asynchrony), and invasive thoracic procedures (e.g., subclavian catheter insertion, bronchoscopy, thoracentesis). Barotrauma from PPV may be prevented by controlling peak and plateau pressures, optimizing PEEP, preventing auto-PEEP, ensuring patient-ventilator synchrony, and ensuring proper artificial airway position.

EQUIPMENT

- Endotracheal tube (see Procedures 2 and 3) or tracheostomy
- Electrocardiogram and pulse oximetry
- Manual self-inflating resuscitation bag (with PEEP valve if PEEP level is greater than 5 cm H_2O)
- Appropriately sized resuscitation facemask
- Ventilator
- Suction equipment

Additional equipment to have available (depending on patient need) includes the following:
- End-tidal carbon dioxide monitor

PATIENT AND FAMILY EDUCATION

- Explain the procedure to the patient and family and why PPV is being initiated. ➔*Rationale:* Communication and explanations for therapy are cited as important needs of patients.
- Discuss the potential sensations the patient will experience, such as relief of dyspnea, lung inflations, noise of ventilator operation, and alarm sounds. ➔*Rationale:* Knowledge of anticipated sensory experiences reduces anxiety and distress.
- Encourage the patient to relax. ➔*Rationale:* This encouragement promotes general relaxation, oxygenation, and ventilation.
- Explain that the patient will be unable to speak. Establish a method of communication in conjunction with the patient and family before initiating mechanical ventilation, if necessary. ➔*Rationale:* Ensuring the patient's ability to communicate is important to alleviate anxiety.
- Teach the family how to perform desired and appropriate activities of direct patient care, such as pharyngeal suction with the tonsil-tip suction device, range-of-motion exercises, and reconnection to ventilator if inadvertent disconnection occurs. Demonstrate how to use call bell. ➔*Rationale:* Family members have identified the need and desire to help in the patient's care.
- Provide the patient and family with information on the critical nature of the patient's dependence on PPV. ➔*Rationale:* Knowing the prognosis, probable outcome, or chance for recovery is cited as an important need of patients and families.
- Offer the opportunity for the patient and family to ask questions about PPV. ➔*Rationale:* Asking questions and having questions answered honestly are cited consistently as the most important need of patients and families.

PATIENT ASSESSMENT AND PREPARATION

Patient Assessment

- Assess for the following signs and symptoms of acute ventilatory failure and fatigue.
  - ❖ Rising arterial carbon dioxide tension
  - ❖ Chest-abdominal dyssynchrony
  - ❖ Shallow or irregular respirations
  - ❖ Tachypnea, bradypnea, or dyspnea
  - ❖ Decreased mental status
  - ❖ Restlessness, confusion, or lethargy
  - ❖ Increasing or decreasing arterial blood pressure
  - ❖ Tachycardia
  - ❖ Atrial or ventricular dysrhythmias
  ➔*Rationale:* Ventilatory failure indicates the need for initiation of PPV. While PPV is being considered and assembled, support ventilation via a manual self-inflating resuscitation bag, if necessary.
- Determine arterial carbon dioxide tension and pH. ➔*Rationale:* Acute ventilatory failure is confirmed by an uncompensated respiratory acidosis. Ventilatory failure is an indication for PPV.
- Assess for the following signs and symptoms of inadequate oxygenation.
  - ❖ Decreasing arterial oxygen tension
  - ❖ Tachypnea
  - ❖ Dyspnea
  - ❖ Central cyanosis

❖ Restlessness
❖ Confusion
❖ Agitation
❖ Tachycardia
❖ Bradycardia
❖ Dysrhythmias
❖ Intercostal and suprasternal retractions
❖ Increasing or decreasing arterial blood pressure
❖ Adventitious breath sounds
❖ Decreasing urine output
❖ Metabolic acidosis

➼***Rationale:*** Hypoxemia may indicate the need for PPV. While PPV is being considered and assembled, provide 100% oxygen via manual resuscitation bag and mask or via an oxygen delivery device, such as a nonrebreather mask.

• Determine PaO_2 or arterial oxygen saturation (SaO_2).
➼***Rationale:*** Hypoxemia is confirmed by PaO_2 of less than 60 mm Hg or SaO_2 of less than 90% on supplemental oxygen. Hypoxemia may indicate the need for PPV.

• Signs and symptoms of inadequate breathing pattern include the following.
❖ Dyspnea
❖ Chest-abdominal dyssynchrony
❖ Rapid-shallow breathing pattern
❖ Irregular respirations
❖ Intercostal or suprasternal retractions

➼***Rationale:*** Respiratory distress is an indication for PPV. A comfortable breathing pattern is a goal of PPV. An inadequate breathing pattern can be corrected by adjusting the ventilator parameters or by finding and treating the underlying acute cause (e.g., malpositioned endotracheal tube, leak in the endotracheal tube cuff, improper assembly of ventilator components).

• Signs of atelectasis include the following.
❖ Localized changes in auscultation (decreased or bronchial breath sounds)
❖ Localized dullness to percussion
❖ Increased breathing effort
❖ Tracheal deviation toward the side of abnormal findings
❖ Increased peak and plateau pressures
❖ Decreased compliance
❖ Decreased PaO_2 or SaO_2 (with constant ventilator parameters)
❖ Localized consolidation ("white out," opacity) on chest radiograph

➼***Rationale:*** Early detection of atelectasis indicates the need for altering interventions to promote resolution (e.g., hyperinflation techniques, PEEP adjustments).

• Signs and symptoms of pulmonary barotrauma (i.e., pneumothorax) include the following.
❖ Acute, increasing, or severe dyspnea
❖ Restlessness
❖ Agitation
❖ Localized changes in auscultation (decreased or absent breath sounds)
❖ Localized hyperresonance or tympany to percussion
❖ Increased breathing effort

❖ Tracheal deviation away from the side of abnormal findings
❖ Increased peak and plateau pressures
❖ Decreased compliance
❖ Decreased PaO_2 or SaO_2
❖ Subcutaneous emphysema
❖ Localized increased lucency with absent lung markings on chest radiograph

➼***Rationale:*** Early detection of pneumothorax is essential to minimize progression and the adverse effects on the patient. Tension pneumothorax requires immediate emergency decompression with a large-bore needle (i.e., 14-gauge) into the second intercostal space, midclavicular line on the affected side, or immediate chest tube placement (see Procedure 18).

• Signs of cardiovascular depression (particularly after an increase in Vt, PEEP, or continuous positive airway pressure [CPAP], or with hyperinflation) include the following.
❖ Acute or gradual decrease in arterial blood pressure
❖ Tachycardia, bradycardia, or dysrhythmias
❖ Weak peripheral pulses, pulsus paradoxus, or decreased pulse pressure
❖ Acute or gradual increase in pulmonary capillary wedge pressure
❖ Decreased mixed venous oxygen tension

➼***Rationale:*** PPV can cause decreased venous return and afterload because of the increase in intrathoracic pressure. This mechanism often is manifested immediately after initiation of mechanical ventilation and with large Vt, increases in PEEP or CPAP levels, and manual hyperinflation techniques. Cardiovascular depression associated with manual or periodic ventilator hyperinflation is immediately reversible with cessation of hyperinflation. Decreases in blood pressure with PPV also may be seen with hypovolemia.

• Signs and symptoms of inadvertent extubation include the following.
❖ Vocalization
❖ Activated low-pressure ventilator alarm
❖ Decreased or absent breath sounds
❖ Gastric distention
❖ Signs and symptoms of inadequate ventilation, oxygenation, and breathing pattern

➼***Rationale:*** Inadvertent extubation is sometimes obvious (e.g., the endotracheal tube is in the patient's hand). Often the tip of the endotracheal tube is in the hypopharynx or in the esophagus, however, and inadvertent extubation is not immediately apparent. Reintubation may be required, although some patients may not require reintubation. If reintubation is necessary, ventilation and oxygenation are assisted with a self-inflating manual resuscitation bag and facemask.

• Signs and symptoms of a malpositioned endotracheal tube include the following.
❖ Dyspnea
❖ Restlessness or agitation
❖ Unilateral decreased or absent breath sounds

❖ Unilateral dullness to percussion
❖ Increased breathing effort
❖ Asymmetric chest expansion
❖ Increased peak inspiratory pressure (PIP)
❖ Radiographic evidence of malposition
➨*Rationale:* Early detection and correction of a malpositioned endotracheal tube can prevent inadvertent extubation, atelectasis, barotrauma, and problems with gas exchange.
• Evaluate the patient's need for long-term mechanical ventilation. ➨*Rationale:* This evaluation allows the nurse to anticipate patient and family needs for the patient's discharge to an extended care facility, rehabilitation center, or home on PPV.

Patient Preparation

• Ensure that the patient understands preprocedural teaching. Answer questions as they arise, and reinforce information as needed. ➨*Rationale:* This communication evaluates and reinforces understanding of previously taught information.
• Premedicate as needed. ➨*Rationale:* Administration of sedatives, narcotics, or muscle relaxants may be necessary to provide adequate oxygenation and ventilation in some patients.

Procedure for Ventilatory Management—Volume and Pressure Modes

Steps	Rationale	Special Considerations
Volume Modes		
1. Select mode (see Table 32-1). *(Level V: Clinical studies in more than one patient population and situation.)*	Mode selection varies depending on the clinical goal and clinician preference. Either IMV or AC mode can be used to provide total ventilatory support. To do so requires, however, that the rate be high enough or the patient sedated so that spontaneous effort is not present.[30,40]	Intermittent mandatory ventilation (IMV) often is used in conjunction with PSV (to overcome circuit resistance and to decrease the work of breathing associated with spontaneous effort). If respiratory muscle rest is the goal using IMV plus PSV, the level of PSV should be high enough to provide a Vt of 8-12 ml/kg and to maintain the total rate (IMV plus PSV breaths) of less than or equal to 20.[7,8,25,40]
2. Set Vt between 8 and 12 ml/kg. *(Level V: Clinical studies in one or more different populations. Expert consensus also exists.)*	Vt is selected in conjunction with rate (fx) to attain a MV 5-10 liters/min with a $Paco_2$ 35-45 mm Hg.[18] Large Vt values have been associated with lung injury, especially in patients with ARDS. In patients with poor lung compliance, Vt may be set at volumes of 6 ml/kg to protect the lung from high distending pressures; hypercarbia results.[5,13,18,19,35,40,42,45]	When lower Vt values are used in an attempt to reduce lung injury, the patient requires heavy sedation and often muscle relaxants to prevent spontaneous effort; hypercarbia is an expected outcome of low Vt values. Permissive hypercarbia is generally well tolerated in patients if the pH is reduced gradually (over 24-48 hours); pH around 7.2 is cited as an end point. Occasionally, bicarbonate infusions are used to keep the pH within an acceptable range. Permissive hypercarbia should not be attempted in patients with elevated intracranial pressure or patients with myocardial ischemia, myocardial injury, or dysrhythmias. Patients who are allowed to become hypercarbic require sedation and often muscle relaxants (paralytic agents) to control ventilation.

Procedure continues on the following page

Procedure for **Ventilatory Management—Volume and Pressure Modes**—*Continued*

Steps	Rationale	Special Considerations
3. Select respiratory frequency between 10 and 20 breaths/min.	Vt and fx are selected to maintain an acceptable $Paco_2$ with an MV between 5 and 10 liters/min. Generally, when Vt is selected, fx is the parameter adjusted to attain a desired $Paco_2$; the rate selected depends on whether or not the clinical goal is to rest or work the respiratory muscles.	
4. For I:E times, select inspiratory time (this parameter is different depending on the ventilator). Examples include percent inspiratory time, inspiratory time, flow rate, and peak flow. Adjust as necessary to attain patient ventilator synchrony. *(Level V: Clinical studies in one or more different populations. Expert consensus also exists.)*	*Inspiratory flow* refers to the speed with which Vt is delivered during inspiration. Achieves the desired I:E ratio and comfortable breathing patterns.[30,31,39]	Generally, flow rates of 50 liters/min are used initially and adjusted to provide an inspiratory time that synchronizes with patient effort. I:E ratios are usually 1:2 or 1:3. Longer expiratory times are necessary in patients with obstructive lung diseases (e.g., emphysema, asthma). A typical inspiratory time for an adult is in the range of 0.75-1 second.
5. Set the sensitivity (trigger sensitivity) between –1 and –2 cm H_2O pressure. *(Level VI: Clinical studies in a variety of patient populations and situations.)* Most ventilators have pressure-sensing sensitivity mechanisms that trigger flow. This means that the patient generates a decrease in the system pressure with an inspiratory effort. If the ventilator has a flow-triggering option, select the flow trigger in liters/min. The smaller the number, the more sensitive the ventilator. Flow triggering is set in conjunction with a base flow (flow in liters/min that is provided between ventilator breaths). Flow rate is monitored in the expiratory limb of the ventilator. When flow is disrupted during a spontaneous breath, a decrease in flow downstream is sensed; additional flow is added to the inspiratory circuit.	The more negative the number, the less sensitive the ventilator is to patient effort; this increases the patient respiratory workload and may lead to dyssynchrony.[3] Flow triggering has been associated with faster ventilator response times and less work of breathing than pressure sensing.[39]	When auto-PEEP is present, the patient has to generate a negative pressure equal to the set sensitivity plus the level of auto-PEEP.[35] Auto-PEEP is common in patients with asthma, chronic obstructive pulmonary disease, and high respiratory rates and minute ventilation. This additional work may fatigue the patient.[26] Patient ventilator dyssynchrony is likely.
6. Set fraction of inspired oxygen (Fio_2) to 0.60-1.0 (60-100%) if Pao_2 is unknown. *(Level VI: Clinical studies in a variety of patient populations and situations.)* Adjust down as tolerated using Sao_2 and arterial blood gas values.	Initiating PPV with maximal oxygen concentration avoids hypoxemia while optimal ventilator settings are being determined and evaluated. Additionally, it permits measurement of the percentage of venous admixture (shunt), which provides an estimate of the severity of the gas-exchange abnormality (see Procedures 30 and 31).	

Procedure **for Ventilatory Management—Volume and Pressure Modes**—*Continued*

Steps	Rationale	Special Considerations
	Goal is F_{IO_2} less than or equal to 0.5; high levels of F_{IO_2} result in increased risk of oxygen toxicity, absorption atelectasis, and reduction of surfactant synthesis.[10,16,21]	
7. Select PEEP level. Initial setting is often 5 cm H_2O. PEEP may be adjusted as needed after evaluation of tolerance (e.g., SaO_2, PaO_2, physical assessment). PEEP levels are increased to restore FRC and allow for reduction of F_{IO_2} to safe levels (i.e., less than or equal to 0.5) to decrease the risk of developing oxygen toxicity. *(Level V: Clinical studies in more than one patient population and situation.)*	A PEEP level of 5 cm H_2O is considered physiologic (essentially the amount of pressure at end exhalation normally provided by the glottis). The work of breathing imposed by the artificial airway is offset by 5 cm H_2O.	High levels of PEEP greater than or equal to 10 cm H_2O rarely should be interrupted because it may take hours to reestablish FRC (and PaO_2). Super-PEEP levels (i.e., greater than or equal to 20 cm H_2O) may be necessary in patients with noncompliant lungs (e.g., patients with ARDS) to prevent lung injury. It is thought that the repetitive opening and closing of stiff alveoli result in alveolar damage; to that end, the use of high PEEP levels to maintain alveolar distention and to prevent injury during PPV is considered a protective lung strategy.[2,13,24,38] In general, when high PEEP levels are used, Vt values are lower than normal, and hypercarbia is anticipated. Use of muscle relaxants, sedatives, and narcotics often is necessary.
Pressure Modes (Invasive) 1. Select mode: PSV, pressure-controlled/inverse ratio ventilation (PC/IRV), volume-assured pressure support option (VAPS), pressure release ventilation (PRV), high-frequency oscillation (HFO). *(Level VI: Clinical studies in a variety of patient populations and situations.)*	Mode selection depends on clinical goals and clinician preference. If spontaneous breathing is desired, PSV is selected. If a controlled rate and inspiratory time are desired, PC/IRV or another pressure mode may be chosen.	PSV sometimes is used between IMV breaths to offset the work of breathing associated with artificial airways and circuits during spontaneous breathing.[8,15,25] Some ventilators have VAPS (i.e., pressure modes with volume guarantees). Refer to specific ventilator operating manuals for details.
2. For PSV, adjust level to attain Vt between 8 and 12 ml/kg with spontaneous respiratory rate (RR) less than or equal to 20/min (if respiratory muscle rest is desired; this is called *PSVmax*). Decrease PSV level during weaning trials as tolerated by patient. Tolerance criteria for trials may be predetermined by protocols or on an individual basis. Often during trials, Vt values are allowed to be lower (i.e., 5-8 ml/kg) and RR higher (i.e., 25-30/min) than when rest is the goal. Follow these steps: A. Set sensitivity (as with volume ventilation).	Pressure level in conjunction with compliance and resistance determine delivered Vt.	PSV generally is considered a weaning mode of ventilation, necessitating patient stability. PSV may be used in less stable patients, provided that close attention is given to changes in Vt and RR. With changes in resistance and compliance, Vt is affected.

Procedure continues on the following page

Procedure for Ventilatory Management—Volume and Pressure Modes—*Continued*

Steps	Rationale	Special Considerations
B. Set PEEP (as with volume ventilation).		
C. Set FIO_2 (as with volume ventilation).		
3. For PC/IRV, follow these steps: A. Select inspiratory pressure support level (IPS). In this pressure mode, the level of pressure support often is identified as IPS versus PSV (as in pressure support). B. Select rate.	Absolute pressure level is the sum of IPS level and PEEP; this is a controlled mode. Rate and IPS level determine MV.	If clinical goal is to ensure plateau pressure of less than or equal to 30 cm H_2O, the pressure level may be lowered gradually over 24-48 hours to prevent sudden changes in $PaCO_2$ and pH.[5,19,40,42]
C. Select inspiratory time or inverse I:E ratio (ventilators vary).	I:E ratios are set at 1:1, 2:1, 3:1, or 4:1 by selecting the appropriate inspiratory time. Ratios are adjusted upward to improve shunt and oxygenation. Blood pressure may be adversely affected.	Generally, clinicians start with 1:1 ratios and increase as necessary to improve oxygenation. A limiting factor related to prolonged inspiratory times is hemodynamic compromise and hypotension; this is generally why the use of ratios greater than 2:1 rarely is seen clinically. Auto-PEEP is common and may be a desired outcome of PC/IRV.
D. Select PEEP level. When transitioning from volume ventilation to PC/IRV, the PEEP initially is maintained at the level used previously until the effect of the IRV is assessed. E. Select FIO_2 (as with volume ventilation).	Because IRV may result in auto-PEEP, it is important to evaluate the total amount of PEEP present.	The goal of PC/IRV is to improve oxygenation and allow for reduction of FIO_2 to less than or equal to 0.5.[20]
F. Set sensitivity (as with volume ventilation).	Always set sensitivity so that the patient can get a breath if needed. If controlled ventilation is the goal, chemical relaxation may be necessary in conjunction with sedatives and narcotics. It is unlikely that the patient would tolerate IRV (i.e., the prolonged inspiratory times) without such interventions.	
4. For volume-guaranteed pressure support options, parameter selection (i.e., pressure, volume, rate) is specific to the ventilator; however, selection of desired (or guaranteed) Vt is required. Some ventilators also require selection of the pressure level. Spontaneous breathing modes and controlled modes are available. Parameters including inspiratory time, rate, FIO_2, and PEEP are	Specific names vary depending on ventilator manufacturer. Examples include Pressure Augmentation (Bear Medical Systems, Riverside, CA), Volume Support (Siemens Medical, Iselin, NJ), and Pressure Regulated Volume Control (Siemens Medical, Iselin, NJ)[1]; similar modes are available on other manufacturers' ventilators.	These modes are complex; concurrent use of pressure, flow, and volume waveform displays may be necessary to assess the modes accurately. Refer to specific ventilator operating manuals.

Procedure for Ventilatory Management—Volume and Pressure Modes—*Continued*

Steps	Rationale	Special Considerations
selected accordingly, but principles are similar to volume ventilation. *(Level IV: Limited clinical studies to support recommendations.)*		
5. PRV and biphasic ventilation are relatively new modes appearing on selected ventilators. Used most commonly for patients with ARDS, the modes use a high level of CPAP to recruit the lung (restore FRC). With PRV, a high level of CPAP is selected, and brief expiratory "releases" are provided at set intervals (similar to setting a RR); the releases are very brief (less than or equal to 1.5 seconds).	The high level of CPAP helps "recruit" the lung. Filling and emptying time constants in the ARDS lung vary; the brief expiratory releases provided with PRV allow for more uniform emptying throughout the lung and ultimately improved gas distributions. An additional benefit of periodic airway pressure releases is that they may decrease the potential negative effect on venous return that is common with traditional high-level ventilatory support.[17,37,41]	This form of ventilation requires a steep learning curve on the part of the physicians, advanced practice nurses, respiratory therapists, and nurses who care for the patients; as with most new forms of ventilation, education of staff should occur before the mode is used.
With the biphasic mode (Puritan Bennett, Pleasanton, CA), two different levels of CPAP are selected and are called *Hi-PEEP* and *Low-PEEP*. A rate is set, and the cycles look similar to PC/IRV ventilation. The major difference is that flow is available to the patient for spontaneous breathing at both pressure levels. In addition, PS may be added to assist in decreasing the work associated with spontaneous breathing.[28]	The theoretical advantage of this mode over traditional PC/IRV, is that the mode may fully support lung recruitment, while still allowing for spontaneous breathing at the two pressure levels. In contrast to traditional PC/IRV, the patient receives additional flow adequate to meet inspiratory demands. Deterioration with spontaneous effort is less likely; as a result, heavy sedation and paralytics may be avoided.	
6. HFO differs significantly from conventional ventilator modes or mode options. HFO does not require bulk movement of volume in and out of the lungs; rather, a bias flow of gases is provided, and an oscillator disperses the gases throughout the lung in what has been called *augmented dispersion* at high frequencies.[11,27] Some parameters are different than with conventional ventilation. They include the following: *(Level IV: Limited clinical studies to support recommendations.)*	Studies are in progress to determine the efficacy of HFO in adults with ARDS; current data are promising, but as yet do not show a clear advantage over traditional modes (and especially the low Vt approach described by the ARDS network). The method achieves oscillation of the lung around a constant airway pressure (essentially opening the lung and "keeping it open").	
Bias flow: this is flow in liters/min (somewhere around 40-50 liters/min). *Oscillatory frequency (fx):* this is in Hz (5 is cited in one study as a starting point).[11] *Mean airway pressure:* generally slightly greater than conventional ventilation initially. ΔP: this is the change in pressure or pressure amplitude (generally adjusted to achieve chest wall vibration).	The bias flow combined with the oscillatory activity (extremely rapid pulses in a back and forth motion) result in the constant infusion of fresh gases and evacuation of old gases. ΔP and Hz are adjusted to achieve $Paco_2$ within a target range.	

Procedure continues on the following page

Procedure for Ventilatory Management—Volume and Pressure Modes—*Continued*

Steps	Rationale	Special Considerations
FiO₂ level and PEEP level: as in conventional ventilation (generally PEEP is greater than 10). *Percent inspiratory time:* this controls the percentage of time the oscillator spends in the inspiratory phase. A starting place is 33%.		
Ensure activation of alarms (Table 32-2).	Safety of the patient is paramount.	
Humidity	Inspired gases may be humidified with the use of standard cascade or high-volume humidifiers. Many institutions use disposable heat and moisture exchanges (HMEs) in place of conventional humidifiers.	HMEs are becoming increasingly more popular because they decrease the risk of infection and they are inexpensive (see later).
1. For conventional humidifiers, ensure that the humidifier has adequate fluid (sterile distilled water) and that the thermostat setting is adjusted according to manufacturer's recommendations. *(Level V: Clinical studies in one or more different populations. Expert consensus also exists.)*	Gases generally are humidified before entering the artificial airway. Temperature is measured at the patient wye; temperatures between 35°C and 37°C (95°F and 98°F) are considered optimal.[32]	Cool circuits may be tolerated well in patients without secretions. In patients with thick or tenacious secretions, attention to inspired temperature is important to prevent mucus plugging; circuit temperatures may need to be closer to body temperature (37°C versus 35°C) in these cases.
2. HMEs are placed between the airway and the patient wye. *(Level V: Clinical studies in more than one patient population and situation.)*	The moisture in warmed, exhaled gases passes through the vast surface area of the HME and condenses. With inspiration, dry gases pass through the HME and become humidified.	

TABLE 32-2 Ventilator Alarms

Disconnect Alarms (Low-Pressure or Low-Volume Alarms)

It is essential that when disconnection occurs, the clinician be immediately notified. Generally, this alarm is a continuous one and is triggered when a preselected inspiratory pressure level or minute ventilation is not sensed. With circuit leaks, this same alarm may be activated even though the patient may still be receiving a portion of the preset breath. Physical assessment, digital displays, and manometers are helpful in troubleshooting the cause of the alarms.

Pressure Alarms

High-pressure alarms are set with volume modes of ventilation to ensure notification of pressures exceeding the selected threshold. These alarms are usually set 10-15 cm H₂O above the usual peak inspiratory pressure (PIP). Some causes for alarm activation (generally an intermittent alarm) include secretions, condensate in the tubing, biting on the endotracheal tubing, increased resistance (i.e., bronchospasm), decreased compliance (e.g., pulmonary edema, pneumothorax), and tubing compression.

Low-pressure alarms are used to sense disconnection, circuit leaks, and changing compliance and resistance. They are generally set 5-10 cm H₂O below the usual PIP or 1-2 cm H₂O below the PEEP level or both.

Minute ventilation alarms may be used to sense disconnection or changes in breathing pattern (rate and volume). Generally, low–minute ventilation and high–minute ventilation alarms are set (usually 5-10 liters/min above and below usual minute ventilation). When stand-alone pressure support ventilation (PSV) is in use, this alarm may be the only audible alarm available on some ventilators.

FiO₂ alarms. Most new ventilators provide FiO₂ alarms that are set 5-10% above and below the selected FiO₂ level.

Alarm silence or pause. Because it is essential that alarms stay activated at all times, ventilator manufacturers have built-in silence or pause options so that clinicians can temporarily silence alarms for short periods (i.e., 20 seconds). The ventilators "reset" the alarms automatically. Alarms provide important protection for ventilated patients. However, inappropriate threshold settings decrease usefulness. When threshold gradients are set too narrowly, alarms occur needlessly and frequently. Conversely, alarms that are set too loosely (wide gradients) do not allow for accurate and timely assessments.

From Burns, S. M. (1998). Mechanical ventilation and weaning. In: Kinney, M.R., et al., editors. *AACN Clinical Reference for Critical Care Nursing.* 4th ed. St. Louis: Mosby.

Procedure **for Ventilatory Management—Volume and Pressure Modes**—*Continued*		
Steps	**Rationale**	**Special Considerations**
A. Change HMEs per manufacturer's instructions. *(Level IV: Limited clinical studies to support recommendations.)*	The use of HMEs has been associated with decreased incidence of ventilator-associated pneumonias in ventilated patients.[6,12,22,44] The longer the HME is in line, the more efficient the humidification; however, inspiratory resistance increases over time. HMEs are often changed every 2-3 days (refer to manufacturer's instructions). In weaning patients, the additional resistive load added by these humidifiers may preclude their use.[23,29,34,36]	
B. Do not use if secretions are copious or bloody.	Obstruction is possible, and HMEs are not indicated in these conditions.	

Pressure Modes (Noninvasive): Positive Pressure Delivered by Nasal Mask, Pillows, or Full Facemask

Steps	Rationale	Special Considerations
1. Select mode: bilevel noninvasive ventilation (i.e., Bi-PAP). The names of specific modes vary with the ventilator manufacturer. Regardless, an understanding of the inherent principles related to the modes makes application easier.	PSV and PEEP have been described in specific sections (see earlier). Mode parameters, such as F_{IO_2}, inspiratory time, inspiratory and expiratory ratios, and sensitivity, all have been described previously. The concepts as applied to the application of Bi-PAP are similar; differences are highlighted in this section.	Refer to specific ventilator manufacturer information for specific names of the modes.
2. Bi-PAP is delivered by a full facemask, nasal mask (most common), or nasal pillows. The ventilator is designed to compensate for leaks because they are assumed with this type of ventilation. Sometimes a chin strap is used if necessary to prevent excessive leaks through the mouth. Mask fit is important, as is the creative application of Bi-PAP. This form of therapy may be labor intensive, especially when used to prevent reintubation after extubation.	Bi-PAP has been used successfully in critically ill ICU patients. Bi-PAP has been shown to be especially helpful in patients with COPD, congestive heart failure, and immunocompromised states.[20,33,36]	Obtunded patients and patients with excessive secretions are not good choices for Bi-PAP ventilation. The potential for aspiration is high. Full facemask ventilation should be used cautiously. The patient should be able to remove the mask quickly if nausea and vomiting are imminent.
3. The name *Bi-PAP* was coined initially by Respironics (Pleasanton, CA) and has been applied since to similar bilevel noninvasive modes provided by different vendors. The modes are designed to be delivered via a facemask, nasal mask, or nasal pillows. Bi-PAP		

Procedure continues on the following page

Procedure for Ventilatory Management—Volume and Pressure Modes—*Continued*

Steps	Rationale	Special Considerations
provides two levels of pressure—PEEP and PSV. Mode options include the following: A. A spontaneous mode, whereby the patient initiates all breaths (similar to PSV in the "stand-alone" mode). B. A spontaneous-timed option, which is similar to PSV with a backup rate (some vendors call this *A/C*). C. A control mode. In contrast to the spontaneous and spontaneous-timed modes, the control mode requires that a control rate and inspiratory time be selected.		
4. FIO_2 generally is delivered by means of an oxygen source (oxygen tubing connected to a flowmeter) that is connected into the mask or in the inspiratory line at the junction of the ventilator and ventilator interface. As a result, high levels of FIO_2 may not be delivered. Each ventilator has specifications that dictate the maximal flows allowed.	Ventilator function may be adversely affected if the manufacturer recommendations are not followed.	If the patient has high FIO_2 requirements, Bi-PAP may not be a good option. Instead, if noninvasive ventilation is still the desired intervention, consider providing the noninvasive ventilation via a traditional ventilator. If this is done, PSV may not be the best mode to use because the cycle offmechanism would be impeded by mask leaks (see PSV earlier). Generally the A/C mode is used in these cases (exceptions exist and are ventilator specific).

Expected Outcomes

- Maintenance of adequate pH and $Paco_2$
- Maintenance of adequate Pao_2
- Maintenance of adequate breathing pattern
- Respiratory muscle rest

Unexpected Outcomes

- Unacceptable pH, $Paco_2$, and Pao_2
- Hemodynamic instability
- Pulmonary barotrauma
- Inadvertent extubation
- Malpositioned endotracheal tube
- Nosocomial lung infection
- Acid-base disturbance
- Respiratory muscle fatigue

Patient Monitoring and Care

Steps	Rationale	Reportable Conditions
		These conditions should be reported if they persist despite nursing interventions.
1. Ensure activation of all alarms each shift (see Table 32-2).	Ensures patient safety.	• Continued activation of alarms
2. Check for secure stabilization and maintenance of endotracheal tube (see Procedure 4).	Reduces risk of inadvertent extubation.	• Unplanned extubation • Dislodgment of airway

Patient Monitoring and Care—*Continued*

Steps	Rationale	Reportable Conditions
3. Monitor in-line thermometer to maintain inspired gas temperature (in the range 35-37°C [95-98°F]).	Reduces risk of thermal injury from overheated inspired gas and risk of poor humidity from underheated inspired gas.	• Temperature less than 35°C or greater than 37°C
4. Keep ventilator tubing clear of condensation (drain tubing from clean to dirty).	Reduces risk of respiratory infection by decreasing inhalation of contaminated water droplets.	• Continued condensation
5. Ensure availability of manual self-inflating resuscitation bag with supplemental oxygen at the head of the bed. Attach or adjust PEEP valve if the patient is on greater than 5 cm H_2O.	Provides capability for immediately delivering ventilation and oxygenation to relieve acute respiratory distress caused by hypoxemia or acidosis.	
6. Check ventilator for baseline FIO_2, PIP, Vt, and alarm activation with initial assessment and after removal of ventilator from patient for suctioning, bagging, or draining ventilator tubing.	Ensures that prescribed ventilator parameters are used (e.g., 100% oxygen used for suctioning is not inadvertently delivered after suctioning procedure), provides diagnostic data to evaluate interventions (e.g., PIP is reduced after suctioning or bagging), and ensures that the monitoring and warning functions of the ventilator are functional (i.e., alarms).	• FIO_2, PIP, Vt, or fx settings different from prescribed
7. Explore any changes in peak inspiratory pressure greater than 4 cm H_2O or decreased (sustained) Vt on PSV. Immediately explore the cause of high-pressure alarms.	Acute changes in PIP or Vt may indicate mechanical malfunction, such as tubing disconnection, cuff or connector leaks, tubing or airway kinks, or changes in resistance and compliance. Always consider possibility of tension pneumothorax. Have equipment readily available (see Procedure 18).	• Unexplained high-pressure alarms
8. Place bite-block between the teeth if the patient is biting on the oral endotracheal tube (see Procedure 4).	An oral airway serves the same purpose but may not be tolerated as well as the bite-block because it may induce gagging.	• Biting on tube
9. Change the patient's body position as often as possible, but at least every 2 hours.	Frequent position changes are indicated to reduce the potential for atelectasis and pneumonia caused by secretion stasis. Promotes airway clearance.	
10. Evaluate patient-ventilator dyssynchrony by manually ventilating the patient with a self-inflating resuscitation bag (see Procedure 29).	By taking the patient off the ventilator for manual ventilation, synchrony may be accomplished more quickly than on the ventilator. This intervention may reduce risk of barotrauma and cardiovascular depression. If patient breathes in synchrony with bagging, consider changes in ventilatory parameters. If patient does not breathe synchronously with bagging, explore differential diagnoses of problems distal to the airway. Physician consultation may be required.	• Patient-ventilator dyssynchrony

Procedure continues on the following page

Patient Monitoring and Care—*Continued*

Steps	Rationale	Reportable Conditions
11. Observe for hemodynamic changes associated with increased Vt or PEEP.	May indicate functional changes in circulating volume caused by positive intrathoracic pressure. Always consider potential for pneumothorax with acute changes. Equipment used for rapid release of tension pneumothorax should be at bedside at all times (i.e., 14-gauge needle) (see Procedure 23). Chest tube insertion equipment should be readily available.	• Decreased blood pressure • Change in heart rate (increase or decrease of greater than 10% of baseline) • Decreased cardiac output • Decreased mixed venous oxygen tension • Increased arterial-venous oxygen difference (see Procedure 26)
12. Monitor for signs and symptoms of acute respiratory distress, hypoxemia, hypercarbia, and fatigue.	Respiratory distress indicates the need for changes in PPV. While troubleshooting the difficulties, support ventilation via a manual self-inflating resuscitation bag (see Procedure 29), if necessary.	• Rising arterial carbon dioxide tension • Chest-abdominal dyssynchrony • Shallow or irregular respirations • Tachypnea, bradypnea, or dyspnea • Decreased mental status • Restlessness, confusion, lethargy • Increasing or decreasing arterial blood pressure • Tachycardia • Atrial or ventricular dysrhythmias • Significant changes in pH, PaO_2, $PaCO_2$, or SaO_2

Documentation

Documentation should include the following:

- Patient and family education
- Date and time ventilatory assistance was instituted
- Ventilator settings, including the following: FiO_2, mode of ventilation, Vt, respiratory frequency (total and mandatory), PEEP level, I:E ratio or inspiratory time, PIP, C_{dyn}, and C_{stat}
- Arterial blood gas results
- SaO_2 readings
- Reason for initiating PPV

- Patient responses to PPV (including the patient's indication of level of comfort and respiratory complaints)
- Hemodynamic values
- Vital signs
- Respiratory assessment findings
- Unexpected outcomes
- Nursing interventions

References

1. Amato, M.B.P., et al. (1992). Volume-assured, pressure support ventilation (VAPSV): A new approach for reducing muscle workload during acute respiratory failure. *Chest, 102,* 1225-34.
2. Amato, M.B.P., et al. (1995). Beneficial effects of the "open lung approach" with low distending pressures in acute respiratory distress syndrome. *Am J Respir Crit Care Med, 152,* 1835-46.
3. Banner, M.J., Blanch, P.B., and Kirby, R.R. (1993). Imposed work of breathing and methods of triggering a demand-flow continuous positive airway system. *Crit Care Med, 21,* 183-90.
4. Bellemare, F., and Grassino, A. (1982). Evaluation of human diaphragm fatigue. *J Appl Physiol, 53,* 1196-206.
5. Bidani, A., et al. (1994). Permissive hypercapnia in acute respiratory failure. *JAMA, 272,* 957-62.
6. Boots, R.J., et al. (1997). Clinical utility of hygroscopic heat and moisture exchanges in intensive care patients. *Crit Care Med, 25,* 1707-12.
7. Brochard, L., et al. (1989). Inspiratory pressure support prevents diaphragmatic fatigue during weaning from mechanical ventilation. *Am Rev Respir Dis, 139,* 513-21.
8. Brochard, L., Pluskwa, F., and Lemaire, R. (1987). Improved efficacy of spontaneous breathing with inspiratory pressure support. *Am Rev Respir Dis, 136,* 411-5.
9. Cohen, C.A., et al. (1982). Clinical manifestations of inspiratory muscle fatigue. *Am J Med, 73,* 308-16.
10. Davis, W.B., et al. (1983). Pulmonary oxygen toxicity: early reversible changes in human alveolar structures induced by hyperoxia. *N Engl J Med, 309,* 878-83.
11. Derak, S., et al., and the Multicenter Oscillatory Ventilation for Acute Respiratory Distress Syndrome Trial (MOAT) study investigators. (2002). High-frequency oscillatory ventilation for acute respiratory distress syndrome in adults: a randomized controlled trial. *Am J Respir Crit Care Med, 166,* 801-8.
12. Djedaini, K., et al. (1995). Changing heat and moisture exchanges every 48 hours rather than 24 hours does not alter their efficacy and the incidence of nosocomial pneumonia. *Am J Respir Crit Care Med, 152,* 1562-9.
13. Dreyfuss, D., and Saumon, G. (1993). The role of Vt, FRC, and end-inspiratory volume in the development of pulmonary edema following mechanical ventilation. *Am Rev Respir Dis, 148,* 1194-203.

14. Dreyfuss, D., et al. (1988). High inflation pressure pulmonary edema: Respective effects of high airway pressure, high Vt, and positive end-expiratory pressure. *Am Rev Respir Dis,* 137, 1159-64.

15. Fiastro, J.F., Habib, M.P., and Quan, S.F. (1998). Pressure support compensation for respiratory work due to endotracheal tubes and demand continuous positive airway pressure. *Chest,* 93, 499-505.

16. Fisher, A.B. (1980). Oxygen therapy: Side effects and toxicity. *Am Rev Respir Dis,* 122, 61-9.

17. Frawley, P.M., and Habashi, N. (2001). Airway pressure release ventilation: Theory and practice. *AACN Clinical Issues,* 12, 234-46.

18. Fu, Z., et al. (1992). High lung volume increases stress failure in pulmonary capillaries. *J Appl Physiol,* 73, 123-33.

19. Hickling, K.G., et al. (1994). Low mortality rate in acute respiratory distress syndrome using low volume, pressure limited ventilation with permissive hypercapnia: A prospective study. *Crit Care Med,* 22, 1568-78.

20. Hilbert, G., et al. (2001). Noninvasive ventilation in immunosuppressed patients with pulmonary infiltrates, fever and acute respiratory failure. *N Engl J Med,* 344, 481-7.

21. Holm, B.A., et al. (1985). Pulmonary physiological and surfactant changes during injury and recovery from hyperoxia. *J Appl Physiol,* 59, 1402-9.

22. Iotti, G.A., et al. (1997). Unfavorable mechanical effects of heat and moisture exchangers in ventilated patients. *Intensive Care Med,* 23, 399-405.

23. Johnson, P.A., Raper, R.F., and Fisher, M. (1995). The impact of heat and moisture exchanging humidifiers on work of breathing. *Anaesth Intensive Care,* 23, 697-701.

24. Lachman, B. (1992). Open up the lung and keep the lung open. *Intensive Care Med,* 18, 319-21.

25. MacIntyre, N.R. (1986). Respiratory function during pressure support ventilation. *Chest,* 89, 677-83.

26. MacIntyre, N.R., Cheng, K.-C.G., and McConnell, R. (1997). Applied PEEP during pressure support reduces the inspiratory threshold load of intrinsic PEEP. *Chest,* 111, 188-93.

27. MacIntyre, N.R. (1998). High-frequency ventilation (Editorial). *Crit Care Med,* 26, 1955-6.

28. Mallinckrodt, Inc. (1999). *Two Ventilating Strategies in One Mode: BiLevel.* St Louis: Author.

29. Manthous, C.A., and Schmidt, G.A. (1994). Resistive pressure of a condenser humifier in mechanically ventilated patients. *Crit Care Med,* 22, 1792-5.

30. Marini, J.J., Rodriguez, M., and Lamb, V. (1986). The inspiratory workload of patient-initiated mechanical ventilation. *Am Rev Respir Dis,* 134, 902-9.

31. Marini, J.J., Smith, T.C., and Lamb, V.J. (1998). External work output and force generation during synchronized intermittent mechanical ventilation: Effect of machine assistance on breath effort. *Am Rev Respir Dis,* 138, 1169-79.

32. McEvoy, M.T., and Carey, T.J. (1995). Shivering and rewarming after cardiac surgery: Comparison of ventilator circuits with humidifier and heated wires to heat and moisture exchangers. *Am J Crit Care,* 4, 293-9.

33. Mehta, S., and Hill, N.S. (2001). State of the art: Non-invasive ventilation. *Am J Respir Crit Care Med,* 163, 540-77.

34. Nishimara, M., et al. (1990). Comparison of flow-resistive work load due to humidifying devices. *Chest,* 97, 600-4.

35. Parker, J.C., Hernandez, L.A., and Peevy, K.J. (1993). Mechanisms of ventilator-induced lung injury. *Crit Care Med,* 21, 131-43.

36. Pepe, P.E., and Marini, J.J. (1994). Occult positive end-expiratory pressure in mechanically ventilated patients with airflow obstruction. *Am Rev Respir Dis,* 126, 166-73.

37. Peter, J.V., et al. (2002). Noninvasive ventilation in acute respiratory failure—a meta analysis update. *Crit Care Med,* 30, 555-62.

38. Putensen, C., et al. (2001). Long-term effects of spontaneous breathing during ventilatory support in patients with acute lung injury. *Am J Respir Crit Care Med,* 164, 43-9.

39. Ranieri, V.M., et al. (1991). Effects of positive end-expiratory pressure on alveolar recruitment and gas exchange in patients with the adult respiratory distress syndrome. *Am Rev Respir Dis,* 144, 544-51.

40. Sassoon, C.S.H., et al. (1993). Inspiratory muscle work of breathing during flow-by, demand-flow and continuous-flow systems in patients with chronic obstructive pulmonary disease. *Am Rev Respir Dis,* 143, 860-6.

41. Slutsky, A.S. (1994). Consensus Conference on Mechanical Ventilation, January 28-30, 1993 at Northbrook, Il, USA: Parts 1 and 2. *Intensive Care Med,* 20, 64-79, 150-62.

42. Stock, M., and Downs, J.B. (1987). Airway pressure release ventilation: A new approach to ventilatory support during acute lung injury. *Respir Care,* 32, 517-24.

43. The Acute Respiratory Distress Syndrome Network. (2000). Ventilation with lower tidal volumes as compared with traditional tidal volumes for acute lung injury and the acute respiratory distress syndrome. *N Engl J Med,* 342, 1301-7.

44. Tobin, M.J., et al. (1987). Konno-Mead analysis of ribcage-abdominal motion during successful and unsuccessful trials of weaning from mechanical ventilation. *Am Rev Respir Dis,* 135, 1320-8.

45. Unal, N., et al. (1998). A novel method of evaluation of three heat-moisture exchangers in six different ventilator settings. *Intensive Care Med,* 24, 138-46.

46. West, J.B., et al. (1991). Stress fracture in pulmonary capillaries. *J Appl Physiol,* 70, 1731-42.

Additional Readings

Burns, S.M. (In press). Advanced respiratory concepts. In: Chulay, M., and Burns, S.M., editors. *AACN Essentials of Critical Care Nursing.* New York: McGraw-Hill.

Burns, S.M. (1998). Mechanical ventilation and weaning. In: Kinney, M.R., et al., editors. *AACN Clinical Reference for Critical Care Nursing.* 4th ed. St. Louis: Mosby-Yearbook, 607-33.

Chulay, M. (In press). Airway and ventilatory management. In: Chulay, M., and Burns, S.M., editors. *AACN Handbook of Critical Care Nursing.* New York: McGraw-Hill.

Pierce, L.N.B. (1995). *Mechanical Ventilation and Intensive Respiratory Care.* Philadelphia: W.B. Saunders.

Pierce, L.N.B. (In press). Traditional and non-traditional modes of mechanical ventilation. In: MacArthur, B., executive editor, and Burns, S.M., series editor. *Protocols for Practice: Care of the Mechanically Ventilated Patient. AACN Critical Care.* Aliso Viejo, CA: American Association of Critical-Care Nurses.

PROCEDURE 33

Weaning Criteria—Negative Inspiratory Pressure, Positive End-Expiratory Pressure, Spontaneous Tidal Volume, and Vital Capacity Measurement

PURPOSE: Standard weaning criteria are measured to evaluate *respiratory muscle strength* (negative inspiratory pressure [NIP] and positive expiratory pressure [PEP]) and *endurance* (spontaneous tidal volume [SVt] and vital capacity [VC]). The results may help determine the need for intubation, the ability of the patient to tolerate weaning trials, and the potential for extubation.

Suzanne M. Burns

PREREQUISITE NURSING KNOWLEDGE

- NIP also is called *negative inspiratory force* or sometimes *maximal inspiratory pressure*. The measurement of NIP is *effort independent* (meaning that the patient does not have to actively cooperate), and it is considered the most reliable of the standard weaning criteria (SWC). NIP is a measure of inspiratory respiratory muscle strength. It is a strong negative predictor but a poor positive predictor.[2,4,9-12] The most common threshold cited for NIP is less than or equal to –20 cm H_2O.

- PEP, also called *positive expiratory force,* is *effort dependent,* requiring that the patient cooperate fully to obtain a reliable value. PEP is a measure of expiratory muscle strength and ability to cough. The threshold for PEP is greater than or equal to 30 cm H_2O.

- SVt is a measure of respiratory muscle endurance. The threshold for SVt is greater than or equal to 5 ml/kg. When muscles fatigue, the compensatory breathing pattern is rapid and shallow. As a result, investigators have combined SVt and spontaneous respiratory rate (fx) in a ratio called the *rapid: shallow breathing index* or *fx:Vt.*[12]

- VC is also a measure of respiratory muscle endurance or reserve or both. A fatigued patient would be unable to triple or even double the size of a breath. The threshold

for VC is greater than or equal to 15 ml/kg (at least three times SVt).

- All SWC are best used in combination with other assessment data to determine the appropriateness of weaning trials or extubation.[2-4,7-8,12]

- It may be that weaning trials, such as short-duration "sprints" on continuous positive airway pressure or t-piece, provide enough information about extubation potential that SWC are not required.[10-12] Regardless, the SWC do provide information about respiratory muscle strength and endurance. They may be especially helpful in following trends in gains in strength and endurance in debilitated, weak patients or patients with myopathies. They also may help to evaluate respiratory muscle fatigue (see Procedure 34).

EQUIPMENT*

- An aneroid manometer (also called a *force meter*)
- A respirometer (to measure volumes)
- Appropriate adapters and one-way valves

---

*Some ventilators allow for measurement of these parameters while the patient is on the ventilator. Refer to specific ventilator guidelines for measurement.

PATIENT AND FAMILY EDUCATION

- Inform the patient and family about the patient's respiratory status, changes in therapy, and how to interpret the changes. If the patient or a family member requests specific information about the measurements, explain the relationship between these measurements and respiratory muscle strength and endurance. ➤*Rationale:* Most patients and families are less concerned with the diagnostic and therapeutic details and more concerned with how the patient is progressing overall. Patients and families readily grasp the concepts of muscle strength and endurance, however. They may wish to follow the patient's progress by monitoring the results of the tests over time. If so, the family can be recruited to help the patient provide a maximal effort during measurements.
- Discuss the sensations the patient may experience, such as transient shortness of breath and fatigue. ➤*Rationale:* Knowledge of anticipated sensory experiences reduces anxiety and distress.
- Explain to the patient the importance of cooperation and maximal effort to achieve valid and reliable measurements. ➤*Rationale:* Information about the patient's therapy, including the rationale, is cited consistently as an important need of patients and family members.

PATIENT ASSESSMENT AND PREPARATION

Patient Assessment

- Assess for the following signs and symptoms of inadequate ventilation.

- ❖ Increasing arterial carbon dioxide tension
- ❖ Chest-abdominal dyssynchrony
- ❖ Shallow or irregular respirations
- ❖ Tachypnea or bradypnea
- ❖ Dyspnea
- ❖ Restlessness, confusion, lethargy
- ❖ Increasing or decreasing arterial blood pressure
- ❖ Tachycardia/bradycardia
- ❖ Atrial or ventricular dysrhythmias

➤*Rationale:* Inadequate ventilation may indicate the need for positive-pressure ventilation. If signs and symptoms suggest inadequate ventilation, measurement of SWC may be helpful in determining respiratory muscle strength and endurance and the potential need for positive-pressure ventilation. Conversely, if no signs and symptoms of inadequate ventilation are present in a patient on positive-pressure ventilation, SWC measurements (in conjunction with other patient data) are useful to determine the patient's ability to tolerate weaning trials and possibly extubation.

- Assess patient's need for a long-term artificial airway and mechanical ventilatory assistance. ➤*Rationale:* Consistently low measurements in conjunction with overall patient status (e.g., mental status, hemodynamics, fluid and electrolyte balance, comfort, mobility) may suggest the need for permanent complete or partial ventilator support.

Patient Preparation

- Ensure that the patient understands preprocedural teaching. Answer questions as they arise, and reinforce information as needed. ➤*Rationale:* This communication evaluates and reinforces understanding of previously taught information.

Procedure for Weaning Criteria		
Steps	**Rationale**	**Special Considerations**
Level IV: Limited clinical studies to support recommendations; problems with reproducibility of data obtained from measurement of SWC make attention to exact procedure essential.[1,3,5-8]		
1. Wash hands.	Reduces the transmission of microorganisms.	
2. Don examination gloves.	Standard precautions.	
3. Attach portable respirometer to airway via adapter and series of one-way valves. *Note:* If patient is on positive-pressure ventilation, place patient back on ventilator to rest for a few minutes between all measurements.	Respirometer is used to measure SVt and VC. Depending on institutional standard and specific ventilator, volumes and pressures may be measured while patient is on the ventilator.	Generally, a series of one-way valves are used for attachment of the respirometer and aneroid manometer.
4. *SVt:* Instruct the patient to breathe normally for 1 minute. Count the fx and record the minute ventilation.		If patient's saturation decreases or other signs of intolerance of the procedure emerge, the test is aborted

Procedure continues on the following page

Procedure for Weaning Criteria—*Continued*

Steps	Rationale	Special Considerations
Divide minute ventilation by fx to obtain average SVt.		or may be done for a shorter interval (i.e., test for 15 seconds, and multiply result by 4 for calculation of full minute).
5. For VC, instruct patient to inhale as deeply as possible, zero respirometer, and instruct patient to exhale as completely as possible. The VC may be tested more than once to obtain the best effort.	A good VC effort mandates a maximal inspiration followed by a maximal expiration.	
6. Measure NIP as follows: A. The inspiratory one-way valve should be closed or capped, ensuring a closed system for measurement of inspiratory effort. Attach pressure manometer to airway with adapter and one-way valves.	Ensures best effort and evaluation reproducibility. Pressure manometer is used to measure NIP. Some ventilators allow for the measurement to be accomplished with the patient on the ventilator.	The pressure manometer is usually attached to the airway via a series of one-way valves (Fig. 33-1). The valves (one is for inspiration and one is for expiration) are capped as necessary to ensure a closed system and a clean measurement device for attachment to the patient's artificial airway.
B. Instruct the patient to inhale as deeply as possible. Observe the manometer needle during inspiration. This test can be done for 20 seconds with multiple attempts by patient.	The goal is to obtain the patient's best effort.	NIP can be frightening for patients because it is impossible to get a breath during the maneuver. Coaching should include warning the patient that this test renders him or her temporarily unable to take a breath. Watch the manometer as the 20 seconds elapse; stop the procedure if the NIP measurements begin to get weaker as time elapses or if the patient does not tolerate the procedure (e.g., experiences agitation, bradycardia, desaturation).
7. Measure PEP as follows: A. The expiratory valve should be closed or capped. This ensures that the patient is able to take a breath in but must exhale against a closed system. Attach the pressure manometer to the airway via adapter and one-way valves.		
B. Instruct the patient to exhale forcefully after taking a deep breath. Do this a number of times (not to exceed 20 seconds). Take the greatest positive number.	Obtains patient's best effort.	As with NIP, any deterioration of the patient indicates that the test should be aborted.
8. Encourage the patient throughout all measurements.	Provides incentive.	
9. Document findings and discuss with team.	Decisions related to weaning trials, intubation, or extubation are made with the results of these tests in conjunction with others.	

Negative Inspiratory Pressure

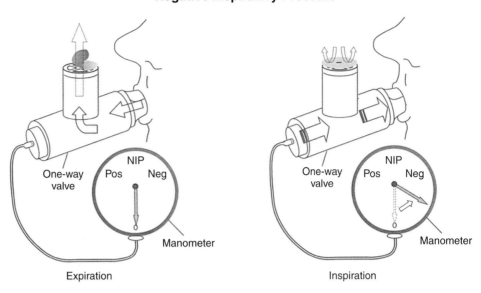

Positive Expiratory Pressure

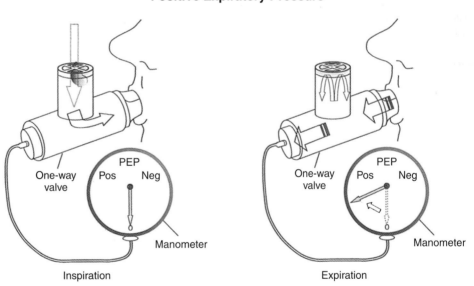

FIGURE 33-1 Negative inspiratory pressure (NIP) and positive expiratory pressure (PEP).

Expected Outcome	Unexpected Outcomes
• Valid and reliable measurements	• Invalid and unreliable measurements • Untoward physical, emotional, or hemodynamic changes

Patient Monitoring and Care

Steps	Rationale	Reportable Conditions
1. Compare the SWC measurements with the desired patient goals.	If the measurements are less than anticipated, the patient may need either initiation of positive-pressure ventilation or continuance of mechanical ventilation.	*These conditions should be reported if they persist despite nursing interventions.* • NIP greater than –20 cm H_2O (e.g., –10 cm H_2O) • PEP less than +30 cm H_2O (e.g., +10 cm H_2O) • SVt less than 5 ml/kg

Patient Monitoring and Care—*Continued*

Steps	Rationale	Reportable Conditions
	If the measurements equal or exceed the goals, initiation of weaning trials or extubation may be possible.	• VC less than 10 ml/kg • Any deterioration of patient during measurements that does not immediately respond by returning to mechanical ventilator or bagging

Documentation

Documentation should include the following:

- Patient and family education
- Best values obtained
- How the patient tolerated the tests

- Unexpected outcomes
- Nursing interventions

References

1. Brochard, L., et al. (1994). Comparison of three methods of gradual withdrawal from ventilatory support during weaning from mechanical ventilators. *Am Respir Crit Care Med,* 150, 896-903.
2. Burns, S.M., Burns, J.E., and Truwit, J.D. (1994). Comparison of five clinical weaning indices. *Am J Crit Care,* 3, 342-52.
3. Burns, S.M., et al. (1995). Weaning from long term mechanical ventilation. *Am J Crit Care,* 4, 4-22.
4. Cook, D., et al. (1999). *Evidence Report on Criteria for Weaning From Mechanical Ventilation.* Contract No. 290-97-0017. Rockville, MD: Agency for Health Care Policy and Research.
5. Ely, E.W., et al. (1996). Effect on the duration of mechanical ventilation of identifying patients capable of breathing spontaneously. *N Engl J Med,* 335, 1964-9.
6. Esteban, A., et al. (Spanish Lung Failure Collaborative Group). (1995). A comparison of four methods of weaning patients from mechanical ventilation. *N Engl J Med,* 332, 345-50.
7. Hanneman, S.K.G. (1994). Multidimensional predictors of success or failure with early weaning from mechanical ventilation after cardiac surgery. *Nurs Res,* 43, 4-10.
8. Hanneman, S.K., et al. (1994). Weaning from short term mechanical ventilation: A review. *Am J Crit Care,* 3, 421-43.
9. MacIntyre, N.R., et al. (2001). Evidence-based Guidelines for Weaning and Discontinuing Ventilatory Support: A collective task force facilitated by the American College of Chest Physicians; the American Association for Respiratory Care; and the American College of Critical Care Medicine. *Chest,* 120(6 Suppl), 375S-95S.
10. Mador, M.J. (1992). Weaning parameters: Are they clinically useful? *Chest,* 102, 1642.
11. Yang, K.L. (1992). Reproducibility of weaning parameters: A need for standardization. *Chest,* 102, 1829-32.
12. Yang, K.L., and Tobin, M.J. (1991). A prospective study of indexes predicting the outcome of trials of weaning from mechanical ventilation. *N Engl J Med,* 324, 1445-50.

Additional Readings

Burns, S.M. (1998). Mechanical ventilation and weaning. In: Kinney, M.R., et al., editors. *AACN's Clinical Reference for Critical Care Nursing.* 4th ed. St. Louis: Mosby-Yearbook, 624-7.
Burns, S.M. (In press). Weaning from long-term mechanical ventilation. In: MacArthur, B., executive editor, and Burns, S.M., series editor. *AACN Protocols for Practice: Care of the Mechanically Ventilated Patient.* Aliso Viejo, CA: American Association of Critical-Care Nurses.

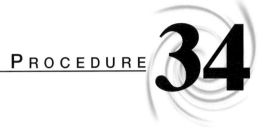

PROCEDURE **34**

Weaning Process

PURPOSE: The purposes of weaning patients from mechanical ventilation are liberation from ventilatory support and removal of artificial airways.

Suzanne M. Burns

PREREQUISITE NURSING KNOWLEDGE

- Knowledge and skills related to the care of patients on mechanical ventilation (e.g., airway management, suctioning, mechanical ventilator modes, blood gas interpretation) are necessary.
- The weaning process is markedly different between short-term mechanical ventilation (STMV) and long-term mechanical ventilation (LTMV).[8,22] In STMV (less than or equal to 3 days), the weaning progress is linear, whereas in LTMV (greater than 3 days), progress generally is manifested by peaks and valleys.[25]
- Weaning may be viewed as a continuum with distinct stages: prewean, weaning, and outcome (Fig. 34-1).[3] Some authors also add an acute stage to describe the time when a patient experiences severe cardiopulmonary instability.[11]
- Weaning readiness in STMV is determined by the patient's level of consciousness, hemodynamic stability, adequacy of gas exchange, and pulmonary mechanics.[14,30]
- LTMV weaning readiness is assessed with a wide variety of factors, including physiologic, psychological, and pulmonary impediments. To date, no single factor or impediment has been identified that determines ventilator dependence or independence. Instead, a combination of factors is responsible.[7,14,21,30,31,36]
- Weaning indices have proved to be disappointing predictors of a patient's ability to wean.[14,30] Most predictors focus on pulmonary-specific factors. Some investigators have combined indices and pulmonary factors, however, to enhance the comprehensive nature of the indices and their predictive potential. In general, the indices are poor positive predictors (they do not tell us the patient *will* wean), but they are strong negative predictors (they tell us the patient *will not* wean).[7,14,30] The various weaning indices are best used to evaluate the components important

to the weaning process and to track progress over time. This type of approach prevents lapses in care and may result in shorter ventilator durations. Table 34-1 describes standard or traditional weaning parameters, and Tables 34-2 and 34-3 are examples of integrated weaning indices.

- Studies about weaning suggest that weaning progress in patients requiring prolonged ventilation is more likely when rigorous attention is paid to the correction of impediments and a standardized comprehensive approach

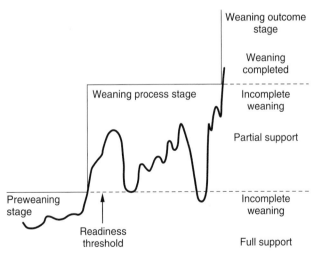

FIGURE 34-1 Weaning continuum model, a refined model of weaning in which stages and forward progression are represented by a stair-step configuration. The trajectory shown is only one theoretical possibility. Testing of the model is required to determine the actual trajectory of individual patients. The length of the steps is not intended to represent the actual duration of each stage. For clarity, relevant elements of the original model (e.g., factors affecting weaning, decisions about weaning) have been omitted. *(From Knebel, A.R., et al. [1998]. Weaning from mechanical ventilatory support: refinement of a model.* Am J Crit Care, *7, 151.)*

TABLE 34-1	**Standard Weaning Criteria**

Negative inspiratory pressure less than or equal to −20 cm H$_2$O
Positive expiratory pressure greater than or equal to +30 cm H$_2$O
Spontaneous tidal volume greater than or equal to 5 ml/kg
Vital capacity greater than or equal to 10-15 ml/kg
Fraction of inspired oxygen less than or equal to 50%
Minute ventilation less than or equal to 10 liters/min

Modified from Burns, S.M. (1998). Mechanical ventilation and weaning.
In: Kinney, M.R., et al., editors. *AACN Clinical Reference for Critical Care
Nursing.* 4th ed. St. Louis: Mosby.

TABLE 34-2	**Rapid Shallow Breathing (fx/Vt) and Compliance, Rate, Oxygenation, and Pressure (CROP) Indices**

fx/Vt	CROP
Spontaneous respiratory frequency in 1 min divided by Vt in liters	Dynamic characteristic × NIP × (Pao$_2$/Pao$_2$) divided by respiratory rate
fx/Vt less than 105 = weaning success	greater than 13 = weaning success
fx/Vt greater than 105 = weaning failure	less than 13 = weaning failure

fx, frequency; *NIP*, negative inspiratory pressure; *Pao$_2$*, partial pressure of arterial
oxygen; *Pao$_2$*, partial pressure of alveolar oxygen; *Vt*, tidal volume.
Data from Yang, K.L., and Tobin, J.M. (1991). A prospective study of indexes
predicting the outcome of trials of weaning from mechanical ventilation.
N Engl J Med, 324, 1445-50.

TABLE 34-3	**Burns Weaning Assessment Program (BWAP)***

Patient name_____
Patient history number_____

Yes	No	Not Assessed	
			General Assessment
—	—	—	1. Hemodynamically stable (pulse rate, cardiac output)?
—	—	—	2. Free from factors that increase or decrease metabolic rate (seizures, temperature, sepsis, bacteremia, hypothyroid, hyperthyroid)?
—	—	—	3. Hematocrit >25% (or baseline)?
—	—	—	4. Systemically hydrated (weight at or near baseline, balanced intake and output)?
—	—	—	5. Nourished (albumin >2.5, parenteral/enteral feedings maximized)? (If albumin is low and anasarca or third spacing is present, score for hydration should be "No")
—	—	—	6. Electrolytes within normal limits (including Ca^{++}, Mg$^+$, PO$_4$)? Correct Ca^{++} for albumin level
—	—	—	7. Pain controlled? (subjective determination)
—	—	—	8. Adequate sleep/rest? (subjective determination)
—	—	—	9. Appropriate level of anxiety and nervousness? (subjective determination)
—	—	—	10. Absence of bowel problems (diarrhea, constipation, ileus)?
—	—	—	11. Improved general body strength/endurance (i.e., out of bed in chair, progressive activity program)?
—	—	—	12. Chest roentgenogram improving?
			Respiratory Assessment
			Gas Flow and Work of Breathing
—	—	—	13. Eupneic respiratory rate and pattern (spontaneous respiratory rate <25, without dyspnea, absence of accessory muscle use). This is assessed off the ventilator while measuring #20-23.
—	—	—	14. Absence of adventitious breath sounds (rhonchi, rales, wheezing)?
—	—	—	15. Secretions thin and minimal?
—	—	—	16. Absence of neuromuscular disease/deformity?
—	—	—	17. Absence of abdominal distention/obesity/ascites?
—	—	—	18. Oral endotracheal tube >7.5 Fr or tracheotomy >6.0 Fr
			Airway Clearance
—	—	—	19. Cough and swallow reflexes adequate?
			Strength
—	—	—	20. Negative inspiratory pressure <−20?
—	—	—	21. Positive expiratory pressure >+30?
			Endurance
—	—	—	22. Spontaneous tidal volume >5 ml/kg?
—	—	—	23. Vital capacity >10-15 ml/kg?
			Arterial Blood Gases
—	—	—	24. pH 7.30-7.45?
—	—	—	25. Paco$_2$ approximately 40 mm Hg (or baseline) with minute ventilation <10 liters/min (evaluated while on ventilator)?
—	—	—	26. Pao$_2$ 60 or Fio$_2$ <40%?

*To score the BWAP: divide the number of "Yes" responses by 26. Threshold: >65% = weaning probable; <65% = weaning improbable.
Ca^{++}, calcium; *Fio$_2$*, fraction of inspired oxygen; *Mg$^+$*, magnesium; *Paco$_2$*, arterial partial pressure of carbon dioxide; *Pao$_2$*, arterial partial pressure of oxygen; *PO$_4$*, phosphate.
Copyright © S. M. Burns, 1990.

is used.[7,9,10,12,15,23,24,26,30,31,33,34] Decreasing system variation in care provision is the goal.

- No weaning modes or methods of weaning seem to be superior[8,14,30]; however, attention to early testing of ability to wean combined with distinct trials that balance respiratory muscle work and rest may result in shorter weaning durations.[6,15,16]
- The concept of respiratory muscle fatigue must be understood if it is to be prevented in the ventilated weaning patient. All muscles may fatigue if work exceeds energy stores. Signs and symptoms of impending fatigue include dyspnea, tachypnea, chest-abdominal asynchrony, and increasing arterial partial pressure of carbon dioxide ($PaCO_2$) (a late sign).[2,13,35] Generally, fatigue may be prevented by avoiding premature trials or excessively long or difficult weaning trials.
- Protocols for weaning have been noted to improve weaning outcomes in STMV and LTMV patients.[6,15,16,26] In general, these protocols consist of three components: entry criteria, definition of weaning trial tolerance (when to initiate and when to stop trials), and distinct steps for progression of the specific modes or methods to be used (Tables 34-4 and 34-5).
- The concepts of work, rest, and conditioning are integrated into many protocols. The use of two classifications—high-pressure, low-volume work and low-pressure, high-volume work—may help with practical applications of specific modes and methods.
  - ❖ *High-pressure, low-volume work* is found with the use of a t-piece, continuous positive airway pressure (CPAP), and low intermittent mandatory ventilation (IMV) rates. Generally, any method that requires that the patient breathe spontaneously (without inspiratory support) results in high-pressure, low-volume work. This form of muscle conditioning is thought to build sarcomeres because it employs maximal muscle loading.[27,29] Conditioning episodes are generally of short duration with full muscle rest between episodes. This type of conditioning is referred to as *strengthening training*.
  - ❖ *Low-pressure, high-volume work* is found with the use of pressure support ventilation (PSV), in which inspiration is augmented. For any given pressure level, workload is less than if the patient were breathing spontaneously. At high levels of PSV, little work occurs, but as the level is reduced, muscle workload increases. Conditioning with PSV often is referred to as *endurance conditioning*; muscles are not worked to maximal effort. Instead, training focuses on maintaining a specific level of work for progressively longer intervals.[27,29]
- With both types of conditioning, the goal is to progress the trials without inducing fatigue. Noninvasive criteria that define intolerance (see Tables 34-4 and 34-5, section D) may result in cessation of the trial and a return to full rest. Rest and fatigue are described in Procedure 32 and in sample protocols (see Tables 34-4 and 34-5, sections C-1 and D).
- Weaning is the process of gradual reduction of ventilatory support. To that end, a plan for weaning is essential. The plan, whether it means employing a protocol or

---

TABLE 34-4 | **Example CPAP Protocol**

A. Mode

CPAP (0, or level of current mechanical ventilator settings)

B. Entry Criteria

BWAP score greater than or equal to 50%
FIO_2 less than or equal to 0.5
PEEP less than or equal to 8 cm H_2O

C. Protocol Steps

1. Ensure complete rest the previous night and until the trial begins. (Complete respiratory muscle rest is defined as total cessation of respiratory effort when in assist-control or IMV modes; respiratory rate less than 20 breaths/min with inspiratory Vt of 8-12 ml/kg in PSV mode)
2. Place the patient on a CPAP level of 0 (or level determined by team) at the same FIO_2 as when ventilated
3. Maintain CPAP at 0 for 2 hours unless signs of intolerance develop. Trial is done once daily.
4. If signs of intolerance develop at any time during the trial, place the patient back on the previous ventilator settings. Make adjustments as necessary to achieve complete respiratory muscle rest. Total rest continues until the next day or another trial is attempted that day (this is only if there is a compelling reason that explains the patient's inability to sustain the earlier trial)
5. If the patient tolerates 2 hours of CPAP trial, consider extubation

D. Intolerance Criteria

1. Respiratory rate increase to 30 breaths/min (sustained)
2. Heart rate increase by 20% (sustained)
3. Oxygen saturation decreases to less than 91% or 2% below baseline (sustained)
4. Systolic blood pressure greater than 180 mm Hg or less than 90 mm Hg
5. Agitation
6. Diaphoresis
7. Anxiety
8. Vt less than 5 ml/kg (sustained)
9. Excessive dyspnea (new or unrelated to activity)
10. Patients are also "rested" and the weaning process held if any of the following conditions apply:
    a. During acute events (e.g., hypotension, bronchospasm)
    b. Intrahospital transports
    c. Temperature spikes
    d. Decreased weaning indices scores (BWAP less than 50%, WI greater than 4.5)
    e. Trendelenburg position required (e.g., for line placement)

BWAP, Burns Weaning Assessment Program; *CPAP,* continuous positive airway pressure; *FIO2,* fraction of inspired oxygen; *IMV,* intermittent mechanical ventilation; *PEEP,* positive end-expiratory pressure; *PSV,* pressure support ventilation; *Vt,* tidal volume.
Adapted from University of Virginia, MICU Weaning Protocols.

---

consists of an individualized written plan, should be available to all health care workers involved in the weaning process. Assessment of weaning potential may include checklists of factors important to weaning, such as the Burns Weaning Assessment Program (BWAP) (see Table 34-3), and the measurement and application of various weaning indices, such as standard weaning criteria (see Procedure 33 and Table 34-1), frequency/tidal volume (Vt) (see Table 34-2), and BWAP (see Table 34-3).

EQUIPMENT

- If t-piece or tracheotomy collar setup is required, a flowmeter with a functional heated aerosol humidifier for the trials is necessary. The setup should have an in-line thermometer and a water trap.

TABLE 34-5	Example PSV Protocol

A. Mode

Pressure support wean/pressure support rest

B. Entry Criteria

BWAP score greater than or equal to 50%
F_{IO_2} less than or equal to 0.5
PEEP less than or equal to 6 cm H_2O

C. Protocol Steps

1. The baseline (resting) PSV level is set to achieve Vt of 8-12 ml/kg, while ensuring a respiratory rate of less than or equal to 20 breaths/min
2. The PSV level is decreased by 2-5 cm H_2O/day. If the patient successfully maintains the previous day's PSV level for 10-14 hours, the PSV level is decreased by 2-5 cm H_2O again. This process is continued until the patient reaches a PSV level of 3-5 cm H_2O. (If the team wishes to advance weaning based on rapid improvements in the patient's physical status, the PSV level may be decreased more rapidly)
3. The patient is rested at night or with any acute events (see "baseline" definition above)
4. If a patient exhibits signs of fatigue during a PSV trial, the patient is returned to the previous day's PSV level. After 30 minutes, if the patient continues to be fatigued, the patient is returned to the resting level of PSV
5. The patient is progressed to a lower PSV level the following day only if 10-14 hours of PSV is achieved on the current setting
6. When the patient reaches a PSV of 3-5 cm H_2O and can maintain this level for the required time, the team is approached for extubation orders. For some patients (e.g., obese patients), the lowest level of PSV may need to be higher

D. Intolerance Criteria (as for CPAP protocol)

BWAP, Burns Weaning Assessment Program; F_{IO_2}, fraction of inspired oxygen; *PEEP*, positive end-expiratory pressure; *PSV*, pressure support ventilation.
Adapted from University of Virginia, MICU Weaning Protocols.

- Tracheotomy collar or t-piece adapters
- Pressure manometers
- Weaning protocol or wean plan
- Extubation equipment (see Procedures 5 and 6)

PATIENT AND FAMILY EDUCATION

- Explain the procedures and why weaning is being initiated. ➺*Rationale:* Anxiety is reduced when patients are prepared for the sensations they may experience during procedures.
- Reassure the patient of the nurse's or the therapist's presence during initiation of weaning (especially when tracheostomy collar, t-piece, and CPAP trials are used). ➺*Rationale:* Assurance of the caregiver's support and monitoring decreases anxiety.
- Discuss the sensations the patient may experience, such as smaller lung inflations, dyspnea, and change or absence of ventilator sounds. Describe that weaning trials are a form of conditioning and do require effort. Some dyspnea is to be expected. ➺*Rationale:* Patients (in particular patients who have been on prolonged positive-pressure ventilation [PPV] support) may report discomfort with resumption of spontaneous breathing.
- Encourage the patient to relax and breathe comfortably. ➺*Rationale:* Relaxation decreases muscle tension.
- Assure the patient and family that rapid return to ventilatory support will be accomplished if patient becomes excessively dyspneic, becomes anxious, or exhibits untoward

physiologic changes (e.g., desaturation; blood pressure, heart rate, and rhythm changes; diaphoresis). ➺*Rationale:* To develop trust, the patient and family must believe that the nurse will not allow the trials to harm the patient.

PATIENT ASSESSMENT AND PREPARATION

Patient Assessment

- Regular evaluation of factors that impede weaning in conjunction with factors that measure respiratory muscle strength, endurance, and gas exchange is necessary to determine when to begin weaning trials (see Tables 34-1, 34-2, and 34-3). ➺*Rationale:* Premature attempts at weaning may be harmful physiologically and psychologically.
- Assess progress toward achievement of individual short-term goals every 5 to 30 minutes, as appropriate. ➺*Rationale:* Successful weaning may be achieved within several hours if patient response is monitored closely and interventions are applied in tandem with patient response.
- In patients who are ventilator dependent, assess daily progress toward achievement of individual long-term goals, in collaboration with the physician, respiratory therapist, patient, and family, as appropriate. ➺*Rationale:* Successful weaning may be achieved within days to weeks in these patients if patient response is methodically evaluated and interventions are applied in tandem with patient response.
- Observe breathing pattern, and note complaints of dyspnea in response to decrements in PPV support. Other signs of fatigue include the following:
  - ❖ Accessory muscle use
  - ❖ Chest or abdominal asynchrony
  - ❖ Retractions
  - ❖ Rapid shallow breathing pattern
  ➺*Rationale:* These are signs and symptoms of potential or actual respiratory muscle fatigue. Interventions to offset the work of breathing are necessary.
- Note if the patient experiences changes in level of consciousness or nonverbal behavior and complains of dyspnea or fatigue. ➺*Rationale:* Work of breathing may be such that the patient is maintaining an adequate breathing pattern and gas exchange at the moment but does not have sufficient reserves to continue expending energy to breathe. Patient exhaustion during weaning results in psychological and physiologic delays in the weaning progress.
- Assess arterial blood gases as needed. ➺*Rationale:* Although frequent arterial blood gas assesssments are rarely necessary during weaning if active attention is paid to signs and symptoms of intolerance, arterial blood gases are the only definitive method of evaluating efficiency of gas exchange. It is especially important to evaluate $Paco_2$ with spontaneous breathing if rapid return to increased ventilatory settings is not part of the plan or if there are dramatic changes in the patient's condition. $Paco_2$ is the definitive indicator of the adequacy of ventilation. $Paco_2$ within the patient's normal physiologic range indicates that the patient's ventilation is

adequate with spontaneous breathing. The advantage to the use of weaning protocols is that criteria that identify intolerance are clearly defined and result in a return to ventilatory support. Arterial blood gases are often not required to evaluate weaning trials.

- Assess oxygenation indices (see Procedure 30)—arterial oxygen saturation (SaO_2) or arterial partial pressure of oxygen (PaO_2) during trials. ➡️*Rationale:* SaO_2 is a real-time continuous indicator of oxygenation during weaning trials and should be monitored continually. A saturation of greater than or equal to 90% generally indicates oxygenation adequacy. PaO_2 is the definitive indicator of the adequacy of oxygenation and in some cases is required. A PaO_2 within the patient's normal physiologic range indicates that the patient's oxygenation is adequate with spontaneous breathing. Generally, PaO_2 greater than 60 mm Hg and SaO_2 greater than or equal to 90% on a fraction of inspired oxygen (FiO_2) of less than or equal to 0.4 is acceptable during trials.
- Assess patient anxiety level. ➡️*Rationale:* Resumption of spontaneous breathing may cause anxiety, particularly in patients who have been on prolonged PPV support. Encouragement is necessary in addition to assurance that prompt return to ventilatory support will be accomplished if the patient becomes excessively tired, anxious, or otherwise distressed. Patients must trust that the health care workers will address their concerns competently and rapidly during weaning trials.

Patient Preparation

- Ensure that the patient understands preprocedural teaching. Answer questions as they arise, and reinforce information as needed. ➡️*Rationale:* This communication evaluates and reinforces understanding of previously taught information.
- Address all factors that are impeding wean potential. In STMV, this may include factors such as pH level, hemodynamic stability, electrolytes, strength, and endurance. In a patient who requires LTMV, other factors, such as mobility, nutrition, and fluid status, may be more significant. ➡️*Rationale:* Weaning of STMV and LTMV patients has been associated with the correction of a myriad of physiologic factors. Weaning is not solely dependent on respiratory muscle strength and endurance. Frequency and timing of measurement of weaning criteria depend on whether the patient requires STMV or LTMV.
- Establish weaning criteria. ➡️*Rationale:* Weaning criteria (pulmonary and nonpulmonary) are helpful to determine a patient's weaning potential, track progress, and determine when extubation is appropriate.

Procedure for Weaning Process

Steps	Rationale	Special Considerations
1. Communicate with the patient and family throughout the weaning process.	Attention is given to the patient's subjective response to weaning. The nurse remains with the patient (especially at the beginning of the trial); monitors frequently during trials; coaches the patient; reinforces the goals and desired outcomes; reminds the patient that talking, eating, self-care activities, and mobilization are facilitated by successful weaning and extubation; and celebrates weaning progress with the patient and family.	
T-Piece or Tracheotomy Collar Trials 1. Wash hands, and don gloves.	Reduces transmission of microorganisms; standard precautions.	
2. Connect patient to heated aerosol via t-piece or tracheotomy collar. Instruct patient to breathe normally, and monitor frequency, breathing pattern, heart rate, cardiac rhythm, SaO_2, and general appearance of patient. (*Level V: Clinical studies in*	Heated aerosol replaces water that normally would be added by the upper airway if it were not bypassed by the endotracheal or tracheostomy tube. This method of weaning employs high-pressure, low-volume work.	Abort weaning for any signs of patient intolerance and place patient back on PPV support.

Procedure continues on the following page

Procedure for Weaning Process—*Continued*

Steps	Rationale	Special Considerations
more than one patient population and situation.)	Signs and symptoms of tolerance must be heeded if respiratory muscle fatigue is to be prevented.[6,15,16,26]	
3. After a predetermined time interval or with the emergence of signs of intolerance, place patient back on resting ventilator settings. *(Level V: Clinical studies in more than one patient population and situation.)*	To ensure respiratory muscle conditioning and forward progress during weaning trials, the work of breathing must not be excessive; do not exceed predetermined wean trial duration. Adequate rest between trials and at night offsets fatigue and encourages effective respiratory muscle conditioning. Patient is placed back on the ventilator to rest until all data regarding weaning response can be assessed.[6,15,16,26]	
4. If patient successfully meets full trial criteria, notify physician, advanced practice nurse, or team of patient's response and consider extubation. If a protocol is in place, extubation may be the next step and may not require such notification.		

CPAP Trials (Levels 0-10 cm H₂O) (With or Without Flow-By Option)

1. Explain purpose and procedure of CPAP trials to patient and family, and switch patient from resting settings to CPAP level. Instruct the patient to breathe normally, and monitor for signs and symptoms of intolerance (described earlier). If using protocol, refer to specific criteria. *(Level V: Clinical studies in more than one patient population and situation.)*	As with the t-piece, this method employs high-pressure, low-volume work. Prompt return to the ventilator is necessary if excessive work and fatigue are to be prevented.[6,15,16,26]	An advantage of CPAP over t-piece trials is that Vt and respiratory rate are monitored easily throughout the trial by means of the digital display on the ventilator. Alarms, such as a low minute ventilation alarm, may be set with a *CPAP trial.*
2. After predetermined time interval on CPAP or with signs or symptoms of intolerance, place patient back on resting ventilator settings. *(Level V: Clinical studies in more than one patient population and situation.)*	Do not exceed predetermined wean trial duration. Adequate rest between trials and at night offsets fatigue and encourages effective respiratory muscle conditioning. The patient is placed back on the ventilator to rest until all data regarding weaning response can be assessed.[6,15,16,26]	
3. Notify physician, advanced practice nurse, or team of results of trials. If last step of wean plan or protocol has been attained, extubation should be considered. (If protocol is used, this step may be automatic.)		

IMV and Synchronized Intermittent Mandatory Ventilation (SIMV) Weaning Method

1. Gradually and progressively decrease IMV/SIMV breaths.	This method of weaning provides gradual decrements or full PPV support by permitting spontaneous	Some IMV/SIMV demand valves offer high resistance to breathing and produce a lag between the patient's

Procedure for Weaning Process—*Continued*

Steps	Rationale	Special Considerations
(Level V: Clinical studies in more than one patient population and situation.)	breathing between periodic preset ventilator breaths. The preset breaths are progressively decreased as the patient assumes a greater proportion of the minute volume with spontaneous breathing.	initiation of a breath and delivery of the inspired gas during spontaneous breathing; these factors may increase the work of breathing and result in subsequent fatigue.[1,3,18-20] To avoid this, some use PSV between IMV breaths to offset the work associated with small tube sizes, circuit resistance, and high breathing rates.[4,5,17,28] This method of weaning has been associated with prolonged weaning trial duration in at least one study.[17] It is essential that a plan be in place for progressive weaning and that a clinical end point be predetermined (e.g., IMV of 4). Another method used to decrease work between IMV breaths is the use of flow-by and a flow-triggering option (see Procedure 32).[32]
2. Assess the patient for signs and symptoms of fatigue, inadequate gas exchange, and impaired breathing pattern with each decrement in IMV/SIMV support.[2,13,28,35] *(Level IV: Limited clinical studies to support recommendations.)*	Determines patient response to weaning. A plan that clearly describes the end point of this method is essential. The multidisciplinary team may more readily determine when extubation is appropriate.[9-10,12,14,15,23,24,26,30,34] *(Level V: Clinical studies in more than one patient population and situation.)*	Lower levels of IMV (i.e., less than or equal to 4), when not used with PSV or flow-by, are similar to strength-conditioning trials. Adequate rest times should be ensured between trials and especially at night.
Pressure Support Weaning Method 1. Start at pressure support maximum (PSVmax) and decrease level according to the protocol or as clinically indicated (i.e., no signs of intolerance). *(Level IV: Limited clinical studies to support recommendations.)*	This weaning method provides for endurance conditioning; to that end, the level is decreased gradually as patient's endurance increases. PSVmax is the level that attains a spontaneous respiratory rate of less than or equal to 20, absence of accessory muscle use, and a Vt of 8-12 ml/kg. Higher respiratory rates and smaller Vt values are generally acceptable during trials. Because the mode employs low-pressure, high-volume work, weaning intervals may be longer than with strengthening modes. Regardless, full support should be ensured at night and for rest, especially early in the weaning stage.[4,5,28,32]	With PSV, the selected level should not be determined arbitrarily. The pressure level should be increased if any sustained signs of intolerance occur. Work is increased gradually by lowering the level of PSV in increments.
2. Monitor patient responses to weaning. Return to full ventilatory support if signs of intolerance occur and when intended duration of trial has been reached. *(Level V: Clinical studies in more than one patient population and situation.)*	PSV, despite requiring spontaneous effort, reduces the work of breathing associated with circuits, endotracheal tubes, and high breathing rates.[18]	An incompletely inflated artificial airway cuff can create a leak that prevents the PSV cycle-off mechanism from activating (i.e., the ventilator cycles off when it senses that flow is one fourth the original flow).

Procedure continues on the following page

Procedure for Weaning Process—*Continued*

Steps	Rationale	Special Considerations
	Fatigue is possible if the level is not high enough.[4,5] PSVmax is used as a respiratory muscle rest level.	If this decrement of flow is not recognized, the result is an inappropriately long inspiratory time.
3. When the clinical goal for PSV wean is accomplished (e.g., 12 hours at lowest level), extubation or an additional step is discussed with the team. (*Level V: Clinical studies in more than one patient population and situation.*)	If protocol is used, the next step may be automatic.[15,26]	

Expected Outcomes

- Timely and successful discontinuance of PPV
- Comfortable and adequate breathing pattern during the weaning process

Unexpected Outcomes

- Tracheal injury
- Pulmonary barotrauma
- Cardiovascular depression
- Fatigue
- Hypoxemia
- Hypercapnia
- Dyspnea
- Unsuccessful, demoralizing weaning trials

Patient Monitoring and Care

Steps	Rationale	Reportable Conditions
		These conditions should be reported if they persist despite nursing interventions.
1. Evaluate overall patient stability (i.e., physiologic, psychological, and mechanical) in a systematic manner. Frequency of evaluation may vary depending on whether the patient requires STMV or LTMV. A multidisciplinary approach is encouraged.	Patient stability and overall condition must be considered before initiating active weaning trials. Premature attempts may be a harmful and frustrating for all involved. A multidisciplinary team approach ensures active attention to the diverse factors that affect weaning readiness. See Tables 34-1, 34-2, and 34-3 for pulmonary-specific and comprehensive weaning assessment tools.	- Changes in weaning indices (pulmonary-specific and integrated) along with general factors that affect weaning
2. During weaning trials, pay attention to signs and symptoms of intolerance and respiratory muscle fatigue. If signs of intolerance occur, prompt return to PPV is required.	Trials continued despite emergence of signs of intolerance lead to fatigue and failure. Cardiopulmonary failure and collapse are potential outcomes.	- Signs of weaning trial intolerance (tachypnea, dyspnea, chest and abdominal asynchrony) - Agitation - Mental status changes - Significant decrease in SaO_2 (SaO_2 less than 90% or 10% decrease) - Changes in pulse rate or rhythm - Blood pressure increase or decrease
3. If no signs of intolerance occur during trials, continue until the patient achieves the trial criteria, and report to team so that additional planning can occur (e.g., extubation) or follow protocol steps to extubation.		

Documentation

Documentation should include the following:

- Patient and family education
- Individualized goals for weaning
- Procedure used for weaning (e.g., t-piece, decreasing IMV/SIMV support, pressure support, flow-by positive end-expiratory pressure, or CPAP)
- Parameters used to assess patient readiness to wean and weaning trial tolerance, such as arterial blood gases, oximetry readings, BWAP score, negative inspiratory pressure, positive expiratory pressure, spontaneous Vt, vital capacity, mechanical ventilation,

dynamic characteristics, static compliance measurements, airway resistance measurement, breathing pattern, and accessory muscle use
- Patient response to decrements in mechanical ventilation support
- Mode or method of weaning
- Duration of trial
- Level of support (if appropriate, as in PSV, flow-by, or CPAP)
- Unexpected outcomes
- Nursing interventions

References

1. Banner, M.J., Blanch, P.B., and Kirby, R.R. (1993). Imposed work of breathing and methods of triggering a demand-flow continuous positive airway system. *Crit Care Med, 21*, 183-90.
2. Bellemare, F., and Grassino, A. (1982). Evaluation of human diaphragm fatigue. *J Appl Physiol, 53*, 1196-206.
3. Beydon, L., et al. (1988). Inspiratory work of breathing during spontaneous ventilation using demand values and continuous flow systems. *Am Rev Respir Dis, 138*, 300-4.
4. Brochard, L., et al. (1989). Inspiratory pressure support prevents diaphragmatic fatigue during weaning from mechanical ventilation. *Am Rev Respir Dis, 139*, 513-21.
5. Brochard, L., Pluskwa, F., and Lemaire, F. (1987). Improved efficacy of spontaneous breathing with inspiratory pressure support. *Am Rev Respir Dis, 136*, 411-5.
6. Brochard, L., et al. (1994). Comparison of three methods of gradual withdrawal from ventilatory support during weaning from mechanical ventilation. *Am J Respir Crit Care, 150*, 896-903.
7. Burns, S.M., Burns, J.E., and Truwit, J.D. (1994). Comparison of five clinical weaning indices. *Am J Crit Care, 3*, 342-52.
8. Burns, S.M., et al. (1995). Weaning from long-term mechanical ventilation. *Am J Crit Care, 4*, 4-22.
9. Burns, S.M., et al. (2003). Implementation of an institutional program to improve clinical and financial outcomes of patients requiring mechanical ventilation: one year outcomes and lessons learned. *Crit Care Med, 31*, 2752-63.
10. Burns, S.M., et al. (1998). Design, testing and results of an outcomes-managed approach to patients requiring prolonged ventilation. *Am J Crit Care, 7*, 45-7.
11. Burns, S.M., Ryan, B., and Burns, J.E. (2000). The weaning continuum: Use of APACHE III, BWAP, TISS, and WI scores to establish stages of weaning. *Crit Care Med, 28*, 2259-67.
12. Cohen, I.L., et al. (1991). Reduction of duration and cost of mechanical ventilation in an intensive care unit by use of a ventilatory management team. *Crit Care Med, 19*, 1278-84.
13. Cohen, C.A., et al. (1982). Clinical manifestations of inspiratory fatigue. *Am J Med, 73*, 308-16.
14. Cook, D., et al. (1999). *Evidence Report on Criteria for Weaning From Mechanical Ventilation.* Contract No. 290-97-0017. Rockville, MD: Agency for Health Care Policy and Research.
15. Ely, E.W., et al. (1998). Effect on the duration of mechanical ventilation of identifying patients capable of breathing spontaneously. *N Engl J Med, 335*, 1864-9.
16. Esteban, A., et al. (1995). A comparison of four methods of weaning patients from mechanical ventilation. *N Engl J Med, 332*, 345-50.
17. Esteban, A., et al., and the Spanish Lung Failure Collaborative Group. (1994). Modes of mechanical ventilation and weaning: A national survey of Spanish hospitals. *Chest, 106*, 1188-93.

18. Fiastro, J.F., et al. (1988). Comparison of standard weaning parameters and the work of breathing in mechanically ventilated patients. *Chest, 93*, 499-505.
19. Gibney, N.R.T., Wilson, R.S., and Pontoppidan, H. (1982). Comparison of work of breathing on high gas flow and demand valve continuous positive airway pressure systems. *Chest, 82*, 692-5.
20. Gurevitch, M.J., and Gelmont, D. (1989). Importance of trigger sensitivity in ventilator response delay in advanced chronic obstructive pulmonary disease with respiratory failure. *Crit Care Med, 17*, 354-9.
21. Hanneman, S.K.G. (1994). Multidimensional predictors of success or failure with early weaning from mechanical ventilation after cardiac surgery. *Nurs Res, 43*, 4-10.
22. Hanneman, S.K., et al. (1994). Weaning from short-term mechanical ventilation: A review. *Am J Crit Care, 3*, 421-43.
23. Henneman, E., et al. (2001). Effect of a collaborative weaning plan on patient outcome in the critical care setting. *Crit Care Med, 29*, 297-303.
24. Henneman, E., et al. (2002). Using a collaborative weaning plan to decrease duration of mechanical ventilation and length of stay in the intensive care unit for patients receiving long-term mechanical ventilation. *Am J Crit Care, 11*, 132-40.
25. Knebel, A.R., et al. (1998). Weaning from mechanical ventilatory support: Refinement of a model. *Am J Crit Care, 7*, 149-52.
26. Kollef, M.H., et al. (1997). A randomized, controlled trial of protocol-directed versus physician-directed weaning from mechanical ventilation. *Crit Care Med, 25*, 557-74.
27. MacIntyre, N.R. (1986). Respiratory function during pressure support ventilation. *Chest, 89*, 677-83.
28. MacIntyre, N.R. (1988). Weaning from mechanical ventilatory support: Volume-assisting intermittent breaths versus pressure assisting every breath. *Respir Care, 33*, 121-5.
29. MacIntyre, N.R. (1997). Ventilatory modes and mechanical ventilatory support. *Crit Care Med, 25*, 1106-7.
30. MacIntyre, N.R., et al. (2001). Evidence-based guidelines for weaning and discontinuing ventilatory support: A collective task force facilitated by the American College of Chest Physicians; the American Association for Respiratory Care; and the American College of Critical Care Medicine. *Chest, 120*(6 Suppl), 375S-95S.
31. Morganroth, M.L., et al. (1984). Criteria for weaning from prolonged mechanical ventilation. *Am J Crit Care, 144*, 1012-6.
32. Sassoon, C.S.H., et al. (1992). Inspiratory muscle work of breathing during flow-by, demand-flow, and continuous-flow systems in patients with chronic obstructive pulmonary disease. *Am Rev Respir Dis, 145*, 1219-22.

33. Scheinhorn, D.J., Artinian, B.M., and Catlin, J.L. (1994). Weaning from prolonged, mechanical ventilation: The experience at a regional weaning center. *Chest,* 105, 534-9.

34. Smyrnios, N.A., et al. (2002). Effects of a multifaceted, multidisciplinary, hospital-wide quality improvement program on weaning from mechanical ventilation. *Crit Care Med,* 30, 1224-30.

35. Tobin, M.J., et al. (1987). Konno-Mead analysis of ribcage-abdominal motion during successful and unsuccessful trials of weaning from mechanical ventilation. *Am Rev Respir Dis,* 135, 1320-8.

36. Yang, K.L., and Tobin, J.M. (1994). A prospective study of indexes predicting the outcome of trials of weaning from mechanical ventilation. *N Engl J Med,* 324, 1445-50.

Additional Readings

Burns, S.M. (1998). Mechanical ventilation and weaning. In: Kinney, M.R., et al., editors. *AACN's Clinical Reference for Critical Care Nursing.* 4th ed. St. Louis: Mosby-Yearbook, 624-7.

Burns, S.M. (In press). Weaning from long-term mechanical ventilation. In: MacArthur B., executive editor, and Burns, S.M., series editor. *AACN Protocols for Practice: Care of the Mechanically Ventilated Patient.* Aliso Viejo, CA: American Association of Critical-Care Nurses.

MacIntyre, N.R. (1995). Weaning mechanical ventilatory support. In: Dantzker, D.R., MacIntyre, N.R., and Bakow, E.D., editors. *Comprehensive Respiratory Care.* Philadelphia: W.B. Saunders, 735-42.

Tobin, M.J., and Alex, C.G. (1994). Discontinuation of mechanical ventilation. In: Tobin, M.J., editor. *Principles and Practice of Mechanical Ventilation.* New York: McGraw-Hill, 1177-206.

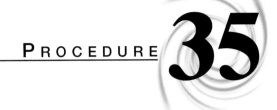

PROCEDURE **35**

Automated External Defibrillation

PURPOSE: An automated external defibrillator (AED) is a defibrillator that, by use of a computerized detection system, analyzes cardiac rhythms, distinguishes between rhythms that require defibrillation and rhythms that do not, and delivers a series of preprogrammed electric shocks. The AED is designed to allow early defibrillation by providers who have minimal or no training in rhythm recognition or manual defibrillation.

Charlotte A. Green
Karen K. Carlson

PREREQUISITE NURSING KNOWLEDGE

- Defibrillation is the therapeutic use of an electric shock that temporarily stops or stuns an irregularly beating heart and allows more coordinated electrical activity to resume. Physiologically, it is thought that the shock depolarizes the myocardium, terminates ventricular fibrillation (VF) or ventricular tachycardia (VT), and allows normal electric activity to occur. VF and pulseless VT are the only two rhythms amenable to conversion by an AED.

- Time is the major determining factor in the success rates of defibrillation. For every minute defibrillation is delayed, the chance of success decreases by 7% to 10%.[3-5]

- The AED (Fig. 35-1) is attached to the patient using adhesive electrode pads. Through these pads, the rhythm is analyzed and shock delivered, if indicated. If the AED

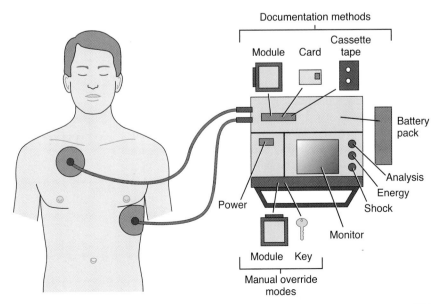

FIGURE 35-1 Generic AED control panel.

recognizes VF or VT, visual and verbal prompts guide the operator to deliver a shock to the patient. The AED, not the operator, makes the decision about whether the rhythm is appropriate for defibrillation.

- The chance of the AED shocking inappropriately is minimal.[7] The AED should be applied only to unresponsive, nonbreathing, and pulseless patients. To keep artifact interference to a minimum, the patient should not be touched or moved during the analysis time. Equipment that emits strong electromagnetic frequency or radiofrequency could affect analysis. Radiofrequency interference may cause electrocardiogram (ECG) distortion and failure to detect a shockable rhythm. Keep equipment such as cellular phones, CB radios, and emergency medical system (EMS) radios at least 6 feet away from the AED while analysis is occurring.

- Although defibrillation is the definitive treatment for pulseless VT and VF, the use of the AED is not a stand-alone skill; it is used in conjunction with cardiopulmonary resuscitation (CPR).

- The AED is now recommended for use in children age 1 through 8 years if the child shows no signs of circulation and if the defibrillator shows high specificity for pediatric shockable rhythms (check with the manufacturer). It is best if the defibrillator has pediatric pads, which have an attenuator in the cord that decreases the amount of energy delivered. If using adult pads, ensure that they do not overlap or touch each other or other things because doing so may cause electrical arching and skin burns and divert defibrillation energy; they should be at least 1 inch apart. If you cannot fit them on the child's chest in a lead two position, use an anterior/posterior pad placement. Never use pediatric pads on an adult or large child because the reduced energy levels delivered by these electrodes may not be effective for treating VF.[1-3,5,6,9]

- The use of AEDs in prehospital settings has increased the success of defibrillation. It is recommended that AEDs be placed on any nonmonitored unit where the response time of the resuscitation (i.e., code) team is greater than 1 minute.[5,8] It also is recommended that AEDs be placed in freestanding health care settings where health care providers are not familiar with rhythm recognition or defibrillation.

- Many manual defibrillators can be purchased that have AED capability allowing a tiered response (i.e., individuals with different skill levels can use the same defibrillator).

- Most AEDs in use in EMS or in the hospital have a method of recording the event. These can be in the form of rhythm strip printouts, audio and event recording devices, data cards, or computer chips that can print an event summary.[5]

- AEDs can be purchased with and without monitor screens. AEDs with screens may allow the provider with rhythm recognition skills to override the AED's analysis and recommendations.

- An important safety issue an AED operator must address is the possibility of inadvertently shocking a bystander or other provider at the scene. It is imperative that the operator clear the patient verbally and visibly, by looking at the patient from head to toe, before discharging energy to the patient.

- All defibrillation programs need to include training for the potential operators. Training should include psychomotor skills, troubleshooting, equipment maintenance, and how to interface with advanced cardiac life support (ACLS) providers.[4,5,9]

- Specific information regarding the use of an institution's AED, including monitoring, recording, overriding, troubleshooting, and safety features, is available from the manufacturer. It is each provider's responsibility to be familiar with this information before using the AED.

- When a resuscitation team (e.g., 911 responders, code team, ACLS providers) arrives, they assume responsibility for monitoring and treating the patient. Ideally, they should continue to use the AED to monitor and shock, if possible, allowing the AED provider to operate the AED.[4,5] There are two reasons to change to a standard monitor and defibrillator: if the AED does not have a monitoring screen and if transport would interfere with the AED's ability to analyze. Some manufacturers have AEDs and manual defibrillators with compatible cables allowing a quick, smooth transition from one device to the other.[4,5]

EQUIPMENT

- AED
- Disposable gloves
- Barrier device or airway management equipment
- Spare sets of gauze pads in sealed packages
- Hand towel
- Scissors
- Razor

Additional equipment, which varies based on the model and abilities of the device, includes the following:

- One or two spare sets of adhesive electrode pads
- Spare charged battery if appropriate for the machine
- Adequate ECG paper
- Spare data card

PATIENT AND FAMILY EDUCATION

- AEDs are used in emergency situations. There is limited or no time to educate the family about the equipment and its uses. Occasionally, after a sudden cardiac event, a patient may be discharged from an institution with an AED. In these situations, patient and family education would be essential.[5]

PATIENT PREPARATION AND ASSESSMENT

Patient Assessment

- Establish that patient is unresponsive, nonbreathing, and pulseless. ➤➤*Rationale:* AEDs are indicated for the treatment of patients in cardiac arrest.

Patient Preparation

- Remove clothing from the chest, ensure that skin is dry where electrodes or pads will be placed, and remove any medication patches from the chest if located where electrode pads need to be placed. If excessive hair interferes with good contact, either shave the area before applying the pad or apply the pad, then immediately remove the pad and hair and apply a new pad in the same area.[3-5,9] ➤➤*Rationale:* Good contact must be ensured to analyze the rhythm and to defibrillate most effectively.

Procedure for Automated External Defibrillation

Steps	Rationale	Special Considerations
1. Establish that patient is unresponsive, not breathing, and pulseless.	AEDs are indicated for the treatment of patients in cardiac arrest.	
2. Call for AED; activate emergency response procedures for your settings.	Defibrillation is the definitive treatment for VF. Time is crucial.	Knowing how to activate the emergency response team in your setting is vital.
3. Perform CPR until the AED arrives.	CPR helps keep the patient in a rhythm amenable to defibrillation longer, increasing the chance that defibrillation will be effective.	Personal protective equipment is used in all settings, including gloves and a mask-valve device or a barrier device.
4. Press the *on* button.	When the AED is on, the prompts tell you what to do.	
5. Attach the pads to the patient (Fig. 35-2): one pad below the right clavicle to the right of the sternum and the other to the left of the left nipple on the midaxillary line. An alternative pad position would be anterior/posterior placement, where one patch is anterior over the left apex and the other is posterior behind the heart in the infrascapular location.	This placement also ensures that the heart is between the two patches, maximizing the current flow through the heart.	Placing the sternal pad on the sternum decreases the effectiveness of the shock because the defibrillating energy is going through bone to reach the heart.[5] Place the apex pad down on the midaxillary line to ensure that the energy is delivered to the heart, increasing your effectiveness.[5] Ensure that the patches are directly above and below each other.[6]
6. Place pads firmly to eliminate air pockets and to form a complete seal.	The AED uses the electrode pads to monitor and to shock.	Some models require attaching cables to the pads before placing them on the patient. Polarity of the pads is interchangeable for defibrillation purposes.[1]

Procedure continues on the following page

Procedure for Automated External Defibrillation—*Continued*

Steps	Rationale	Special Considerations
A. Do not place the pads over any medication or monitoring patches. Remove any medication pads from the chest.	Good contact must be ensured to defibrillate most effectively; air pockets under the electrode can cause electrical sparks and skin burns and divert defibrillating energy away from the heart.	If ECG monitoring is being done, the QRS complex is inverted if the positive and negative pads are reversed.
B. Do not place an AED pad directly over an implanted device (see Fig. 35-2). Try to stay at least 1 inch to the side of the power source of the pacemaker or internal cardiac defibrillator	Placing electrodes directly over an implanted device can divert defibrillating energy away from the heart.	After successfully defibrillating a patient with an implanted pacemaker or defibrillator, the device should be checked by an appropriate health care provider for programmed performance.[3-5]
7. Press the analyze button to analyze the patient's rhythm. Some AEDs automatically analyze the rhythm when they sense a patient connection or when the electrode pads are applied.	The machine needs to analyze the rhythm to determine if the heart rhythm is amenable to defibrillation.	Avoid CPR, transport, or any contact with the patient during the analyze mode. Radio transmitters and receivers and cell phones should be off or at least 6 feet from the AED.[3-5]
8. If a shock is advised, clear the patient visually and verbally.	The AED has determined that the rhythm is either VF or VT; defibrillation is needed. Maintain safety for everyone around the patient. If anyone is touching the patient or any conductive apparatus that is in contact with the patient (e.g., stretcher frame, intubation stylet) when the energy is discharged, he or she also may receive that shock.	Use a mnemonic such as "I'm clear, you're clear, we're all clear," and look at the patient head to toe while talking to ensure that no one is touching the patient. Another mnemonic is "Shocking on three. One, I am clear. Two, you are clear. Three, we are all clear. Shocking now."

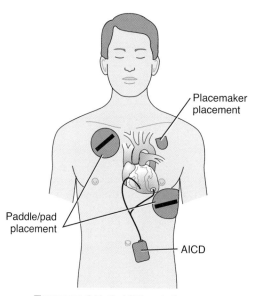

Placemaker placement

Paddle/pad placement

AICD

FIGURE 35-2 AED pad placement.

Procedure for Automated External Defibrillation—*Continued*

Steps	Rationale	Special Considerations
9. Push the shock button or buttons, as prompted.	Delivering the shock quickly is the best way to convert the fatal rhythm.	The energy levels for AEDs are preset; the shocks are delivered in sets of three as long as a shockable rhythm is detected. A CPR time interval usually occurs between the sets of shocks. Some AEDs are fully automatic and deliver a shock if needed without user interaction. In this case, the AED warns the user to stand clear before delivering the shock.
10. Reanalyze the rhythm.	The rhythm must be analyzed to determine if a shockable rhythm still persists. Shocks are delivered in sets of three only if the AED determines that another shock is indicated.	Remember to clear the patient for analysis. Some AEDs are fully automatic and deliver a shock if needed without user interaction. In this case, the AED warns the user to stand clear before delivering the shock.
11. If a shock is advised, clear the patient, and push the shock button.	The AED now delivers shocks according to preprogrammed energy settings, appropriate to the AED's technology and typically based on the American Heart Association (AHA) AED algorithm (a series of three shocks at 200, 300, and 360 J, or equivalent biphasic).[4,5]	
12. Repeat **Steps 10 and 11,** as needed.	No pulse check is needed between shocks.	Be sure to clear the patient for analysis and shocking.
13. After the third shock, or if a "no shock advised" message occurs, check the pulse.	Checking the pulse determines whether the last shock restored a perfusing rhythm and determines the need for continued CPR.	
14. If no pulse, do CPR for 1 minute or as per your protocol.	Provides oxygen and circulation.	Most AEDs have a CPR timer that counts down and alerts you when the time for CPR is complete. Time interval is usually 1 minute based on AHA guidelines[4,5,9] but can be configured to meet local protocols.
15. Repeat **Steps 7 to 14** if so advised until ACLS team arrives.[4]	Algorithm is series of three shocks followed by 1 minute of CPR with the series repeated until resuscitation units arrive.	
16. If at any time a "no shock advised" message occurs, check the pulse.	If the "no shock advised" message is given, the patient is not in a rhythm appropriate for defibrillation. A pulse always must be checked after a "no shock advised" message.	A "no shock advised" message does not imply that the patient has been resuscitated.

Procedure continues on the following page

Procedure for Automated External Defibrillation—*Continued*

Steps	Rationale	Special Considerations
17. If a "no shock advised" message occurs and there is no pulse, begin CPR.	CPR needs to be initiated to maintain circulation in the absence of a pulse.	
18. If a "no shock advised" message occurs and the patient has a pulse, check for breathing. If the patient is not breathing, begin rescue breathing, 12-15 breaths/min.	Defibrillation has been successful in restoring the patient to a perfusing rhythm, but spontaneous respirations are not present.	
19. Check blood pressure and treat as needed.	A perfusing rhythm has been restored. The patient needs to be evaluated and monitored until the resuscitation team arrives.	Be aware that patients could return to their original, pulseless rhythm. Patients need to be monitored closely. If at any time patients lose their pulse, begin again at **Step 7**.

Expected Outcomes

- Restoration of perfusing rhythm
- Restoration of spontaneous respirations

Unexpected Outcomes

- Operator or bystander shocked
- Skin burns

Patient Monitoring and Care

Steps	Rationale	Reportable Conditions
		These conditions should be reported if they persist despite nursing interventions.
1. Monitor vital signs and rhythm after resuscitation.	A patient experiencing VF or VT is at risk for development of arrhythmias, including further cardiac instability and recurrence of VF or VT.	• Change in vital signs from baseline • Arrhythmias
2. Administer appropriate antiarrhythmic agents as indicated.	Antiarrhythmic agents decrease the risk of development of further arrhythmias.	• Arrhythmias • Adverse effects of antiarrhythmics (e.g., hypotension, bradycardia)
3. Transport patient into appropriate follow-up care.	Hospitalized patients are transferred to a critical care unit; nonhospitalized patients should be transferred to an emergency department for follow-up care.	

Documentation

Documentation should include the following:

- Type of arrest (witnessed or unwitnessed)
- Time from patient collapse to first shock (only if witnessed)
- CPR information (including start and stop times)
- CPR performed before AED application: yes/no
- Application of AED
- Time from activation of AED to first shock
- Number of times patient was defibrillated

- Level of energy for each shock
- Preshock and postshock rhythms
- Any complications
- Assessment after resuscitation (if applicable)
- Unexpected outcomes
- Nursing interventions
- Patient and family education

References

1. Atkinson, E., et al. (2003). Specificity and sensitivity of automated external defibrillator rhythm analysis in infant and children. *Ann Emerg Med,* 42, 185-96.
2. Cecchin, F., et al. (2001). Is arrhythmia detection by automatic external defibrillator accurate for children? *Circulation,* 103(20):2438-8.
3. Chameides, L., editor. (2002). *Heartsaver First Aid with CPR and AED.* Dallas: American Heart Association, 84-6.
4. Cummins, R.O., editor. (2001). *ACLS Provider Manual.* Dallas: American Heart Association, 63-95.
5. Cummins, R.O., editor. (2003). *ACLS—The Reference Textbook, ACLS: Principles and Practice.* Dallas: American Heart Association, 89-133.
6. Jorgenson, D., et al. (2002). Energy attenuator for pediatric application of an automated external defibrillator. *Crit Care Med,* 30(Suppl 8), S145-7.
7. Martinez-Rubio, A., et al. (2003). Advances for treating in-hospital cardiac arrest: Safety and effectiveness of a new automatic external cardioverter-defibrillator. *J Am Coll Cardiol,* 41, 627-32.
8. Powers, C., and Martin, N. (2002). When seconds count, use an AED. *Am J Nurs,* May(Suppl), 102,8-10.
9. Samson, R., Berg, R., Bingham, R., and PALS Task Force. (2003). Use of automated external defibrillators for children: an update. An advisory statement from the Pediatric Advanced Life Support Task Force, International Liaison Committee on Resuscitation. *Resuscitation,* 57, 237-43.
10. Stapelton, E., (editor) (2001). *BLS for Healthcare Providers.* Dallas: American Heart Association, 91-121.

Additional Readings

Henderson, S., and Ballesteros, D. (2001). Evaluation of a hospital-wide resuscitation team: Does it increase survival for in-hospital cardiopulmonary arrest? *Resuscitation,* 48, 111-6.

Hernandez, B., and Christensen, J. (2001). Automatic external defibrillator intervention in the workplace: A comprehensive approach to program development. *AAOHN,* 49, 96-108.

White, R. (2002). New concepts in transthorasic defibrillation. *Emerg Med Clin North Am,* 20.

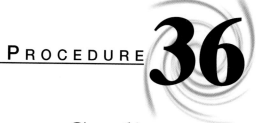
PROCEDURE **36**

Cardioversion

P U R P O S E :   Cardioversion is the therapy of choice for termination of hemodynamically unstable tachydysrhythmias. It also may be used to convert hemodynamically stable atrial fibrillation or atrial flutter into normal sinus rhythm.

Cynthia Hambach

PREREQUISITE NURSING KNOWLEDGE

- Understanding of the anatomy and physiology of the cardiovascular system, principles of cardiac conduction, basic dysrhythmia interpretation, and electric safety is needed.
- Advanced cardiac life support knowledge and skills are needed.
- Clinical and technical competence in the use of the defibrillator is needed.
- Synchronized cardioversion is recommended for termination of unstable paroxysmal supraventricular tachycardia, atrial fibrillation, atrial flutter, and unstable ventricular tachycardia with a pulse.[6,7,18,19,33,46,50] Because ventricular tachycardia is often a precursor to ventricular fibrillation, cardioversion has the potential to prevent this life-threatening dysrhythmia.[50]
- The electric current delivered with cardioversion depolarizes the myocardium in an attempt to restore the heart's coordinated impulse conduction as a single source of impulse generation. A countershock synchronized to the QRS complex allows for the electric current to be delivered outside the heart's vulnerable period.[6,7,18,19,33,41,46,50] This synchronization occurs a few milliseconds after the highest part of the R wave, but before the vulnerable period associated with the T wave.[18,33,41,50]
- Cardioversion may be implemented in the patient with an emergent condition. The aforementioned dysrhythmias are converted by synchronized cardioversion when the patient develops symptoms from the rapid ventricular response.[46] Symptoms may include the following: hypotension, chest pressure, shortness of breath, dyspnea

on exertion, decreased level of consciousness, pulmonary edema, rales, rhonchi, jugular vein distention, peripheral edema, and ischemic electrocardiogram (ECG) changes.[7]
- Elective cardioversion may be used to convert hemodynamically stable atrial fibrillation or atrial flutter into normal sinus rhythm.[2,33,46] When used to convert atrial fibrillation or atrial flutter, anticoagulation is considered for 3 weeks before cardioversion to decrease the risk of thromboembolism.[2,7,12,14,21,28,33,41,46] Anticoagulation may not be necessary if atrial fibrillation or atrial flutter has been present for less than 48 hours.[7,12,14,21,33] A physician may choose to perform a transesophageal echocardiogram to exclude the possibility of an atrial thrombus before cardioversion for patients at high risk for thromboembolism, even if the duration is near the 48-hour time frame. The patient is started on intravenous heparin, and the cardioversion is performed within 24 to 48 hours.[2,7,14,28,46] Anticoagulation should be continued for 4 weeks after cardioversion because of the possibility of delayed embolism.[2,7,12,14,21,28,46] Thromboembolism is less likely to occur with atrial flutter.[21,33,46]
- Elective cardioversion also may be used in patients with hemodynamically stable ventricular or supraventricular tachydysrhythmias unresponsive to medication therapy.[7,46,50]
- If time and clinical condition permit, the patient should be given a combination of analgesia and sedation to minimize discomfort.[2,7,20,33,47]
- Defibrillators deliver energy or current in waveform patterns. Delivered energy levels may differ among the various defibrillators and waveforms. Various types of monophasic waveforms are used in most defibrillators. Biphasic waveforms have been designed more recently

and are used in implantable defibrillators, automatic external defibrillators, and some manual defibrillators.

- ❖ Monophasic waveforms deliver energy in one direction. The energy travels through the heart from one paddle or pad to the other.[18,34]
- ❖ Biphasic waveforms deliver energy in two directions. The energy travels through the heart in a positive direction, then it reverses itself and flows back through the heart in a negative direction.[18,34] Biphasic waveform technology is able to decrease the amount of current needed to terminate the dysrhythmia, decreasing the amount of potential damage to the myocardium.[16,32,40,48] In more recent studies, atrial fibrillation was successfully cardioverted with biphasic waveform shocks ranging from 100 to 150 J.[18,35,38,42] More research is needed to determine a specific recommendation for biphasic waveform cardioversion.[16,18] For that reason, the American Heart Association states that biphasic waveform shocks are acceptable if documented as clinically equivalent to reports of monophasic shocks.[7]
- Some biphasic defibrillators measure and compensate for transthoracic impedance before the delivery of the shock. This allows the defibrillator to deliver the actual amount of energy selected by the rescuer.[32,40]

EQUIPMENT

- Defibrillator/monitor with ECG oscilloscope/recorder capable of delivering a synchronized shock
- ECG cable
- Conductive gel or paste, prepackaged gelled conduction pads or self-adhesive defibrillation pads connected directly to the defibrillator
- Intravenous sedative or analgesic pharmacologic agents as prescribed
- Bag-valve-mask oxygen delivery device
- Flowmeter for oxygen administration, oxygen source
- Emergency suction and intubation equipment
- Blood pressure monitoring equipment
- Intravenous infusion pumps
  Additional equipment to have available as needed includes the following:
- Cardiac board
- Emergency medications
- Emergency pacing equipment

PATIENT AND FAMILY EDUCATION

- Assess patient and family understanding of the etiology of the dysrhythmia. ➤*Rationale:* This assessment determines the patient and family understanding of the condition and additional educational needs.
- Explain the procedure to the patient and family. ➤*Rationale:* This decreases anxiety and promotes patient cooperation.
- Explain the signs and symptoms of hemodynamic compromise associated with the preexisting cardiac dysrhythmias to the patient and family. ➤*Rationale:* This explanation enables the patient and family to recognize when the patient needs to notify the nurse or physician.
- Evaluate and discuss with the patient the need for long-term pharmacologic support. ➤*Rationale:* This allows the nurse to anticipate educational needs of the patient and family regarding specific discharge medications.
- Assess and discuss with the patient the need for lifestyle changes. ➤*Rationale:* The underlying pathophysiology may necessitate alterations in the patient's current lifestyle and require a plan for behavioral changes.

PATIENT ASSESSMENT AND PREPARATION

Patient Assessment

- Assess the patient's ECG for tachydysrhythmias, including paroxysmal supraventricular tachycardia, atrial fibrillation, atrial flutter, and ventricular tachycardia, which could require synchronized cardioversion. ➤*Rationale:* Tachydysrhythmias may precipitate deterioration of hemodynamic stability.[7]
- Assess the patient's vital signs and any associated symptoms of hemodynamic compromise with each significant change in ECG rate and rhythm. ➤*Rationale:* Deterioration of vital signs or the presence of associated symptoms indicates hemodynamic compromise that could become life-threatening.[7]
- Assess for the presence or absence of peripheral pulses and the patient's level of consciousness. ➤*Rationale:* This baseline determination assists in the detection of cardioversion-induced peripheral embolization.[12,14,28,33,41,46,47]
- Obtain the patient's serum potassium, magnesium, and digitalis levels and arterial blood gas results. ➤*Rationale:* Electrolyte imbalances, acid-base disturbances, and digitalis toxicity significantly contribute to electrical instability and may potentiate postconversion dysrhythmias.[41,46,47] Hypokalemia should be corrected to prevent postconversion dysrhythmias. Although cardioversion is considered a safe practice in patients taking digitalis glycosides, they generally are held on the day of cardioversion.[33]

Patient Preparation

- Ensure that the patient and family understand preprocedural teaching. Answer questions as they arise, and reinforce information as needed. ➤*Rationale:* This communication evaluates and reinforces understanding of previously taught information.
- Validate that informed consent has been obtained according to institutional policy. ➤*Rationale:* Informed consent is advised before performing cardioversion unless the patient presents in a life-threatening state.[51]
- Establish a patent intravenous access. ➤*Rationale:* Medication administration may be required.[7]
- Assist the patient to a supine position. ➤*Rationale:* Supine positioning provides the best access for procedure initiation, intervention, and management of possible adverse effects.

- Remove all metallic objects from the patient. ➤*Rationale:* Metallic objects are excellent conductors of electric current and could result in burns.
- Remove transdermal medication patches from the patient's chest or ensure the defibrillator pad or paddle does not touch the patch.[7,31,40] ➤*Rationale:* Transdermal nitroglycerin patches may produce a chest burn when the paddle is placed over it.[18,39]
- Ensure that the patient is in a dry environment, and dry the patient's chest, if it is wet. ➤*Rationale:* Water is a conductor of electricity. If the patient and rescuer are in contact with water, the rescuer may receive a shock or the patient may receive skin burn.[18,40] Also, if the patient's chest is wet, the current may travel from one paddle across the water to the other, resulting in a decreased amount of energy to the myocardium.[6,7,18,40]
- Give the patient nothing by mouth per institution policy. ➤*Rationale:* This decreases the risk of aspiration.

- Remove loose-fitting dentures, partial plates, or other mouth prostheses. ➤*Rationale:* This decreases the risk of airway obstruction during the procedure. Evaluate each individual situation (e.g., dentures may facilitate a tighter seal for airway management).
- Preoxygenate the patient as appropriate to the condition. ➤*Rationale:* Adequate oxygenation of cardiac tissue diminishes the risk of cerebral and cardiac complications.[7,18]
- Maintain a patent airway with oxygenation throughout the procedure. ➤*Rationale:* Respiratory depression and hypoventilation can occur after administration of sedatives and analgesics.[51]
- If time allows, consider administering sedation and analgesia. ➤*Rationale:* These medications provide amnesia and decrease pain during the procedure.[2,7,47]

Procedure   for Cardioversion

Steps	Rationale	Special Considerations
1. Wash hands.	Reduces the transmission of microorganisms; standard precautions.	
2. Connect the patient to the lead wires.	The R wave must be sensed by the defibrillator to achieve synchronization for cardioversion.[7,33,41,50]	
3. Select a monitor lead displaying an R wave of sufficient amplitude to activate the synchronization mode of the defibrillator. In most models, synchronization is achieved when the monitoring lead produces a tall R wave. *(Level VI: Clinical studies in a variety of patient populations and situations to support recommendations.)*	Synchronized cardioversion must sense the R wave to deliver the current outside the heart's vulnerable period.[6,18,33,41,46,50] Lead II generally produces a large R wave.[41]	If a combination defibrillator/ monitor is not being used, a converter cable must connect the monitor to the defibrillator to achieve synchronization.
4. Place the defibrillator in the synchronization mode. Ensure that the patient's QRS complexes appear with a marker to signify correct synchronization of the defibrillator with the patient's ECG rhythm (Fig. 36-1). To confirm that the synchronization has been achieved, observe for visual flashing on the screen or listen for auditory beeps. If necessary, adjust the R wave gain until the synchronization marker appears on each R wave. *(Level VI: Clinical studies in a variety of patient populations and situations to support recommendations.)*	Synchronization prevents the random delivery of an electric charge, which may cause ventricular fibrillation.[6,18,33,41,46,50]	

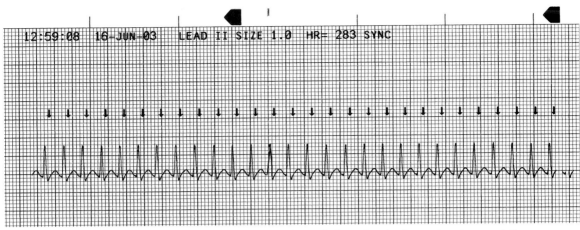

FIGURE 36-1 R wave synchronization. Note the vertical synchronization marker above each R wave.

Procedure	**for Cardioversion**—*Continued*	
Steps	**Rationale**	**Special Considerations**
5. If the defibrillator is unable to distinguish between the peak of the QRS complex and the peak of the T wave, as in polymorphic ventricular tachycardia, proceed with unsynchronized defibrillation (see Procedure 37).	This avoids a delay or failure of shock delivery in the synchronized mode.[18,50]	
6. Prepare the patient or paddles or both with the proper conductive agent. *(Level VI: Clinical studies in a variety of patient populations and situations to support recommendations.)*	Reduces transthoracic resistance, enhancing electric conduction through subcutaneous tissue.[5,6,10,17-20,33,40,41,43,50] Minimizes erythema from the electric current.[19,41]	Prepackaged gelled conductive pads are available for placement in the area of the paddle.[50] Gel pads should be replaced if they appear to be drying out or after three countershocks.[19] Never use alcohol-soaked pads because they are combustible when in contact with electric current. Conductive gel should be evenly dispersed on the defibrillator paddles and should adequately cover the surface; be careful not to smear gel between paddles because current may follow through the alternate pathway over the chest wall and avoid the heart.[4,6,18-20,24,33,40,46] Do not use inappropriate gel (i.e., ultrasound gel) because it increases the transthoracic resistance and decreases the current given to the patient[17,43]; it also may cause burns or sparks, which can increase the risk of fire.[17] Self-adhesive defibrillation pads connected directly to the defibrillator have been found to be as effective as paddles.[8,9,20,24,44,49,50] Advantages of "hands-free" cardioversion are safety and convenience of use in any of the appropriate locations.[8,24,44,49,50]

Procedure continues on the following page

Procedure for Cardioversion—*Continued*

Steps	Rationale	Special Considerations
7. Ensure that the defibrillator cables are positioned to allow for adequate access to the patient.	Allows cardioversion to occur without excessive tension on the cables.	
8. Turn on the ECG recorder for a continuous printout.	Establishes a visual recording of the patient's current ECG status and response to intervention and provides a permanent record of the patient response to intervention.	
9. Follow these steps for paddle placement. A. Place one paddle at the heart's apex just to the left of the nipple at the midaxillary line. Place the other paddle just below the right clavicle to the right of the sternum (Fig. 36-2). *(Level VI: Clinical studies in a variety of patient populations and situations to support recommendations.)*	Cardioversion is achieved by passing an electric current through the cardiac muscle mass to restore a single source of impulse generation; this pathway maximizes current flow through the myocardium.[6,7,10,18-20,33,41,46,50]	A larger paddle size (12-13 cm) decreases the transthoracic resistance and improves current flow.[5,9,10,20,25,45] Most paddles are 8-12 cm in diameter and are effective.[6,18,20,22,46,50] Avoid placing paddles over lead wires.[31]
B. In women, the apex paddle is placed at the fifth to sixth intercostal space with the center of the paddle at the midaxillary line.	Placement over a woman's breast should be avoided to reduce transthoracic resistance.[8,44]	
C. Anterior-posterior placement also may be used. *(Level VI: Clinical studies in a variety of patient populations and situations to support recommendations.)*	All methods of paddle placement are effective.[13,18,20,22,24,33,36,50] Some investigators have found the anterior-posterior placement to be more effective.[3,27]	

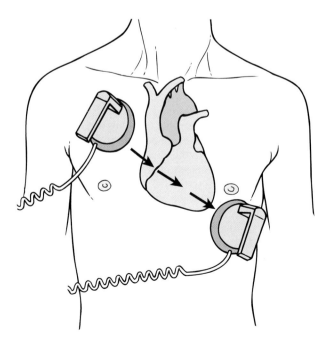

FIGURE 36-2 Paddle placement and current flow in cardioversion and defibrillation. *(From Lewis, S., Heitkemper, M., and Dirksen, M. [2004]. Medical Surgical Nursing: Assessment and Management of Clinical Problems. 6th ed. St. Louis: Mosby.)*

Procedure for Cardioversion—*Continued*

Steps	Rationale	Special Considerations
(1) Self-adhesive defibrillation pads are used for this approach. (2) The anterior pad is placed in the anterior left precordial area (Fig. 36-3). (3) The posterior pad is placed posteriorly behind the heart in the right or left infrascapular area (see Fig. 36-3). (4) An alternative approach is to place the anterior pad in the right infraclavicular area and the posterior pad in the left infrascapular position.		
D. In a patient with a permanent pacemaker, do not place paddles directly over the pulse generator. *(Level IV: Limited clinical studies to support recommendations.)*	Cardioversion over an implanted pacemaker may impair passage of current to the patient and may cause the device to malfunction or become damaged.[7,10,15,18,20,30,37] Myocardial injury also may occur if the current flows down the lower resistance pathway of the lead wire(s).[30,33,37]	Some authors recommend paddle placement at least 5 inches (10-13 cm) from the pulse generator and lead wire(s).[10,15,33,37,50] Anterior-posterior placement also is suggested.[15,30,37] The pacemaker should be assessed after any electric countershock.[10,15,18,20,30,33,37] Standby emergency pacing equipment should be available should pacemaker failure occur.[15,29,37]
E. Paddle placement in the patient with an implantable cardioverter-defibrillator (ICD) is the same as standard paddle placement for cardioversion (see Fig. 36-2). Paddles should not be placed over the device.	Cardioversion over an implanted pacemaker may impair passage of current to the patient and cause the device to malfunction or become damaged.[7,18,50]	The ICD should be checked after external countershock.[18,40,50]
10. Charge defibrillator paddles as prescribed or in accordance with the recommendations of the American Heart Association (Table 36-1). *(Level VI: Clinical studies in a variety of patient populations and situations to support recommendations.)*	The defibrillator is charged with the lowest energy level required to convert the tachydysrhythmia.[16,18,23,26,40]	

Procedure continues on the following page

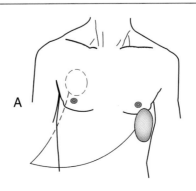
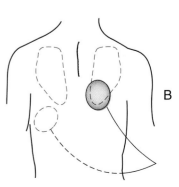

A   B

FIGURE 36-3 Anterior-posterior placement of self-adhesive defibrillation pads. **A,** Anterior pad placed over the left precordium. **B,** Posterior pad placed under the right scapula.

TABLE 36-1	American Heart Association Energy Level Recommendations for Treating Tachydysrhythmias		
Ventricular Tachycardia with Pulse	Paroxysmal Supraventricular Tachycardia	Atrial Fibrillation	Atrial Flutter
First Attempt			
Cardiovert with 100 J	Cardiovert with 50 J	Cardiovert with 100 J	Cardiovert with 50 J
Second Attempt			
Cardiovert with 200 J	Cardiovert with 100 J	Cardiovert with 200 J	Cardiovert with 100 J
Subsequent Attempts			
Cardiovert with 300 J, then 360 J	Cardiovert with 200 J, then 300 J, then 360 J	Cardiovert with 300 J, then 360 J	Cardiovert with 200 J, then 300 J, then 360 J

Note: These are recommendations for monophasic energy dose. It is acceptable to use clinically equivalent biphasic energy dose. Polymorphic ventricular tachycardia should be treated as ventricular fibrillation.
From Cummins, R.O. (2001). *ACLS Provider Manual.* Dallas: American Heart Association.

Procedure for Cardioversion—*Continued*

Steps	Rationale	Special Considerations
11. Disconnect the oxygen source during actual cardioversion.[19]	Decreases the risk of combustion in the presence of electric current.[6,17,19]	Arcing of electric current in the presence of oxygen could precipitate an explosion and subsequent fire hazard.[17,19]
12. Apply 25 lb/in^2 pressure to each paddle against the chest wall.[7]	Firm paddle pressure decreases transthoracic resistance, improving the flow of current across the axis of the heart.[6,10,18,20,25,33,40,43,46,50]	This application of pressure is not necessary for defibrillator models with newer hands-free and automatic transthoracic impedance sensing/correction options built in.
13. State "all clear" or similar wording three times, and visually verify that everyone is clear of contact with the patient, bed, and equipment.	Maintains safety to caregivers because electric current can be conducted from the patient to another individual if contact occurs.[19,33]	When using hands-free cardioversion, take special care to clear other personnel from patient contact because they will not have the visual cue of the paddles being placed on the patient's chest.
14. Verify that the defibrillator is in synchronization mode and that the patient's QRS complexes appear with a marker to signify correct synchronization of the defibrillator with the patient's ECG rhythm (see Fig. 36-1). *(Level VI: Clinical studies in a variety of patient populations and situations to support recommendations.)*	Synchronization prevents the randomdelivery of an electric charge, which may ventricular potentiate fibrillation.[6,18,19,33,41,46,50]	
15. Depress both buttons on the paddles simultaneously, and hold until the defibrillator fires. In the synchronized mode, there is a delay before the charge is released; this allows the sensing mechanism to detect the QRS complex.[7,41,50]	Depolarizes the cardiac muscle.[7]	If self-adhesive, hands-free defibrillation pads are used, the charge is delivered by depressing the discharge button on the defibrillator.
16. Observe the monitor for conversion of the tachydysrhythmia, and	Simultaneous depolarization of the myocardial muscle cells	If unsuccessful in converting the rhythm, proceed with repeated

Procedure for Cardioversion—*Continued*

Steps	Rationale	Special Considerations
assess the patient's pulse. If a pulse is noted, assess the patient's vital signs and level of consciousness.	should reestablish a single source of impulse generation.[6,7,18,19,33,41,46,50]	energy recommendations (see Table 36-1). Ensure that the defibrillator is still in the synchronization mode; many defibrillators revert back to the unsynchronized mode after cardioversion. Ventricular fibrillation may develop after cardioversion. If so, deactivate the synchronizer and follow the procedure for defibrillation (see Procedure 37).[7,41,50]
17. Clean the defibrillator, and remove any gel from the paddles.	Conductive gel accumulated on the defibrillator paddles impedes surface contact and increases transthoracic resistance. Self-adhesive defibrillation pads may crimp, crack, or fold with loss of adhesiveness.	Loss of adhesive integrity in self-adhesive defibrillation pads may occur in restless or diaphoretic patients.
18. Discard supplies in appropriate receptacle.	Standard precautions.	
19. Wash hands.	Reduces the transmission of microorganisms; standard precautions.	

Expected Outcomes

- Reestablishment of a single source of impulse generation for the cardiac muscle
- Hemodynamic stability

Unexpected Outcomes

- Continued tachydysrhythmias
- Ventricular fibrillation progressing to cardiopulmonary arrest
- Bradycardia
- Asystole
- Pulmonary edema
- Systemic embolization
- Respiratory complications
- Hypotension
- Pacemaker or ICD dysfunction
- Skin burns

Patient Monitoring and Care

Steps	Rationale	Reportable Conditions
		These conditions should be reported if they persist despite nursing interventions.
1. Evaluate neurologic status before and after cardioversion. Reorient as needed to person, place, and time.	An altered level of consciousness may occur after hemodynamically unstable dysrhythmias.[7,18] Cerebral emboli may develop as a postprocedure complication.[12,14,28,33,41,46,47]	• Change in level of consciousness • Sensory or motor changes
2. Monitor pulmonary status before and after cardioversion.	Hemodynamically unstable tachydysrhythmias may cause respiratory complications, such as pulmonary edema.[7,50]	• Dyspnea • Rales • Rhonchi • Slow, shallow respirations

Procedure continues on the following page

Patient Monitoring and Care—*Continued*

Steps	Rationale	Reportable Conditions
	Respiratory depression and hypoventilation can occur after administration of sedatives and analgesics.[51]	• Decrease in oxygen saturation as measured by pulse oximetry
3. Monitor cardiovascular status (blood pressure, heart rate, and rhythm) before and after cardioversion.	Dysrhythmias may develop after cardioversion.[2,11,33,41,46,47]	• Hypotension • Supraventricular dysrhythmias • Ventricular dysrhythmias • Bradycardia • Asystole
4. Continue to monitor the ECG after the procedure.	Dysrhythmias may develop after cardioversion.[2,11,33,41,46,47]	• Supraventricular dysrhythmias • Ventricular dysrhythmias • Bradycardia • Asystole
5. Prepare for possible intravenous antidysrhythmic medication.	Dysrhythmias may develop after cardioversion.[2,11,33,41,46,47]	• Supraventricular dysrhythmias • Ventricular dysrhythmias • Bradycardia • Asystole
6. Evaluate for burns.	Erythema at the electrode sites may be seen secondary to local hyperemia in the current pathway.[19] Skin burns may be minimized by use of gel pads or applying appropriate paste or gel to the paddles.[19,41]	• Skin burns

Documentation

Documentation should include the following:

- Patient and family education
- Neurologic, pulmonary, and cardiovascular assessment before and after cardioversion
- Interventions to prepare the patient for cardioversion
- The joules (J) used and the number of cardioversion attempts made
- Printout of the ECG tracing depicting the cardiac rhythm before and after cardioversion (before and after each attempt if more than one attempt is used)
- Condition of the skin of the chest wall
- Unexpected outcomes and nursing interventions
- Serum electrolytes, digoxin level, and coagulation laboratory results

References

1. Altamura, G., et al. (1995). Transthoracic DC shock may represent a serious hazard in pacemaker dependent patients. *Pacing Clin Electrophysiol*, 18(part II), 194-8.
2. American College of Cardiology/American Heart Association/American College of Physicians-American Society of Internal Medicine Task Force on Clinical Competence. (2000). American College of Cardiology/American Heart Association Clinical Competence Statement on Invasive Electrophysiology Studies, Catheter Ablation and Cardioversion. *Circulation*, 102, 230-920.
3. Botto, G.L., et al. (1999). External cardioversion of atrial fibrillation: Role of paddle position on technical efficacy and energy requirements. *Heart*, 82, 726-30.
4. Caterine, M.R., et al. (1997). Effect of electrode position and gel-application technique on predicted transcardiac current during transthoracic defibrillation. *Ann Emerg Med*, 29, 588-95.
5. Connell, P.N., et al. (1973). Transthoracic impedance to defibrillator discharge: Effect of electrode size and electrode-chest wall interface. *J Electrocardiol*, 6, 313-7.
6. Cooper, M., et al. (1998). A guide to defibrillation. *Emerg Nurse*, 6, 16-21.
7. Cummins, R.O., editor. (2001). *ACLS Procedure Manual*. Dallas: American Heart Association.
8. Dalzell, G.W. (1998). Determinants of successful defibrillation. *Heart*, 80, 405-7.
9. Dalzell, G.W., et al. (1989). Electrode pad size, transthoracic impedance and success of external ventricular defibrillation. *Am J Cardiol*, 64, 741-4.
10. Ewy, G.A. (1986). Electrical therapy for cardiovascular emergencies. *Circulation*, 74(Suppl IV), IV-111-6.
11. Eysmann, S.B., et al. (1986). Electrocardiographic changes after cardioversion of ventricular arrhythmias. *Circulation*, 73, 73-81.
12. Gallagher, M.M., et al. (2002). Embolic complications of direct current cardioversion of atrial arrhythmias: Association with low intensity of anticoagulation at the time of cardioversion. *J Am Coll Cardiol*, 40, 926-33.
13. Garcia, L.A., and Kerber, R.E. (1998). Transthoracic defibrillation: Does electrode adhesive pad position alter transthoracic impedance? *Resuscitation*, 37, 139-43.

14. Gentile, F., et al. (2002). Safety of electrical cardioversion in patients with atrial fibrillation. *Mayo Clin Proc, 77,* 897-904.
15. Gould, L., et al. (1981). Pacemaker failure following external defibrillation. *Pacing Clin Electrophysiol, 4,* 575-7.
16. Harris, J. (2002). Biphasic defibrillation. *Emerg Nurs, 10,* 33-7.
17. Hummel, R.S., et al. (1988). Spark-generating properties of electrode gels used during defibrillation: A potential fire hazard. *JAMA, 260,* 3021-4.
18. International Consensus on Science. (2000). Guidelines 2000 for cardiopulmonary resuscitation and emergency cardiovascular care. *Circulation, 102*(Suppl I), I-90-4.
19. Inwood, H., and Cull, C. (1997). Defibrillation. *Prof Nurse, 13,* 165-8.
20. Kerber, R.E. (1993). Electrical treatment of cardiac arrhythmias: Defibrillation and cardioversion. *Ann Emerg Med, 22*(Part 2), 296-301.
21. Kerber, R.E. (1996). Transthoracic cardioversion of atrial fibrillation and flutter: Standard technique and new advances. *Am J Cardiol, 78*(Suppl 8), 22-6.
22. Kerber, R.E., et al. (1981). Elective cardioversion: Influence of paddle-electrode location and size on success rates and energy requirements. *N Engl J Med, 305,* 658-62.
23. Kerber, R.E., et al. (1988). Energy, current and success in defibrillation and cardioversion: Clinical studies using an automated impedance-based method of energy adjustment. *Circulation, 77,* 1038-46.
24. Kerber, R.E., et al. (1984). Self-adhesive preapplied electrode pads for defibrillation and cardioversion. *J Am Coll Cardiol, 3,* 815-20.
25. Kerber, R.E., et al. (1981). Transthoracic resistance in human defibrillation: Influence of body weight, chest size, serial shocks, paddle size and paddle contact pressure. *Circulation, 3,* 676-82.
26. Kerber, R.E., et al. (1992). Ventricular tachycardia rate and morphology determine energy and current requirements for transthoracic cardioversion. *Circulation, 85,* 158-63.
27. Kirchhof, P., et al. (2002). Anterior-posterior versus anterior-lateral electrode positions for external cardioversion of atrial fibrillation: A randomized trial. *Lancet, 360,* 1275-9.
28. Klein, A.L., et al. (2001). Use of transesophageal echocardiography to guide cardioversion in patients with atrial fibrillation. *N Engl J Med, 344,* 1411-20.
29. Lau, F.Y., Bilitch, M., and Wintroub, H.J. (1969). Protection of implanted pacemakers from excessive electrical energy of DC shock. *Am J Cardiol, 23,* 244-9.
30. Levine, P.A., et al. (1983). Adverse acute and chronic effects of electrical defibrillation and cardioversion on implanted unipolar cardiac pacing systems. *J Am Coll Cardiol, 1,* 1413-22.
31. Lezon, K. (1998). Code blue: Defibrillate. *Nursing, 28,* 58-60.
32. Low-energy biphasic waveform defibrillation: Evidence-based review applied to emergency cardiovascular care guidelines. A statement for healthcare professionals from the American Heart Association Committee on Emergency Cardiovascular Care and the Subcommittees on Basic Life Support, Advanced Cardiac Life Support and Pediatric Resuscitation. (1998). *Circulation, 97,* 1654-67.
33. Lown, B., and deSilva, R.A. (1998). External cardioversion and defibrillation. In: Alexander, R.W., Schlant, R.C., and Fuster, V, editors. *Hurst's the heart: arteries and veins.* 9th ed. New York: McGraw-Hill.
34. Mair, M. (2003). Monophasic and biphasic defibrillators: The evolving technology of cardiac defibrillation. *Am J Nurs, 103,* 58-60.
35. Marinsek, M., et al. (2003). Efficacy and impact of monophasic versus biphasic countershocks for transthoracic cardioversion of persistent atrial fibrillation. *Am J Cardiol, 92,* 988-91.
36. Mathew, T.P., et al. (1999). Randomised comparison of electrode positions for cardioversion of atrial fibrillation. *Heart, 81,* 576-9.
37. Owen, P.M. (1983). The effects of external defibrillation on permanent pacemakers. *Heart Lung, 12,* 274-7.
38. Page, R.L., et al. (2002). Biphasic versus monophasic shock waveform for consversion of atrial fibrillation. *J Am Coll Cardiol, 39,* 1956-63.
39. Panacek, E.A., et al. (1992). Report of nitropatch explosions complicating defibrillation. *Am J Emerg Med, 10,* 128-9.
40. Peberdy, M.A. (2002). Defibrillation. *Cardiol Clin, 20,* 13-21.
41. Riley, M. (1997). Elective cardioversion: Who, when, and how. *RN, 60,* 27-9.
42. Scholten, M., et al. (2003). Comparison of monophasic and biphasic shocks for transthoracic cardioversion of atrial fibrillation. *Heart, 89,* 1032-4.
43. Sirna, S.J., et al. (1988). Factors affecting transthoracic impedance during electrical cardioversion. *Am J Cardiol, 62,* 1048-52.
44. Stults, K.R., et al. (1987). Self-adhesive monitor/defibrillation pads improve prehospital defibrillation success. *Ann Emerg Med, 16,* 872-7.
45. Thomas, E.D., et al. (1977). Effectiveness of direct current defibrillation: role of paddle electrode size. *Am Heart J, 93,* 463-7.
46. Trohman, R.G., and Parillo, J.E. (2000). Direct current cardioversion: Indications, techniques and recent advances. *Crit Care Med, 28*(Suppl), N170-N173.
47. Walker, J.R. (1999). Anesthesia for cardioversion. *J Perianesth Nurs, 14,* 35-8.
48. White, R.D. (2002). New concepts in transthoracic defibrillation. *Emerg Med Clin North Am, 20,* 785-807.
49. Wilson, R.F., et al. (1987). Defibrillation of high-risk patients during coronary angiography using self-adhesive, preapplied electrode pads. *Am J Cardiol, 60,* 380-2.
50. Woods, S.L., Sivarajan Froelicher, E.S., and Motzer, S.W., editors. (2000). *Cardiac Nursing.* 4th ed. Philadelphia: Lippincott Williams & Wilkins.
51. Yaney, L.L. (1998). Intravenous conscious sedation: Physiologic, pharmacologic and legal implications for nurses. *J Intravenous Nurs, 21,* 9-19.

Additional Reading

Lown, B. (2002). Defibrillation and cardioversion. *Cardiovasc Res, 55,* 220-4.

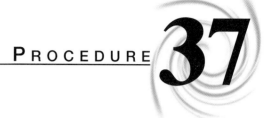

Defibrillation (External)

P U R P O S E : External defibrillation is performed to eradicate life-threatening ventricular fibrillation or pulseless ventricular tachycardia. The goal for defibrillation is to restore coordinated cardiac electrical and mechanical pumping action, resulting in restored cardiac output, tissue perfusion, and oxygenation.

Cynthia Hambach

PREREQUISITE NURSING KNOWLEDGE

- Understanding of the anatomy and physiology of the cardiovascular system, principles of cardiac conduction, basic dysrhythmia interpretation, and electric safety is needed.
- Advanced cardiac life support knowledge and skills are required.
- Clinical and technical competence in the use of the defibrillation is needed.
- Ventricular fibrillation and pulseless ventricular tachycardia are lethal dysrhythmias. Early emergent defibrillation is the treatment of choice to restore normal electrical activity and coordinated contractile activity within the heart.[4-6,13,15,16,28,32,38]
- The electric current delivered with defibrillation depolarizes the myocardium in an attempt to restore the heart's coordinated impulse conduction as a single source of impulse generation.[4,5,13,16,38] Defibrillator paddles placed over the patient's chest wall surface in the anterior-apex or anterior-posterior position maximize the current flow through the myocardium.[4,5,15,16,21]
- Defibrillators deliver energy or current in waveform patterns. Delivered energy levels may differ between different defibrillators and waveforms. Various types of monophasic waveforms are used in most current defibrillators. Biphasic waveforms have been designed more recently and are used currently in implantable defibrillators, automatic external defibrillators and some manual defibrillators.
  - ❖ Monophasic waveforms deliver energy in one direction. The energy travels through the heart from one paddle or pad to the other.

- ❖ Biphasic waveforms deliver energy in two directions. The energy travels through the heart in a positive direction, then it reverses itself and flows back through the heart in a negative direction.[15,29] Researchers have found that biphasic waveform technology is able to decrease the amount of current needed to terminate the dysrhythmia (less than or equal to 200 J), decreasing the amount of potential damage to the myocardium.[10,36] Researchers found that 115- to 130-J biphasic waveform shocks achieved the same first shock success rate as 200-J monophasic waveform shocks. These shocks also produced less ST-segment change than the monophasic shocks.[10,15,27] Investigators from in-hospital and out-of-hospital studies concluded that repetitive lower energy biphasic waveform shocks had equal or higher success rates for eradicating ventricular fibrillation than defibrillators that increase the current with each shock (200 J, 300 J, 360 J).[15,27] More research is needed to determine a specific recommendation for the optimal energy level for biphasic waveform defibrillation.[5,10,13,15,27] For that reason, the American Heart Association states that biphasic waveform shocks are acceptable if documented as clinically equivalent to reports of monophasic shocks.[5]
- Some biphasic defibrillators measure and compensate for transthoracic impedance before the delivery of the shock. This allows the defibrillator to deliver the actual amount of energy selected by the rescuer.[27,32]

EQUIPMENT

- Defibrillator with electrocardiogram (ECG) oscilloscope/recorder

- ECG cable
- Conductive gel, paste, or prepackaged gelled conduction pads or self-adhesive defibrillation pads connected directly to the defibrillator
- Bag-valve-mask oxygen delivery device
- Flowmeter for oxygen administration, oxygen source
- Emergency suction and intubation equipment
- Blood pressure monitoring equipment
- Intravenous infusion pumps

Additional equipment to have available as needed includes the following:
- Cardiac board
- Emergency medications
- Emergency pacing equipment

PATIENT AND FAMILY EDUCATION

- Teaching may need to be performed after the procedure. ➤➤*Rationale:* If the emergent defibrillation is performed in the face of hemodynamic collapse, education may be impossible until after the procedure has been performed.
- Assess patient and family understanding of the etiology of the dysrhythmia. ➤➤*Rationale:* This assessment determines the patient and family understanding of the condition and additional educational needs.[38]
- Explain the procedure to the patient and the family. ➤➤*Rationale:* This explanation decreases anxiety and promotes understanding.
- Explain to the patient and the family the signs and symptoms of hemodynamic compromise associated with preexisting cardiac dysrhythmias. ➤➤*Rationale:* This enables the patient and the family to recognize when to contact the nurse or physician.[38]
- Evaluate and discuss with the patient the need for long-term pharmacologic support. ➤➤*Rationale:* This allows the nurse to anticipate educational needs of the patient and family regarding specific discharge medications.[38]
- Assess and discuss with the patient the need for lifestyle changes. ➤➤*Rationale:* Underlying pathophysiology may necessitate alterations in the patient's current lifestyle and require a plan for behavioral changes.[38]
- Assess and discuss with the patient the need as applicable for an automatic implantable cardioverter-defibrillator. ➤➤*Rationale:* Life-threatening dysrhythmias may persist after initial defibrillation and pharmacologic interventions. Recurrent ventricular dysrhythmias may represent a chronic condition for the patient.[4,38]
- Assess and discuss with the patient the need as applicable for an emergency communication system. ➤➤*Rationale:* People with recurrent life-threatening dysrhythmias are at risk for cardiac arrest.[38]

PATIENT ASSESSMENT AND PREPARATION

Patient Assessment

- Assess the ECG for tachydysrhythmias, including paroxysmal supraventricular tachycardia, atrial fibrillation, atrial flutter, atrial tachycardia, and ventricular tachycardia. ➤➤*Rationale:* Tachydysrhythmias often precede ventricular fibrillation, can be life-threatening, and can precipitate deterioration of hemodynamic stability.[5,15,38]
- Assess the ECG for ventricular fibrillation. ➤➤*Rationale:* Ventricular fibrillation is life-threatening; if not terminated immediately, death ensues.[5,15,16,38]
- Assess vital signs. ➤➤*Rationale:* Blood pressure and pulse are absent in the presence of ventricular fibrillation because of the loss of cardiac output.[16]

Patient Preparation

- Ensure that the patient and family understand preprocedural teaching (if time is available). Answer questions as they arise, and reinforce information as needed. ➤➤*Rationale:* This communication evaluates and reinforces understanding of previously taught information.
- If possible, ask a member of pastoral care or the clergy to provide support for family members during the procedure. ➤➤*Rationale:* Pastoral care team members or the clergy may provide support to ease family members' anxiety during the procedure.
- Remove all metallic objects from the patient. ➤➤*Rationale:* Metallic objects are excellent conductors of electric current and could result in burns.
- Remove transdermal medication patches from the patient's chest or ensure the defibrillator pad or paddle does not touch the patch. ➤➤*Rationale:* The patch may impede transmission of the current.[5,15,26,32] Transdermal nitroglycerin patches may produce a chest burn when the paddle is placed over it.[15,31]
- Ensure that the patient is in a dry environment, and dry the patient's chest, if it is wet. ➤➤*Rationale:* Water is a conductor of electricity. If the patient and rescuer are in contact with water, the rescuer may receive a shock or the patient may receive a skin burn.[15,32] Also, if the patient's chest is wet, the current may travel from one paddle across the water to the other, resulting in a decreased amount of energy to the myocardium.[5,15,32]
- Initiate basic life support if immediate defibrillation is not available. ➤➤*Rationale:* Basic life support maintains cardiac output to diminish irreversible organ and tissue damage.[5,15]
- Oxygenate the patient with a bag-valve-mask device and 100% oxygen. ➤➤*Rationale:* Adequate oxygenation diminishes the risk of cerebral and cardiac complications.[5,15]
- Place the defibrillator in the defibrillation mode. ➤➤*Rationale:* The defibrillation mode must be set to disperse the electric charge randomly because the synchronization mode does not fire in the absence of a QRS complex.

Procedure for Defibrillation (External)

Steps	Rationale	Special Considerations
1. Wash hands.	Reduces the transmission of microorganisms; standard precautions.	
2. Prepare the patient or paddles or both with proper conductive agent. *(Level VI: Clinical studies in a variety of patient populations and situations to support recommendations.)*	Reduces transthoracic resistance, enhancing electric conduction through subcutaneous tissue.[3,4,8,14-17,28,32,33,38] Minimizes erythema from the electric current.[16]	Prepackaged gelled conductive pads are available for placement in area of paddle.[16,38] Gel pads should be replaced if they appear to be drying out or after three countershocks.[20] Never use alcohol-soaked pads because they are combustible when in contact with electric current. Conductive gel should be dispersed evenly on the defibrillator paddles and should cover the surface adequately. Be careful not to smear gel between paddles because current may follow an alternate pathway over the chest wall and avoid the heart.[2,4,15-17,21,28,32] Do not use inappropriate gel (i.e., ultrasound gel) because it increases the transthoracic resistance and decreases the current given to the patient[14,33]; it also may cause burns or sparks, which can increase the risk of fire.[14,32] Self-adhesive defibrillation pads connected directly to the defibrillator have been found to be as effective as paddles.[6,7,15,17,21,32,34,37,38] Advantages of "hands-free" defibrillation are safety and convenience of use in any of the appropriate locations.[6,21,34,37,38]
3. Ensure that the defibrillator cables are positioned to allow for adequate access to the patient.	Allows defibrillation to occur without excessive tension on the cables.	
4. Turn on the ECG recorder for a continuous printout.	Establishes a visual recording of the patient's current ECG, verifies the response to the intervention, and provides a permanent record of the response to defibrillation.	
5. Follow these steps for paddle placement. A. Place one paddle at the heart's apex just to the left of the nipple at the midaxillary line. Place the other paddle below the right clavicle to the right of the sternum (see Fig. 36-2). *(Level VI: Clinical studies in a variety of patient populations and situations to support recommendations.)*	Defibrillation is achieved by passing an electric current through the cardiac muscle mass to restore a single source of impulse generation; this pathway maximizes current flow through the myocardium.[4-6,8,15-17,28,38]	A larger paddle size (12-13 cm) decreases the transthoracic resistance and improves current flow.[3,7,8,17,22,35] Most paddles range from 8-12 cm in diameter and are effective.[4,15,17,19,38] Avoid placing paddles over lead wires.[26]

Procedure **for Defibrillation (External)**—*Continued*

Steps	Rationale	Special Considerations
B. In women, the apex paddle is placed at the fifth to sixth intercostal space with the enter of the paddle at the midaxillary line.	Placement over a woman's breast should be avoided to reduce transthoracic resistance.[4,6,18]	
C. Anterior-posterior placement also may be used. *(Level VI: Clinical studies in a variety of patient populations and situations to support recommendations.)*	All methods of paddle placement are effective.[4,6,11,15,17,19,28,38]	
(1) Self-adhesive defibrillation pads are used for this approach.		
(2) The anterior pad is placed in the anterior left precordial area (see Fig. 36-3).		
(3) The posterior pad is placed posteriorly behind the heart in the right or left infrascapular area (see Fig. 36-3).		
(4) An alternative approach is to place the anterior pad in the right infraclavicular area and the posterior pad in the left infrascapular position.		
D. In a patient with a permanent pacemaker, do not place paddles directly over the pulse generator. *(Level IV: Limited clinical studies to support recommendations.)*	Defibrillation over an implanted pacemaker may impair passage of current to the patient and may cause the device to malfunction or become damaged.[1,5,8,12,15,17,24,25,28,30,32] Myocardial injury also may occur if the current flows down the lower resistance pathway of the lead wire.[25,28,30]	Some authors recommend paddle placement at least 5 inches (10-13 cm) from the pulse generator and lead wire.[8,12,28,30,38] Anterior-posterior placement also is suggested.[12,25,30] The pacemaker should be assessed after any electric countershock.[8,12,15,17,25,28,30,32] Standby emergency pacing equipment should be available in the event that pacemaker failure occurs.[12,24]
E. Paddle placement in a patient with an implantable cardioverter-defibrillator (ICD) is the same as standard paddle placement for defibrillation (see Fig. 36-2). Paddles should not be placed over the device.	Defibrillation over an implanted ICD may impair passage of current to the patient and cause the device to malfunction or become damaged.[4,5,15,32,38]	The ICD should be checked after external countershock.[15,32,38]
6. Charge the defibrillator paddles as prescribed or in accordance with recommendations of the American Heart Association (AHA). *(Level VI: Clinical studies in a variety of patient populations and situations to support recommendations.)*	The defibrillator is charged with the lowest energy level required to convert ventricular fibrillation or pulseless ventricular tachycardia.[13,15,20,23,32]	Monophasic energy recommendations by the AHA for adults: first attempt, 200 J; second attempt, 200-300 J; subsequent attempts, 360 J.[5,15] Researchers have found that 115-130 J biphasic waveform shocks achieved the same first shock success rate as 200 J monophasic waveform shocks.[10,15,27] Further studies concluded that repetitive lower energy biphasic waveform shocks had equal or higher success rates for eradicating

Procedure continues on the following page

Procedure for Defibrillation (External)—*Continued*

Steps	Rationale	Special Considerations
		ventricular fibrillation than defibrillators that increase the current with each shock (200 J, 300 J, 360 J).[15,27] More research is needed to determine a specific recommendation for the optimal energy level for biphasic waveform defibrillation.[5,13,15,27] For that reason, the AHA states that biphasic waveform shocks are acceptable if documented as clinically equivalent to reports of monophasic shocks.[5]
7. Disconnect the oxygen source during actual defibrillation.[16]	Decreases the risk of combustion in the presence of electric current.[4,14,16]	Arcing of electric current in the presence of oxygen could precipitate an explosion and subsequent fire hazard.[14,16]
8. Apply 25 lb/in^2 pressure to each paddle against the chest wall.[4,5,38]	Firm paddle pressure decreases transthoracic resistance, improving the flow of current across the axis of the heart.[4,8,15,17,22,28,33,38]	This application of pressure is not necessary for defibrillator models with newer hands-free and automatic transthoracic impedance sensing/correction options built in.
9. State "all clear" or similar wording three times, and visually verify that all personnel are clear of contact with the patient, bed, and equipment.	Maximizes safety to self and caregivers because electric current can be conducted from the patient to another person if contact occurs.[4,5,15,16,28]	When using hands-free defibrillation, take special care to clear other personnel from patient contact because they do not have the visual cue of the paddles being placed on the patient's chest.
10. Verify that the patient is still in ventricular fibrillation or pulseless ventricular tachycardia.	Ensures that defibrillation is necessary.[5,15]	
11. Depress both buttons on the paddles simultaneously, and hold until the defibrillator fires. In the defibrillation mode, there is an immediate release of the electric charge.[4]	Depolarizes the cardiac muscle.[4,5,15,16,38]	If self-adhesive, hands-free defibrillation pads are used, the charge is delivered by depressing the discharge button on the defibrillator.
12. Observe the monitor for conversion of the dysrhythmia. If a stable rhythm is noted, assess for the presence of a carotid pulse. If a pulse noted, assess vital signs and level of consciousness.	Simultaneous depolarization of the myocardial muscle cells should reestablish a single source of impulse generation.[4,5,15,16,38]	
13. If unsuccessful, immediately charge the paddles to 200-300 J, and repeat **Steps 5 to 12**.	Immediate action increases the chance of successful depolarization of cardiac muscle.[4,5,15,38]	Transthoracic resistance decreases with repeated shocks.[4,15,21,38]
14. If the second attempt is unsuccessful, immediately charge the paddles to 360 J, and repeat **Steps 5 to 12**.	Immediate action increases the chance of successful depolarization of cardiac muscle.[4,5,15,38]	Transthoracic resistance decreases with repeated shocks.[4,15,21,38]
15. If the third attempt is unsuccessful, initiate advanced cardiac life support. (*Level VI: Clinical studies in a variety of patient populations and situations to support recommendations.*)	Actions necessary to maintain the delivery of oxygenated blood to vital organs.[5]	Basic life support must be continued throughout resuscitation.[5]

Procedure for Defibrillation (External)—*Continued*

Steps	Rationale	Special Considerations
16. Clean the defibrillator and remove any gel. If self-adhesive defibrillation pads were used, evaluate the placement and integrity of the pads.	Conductive gel accumulated on the defibrillator paddles impedes surface contact and increases transthoracic resistance. Self-adhesive defibrillation pads may crimp, crack, or fold with loss of adhesiveness.	Loss of adhesive integrity in self-adhesive defibrillator pads occurs in restless or diaphoretic patients.
17. Discard used supplies in the appropriate receptacle.	Standard precautions.	
18. Wash hands.	Reduces the transmission of microorganisms; standard precautions.	

Expected Outcomes

- Reestablishment of a single source of impulse generation for the cardiac muscle
- Hemodynamic stability

Unexpected Outcomes

- Continued ventricular fibrillation
- Cardiopulmonary arrest
- Asystole
- Respiratory complications
- Cerebral anoxia and brain death
- Systemic embolization
- Hypotension
- Pacemaker or ICD dysfunction
- Skin burn

Patient Monitoring and Care

Steps	Rationale	Reportable Conditions
		These conditions should be reported if they persist despite nursing interventions.
1. Evaluate the patient's neurologic status before and after defibrillation. Reorient as necessary to person, place, and time.	An altered level of consciousness may occur after ventricular fibrillation.[5,15,38]	- Change in level of consciousness
2. Monitor the patient's pulmonary status after defibrillation.	The goal is to support cardiac and pulmonary function to optimize tissue perfusion to the vital organs.[5,15,38]	- Change in respirations - Change in breath sounds - Decreased oxygen saturation as measured by pulse oximetry - Abnormal arterial blood gas results
3. Maintain a patent airway and provide oxygen and mechanical ventilation as needed.	The goal is to support cardiac and pulmonary function to optimize tissue perfusion to the vital organs.[5,15,38]	- Change in respirations - Change in breath sounds - Decreased oxygen saturation as measured by pulse oximetry - Abnormal arterial blood gas results
4. Monitor cardiovascular status (blood pressure, heart rate, and rhythm) immediately after defibrillation and every 15 minutes until stable.	Dysrhythmias may develop after defibrillation.[5,9,15,38] Vital signs should stabilize after achieving a normal heart rate and rhythm.	- Dysrhythmias - Hypotension - Hypertension

Procedure continues on the following page

Patient Monitoring and Care—*Continued*

Steps	Rationale	Reportable Conditions
5. Administer intravenous fluids or medications to maintain normal blood pressure.	The goal is to support cardiac and pulmonary function to optimize tissue perfusion to vital organs.[5,15,38]	• Hypotension • Hypertension
6. Continue to monitor the ECG after defibrillation.	Postdefibrillation dysrhythmias may occur.[5,9,15,38]	• Dysrhythmias
7. Initiate intravenous antidysrhythmic pharmacologic therapy as prescribed.	Ventricular fibrillation is indicative of the myocardium's state of irritability. If antidysrhythmic therapy is not administered, recurrence of ventricular fibrillation is probable.[5,15,38]	• Dysrhythmias despite antidysrhythmic therapy
8. Evaluate for burns.	Erythema at the electrode sites may be seen secondary to local hyperemia in the current pathway.[16] Skin burns may be minimized by use of gel pads or placing appropriate paste or gel to the paddles.[16]	• Skin burns
9. Monitor electrolytes.	Abnormal electrolytes may have contributed to the development of ventricular dysrhythmias.[15,28,38]	• Abnormal electrolyte results
10. Consider other possible causes for ventricular fibrillation or pulseless ventricular tachycardia.	Interventions may be aimed at correcting underlying pathophysiology and preventing reoccurrence of lethal dysrhythmias.[5]	

Documentation

Documentation should include the following:

- Neurologic, pulmonary, and cardiovascular assessments before and after defibrillation
- Interventions to prepare the patient for defibrillation
- The Joules used and the number of defibrillation attempts made
- Printout ECG tracing depicting the cardiac rhythm before and after defibrillation
- Patient response to defibrillation
- Condition of skin of the chest wall
- Unexpected outcomes and nursing interventions
- Patient and family education

References

1. Altamura, G., et al. (1995). Transthoracic DC shock may represent a serious hazard in pacemaker dependent patients. *Pacing Clin Electrophysiol,* 18(Part II), 194-8.
2. Caterine, M.R., et al. (1997). Effect of electrode position and gel-application technique on predicted transcardiac current during transthoracic defibrillation. *Ann Emerg Med,* 29, 588-95.
3. Connell, P.N., et al. (1973). Transthoracic impedance to defibrillator discharge: Effect of electrode size and electrode-chest wall interface. *J Electrocardiol,* 6, 313-7.
4. Cooper, M., et al. (1998). A guide to defibrillation. *Emerg Nurse,* 6, 16-21.
5. Cummins, R.O., editor. (2001). *ACLS Procedure Manual.* Dallas: American Heart Association.
6. Dalzell, G.W. (1998). Determinants of successful defibrillation. *Heart,* 80, 405-7.
7. Dalzell, G.W., et al. (1989). Electrode pad size, transthoracic impedance and success of external ventricular defibrillation. *Am J Cardiol,* 64, 741-4.
8. Ewy, G.A. (1986). Electrical therapy for cardiovascular emergencies. *Circulation,* 74(Suppl IV), IV-111-6.
9. Eysmann, S.B., et al. (1986). Electrocardiographic changes after cardioversion of ventricular arrhythmias. *Circulation,* 73, 73-81.
10. Faddy, S.C., et al. (2003). Biphasic and monophasic shocks for transthoracic defibrillation: A meta analysis of randomized controlled trials. *Resuscitation,* 58, 9-16.
11. Garcia, L.A., and Kerber, R.E. (1998). Transthoracic defibrillation: Does electrode adhesive pad position alter transthoracic impedance? *Resuscitation,* 37, 139-43.
12. Gould, L., et al. (1981). Pacemaker failure following external defibrillation. *Pacing Clin Electrophysiol,* 4, 575-7.
13. Harris, J. (2002). Biphasic defibrillation. *Emerg Nurs,* 10, 33-7.
14. Hummel, R.S., et al. (1988). Spark-generating properties of electrode gels used during defibrillation: A potential fire hazard. *JAMA,* 260, 3021-4.
15. International Consensus on Science. (2000). Guidelines 2000 for Cardiopulmonary Resuscitation and Emergency Cardiovascular Care. *Circulation,* 102(Suppl I), I-90-4.
16. Inwood, H., and Cull, C. (1997). Defibrillation. *Prof Nurse,* 13, 165-8.
17. Kerber, R.E. (1993). Electrical treatment of cardiac arrhythmias: Defibrillation and cardioversion. *Ann Emerg Med,* 22(Part 2), 296-301.
18. Kerber, R.E. (1996). Transthoracic cardioversion of atrial fibrillation and flutter: Standard technique and new advances. *Am J Cardiol,* 78(Suppl 8), 22-6.

19. Kerber, R.E., et al. (1981). Elective cardioversion: Influence of paddle-electrode location and size on success rates and energy requirements. *N Engl J Med,* 305, 658-62.

20. Kerber, R.E., et al. (1988). Energy, current and success in defibrillation and cardioversion: Clinical studies using an automated impedance-based method of energy adjustment. *Circulation,* 77, 1038-46.

21. Kerber, R.E., et al. (1984). Self-adhesive preapplied electrode pads for defibrillation and cardioversion. *J Am Coll Cardiol,* 3, 815-20.

22. Kerber, R.E., et al. (1981). Transthoracic resistance in human defibrillation: Influence of body weight, chest size, serial shocks, paddle size and paddle contact pressure. *Circulation,* 3, 676-82.

23. Kerber, R.E., et al. (1992). Ventricular tachycardia rate and morphology determine energy and current requirements for transthoracic cardioversion. *Circulation,* 85, 158-63.

24. Lau, F.Y., Bilitch, M., and Wintroub, H.J. (1969). Protection of implanted pacemakers from excessive electrical energy of DC shock. *Am J Cardiol,* 23, 244-9.

25. Levine, P.A., et al. (1983). Adverse acute and chronic effects of electrical defibrillation and cardioversion on implanted unipolar cardiac pacing systems. *J Am Coll Cardiol,* 1, 1413-22.

26. Lezon, K. (1998). Code blue: Defibrillate. *Nursing,* 28, 58-60.

27. Low-energy biphasic waveform defibrillation: Evidence-based review applied to emergency cardiovascular care guidelines. A statement for healthcare professionals from the American Heart Association Committee on Emergency Cardiovascular Care and the Subcommittees on Basic Life Support, Advanced Cardiac Life Support and Pediatric Resuscitation. (1998). *Circulation,* 97, 1654-67.

28. Lown, B., and deSilva, R.A. (1998). External cardioversion and defibrillation. In: Alexander, R.W., Schlant, R.C., and Fuster, V., editors. *Hurst's the Heart: Arteries and Veins.* 9th ed. New York: McGraw-Hill.

29. Mair, M. (2003). Monophasic and biphasic defibrillators: The evolving technology of cardiac defibrillation. *Am J Nurs,* 103, 58-60.

30. Owen, P.M. (1983). The effects of external defibrillation on permanent pacemakers. *Heart Lung,* 12, 274-7.

31. Panacek, E.A., et al. (1992). Report of nitropatch explosions complicating defibrillation. *Am J Emerg Med,* 10, 128-9.

32. Peberdy, M.A. (2002). Defibrillation. *Cardiol Clin,* 20, 13-21.

33. Sirna, S.J., et al. (1988). Factors affecting transthoracic impedance during electrical cardioversion. *Am J Cardiol,* 62, 1048-52.

34. Stults, K.R., et al. (1987). Self-adhesive monitor/defibrillation pads improve prehospital defibrillation success. *Ann Emerg Med,* 16, 872-7.

35. Thomas, E.D., et al. (1977). Effectiveness of direct current defibrillation: Role of paddle electrode size. *Am Heart J,* 93, 463-7.

36. White, R.D. (2002). New concepts in transthoracic defibrillation. *Emerg Med Clin North Am,* 20, 785-807.

37. Wilson, R.F., et al. (1987). Defibrillation of high-risk patients during coronary angiography using self-adhesive, preapplied electrode pads. *Am J Cardiol,* 60, 380-2.

38. Woods, S.L., Sivarajan Froelicher, E.S., and Motzer, S.W., editors. (2000). *Cardiac Nursing.* 4th ed. Philadelphia: Lippincott Williams & Wilkins.

Additional Readings

Cook, L. (2003). Staying current on defibrillator safety. *Nursing,* 33(11 Part 1), 44-6.

Lown, B. (2002). Defibrillation and cardioversion. *Cardiovasc Res,* 55, 220-4.

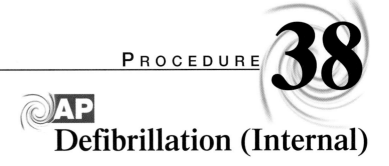

PROCEDURE **38**

AP Defibrillation (Internal)

PURPOSE: Internal defibrillation is achieved by delivering an electric current directly to the myocardial surface via an open thoracotomy approach or open sternotomy, as in a postoperative cardiovascular surgery patient.

Christine Shamloo

PREREQUISITE NURSING KNOWLEDGE

*   Understanding of cardiovascular anatomy and physiology, principles of cardiac conduction, basic dysrhythmia interpretation, and electric safety.
*   Advanced cardiac life support knowledge and skills are needed.
*   Knowledge of sterile technique is required.
*   Clinical and technical competence related to use of the defibrillator is needed.
*   Knowledge of internal paddle placement and energy requirements for internal defibrillation is required.
*   Internal paddle placement ensures that the axis of the heart is situated between the sources of current.
*   Energy requirements for internal defibrillation range from 5 to 60 J. Ideal energy requirements that cause minimal damage to the myocardium and are effective for defibrillation have not been established.
*   Geddes and colleagues[2] reported that an energy level of 5 J was sufficient in 50% of human hearts internally defibrillated. Energy levels of 10 to 20 J were successful in terminating the dysrhythmias without myocardial necrosis developing in 90% of the patients studied.

*   Emergent open sternotomy precedes internal defibrillation (see Procedures 39 and 40).

EQUIPMENT

*   Sterile gloves, goggles or face shield, gowns, and masks
*   Open thoracotomy or sternotomy tray
*   Sterile internal paddles (ensure their compatibility with the defibrillator)
*   Defibrillator with electrocardiogram (ECG) oscilloscope and recorder
*   Antiseptic solution (e.g., 2% chlorhexidine–based preparation)
*   Large sterile suction catheter and tubing
*   Flowmeter for oxygen administration
*   Bag-valve-mask device capable of delivering 100% oxygen and large inflation volumes
*   Intubation equipment
*   Intravenous access and fluids
    Additional equipment as needed includes the following:
*   Emergency medications
*   Emergency pacemaker equipment

PATIENT AND FAMILY EDUCATION

*   Teaching may need to be performed after the procedure.
    ➤➤*Rationale:* Internal defibrillation usually is performed in the face of hemodynamic collapse.

- Explain to the family the need for internal defibrillation. ➥*Rationale:* This explanation keeps the family informed.
- Assess and discuss, as applicable, with the patient and family the need for follow-up electrophysiologic studies (EPS). ➥*Rationale:* This communication enables the patient and family to understand the importance of EPS.
- Assess patient and family understanding of the underlying disease pathology. ➥*Rationale:* This prepares the patient and family for expected and unexpected outcomes.
- Explain to the patient and family the signs and symptoms of hemodynamic compromise associated with preexisting cardiac dysrhythmias. ➥*Rationale:* This explanation enables the patient and family to recognize when the patient needs to contact health care providers.
- Evaluate the patient's need for long-term antidysrhythmic support. ➥*Rationale:* This evaluation allows the nurse to anticipate educational needs of the patient and family regarding specific discharge medications.
- Assess and discuss with the patient the need as applicable for lifestyle changes. ➥*Rationale:* Underlying pathophysiology may necessitate alterations in the patient's current lifestyle and require a plan for behavioral changes.
- Assess and discuss with the patient the need as applicable for an emergency communication plan. ➥*Rationale:* Patients with recurrent life-threatening ventricular dysrhythmias are at risk for cardiac arrest.

PATIENT ASSESSMENT AND PREPARATION

Patient Assessment

- Assess the ECG for dysrhythmias, including ventricular ectopy and ventricular tachycardia. ➥*Rationale:* Ventricular dysrhythmias often precede ventricular fibrillation and precipitate deterioration of hemodynamic stability.
- Assess the ECG for ventricular fibrillation. ➥*Rationale:* The development of ventricular fibrillation is life-threatening, and if it is not terminated immediately, death ensues.
- Assess vital signs with each significant change in the ECG rate and rhythm. ➥*Rationale:* The hemodynamic response to ECG changes needs to be assessed.

Patient Preparation

- Place the patient in a flat supine position. ➥*Rationale:* Provides the best access during the procedure and during intervention for management of adverse effects.
- Remove all metallic objects from the patient. ➥*Rationale:* Metallic objects are conductors of electric current and can cause burns.
- Prepare the patient's skin with antibacterial solution, and drape the patient. ➥*Rationale:* Decreases the potential for infection.
- Ensure that the patient is intubated, sedated, and ventilated before the initiation of the procedure. ➥*Rationale:* Maintains adequate oxygenation.

Procedure for Defibrillation (Internal)

Steps	Rationale	Special Considerations
1. Initiate basic life support.	Decreases the risk of airway obstruction during the procedure; maintains oxygenation and perfusion.	External defibrillation should be attempted first whenever possible (see Procedure 37).
2. Assist the physician or advanced practice nurse with donning sterile gloves, masks, gown, and goggles and with opening the chest as needed (see Procedure 40).	Maintains sterility; standard precautions.	
3. Set up the sterile suction.	Prepares the equipment.	
4. Assist with suctioning as needed.	If drainage or bleeding is present, suctioning around the heart may be necessary before defibrillating.	
5. Ensure that the defibrillator electric cord is inserted into a grounded electric wall outlet.	Prepares the equipment.	Not necessary for all defibrillators.

Procedure continues on the following page

Procedure for Defibrillation (Internal)—*Continued*

Steps	Rationale	Special Considerations
6. Ensure that the defibrillator is in the defibrillation mode.	The defibrillation mode must be selected to deliver the electric charge immediately. The synchronization mode does not fire in the absence of a QRS complex.	The defibrillation mode may be the default setting of the defibrillator; always confirm the setting.
7. Turn on the ECG recorder for a continuous printout.	Establishes a visual recording of the patient's current ECG status and provides a permanent record of the patient's response to the intervention.	
8. When the physician or advanced practice nurse has positioned the internal paddles on the heart, connect the other end of the internal paddles to the defibrillator.	Prepares the equipment.	One paddle is placed over the right atrium or right ventricle; the other paddle is placed over the apex (Fig. 38-1).
9. Charge the defibrillator paddles as prescribed (usually 5-20 J). *(Level IV: Limited clinical studies to support recommendations.)*	The defibrillator is charged with the lowest energy level required to convert ventricular fibrillation and prevent any damage to the heart muscle.	Usually 5-20 J is sufficient to convert ventricular fibrillation.[3] Refer to the defibrillator manufacturer's operation guidelines for specific recommendations.
10. Ensure that the physician or advanced practice nurse states "all clear" three times, and visually verifies that all personnel are clear of contact with the patient, bed, and equipment.	Electric current can be conducted from the patient to another person if contact occurs.	

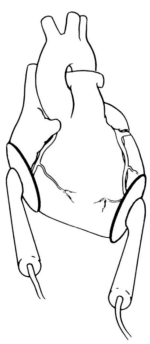

FIGURE 38-1 Paddle placement for internal defibrillation.
(From Kinkade, S., and Lohrman, J.E. [1990]. Critical Care Nursing Procedures: A Team Approach. *Philadelphia: B.C. Decker.)*

Procedure for Defibrillation (Internal)—*Continued*

Steps	Rationale	Special Considerations
11. The physician or advanced practice nurse depresses both buttons on the paddles simultaneously and holds until the defibrillator fires. In the defibrillation mode, there is an immediate release of the electric charge.	Depolarizes the cardiac muscle. Simultaneous depolarization of the myocardial muscle cells may reestablish a single source of impulse generation.	The charge also may be delivered by depressing the discharge button on the defibrillator until the charge is delivered. Some internal paddles can be discharged only by depressing the "discharge button" on the defibrillator.
12. Observe for conversion of the dysrhythmia, and assess for the presence of a pulse. A. If the first attempt is unsuccessful, immediately charge the paddles and repeat **Steps 9 to 11** two additional times. If the third attempt is unsuccessful, initiate advanced cardiac life support. B. If successful, obtain vital signs and assess the patient.	Immediate action increases the chance for successful depolarization of cardiac muscle. Actions are necessary to maintain the delivery of oxygenated blood to vital organs. Assesses the patient's response to defibrillation.	Open-chest compression must be resumed after the third attempt, if not successful. Consider the need for pacing if the rhythm converts to asystole.
13. Prepare the patient for transport to the operating room, or prepare to assist with closing the incision and sternum at the beside.	Surgical intervention is necessary when the open-chest technique is used.	Notify the operating room staff before transporting the patient.
14. Clean the defibrillator with a cleansing solution, and remove blood or body fluid from paddles. Send used paddles for resterilization. Obtain sterile paddles to restock emergency supplies.	Reduces the transmission of microorganisms; sterile precautions; standard precautions.	
15. Discard used disposable supplies and wash hands.	Reduces the transmission of microorganisms; standard precautions.	

Expected Outcomes

- Reestablishment of a single source of impulse generation for the cardiac muscle
- Hemodynamic stability

Unexpected Outcomes

- Cardiopulmonary arrest and death
- Cerebral anoxia and brain death
- Infection
- Myocardial damage caused by defibrillation

Patient Monitoring and Care

Steps	Rationale	Reportable Conditions
		These conditions should be reported if they persist despite nursing interventions.
1. Continue to monitor the ECG after defibrillation.	Dysrhythmias may develop after defibrillation.[1]	• Dysrhythmias

Procedure continues on the following page

Patient Monitoring and Care—*Continued*

Steps	Rationale	Reportable Conditions
2. Evaluate the patient's neurologic status after defibrillation. Reorient as necessary to person, place, and time.	Temporary altered level of consciousness may occur after defibrillation.[1]	• Change in level of consciousness
3. Monitor the patient's pulmonary status after defibrillation.	Respiratory centers of the brain may be depressed as a result of hypoxia.[1]	• Change in respirations • Decrease in oxygen saturation • Abnormal arterial blood gas results
4. Monitor the patient's cardiovascular status (blood pressure, heart rate, and rhythm) immediately after defibrillation and at least every 15 minutes until stable.	Vital signs should stabilize after achieving a normal heart rate and rhythm.	• Abnormal vital signs • Dysrhythmias
5. Initiate intravenous antidysrhythmic pharmacologic therapy as prescribed.	Ventricular fibrillation is indicative of the myocardium's state of irritability. If antidysrhythmic therapy is not administered, ventricular fibrillation may reoccur.	• Dysrhythmias despite antidysrhythmic therapy
6. Notify blood bank as needed.	Ensures blood availability if needed during or after the procedure.	
7. Monitor electrolytes.	Abnormal electrolytes may contribute to the development of ventricular dysrhythmias. Cellular and tissue perfusion returns with restoration of a pulse and blood pressure, but intracellular acidosis may remain after resuscitation.[2]	• Abnormal electrolyte results
8. Monitor for signs and symptoms of infection.	Disruption of skin integrity and introduction of foreign material into the thoracic cavity predisposes the patient to the risk of infection.	• Elevated white blood cell count • Elevated or depressed temperature • Pain at incisional site • Erythema • Drainage from the incisional site

Documentation

Documentation should include the following:

• Neurologic, respiratory, and cardiovascular assessments before and after defibrillation
• Joules used and number of defibrillations
• Printout of ECG tracings depicting defibrillation and cardiac events before and after defibrillation

• Amount of chest drainage
• Patient response to defibrillation
• Any unexpected outcomes and interventions taken
• Time patient transferred to the operating room
• Patient and family education

References

1. Cummins, R.O., editor. (2001). *ACLS Procedure Manual.* Dallas: American Heart Association.
2. Geddes, L.A., et al. (1974). The electrical dose for ventricular defibrillation with electrodes applied directly to the heart. *J Thorac Cardiovasc Surg,* 68, 593-602.
3. Moore, S. (1986). Jump-starting the heart: A current review of defibrillation techniques and equipment. *JAMA,* 12, 213-7.

Additional Readings

Proehl, J.A., et al. (2000). Open thoracotomy and internal defibrillation. *Int J Trauma Nurs,* 6, 128, 132.
Pugsley, W.B., et al. (1989). Low energy level internal defibrillation during cardiopulmonary bypass. *Eur J Cardiothorac Surg,* 3, 273-5.
Seifert, P.C. (1994). *Cardiac Surgery.* St. Louis: Mosby-Yearbook.

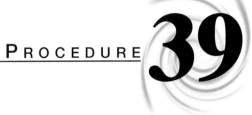

PROCEDURE **39**

Emergent Open Sternotomy (Perform)

PURPOSE: Emergent open sternotomy in a postoperative patient after cardiac surgery is designed to identify and eliminate areas of persistent hemorrhage, relieve pericardial tamponade, and provide access for open cardiac massage.

Deborah G. Lamarr

PREREQUISITE NURSING KNOWLEDGE

- Knowledge of anatomy and physiology of the cardiovascular system is required.
- Advanced cardiac life support knowledge and skills are required.
- Knowledge and clinical competence related to sterile technique, suturing, sternal opening, sternal wiring, surgical instrumentation, and sternal exploration are needed.
- This procedure is designed for postoperative patients after cardiac surgeries who have undergone the median sternotomy approach.
- Knowledge of signs and symptoms of cardiac tamponade is required.
- Emergent open sternotomy in a postoperative patient after cardiac surgery is indicated for exanguinating hemorrhage or cardiac tamponade with imminent cardiac arrest.
- Early reexploration for persistent hemorrhage may reduce the requirement for homologous transfusions and may lower the wound infection rate associated with an undrained mediastinal hematoma.
- Mediastinal reexploration for cardiac tamponade decreases ventricular diastolic pressure. This decreased pressure allows for increased ventricular filling, which should increase stroke volume and cardiac output and globally improve systemic perfusion.
- Mechanical ventilation and sedation are prerequisites to sternal reexploration.

- Paralytic agents may be a necessary adjunct to sedation to improve oxygenation, diminish muscle activity, and enhance visualization in the operative field.
- Internal defibrillation may be necessary if life-threatening dysrhythmias occur (see Procedure 38).

EQUIPMENT

- Antiseptic solution (e.g., 2% chlorhexidine–based preparation)
- Caps, masks, goggles, sterile gloves, and sterile drapes
- Sterile staple remover
- Sterile open-chest set
  ❖ Rib spreader
  ❖ Kelly clamps and skin snaps
  ❖ Knife handle
  ❖ Wire cutter
  ❖ Scissors
- Electrocautery equipment: generator, cautery, grounding pad
- Large sterile suction catheter (e.g., Yankauer)
- Suction container and tubing
- Polypropylene (Prolene) suture (cutting needle), other suture material according to preference
- Clip applicator and clips
- Syringes: 3 ml, 5 ml, 10 ml, 20 ml
- Knife blades: No. 10, No. 11, No. 15
- Sternal wires
- Sterile stapler and staples
- Sterile dressing supplies
- Emergency medication and resuscitation equipment
  Additional equipment as needed includes the following:
- Analgesia or sedation as prescribed
- Blood products and intravenous solutions as prescribed
- Chest tubes and chest tube drainage system

This procedure should be performed only by physicians, advanced practice nurses, and other health care professionals (including critical care nurses) with additional knowledge, skills, and demonstrated competence per professional licensure or institutional standard.

- Epicardial wires
- Intraaortic balloon pump or other mechanical assist device

PATIENT AND FAMILY EDUCATION

- Teaching may be necessary after the procedure. ➤➤*Rationale:* If the emergent sternotomy is performed in the face of hemodynamic collapse, education of the patient and family may be impossible until after the procedure has been performed.
- Explain the reason that the open sternotomy procedure was performed and its outcome or anticipated outcome. ➤➤*Rationale:* This explanation clarifies information and encourages the patient and family to ask questions and voice specific concerns about the procedure.

PATIENT ASSESSMENT AND PREPARATION

Patient Assessment

- Assess hemodynamic and neurologic status. ➤➤*Rationale:* Identifies baseline data that may indicate the need for emergent open sternotomy and provides comparison data.
- Assess the patient's medical history, specifically that relates to coagulation disorders, renal disease with coexistent uremia, and functional status of the right and left ventricle. ➤➤*Rationale:* Provides baseline data.
- Assess current laboratory data, specifically complete blood cell count, platelet count, prothrombin time, activated partial thromboplastin time, fibrinogen, and international normalized ratio. ➤➤*Rationale:* Baseline coagulation studies need to be near-normal to be eliminated as possible causes for ongoing hemorrhage.
- Assess for signs and symptoms of cardiac tamponade.
  - ❖ Sudden decrease or cessation in chest tube drainage
  - ❖ Hypotension (mean arterial blood pressure less than 60 mm Hg)
  - ❖ Altered mental status
  - ❖ Apical heart rate greater than 110 beats/min
  - ❖ Narrowing of pulse pressure
  - ❖ Distended neck veins
  - ❖ Distant heart sounds
  - ❖ Equilibrium of intracardiac pressures with right atrial, pulmonary artery wedge, and (if measured) left atrial pressures being equal
  - ❖ Decreased cardiac output and cardiac index
  - ❖ Pulsus paradoxus
  - ➤➤*Rationale:* This determines the need for chest exploration.
- Assess for excessive chest tube drainage[1] (e.g., 500 ml for 1 hour, 400 ml for 2 consecutive hours, or 300 ml for 3 consecutive hours). ➤➤*Rationale:* This determines the need for chest exploration.

Patient Preparation

- Ensure that the patient and family understand procedural teaching (if time available). Answer questions as they arise, and reinforce information as needed. ➤➤*Rationale:* This communication evaluates and reinforces understandings of previously taught information.
- If time allows, obtain a chest radiograph to assess for evidence of a widened mediastinum. ➤➤*Rationale:* Widening of the mediastinum on chest radiograph, especially the right heart border, could indicate mediastinal blood.
- If time allows, obtain a transthoracic echocardiogram in an attempt to identify a mediastinal clot. ➤➤*Rationale:* An echocardiogram aids in the diagnosis and confirms the necessity for the open sternotomy procedure.
- Obtain informed consent (this may not be possible if the procedure is an acute emergency). ➤➤*Rationale:* This protects the rights of the patient and ensures a competent decision for the patient and the family.
- Ensure that the patient's ventilation is maintained. ➤➤*Rationale:* This ensures that the patient's airway is protected and that oxygen needs are met.
- Position the patient in the supine position with the head of the bed flat. ➤➤*Rationale:* This positioning ensures visualization of the chest.
- Prescribe analgesics or sedatives: ➤➤*Rationale:* Analgesics or sedatives promote comfort.

Procedure | for Performing Emergent Open Sternotomy

Steps	Rationale	Special Considerations
1. Call the physician and operative team.	The physician can reassess the need for further surgical intervention. The operative team may be needed to assist at the bedside or to prepare the operating room if further exploration is needed.	Follow hospital standard.
2. Prepare the electrocautery device for possible use: Apply the ground pad to the patient's skin, and attach the grounding and cautery cables.	This device is used to terminate capillary oozing or bleeding.	

Procedure for Performing Emergent Open Sternotomy—*Continued*

Steps	Rationale	Special Considerations
3. Ensure that a new sterile suction system is set up.	This system is used to suction the mediastinum during the procedure.	
4. Wash hands, and don nonsterile gloves.	Reduces the transmission of microorganisms; standard precautions.	
5. Remove the sternal dressing, and cleanse the chest with the antiseptic solution.	Inhibits microorganism transmission.	Prepare the skin from the sternal notch to the midabdomen and from one anterior axillary line to the other.
6. Wash hands, and don caps, goggles, masks, sterile gowns, and sterile gloves for all members of the health care team involved with the procedure.	Reduces the transmission of microorganisms; sterile precautions; standard precautions.	All personnel in the room must don masks and caps.
7. Drape off each side of the sternotomy incision with a half drape.	A large sterile field supplies room for placement of instruments.	Allows good view of the sternal notch.
8. Hand off the electrocautery cable to the assisting critical care nurse.	Cautery is used to stop bleeding from small vessels.	
9. With the scalpel, open the wound down to the sternum, exposing the sternal wires.	Ensures visualization of the sternal wires.	Staples can be removed with the staple remover.
10. Cauterize oozing bleeding sites as needed.	Minimizes blood loss and enhances visualization of the surgical field.	
11. Cut the sternal wires from the top to the bottom with the wire cutter, or untwist the wires with the heavy needle holder.	Provides access to the mediastinum. The sternal wires fatigue and break when untwisted with the heavy needle holders.	Use care when removing the sternal wires to minimize damage to the heart and underlying equipment (e.g., epicardial pacing wires, chest tubes) and bypass grafts.
12. Using your hands, gently separate the sternum.	Caution must be taken to separate the sternum gently because the heart, pacing wires, and grafts rest just under the sternal bone.	
13. Place the sternal retractor under the sternal bone and crank it open.	Exposes the heart.	Blades can trap and tear grafts and wires if caught and pulled apart when the retractor is cranked open. Continuously palpate the edges of the retractor for potential caught grafts or wires.
14. Place a finger over the bleeding site, and suction the remainder of the chest, evacuating any clots.	Pressure on the bleeding site may minimize blood loss.	Resuscitate with intravenous fluids, inotropic medications, and blood products as necessary.
15. Assist the physician with control and ligation of major and minor bleeding sites, enhance sternal retraction, and provide suctioning and electrocautery as needed.	May eliminate the need for further reexploration and allows for full visualization of the surgical field.	The physician determines if the patient needs to be transferred to the operating room for further surgical intervention.

Procedure continues on the following page

Procedure for Performing Emergent Open Sternotomy—*Continued*

Steps	Rationale	Special Considerations
16. Assist the physician with the placement of chest tubes or pacing wires as needed.	Pacing leads and chest tubes can be displaced during sternal retraction.	
17. Assist with the placement of mechanical assist devices if needed.	Cardiac tamponade can conceal right or left ventricular dysfunction; mechanical assistance may be necessary to improve cardiac output.	
18. Assist with patient transport to the operating room if necessary.	The patient may need surgical repair of coronary artery bypass grafts, cardiac valves, or the myocardium.	Ensure that the patient's chest is covered with sterile drapes during transportation.
19. If the patient does not need to return to the operating room, assist the physician with reinsertion of sternal wires as follows: A. Grasp the sternal wire with the needle holder. B. Push through the sternum, anterior to posterior, on one side. C. Pull the wire through to the other sternal edge, pushing through the sternum posterior to anterior. D. Twist the edges of the wires together with the needle holder. E. Cut off the excess wire.	Ensures sternal closure.	Caution must be taken not to penetrate the heart, pericostal vessels, lungs, or grafts with the sternal wires. Occasionally, if severe right and left ventricular dysfunction persists, the chest may need to be left open and covered with a sterile occlusive surgical dressing (e.g., Gore-Tex patch).
20. Repeat the sternal wire reinsertion as described in **Step 19,** placing each insertion 4-5 cm apart until the sternum is closed.	Ensures sternal closure.	
21. Assist the physician with skin closure, according to preference.	Promotes wound healing.	The patient's chest may be left open and covered with a sterile occlusive dressing if severe ventricular dysfunction exists.
22. Apply an occlusive dressing to the sternal incision, epicardial pacing wires, and chest tube sites.	Promotes aseptic management of the surgical incision and wound sites.	
23. Remove and discard personal protective equipment, discard used supplies and package instruments for sterilization, and wash hands.	Reduces the transmission of microorganisms and body secretions; standard precautions.	

Expected Outcomes

- Increased cardiac output
- Increased tissue perfusion, including cerebral, renal, and peripheral perfusion
- Standard chest tube drainage
- Decreased need for transfusions

Unexpected Outcomes

- Severe right or left ventricular dysfunction
- Continued bleeding or coagulation disorders
- Myocardial or aortic perforation
- Cardiac arrest
- Pneumothorax
- Myocardial infection
- Atrial and ventricular dysrhythmias
- Pain

Patient Monitoring and Care

Steps	Rationale	Reportable Conditions
		These conditions should be reported if they persist despite nursing interventions.
1. Perform cardiovascular, peripheral vascular, and hemodynamic assessments every 15-30 minutes as patient status requires, including level of consciousness; vital signs, cardiac index, pulmonary artery pressures and urine output.	Determine the adequacy of cerebral perfusion; hemodynamic instability can lead to cerebral anoxia. Evaluates hemodynamic stability and volume status; recurrent tamponade may develop during and after sternotomy. Validates adequate perfusion to the kidneys.	• Change in levels of consciousness • Decrease in cardiac output and cardiac index • Abnormal pulmonary artery pressures • Equalizing pulmonary artery pressures • Mean arterial blood pressures less than 60 mm Hg • Changes in heart rate • Urine output less than 0.5 ml/kg/hr
2. Assess heart and lung sounds every 2 hours and as needed.	Abnormal heart and lung sounds may indicate the need for additional treatment.	• Distant heart sounds or additional changes in heart and lung sounds
3. Monitor coagulation and hematologic studies.	Coagulation and hematologic profiles provide data that indicate the risk of bleeding and indicate the need for additional treatment.	• Abnormal hemoglobin and hematocrit, prothrombin time, activated partial thromboplastin time, international normalized ratio, platelets, fibrinogen
4. Monitor chest tube drainage.	Determines functioning of the chest tube drainage system and the amount of chest drainage.	• Cessation of chest tube drainage • Increased chest tube drainage • Clots in chest tube drainage system

Documentation

Documentation should include the following:

- Patient and family education
- Indications for the procedure and the procedure performed
- Inform consent obtained
- Amount of blood collected from chest suctioning
- Estimated blood loss

- Unexpected outcomes
- Additional interventions
- Patient therapies and response, including hemodynamics, inotropic or vasopressor agents, ventilation, and neurologic status

Reference

1. Lyerly, H. (1995). *Handbook of Surgical Care.* Chicago: Year Book Medical Publishers, 83-6.

Additional Readings

Bojar, R., Mathisen, D., and Warner, K. (1994). *Manual of Perioperative Care in Cardiac and Thoracic Surgery.* Boston: Blackwell Scientific Publications, 989-99.

Borkon, M., et al. (1981). Diagnosis and management of postoperative pericardial effusions and late cardiac tamponade following open-heart surgery. *Ann Thorac Surg,* 31, 512-8.

Fairman, R., and Edmunds, H. (1981). Emergency thoracotomy in the surgical care unit after open cardiac operation. *Ann Thorac Surg,* 32, 386-91.

Sabiston, D., and Spencer, F. (1995). *Surgery of the Chest.* Philadelphia: W.B. Saunders, 220-2.

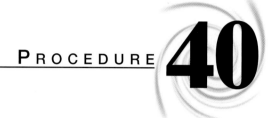 http://evolve.elsevier.com

PROCEDURE **40**

Emergent Open Sternotomy (Assist)

PURPOSE: Emergent open sternotomy in a postoperative patient after cardiac surgery is designed to identify and eliminate areas of persistent hemorrhage, relieve pericardial tamponade, and provide access for open cardiac massage.

Deborah G. Lamarr

PREREQUISITE NURSING KNOWLEDGE

- Knowledge of anatomy and physiology of the cardiovascular system is required.
- Advanced cardiac life support knowledge and skills are required.
- This procedure is designed for postoperative patients after cardiac surgeries who have undergone the median sternotomy approach.
- Knowledge of signs and symptoms of cardiac tamponade is required.
- Emergent open sternotomy in a postoperative patient after cardiac surgery is indicated for exanguinating hemorrhage or cardiac tamponade with imminent cardiac arrest.
- Early reexploration for persistent hemorrhage may reduce the requirement for homologous transfusions and may lower the wound infection rate associated with an undrained mediastinal hematoma.
- Mediastinal reexploration for cardiac tamponade decreases ventricular diastolic pressure. This decreased pressure allows for increased ventricular filling, which should increase stroke volume and cardiac output and globally improve systemic perfusion.
- Mechanical ventilation and sedation are prerequisites to sternal reexploration.
- Paralytic agents may be a necessary adjunct to sedation to improve oxygenation, diminish muscle activity, and enhance visualization in the operative field.
- Internal defibrillation may be necessary if life-threatening dysrhythmias occur (see Procedure 38).

EQUIPMENT

- Antiseptic solution (e.g., 2% chlorhexidine–based preparation)
- Caps, masks, goggles, sterile gloves, and sterile drapes
- Sterile staple remover
- Sterile open-chest set
  - ❖ Rib spreader
  - ❖ Kelly clamps and skin snaps
  - ❖ Knife handle
  - ❖ Wire cutter
  - ❖ Scissors
- Electrocautery equipment: generator, cautery, grounding pad
- Large sterile suction catheter (e.g., Yankauer)
- Suction container and tubing
- Polypropylene (Prolene) suture (cutting needle), other suture material according to preference
- Clip applicator and clips
- Syringes: 3 ml, 5 ml, 10 ml, 20 ml
- Knife blades: No. 10, No. 11, No. 15
- Sternal wires
- Sterile stapler and staples
- Sterile dressing supplies
- Emergency medication and resuscitation equipment
Additional equipment as needed includes the following:
- Analgesia or sedation as prescribed
- Blood products and intravenous solutions as prescribed
- Chest tubes and chest tube drainage system
- Epicardial wires
- Intraaortic balloon pump or other mechanical assist device

PATIENT AND FAMILY EDUCATION

- Teaching may be necessary after the procedure. ➤*Rationale:* If the emergent sternotomy is performed in the face of hemodynamic collapse, education of the patient and family may be impossible until after the procedure has been performed.
- Explain the reason that the open sternotomy procedure was performed and its outcome or anticipated outcome. ➤*Rationale:* This explanation clarifies information and encourages the patient and family to ask questions and voice specific concerns about the procedure.

PATIENT ASSESSMENT AND PREPARATION

Patient Assessment

- Assess hemodynamic and neurologic status. ➤*Rationale:* Identifies baseline data that may indicate the need for emergent open sternotomy and provides comparison data.
- Assess the patient's medical history, specifically that relates to coagulation disorders, renal disease with coexistent uremia, and functional status of the right and left ventricle. ➤*Rationale:* Provides baseline data.
- Assess current laboratory data, specifically complete blood cell count, platelet count, prothrombin time, activated partial thromboplastin time, fibrinogen, and international normalized ratio. ➤*Rationale:* Baseline coagulation studies need to be near-normal to be eliminated as possible causes for ongoing hemorrhage.
- Assess for signs and symptoms of cardiac tamponade.
  - ❖ Sudden decrease or cessation in chest tube drainage
  - ❖ Hypotension (mean arterial blood pressure less than 60 mm Hg)
  - ❖ Altered mental status
  - ❖ Apical heart rate greater than 110 beats/min
  - ❖ Narrowing of pulse pressure
  - ❖ Distended neck veins
  - ❖ Distant heart sounds
  - ❖ Equilibrium of intracardiac pressures with right atrial, pulmonary artery wedge, and (if measured) left atrial pressures being equal
  - ❖ Decreased cardiac output and cardiac index
  - ❖ Pulsus paradoxus
  - ➤*Rationale:* This determines the need for chest exploration.
- Assess for excessive chest tube drainage[1] (e.g., 500 ml for 1 hour, 400 ml for 2 consecutive hours, or 300 ml for 3 consecutive hours). ➤*Rationale:* This determines the need for chest exploration.

Patient Preparation

- Ensure that the patient and family understand procedural teaching (if time available). Answer questions as they arise, and reinforce information as needed. ➤*Rationale:* This communication evaluates and reinforces understandings of previously taught information.
- If time allows, obtain a chest radiograph to assess for evidence of widened mediastinum. ➤*Rationale:* Widening of the mediastinum on chest radiograph, especially the right heart border, could indicate mediastinal blood.
- If time allows, obtain a transthoracic echocardiogram in an attempt to identify a mediastinal clot. ➤*Rationale:* An echocardiogram aids in the diagnosis and confirms the necessity for the open sternotomy procedure.
- Ensure that informed consent was obtained (this may not be possible if the procedure is an acute emergency). ➤*Rationale:* This protects the rights of the patient and ensures a competent decision for the patient and the family.
- Ensure that the patient's ventilation is maintained. ➤*Rationale:* This ensures that the patient's airway is protected and that oxygen needs are met.
- Position the patient in the supine position with the head of the bed flat. ➤*Rationale:* This positioning ensures visualization of the chest.
- Prescribe analgesics or sedatives: ➤*Rationale:* Analgesics or sedatives promote comfort.

Procedure | for Assisting With Emergent Open Sternotomy

Steps	Rationale	Special Considerations
1. Call the physician and operative team.	The physician can reassess the need for further surgical intervention. The operative team may be needed to assist at the bedside or to prepare the operating room if further exploration is needed.	Follow hospital standard.
2. Assist with preparation of the electrocautery device for possible use: Apply the ground pad to the patient's skin, and attach the grounding and cautery cables.	This device is used to terminate capillary oozing or bleeding.	

Procedure continues on the following page

Procedure for Assisting With Emergent Open Sternotomy—*Continued*

Steps	Rationale	Special Considerations
3. Set up a new sterile suction system.	This system is used to suction the mediastinum during the procedure.	
4. Wash hands, and don nonsterile gloves.	Reduces the transmission of microorganisms; standard precautions.	
5. Assist with removing the sternal dressing and cleansing the chest with antiseptic solution.	Inhibits microorganism transmission.	Prepare the skin from the sternal notch to the midabdomen and from one anterior axillary line to the other.
6. Wash hands, and don caps, masks, goggles, sterile gowns, and sterile gloves for all members of the health care team involved with the procedure.	Reduces the transmission of microorganisms; sterile precautions; standard precautions.	All personnel in the room must don masks and caps.
7. Assist with placement of the sterile drapes.	A large sterile field supplies room for placement of instruments.	
8. Assist with electrocautery as needed.	Cautery is used to stop bleeding from small vessels.	
9. Assist as needed by supplying the wire cutters and aiding in the removal of cut wires from the surgical field.	Assists with procedure and ensures that wires are adequately removed.	If staples are present, the staple remover is needed.
10. Assist with cauterization of oozing bleeding sites as needed.	Minimizes blood loss and enhances visualization of the surgical field.	
11. Assist with controling bleeding, enhancing sternal retraction, and suctioning as needed.	May eliminate the need for further exploration and allows for full visualization of the surgical field. Suction is necessary to clear blood from the field.	
12. Assist with the placement of chest tubes or pacing wires as needed.	Pacing leads and chest tubes can be displaced during sternal retraction.	
13. Assist with placement of mechanical assist devices if needed.	Cardiac tamponade can conceal right or left ventricular dysfunction; mechanical assistance may be necessary to improve cardiac output.	
14. Assist with patient transport to the operating room if necessary.	The patient may need surgical repair of coronary artery bypass grafts, cardiac valves, or the myocardium.	Ensure that the patient's chest is covered with sterile drapes during transportation.
15. If the patient does not need to return to the operating room, assist the physician or advanced practice nurse with reinsertion of the sternal wires as needed.	Ensures sternal closure.	
16. Assist as needed with skin closure.	Provides assistance as needed.	
17. Apply an occlusive dressing to the sternal incision, epicardial pacing wires, and chest tube sites.	Promotes aseptic management of the surgical incision and wound sites.	The patient's chest may be left open and covered with a sterile, occlusive surgical dressing if severe ventricular dysfunction exists.
18. Remove and discard personal protective equipment, discard used supplies, package instruments for sterilization, and wash hands.	Reduces the transmission of microorganisms and body secretions; standard precautions.	

Expected Outcomes	Unexpected Outcomes
• Increased cardiac output • Increased tissue perfusion, including cerebral, renal, and peripheral perfusion • Standard chest tube drainage • Decreased need for homologous transfusion	• Severe right or left ventricular dysfunction • Continued bleeding or coagulation disorders • Myocardial or aortic perforation • Cardiac arrest • Pneumothorax • Myocardial infarction • Atrial and ventricular dysrhythmias • Pain

Patient Monitoring and Care

Steps	Rationale	Reportable Conditions
		These conditions should be reported if they persist despite nursing interventions.
1. Perform cardiovascular, peripheral vascular, and hemodynamic assessments every 15-30 minutes as patient status requires. 　A. Assess level of consciousness.	Assesses for adequacy of cerebral perfusion; hemodynamic instability can lead to cerebral anoxia.	• Change in level of consciousness
B. Assess vital signs, cardiac index, and pulmonary artery pressures.	Evaluates hemodynamic stability and volume status; recurrent tamponade may develop during and after sternotomy.	• Decrease in cardiac output and cardiac index • Abnormal pulmonary artery pressures • Equalizing pulmonary artery pressures • Mean arterial blood pressure less than 60 mm Hg • Changes in heart rate
C. Measure urine output.	Validates adequate perfusion to the kidneys.	• Urine output less than 0.5 ml/kg/hr
2. Assess heart and lung sounds every 2 hours and as needed.	Abnormal heart and lung sounds may indicate the need for additional treatment.	• Distant heart sounds or additional changes in heart and lung sounds
3. Monitor coagulation and hematologic studies.	Coagulation and hematologic profiles provide data that indicate the risk of bleeding and indicate the need for additional treatment.	• Abnormal hemoglobin and hematocrit, prothrombin time, activated partial thromboplastin time, international normalized ratio, platelets, fibrinogen
4. Monitor chest tube drainage.	Determines functioning of the chest tube drainage system and the amount of chest drainage.	• Cessation of chest tube drainage • Increased chest tube drainage • Clots in chest tube drainage system

Documentation

Documentation should include the following:

- Patient and family education
- Indications for procedure and the procedure performed
- Amount of blood collected from chest suctioning
- Estimated blood loss
- Patient therapies and response, including hemodynamics, inotropic or vasopressor agents, ventilation, and neurologic status
- Unexpected outcomes
- Additional interventions

Reference

1. Lyerly, H. (1995). *Handbook of Surgical Care*. Chicago: Year Book Medical Publishers, 83-6.

Additional Readings

Bojar, R., Mathisen, D., and Warner, K. (1994). *Manual of Perioperative Care in Cardiac and Thoracic Surgery*. Boston: Blackwell Scientific Publications, 989-99.

Borkon, M., et al. (1981). Diagnosis and management of postoperative pericardial effusions and late cardiac tamponade following open-heart surgery. *Ann Thorac Surg, 31*, 512-8.

Fairman, R., and Edmunds, H. (1981). Emergency thoracotomy in the surgical care unit after open cardiac operation. *Ann Thorac Surg, 32*, 386-91.

Sabiston, D., and Spencer, F. (1995). *Surgery of the Chest*. Philadelphia: W.B. Saunders, 220-2.

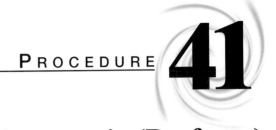
PROCEDURE **41**

AP
Pericardiocentesis (Perform)

PURPOSE: Pericardiocentesis is performed to remove fluid from the pericardial sac, to obtain a specimen for the differential diagnosis of the etiology of pericardial effusion, and to prevent or treat cardiac tamponade. Cardiac output usually is improved after pericardiocentesis.

Deborah E. Becker

PREREQUISITE NURSING KNOWLEDGE

- Advanced cardiac life support knowledge and skills are needed.
- Knowledge of sterile technique is required.
- Clinical and technical competence in the performance of pericardiocentesis is required.
- Knowledge of cardiovascular anatomy and physiology is needed.
- Pericardial effusion is the abnormal accumulation of greater than 50 ml of serosanguineous fluid within the pericardial sac.
- A pericardial effusion can be noncompressive or compressive. With a compressive effusion, there is increased pressure within the pericardial sac, which results in cardiac tamponade and resistance to cardiac filling.
- The presentation of acute and chronic fluid accumulation varies. A rapid collection of fluid (over minutes to hours) may result in hemodynamic compromise with volumes of less than 250 ml. Chronically developing effusions (over days to weeks) allow for hypertrophy and distention of the fibrous parietal membrane.[1] A patient may accumulate greater than or equal to 2000 ml of fluid before exhibiting symptoms of hemodynamic compromise.[2,4]
- Symptoms of cardiac tamponade are not specific. Patients may exhibit signs and symptoms of an associated disease. With a decrease in cardiac output, the patient often develops tachycardia, tachypnea, pallor, cyanosis, impaired cerebral and renal function, sweating, hypotension, neck vein distention, and pulsus paradoxus.[5]
- The presence and amount of fluid in the pericardium are evaluated through chest radiograph, two-dimensional echocardiogram, and clinical findings.
- When cardiac tamponade or a large enough effusion to warrant drainage is verified, a pericardiocentesis is performed to remove fluid from the pericardial sac. An acute tamponade resulting in hemodynamic instability necessitates an emergency procedure.
- Pericardiocentesis commonly is performed using a subxiphoid approach.
- Two-dimensional echocardiography is recommended to assist in guiding the needle during the pericardiocentesis.[7]
- Inability to obtain pericardial drainage, reaccumulation of pericardial fluid, or cardiac injury may progress into cardiac tamponade requiring urgent or emergent chest exploration.

EQUIPMENT

- Pericardiocentesis tray (or thoracentesis tray)
- 16-gauge or 18-gauge, 3-inch cardiac needle or catheter over the needle
- Antiseptic solution (e.g., 2% chlorhexidine–based preparation)
- Two packs of 4 × 4 gauze sponges
- No. 11 knife blade with handle (scalpel)
- Sterile 50-ml, 10-ml, 5-ml, and 3-ml syringes
- Sterile drapes and towels
- Masks, goggles or face shields, surgical caps, sterile gowns, and gloves for all personnel
- Sterile alligator clip cable
- Two three-way stopcocks
- 1% lidocaine (injectable)
- 12-lead electrocardiogram (ECG) machine

- Culture bottles and specimen tubes for fluid analysis
- 2-inch and 3-inch tape
  Additional equipment as needed includes the following:
- Emergency cart (defibrillator, emergency respiratory equipment, emergency cardiac medications, and temporary pacemaker)
- Two-dimensional echocardiography equipment
- If continuous drainage is required:
  - J guidewire, 0.035 diameter
  - Vessel dilator, 7 Fr
  - Pigtail catheter, 7 Fr
  - Tubing and drainage bag or bottle

PATIENT AND FAMILY EDUCATION

- Instruct the patient and family regarding the reason the pericardiocentesis is needed; describe the procedure; and explain expected outcomes, alternatives, and possible complications. ➤*Rationale:* This communication helps the patient and family to understand the procedure. Information about the procedure reduces anxiety and apprehension.
- Instruct the patient and family about potential signs and symptoms of recurrent pericardial effusion (e.g., dyspnea, dull ache or pressure within the chest, dysphagia, cough, tachypnea, hoarseness, hiccups, or nausea).[3,6] ➤*Rationale:* Early detection of pericardial effusion may prevent complications from heart compression.
- Instruct the patient and family about the patient's risk for recurrent pericardial effusion. ➤*Rationale:* Predicting pericardial effusion may allow early detection of a potentially life-threatening problem.

PATIENT ASSESSMENT AND PREPARATION

Patient Assessment

- Determine the history of the present illness and mechanism of injury (if applicable), past medical history, and current medical therapies. ➤*Rationale:* The history is needed to determine the patient's present health, to identify potential risk factors, and to provide an opportunity for the nurse to establish a relationship with the patient.
- Assess the patient's heart rate, cardiac rhythm, heart sounds (S_1, S_2, rubs), venous pressure (noninvasive or invasive), blood pressure, pulse pressure, oxygen saturation by pulse oximetry (SpO_2), respiratory status, and neurologic status. ➤*Rationale:* These data are needed to compare baseline data to assess for changes during or after the procedure.
- Assess current laboratory values, including the complete blood cell count, electrolytes, and coagulation profile. ➤*Rationale:* These data are needed to identify the potential for cardiac dysrhythmias or abnormal bleeding. If the international normalized ratio or partial thromboplastin time or both are elevated, consider reversing the level of anticoagulation before performing or deferring the procedure until the levels indicate a reduced possibility of bleeding.

Patient Preparation

- Ensure that the patient and family understand preprocedural teaching. Answer questions as they arise, and reinforce information as needed. ➤*Rationale:* This communication evaluates and reinforces understanding of previously taught information.
- Obtain informed consent. ➤*Rationale:* Informed consent protects the rights of the patient and makes competent decision making possible for the patient; however, under emergency circumstances, time may not allow the consent form to be signed.
- Coordinate the procedure with the echocardiogram technician to assist with the two-dimensional echocardiogram if this approach is being taken. ➤*Rationale:* Echocardiogram-directed pericardiocentesis allows for more precise localization of the effusion and may help to prevent complications from occurring.
- Position the patient comfortably in the supine position with the head of the bed elevated 30 to 60 degrees. ➤*Rationale:* The supine position facilitates the aspiration of pericardial fluids and ease of breathing.
- Prescribe sedatives. ➤*Rationale:* Sedatives reduce anxiety, promote comfort, and decrease myocardial workload.
- Apply the limb leads and connect the leads to the cardiac bedside monitoring system or to the 12-lead ECG machine. ➤*Rationale:* The ECG is analyzed during the procedure (V lead) to indicate when the pericardial needle is in contact with the myocardium and after the procedure to monitor the patient for changes that may indicate cardiac injury.

Procedure for Performing Pericardiocentesis

Steps	Rationale	Special Considerations
1. Wash hands and don nonsterile gloves.	Reduces the transmission of microorganisms; standard precautions.	
2. Open the pericardiocentesis tray and appropriate supplies using aseptic technique, and prepare the tray for the procedure (other supplies are opened as needed).	Minimizes the potential for infection.	

Procedure for Performing Pericardiocentesis—*Continued*

Steps	Rationale	Special Considerations
3. Ensure that the patient is positioned comfortably in the supine position (with the head of the bed elevated 60 degrees).	Facilitates aspiration of fluids (elevated head of bed facilitates ease of breathing).	
4. Prepare the skin by applying the antiseptic solution (e.g., 2% chlorhexidine–based preparation).	Minimizes the potential for infection.	Clipping the hair may be necessary before applying antiseptic solution.
5. If two-dimensional echocardiogram is being used, skip to **Step 13**.		
6. Don mask, goggles or face shield, surgical cap, sterile gown, and sterile gloves.	Maintains aseptic technique.	
7. Attach a three-way stopcock to a 3-inch cardiac needle, and attach to a 50-ml syringe.	Provides the mechanism to aspirate fluid.	
8. Attach a syringe with 1% lidocaine to one side of the stopcock.	Reduces patient's discomfort.	As the needle is introduced, the provider may insert a small amount of 1% lidocaine to add analgesic effect.
9. Connect one end of an alligator clip to the proximal portion of the needle (closest to the syringe or hub of a sheathed needle), and have the nurse attach the other end to the V_1 lead of the ECG. The bedside monitor or a 12-lead ECG machine can be used to obtain the ECG (Fig. 41-1).	Provides the mechanism to identify myocardial contact or injury.	
10. Continuously monitor the bedside ECG or the 12-lead ECG, vital signs, SpO$_2$, and venous pressure during needle aspiration, fluid withdrawal, and withdrawal of the needle.[2,4,8]	Detects myocardial contact or injury; monitors the results of the procedure. If the needle contacts the ventricle, ST-segment depression is seen. With atrial contact, PR-segment elevation occurs.	If ST-segment depression or PR-segment elevation is noted, the needled should be withdrawn and reinserted slowly in a different direction until fluid is aspirated. Emergent chest exploration may be necessary if aspiration is unsuccessful, pericardial fluid repeatedly accumulates, or complications develop.
11. Slowly insert the needle while aspirating with the 50-ml syringe into the skin just under the xiphoid at a 30-degree angle. The needle moves into the pericardial sac until fluid is aspirated. If using a sheathed needle, when fluid is obtained, advance the needle approximately 2 mm further, then	Minimizes the risk of cardiac injury. If the pericardiocentesis is performed blindly, fluid received may be placed in a bowl and observed for clotting. If clotting does not occur, it can be assumed that this fluid is from the effusion.	The movement of the heart usually defibrinates blood in the pericardial space so that it cannot clot. Clotting usually indicates penetration of the heart chamber and blood obtained from within a ventricle or atrium.[8]

Procedure continues on the following page

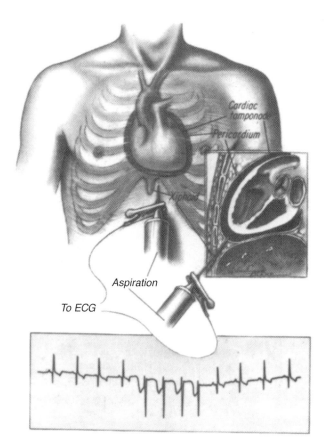

FIGURE 41-1 Subxiphoid pericardiocentesis with ECG monitoring. Note the negative QRS deflection indicating myocardial contact. *(From Sellke, F., Swanson, S., and del Nido, P.J. [2005]. Sabiston and Spencer Surgery of the Chest. 7th ed. Philadelphia: W.B. Saunders.)*

Procedure for Performing Pericardiocentesis—*Continued*

Steps	Rationale	Special Considerations
remove the needle and maintain the sheath in the fluid space while draining the effusion.[7] If two-dimensional echocardiogram is used, go to **Step 15**.		If clotting occurs with the fluid obtained, withdraw the needle and reinsert slowly in a different direction.
12. When the needle position is confirmed, obtain samples of fluid, remove the needle, and send the samples to the laboratory for evaluation. If continuous drainage is warranted, go to **Step 16**. If not, skip to **Step 22**.	Provides diagnosis of the organism involved in the pericardial effusion.	Usual tests include body fluid cytology, cell count, electrolytes, routine aerobic and anaerobic cultures, acid-fast bacilli cultures, and other tests as indicated.
When Two-Dimensional Echocardiogram Is Used		
13. If available, perform a two-dimensional echocardiogram (or have a technician perform one). Determine the location and size of the effusion and the ideal entry site and needle trajectory for the pericardiocentesis.	Two-dimensional echocardiogram allows for more accurate identification of the location and size of the pericardial effusion. The ideal entry site is the point where the effusion is closest to the transducer and fluid accumulation is maximal.[2,4,7]	A straight trajectory that best avoids vital structures, including the liver, myocardium, and lung, should be chosen. The internal mammary artery also should be avoided. Mark the skin with a small pen mark (which stays on the skin when ready to perform the procedure to assist in guiding the needle), and make special note of the trajectory to be taken.[5,8]

Procedure for Performing Pericardiocentesis—*Continued*

Steps	Rationale	Special Considerations
		If two-dimensional echocardiogram is not available, skip this step and continue on from **Step 5**.
14. Return to **Step 5** and follow the procedural steps.		
15. If bloody fluid is aspirated, a few milliliters of echocontrast medium are infused to confirm position.[1,7] When it is determined that the fluid, is pericardial, return to **Step 12**.	If the contrast material appears in the pericardial space, the procedure can be continued. If the contrast material disappears, the needle may be in one of the heart chambers and must be withdrawn and repositioned.	Two-dimensional echocardiogram assists in determining position of the needle. Echocontrast is agitated saline that is injected via the side port of the stopcock.[7]
When Continuous Drainage Is Desired 16. When the needle tip position is confirmed to be within the pericardial space, remove the steel needle and insert a soft, floppy-tipped guidewire through the needle. The guidewire is passed so that it wraps around the heart within the pericardial space.[2,4,8]	Minimizes the risk of cardiac injury. Allows for the passage of the guidewire and placement within the pericardial space.	
17. A pigtail or straight soft catheter is passed over the guidewire.	A flexible-tipped, soft catheter with multiple holes in the tip is used to facilitate drainage of the effusion. Using a soft-tipped catheter reduces the chances of causing myocardial injury and dysrhythmias during the procedure.[2]	Either a pigtail catheter or a straight catheter with multiple holes can be used for better drainage. The soft catheter can remain in place for 24 hours.
18. Remove the guidewire and connect the end of the catheter to the three-way stopcock and the drainage collection bag.[2,4,8]	Maintains asepsis; allows for continual drainage of the effusion.	If the effusion is small, when fluid is drained, remove the catheter.
19. If an indwelling catheter is placed to continuously drain a large pericardial effusion, attach the catheter to the sterile bag or bottle using aseptic technique (see Procedure 77).	Facilitates fluid drainage; minimizes the potential for infection.	
20. If an indwelling catheter is to remain in place, secure the catheter by taping the catheter securely to the patient's chest wall.	Prevents dislodging or accidental discontinuation of drainage.	A purse-string suture also can be used to prevent dislodging the catheter.
21. Instruct the nurse to cleanse the area with antiseptic solution and apply an occlusive, sterile dressing.	Minimizes skin breakdown and minimizes infection.	
22. Continue bedside ECG monitoring, and discontinue 12-lead ECG (if used).	Allows monitoring of cardiac rate and rhythm.	

Procedure continues on the following page

Procedure for Performing Pericardiocentesis—*Continued*

Steps	Rationale	Special Considerations
23. Dispose of used supplies.	Standard precautions.	
24. Wash hands.	Reduces the transmission of microorganisms; standard precautions.	
25. If an indwelling catheter is placed, consider prescribing antibiotics.	Reduces the risk of infection.	

Expected Outcomes

- Fluid removed from the pericardial sac
- Relief of pain, discomfort, or other symptoms that indicated need for the procedure
- Improved cardiac output
- Patient's blood pressure, venous pressure, heart sounds, pulse pressure, and cardiac rhythm within normal limits

Unexpected Outcomes

- Decrease in blood pressure, increase in venous pressure, cardiac dysrhythmias, or excessive bleeding
- Hemodynamic instability
- ST-segment depression
- PR-segment elevation
- Cardiac tamponade

Patient Monitoring and Care

Steps	Rationale	Reportable Conditions
		These conditions should be reported if they persist despite nursing interventions.
1. Continuously monitor ECG; evaluate venous pressure, systemic blood pressure, heart sounds, SpO_2, and neurologic status before, during, and every 15 minutes immediately postprocedure until stable (if available, continuously monitor cardiac index and systemic vascular resistance).	A change in these signs may indicate cardiac tamponade, cardiac injury, or hemodynamic instability.	- Increasing venous pressure, decreasing arterial pressure, decrease in intensity of heart sounds, change in level of consciousness, or pulsus paradoxus; if applicable, abnormal cardiac index or systemic vascular resistance
2. Treat dysrhythmias if they occur.	Dysrhythmias may lead to cardiac decompensation.	- Persistent dysrhythmias despite appropriate intervention
3. Auscultate heart and lung sounds immediately before and after the procedure.	Evaluates potential fluid reaccumulation or puncture of the lung.	- Asymmetrical breath sounds, dyspnea, tachypnea, abrupt change in SpO_2, or decreased or muffled heart sound intensity
4. Obtain a portable chest radiograph immediately postprocedure.	Assesses for pneumothorax and hemothorax.	- Pneumothorax or hemothorax
5. Obtain a two-dimensional echocardiogram within several hours after the procedure.	Shows effectiveness of the pericardial drainage.	- Pericardial effusion
6. Monitor the pericardiocentesis site for bleeding every 15 minutes after the procedure is completed until the patient is stable, then every 4 hours for 24 hours. If an indwelling catheter is present, continue to monitor the site every 4 hours until the catheter has been removed for a total of 24 hours.	Assesses for postprocedural hemostasis.	- Bleeding or hematoma at site

Patient Monitoring and Care—*Continued*

Steps	Rationale	Reportable Conditions
7. Monitor hemoglobin, hematocrit, and coagulation studies every 8 hours postprocedure for 24 hours and then as indicated.	Assesses for potential of effusion recurrence or bleeding at the site.	• Bleeding or hematoma at site • Decrease in hemoglobin or hematocrit • Changes in coagulation studies
8. Assess pericardiocentesis site for signs of infection.	Identifies presence or absence of infection. If indwelling catheter, potential for catheter-related sepsis exists.	• Erythema • Edema • Purulent drainage • Foul odor of site • Temperature greater than 100.5°F (greater than 38°C)
9. Prescribe dressing changes daily and as needed.	Minimizes the potential for infection.	
10. Evaluate the size of the effusion within 24 hours of the indwelling catheter placement by the use of a two-dimensional echocardiogram.	Records how effective drainage was and whether the need for the indwelling catheter continues to exist.	
11. Remove the indwelling catheter when no longer needed using aseptic technique.	Minimizes the potential for infection.	
12. Be prepared for chest exploration if deterioration in the patient's condition occurs.	Deterioration may indicate development of further cardiac tamponade.	• Decreased blood pressure • Presence of dysrhythmias • Increased venous pressure • Change in mental or respiratory status • Diaphoresis • Distant heart sounds
13. Provide emotional support to the patient throughout the procedure.	Minimizes apprehension and anxiety.	
14. Keep the patient and family informed about the patient's condition. Be available to answer patient and family's questions and facilitate meeting their needs as appropriate.	The unknown increases the anxiety and apprehension of the patient and family.	

Documentation

Documentation should include the following:

- Preprocedure instruction and patient and family's response
- Signed informed consent form
- Preprocedure and postprocedure blood pressure, venous pressures, pulmonary arterial pressures, cardiac index/cardiac output/systemic vascular resistance if available, heart sounds, level of consciousness, respiratory status, cardiac rhythm
- Preprocedural hemoglobin, hematocrit, and coagulation results if performed
- Medications administered
- Placement of indwelling catheter if used

- Removal of indwelling catheter if used
- Assessment of pericardiocentesis fluid
- Amount and consistency of postprocedure drainage
- Occurrence of unexpected outcomes
- Preprocedural and postprocedural evaluation and location of effusion by two-dimensional echocardiogram (if used)
- ECG rhythm strips
- Emergency interventions required
- Specimens sent to the laboratory

References

1. Douglas, J.M. (1995). The pericardium. In: Sabiston, J.R., and Spencer, F.C., editors. *Surgery of the Chest.* Philadelphia: W.B. Saunders, 1379-80.
2. Focht, G., and Becker, R.C. (1996). Pericardiocentesis. In: Rippe, J.M., et al, editors. *Intensive Care Medicine.* Boston: Little, Brown, 111-6.
3. Muirhead, J. (1989). Pericardial disease. In: Underhill, S.L., et al, editors. *Cardiac Nursing.* Philadelphia: J.B. Lippincott, 111-6.
4. Shabetai, R. (1996). Treatment of pericardial disease. In: Smith, T.W., editor. *Cardiovascular Therapeutics: A Companion to Braunwald's Heart Disease.* Philadelphia: W.B. Saunders, 742-6.
5. Spodick, D. (1989). Percarditis, pericardial effusion, cardiac tamponade, and constriction. *Crit Care Clin,* 5, 455-76.
6. Suddarth, D.S. (1991). *Lippincott Manual of Nursing Practice.* Philadelphia: J.B. Lippincott, 310-1.
7. Tsang, T.S., et al. (1998). Echocardiographically guided pericardiocentesis: Evolution and state-of-the-art technique. *Mayo Clin Proc,* 73, 647-52.
8. Yeston, N., Grotz, R., and Loiacono, L. (1997). Pericardiocentesis. In: Civetta, J.M., Taylor, J.W., and Kirby, R.R., editors. *Critical Care.* Philadelphia: Lippincott-Raven, 577-8.

Additional Readings

Loeb, S., McCloskey, P.W., and Tryniszewski, C. (1994). *Critical Care Procedures.* Springhouse, PA: Springhouse, 225-9.

Lorell, B. (1997). Pericardial disease. In: Braunwald, A.B., editor. *Heart Disease: A Textbook of Cardiovascular Medicine.* Philadelphia: W.B. Saunders, 1478-524.

Mavroukakis, S., and Stine, A. (1998). Nursing management of adults with disorders of the coronary arteries, myocardium, or pericardium. In: Beare, P.G., and Myers, J.L., editors. *Adult Health Nursing.* St. Louis: Mosby, 597-603.

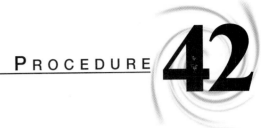
PROCEDURE **42**

Pericardiocentesis (Assist)

PURPOSE: Pericardiocentesis is performed to remove fluid from the pericardial sac, to obtain a specimen for the differential diagnosis of the etiology of pericardial effusion, and to prevent or treat cardiac tamponade. Cardiac output usually is improved after pericardiocentesis.

Deborah E. Becker

PREREQUISITE NURSING KNOWLEDGE

- Advanced cardiac life support knowledge and skills are needed.
- Knowledge of sterile technique is required.
- Knowledge of cardiovascular anatomy and physiology is needed.
- Pericardial effusion is the abnormal accumulation of greater than 50 ml of serosanguineous fluid within the pericardial sac.
- A pericardial effusion can be noncompressive or compressive. With a compressive effusion, there is increased pressure within the pericardial sac, which results in cardiac tamponade and resistance to cardiac filling.
- The presentation of acute and chronic fluid accumulation varies. A rapid collection of fluid (over minutes to hours) may result in hemodynamic compromise with volumes of less than 250 ml. Chronically developing effusions (over days to weeks) allow for hypertrophy and distention of the fibrous parietal membrane.[1] A patient may accumulate greater than or equal to 2000 ml of fluid before exhibiting symptoms of hemodynamic compromise.[2,4]
- Symptoms of cardiac tamponade are not specific. Patients may exhibit signs and symptoms of an associated disease. With a decrease in cardiac output, the patient often develops tachycardia, tachypnea, pallor, cyanosis, impaired cerebral and renal function, sweating, hypotension, neck vein distention, and pulsus paradoxus.[5]
- The presence and amount of fluid in the pericardium are evaluated through chest radiograph, two-dimensional echocardiogram, and clinical findings.

- When cardiac tamponade or a large enough effusion to warrant drainage is verified, a pericardiocentesis is performed to remove fluid from the pericardial sac. An acute tamponade resulting in hemodynamic instability necessitates an emergency procedure.
- Pericardiocentesis commonly is performed using a subxiphoid approach.
- Two-dimensional echocardiography is recommended to assist in guiding the needle during the pericardiocentesis.[7]
- Inability to obtain pericardial drainage, reaccumulation of pericardial fluid, or cardiac injury may progress into cardiac tamponade requiring urgent or emergent chest exploration.

EQUIPMENT

- Pericardiocentesis tray (or thoracentesis tray)
- 16-gauge or 18-gauge, 3-inch cardiac needle or catheter over the needle
- Antiseptic solution (e.g., 2% chlorhexidine–based preparation)
- Two packs of 4 × 4 gauze sponges
- No. 11 knife blade with handle (scalpel)
- Sterile 50-ml, 10-ml, 5-ml, and 3-ml syringes
- Sterile drapes and towels
- Masks, goggles or face shields, surgical caps, sterile gowns, and gloves for all personnel
- Sterile alligator clip cable
- Two three-way stopcocks
- 1% lidocaine (injectable)
- 12-lead electrocardiogram (ECG) machine
- Culture bottles and specimen tubes for fluid analysis
- 2-inch and 3-inch tape

Additional equipment as needed includes the following:
- Emergency cart (defibrillator, emergency respiratory equipment, emergency cardiac medications, and temporary pacemaker)
- Two-dimensional echocardiography equipment
- If continuous drainage is required:
  ❖ J guidewire, 0.035 diameter
  ❖ Vessel dilator, 7 Fr
  ❖ Pigtail catheter, 7 Fr
  ❖ Tubing and drainage bag or bottle

PATIENT AND FAMILY EDUCATION

- Instruct the patient and family regarding the reason the pericardiocentesis is needed; describe the procedure; and explain the expected outcomes, alternatives, and possible complications. ➽*Rationale:* This communication helps the patient and family to understand the procedure. Information about the procedure reduces anxiety and apprehension.
- Instruct the patient and family about potential signs and symptoms of recurrent pericardial effusion (e.g., dyspnea, dull ache or pressure within the chest, dysphagia, cough, tachypnea, hoarseness, hiccups, or nausea).[3,6] ➽*Rationale:* Early detection of pericardial effusion may prevent complications from heart compression.
- Instruct the patient and family about the patient's risk for recurrent pericardial effusion. ➽*Rationale:* Predicting pericardial effusion may allow early detection of a potentially life-threatening problem.

PATIENT ASSESSMENT AND PREPARATION

Patient Assessment
- Determine the history of the present illness and mechanism of injury (if applicable), past medical history, and current medical therapies. ➽*Rationale:* The history is needed to determine the patient's present health, to identify potential risk factors, and to provide an opportunity for the nurse to establish a relationship with the patient.

- Assess the patient's heart rate, cardiac rhythm, heart sounds (S_1, S_2, rubs), venous pressure (noninvasive or invasive), blood pressure, pulse pressure, oxygen saturation by pulse oximetry (SpO_2), respiratory status, and neurologic status. ➽*Rationale:* These data are needed to compare baseline data to assess for changes during or after the procedure.
- Assess the current laboratory values, including the complete blood cell count, electrolytes, and coagulation profile. ➽*Rationale:* These data are needed to identify the potential for cardiac dysrhythmias or abnormal bleeding.

Patient Preparation
- Ensure that the patient and family understand preprocedural teaching. Answer questions as they arise, and reinforce information as needed. ➽*Rationale:* This communication evaluates and reinforces understanding of previously taught information.
- Ensure that informed consent is obtained. ➽*Rationale:* Informed consent protects the rights of the patient and makes competent decision making possible for the patient; however, under emergency circumstances, time may not allow the consent form to be signed.
- Coordinate the procedure with the echocardiogram technician to assist with the two-dimensional echocardiogram if this approach is being taken. ➽*Rationale:* The echocardiogram technician will locate the fluid accumulation, making it easier to perform the pericardiocentesis.
- Position the patient comfortably in the supine position with the head of bed elevated 30 to 60 degrees. ➽*Rationale:* The supine position facilitates aspiration of pericardial fluids and ease of breathing.
- Administer the sedatives as prescribed. ➽*Rationale:* Sedatives reduce anxiety, promote comfort, and decrease myocardial workload.
- Apply the limb leads and connect the patient to the cardiac bedside monitoring system or to the 12-lead ECG machine. ➽*Rationale:* The ECG is analyzed during the procedure (V lead) to indicate when the pericardial needle is in contact with the myocardium and after the procedure to monitor the patient for changes that may indicate cardiac injury.

Procedure for Assisting With Pericardiocentesis

Steps	Rationale	Special Considerations
1. Wash hands and don nonsterile gloves.	Reduces the transmission of microorganisms; standard precautions.	
2. Assist as needed with opening the pericardiocentesis tray and the appropriate supplies using aseptic technique (other supplies are opened as needed).	Minimizes the potential for infection.	

Procedure for Assisting With Pericardiocentesis—*Continued*		
Steps	**Rationale**	**Special Considerations**
3. Ensure that the patient is positioned comfortably in the supine position (with the head of the bed elevated 60 degrees).	Facilitates the aspiration of fluids (elevated head of bed facilitates the ease of breathing).	
4. Assist the health care provider (e.g., physician, advance practice nurse) to prepare the skin by applying an antiseptic solution (e.g. 2% chlorhexidine–based preparation).	Minimizes the potential for infection.	Clipping hair from the area may be necessary before applying the antiseptic solution.
5. If two-dimensional echocardiogram is being used, skip to **Step 13**.		
6. Assist personnel as needed with donning masks, surgical caps, sterile gowns, and sterile gloves.	Maintains aseptic technique.	
7. Assist with attaching a three-way stopcock to a 3-inch cardiac needle and attach to a 50-ml syringe.	Provides the mechanism to aspirate fluid.	
8. Assist with preparing a syringe with 1% lidocaine.	Reduces patient's discomfort.	As the needle is introduced, the provider may insert a small amount of 1% lidocaine to add analgesic effect.
9. Assist with connecting one end of an alligator clip to the proximal portion of the needle (closest to the syringe or hub of a sheathed needle) and the other end to the V_1 lead of the ECG machine (see Fig. 41-1).	Provides mechanism to identify myocardial injury.	The bedside monitor or the 12-lead ECG can be used.
10. Continuously monitor the bedside ECG or 12-lead ECG, vital signs, SpO_2, and venous pressure during needle aspiration, fluid withdrawal, and withdrawal of the needle.[2,4,8]	The ECG detects myocardial contact or injury; monitors results of the procedure. If the needle contacts the ventricle, ST-segment depression is seen; with atrial contact, PR-segment elevation occurs. Vital signs and other assessments may indicate patient stability or signs of complications.	Emergent chest exploration may be necessary if aspiration is unsuccessful, pericardial fluid repeatedly accumulates, or complications develop.[4]
11. Observe as the health care provider slowly inserts the needle while aspirating with the 50-ml syringe into the skin just under the xiphoid at a 30-degree angle until pericardial fluid is aspirated.[6] If two-dimensional echocardiogram is used, go to **Step 15**. Assist the health care provider with placing aspirate into a bowl to determine if the fluid clots or not.	Minimizes the risk of cardiac injury. If the pericardiocentesis is performed blindly, fluid obtained may be placed in a bowl and observed for clotting. If clotting does not occur, it can be assumed that this fluid is from the effusion.	The movement of the heart usually defibrinates blood in the pericardial space so that it cannot clot. Clotting usually indicates penetration of the heart chamber and blood obtained from within a ventricle or atrium.[8]
12. When the needle position is confirmed, assist the health care provider with obtaining samples of fluid and sending the samples to the laboratory for evaluation. If continuous drainage is warranted, go to **Step 16**. If not, go to **Step 20**.	Provides diagnosis of organism involved in pericardial effusion.	Usual tests include body fluid cytology, cell count, electrolytes, routine aerobic and anaerobic cultures, acid-fast bacilli cultures, and other tests as indicated.

Procedure continues on the following page

Procedure for Assisting With Pericardiocentesis—*Continued*

Steps	Rationale	Special Considerations
When Two-Dimensional Echocardiogram Is Used		
13. If available, assist the health care provider and the echocardiogram technician in performing a two-dimensional echocardiogram to determine the location and size of the effusion and the ideal entry site and needle trajectory for the pericardiocentesis.	Two-dimensional echocardiogram allows for more accurate identification of the location and the size of the pericardial effusion. The ideal entry site is the point where the effusion is closest to the transducer and fluid accumulation is maximal.[2,4,7]	A straight trajectory that best avoids vital structures, including the liver, myocardium, and lung, is chosen. The internal mammary artery also is avoided. Assist if needed with marking the skin with a small pen mark (which stays on the skin when ready to perform the procedure to assist in guiding the needle), and make special note of the trajectory to be taken.[5,8] If two-dimensional echocardiogram is not available, skip this step, and continue on from **Step 5**.
14. Return to **Step 5**, and proceed.		
15. If bloody fluid is aspirated, be prepared to assist the health care provider in infusing a few milliliters of echocontrast medium into the space where the needle is to confirm position.[1,7] When it is determined that this is pericardial fluid, return to **Step 12**.	If contrast material appears in the pericardial space, the procedure can be continued. If the contrast material disappears, the needle may be in one of the heart chambers and must be withdrawn and repositioned.	Two-dimensional echocardiogram assists in determining the position of the needle. Echocontrast is agitated saline that is injected via the side port of the stopcock.[7]
When Continuous Drainage Is Desired		
16. When the needle tip position is confirmed to be within the pericardial space, assist the health care provider with removing the steel needle and inserting a soft, floppy-tipped guidewire through the needle. The guidewire is passed so that it wraps around the heart within the pericardial space.[2,4,8]	Minimizes the risk of cardiac injury. Allows for the passage of the guidewire and placement within the pericardial space.	
17. Assist the health care provider with removing the guidewire and connecting the end of the catheter to the three-way stopcock and the drainage collection bag.[2,4,8]	Maintains asepsis; allows for continual drainage of the effusion.[2]	
18. If an indwelling catheter is placed to drain continuously a large pericardial effusion, assist the health care provider with attaching the sterile bag or bottle using aseptic technique (see Procedure 77).	Facilitates fluid drainage; minimizes the potential for infection.	
19. If an indwelling catheter is to remain in place, secure it by taping the catheter securely to the patient's chest wall.	Prevents dislodging or accidental discontinuation of the drainage.	It may be necessary to assist the health care provider in placing a purse-string suture to prevent dislodging the catheter.
20. Cleanse the area with antiseptic solution and apply an occlusive, sterile dressing.	Minimizes skin breakdown and minimizes infection.	

Procedure for Assisting With Pericardiocentesis—*Continued*

Steps	Rationale	Special Considerations
21. Continue bedside ECG monitoring, and discontinue the 12-lead ECG (if used).	Allows monitoring of cardiac rate and rhythm.	
22. Dispose of used supplies.	Standard precautions.	
23. Wash hands.	Reduces the transmission of microorganisms; standard precautions.	

Expected Outcomes

- Fluid removed from the pericardial sac
- Relief of pain, discomfort, or other symptoms that indicated the need for the procedure
- Improved cardiac output
- Patient's blood pressure, venous pressure, heart sounds, pulse pressure, and cardiac rhythm within normal limits

Unexpected Outcomes

- Decrease in blood pressure, rise in venous pressure, cardiac dysrhythmias, or excessive bleeding
- Hemodynamic instability
- ST-segment depression
- PR-segment elevation
- Cardiac tamponade

Patient Monitoring and Care

Steps	Rationale	Reportable Conditions
		These conditions should be reported if they persist despite nursing interventions.
1. Continuously monitor the patient's ECG; evaluate venous pressure, systemic blood pressure, heart sounds, SpO_2, and neurologic status before, during, and every 15 minutes immediately postprocedure until stable (if available, continuously monitor cardiac index and systemic vascular resistance).	A change in these signs may indicate cardiac tamponade, cardiac injury, or hemodynamic instability.	• Increasing venous pressure • Decreasing arterial pressure • Decrease in intensity of heart sounds • Change in level of consciousness • Pulsus paradoxus • Abnormal cardiac index or systemic vascular resistance
2. Treat dysrhythmias as prescribed.	Dysrhythmias may lead to cardiac decompensation.	• Persistent dysrhythmias despite appropriate intervention
3. Auscultate heart and lung sounds immediately before and after the procedure.	Evaluates potential fluid reaccumulation or puncture of the lung.	• Asymmetric breath sounds • Dyspnea • Tachypnea • Abrupt change in SpO_2 • Decrease in heart sound intensity
4. Ensure a portable chest radiograph is obtained immediately postprocedure.	Assesses for pneumothorax and hemothorax.	• Pneumothorax • Hemothorax
5. Ensure a two-dimensional echocardiogram is obtained within several hours after the procedure.	Shows the effectiveness of the pericardial drainage.	• Pericardial effusion
6. Monitor the pericardiocentesis site for bleeding every 15 minutes after the procedure is completed until the patient is stable, then every 4 hours for 24 hours. If an indwelling catheter is present, continue to monitor the site every 4 hours until the catheter has been discontinued for a total of 24 hours.	Assesses for postprocedural hemostasis.	• Bleeding or hematoma at the site

Procedure continues on the following page

Patient Monitoring and Care—*Continued*

Steps	Rationale	Reportable Conditions
7. Monitor hemoglobin, hematocrit, and coagulation studies every 8 hours postprocedure for 24 hours and then as indicated.	Assesses for potential of effusion recurrence or bleeding at the site.	• Bleeding or hematoma at site • Decrease in hemoglobin or hematocrit • Changes in coagulation studies
8. Assess the pericardiocentesis site for signs or symptoms of infection.	Identifies the presence or absence of infection. If an indwelling catheter, the potential for catheter-related sepsis exists.	• Erythema • Edema • Purulent drainage • Foul odor of site • Temperature greater than 100.5°F (greater than 38°C)
9. Change the dressing daily and as needed.	Minimizes the potential for infection.	• Signs and symptoms of infection
10. Be prepared for chest exploration if the patient's status deteriorates.	Deterioration in the patient's hemodynamic status may indicate an increasing effusion and the need for immediate surgical intervention.	• Decreased blood pressure • Dysrhythmias • Increased venous pressure • Change in mental or respiratory status • Diaphoresis • Distant heart sounds
11. Keep the patient and family informed about the patient's condition. Be available to answer patient and family's questions, and facilitate meeting their needs as appropriate.	The unknown increases the anxiety and apprehension of the patient and family.	

Documentation

Documentation should include the following:

- Preprocedure instruction and patient and family's response
- Preprocedure and postprocedure blood pressure, venous pressures, pulmonary arterial pressures, cardiac index/cardiac output/systemic vascular resistance if available, heart sounds, level of consciousness, respiratory status, cardiac rhythm
- Preprocedural hemoglobin, hematocrit, and coagulation results if performed
- Medications administered
- Placement of the indwelling catheter if used
- Removal of the indwelling catheter if used
- Assessment of pericardiocentesis fluid
- Amount and consistency of postprocedure drainage
- Occurrence of unexpected outcomes
- Preprocedural and postprocedural evaluation and location of effusion by two-dimensional echocardiogram (if used)
- ECG rhythm strips
- Emergency interventions required
- Specimens sent to the laboratory

References

1. Douglas, J.M. (1995). The pericardium. In: Sabiston, J.R., and Spencer, F.C., editors. *Surgery of the Chest.* Philadelphia: W.B. Saunders, 1379-80.
2. Focht, G., and Becker, R.C. (1996). Pericardiocentesis. In: Rippe, J.M., et al, editors. *Intensive Care Medicine.* Boston: Little, Brown, 111-6.
3. Muirhead, J. (1989). Pericardial disease. In: Underhill, S.L., et al, editors. *Cardiac Nursing.* Philadelphia: J.B. Lippincott, 111-6.
4. Shabetai, R. (1996). Treatment of pericardial disease. In: Smith, T.W., editor. *Cardiovascular Therapeutics:*
A Companion to Braunwald's Heart Disease. Philadelphia: W.B. Saunders, 742-6.
5. Spodick, D. (1989). Percarditis, pericardial effusion, cardiac tamponade, and constriction. *Crit Care Clin,* 5, 455-76.
6. Suddarth, D.S. (1991). *Lippincott Manual of Nursing Practice.* Philadelphia: J.B. Lippincott, 310-1.
7. Tsang, T.S., et al., (1998). Echocardiographically guided pericardiocentesis: Evolution and state-of-the-art technique. *Mayo Clin Proc,* 73, 647-52.
8. Yeston, N., Grotz, R., and Loiacono, L. (1997). Pericardiocentesis. In: Civetta, J.M., Taylor, J.W., and Kirby, R.R., editors. *Critical Care.* Philadelphia: Lippincott-Raven, 577-8.

Additional Readings

Loeb, S., McCloskey, P.W., and Tryniszewski, C. (1994). *Critical Care Procedures.* Springhouse, PA: Springhouse, 225-9.

Lorell, B. (1997). Pericardial disease. In: Braunwald, A.B., editor. *Heart Disease: A Textbook of Cardiovascular Medicine.* *Philadelphia:* W.B. Saunders, 1478-524.

Mavroukakis, S., and Stine, A. (1998). Nursing management of adults with disorders of the coronary arteries, myocardium, or pericardium. In: Beare, P.G., and Myers, J.L., editors. *Adult Health Nursing.* St. Louis: Mosby, 597-603.

PROCEDURE **43**

Atrial Electrogram

P U R P O S E : An atrial electrogram (AEG) is obtained to determine the presence of atrial activity in a dysrhythmia or to identify the relationship between atrial and ventricular depolarizations.

Teresa Preuss
Debra Lynn-McHale Wiegand

PREREQUISITE NURSING KNOWLEDGE

- Understanding of the anatomy and physiology of the cardiovascular system, principles of cardiac conduction, and basic dysrhythmia interpretation is required.
- Principles of general electrical safety apply when using temporary invasive pacing. Gloves should always be worn when handling pacing electrodes to prevent microshock because even small amounts of electric current can cause serious dysrhythmias if transmitted to the heart.
- Advanced cardiac life support knowledge and skills are needed.
- Indications for AEG are as follows:
  ❖ When atrial activity is not clearly detected on electro-cardiogram (ECG) monitoring
  ❖ To determine the relationship between atrial and ventricular activity
  ❖ To differentiate wide-complex rhythms (i.e., ventricular tachycardia and supraventricular tachycardia with aberrant ventricular conduction)
  ❖ To differentiate narrow-complex supraventricular tachycardias (i.e., sinus tachycardia, atrial tachycardia, paroxysmal supraventricular tachycardia, atrial flutter, atrial fibrillation with relatively regular R-R intervals, or junctional tachycardia)
- AEGs can be performed by using a multichannel bedside ECG monitor that allows for simultaneous display of the AEG along with the surface ECG. A 12-lead ECG machine also can be used to obtain an AEG.
- AEG is a method of recording electrical activity originating from the atria by using temporary atrial epicardial wires placed during cardiac surgery. Standard ECG monitoring records electrical events from the heart using electrodes

located on the surface of the patient's body, which is a considerable distance from the myocardium. One limitation of ECG monitoring may be its inability to detect P waves effectively.
- AEGs detect electrical events directly from or in close proximity to the atria, providing a greatly enhanced tracing of atrial activity. This enhanced tracing allows for comparison of atrial events with ventricular events and determination of the relationship between the two.
- It is important to identify accurately the epicardial atrial pacing wire or wires.
- The two types of AEGs that can be obtained from epicardial pacing wires are unipolar and bipolar.
  ❖ A *unipolar electrogram* measures electrical activity between one atrial epicardial wire and a surface ECG electrode. The *unipolar* AEG detects atrial and ventricular activity.
  ❖ A *bipolar electrogram* detects electrical activity between the two atrial epicardial wires attached to the myocardium. The *bipolar* AEG predominantly detects atrial activity because both electrodes are attached to the atria.

EQUIPMENT

- Nonsterile gloves
- Temporary atrial epicardial pacing wires placed during cardiac surgery
- Alligator clips, wires with connector pins, or AEG-modified patient lead wires
- Bedside multichannel ECG monitor and recorder or 12-lead ECG machine (ensure that biomedical safety standards are met and safe for use with epicardial wires)
- Sterile dressings and materials needed for site care

PATIENT AND FAMILY EDUCATION

• Provide information about the normal conduction system, normal and abnormal heart rhythms, and symptoms of abnormal heart rhythms. ➤*Rationale:* This information helps the patient and family to understand the patient's condition and encourages the patient and family to ask questions.
• Provide information about the AEG, reason for the AEG, and explanation of the equipment. ➤*Rationale:* This communication decreases patient anxiety and helps the patient and family to understand the procedure, why it is needed, and how it will help the patient.
• Explain the patient's expected participation during the procedure. ➤*Rationale:* This encourages patient assistance.

PATIENT ASSESSMENT AND PREPARATION

Patient Assessment

• Assess the patient's cardiac rhythm strip or 12-lead ECG for the presence of atrial activity. ➤*Rationale:* This assessment determines the presence or absence of P waves and the potential need for an AEG.

• Assess the patient's cardiac rhythm for the relationship between atrial and ventricular activity. ➤*Rationale:* This assessment determines the relationship between P waves and QRS complexes and the potential need for an AEG.
• Assess for dysrhythmias. ➤*Rationale:* This assessment determines the patient's baseline cardiac rhythm.
• Assess for compromise of the patient's hemodynamic status (e.g., systolic blood pressure less than 90 mm Hg; mean arterial pressure less than 60 mm Hg; altered level of consciousness; dizziness, shortness of breath, nausea, vomiting, cool or clammy skin, or chest pain). ➤*Rationale:* Clinical parameters that reflect a decreased cardiac output indicate a need for immediate intervention.

Patient Preparation

• Ensure that the patient understands preprocedure teaching. Answer questions as they arise, and reinforce information as needed. ➤*Rationale:* This communication evaluates and reinforces understanding of previously taught information.
• Expose the patient's chest, and identify the epicardial pacing wires. ➤*Rationale:* This provides access to the atrial pacing wires.

Procedure for Atrial Electrogram

Steps	Rationale	Special Considerations
1. Wash hands, and don nonsterile gloves.	Reduces the transmission of microorganisms and body secretions; standard precautions.	Use of gloves prevents microshocks when handling epicardial wires.
2. Expose and identify the atrial epicardial pacing wires.	It is important to differentiate the atrial from ventricular wires to ensure that the appropriate epicardial wires are used.	Typically the atrial wires exit the chest to the right of the patient's sternum and the ventricular wires exit to the left of the patient's sternum (Fig. 43-1).

Procedure continues on the following page

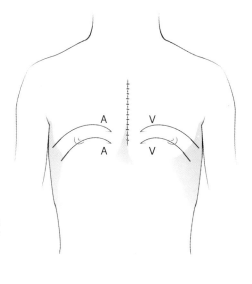

FIGURE 43-1 Atrial wires exit the chest to the right of the patient's sternum. Ventricular wires exit the chest to the left of the patient's sternum. *(Drawing by Todd Sargood.)*

Procedure for Atrial Electrogram—*Continued*		
Steps	**Rationale**	**Special Considerations**
Obtaining a Unipolar AEG Using a Multichannel Bedside ECG Monitor—Lead I		
1. Attach one atrial pacing wire to the alligator clip of the AEG-modified patient lead wire (Fig. 43-2).	One atrial pacing wire is used when obtaining a unipolar AEG.	A lead wire with alligator clips at both ends or a lead wire with connector pins also can be used.
2. Disconnect the surface ECG standard lead wire from the right arm (RA) port of the trunk of the ECG bedside monitor cable (see Fig. 43-2).		
3. Plug the AEG-modified patient lead wire into the RA port of the trunk of the ECG bedside monitor cable.	Connects the atrial pacing wire to the ECG bedside monitoring system.	Determine that the ECG bedside monitoring system meets all safety requirements.
4. Select lead I on the bedside ECG monitor.	Lead I detects electrical activity between the RA limb lead and the left arm (LA) limb lead. Because the atrial pacing wire is connected into the RA port, lead I detects the electrical activity between the atrial wire and the surface LA limb lead.	
5. Record a dual-channel strip.	Displays the AEG for analysis.	A dual-channel recorder permits the comparison of the surface ECG and the AEG.
6. Analyze the AEG strip and compare the surface ECG with the AEG (Fig. 43-3).	Identifies P waves and QRS complexes, and determines the relationship between the P waves and the QRS complexes.	
Obtaining a Unipolar AEG Using a Multichannel Bedside ECG Monitor—Lead V		
1. Attach one atrial pacing wire to the alligator clip of the AEG-modified patient lead wire.	One atrial pacing wire is used when obtaining a unipolar AEG.	A lead wire with alligator clips at both ends or a lead wire with connector pins also can be used.

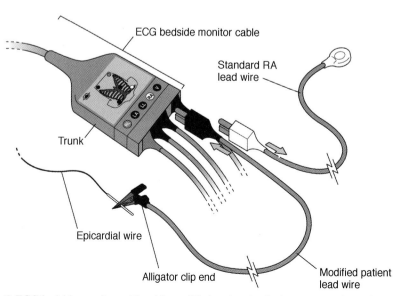

FIGURE 43-2 ECG bedside monitor cable with modified patient lead wire connected to epicardial wire. *(Drawing by Todd Sargood.)*

Procedure for Atrial Electrogram—*Continued*

Steps	Rationale	Special Considerations
2. Disconnect the surface ECG standard lead wire from the lead V port of the trunk of the ECG bedside monitor cable.		
3. Plug the AEG-modified patient lead wire into the lead V port of the trunk of the ECG bedside monitor cable.	Connects the atrial pacing wire to the ECG bedside monitoring system.	Determine that the ECG bedside monitoring system meets all safety requirements.
4. Select lead V on the bedside ECG monitor.	Use of the precordial lead allows for detection of atrial electrical activity between lead V and an indifferent limb lead in a unipolar configuration.	
5. Record a dual-channel strip.	Displays the AEG for analysis.	
6. Analyze the AEG strip and compare the surface ECG with the AEG (Fig. 43-4).	Identifies P waves and QRS complexes, and determines the relationship between the P waves and the QRS complexes.	

Obtaining a Bipolar AEG Using a Multichannel Bedside ECG Monitor

1. Attach both atrial pacing wires to alligator clips of two separate AEG-modified patient lead wires.	Two atrial pacing wires are used when obtaining a bipolar AEG.	A lead wire with alligator clips at both ends or a lead wire with connector pins also can be used.

Procedure continues on the following page

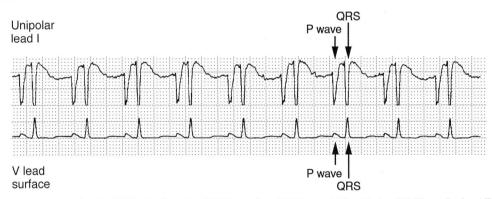

FIGURE 43-3 Unipolar AEG strip from lead I. The surface ECG was obtained in lead V. The unipolar AEG was obtained in lead I. The atrial activity is magnified in lead I.

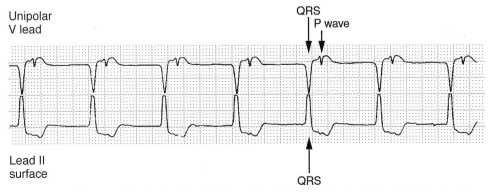

FIGURE 43-4 Unipolar AEG strip from lead V. The surface ECG was obtained in lead II. Based on the surface ECG, the rhythm appears to be junctional with no evidence of P waves or atrial activity. The unipolar AEG shows retrograde P waves that follow the QRS complex, confirming the junctional rhythm interpretation.

Procedure **for Atrial Electrogram**—*Continued*

Steps	Rationale	Special Considerations
2. Disconnect the surface ECG standard lead wire from the RA and LA lead ports of the trunk of the ECG bedside monitor cable.		
3. Plug the AEG-modified patient lead wires into the RA and LA ports of the trunk of the ECG bedside monitor cable.	Connects the atrial pacing wires to the ECG bedside monitoring system.	Determine that the ECG bedside monitoring system meets all safety requirements.
4. Select lead I on the bedside ECG monitor.	Lead I detects electrical activity between the RA limb lead and the LA limb lead. Because the atrial pacing wires are connected into the RA and LA ports, lead I detects the electrical activity between the two atrial wires.	
5. Record a dual-channel strip.	Displays the AEG for analysis.	
6. Analyze the AEG strip and compare the surface ECG with the AEG (Fig. 43-5).	Identifies P waves and QRS complexes, and determines the relationship between the P waves and the QRS complexes.	A dual-channel recorder permits the comparison of the surface ECG and the AEG. Bipolar tracings usually magnify atrial activity and minimize ventricular activity.
Obtaining a Unipolar AEG Using a 12-Lead ECG Machine 1. Connect the patient to the 12-lead ECG machine (see Procedure 57).	Provides another method of obtaining an AEG.	Determine that the 12-lead ECG machine meets all safety requirements.
2. Attach one atrial epicardial pacing wire to the clip of the RA lead wire of the 12-lead ECG machine (Fig. 43-6).		
3. Run a 12-lead ECG.	Lead I measures the electrical activity between the RA and LA. Because the atrial pacing wire is connected to the RA lead, lead I detects the electrical activity between the atrial wire and the surface LA limb lead. Lead II measures the electrical activity between the RA and left leg (LL). Because the atrial	

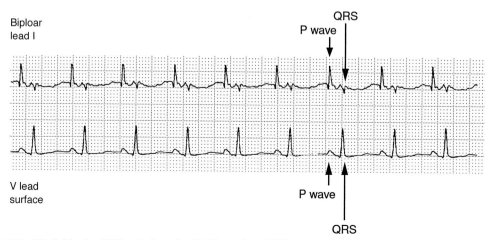

Bipolar
lead I

QRS

P wave

V lead
surface

P wave

QRS

FIGURE 43-5 Bipolar AEG strip from lead I. The surface ECG was obtained in lead V. The bipolar AEG was obtained in lead I. The atrial activity is magnified in lead I. Also note how small the ventricular activity is in lead I.

Procedure | for **Atrial Electrogram**—*Continued*

Steps	Rationale	Special Considerations
	pacing wire is connected to the RA lead, lead II detects the electrical activity between the atrial wire and the surface LL lead.	
4. Analyze leads I and II.	Identifies P waves and QRS complexes, and determines the relationship between the P waves and the QRS complexes.	
Obtaining a Bipolar AEG **Using a 12-Lead ECG Machine** 1. Connect the patient to the 12-lead ECG machine (see Procedure 57).	Provides another method of obtaining an AEG.	Determine that the 12-lead ECG machine meets all safety requirements.
2. Attach one atrial epicardial pacing wire to the RA limb lead and the other atrial epicardial pacing wire to the LA limb lead of the 12-lead ECG machine.	Connection to the limb leads of the ECG machine allows for the detection and recording of atrial electrical activity.	
3. Run a 12-lead ECG (Fig. 43-7).	Lead I measures the electrical activity between the RA and LA limb leads, which sense atrial activity from both epicardial wires, to provide a bipolar tracing.	
4. Analyze lead I (see Fig. 43-7).	Displays bipolar AEG for analysis. Identifies P waves and QRS complexes, and determines the relationship between the P waves and the QRS complexes.	Bipolar tracings usually magnify atrial activity and minimize ventricular activity. Using this method, unipolar AEGs also are obtained in lead II and lead III.
After AEG Is Obtained 1. Disconnect the atrial pacing wires from the alligator clips.	Removes equipment used for obtaining the AEG.	
2. Reconnect the bedside ECG lead wires.	Reestablishes continuous ECG monitoring.	

Procedure continues on the following page

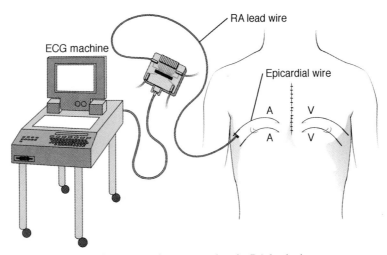

FIGURE 43-6 Attach 12-lead ECG per procedure except that the RA lead wire connects to one of the atrial epicardial pacing wires. *(Drawing by Todd Sargood.)*

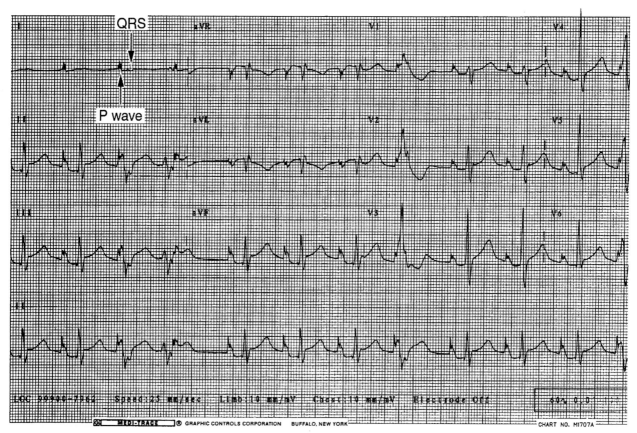

FIGURE 43-7 A 12-lead ECG obtained with two atrial pacing wires connected to the RA and LA lead wires. Lead I shows a bipolar AEG. The P wave is greater in size than the QRS complex. Leads II and III show unipolar AEGs. In leads II and III, atrial activity is enhanced. Throughout, the 12-lead ECG atrial activity is enhanced.

Procedure   for Atrial Electrogram—*Continued*

Steps	Rationale	Special Considerations
3. Apply a dry sterile dressing to the epicardial wire exit sites.	Reduces the transmission of microorganisms; sterile precautions.	Follow institution guidelines for site care.
4. Place the uninsulated portion of the epicardial wires in an insulated material.	Prevents microshock.	
5. Discard disposable supplies, and wash hands.	Reduces the transmission of microorganisms; standard precautions.	

Expected Outcomes	Unexpected Outcomes
• Atrial activity is identified. • The relationship between atrial and ventricular activity is determined.	• Hemodynamically significant dysrhythmias • Dysrhythmias in which atrial activity is unclear or the relationship between atrial and ventricular activity is unclear • Microschocks causing dysrhythmias

Patient Monitoring and Care

Steps	Rationale	Reportable Conditions
		These conditions should be reported if they persist despite nursing interventions.
1. Evaluate the AEG for the presence of atrial activity and its relationship to ventricular activity. Compare with the surface ECG for interpretation.	AEG determines the presence or absence of atrial activity.	• Inability to identify atrial activity
2. Monitor the ECG rhythm for changes.	The underlying dysrhythmia may change during the AEG.	• Altered hemodynamic status caused by change in ECG rhythm
3. Monitor vital signs and level of consciousness during the AEG and as needed.	Ensures adequate tissue perfusion.	• Hemodynamic instability or decrease in level of consciousness
4. Evaluate and treat dysrhythmias.	Identification and treatment of dysrhythmias may improve patient outcome.	• Return of rhythm stability • Change in cardiac rate or rhythm
5. Site care should be as follows: A. Cleanse the area surrounding the epicardial pacing wires with an antiseptic solution (e.g., 2% chlorhexidine–based preparation).	Reduces infection. The Centers for Disease Control and Prevention does not have a specific recommendation for care of epicardial pacing wires or site care.	• Any signs or symptoms of infection
B. Apply a dry sterile dressing with the date and time of the dressing change. Institution standard should be followed for frequency and type of dressing.	The Centers for Disease Control and Prevention recommends replacing the dressing when the dressing becomes damp, loosened, or soiled or when inspection of the site is necessary.[1]	
C. Protect the exposed, uninsulated portion of the epicardial pacing wires in an insulated environment according to institution standards (e.g., closed container, finger cots, insulated gloves).	Prevents microshocks and potentially lethal dysrhythmias.	

Documentation

Documentation should include the following:

- Patient and family education
- ECG tracings before, during, and after the AEG
- AEG tracing with interpretation
- Hemodynamic status and level of consciousness
- Patient tolerance of the procedure
- Occurrence of unexpected outcome

Reference

1. O'Grady, N.P., et al. (2002). Guidelines for prevention of intravascular catheter-related infections. *Am J Infect Control*, 30, 476-89.

Additional Readings

Bass, L.S., and Schneider, C.L. (1986). Temporary epicardial electrodes. *Dimens Crit Care Nurs*, 5, 80-90.

Bumgarner, L.I. (1992). Diagnostic uses of epicardial electrodes after cardiac surgery. *Prog Cardiovasc Nurs*, 7, 21-4.

Dziadulewicz, L., and Lang, R. (1992). The use of atrial electrograms in the diagnosis of supraventricular dysrhythmias. *AACN Clin Issues*, 3, 203-8.

Finkelmeier, B.A., and Salinger, M.H. (1984). The atrial electrogram: Its diagnostic use following cardiac surgery. *Crit Care Nurse*, 4, 42-6.

Lombness, P.M. (1992). Taking the mystery out of rhythm interpretation: Atrial electrograms. *Heart Lung*, 21, 415-26.

Lynn-McHale, D.J., Riggs, K.L., and Thurman, L. (1991). Epicardial pacing after cardiac surgery. *Crit Care Nurse*, 11, 62-77.

Schultz, C.K., and Woodall, C.E. (1989). Using epicardial pacing electrodes. *J Cardiovasc Nurs*, 3, 25-33.

Sulzbach, L.M. (1985). The use of temporary atrial wire electrodes to record atrial electrograms in patients who had cardiac surgery. *Heart Lung*, 14, 540-8.

Sulzbach, L.M., and Lansdowne, L.M. (1991).Temporary atrial pacing after cardiac surgery. *Focus Crit Care*, 18, 65-74.

Young, L.C. (1981). Atrial electrogram: An asset to ECG monitoring. *Crit Care Nurse*, 1, 14-8.

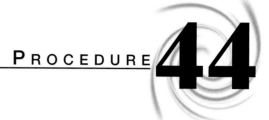
PROCEDURE **44**

@AP

Atrial Overdrive Pacing (Perform)

PURPOSE: Atrial overdrive pacing is used in an attempt to terminate reentrant atrial dysrhythmias, especially atrial flutter, and allow restoration of sinus rhythm. Sinus rhythm enhances cardiac output by allowing atrial contraction to contribute to ventricular filling.

Carol Jacobson

PREREQUISITE NURSING KNOWLEDGE

- Knowledge of the anatomy and physiology of the cardiovascular system, principles of cardiac conduction, and basic and advanced dysrhythmia interpretation is required.
- Knowledge of pacemakers is required to evaluate pacemaker function and patient response to pacemaker therapy.
- Principles of general electrical safety apply when using temporary invasive pacing. Gloves always should be worn when handling pacing electrodes to prevent microshock because even small amounts of electrical current can cause serious dysrhythmias if they are transmitted to the heart.
- Clinical and technical competence related to use of an atrial pacing pulse generator or the rapid atrial pacing feature of a standard pulse generator is needed.
- Advanced cardiac life support knowledge and skills are required.
- Supraventricular dysrhythmias, such as atrial flutter, reentrant atrial tachycardia, atrioventricular (AV) nodal reentry tachycardia, and reentrant tachycardias that use an accessory pathway in Wolff-Parkinson-White (WPW) syndrome, sometimes can be terminated by overdrive atrial pacing.

- Atrial fibrillation occasionally terminates with overdrive atrial pacing, but this is not a reliable therapy for atrial fibrillation.
- Overdrive atrial pacing is performed most commonly using epicardial atrial pacing wires placed during cardiac surgery. A transvenous atrial pacing lead with an active fixation tip to help keep the lead in the atrium also can be used.
- A pulse generator that is capable of overdrive atrial pacing should be selected. An atrial pacing pulse generator can be used to perform rapid atrial pacing. Some newer temporary pulse generators have a feature that can be used to perform rapid atrial pacing (Fig. 44-1).
- Overdrive atrial pacing involves the delivery of short bursts of rapid pacing stimuli through an epicardial atrial pacing wire or a transvenous lead in the atrium. The physician or advanced practice nurse usually determines the duration and rate of the burst.
  ❖ Typically a 10- to 30-second burst at a rate 20% to 30% faster than the intrinsic atrial rate is used initially (e.g., begin at a rate of 375 pulses/minute for atrial flutter at a rate of 300 beats/minute).[1] An alternative approach is to initiate atrial pacing at a rate 10 beats/minute faster than the intrinsic atrial rate.[1]
  ❖ Successive bursts usually are performed at gradually increasing rates (maximal capability of the pulse generator for overdrive atrial pacing is 800 pulses/minute) and may be delivered for longer periods (up to 1 minute).
- It is extremely important that the atrial pacing wire or atrial pacing lead be identified correctly when initiating overdrive

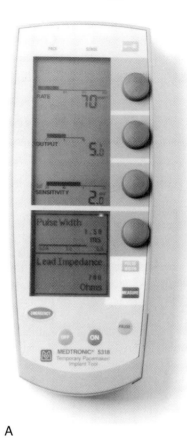

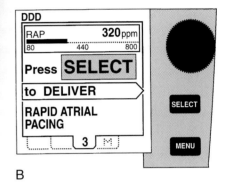

FIGURE 44-1 **A,** Temporary dual-chamber pulse generator with overdrive atrial pacing capability. **B,** Enlargement of lower screen on the pacemaker showing rapid atrial pacing controls. *(Courtesy Medtronic, Inc.)*

A

B

pacing because pacing the ventricle at rapid rates may result in ventricular tachycardia or ventricular fibrillation.
- Rapid atrial pacing may result in degeneration of the atrial rhythm to atrial fibrillation with a rapid ventricular response.
- If an accessory pathway is present, rapid atrial pacing can result in conduction to the ventricles over the accessory pathway, leading to ventricular fibrillation.
- Overdrive suppression of the sinus node can result in periods of bradycardia, asystole, junctional or ventricular escape rhythms, or polymorphic ventricular tachycardia on termination of the atrial tachydysrhythmia.
- Conversion of an atrial tachydysrhythmia can result in dislodgment of thrombus and embolization of clots to the pulmonary or systemic circulation.

EQUIPMENT

- Nonsterile gloves
- External pulse generator capable of rapid atrial pacing
- Connecting cable
- Cardiac monitor and recorder

- Electrocardiogram (ECG) electrodes
- Double alligator clip or wire with connector pins (if needed to create a ground wire)
- Materials for epicardial pacing wire site care
  - ❖ Antiseptic pads or swab sticks (e.g., 2% chlorhexidine–based preparation)
  - ❖ Gauze pads
  - ❖ Tape
- Insulating material for epicardial pacing wires or trans-venous pacing electrode connector pins (e.g., finger cots, glove, needle caps)

Additional equipment to have available as needed includes the following:
- Defibrillator
- Emergency medications
- Airway management equipment
- Standard pulse generator or transcutaneous pacemaker

PATIENT AND FAMILY EDUCATION

- Explain the procedure and its purpose to the patient and family. ➤*Rationale:* This explanation decreases patient and family anxiety and promotes cooperation with the procedure.
- Reassure the patient that the pacing probably will not be felt and that any sensation felt most likely will be a "fluttering"

feeling in the chest. ➥*Rationale:* This prepares the patient and may decrease the patient's anxiety.

PATIENT ASSESSMENT AND PREPARATION

Patient Assessment

- Assess the patient's ECG rhythm and intervals, noting atrial and ventricular rates. ➥*Rationale:* This assessment determines baseline cardiac conduction.
- Assess the patient's vital signs, hemodynamic oxygenation parameters. ➥*Rationale:* This determines baseline cardiovascular function.
- Assess signs and symptoms that might be caused by the dysrhythmia (e.g., shortness of breath, dizziness, nausea, chest pain, signs of poor peripheral perfusion). ➥*Rationale:* This determines the patient's response to the dysrhythmia.
- Assess the patency of the intravenous access. ➥*Rationale:* This assessment ensures a functional intravenous access.
- Note any medications that might have an effect on the patient's rhythm or hemodynamic parameters (e.g., β-blockers, calcium channel blockers, antidysrhythmics, digoxin). ➥*Rationale:* Knowing the effects of medication therapy can alert the health care team to potential problems after successful conversion to sinus rhythm (e.g., bradycardia or AV block caused by β-blocker or calcium channel blocker therapy).

- Check the patient's prothrombin time or international normalized ratio if the patient has been taking wafarin (Coumadin) for treatment of atrial tachydysrhythmias. ➥*Rationale:* This assesses the effectiveness of the anticoagulant therapy in decreasing the risk of embolization.

Patient Preparation

- Ensure that the patient and family understand preprocedural teaching. Answer questions as they arise, and reinforce information as needed. ➥*Rationale:* This communication evaluates and reinforces understanding of previously taught information.
- Initiate continuous bedside cardiac monitoring (if not already in place). ➥*Rationale:* The patient's cardiac rhythm must be visible at the bedside during the procedure to determine atrial capture during pacing and to evaluate the response of the patient's cardiac rhythm to pacing. Immediate detection of adverse outcomes to overdrive atrial pacing is essential to provide safe patient care.
- Assist the patient to a supine position. ➥*Rationale:* Allows easy access to epicardial pacing wires or transvenous atrial pacing lead wire.
- Place the blood pressure cuff on the patient's arm (unless using an arterial line for blood pressure monitoring). ➥*Rationale:* This aids in assessment of the patient's hemodynamic response to atrial overdrive pacing.

Procedure for Performing Atrial Overdrive Pacing		
Steps	**Rationale**	**Special Considerations**
1. Wash hands.	Reduces the transmission of microorganisms; standard precautions.	
2. Don nonsterile gloves.	Protects the patient from microshock while pacing wires are being handled.[1]	
3. Attach the connecting cable to the external pulse generator, making sure that the positive (+) pole of the cable is connected to the (+) terminal of the pulse generator and the negative (−) pole of the cable is connected to the (−) terminal.	The connecting cable provides extra length so that the pulse generator does not have to be placed on the patient's chest or abdomen.	
4. For transvenous atrial pacing: A. Identify the proximal and the distal electrode connector pins on the external portion of the atrial pacing lead.	The pacing stimulus travels from the pulse generator to the negative terminal, and energy returns to the pulse generator via the positive terminal.	
B. Connect the distal (negative) electrode connector pin to the negative terminal of the connecting cable.	Energy from the pulse generator is directed to the distal electrode in contact with the atrium.	
C. Connect the proximal (positive) electrode connecting pin to the positive terminal of the connecting cable.	The pacing circuit is completed as energy reaches the positive electrode.	

Procedure for Performing Atrial Overdrive Pacing—*Continued*

Steps	Rationale	Special Considerations
5. For epicardial atrial pacing: A. Expose the atrial epicardial pacing wires.	The atrial epicardial wires exit the chest to the right of the patient's sternum (see Fig. 43-1).	The atrial epicardial pacing wires can be verified by performing an atrial electrogram (see Procedure 43) or by atrial pacing (see Procedure 50).
B. Connect an atrial epicardial pacing wire to the negative terminal of the connecting cable.	The pacing current is delivered through the negative terminal of the pulse generator; an epicardial pacing wire on the atrium must be connected to the negative terminal for the atrium to receive pacing impulses.	
C. Connect a second epicardial pacing wire or a ground wire to the positive terminal of the connecting cable.	The pacing circuit is completed as energy reaches the positive electrode.	Additional options for a ground wire include a subcutaneous needle in the tissue on the chest or an ECG monitoring electrode on the chest near the epicardial wire exit site. The positive terminal of the connecting cable is connected to the subcutaneous needle hub or to the metal snap of the monitoring electrode with a double alligator clip.
6. Set the rate and the milliampere (mA/output) controls on the pulse generator.	Settings are based on the characteristics of the patient's dysrhythmia and the threshold required for atrial capture.	The pacing rate is set initially at least 10 beats/minute higher than the intrinsic atrial rate (often 20-30% higher) for atrial tachycardia or atrial flutter. If the rhythm is atrial fibrillation, the pacing rate usually is set at 300-350 pulses/minute initially and may be increased to the maximum of 800 pulses/minute. An output of at least 10 mA is recommended, and outputs up to 20 mA are sometimes necessary.[2]
7. Pace the atrium for a brief period (several beats or for several seconds), then abruptly terminate pacing (Figs. 44-2 and 44-3).	Short bursts of pacing stimuli at a rapid rate are intended to create refractory tissue in the atrium and interrupt the reentry circuit responsible for the tachydysrhythmia.[2] These bursts can be repeated at faster rates and for longer intervals until the dysrhythmia terminates or changes.	Refer to the pulse generator's technical manual for instructions on how to initiate rapid atrial pacing. On termination of the dysrhythmia, the sinus node may be suppressed for a period, resulting in bradycardia, asystole, junctional or ventricular escape rhythms, or polymorphic ventricular tachycardia. It may be necessary to initiate temporary ventricular pacing or transcutaneous pacing for a period until normal sinus function returns.

Procedure continues on the following page

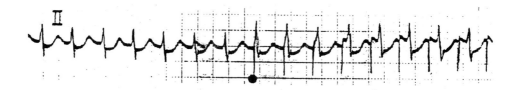

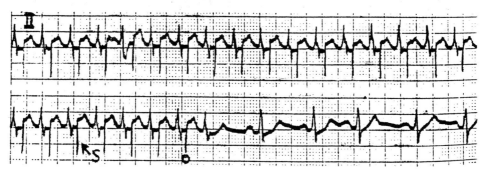

FIGURE 44-2 The top trace shows ECG lead II recorded during an episode of paroxysmal atrial tachycardia at a rate of 150 beats/min. Beginning with the eighth beat in this trace (*black dot*), rapid atrial pacing at a rate of 165 beats/min was initiated. In the middle trace, which begins 12 seconds after the top trace, atrial capture is shown clearly. In the bottom trace, which is continuous with the middle trace, sinus rhythm appears when atrial pacing is terminated abruptly (*open circle*). S, stimulus artifact. Paper recording speed 25 mm/sec. *(From Cooper, T.B., MacLean, W.A.H., and Waldo, A.L. [1978]. Overdrive pacing for supraventricular tachycardia: A review of theoretical implications and therapeutic techniques. Pacing Clin Electrophysiol, 1, 200.)*

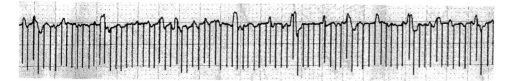

FIGURE 44-3 Rhythm strip showing rapid atrial pacing in an attempt to terminate atrial flutter.

Procedure | for Performing Atrial Overdrive Pacing—*Continued*

Steps	Rationale	Special Considerations
8. If atrial pacing is no longer needed, disconnect the connecting cable from the epicardial pacing wires or from the transvenous pacing electrode connector pins.	Removes the rapid atrial pacemaker.	Standard pacing can be resumed if necessary.
9. Apply a sterile, occlusive dressing to the pacing site if not already in place.	Reduces the incidence of infection.	
10. Protect the exposed pacing electrode connector pins or epicardial wires with an insulating material (e.g., finger cots, needle covers).	Prevents microshock, which can result in significant dysrhythmias.[1]	
11. Coil the epicardial pacing wires on top of the gauze dressing, covered with another piece of gauze, and tape in place.	Prevents accidental dislodgment of pacing wires.	
12. Label each wire or dressing to identify atrial and ventricular pacing wires.	Aids identification of pacing wires.	
13. Discard used supplies, and wash hands.	Reduces the transmission of microorganisms; standard precautions.	

Expected Outcomes	Unexpected Outcomes
• Return to normal sinus rhythm • Stable or improved hemodynamic parameters	• Failure to capture the atrium • Conversion to atrial fibrillation • Prolonged period of bradycardia or asystole after termination of the tachydysrhythmia • Rapid conduction of atrial paced impulses to the ventricle through an accessory pathway, resulting in ventricular tachycardia or ventricular fibrillation • Emergence of slow junctional or ventricular escape rhythm or polymorphic ventricular tachycardia after termination of the tachydysrhythmia • Microshock resulting in ventricular tachycardia or fibrillation

Patient Monitoring and Care

Steps	Rationale	Reportable Conditions
		These conditions should be reported if they persist despite nursing interventions. • Rhythm changes • Return of initial tachydysrhythmia • Any significant or hemodynamically unstable dysrhythmia • Need for additional temporary pacing to maintain adequate heart rate after conversion of the tachydysrhythmia
1. Monitor the patient's cardiac rhythm continuously at the bedside during the procedure and after the procedure.	Allows for immediate recognition of rhythm changes or return of initial tachydysrhythmia.	
2. Monitor the patients's vital signs before initiating overdrive pacing, every 5-10 minutes during attempts to overdrive pace, with any significant rhythm change during the procedure, and on termination of the procedure. If the patient is not hemodynamically stable after the procedure, monitor vital signs every 5-10 minutes. Monitor vital signs per unit standards if the patient is stable after the procedure.	Changes in vital signs may indicate significant change in patient's condition. Blood pressure often improves with cessation of the tachydysrhythmia or restoration of normal sinus rhythm; blood pressure may deteriorate if the ventricular rate accelerates because of overdrive pacing. If the patient is receiving antidysrhythmic medications, changes in vital signs may indicate an adverse medication reaction.	• Changes in vital signs
3. Perform site care to the transvenous pacing lead site or the epicardial pacing wire exit site with antiseptic swabs, and apply a sterile gauze dressing to the exit site. Observe the site for signs of infection.	Decreases the incidence of infection.	• Redness or exudate around site • Increased white blood cell count • Elevated temperature
4. Monitor the patient's response to antidysrhythmic medications.	Antidysrhythmic medications may be necessary to prevent recurrence of the initial tachydysrhythmia or to control the ventricular rate.	• Prolongation of Q-T interval • Rhythm changes

Documentation

Documentation should include the following:

- Patient and family education provided and an evaluation of their understanding of the procedure
- Rhythm strip documenting initial cardiac rate and rhythm
- Initial vital signs and other pertinent physical assessment findings
- Pacemaker settings used
- Rhythm strip documenting atrial pacing
- Number of pacing attempts
- Rate and duration of successful pacing burst
- Patient's response to the procedure (e.g., anxiety, pain)
- Postprocedure rhythm strip
- Postprocedure vital signs
- Any medications given during procedure
- Any unexpected outcomes
- Additional interventions

References

1. Baas, L.S., Beery, T.A., and Hickey, C.S. (1997). Care and safety of pacemaker electrodes in intensive care and telemetry nursing units. *Am J Crit Care,* 6, 302-11.
2. Waldo, A.L. (2001). Atrial flutter. In: Podrid, P.J., and Kowey, P.R., editors. *Cardiac Arrhythmia: Mechanisms, Diagnosis, and Management.* 2nd ed. Philadelphia: Lippincott Williams & Wilkins, 501-16.

Additional Readings

Jacobson, C., and Gerity, D. (2004). Pacemakers and implantable defibrillators. In: Woods, S.L., Froelicher, E.S., and Motzer, S., editors. *Cardiac Nursing.* 5th ed. Philadelphia: Lippincott Williams & Wilkins.

Roman-Smith, P. (1991). Pacing for tachydysrhythmia. *AACN Clin Issues Crit Care Nurs,* 2, 132-9.

Sohn, R.H., and Goldschlager, N. (2001). Cardiac pacing in the critical care setting. In: Kusumoto, F.M., and Goldschlager, N.F., editors. *Cardiac Pacing for the Clinician.* Philadelphia: Lippincott Williams & Wilkins.

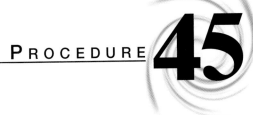

PROCEDURE **45**

Epicardial Pacing Wire Removal

P U R P O S E : Temporary epicardial pacing wires are inserted into the epicardium during cardiac surgery and are removed when pacing therapy is no longer needed.

Christine Shamloo

PREREQUISITE NURSING KNOWLEDGE

- Knowledge of the cardiovascular anatomy and physiology is needed.
- Knowledge of principles of aseptic technique is required.
- Knowledge of concepts related to placement and function of epicardial pacing wires is required.
- Advanced cardiac life support knowledge and skills are needed.
- Knowledge of basic dysrhythmia recognition and treatment of life-threatening dysrhythmias is needed.
- Complications after epicardial pacing wire removal may include cardiac tamponade, myocardial ischemia, graft site disruption, and dysrhythmias.
- Signs and symptoms of cardiac tamponade should be known.
- Relative contraindications to epicardial pacing wire removal include bleeding, abnormal coagulation studies, presence of dysrhythmias requiring pacing assistance, and compromised hemodynamic status.

EQUIPMENT

- Suture removal kit
- Sterile gauze
- Nonsterile gloves, gown, goggles or face shield with mask

Additional equipment that may be needed includes the following:
- Emergency equipment
- Temporary transcutaneous or transvenous pacing equipment

PATIENT AND FAMILY EDUCATION

- Assess patient and family readiness to learn, and identify factors that affect learning. ➤*Rationale:* This assessment allows the nurse to individualize teaching.
- Provide information about the epicardial pacing wires, the reason for their removal, and an explanation of the procedure. ➤*Rationale:* This information helps the patient and family to understand the procedure, why it is needed, and decreases anxiety.
- Explain the patient's expected participation during the procedure. ➤*Rationale:* This encourages patient involvement.
- Explain that the patient may feel a burning or pulling sensation for a few seconds during the procedure. ➤*Rationale:* Prepares the patient for what to expect.

PATIENT ASSESSMENT AND PREPARATION

Patient Assessment

- Assess the patient's baseline cardiovascular, hemodynamic, and peripheral vascular status. ➤*Rationale:* This assessment provides data that can be used for comparison with postremoval assessment data and hemodynamic values.

- Assess the patient's current laboratory data, including electrolyte and coagulation studies. Ensure that the patient is not receiving anticoagulants. ➤**Rationale:** This assessment identifies laboratory abnormalities. Baseline coagulation studies are helpful in determining the patient's risk for bleeding. Electrolyte imbalances may increase cardiac irritability.

Patient Preparation

- Ensure that the patient and family understand preprocedural teaching. Answer questions as they arise, and reinforce information as needed. ➤**Rationale:** This communication evaluates and reinforces understanding of previously taught information.

- Schedule epicardial pacing wire removal at least 24 hours before discharge. ➤**Rationale:** This timing allows for observation for potential complications.
- Administer analgesia medication at least 30 minutes before removing the epicardial pacing wires. ➤**Rationale:** Analgesia administered before the procedure minimizes discomfort during epicardial pacing wire removal.
- Validate the patency of the peripheral intravenous line. ➤**Rationale:** Ensure a patent IV should emergency fluids or medications be needed.
- Ensure that patient has bedside electrocardiogram (ECG) monitoring. ➤**Rationale:** This provides ECG assessment for the presence of potential dysrhythmias during epicardial wire removal.[2,4,5]

Procedure for Epicardial Pacing Wire Removal

Steps	Rationale	Special Considerations
1. Wash hands and don gown and goggles or face shield with mask.	Reduces the transmission of microorganisms and body secretions; maintains standard precautions.	
2. Ask the patient to remain supine.	Supine positioning provides the best access during the procedure and during intervention for management of adverse effects.	
3. Apply nonsterile gloves.	Minimizes the possibility of microshock when in contact with the epicardial pacing wires.	
4. Remove the dressing and tape over the epicardial wires.	Exposes the epicardial wire exit sites.	
5. Untie or cut the suture/first knot of the pacing wires at the skin, using the epicardial suture removal kit.	Prepares for epicardial pacing wire removal.	
6. Remove the pacing wires by pulling each with a steady, slow gentle tension.	A steady, slow gentle tension uncoils the pacing lead on the epicardial surface of the heart.	Observe the patient's ECG monitor while removing the epicardial wires. If a steady, slow gentle tension does not remove the wires, stop the procedure, and notify the physician.
7. Inspect each epicardial pacing wire for the presence of tissue.	Ensures that each epicardial wire extracted is completely intact.	If bleeding occurs at the epicardial pacing wire site, apply direct pressure until bleeding stops. Notify the physician if bleeding or oozing continues.
8. Apply a sterile, occlusive dressing over the epicardial exit sites.	Decreases the risk of infection until the exit sites heal.	
9. Discard used supplies and wash hands.	Reduces the transmission of microorganisms and body secretions; maintains standard precautions.	

Expected Outcomes

- Removal of the epicardial pacing wires
- Stable vital signs
- Stable ECG rhythm

Unexpected Outcomes

- Cardiac tamponade
- Infection
- Hemorrhage
- Hematoma
- Dysrhythmias
- Hemodynamic instability

Patient Monitoring and Care

Steps	Rationale	Reportable Conditions
		These conditions should be reported if they persist despite nursing interventions. • Changes in vital signs
1. Obtain the patient's vital signs every 15 minutes × 4, every 30 minutes × 2, and every 1 hour × 2.	Determines the patient's hemodynamic status.	
2. Obtain an ECG strip during removal of the epicardial wires.	Determines the presence of dysrhythmias	• Dysrhythmias • ECG changes
3. When obtaining vital signs, assess for signs and symptoms of cardiac tamponade.	Early detection is important because cardiac tamponade is a potentially fatal complication.	• Beck triad (jugular venous distention, hypotension, and muffled heart sounds) • Hypotension and tachycardia • Pulsus paradoxus • Cyanosis • Altered level of consciousness

Documentation

Documentation should include the following:

- Patient and family education
- Removal of epicardial pacing wires
- Patient tolerance of the procedure
- Site assessment
- Vital signs and ECG strip
- Occurrence of unexpected outcomes and interventions

References

1. Boyle, J., and Rost, M.K. (2000). Present status of cardiac pacing: A nursing perspective. *Crit Care Nurse Q,* 1, 1-19.
2. Caroll, K.C., et al. (1998). Risks associated with removal of ventricular epicardial pacing wires after cardiac surgery. *Am J Crit Care,* 7, 444-9.
3. Johnson, L.G., Brown, O.F., and Alligood, M.R. (1993). Complications of epicardial pacing wire removal. *J Cardiovasc Nurs,* 7, 32-40.
4. Meier, J.D., Tamirisa, K.P., and Eitzman, D.T. (2004). Ventricular tachycardia associated with transmyocardial migration of an epicardial pacing wire. *Soc Thorac Surg,* 77, 1077-9.
5. Wollan, D.L. (1995). Removal of epicardial pacing wires: An expanded role for nurses. *Prog Cardiovasc Nurs,* 10, 21-6.

PROCEDURE **46**

Implantable Cardioverter-Defibrillator

P U R P O S E : The implantable cardioverter-defibrillator (ICD) is an implanted electronic device that is used to prevent sudden cardiac death (SCD) caused by malignant ventricular dysrhythmias. The ICD continuously monitors a patient's rhythm and attempts to convert ventricular tachycardia (VT) or ventricular fibrillation (VF) via antitachycardia pacing, cardioversion, defibrillation, or some combination of these. The ICD has the capability for backup bradycardia pacing and dual-chamber pacing.

Deborah Nolan Reilly
Patricia Gonce Morton
Karen Vojtko

PREREQUISITE NURSING KNOWLEDGE

- Knowledge of the anatomy and physiology of the cardiovascular system, principles of cardiac conduction, and basic dysrhythmia interpretation is needed.
- Knowledge of basic functioning of ICDs and patient response to ICD therapy is needed.
- Knowledge of principles of defibrillation threshold, antidysrhythmic medication, alteration in electrolytes, and how they may affect the defibrillation threshold is required.
- Advanced cardiac life support (ACLS) knowledge and skills are needed.
- Clinical and technical competence related to use of the external defibrillator is required.
- Knowledge of indications for use of the ICD as a long-term therapy for patients at risk for SCD is required.[19,49]
- Outcome data support the efficacy of the ICD in prolonging the overall survival of patients and preventing SCD.[3,10,18,21,33,34,41,50,51]
- The American College of Cardiology/American Heart Association Task Force revised the guidelines for the use of ICDs in 2002.[19] ICDs are most effective in patients who have had a cardiac arrest caused by VF or VT not caused by a transient or reversible cause.[19]
- The ICD system is composed of a pulse generator and a lead system (Fig. 46-1).
- The pulse generator contains capacitors, circuits, and a lithium battery. The battery usually lasts 3 to 8 years before requiring replacement.[6,24,36,43,44]

- Battery life depends on the number of times therapies are delivered or pacing modes are used.[36]
- The ICD system monitors the heart rate and cardiac rhythm and provides the energy for treating the life-threatening dysrhythmia by antitachycardia pacing, cardioversion, or defibrillation. The pulse generator also may provide postshock bradycardia pacing if the patient is converted to a bradydysrhythmia. The postshock bradycardia pacing rate may be faster than the backup bradycardia rate (i.e., postshock bradycardia pacing rate is 60 beats/min, but the backup bradycardia rate is 40 beats/min). The postshock pacing rate is faster to restore adequate hemodynamics more quickly.

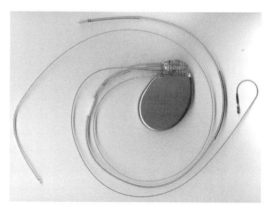

FIGURE 46-1 ICD and lead system (including superior vena cava lead, right ventricular lead, and coronary sinus lead). *(Courtesy Guidant Corporation.)*

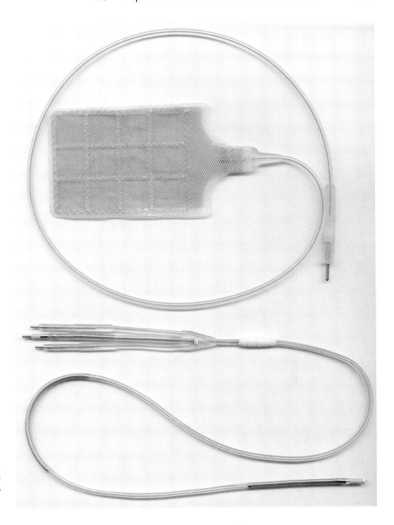

FIGURE 46-2 *Top,* ICD patch that is placed on the right ventricle. *Bottom,* Superior vena cava lead. *(Courtesy Guidant Corporation.)*

- Early ICDs were implanted surgically using the sternotomy, thoracotomy, or subxiphoid approach.[4,22]
- Early ICD models used two sets of leads. The first lead was placed in the superior vena cava. The second lead was a ventricular patch, which was made of titanium mesh and rubber insulation and was sewn onto the epicardial surface of the ventricle. A two-patch system could be used as an alternative, and the patches typically were placed on the anterior right ventricle and the posterior left ventricle. On chest radiography the patch leads can be identified by their mesh perimeter, (Fig. 46-2) and the manufacturer's model number can be read.[4,22] For early-model ICDs, the generator was implanted in the abdominal area because of its large size (Fig. 46-3).
- Current-generation ICD generators are implanted subcutaneously in the pectoral region. The lead system is in contact with the endocardial surface and consists of single, double, or triple leads. Current systems use a single tripolar endocardial lead that is capable of sensing the patient's heart rate and rhythm and delivering the shock.[39,43,44] These lead systems are inserted transvenously through the subclavian, cephalic, or axillary vein and are positioned at the apex of the right ventricle and the superior vena cava.[4] This placement technique has

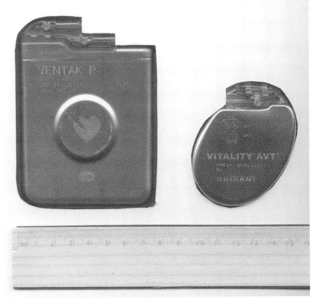

FIGURE 46-3 *Left,* Ventak P, one of the earliest ICDs. *Right,* Vitality AVT, one of the currently used ICDs. *(Courtesy Guidant Corporation.)*

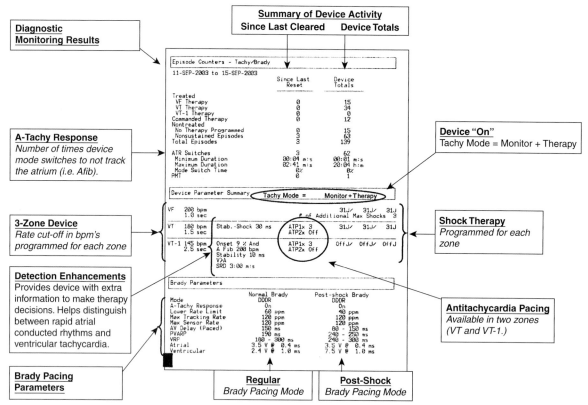

Diagnostic Monitoring Results

Summary of Device Activity
Since Last Cleared   Device Totals

A-Tachy Response
Number of times device mode switches to not track the atrium (i.e. Afib).

3-Zone Device
Rate cut-off in bpm's programmed for each zone

Detection Enhancements
Provides device with extra information to make therapy decisions. Helps distinguish between rapid atrial conducted rhythms and ventricular tachycardia.

Brady Pacing Parameters

Device "On"
Tachy Mode = Monitor + Therapy

Shock Therapy
Programmed for each zone

Antitachycardia Pacing
Available in two zones (VT and VT-1.)

Regular
Brady Pacing Mode

Post-Shock
Brady Pacing Mode

FIGURE 46-4 Printout from ICD interrogation. The interrogation determines the ICD settings and determines if the ICD has been used (e.g., ICD defibrillation). *(Courtesy Guidant Corporation.)*

decreased recovery time, perioperative complications, length of stay, and mortality.[26] Complications of the endocardial technique include lead dislodgment, lead fracture, and venous thrombosis.[7,9,11,16,23,29,31,32,42]

- Current ICDs offer enhanced capabilities. On recognition of VT or VF, the newer ICDs provide tiered therapy, a type of multilevel therapy, to terminate the dysrhythmia. The first tier is usually antitachycardia pacing, and if it is ineffective, the second tier of therapy involves a low-energy cardioversion. The third tier is defibrillation and is used if the second tier fails to convert the rhythm. The fourth tier of therapy is ventricular demand pacing, and it is used if the previous tiers convert the rhythm to asystole or bradycardia.[4,24]
- A patient who needs a permanent pacemaker may receive an ICD with dual-chamber pacing.
- The ICD can be programmed from one to three zones. Each zone (heart rate range) may include several tiered therapies (Fig. 46-4).[24,36]
- ICD devices have various programmable features, including antitachycardia pacing, low-energy cardioversion, defibrillation, antibradycardia pacing, set time to therapy, stored data, noninvasive electrophysiologic stimulation, variable energy outputs, and redetection algorithms. These features allow therapy to be individualized for each patient.[24,36]
- The newest ICD may include cardiac resynchronization therapy (CRT-D), which is able to antitachycardia pace,

cardiovert, defibrillate, and backup antibradycardia pace and has the capability to pace the right and left ventricle synchronously. CRT-D is used in the treatment of patients with New York Heart Association class III/IV heart failure who have an ejection fraction less than 30% and prolonged QRS duration. The device needs to pace 100% of the time to be effective. Leads are placed in the right atrium, in the right ventricle, and in an epicardial vein on the surface of the left ventricle accessed through the coronary sinus.[1,2]

- A defibrillator code was developed in 1993 by the North American Society of Pacing and Electrophysiology and the British Pacing and Electrophysiology Group to describe the capabilities and operation of ICDs.[5] The defibrillator code is patterned after the pacemaker code; however, it has some important differences (Table 46-1).[5] The defibrillator code offers less information about the ICD's antibradycardia pacing function, but it offers more specific information about the shock functions.
- Magnet mode is an ICD feature that varies among manufacturers. If available on individual models, the magnet mode allows for suppression of therapy in an emergency. All health care providers caring for patients with an ICD must be trained in the proper use of this mode. The magnet mode deactivates the defibrillator capability of the ICD; however, the magnet mode does not interfere with the backup pacing mode.[37] Confirmation of reactivation of therapy can be accomplished only with the appropriate manufacturer's programmer.

TABLE 46-1	NASPE/BPEG Defibrillator Code		
Position I	**Position II**	**Position III**	**Position IV**
Shock Chamber	*Antitachycardia Pacing Chamber*	*Tachycardia Detection*	*Antibradycardia Pacing Chamber*
O = None	O = None	E = Electrogram	O = None
A = Atrium	A = Atrium	H = Hemodynamic	A = Atrium
V = Ventricle	V = Ventricle		V = Ventricle
D = Dual (A + V)	D = Dual (A + V)		D = Dual (A + V)

NASPE/BPEG, North American Society of Pacing and Electrophysiology/British Pacing and Electrophysiology Group.
From Bernstein, A.D., et al. (1993). The NASPE/BPEG defibrillator code (NBD Code). *Pacing Clin Electrophysiol,* 16, 1776.

- Emotional adjustments vary with each patient and family. Patients may exhibit depression, anxiety, fear, and anger. Some patients view the device as an activity restriction, and others see it as a lifesaving device that allows them to resume a normal life. Phantom shock is a condition in which a patient's anxiety and concern about the delivery of a shock is so great that it affects the patient's daily activity. Support groups should be encouraged for patients receiving ICD therapy.[8,14,15,40,46,47]

EQUIPMENT

- Electrocardiogram (ECG) monitor and recorder
- ECG electrodes
  Additional equipment to have available as needed includes the following:
- ICD interrogator or programmer (commonly obtained from the electrophysiology department and specific to each manufacturer; contact specific manufacturer)
- Magnet (doughnut or bar type)
- 12-lead ECG machine
- Analgesics as prescribed
- Emergency medications and resuscitation equipment
- Antidysrhythmics as prescribed

PATIENT AND FAMILY EDUCATION

- Assess learning needs, readiness to learn, and factors that influence learning. ➨*Rationale:* This assessment allows the nurse to individualize teaching in a meaningful manner.
- Assess patient and family understanding of ICD therapy and the reason for its use. ➨*Rationale:* This assessment provides information regarding knowledge level and necessity of additional teaching.
- Provide information about the normal conduction system, such as structure of the conduction system, source of the heart beat, normal and abnormal heart rhythms, and symptoms of abnormal heart rhythms. ➨*Rationale:* Understanding of the normal conduction system assists the patient and family in recognizing the seriousness of the patient's condition and the need for ICD therapy.
- Provide information about ICD therapy, including the reason for the ICD, explanation of the equipment, what to expect during activation of the ICD, precautions and restrictions in activities of daily living (e.g., first 4 to 8 weeks do not raise the arm on the battery insertion side above the head), signs and symptoms of infection and complications, and instructions on when to call the physician, and information on expected follow-up.[12] ➨*Rationale:* Understanding of ICD functioning and expectations after discharge assists the patient and family in developing realistic perceptions of ICD therapy. Limiting usage of the affected arm helps to prevent dislodgment of the lead system.

- Provide patient registration and identification card. Encourage the patient to wear Medic Alert identification and to carry an identification card at all times. ➨*Rationale:* This reinforces the seriousness of the patient's condition and ensures that appropriate identifying information is available to other health care providers if needed.
- Inform the patient and family of the need to continue antidysrhythmic medication therapy. ➨*Rationale:* Antidysrhythmic medication suppresses dysrhythmias and limits the potential of frequent ICD shocks.
- Discuss the need for the patient to keep a current list of medications in his or her wallet. ➨*Rationale:* The patient or other family members should be prepared to provide necessary information to health care providers in an emergency situation.
- Discuss the need for family members to learn cardiopulmonary resuscitation (CPR). ➨*Rationale:* Family members should be prepared for an emergency situation (e.g., if ICD does not convert life-threatening rhythm or ICD malfunctions).
- Inform the patient to activate the emergency medical services (EMS) system when having any symptoms, such as dizziness, extreme fatigue, heart palpitations, or light-headedness.[47] ➨*Rationale:* Activation of the EMS system provides trained personnel to initiate ACLS.
- Teach the patient and family members to remain calm in the event of a shock. Instruct them to move the patient to a safe place to lie down. Have someone stay with the patient if possible throughout the event. If multiple shocks occur or if the patient becomes unresponsive, someone should activate the EMS system or call 911 (inform patient and family not to contact the physician, but to activate the EMS system immediately). ➨*Rationale:* Activation of the EMS system provides trained personnel to initiate ACLS.
- Instruct the patient to keep a log of all the events surrounding a shock (time of day, number of shocks, any symptoms felt before or after the shock, activity before the shock, any action taken by the patient or bystanders).[45] ➨*Rationale:* This information helps the

physician to evaluate the functioning of the ICD and the patient's response to the therapy.

- Instruct the patient to notify the health care provider whenever he or she receives a shock. ➥*Rationale:* The healthcare provider may want to interrogate the ICD to determine if the device detected and responded appropriately.
- Inform the patient about the ICD and reason for the tones that may be emitted from the device. An audible tone may indicate battery depletion. Electromagnetic interference (EMI) may deactivate the ICD. If this occurs, the patient may hear an audible tone *(no louder than the alarm on a wristwatch)* from the device indicating deactivation. The patient should move away from the source of EMI and notify the physician immediately if he or she hears a tone from the ICD.[17,20,25,28,38] ➥*Rationale:* The patient needs to be seen by the physician and have the ICD interrogated to determine whether or not the ICD is activated.
- Inform the patient and family that family members will not be harmed if they touch the patient when a shock is delivered. ➥*Rationale:* This information prepares the patient and family, encourages verbalization of feelings, and may decrease anxiety.
- Driving restrictions vary from state to state and among physicians. The patient should discuss plans for long trips and driving restrictions with the physician.[22] ➥*Rationale:* These restrictions may help to prevent lead fracture, generator migration, and motor vehicle accidents.
- Inform the patient when going on vacation that he or she should obtain the name of an electrophysiology physician in the area where he or she is traveling. ➥*Rationale:* In case of an emergency, the patient and family have contact with trained personnel to ensure proper functioning of the ICD.
- Teach the patient and family members that the terms *BOL* (beginning of life), *MOL* (middle of life), *ERI* (elective replacement indicator), and *EOL* (end of life) are used to describe the status of the battery (ICD generator). ➥*Rationale:* This teaching prepares the patient and family for generator changes, encourages verbalization of feelings, alleviates misunderstanding, may decrease anxiety, and reinforces ICD teaching.
- Inform the patient and family members of the importance of having the ICD checked every 4 to 6 months. ➥*Rationale:* This maintains optimal functioning of the ICD.
- Instruct the patient to notify the physician's office of a change in address. ➥*Rationale:* This is done so that the physician can notify the patient of any potential advisories related to the ICD and lead system.[30]
- Instruct the patient to inform his or her dentist about the ICD. ➥*Rationale:* For the first 6 months after initial implant, the patient should take antibiotics prophylactically.[35]
- Inform the patient and family of potential sources of EMI to the ICD. In the hospital, these include magnetic resonance imaging, diathermy, computed tomography, lithotripsy, electrocautery, radiation therapy, and nerve stimulators. Outside of the hospital, these include hand-held wands used by airport security, arc welders, large transformers or motors, antitheft devices at stores or libraries, cellular phones less than 6 inches away from the pulse generator, the antenna of an operating citizens' band or ham radio, improperly grounded electric equipment, and hand-held tools less than 12 inches away from the pulse generator.[17,20,25,27,28] ➥*Rationale:* EMI can deactivate the ICD, deplete the battery of the ICD, or inhibit the pulse generator of the ICD. Cellular phones may temporarily inhibit functioning of the ICD; the phone should be positioned on the opposite side of device.
- Teach the patient to notify the physician if the device appears to wear through the skin or the device site becomes reddened, warm, or has a discharge. ➥*Rationale:* These signs identify problems (e.g., infection).

PATIENT ASSESSMENT AND PREPARATION

Patient Assessment

- Assess the patient's ECG for cardiac rate and rhythm. ➥*Rationale:* This assessment establishes baseline data.
- Assess the patency of the patient's intravenous access. ➥*Rationale:* Intravenous access should be ensured in case emergency medications are needed.
- Ensure a radiograph is prescribed and obtained before the patient is sent home. ➥*Rationale:* A radiograph provides essential data to determine lead position and integrity,[32] confirms the absence of pneumothorax, and provides a baseline to compare lead position in the future.
- Identify whether the ICD is activated or deactivated. ➥*Rationale:* This provides essential data regarding the functioning of the ICD and treatment of VT and VF.
- Identify the type of ICD, the mode of function, how it is programmed, and the manufacturer. ➥*Rationale:* This information aids in assessment of what rate and rhythm activate the device; whether antitachycardia pacing, cardioversion, defibrillation, and backup pacing capabilities are present; and how they are set. This information determines what programmer is necessary to interrogate the device.
- Determine the patient's ICD history: date of insertion, last battery change, most recent ICD check, how often the device is used, if the patient has experienced any problems with the ICD or ICD site, and any unexpected symptoms.[12,45,49] ➥*Rationale:* The ICD history provides baseline information and may aid in determining any problems that might be occurring.
- Explore issues such as body image, lifestyle changes, and sexual concerns. ➥*Rationale:* Patients with ICDs may develop emotional, physical, and social changes. Referral for counseling may be necessary.
- Assess for postprocedure pain. ➥*Rationale:* The procedure is generally well tolerated with oral analgesics containing acetaminophen and codeine.

Patient Preparation

- Ensure that the patient and family understand teaching. Answer questions as they arise, and reinforce information as needed. ➤➤*Rationale:* This communication evaluates and reinforces understanding of previously taught information.

- Provide analgesics or sedatives as prescribed and needed. ➤➤*Rationale:* These medications decrease discomfort or anxiety related to ICD therapy.

Procedure for Implantable Cardioverter-Defibrillator

Steps	Rationale	Special Considerations
1. Wash hands.	Reduces the transmission of microorganisms; standard precautions.	
2. Cleanse the skin for application of the ECG electrodes with cleansing pads or soap and water (see Procedure 54).	Proper skin preparation is essential to maintain appropriate skin-to-electrode contact.	It may be necessary to clip chest hair to ensure good skin contact with the electrodes.
3. Attach the ECG leads to the electrodes, place the electrodes on the patient's chest, and record the ECG (see Procedure 54).	Necessary to assess cardiac rhythm.	
4. If patient experiences VT or VF:		Run a continuous ECG strip of the dysrhythmia from the bedside monitor if possible; record a 12-lead ECG if possible.
A. Assess and stay with the patient.	Ensures patient safety, and provides an opportunity to assess the patient's response to the dysrhythmia.	
B. Wait for the device to function: antitachycardia pacing, cardioversion, defibrillation.	The ICD requires a brief period (8-30 seconds) to assess the VT or VF and to initiate therapy.	
C. If the dysrhythmia continues, wait for the ICD to recharge and defibrillate again if indicated.	The ICD reassesses the cardiac rhythm, recharges, and defibrillates again as preprogrammed.	Time needs to be allotted for the ICD to defibrillate as it is preprogrammed.
D. If the ICD has been functioning as preprogrammed and still does not convert the dysrhythmia, initiate ACLS.[13]	Provides emergency care.	Assess the patient's response to VT; the patient may be hemodynamically stable or unstable. Follow ACLS standards. Remain with the patient. Notify the physician or advanced practice nurse immediately, and prepare emergency equipment.
E. Apply defibrillation paddles in one of the two following ways: Place at the heart's apex just to the left of the nipple in the midaxillary line (at fifth to sixth intercostal space), and place the other paddle just below the right clavicle to the right of the sternum or apply anterior-posterior defibrillation electrodes or paddles. The anterior paddle is placed in the anterior left precordial area, and the posterior paddle is placed posteriorly behind the heart in the left infrascapular area.[13]	The electric current passes through the cardiac muscle.	Defibrillator paddles and defibrillation patches should not be placed over nitroglycerin patches or the ICD generator. The paddles and patches should be a minimum of 2 inches away from the generator when delivering external shocks.

Procedure continues on the following page

Procedure for Implantable Cardioverter-Defibrillator—*Continued*

Steps	Rationale	Special Considerations
F. If indicated, externally defibrillate the patient according to ACLS[13] (see Procedure 37).	Provides efficacious emergency care.	ICDs have preprogrammed pacing capability; cardiac pacing *will* be initiated by the ICD if the result of defibrillation is bradycardia or asystole. If external defibrillation is required, the ICD should be interrogated to assess for potential damage to the device.
5. Deactivation of the ICD:	The ICD may need to be deactivated if it is defibrillating a cardiac rhythm that is not VT or VF, such as atrial fibrillation with rapid ventricular response. If the device is functioning inappropriately, deactivation may be required to prevent harm to the patient. Deactivation response to a magnet varies among manufacturers.	Follow hospital standards to ensure that a nurse can deactivate an ICD. Inform the physician of ICD deactivation. The following circumstances may require ICD deactivation: lead dislodgment, lead migration, lead fracture, inappropriate identification of the rhythm, inappropriate defibrillation threshold, and death.[7,9,11,16,22,23,29,31,32,42] Consider connecting the patient to an external defibrillator. Per manufacturers' guidelines, explant of the ICD is necessary only if it is an investigational device or if the body is to be cremated; if the body is to be buried, removal of the device is the perogative of the family of the deceased. The bradycardia pacing component cannot be turned off; turn the ECG monitor off postmortem to diminish family's anxiety.
A. Place a bar or doughnut magnet over the right upper corner of the pulse generator.	In the newest devices, the magnet inhibits therapy only when it is on the ICD, preventing accidental deactivation of the device. As long as the magnet is in place, the ICD is inactive.	A programmer is needed to deactivate most ICDs.
B. Listen for a synchronous tone that should occur simultaneously with each R wave (the tone lasts for approximately 30 seconds).	A synchronous tone indicates that the ICD is activated.	Know which manufacturers have this ability and if the feature is turned on; not all devices emit a synchronous tone.
(1) Maintain magnet position and listen for a constant tone. (2) Remove the magnet after the constant tone is heard.	A constant tone indicates that the ICD is deactivated.	Know manufacturer's magnet features.
6. Reactivation of an ICD:	Turns the ICD on.	Follow hospital standards to ensure that a nurse can reactivate an ICD. An ICD can be inadvertently deactivated when the pulse generator is exposed to EMI. Some ICDs have audible tones that are emitted if the ICD becomes deactivated. Interrogation is required to determine whether or not the ICD is activated.[12,22,37]

Procedure for Implantable Cardioverter-Defibrillator—*Continued*

Steps	Rationale	Special Considerations
A. Remove the magnet.	When the magnet is removed, the ICD automatically reactivates.	
B. Place a bar or doughnut magnet over the right upper corner of the pulse generator.	The magnet activates and deactivates the ICD.	A programmer is needed to activate most ICDs.
(1) Listen for a constant tone.	A constant tone indicates that the ICD is deactivated.	Know manufacturer's magnet features.
(2) Listen for a synchronous tone that should occur simultaneously with each R wave.	A synchronous tone indicates that the ICD is activated.	
(3) Remove the magnet.		

Expected Outcomes

- ICD detects life-threatening VT or VF.
- ICD delivers appropriate therapy, including defibrillation as necessary.
- Cardiac rhythm is converted to a hemodynamically stable rhythm.
- Hemodynamic stability is achieved.

Unexpected Outcomes

- Failure of the ICD to detect VT or VF
- Failure of the ICD to convert life-threatening dysrhythmia despite appropriate therapy and defibrillation attempts
- Failure of the backup pacing system to pace if bradycardia or asystole is the result of defibrillation
- Inappropriate defibrillation
- Infection at the ICD pulse generator site, tunneled region, or myocardium
- Lead fracture or migration
- Pulse generator migration
- Pulse generator pocket hematoma
- Loosened set screw in device header
- Air embolism
- Venous thrombosis
- Cardiac tamponade
- Skin erosion
- Pneumothorax
- Frozen shoulder on operative side[9]

Patient Monitoring and Care

Steps	Rationale	Reportable Conditions
		These conditions should be reported if they persist despite nursing interventions.
1. Monitor the ECG continuously.	Detects dysrhythmias.	• Dysrhythmias
2. Monitor the ICD for antitachycardia pacing, cardioversion, and defibrillation.	Detects functioning of the ICD.	• Ventricular dysrhythmias • ICD therapy • Defibrillation • ICD malfunction
3. Assess the patient's response to ICD defibrillation, including cardiac rate and rhythm, level of consciousness, and vital signs.	Determines patient status and necessity for additional treatment.	• Cardiac rate and rhythm before and after defibrillation • Level of consciousness • Vital signs
4. Evaluate and treat the patient for pain and anxiety.	ICD defibrillation may cause pain and may increase patient anxiety.	• Pain and anxiety that are not relieved by prescribed analgesic or sedative

Procedure continues on the following page

Patient Monitoring and Care—*Continued*

Steps	Rationale	Reportable Conditions
5. Assess the ICD pulse generator site for evidence of manipulation.	Patient manipulation at the site may affect ICD therapy.	• Evidence of ICD pulse generator manipulation
6. Monitor for signs and symptoms of infection.	Placement of an invasive device may result in infection.	• Signs or symptoms of infection
7. Monitor for signs of bleeding and hematoma.	Placement of an invasive device may result in untoward bleeding.	• Signs or symptoms of bleeding or hematoma.

Documentation

Documentation should include the following:

- ICD history
- Preprogrammed ICD parameters
- Status of the device (i.e., if it is on or off)
- Patient and family education; acceptance of device
- Dysrhythmias
- All rhythm strip recordings

- ICD functioning
- Patient response to ICD therapy
- Occurrence of any unexpected outcomes
- Additional interventions
- Device interrogation (see Fig. 46-4)

References

1. Abraham, W.T., et al. (2002). Cardiac resynchronization in chronic heart failure. *N Engl J Med,* 346, 1845-53.
2. Albert, N.M. (2003). Cardiac resynchronization therapy through biventricular pacing in patients with heart failure and ventricular dyssynchrony. *Crit Care Nurse,* June(Suppl), 2-13.
3. Anderson, J.L., et al. (1999). Design results of the antiarrhythmics vs implantable defibrillators (AVID) registry. *Circulation,* 99, 1692-9.
4. Belott, P.H., and Reynolds, D.W. (2000). Permanent pacemaker and implantable cardioverter-defibrillator implantation. In: Ellenbogen, K.A., et al, editors. *Clinical Cardiac Pacing and Defibrillation.* 2nd ed. Philadelphia: W.B. Saunders.
5. Bernstein, A.D., et al. (1993). The NASPE/BPEG defibrillator code (NBD Code). *Pacing Clin Electrophysiol,* 16, 1776.
6. Block, M., and Breihardt, G. (2004). Implantable cardioverter-defibrillators: Clinical aspects. In: Zipes, D.P., et al, editors. *Cardiac Electrophysiology: From Cell to Bedside.* 4th ed. Philadelphia: W.B. Saunders.
7. Brown, L.A., et al. (2001). Implantable cardioverter-defibrillator endocarditis secondary to *Candida albicans. Am J Med Sci,* 322, 160-2.
8. Burke, J.L., et al. (2003). The psychosocial impact of implantable cardioverter defibrillator: A meta-analytic review. *Br J Health Psychol,* 8, 65-78.
9. Burke, M.C., et al. (1999). Frozen shoulder syndrome associated with subpectoral defibrillator implantation. *J Interv Card Electrophysiol,* 3, 253-6.
10. Buxton, A.E., et al. (1999). A randomized study of the prevention of sudden death in patients with coronary artery disease. *N Engl J Med,* 341, 1882-90.
11. Chua, J.D., et al. (2000). Diagnosis and management of infections involving implantable electrophysiologic cardiac devices. *Ann Intern Med,* 133, 604-8.
12. Crossley, G.H., III. (2000). Follow-up of the patient with a defibrillator. In: Ellenbogen, K.A., et al, editors. *Clinical Cardiac Pacing and Defibrillation.* 2nd ed. Philadelphia: W.B. Saunders.
13. Cummins, R.O., et al. (2001). *ACLS Provider Manual.* Dallas: American Heart Association.
14. Dunbar, S.B., et al. (1999). Factors associated with outcomes 3 months after implantable cardioverter defibrillator insertion. *Heart Lung,* 28, 303-15.
15. Edelman, S., Lemon, J., and Kidman, A. (2003). Psychological therapies for recipients of implantable cardioverter defibrillators. *Heart Lung,* 32, 234-40.
16. Ellenbogen, K.A., et al. (2003). Detection and management of an implantable cardioverter defibrillator lead failure: Incidence and clinical implications. *J Am Coll Cardiol,* 41, 73-80.
17. Garg, A., et al. (2002). Inappropriate implantable cardioverter defibrillator discharge from sensing external alternating current leak. *J Interv Card Electrophysiol,* 7, 181-4.
18. Gotlieb, C., Callans, D., and Marchlinski, F. (1998). Implantable cardioverter defibrillators in the United States: Understanding the benefits and the limitations of implantable cardioverter defibrillator therapy based on clinical trail results. *Pacing Clin Electrophysiol,* 21, 2016-20.
19. Gregoratos, G., et al. (2002). *ACC/AHA/NASPE 2002 Guideline Update for Implantation of Cardiac Pacemakers and Antiarrhythmia Devices: A Report of the ACC/AHA Task Force on Practice Guidelines (Committee on Pacemaker Implantation).* Available at: www.acc.org/clinical/guidelines/pacemaker/pacemaker/pdf.
20. Hayes, D.L., and Strathmore, N.F. (2000). Electromagnetic interference with implantable devices. In: Ellenbogen, K.A., et al, editors. *Clinical Cardiac Pacing and Defibrillation.* 2nd ed. Philadelphia: W.B. Saunders.
21. Heidenreich, P.A., et al. (2002). Overview of randomized trials of antiarrhythmic drugs and devices for prevention of sudden cardiac death. *Am Heart J,* 144, 422-30.
22. Jacobson, C., and Gerity, D. (2000). Pacemakers and implantable defibrillations. In: Woods, S.L., et al, editors. *Cardiac Nursing.* 4th ed. Philadelphia: Lippincott Williams & Wilkins.
23. Joglar, J.A., et al. (2001). The hot can: ICD failure presenting as severe shoulder pain. *Pacing Clin Electrophysiol,* 24, 396-7.
24. Josephson, M.E. (2002). Evaluation of electrical therapy for arrhythmias. In: Josephson, M.E. *Clinical Cardiac Electrophysiology: Techniques and Interpretations.* 3rd ed. Philadelphia: Lippincott Williams & Wilkins.
25. Kolb, C., Schmeider, S., and Schmitt, C. (2002). Inappropriate shock delivery due to interference between a washing machine and an implantable cardioverter defibrillator. *J Interv Card Electrophysiol,* 7, 255-6.
26. Kroll, M.W., and Tchou, P.J. (2000). Testing of implantable defibrillator functions at implantation. In Ellenbogen, K.A.,

et al, editors. *Clinical Cardiac Pacing and Defibrillation.* 2nd ed. Philadelphia: W.B. Saunders.

27. Kron, J., et al. (2001). Lead- and device-related complications in the antiarrhythmics versus implantable defibrillators trial. *Am Heart J, 141,* 92-8.

28. Lee, S.W., Moak, J.P., and Lewis, B. (2002). Inadvertent detection of 60-Hz alternating currents by an implantable cardioverter defibrillator. *Pacing Clin Electrophysiol,* 25, 518-9.

29. Liu, B.C., et al. (2003). Inappropriate shock delivery and biventricular pacing cardiac defibrillators. *Texas Heart Inst J,* 30, 45-9.

30. Maisel, W.H., Stevenson, W.G., and Epstein, L.M. (2002). Changing trends in pacemaker and implantable cardioverter defibrillator generator advisories. *Pacing Clin Electrophysiol,* 25, 1670-8.

31. Mela, T., et al. (2001). Long-term infection rates associated with the pectoral versus abdominal approach to cardioverter-defibrillator implants. *Am J Cardiol,* 88, 750-3.

32. Morishima, I., et al. (2003). Follow-up x-rays play a key role in detecting implantable cardioverter defibrillator lead fracture: A case of incessant inappropriate shocks due to lead fracture. *Pacing Clin Electrophysiol,* 26, 911-3.

33. Moss, A.J., et al. (1996). Improved survival with an implanted defibrillator in patients with coronary disease at high risk for ventricular arrhythmia. *N Engl J Med,* 335, 1933-40.

34. Moss, A.J., et al. (2002). Prophylactic implantation of a defibrillator in patients with myocardial infarction and reduced ejection fraction. *N Engl J Med,* 346, 877-83.

35. Mylonakis, E., and Calderwood, S. (2001). Infective endocarditis in adults. *N Engl J Med,* 345, 1318-29.

36. Niebauer, M.J., and Wilkoff, B.L. (2000). Implantable cardioverter-defibrillators: Technical aspects. In: Zipes, D.P., et al, editors. *Cardiac Electrophysiology: From Cell to Bedside.* 3rd ed. Philadelphia: W.B. Saunders.

37. Pinski, S.L. (2000). Emergencies related to implantable cardioverter-defibrillators. *Crit Care Med,* 28, 174-80.

38. Sabate, X., et al. (2001). Washing machine associated 50 Hz detected as ventricular fibrillation by an implanted cardioverter defibrillator. *Pacing Clin Electrophysiol,* 24, 1281-3.

39. Schaer, B., and Osswald, S. (2000). Methods of minimizing inappropriate implantable cardioverter-defibrillator shocks. *Curr Cardiol Rep,* 2, 346-52.

40. Sears, S.F., and Conti, J.B. (2002). Quality of life and psychological functioning of ICD patients. *Heart,* 87, 488-93.

41. Siebels, J., et al. (1993). Preliminary results of the Cardiac Arrest Study Hamburg (CASH). *Am J Cardiol,* 72, 109F-13F.

42. Sticherling, C., et al. (2001). Prevalence of central venous occlusion in patients with chronic defibrillator leads. *Am Heart J,* 141, 813-6.

43. Swerdlow, C.D., and Zhang, J. (2001). Implantable cardioverter defibrillator shocks: A troubleshooting guide. *Rev Cardiovasc Med,* 2, 61-72.

44. Swygman, C., et al. (2002). Advances in implantable cardioverter defibrillators. *Curr Opin Cardiol,* 17, 24-8.

45. Theuns, D.A., Res, J.C., and Jordaens, L.J. (2003). Home monitoring in ICD therapy: Future perspectives. *Europace,* 5, 139-42.

46. Thomas, S.A., Friedmann, E., and Kelley, F.J. (2001). Living with an implantable cardioverter: A review of the current literature related to psychosocial factors. *AACN Clin Issues,* 12, 156-63.

47. White, M.M. (2002). Psychosocial impact of the implantable cardioverter defibrillator: Nursing implications. *J Cardiovasc Nurs,* 16, 53-61.

48. Wilbur, S.L., and Marchlinski, F.E. (1999). Implantable cardioverter-defibrillator follow-up: What everyone needs to know. *Cardiol Rev,* 7, 176-90.

49. Winters, S.L., et al. (2001). Consensus statement on indications, guidelines for use, and recommendations for follow-up of implantable cardioverter defibrillators. *Pacing Clin Electrophysiol,* 24, 262-9.

50. Wyse, G.D., and Greene, H.L. (2000). Indications for implantable cardioverter defibrillators: Clinical trials. In Ellenbogen, K.A., et al, editors. *Clinical cardiac pacing and defibrillation.* 2nd ed. Philadelphia: W.B. Saunders.

51. Zippes, D.P., et al. (1997). A comparison of antiarrhythmic-drug therapy with implantable defibrillators in patients resuscitated from near-fatal ventricular arrhythmias. *N Engl J Med,* 337, 1576-83.

Additional Readings

Cooper, R.A.S., et al. (2000). The implantable atrial defibrillator: basic development to clinical implementation. In Ellenbogen, K.A., et al, editors. *Clinical Cardiac Pacing And Defibrillation.* 2nd ed. Philadelphia: W.B. Saunders.

Dickerson, S.S., et al. (2000). Therapeutic connection: Help seeking on the internet for persons with implantable cardioverter defibrillators. *Heart Lung,* 29, 248-55.

Sorbera, C.A., and Cusack, E.J. (2002). Indications for implantable cardioverter defibrillator therapy. *Heart Dis,* 4, 166-70.

Sweeney, M.O., et al. (2002). Upgrade of permanent pacemakers and single chamber implantable cardioverter defibrillators to pectoral dual chamber implantable cardioverter defibrillators: Indications, surgical approach, and long-term clinical results. *Pacing Clin Electrophysiol,* 25, 1715-23.

White, E. (2000). Patients with implantable cardioverter defibrillators: Transition to home. *J Cardiovasc Nurs,* 14, 42-52.

Web Sites

http://www.medtronic.com
http://www.guidant.com
http://www.lifebeatonline.com
http://www.biotronic.com
http://www.duff.net/zapper/zap1.htm

Technical Support Numbers

Medtronic (1-800-Medtronic) Tachy Support
Guidant (1-800-Cardiac) Tachy Support

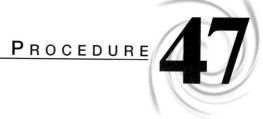

PROCEDURE **47**

Permanent Pacemaker (Assessing Function)

PURPOSE: The purpose of permanent pacing is to establish and maintain an appropriate heart rate or ventricular synchrony when a chronic conduction or impulse formation disturbance exists in the cardiac conduction system that is not reversible.

Fred Williams
Sue Wingate

PREREQUISITE NURSING KNOWLEDGE

- Knowledge of the normal anatomy and physiology of the cardiovascular system, cardiac conduction, and basic dysrhythmia interpretation is required.
- Knowledge of pacemaker function and patient response to pacemaker therapy is needed.
- Advanced cardiac life support knowledge and skills are needed.
- Permanent pacing is indicated for the following clinical conditions:[5]
  - ❖ Acquired atrioventricular (AV) block in adults
  - ❖ Chronic bifascicular and trifascicular block
  - ❖ AV block associated with acute myocardial infarction
  - ❖ Sinus node dysfunction
  - ❖ Prevention and termination of tachydysrhythmias
  - ❖ Hypersensitive carotid sinus and neurocardiogenic syncope
  - ❖ Certain congenital heart defects
  - ❖ Certain clinical features associated with hypertrophic cardiomyopathy, dilated cardiomyopathy, or cardiac transplantation
- Relative contraindications to permanent pacemakers include the following:
  - ❖ Active infection (endocarditis, positive blood cultures)
  - ❖ Bleeding (evidenced by increased blood coagulation studies)
- The pulse generator typically is implanted subcutaneously in a pectoral pocket. The outer casing is made of titanium and contains the electronic components and the battery necessary to sustain pacing for several years (Fig. 47-1).

- A transvenous pacing lead is another component of the permanent pacing system and may be positioned in the right atrium, the right ventricle, or the left ventricle (or combination of these), depending on the type of pacing needed.
- Unipolar pacing involves a relatively large electrical circuit. The distal tip of the pacing lead is the negative electrode and is in contact with the myocardium. The positive electrode encompasses the metallic pacemaker case, located in the soft tissue. Energy is delivered from the negative electrode to the positive electrode causing myocardial depolarization. The electrocardiogram (ECG) tracing shows a large, easily visible spike. Unipolar leads are rarely used in current practice.
- Bipolar pacing uses a smaller electrical circuit in which the distal tip of the pacing lead is the negative electrode

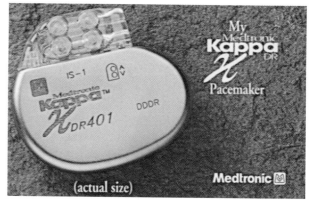

FIGURE 47-1 Permanent pulse generator. *(Courtesy of Medtronic, Inc.)*

TABLE 47-1	Pertinent Definitions Related to Pacemakers
Sensing	Ability of the pacemaker to detect intrinsic myocardial electrical activity
	The pacemaker either is inhibited from delivering a stimulus or initiates an electrical impulse, based on the programmed response
Pulse generation	Occurs when the pacemaker produces a programmed current for a set duration
	This energy travels through the transvenous lead wires to the myocardium—this is known as *pacemaker firing* and usually produces a line or spike on the ECG recording (pacemaker spikes are shown in Fig. 47-2)
Capture	Refers to the successful stimulation of the myocardium by the pacemaker impulse that results in depolarization
	Evidenced on the ECG by a pacemaker spike/stimulus followed by either an atrial or ventricular complex, depending on the chambers being paced (see Fig. 47-3)
Failure of pulse generation	Pacemaker does not discharge a pacing stimulus at its programmed time to the myocardium
	Evidenced by the absence of a pacemaker spike on the ECG where expected (see Fig. 47-4)
Sensing failure	Pacemaker has either detected extraneous signals that mimic intrinsic cardiac activity (oversensing) or did not accurately identify intrinsic activity (undersensing)
	Oversensing is recognized on the ECG by pauses where paced beats were expected and prolongation of the interval between paced beats (see Fig. 47-5)
	Undersensing is recognized on the ECG by inappropriate pacemaker spikes relative to the intrinsic electrical activity (pacemaker spikes occurring within the P wave, QRS complex, or T wave) and shortened distances between paced beats (see Fig. 47-6)
Failure to capture	Pacemaker has delivered a pacing stimulus that was unable to initiate depolarization of the myocardium and subsequent myocardial contraction
	Evidenced on the ECG by pacemaker spikes that are not followed by a P wave for atrial pacing or spikes not followed by a QRS complex for ventricular pacing (see Fig. 47-7)

ECG, Electrocardiogram.

in contact with the myocardium. The pacing lead has a second positive electrode that is located within 1 cm of the negative electrode. Energy is delivered from the negative electrode to the positive electrode, causing myocardial depolarization. The ECG tracing may show small spikes, or the spikes may not be visible on a surface ECG.

- Basic principles of cardiac pacing include sensing, pulse generation, and capture (see Table 47-1 for definitions).
- Depending on the type of pacemaker, the pacemaker may function in the atrium, the right ventricle, or the left ventricle. A standard code exists to describe pacemakers (Table 47-2). The nurse must know the programmed mode using the pacemaker code to determine whether the device is functioning appropriately (Figs. 47-2 through 47-7).

- Inappropriate pacemaker function includes failure of pulse generation, sensing failure, and failure to capture (see Table 47-1 for definitions).
- Dual-chamber or DDD pacemakers contain pacing leads that are located in the atrium and the ventricle. Pacing and sensing occur in both chambers. Pacing is inhibited by sensed atrial or ventricular activity. Sensed or paced atrial activity triggers a ventricular paced response in the absence of intrinsic ventricular activity within a programmed AV interval.
- Biventricular pacemakers (resynchronization therapy) contain a third lead that is on the surface of the left ventricle and simultaneously paces the right and left ventricle (Fig. 47-8).

TABLE 47-2	Revised NASPE/BPEG Generic Code for Antibradycardia Pacing*			
I	II	III	IV	V
Chamber(s) Paced	Chamber(s) Sensed	Response to Sensing	Rate Modulation	Multisite Pacing
O = None	O = None	O = None	O = None	O = None
A = Atrium	A = Atrium	T = Triggered	R = Rate modulation	A = Atrium
V = Ventricle	V = Ventricle	I = Inhibited		V = Ventricle
D = Dual (A+V)	D = Dual (A+V)	D = Dual (T+I)		D = Dual (A+V)
S = Single (A or V)[†]	S = Single (A or V)[†]			

*This code differs from the 1987 version that listed programmability and antitachycardia functions. These functions are described in Bernstein, A.D., et al. (1993). NASPE policy statement: The NASPE/BPEG defibrillator code. *Pacing Clin Electrophysiol,* 16, 1776-80.
[†]Manufacturer's designation only.
From Bernstein, A.D., et al. (2002). The revised NASPE/BPEG generic code for antibradycardia, adaptive-rate, and multisite pacing. *Pacing Clin Electrophysiol,* 25, 261.

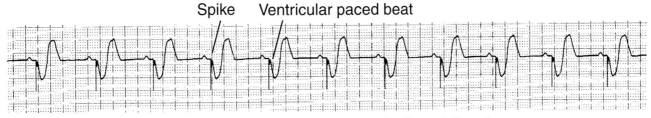

Spike   Ventricular paced beat

FIGURE 47-2 DDD pacing, normal operation: P-sensed, V-paced.

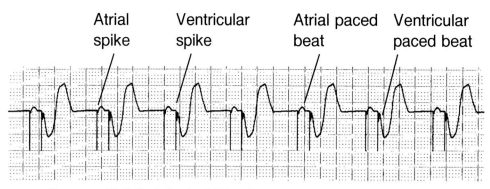

FIGURE 47-3 Dual-chamber DDD pacing, normal operation: A-paced, V-paced.

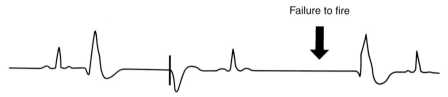

FIGURE 47-4 Failure of pulse generation.

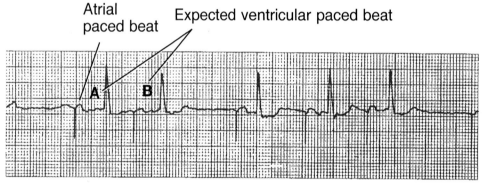

FIGURE 47-5 Ventricular oversensing and possibly ventricular pulse generation failure. Ventricular spike expected at 150 msec. Ventricular spike and corresponding ventricular depolarization did not occur at points *A* and *B*. Also, atrial timing reset by oversensed ventricular activity resulted in erratic atrial pacing (suspicious for fracture of ventricular lead).

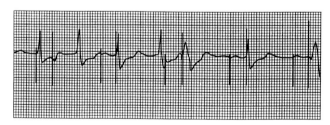

FIGURE 47-6 Ventricular undersensing. Pacemaker appears to be firing asynchronously. The third and sixth ventricular complexes represent concurrent intrinsic ventricular depolarization overlaid by inappropriate pacemaker fire.

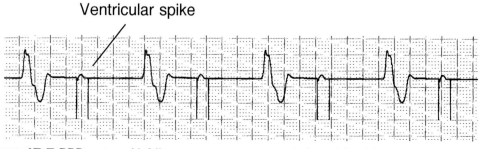

FIGURE 47-7 DDD system with failure to capture or sense ventricular activity. All ventricular spikes show absence of corresponding ventricular depolarization. No timing circuit reset by intrinsic ventricular complexes.

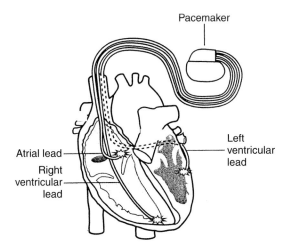

FIGURE 47-8 Biventricular pacemaker (cardiac resynchronization therapy). *(Courtesy Medtronic, Inc.)*

- Some pacemaker systems also include an internal cardioverter defibrillator (ICD) (see Procedure 46).
- Some pacemakers can be programmed to switch modes (e.g., DDD mode to VVI mode) to avoid pacing at the upper rate in patients who experience intermittent atrial dysrhythmias in which rapid atrial rates are generated. This is called *antitachycardia pacing*. There may be other programmed pacemaker interventions also to avoid tachycardias.
- Rate-responsive pacemakers include a sensor and are designed to mimic normal changes in heart rate based on physiologic needs. Most commonly, the sensor reacts to motion and vibration or respirations and initiates an appropriate change in the pacing rate, depending on the metabolic activity. These patients have a pacemaker rate range.
- Electromagnetic interference (EMI) may interfere with pacemaker function. Electrocautery, cardiac electroversion, magnetic resonance imaging (which is contraindicated for pacemaker patients), radiation, diathermy, and extracorporeal shock wave lithotripsy are examples of sources of EMI that may disrupt the pacemaker-initiated electrical circuit.

EQUIPMENT

- ECG monitor and recorder with paper
- ECG cables and electrodes
- Pacemaker magnet
- Pacemaker programmer appropriate for pacemaker make and model*

PATIENT AND FAMILY EDUCATION

- Assess learning needs, readiness to learn, and factors that would influence learning. ➥*Rationale:* This assessment allows the nurse to individualize teaching in a meaningful manner.

---

*Note that some situations may require notification of the device manufacturer to obtain the proper interrogation equipment. Manufacturer information can be found on the patient's pacemaker identification card.

- Provide information about the normal conduction system, such as structure of the conduction system, source of heart beat, normal and abnormal heart rhythms, and symptoms of abnormal heart rhythms. Patients with cardiomyopathy and heart failure require further information about ventricular dyssynchrony. ➥*Rationale:* Understanding of the normal conduction system and pumping function assists the patient and family in recognizing the seriousness of the patient's condition and the need for permanent pacemaker therapy.
- Provide information about permanent pacing, including the reason for pacing; explanation of the equipment; what to expect during permanent pacing; precautions and restrictions in activities of daily living; signs and symptoms of complications; instructions on when to call the physician, advanced practice nurse, or pacemaker clinic; and information on expected follow-up. ➥*Rationale:* Understanding of pacemaker functioning and expectations after discharge assists the patient and family in developing realistic perceptions of permanent pacing therapy. Information may improve cooperation with restrictions and promote effective lifestyle management after discharge.
- Provide information about required device follow-up, including clinic evaluation and transtelephonic monitoring. ➥*Rationale:* Periodic pacemaker checks are essential for routine device monitoring and evaluating any changes in patient condition related to the pacemaker.
- Provide patient registration and identification card. Encourage the patient to wear Medic Alert information and to carry identification card at all times, especially if the patient is admitted to the hospital. ➥*Rationale:* This reinforces the seriousness of the patients condition and ensures that appropriate identifying information is available to other health care providers, if needed.

PATIENT ASSESSMENT AND PREPARATION

Patient Assessment

- Identify the programmed mode of the pacemaker. ➥*Rationale:* Knowledge of how the pacemaker is intended to respond is necessary to detect appropriate and inappropriate function.
- Identify the reason for permanent pacemaker support. ➥*Rationale:* Knowledge of the clinical indication provides the nurse with baseline data when evaluating pacemaker function and patient response.
- Determine the patient's pacemaker history: date of insertion; last battery change; most recent pacemaker check; whether the patient has experienced any problems with the pacemaker or pacemaker site; and any unexpected symptoms, such as dizziness, chest pain, shortness of breath, palpitations, or activity intolerance. ➥*Rationale:* The pacemaker history provides information useful in determining any problems that might be occurring.

- Assess the patient's ECG for appropriate pacemaker function. ➼*Rationale:* Evidence of inappropriate function determines the need for further testing.
- Assess the patient's hemodynamic response to the paced rhythm. ➼*Rationale:* The patient's hemodynamic response indicates how effective the pacemaker is in maintaining an adequate cardiac output in response to the patient's physiologic needs. Evidence of adequate cardiac output is supported by systolic blood pressure greater than 90 mm Hg; mean arterial blood pressure greater than 60 mm Hg; no decrease in level of consciousness; and no complaints of fatigue, dizziness, shortness of breath, pallor, diaphoresis, or chest pain. Patients with biventricular pacemakers on long-term diuretics may overdiurese after pacemaker implantation due to improved circulation and hemodynamics; these patients need focused attention on signs and symptoms of dehydration.

Patient Preparation

- Ensure that the patient and family understand teaching. Answer questions as they arise, and reinforce information as needed. ➼*Rationale:* This communication evaluates and reinforces understanding of previously taught information.
- Assist the patient to a comfortable position. ➼*Rationale:* Proper positioning promotes patient comfort.

Procedure | for Assessing Function of Permanent Pacemaker

Steps	Rationale	Special Considerations
1. Wash hands with cleansing pads or soap and water.	Reduces the transmission of microorganisms; standard precautions.	
2. Inspect equipment for cracks or other abnormalities.	Prevents possible electrical hazard.	
3. Prepare skin with cleansing pads or soap and water for the application of ECG electrodes (see Procedure 54).	Proper skin preparation is essential to maintain appropriate skin-to-electrode contact.	It may be necessary to clip chest hair to ensure good skin contact with the electrode.
4. Attach the ECG leads to the electrodes, and place the electrodes on the patient's chest.	Attaching the leads to the electrodes first and then placing the electrodes on the chest produces less discomfort.	
5. Record a rhythm strip with and without a magnet placed over the pacemaker. To obtain a rhythm strip with the magnet, place the pacemaker magnet on top of the pacemaker generator, and record the rhythm strip, then remove the magnet.	The nonmagnet rhythm strip represents the patient's current status (intrinsic rhythm, paced rhythm, or a combination). A magnet placed over the pacemaker causes the pacemaker to pace at the preprogrammed parameters.	A single-lead rhythm strip showing visible P waves is adequate.[7] Lead II or MCL$_6$ generally provides the best P-wave morphology if ECG lead availability is limited. Follow hospital standards to ensure that a nurse can use the pacemaker magnet.
6. Assess the cardiac rhythm for the presence of pacemaker activity. *(Level I: Manufacturer's recommendations only.)*	Allows for determination of pacemaker function.	Prerequisite knowledge of pacemaker programmed settings is necessary to evaluate the pacemaker function adequately.
A. Identify atrial activity. Is the pacemaker programmed to detect atrial activity? Was the atrial activity sensed? What is the pacemaker programmed to do when atrial activity is sensed? If the pacemaker is programmed to trigger ventricular pacing with sensed atrial activity, is there a ventricular paced complex at the programmed AV interval? If not, is there an intrinsic QRS complex that occurred before the programmed AV interval?	Troubleshoots programming of the pacemaker and the electrical response of the atria and ventricles.	

<table>
<tr><td colspan="3">**Procedure** for Assessing Function of Permanent Pacemaker—*Continued*</td></tr>
<tr><td>Steps</td><td>Rationale</td><td>Special Considerations</td></tr>
</table>

Steps	Rationale	Special Considerations
B. If there is no intrinsic atrial activity present, determine whether the pacemaker is programmed to pace the atrium. If atrial pacing should be occurring, determine the lower rate limit at which the pacemaker stimulates atrial activity (a paced atrial event should occur at the end of a ventricular-atrial interval). Evaluate whether the pacemaker is firing at this rate.	Troubleshoots programming of the pacemaker and atrial response.	If a pacemaker spike is present, but evidence of atrial capture is not present, attempt to assess the presence of atrial contraction by: (1) Looking for the "a" wave in the central venous pressure (or right atrial pressure) waveform (if available). (2) Changing the ECG lead. (3) Listening to the heart sounds (S_1 becomes softer in the absence of atrial contraction because left ventricular contractility affects the loudness of S_1).[3]
C. Look for ventricular activity. Is the pacemaker programmed to detect intrinsic activity? Is it sensed appropriately? What is the pacemaker programmed to do when ventricular activity is sensed? Does inhibition of ventricular pacing occur?	Determines the presence of ventricular activity and response to pacemaker actions.	Failure of ventricular capture can be a life-threatening situation. With biventricular pacing, the loss of capture in one ventricle may be seen only by a change in the patient's condition or a change in the QRS width or appearance.
D. If there is no intrinsic ventricular activity, determine whether the pacemaker is programmed to pace the ventricles. If pacing should occur, identify the lower rate limit, and determine whether ventricular pacing spikes are occurring at this rate. If ventricular pacing spikes are occurring at intervals that are longer than the lower rate limit, evaluate for oversensing of unwanted signals. If ventricular pacing spikes are occurring at intervals that are shorter than the lower rate limit, is the pacemaker in a rate-responsive mode? Is there hidden atrial activity that is triggering a ventricular output? Is there atrial oversensing? Determine whether each ventricular pacing spike is followed by a QRS complex. If the pacemaker has an upper rate limit, determine whether the patient is being paced appropriately when that limit has been reached.	Troubleshoots the relationship between pacemaker programming and ventricular response.	Look for the presence of P waves in the T wave.
E. If antitachycardia pacing is programmed, determine whether the tachycardia detection criterion has been met and if the pacemaker intervened appropriately.	Determines appropriate pacemaker function.	
F. If the patient has a biventricular pacemaker, verify that the patient is consistently being paced in the ventricles. The ventricles should always be paced.	The purpose of biventricular pacing is to pace both ventricles simultaneously to restore ventricular synchrony. If the patient is not consistently being paced in the ventricles, the system is not working properly.	Detailed interrogation of function is required because a basic rhythm strip does not provide enough information to assess proper function adequately. Figure 47-9 illustrates various aspects of biventricular pacing.

Procedure continues on the following page

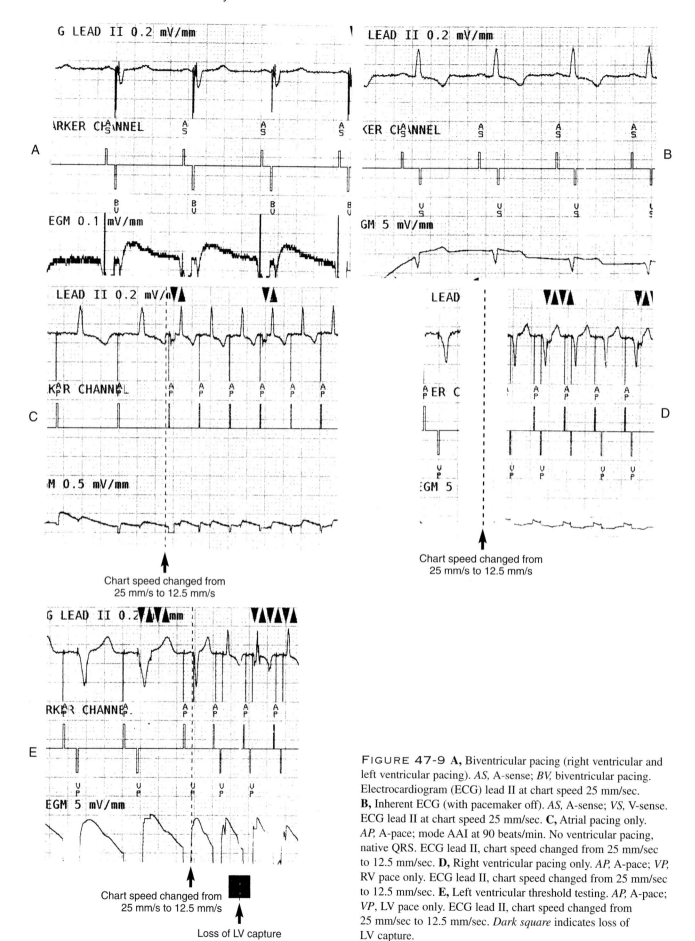

FIGURE 47-9 **A,** Biventricular pacing (right ventricular and left ventricular pacing). *AS,* A-sense; *BV,* biventricular pacing. Electrocardiogram (ECG) lead II at chart speed 25 mm/sec. **B,** Inherent ECG (with pacemaker off). *AS,* A-sense; *VS,* V-sense. ECG lead II at chart speed 25 mm/sec. **C,** Atrial pacing only. *AP,* A-pace; mode AAI at 90 beats/min. No ventricular pacing, native QRS. ECG lead II, chart speed changed from 25 mm/sec to 12.5 mm/sec. **D,** Right ventricular pacing only. *AP,* A-pace; *VP,* RV pace only. ECG lead II, chart speed changed from 25 mm/sec to 12.5 mm/sec. **E,** Left ventricular threshold testing. *AP,* A-pace; *VP,* LV pace only. ECG lead II, chart speed changed from 25 mm/sec to 12.5 mm/sec. *Dark square* indicates loss of LV capture.

Procedure for Assessing Function of Permanent Pacemaker—*Continued*

Steps	Rationale	Special Considerations
7. Assess the patient's hemodynamic response.	It is possible for the patient to have the electrical activity of pacing occurring without the associated mechanical activity of cardiac contraction (pulseless electrical activity).	
8. If inappropriate pacemaker function is detected, notify the physician immediately and implement basic life support/ACLS as needed.	Inappropriate pacemaker function may compromise cardiac output and require immediate adjustment of settings or replacement of malfunctioning components.	
9. Determine the method (transtelephonic monitoring, clinic evaluation) and frequency needed for long-term follow-up of the patient and the device. *(Level II: Theory based, no research data to support recommendations: recommendations from expert consensus group may exist.)*	Regular follow-up is required to assess device parameters and patient tolerance of the device. Transtelephonic monitoring is not recommended for patients with biventricular pacemakers.	Several groups have published guidelines for pacemaker follow-up.[1,4,6]

Expected Outcomes

- Hemodynamically congruent heart rate, proper sensing, and capture shown on the ECG
- Adequate systemic tissue perfusion and cardiac output as evidenced by systolic blood pressure greater than 90 mm Hg; mean arterial blood pressure greater than 60 mm Hg; patient being alert and oriented; and no complaints of dizziness, shortness of breath, nausea, or vomiting because of hypotension or ischemic chest pain
- Absence of hemodynamically significant dysrhythmias

Unexpected Outcomes

- Failure to sense with the possibility of R-on-T phenomenon (initiation of ventricular tachycardia/fibrillation as a result of an improperly timed pacer spike) (this is very rare)
- Oversensing
- Failure to capture (with biventricular pacing the loss of capture in one ventricle may be seen only by a change in patient's condition or a change in the QRS width or appearance)
- Pacemaker-mediated tachycardia: caused when a ventricular paced beat results in retrograde AV nodal conduction and produces a premature P wave. If the premature P wave is sensed, a ventricular output follows, setting up an endless-loop tachycardia[4]; this is often seen with long AV delays or short post–ventricular atrial refractory period. Immediate treatment for this is application of a magnet
- Pacemaker syndrome results from loss of AV synchrony with VVI and nonatrial tracking modes. Symptoms the patient may experience include chest pain, fatigue, dyspnea, palpitations, and a sensation of "heart in throat"
- Diaphragmatic stimulation
- Pacing at an inappropriate rate
- Infection at the site
- Battery end-of life
- Lead fracture (may be suspected with intermittent pacing; an overpenetrated chest x-ray film helps to detect this)

Patient Monitoring and Care

Steps	Rationale	Reportable Conditions
		These conditions should be reported if they persist despite nursing interventions.
1. Monitor the ECG continuously for the presence of a cardiac rate and rhythm that is consistent with the programmed parameters.	Indicates ongoing functioning of the permanent pacemaker.	• Failure of the pacemaker to perform as programmed • Undersensing • Oversensing
2. Evaluate the hemodynamic response to pacemaker therapy.	Provides ongoing assessment of the patient's physiologic response to pacing.	• Deterioration of the patient's condition as evidenced by change in vital signs, hemodynamic parameters, mental status, activity tolerance
3. Assess the insertion site for evidence of manipulation or signs of erosion.	Patient manipulation at the site may affect pacemaker therapy. "Twiddler's" syndrome has been noted to cause lead dislodgment or fracture with resultant loss of pacemaker function.[1]	• Evidence of pacemaker manipulation
4. Monitor for signs and symptoms of infection.	Placement of an invasive device may result in infection.	• Signs or symptoms of local or systemic infection • Pacemaker erosion through the skin

Documentation

Documentation should include the following:

- Device indications and device type
- Patient education and evaluation of patient and family understanding
- Programmed parameters
- ECG rhythm strip recording (with and without magnet)

- Evaluation of pacemaker function
- Physical assessment, including vital signs and hemodynamic response
- Unexpected outcomes
- Interventions required and evaluation of interventions

References

1. Bernstein, A.D., et al. (1994). Report of the NASPE Policy Conference on antibradycardia pacemaker follow-up: Effectiveness, needs, and resources. *Pacing Clin Electrophysiol,* 17, 1714-29.
2. Bernstein, A.D., et al. (1993). NASPE policy statement: The NASPE/BPED defibrillator code. *Pacing Clin Electrophysiol,* 16, 1776-80.
3. Constant, J. (1999). *Bedside Cardiology.* 5th ed. Philadelphia: Lippincott Williams & Wilkins.
4. Fraser, J.D., et al. (2000). Guidelines for pacemaker follow-up in Canada: A consensus statement of the Canadian Working Group on Cardiac Pacing. *Can J Cardiol,* 16, 355-76.
5. Gregoratos, G., et al. (2002). ACC/AHA/NASPE 2002 guideline update for implantation of cardiac pacemakers and antiarrhythmia devices: Summary report. A report of the American College of Cardiology/American Heart Association Task Force on Practice Guidelines (ACC/AHA/NASPE) Committee to update the 1998 pacemaker guidelines. *J Am Coll Cardiol,* 40, 1703-19.
6. *Medicare Coverage Issues Manual.* (1990). Baltimore: U.S. Department of Health and Human Services, Health Care Financing Administration. HCFA publication 6 Thur Rev. 42.
7. Moses, H.W., et al. (1995). *A Practical Guide to Cardiac Pacing.* Boston: Little, Brown, 171-97.

Additional Readings

Abraham, W.T., et al, for the MIRACLE Study Group. (2002). Cardiac resynchronization in chronic heart failure. *N Engl J Med,* 346, 1845-53.
Barbiere, C.C., and Liberatore, K. (1993). From emergent transvenous pacemaker to permanent implant. *Crit Care Nurse,* 13, 39-44.
Busch, M.M., and Haskin, J.B. (1995). Pacemakers and implantable defibrillators. In: Woods, S.L., et al, editors. *Cardiac Nursing.* 3rd ed. Philadelphia: J.B. Lippincott, 618-61.
Gura, M.T., et al. (2003). North American Society of Pacing Electrophysiology: Standards of professional practice for the allied professional in pacing and electrophysiology. *Pacing Clin Electrophysiol,* 26, 127-31.
Hesselson, A.B. (2003). *Simplified Interpretation of Pacemaker ECGs.* Baltimore: Futura/Blackwell Publications.
Morton, P.G. (1997). The pacemaker and defibrillator codes: Implications for critical care nursing. *Crit Care Nurse,* 17, 50-9.
Platt, S., et al. (1996). Transtelephone monitoring for pacemaker follow-up 1981-1994. *Pacing Clin Electrophysiol,* 19(12 Part 1), 2089-98.
Van Orden Wallace, C.J. (1998). Dual-chamber pacemakers in the management of severe heart failure. *Crit Care Nurse,* 18, 57-67.
Vardas, P.E. (1998). *Cardiac Arrhythmias, Pacing and Electrophysiology.* Boston: Kluwer Academic.
Witherall, C.L. (1994). Cardiac rhythm control devices. *Crit Care Nurs Clin North Am,* 6, 85-101.

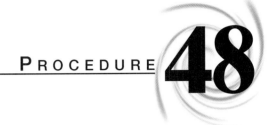

PROCEDURE **48**

Temporary Transcutaneous (External) Pacing

P U R P O S E :   Transcutaneous or external pacing stimulates myocardial depolarization through the chest wall. External pacing is used as a temporary measure when normal cardiac conduction fails to produce myocardial contraction and the patient experiences hemodynamic instability.

Eileen M. Kelly

PREREQUISITE NURSING KNOWLEDGE

- Knowledge of cardiac anatomy and physiology is required.
- Knowledge of cardiac monitoring (see Procedure 54) is necessary.
- Ability to interpret basic dysrhythmias is needed.
- Knowledge of temporary pacemaker function and expected patient responses to pacemaker therapy is needed.
- Clinical and technical competence in the use of the external pacing equipment is required.
- Indications for transcutaneous pacing are as follows:[1]
  - ❖ Asystole, must be performed immediately and combined with medication therapy
  - ❖ Symptomatic bradycardia unresponsive to atropine
  - ❖ Bradycardia with ventricular escape rhythm
  - ❖ Profound bradycardia or pulseless electrical activity due to drug overdose, acidosis, or electrolyte abnormalities
  - ❖ In stand-by mode for the following rhythms in acute myocardial infarction setting:
    - ○ Symptomatic sinus node dysfunction
    - ○ Mobitz type II second-degree heart block
    - ○ Third-degree heart block
    - ○ Newly acquired left, right, or alternating bundle-branch block or bifascicular block
- Temporary transvenous pacing is indicated when prolonged pacing is needed.
- Contraindications for transcutaneous pacing are as follows:[1]
  - ❖ Severe hypothermia
  - ❖ Bradyasystolic cardiac arrest of greater than 20 minutes duration
- External cardiac pacing is a temporary method of stimulating ventricular myocardial depolarization through the

chest wall via two large pacing electrodes. The electrodes are placed on the anterior and posterior chest wall and are attached by a cable to an external pulse generator. The external pulse generator (Fig. 48-1) delivers energy (milliamps) to the myocardium based on the set pacing rate, output, and sensitivity. Some models of external pulse generators are combined with an external defibrillator, and the electrodes of these models may be used for pacing and defibrillation.

- *Sensitivity* refers to the ability of the pacemaker to detect intrinsic myocardial activity. Sensitivity is set in a fixed or demand mode. In the fixed or asynchronous mode, pacing occurs at the set rate regardless of the patient's

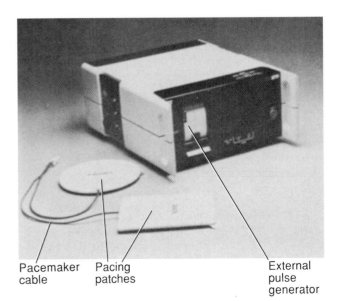

Pacemaker cable

Pacing patches

External pulse generator

FIGURE 48-1 Temporary transcutaneous (external) pacemaker. *(From Zoll Medical Corporation, Burlington, MA.)*

intrinsic rate. In the demand or synchronous mode, the pacemaker senses intrinsic myocardial activity and paces when the intrinsic cardiac rate is lower than the set rate on the external pulse generator.

- *Pacing* occurs when the external pulse generator delivers enough energy through the pacing patches to the myocardium. This is known as pacemaker *firing* and is represented as a *spike* on the electrocardiogram (ECG) tracing (Fig. 48-2).
- *Capture* occurs when the pacemaker delivers enough energy to the myocardium so that depolarization occurs. It is seen on the ECG by a pacemaker spike followed by a ventricular complex. The ventricular complex occurs after the pacemaker spike, and the QRS is wide with the initial and terminal deflections in opposite directions. (In Figure 48-2, complexes 2 and 3 begin with a downward [negative] deflection and end with an upward [positive] direction).
- *Standby pacing* is when the pacing electrodes are applied in anticipation of possible use, but pacing is not needed at the time.
- Pacing is contraindicated in severe hypothermia because cold ventricles are more prone to ventricular fibrillation and are more resistant to defibrillation. Pacing is a relative contraindication in bradyasystolic cardiac arrest of greater than 20 minutes duration because of the poor resuscitation rate for these patients and the high probability that patients who do survive will have profound brain damage.

EQUIPMENT

- Blood pressure monitoring equipment
- External pulse generator
- Pacing cable
- Pacemaker electrodes
- ECG electrodes
- ECG monitor
- ECG cable

  Additional equipment to have available as needed includes the following:
- Emergency cart with medications and other equipment
- Scissors

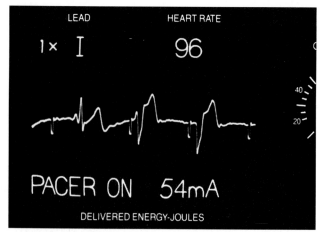

FIGURE 48-2 ECG tracing of external pacing. *ECG,* electrocardiogram. *(From Zoll Medical Corporation, Burlington, MA.)*

PATIENT AND FAMILY EDUCATION

- Assess learning needs, readiness to learn, and factors that influence learning. ➤*Rationale:* This assessment reveals the patient and family's knowledge so that teaching can be individualized to be meaningful to the patient and family.
- Discuss basic facts about the normal conduction system, the reason external cardiac pacing is indicated, and what happens to the patient when pacing occurs. ➤*Rationale:* This discussion assists the patient and family in recognizing the need for external pacing and what to expect when pacing occurs.
- Discuss interventions to alleviate discomfort. ➤*Rationale:* This discussion provides the patient with an opportunity to validate perceptions. It gives the patient and family knowledge that interventions are used to minimize the level of discomfort.
- If indicated, inform patient and family of the possibility of the need for transvenous or permanent pacing support. ➤*Rationale:* This prepares the patient and family for the possibility of additional therapy. If permanent pacing is required, the patient and family would need further instruction about possible lifestyle modifications and follow-up visits and information about the pacemaker to be implanted.

PATIENT ASSESSMENT AND PREPARATION

Patient Assessment

- Maintain bedside ECG monitoring. ➤*Rationale:* External pacing units do not provide central monitoring or dysrhythmia detection.
- Assess the patient's cardiac rhythm for the presence of dysrhythmias that indicate the need for external cardiac pacing. ➤*Rationale:* Recognition of a dysrhythmia is the first step in determining the need for external cardiac pacing or placing the external pacemaker on stand-by.
- Determine the patient's hemodynamic response to the dysrhythmia, such as presence of pulse; systolic blood pressure less than 90 mm Hg; altered level of consciousness; dizziness; shortness of breath; nausea and vomiting; cool, clammy, diaphoretic skin; or the development of chest pain. ➤*Rationale:* The decision to initiate pacing depends on the effect of the dysrhythmia on the patient's cardiac output.

Patient Preparation

- Ensure that the patient and family understand preprocedural teaching. Answer questions as they arise, and reinforce information as needed. ➤*Rationale:* This communication evaluates and reinforces understanding of previously taught information.
- Administer sedative or analgesic medication to a conscious patient before initiating pacing. ➤*Rationale:* External cardiac pacing is uncomfortable.

Procedure for Temporary Transcutaneous (External) Pacing

Steps	Rationale	Special Considerations
1. Wash hands.	Reduces the transmission of microorganisms; standard precautions.	
2. Administer sedation or analgesic to conscious patient.	Decreases discomfort associated with external cardiac pacing.	Not indicated for patients who are unconscious and hemodynamically unstable. Not indicated for stand-by because pacing may not be needed.
3. Turn on the pulse generator and monitor.	Ensures that the equipment is functional.	Many devices work on battery or alternating current (AC) power.
4. Prepare the skin on the patient's chest and back by washing with nonemollient soap and water. Dry thoroughly. Trim body hair with scissors, if necessary.	Removal of skin oils, lotion, and moisture improves electrode adherence and maximizes delivery of energy through the chest wall.	Optional step in an emergency. Avoid use of flammable liquids to prepare the skin (e.g., alcohol, benzoin) because of increased potential for burns. Avoid shaving chest hair because the presence of nicks in the skin under the pacing patches can increase patient discomfort.
5. Apply the ECG electrodes to the ECG leads. Connect the ECG cable to the monitor inlet of the pulse generator. Apply the ECG electrodes to the patient (see Procedure 54).	Displays the patient's intrinsic rhythm on the monitor.	Attachment of the ECG electrodes to the ECG leads and the ECG cable to the monitor is optional in an emergency. The pacemaker electrodes display the rhythm on the monitor.
6. Adjust the ECG lead and size to the maximum R wave size.	Detection of the intrinsic rhythm is necessary for proper demand pacing.	Lead II usually provides the most prominent R wave.
7. Apply the back (posterior, +) pacing electrode between the spine and left scapula at the level of the heart (Fig. 48-3).	Placement of the pacing patches in the recommended anatomic location enhances the potential for successful pacing.	Avoid placement over bone because this increases the level of energy required to pace, increases patient discomfort, and increases the possibility of noncapture.

Procedure continues on the following page

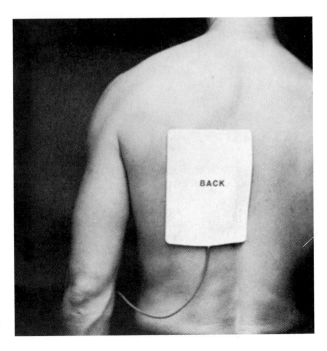

FIGURE 48-3 Location of the posterior (back) pacing electrode. *(From Zoll Medical Corporation, Burlington, MA.)*

Procedure | **for Temporary Transcutaneous (External) Pacing**—*Continued*

Steps	Rationale	Special Considerations
8. Apply the front (anterior, –) pacing electrode at the left, fourth intercostal space, midclavicular line (Fig. 48-4).	Placement of the pacing patches in the recommended anatomic location enhances the potential for successful pacing.	For women, adjust the position of the electrode below and lateral to breast tissue to ensure optimal patch adherence. Avoid placement of the pacing electrodes over the beside monitor ECG electrodes and permanently placed devices, such as implantable cardioverter-defibrillators or permanent pacemakers.
9. If the patient is hemodynamically unstable, the back (posterior) electrode may be placed over the patient's right sternal area at the second or third intercostal space. The front (anterior) electrode is maintained at the apex (fourth or fifth intercostal space, midclavicular line).	Facilitates ease of electrode placement for emergent pacing.	Pacing may be less effective with this method of electrode placement.
10. Connect the pacing electrodes to the pacemaker cable and connect to the external pulse generator.	Necessary for the delivery of electrical energy.	
11. Set the pacemaker rate, level of energy (output, mA), and mode (Fig. 48-5). A. For asystole, set to the highest mA, turn the mA down until there is no capture, and set the mA 20 mA above that number.	Each patient may require different pacemaker settings to provide safe and effective external pacing. Pacing should be maintained at a rate that maintains adequate cardiac output but does not induce ischemia.	Follow hospital standards to ensure that a nurse can initiate external cardiac pacing. Attempt to use the lowest level of energy necessary to pace consistently; the average adult usually can be paced with a current of 40-70 mA.

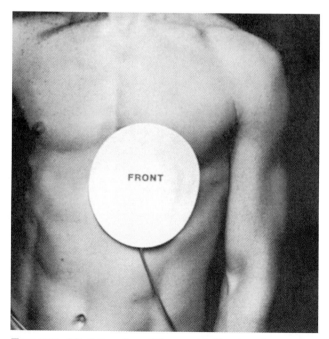

FIGURE 48-4 Location of the anterior (front) pacing electrode.

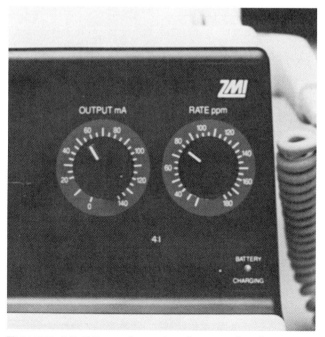

FIGURE 48-5 Pacemaker settings for external pacing. *(From Zoll Medical Corporation, Burlington, MA.)*

Procedure for Temporary Transcutaneous (External) Pacing—*Continued*

Steps	Rationale	Special Considerations
B. For bradydysrhythmias, start at the lowest mA and dial up until capture is present. Set the mA 20 mA above that number.	The demand mode is used to prevent competition from the patient's intrinsic rhythm.	In the fixed mode, the pacemaker fires regardless of the intrinsic rhythm and rate. If firing occurs on the T wave (repolarization), ventricular tachycardia or ventricular fibrillation can occur.
12. Initiate pacing by slowly increasing the energy level (mA) delivered until consistent capture occurs at the prescribed rate.	Use the lowest amount of energy that consistently results in myocardial capture and contraction to minimize discomfort.	
13. When the pacemaker fires, observe that each pacemaker spike is followed by a ventricular complex (complexes 2 and 3 in Fig. 48-2).	Documents adequate functioning of the pacemaker.	If a pacemaker spike occurs and is not followed by a ventricular complex, increase the energy (mA) level. Artifact from muscle twitching may make an ECG tracing difficult to interpret.
14. Palpate the patient's femoral pulse. Do not palpate the carotid pulse because the electrical stimulation from the pacemaker may mimic a pulse.	Ensures adequate blood flow with paced complexes.	It is possible to have electrical activity without associated mechanical contraction.
15. Evaluate the patient's hemodynamic response to pacing.	Hemodynamic response should improve with pacing.	Acidosis and electrolyte abnormalities need to be corrected for an effective response to pacing.
16. Evaluate the patient's response to the initial dose of sedative or analgesic.	Pacing may not be tolerated by the patient.	Administer additional sedatives or analgesics as needed.
17. Discard used supplies, and wash hands.	Reduces the transmission of microorganisms; standard precautions.	

Expected Outcomes	Unexpected Outcomes
• Adequate systemic tissue perfusion and cardiac output as evidenced by blood pressure greater than 90 mm Hg systolic, alert and oriented patient, absence of dizziness or syncope, absence of shortness of breath, absence of nausea and vomiting, and absence of ischemic chest pain • Stable cardiac rhythm • Adequate functioning of the pacemaker	• Failure of the pacemaker to sense the patient's underlying rhythm with the possibility of R-on-T phenomenon (initiation of ventricular tachydysrhythmias as a result of an improperly timed spike on the T wave) • Failure of the pacemaker to capture the myocardium • Failure of the pacemaker to pace • Discomfort, including skin burns from the delivery of high levels of energy through the chest wall, painful sensations, and skeletal muscle twitching

Patient Monitoring and Care

Steps	Rationale	Reportable Conditions
		These conditions should be reported if they persist despite nursing interventions. • Change in vital signs • Hemodynamic deterioration
1. Monitor vital signs hourly and as needed.	Ensures adequate tissue perfusion with paced beats. Adjustments in pacing rate may need to be made based on vital signs.	
2. Monitor level of comfort: A. Assess level of comfort. B. Administer analgesic or sedative as needed. C. Adjust level of energy to the lowest level for capture. D. Evaluate the patient's response to interventions.	External delivery of energy through the chest wall may cause varying degrees of discomfort.	• Pain unrelieved by prescribed medications or interventions • Patient intolerant of the prescribed medications (e.g., severe nausea, hypotension, decreased respirations)
3. Obtain an ECG recording strip to document pacing function every 4-8 hours and as needed.	Documents cardiac rhythm and pacemaker activity.	
4. Evaluate pacemaker function (capturing and sensing) with any change in patient condition or vital signs.	Ensures continued functioning of the pacemaker. Introduction of other variables, such as electrolyte imbalance or metabolic changes, may alter the level of energy required to pace effectively.	• Inability to maintain appropriate sensing and capture • Changes in patient condition that affect appropriate pacemaker function
5. Monitor the patient's cardiac rhythm for resolution of the dysrhythmia requiring pacemaker intervention. This may require turning the pacemaker off to assess the underlying rhythm. *Do not turn the pacemaker off if the patient is 100% paced.*	Indicates if the dysrhythmia has subsided.	• Worsening of the baseline cardiac rhythm (e.g., change from symptomatic second-degree heart block to complete heart block)
6. Evaluate the patient's hemodynamic response to pacing by comparison to the baseline.	Evaluates the patient's physiologic response to pacing and ensures that it is optimal.	• Hemodynamic changes
7. If pacing is not occurring, assess the skin integrity under the pacing electrodes. If the pacemaker is on stand-by, check the adherence of the pacing electrodes to the skin at least every 4 hours. Change the electrodes at least every 24 hours.	Changes in skin integrity caused by burns or skin breaks significantly alters the patient's level of comfort and exposes the patient to possible infection.	• Changes in skin integrity

Documentation

Documentation should include the following:

- Patient and family education
- Patient preparation
- Date and time external cardiac pacing is initiated
- Description of events warranting intervention
- Vital signs and physical assessment before and after external cardiac pacing
- ECG recordings before and after pacing

- Patient comfort level and related interventions
- Medications administered
- Pacing rate, mode, mA
- Percentage of the time the patient is paced if in the demand mode
- Status of skin integrity when the pacing electrodes are changed
- Unexpected outcomes
- Additional interventions

Reference

1. Cummins, R.O. (2001). Bradycardias. In: *ACLS Provider Manual*. Dallas: American Heart Association, 145-52.

Additional Readings

Doukky, R., et al. (2003). Using transcutaneous cardiac pacing to best advantage: How to ensure successful capture and avoid complications. *J Crit Illness*, 5, 219-25.

Waggoner, P.C. (1991). Transcutaneous cardiac pacing. *AACN Clin Issues Crit Care Nurs*, 2, 118-25.

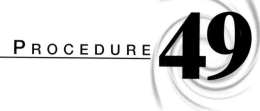

PROCEDURE **49**

Temporary Transvenous Pacemaker Insertion (Perform)

P U R P O S E :   The purpose of temporary cardiac pacing is to ensure or restore an adequate heart rate and rhythm. A transvenous pacemaker is inserted as a temporary measure when the normal conduction system of the heart fails to produce or conduct an electrical impulse, resulting in hemodynamic compromise or other debilitating symptoms in the patient.

Deborah E. Becker

PREREQUISITE NURSING KNOWLEDGE

- Knowledge of the normal anatomy and physiology of the cardiovascular system, principles of cardiac conduction, and basic and advanced dysrhythmia interpretation is required.
- Knowledge of temporary pacemaker function and expected patient responses to pacemaker therapy is necessary.
- Clinical and technical competence in central line insertion, temporary transvenous pacemaker insertion, and suturing is needed.
- Clinical and technical competence related to use of temporary pacemakers is necessary.
- Competence in chest x-ray interpretation is required.
- Advanced cardiac life support knowledge and skills are needed.
- Principles of general electrical safety apply when using temporary invasive pacing methods. Gloves always should be worn when handling electrodes to prevent microshock.

- The insertion of a temporary pacemaker is performed in emergency and elective clinical situations. Temporary pacing may be used to:
  - Stimulate the myocardium to contract in the absence of an intrinsic rhythm
  - Establish adequate cardiac output and blood pressure
  - Ensure tissue perfusion to vital organs
  - Reduce the possibility of ventricular dysrhythmias in the presence of bradycardia
  - Supplement an inadequate rhythm, such as when transient decreases in heart rate occur (e.g., chronotropic incompetence in shock)
  - Allow the administration of medications that may cause a rhythm or conduction abnormality (e.g., β-blockers) when treating ischemia or other dysrhythmias
- Temporary transvenous pacing is indicated for the following:
  - Third-degree atrioventricular (AV) block (symptomatic congenital complete heart block, symptomatic acquired complete heart block)
  - Type II AV block
  - Dysrhythmias complicating acute myocardial infarction (symptomatic bradycardia, complete heart block, new bundle-branch block with transient complete heart block, alternating bundle-branch block)
  - Sinus node dysfunction (symptomatic bradydysrhythmias, treatment of bradycardia-tachycardia syndromes or sick sinus syndrome).

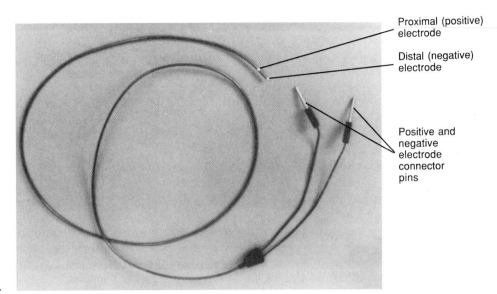

F I G U R E 49-1 Bipolar lead wire.

- ❖ Ventricular standstill or cardiac arrest
- ❖ Long Q-T syndrome with ventricular dysrhythmias
- ❖ Drug toxicity
- ❖ Postoperative cardiac surgery
- ❖ Prophylaxis with cardiac diagnostic or interventional procedures
- ❖ Chronotropic incompetence in the setting of cardiogenic shock
- When temporary transvenous pacing is used, the pulse generator is attached externally to a pacing lead wire that is inserted through a vein into the right atrium or right ventricle.
- Veins used for the insertion of a transvenous pacing lead wire are the subclavian, femoral, brachial, internal jugular, or external jugular.
- Single-chamber ventricular pacing is the most appropriate method in an emergency because the goal is to establish a heart rate as quickly as possible.
- The transvenous pacing lead is an insulated wire with one or two electrodes at the tip of the wire (Fig. 49-1).
- The pacing lead can be a hard-tipped or a balloon-tipped pacing catheter that is placed in direct contact with the myocardium. Most temporary leads are bipolar with the distal tip electrode (seen as a metal ring) separated from the proximal electrode by 1 to 2 cm of pacing catheter (also seen as a metal ring) (see Fig. 49-1).
- Basic principles of cardiac pacing include sensing, pacing, and capture.
  - ❖ *Sensing* refers to the ability of the pacemaker device to detect intrinsic myocardial electrical activity. Sensing occurs if the pulse generator is in the synchronous or demand mode. The pacemaker either is inhibited from delivering a stimulus or initiates an electrical impulse.

- ❖ *Pacing* occurs when the temporary pulse generator is activated and the programmed level of energy travels from the pulse generator through the temporary pacing lead wire to the myocardium. This is known as pacemaker *firing* and is represented as a "line" or "spike" on the electrocardiogram (ECG) recording.
- ❖ *Capture* refers to the successful conduction of the pacemaker impulse through the myocardium, resulting in depolarization. It is evidenced on the ECG by a pacemaker spike followed by either an atrial or a ventricular complex, depending on the chamber being paced. The health care provider can assess whether the electrical depolarization resulted in mechanical activity by observing the right atrial pressure, central venous pressure, left atrial pressure, or pulmonary artery or arterial line waveforms or if the ventricle is paced, by palpating a pulse.
- Temporary pulse generator features include the following:
  - ❖ The temporary pulse generator houses the controls and the energy source for pacing.
  - ❖ Pulse generators can be used for single-chamber pacing with one set of terminals at the top of the pulse generator, into which the pacing wires are inserted (via connecting cable).
  - ❖ A dual-chamber pacemaker requires two sets of terminals, one each for the atrial and ventricular wires.
  - ❖ Different models of pacemakers use either dials or touch pads to change the settings.
  - ❖ The pacing rate is determined by the rate set by the dial or rate pad.
  - ❖ The AV interval dial or pad on a dual-chamber pacemaker controls the amount of time between atrial and ventricular stimulation (electronic P-R interval).
  - ❖ The energy delivered to the myocardium is determined by setting the output (milliamperage [mA]) dial or pad on the pulse generator.
  - ❖ Dual-chamber pacing requires that mAs are set for the atria and the ventricle.

• The ability of the pacemaker to detect the patient's intrinsic rhythm is determined by the pacing mode. In the asynchronous mode, the pacemaker functions as a fixed-rate pacemaker and is not able to sense any of the patient's inherent cardiac activity. In the synchronous mode, the pacemaker is able to sense the patient's inherent cardiac activity.

• The ability of the pacemaker to depolarize the myocardium depends on many variables: position of the electrode and degree of contact with viable myocardial tissue; level of energy delivered through the pacing wire; presence of hypoxia, acidosis, or electrolyte imbalances; fibrosis around the tip of the catheter; and concomitant medication therapy.[2]

• It is important to ensure that all electrical equipment in the patient's room is properly grounded to prevent interference from occurring.

EQUIPMENT

• Antiseptic skin preparation solution (e.g., 2% chlorhexidine–based solution)
• Local anesthetic
• Sterile drapes, towels, masks, goggles or face shields, gowns, gloves, and dressings
• Balloon-tipped pacing catheter and insertion tray
• Pacing lead wire
• Pulse generator
• 9-volt battery for pulse generator
• Connecting cable
• Percutaneous introducer needle or 14-gauge needle
• Introducer sheath with dilator
• Guidewire (per physician or advanced practice nurse choice)
• Alligator clips or wire with connecting pins
• Suture with needle, syringes, needles
• ECG monitor and recorder
• Supplies for dressing at insertion site
  Additional equipment as needed includes the following:
• Emergency equipment
• Fluoroscopy
• Lead aprons or sheets
• 12-lead ECG machine

PATIENT AND FAMILY EDUCATION

• Assess learning needs, readiness to learn, and factors that influence learning. ➠*Rationale:* This assessment enables teaching to be individualized in a manner that is meaningful to the patient and the family.

• Discuss basic facts about the normal conduction system, such as structure and function of the conduction system, normal and abnormal heart rhythms, and symptoms and significance of abnormal heart rhythms. ➠*Rationale:* The patient and family should understand the conduction system and why the procedure is necessary and what potential risks and benefits are associated with undergoing this invasive procedure.

• Provide a basic description of the temporary pacemaker insertion procedure. ➠*Rationale:* The patient and family

should be informed of the invasive nature of the procedure and any risks associated with the procedure. An understanding of the procedure may reduce anxiety associated with the procedure.

• Describe the precautions and restrictions required while the temporary pacemaker is in place, such as limitation of movement, avoiding handling the pacemaker or touching exposed portions of the electrode, and situations in which the nurse should be notified (e.g., if the dressing becomes damp, if the patient experiences dizziness). ➠*Rationale:* Understanding potential limitations may improve the patient's cooperation with restrictions and precautions.

• Discuss with the patient and family the alternatives to this therapy. ➠*Rationale:* The patient and family have the right to know their alternatives to make an informed decision.

• Explain who will be performing the procedure. ➠*Rationale:* Understanding who is performing the procedure may assist in developing trust in the value of having the procedure performed.

PATIENT ASSESSMENT AND PREPARATION

Patient Assessment

• Assess the patient's cardiac rhythm for the presence of the dysrhythmia that necessitates the placement of temporary cardiac pacing. ➠*Rationale:* This assessment determines the need for invasive cardiac pacing.

• Assess the patient's hemodynamic response to the dysrhythmia. Rhythm disturbances may reduce cardiac output significantly, with detrimental effects on perfusion of vital organs. ➠*Rationale:* This assessment determines the urgency of the procedure. It may indicate the need for temporizing measures (e.g., vasopressors or transcutaneous pacing).

• Review current medications. ➠*Rationale:* Medications may be implicated as a cause of the dysrhythmia that led to the need for pacemaker therapy, or medications may need to be held as a result of concomitant effect. Other medications, such as antidysrhythmics, may alter the pacing threshold.

• Review the patient's current laboratory studies, including chemistry, electrolyte profile, arterial blood gases, coagulation profile, platelet count, and cardioactive medication levels. ➠*Rationale:* This review assists in determining if inserting the pacemaker was precipitated by metabolic disturbances or medication toxicity and establishes the pacing milieu. The review provides the health care provider with information regarding the risk for abnormal bleeding during or after the procedure is performed.

• Assess the presence and position of the central venous access (if present). ➠*Rationale:* The temporary transvenous pacing catheter is advanced through the central venous circulation. If access already is established, it is necessary to ensure proper placement before the pacing catheter can be advanced through the circulatory system.

Patient Preparation

- Ensure that the patient and the family understand preprocedural teaching. Answer questions as they arise, and reinforce information as needed. ➤*Rationale:* This communication evaluates and reinforces understanding of previously taught information.
- Obtain informed consent. ➤*Rationale:* Obtaining informed consent protects the rights of the patient and makes a competent decision possible for the patient; however, under emergency circumstances, time may not allow a consent form to be signed.

- Connect the patient to a 5-lead monitoring system or to a 12-lead ECG machine. ➤*Rationale:* This facilitates the placement of the balloon-tipped catheter by indicating the position of the catheter during its placement. Also, it allows for monitoring of the patient's cardiac rhythm during the procedure.
- Prescribe and ensure that pain medication or sedation is administered. ➤*Rationale:* Medication may be indicated depending on the patient's level of anxiety and pain. Sedation or pain medication may not be possible if the patient is hemodynamically unstable.

Procedure for Performing Temporary Transvenous Pacemaker Insertion

Steps	Rationale	Special Considerations
1. Wash hands.	Reduces the transmission of microorganisms; standard precautions.	
2. Connect the patient to the bedside monitoring system, and monitor ECG continuously (see Procedure 54).	Monitors intrinsic heart rate and rhythm during and after the procedure to evaluate for adequate rate and pacemaker function.	If the monitoring system is not a 5-lead system, also connect the patient to the 12-lead ECG machine (see Procedure 57).
3. Assess pacemaker functioning, and insert a new battery into the pulse generator if needed. (see Figs. 50-8 and 50-9).	Ensures functional pacemaker pulse generator.	There are different ways to assess battery function depending on the model and manufacturer; check manufacturer recommendations for specific instructions.
4. Attach the connecting cable to the pulse generator, connecting the "positive" on the cable to the "positive" on the pulse generator and the "negative" on the cable to the "negative" on the pulse generator.	Prepares the pacing system; the pacing stimulus travels from the pulse generator to the negative terminal, and energy returns to the pulse generator via the positive terminal.	Some lead wires are labelled *distal* and *proximal*; distal connects to negative, and proximal connects to positive. Some lead wires may not have *negative* and *positive* marked on them. Polarity is established when the wires are placed in the connecting cable.
5. Check the placement of the central venous access by chest x-ray before starting the procedure. If central venous access is needed, refer to Procedure 80.	Central venous access is needed as the transvenous pacing catheter is passed through the central venous system.	
6. Prepare the insertion site by clipping hair close to the skin in the area surrounding the insertion site.	Reduces the risk of infection.	Shaving should be avoided because nicks in the skin may predispose the patient to infection.
7. All personnel performing and assisting with the procedure should don masks, caps, goggles or face shields, sterile gowns, and gloves.	Minimizes the risk of infection and maintains standard precautions.	Gloves should be worn whenever the pacing electrodes are handled to prevent microshock.

Procedure continues on the following page

Procedure for Performing Temporary Transvenous Pacemaker Insertion—*Continued*

Steps	Rationale	Special Considerations
8. Cleanse the site with antiseptic solution, such as a 2% chlorhexidine–based preparation.	Minimizes the risk of infection.	
9. Drape the site with the sterile drapes.	Provides a sterile field and reduces the transmission of microorganisms.	
10. Administer a local anesthetic to numb the insertion site.	Ensures patient comfort. A large-gauge introducer is used, which causes discomfort during the insertion procedure.	Not necessary if central venous access is already in place.
11. Make a percutaneous puncture through the vein selected for the procedure (e.g., jugular, subclavian, antecubital, or femoral vein) (see Procedure 80).	Allows for direct placement of the introducer.	
12. Insert the balloon-tipped catheter through the introducer, and advance the pacing lead.	The transvenous pacing catheter is threaded through the central venous system.	
13. Inflate the balloon when the tip of the pacing lead is in the vena cava. Transcutaneous ultrasound of the chest during the insertion procedure may assist the practitioner in ensuring proper placement. *(Level II: Theory based, no research data to support recommendations; recommendations from expert consensus group may exist.)*	The air-filled balloon allows the blood flow to carry the catheter tip into the desired position in the right ventricle. Ultrasonographic visualization of the pacing catheter as it is being passed through the central venous system may ensure a quicker and more accurate placement of the pacing electrode within the endocardium of the right ventricle.[1]	
14. Advance the pacing lead. Verify transvenous pacing lead placement by: A. Use the V lead of the bedside monitoring system or the 12-lead ECG machine. B. Connect the patient to the limb leads. C. Use an alligator clip or a wire with connector pins if needed (Fig. 49-2). D. Attach the V lead of the ECG monitoring system or the 12-lead ECG machine to the negative electrode connector pin (distal pin) of the pacing lead wire. E. Set the monitoring system to record the V lead continuously. F. Observe the ECG for ST-segment elevation in the V lead recording (Fig. 49-3). G. Observe for left bundle-branch block pattern and left axis deviation that usually can be identified.	For transvenous, ventricular pacing, the negative pacing electrode is positioned in the endocardium (at the apex) of the right ventricle. The ECG is derived directly from the pacing electrode, and the position of the catheter tip is verified by the internal electrical recording that shows ST-segment elevation indicating contact with the myocardium. As a result of the temporary pacing catheter transmission of impulses from within the right ventricle, conduction of the impulse throughout the ventricles occurs via cellular conduction of the impulse rather than transmission down the bundle branches.	Fluoroscopy may be needed to permit direct visualization of the pacing electrode. If fluoroscopy is used, all personnel must be shielded from the radiation with lead aprons or be positioned behind lead shields. Drape the patient below the waist with a lead sheet or apron. If premature ventricular contractions or runs of ventricular tachycardia occur, deflate the balloon and position the pacing lead with the balloon deflated.

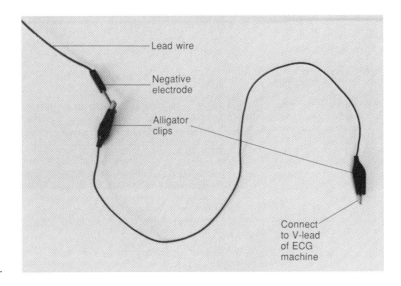

FIGURE 49-2 Alligator clips. *ECG,* electrocardiogram.

FIGURE 49-3 ECG rhythm recorded in the right ventricle: elevated ST segments when pacing electrode is wedged against the endocardial wall of the right ventricle. *(From Meltzer, L.E., Pinneo, R., and Kitchell, J.R. [1983]. Intensive Coronary Care. 4th ed. Bowie, MD: Robert J. Brady Co.)*

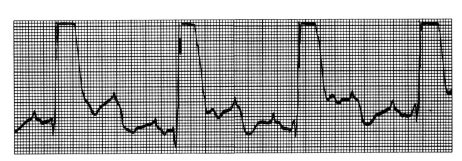

Procedure for Performing Temporary Transvenous Pacemaker Insertion—*Continued*

Steps	Rationale	Special Considerations
15. After the electrodes are properly positioned, deflate the balloon, and connect the external electrode pins to the pulse generator via the connecting cable. Ensure that the positive and negative electrodes are connected to the respective positive and negative terminals on the pulse generator via the connecting cable.	Energy from the pulse generator is directed to the negative electrode in contact with the ventricle. The pacing circuit is completed as energy reaches the positive electrode. The lead wires must be connected securely to the pacemaker to ensure appropriate sensing and capture and to prevent inadvertent disconnection.	It is recommended that a bridging connecting cable be used between the pacing wires and the pulse generator. Some lead wires may not have "negative" and "positive" marked on them. Polarity is established when the wires are placed in the connecting cable.
16. Refer to Procedure 50 for setting pacemaker settings and initiating pacing.		
17. Suture the pacing lead in place.	Minimizes the risk of dislodgment.	
18. Apply a sterile, occlusive dressing over the site.	Minimizes the risk of infection.	

Procedure continues on the following page

Procedure for Performing Temporary Transvenous Pacemaker Insertion—*Continued*

Steps	Rationale	Special Considerations
19. Secure necessary equipment to provide some stability for the pacemaker, such as hanging the pulse generator on an intravenous pole, strapping the pulse generator to the patient's torso, or hanging the pulse generator from a carrying device.	The pulse generator should be protected from falling or becoming inadvertently detached by patient movement. Disconnection or tension on the pacing electrodes may lead to pacemaker malfunction.	Pinning the generator to the patient's sheets or pillow is not recommended because if the patient moves, sits up, or gets out of bed, the pacing lead may be inadvertently disconnected. Keep the pulse generator in clear view so that all are aware it is in use.
20. Discard used supplies, and wash hands.	Reduces the transmission of microorganisms; standard precautions.	
21. Obtain a chest x-ray.	In the absence of fluoroscopy, a chest x-ray is essential to detect potential complications associated with insertion and to visualize lead position.	

Expected Outcomes

- ECG shows paced rhythm consistent with parameters set on the pacemaker, as evidenced by appropriate heart rate, proper sensing, and proper capture.
- Patient exhibits hemodynamic stability, as evidenced by systolic blood pressure greater than 90 mm Hg, mean arterial blood pressure greater than 60 mm Hg, alert and oriented, and no syncope or ischemia.
- Pacemaker leads are isolated from other electrical equipment by maintaining secure connections into the pulse generator.

Unexpected Outcomes

- Inability to achieve proper placement of the pacing catheter
- Failure of the pacemaker to sense, causing competition between the pacemaker-initiated impulses and the patient's intrinsic cardiac rhythm
- Failure of the pacemaker to capture the myocardium
- Pacemaker oversensing causing the pacemaker to be inappropriately inhibited
- Stimulation of the diaphragm causing hiccuping, possibly related to pacing the phrenic nerve, perforation, wire dislodgment, or excessively high pacemaker mA setting
- Development of phlebitis, thrombosis, embolism, or bacteremia
- Ventricular dysrhythmias from manipulation within the cardiac chamber
- Pneumothorax, hemothorax, pneumomediastinum, or development of subcutaneous emphysema from the insertion procedure[2]
- Myocardial perforation, cardiac tamponade, or postpericardiotomy syndrome from the insertion procedure and electrode placement
- Air embolism
- Lead dislodgment

Patient Monitoring and Care

Steps	Rationale	Reportable Conditions
		These conditions should be reported if they persist despite nursing interventions.
1. Monitor vital signs and hemodynamic response to pacing as often as patient condition warrants.	The goal of cardiac pacing is to improve cardiac output by increasing heart rate or by overriding life-threatening dysrhythmias.	- Change in vital signs associated with signs and symptoms of hemodynamic deterioration

Patient Monitoring and Care—*Continued*

Steps	Rationale	Reportable Conditions
2. Evaluate ECG for presence of paced rhythm or resolution of initiating dysrhythmia.	Proper pacemaker functioning is assessed by observing the ECG for pacemaker activity consistent with the parameters set.	• Inability to obtain a paced rhythm • Oversensing • Undersensing

3. Monitor the patient's level of comfort.
  A. Assess level of comfort.
  B. Administer analgesic or sedative as needed.
  C. Evaluate patient response to interventions.
	Discomfort may increase patient's anxiety and decrease tolerance of the procedure, causing hemodynamic compromise.	• Continual hiccups (may indicate wire perforation)
		• Unrelieved discomfort

4. Check and document sensitivity and threshold at least every 24 hours. Threshold may be checked by physicians in high-risk patients.	Ensures proper pacemaker functioning. Prevents unnecessarily high levels of energy delivery to the myocardium. Threshold may be checked more frequently if the patient condition changes or pacemaker function is questioned.	• Problems with sensitivity or threshold

5. Change the dressing as determined by institutional policy depending on the type of dressing used.
  A. Cleanse the surrounding area with antiseptic solution, such as a 2% chlorhexidine–based preparation.
  B. Apply dry, sterile dressing.
  C. Record the date of dressing change.
	Decreases the potential for infection.	• Increased temperature
		• Increased white blood cells
		• Purulent drainage at the insertion site
		• Warmth, redness, discoloration, or pain at the site

6. Monitor for other complications.	Early recognition leads to prompt treatment.	• Embolus • Thrombosis • Perforation of the myocardium • Pneumothorax • Hemothorax • Phlebitis
7. Monitor electrolytes.	Electrolyte imbalances may precipitate dysrhythmias.	• Abnormal electrolyte values
8. Ensure that all connections are secure.	Maintenance of tight connections is necessary to ensure proper sensing, to ensure impulse conduction, and to minimize the risk of microshock conduction to the heart.	• Inability to maintain tight connections with available equipment, jeopardizing pacing therapy

Documentation

Documentation should include the following:

- Description of the events warranting intervention
- Patient and family education and response to education
- Signed informed consent form
- Date and time of insertion
- Date and time of initiation of pacing
- Type of pacing wire inserted and location of insertion
- Pacemaker settings—mode, rate, output, sensitivity setting, threshold measurements, and whether pacemaker is on or off
- ECG monitoring strip recording before and after pacemaker insertion
- Vital signs and hemodynamic parameters before, during, and after the procedure
- Proper placement confirmed by chest x-ray
- Patient response to procedure
- Complications and interventions
- Occurrence of unexpected outcomes and interventions taken
- Medications administered and patient response to medication
- Date and time pacing was discontinued

References

1. Dahlberg, S.T., and Mooradd, M.G. (1994). Temporary cardiac pacing. In: Irwin, R.S., et al, editors. *Procedure and Techniques in Intensive Care Medicine*. 3rd ed. Philadelphia: Lippincott Williams & Wilkins, 67-73.
2. Espiritu, J.D., and Keller, C.A. (2001). Pneumomediastinum and subcutaneous emphysema from pacemaker placement. *Pacing Clin Electrophysiol*, 24, 1041-2.

Additional Readings

Macedo, W., Jr., et al. (1999). Ultrasonographic guidance of transvenous pacemaker insertion in the emergency department: A report of three cases. *J Emerg Med*, 17, 491-6.
Medtronic, Inc. (1997). *Cardiac Pacing and Patient Care*. Minneapolis: Author.
Norman, E.M. (1998). Critical care extra: Critical questions: Avoiding electrical hazards... temporary pacing wires. *Am J Nurs*, 98, 16GG-HH.

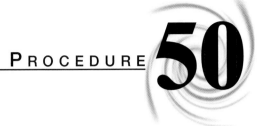
P R O C E D U R E 50

Temporary Transvenous and Epicardial Pacing

P U R P O S E : The purpose of temporary cardiac pacing is to ensure or restore an adequate heart rate and rhythm. Transvenous and epicardial pacing are initiated as temporary measures when there has been a failure of the normal conduction system of the heart to produce an electrical impulse, resulting in hemodynamic compromise or other debilitating symptoms in the patient.

Merrie Jackson
Sandra Schlup Woods

PREREQUISITE NURSING KNOWLEDGE

- Knowledge of the normal anatomy and physiology of the cardiovascular system, principles of cardiac conduction, and basic dysrhythmia interpretation is required.
- Understanding of temporary pacemakers is needed to evaluate pacemaker function and the patient's response to pacemaker therapy.
- Clinical and technical competence related to use of temporary pacemakers is needed.
- Advanced cardiac life support knowledge and skills are required.
- Basic principles of hemodynamic monitoring are essential when assessing the efficacy of temporary pacing therapy.
- Knowledge of the pulmonary artery (PA) catheter function and its use relative to hemodynamic monitoring is a necessity when using a PA catheter with pacing function (see Procedure 72).
- Knowledge of the care of the patient with central venous catheters (see Procedure 66) is required.
- Principles of general electrical safety apply when using temporary invasive pacing methods. Gloves always should be worn when handling electrodes to prevent microshock. In addition, the exposed proximal ends of the pacing wires should be insulated when not in use to prevent microshock.[1]

- The insertion of a temporary pacemaker is performed in emergent and elective clinical situations.
- Temporary pacing may be used to stimulate the myocardium to contract in the absence of an intrinsic rhythm, establish an adequate cardiac output and blood pressure to ensure tissue perfusion to vital organs, reduce the possibility of ventricular dysrhythmias in the presence of bradycardia, supplement an inadequate rhythm with transient decreases in heart rate (e.g., chronotropic incompetence in shock), or allow the administration of medications (e.g., β-blockers) to treat ischemia or tachy-dysrhythmias in the presence of conduction system dysfunction or bradycardia.
- Temporary invasive pacing is indicated for the following:
  - ❖ Third-degree atrioventricular (AV) block
  - ❖ Symptomatic congenital complete heart block
  - ❖ Symptomatic acquired complete heart block
  - ❖ Symptomatic second-degree heart block
  - ❖ Dysrhythmias complicating acute myocardial infarction
  - ❖ Symptomatic bradycardia or bradydysrhythmias
  - ❖ New bundle-branch block with transient complete heart block
  - ❖ Alternating bundle-branch block
  - ❖ Sinus node dysfunction
  - ❖ Treatment of bradycardia-tachycardia syndrome (sick sinus syndrome)
  - ❖ Ventricular standstill or cardiac arrest

❖ Long Q-T syndrome with ventricular dysrhythmias
❖ Medication toxicity
❖ Postoperative cardiac surgery
❖ Low cardiac output states
❖ Prophylaxis with cardiac diagnostic or interventional procedures
❖ Chronotropic incompetence in the setting of cardiogenic shock

• There are three primary methods of invasive temporary pacing: transvenous endocardial pacing, PA catheter pacing, and epicardial pacing.
• Transvenous pacing
  ❖ In temporary transvenous pacing, the pulse generator is externally attached to a pacing lead that is inserted through a vein into the right atrium or ventricle.
  ❖ Veins used for insertion of the pacing lead are the subclavian, femoral, brachial, internal jugular, or external jugular.
  ❖ Single-chamber ventricular pacing is the most common method used in an emergency because the goal is to establish a heart rate as quickly as possible.
  ❖ Temporary atrial or dual-chamber pacing can be initiated if the patient requires atrial contraction for improvement in hemodynamics.
  ❖ The pacing lead is an insulated wire with one or two electrodes at the tip of the wire.
  ❖ The pacing lead can be a hard-tipped or balloon-tipped pacing catheter that is placed in direct contact with the myocardium (Fig. 50-1). Most temporary leads are bipolar, with the distal tip electrode separated from the proximal ring by 1 to 2 cm (see Fig. 49-1).
• Pacing via a PA catheter
  ❖ Temporary atrial or ventricular pacing via a thermodilution PA catheter can be done with combination catheters that are specifically designed for temporary pacing.
  ❖ The newest pacing PA catheter features atrial and ventricular ports for introduction of the pacing lead wires (Fig. 50-2).
  ❖ Use of a PA catheter combines the capabilities of PA pressure monitoring, thermodilution cardiac output

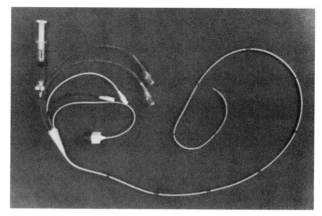

FIGURE 50-2 Pulmonary artery catheter with atrial and ventricular pacing lumens.

measurement, fluid infusion, mixed venous oxygen sampling, and temporary pacing.
  ❖ One limitation of these multifunction catheters is that the simultaneous measurement of pulmonary artery wedge pressure (PAWP) and pacing is usually not possible. Balloon inflation can cause repositioning of the pacing electrode with catheter movement; measurement of the PAWP may cause pacing to become intermittent.
• Temporary epicardial pacing
  ❖ Temporary epicardial pacing is a method of stimulating the myocardium through the use of a Teflon-coated, unipolar stainless steel wires that are sutured loosely to the epicardium after cardiac surgery.
  ❖ The epicardial wires may be attached to the right atrium for atrial pacing, the right ventricle for ventricular pacing, or both for AV pacing (Fig. 50-3).

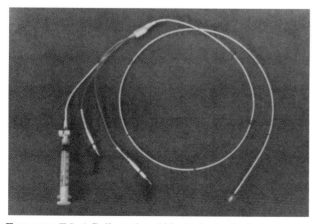

FIGURE 50-1 Balloon-tipped bipolar lead wire for transvenous pacing.

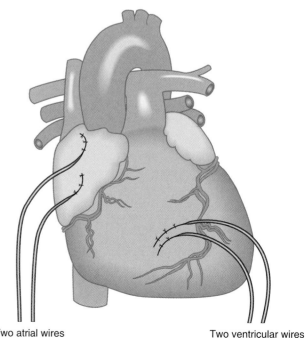

Two atrial wires   Two ventricular wires

FIGURE 50-3 Location of atrial and ventricular epicardial lead wires.

❖ When implanted on the epicardial surface, each pacing wire is brought through the chest wall before the chest is closed.

❖ Typically the atrial wires are located on the right of the sternum, and the ventricular wires exit to the left of the sternum (see Fig. 43-1).

❖ An external temporary pulse generator (Figs. 50-4 and 50-5) is connected to the epicardial pacing wires via a bridging or connecting cable (Fig. 50-6).

• Basic principles of cardiac pacing include sensing, pacing, and capture.

❖ *Sensing* refers to the ability of the pacemaker device to detect intrinsic myocardial electrical activity. Sensing occurs if the pulse generator is in the synchronous or demand mode. The pacemaker either is inhibited from delivering a stimulus or initiates an electrical impulse.

❖ *Pacing* occurs when the temporary pulse generator is activated, and the requisite level of energy travels from the pulse generator through the temporary wires to the myocardium. This is known as pacemaker *firing* and is represented as a line or spike on the electrocardiogram (ECG) recording.

❖ *Capture* refers to the successful stimulation of the myocardium by the pacemaker, resulting in depolarization. It is evidenced on the ECG by a pacemaker spike, followed by either an atrial or a ventricular complex, depending on the chamber being paced.

• Temporary pulse generator

❖ The temporary pulse generator houses the controls and energy source for pacing.

❖ There are pulse generators that can be used for single-chamber pacing that have one set of terminals at the top of the pulse generator into which the pacing wires are inserted (via connecting cable) (see Fig. 50-4).

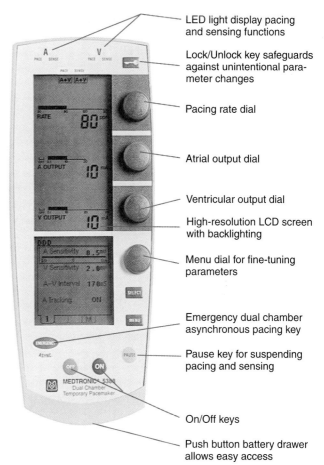

FIGURE 50-5 Dual-chamber temporary pulse generator. *(Courtesy Medtronic USA, Inc.)*

❖ A dual-chamber pacemaker requires two sets of terminals for the atrial and ventricular wires (Fig. 50-7; also see Fig. 50-5).

❖ Different models of pacemakers use either dials or touch pads to change the settings.

❖ The pacing rate is determined by the rate dial or touch pad.

❖ The AV interval dial or pad on a dual-chamber pacemaker controls the amount of time between atrial and ventricular stimulation (electronic P-R interval).

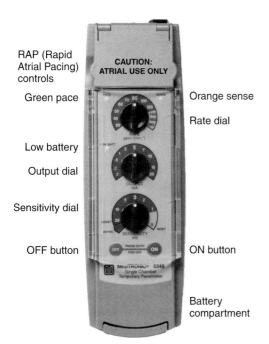

FIGURE 50-4 Single-chamber temporary pulse generator. *(Courtesy Medtronic USA, Inc.)*

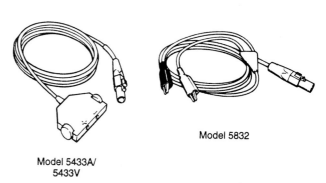

FIGURE 50-6 Connecting cables. *(Courtesy Medtronic USA, Inc.)*

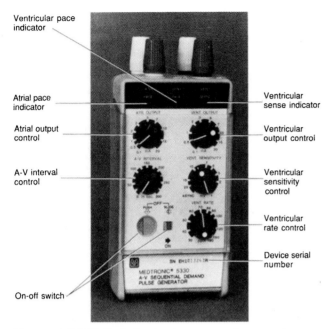

FIGURE 50-7 Dual-chamber temporary pulse generator. *(Courtesy Medtronic USA, Inc.)*

❖ The energy delivered to the myocardium is determined by setting the output (milliampere [mA]) dial or pad on the pulse generator.

❖ Dual-chamber pacing requires that mAs be set for the atria and the ventricle.

• The ability of the pacemaker to detect the patient's intrinsic rhythm is determined by the pacing mode. In the asynchronous mode, the pacemaker functions as a fixed-rate pacemaker and is not able to sense any of the patient's inherent cardiac activity. In the synchronous mode, the pacemaker is able to sense the patient's inherent cardiac activity.

• The ability of the pacemaker to depolarize the myocardium depends on many variables: the position of the electrodes and degree of contact with viable myocardial tissue; the level of energy delivered through the pacing wire; the presence of hypoxia, acidosis, or electrolyte imbalances; fibrosis around the tip of the catheter; and concomitant medication therapy.[3]

EQUIPMENT

• Antiseptic solution (e.g., 2% chlorhexidine–based preparation)
• Nonsterile gloves
• Pacing lead wires
• Pulse generator
• 9-volt battery for pulse generator
• Connecting cables
• ECG monitoring equipment
• Dressing supplies
  Additional equipment to have available includes:
• Central venous catheter insertion supplies (see Procedure 80)
• Alligator clips or wire with connector pins
• Suture with needle, needles, syringes
• Emergency equipment

• Fluoroscopy
• Lead aprons or shields
• Flush solution and pressure line setup, if using PA catheter (see Procedure 75)
• 12-lead ECG machine
• Local anesthetic
• Sterile drapes, towels, masks, goggles or face shields, gowns, caps

PATIENT AND FAMILY EDUCATION

• Assess learning needs, readiness to learn, and factors that influence learning. ➤*Rationale:* This assessment enables teaching to be individualized in a manner that is meaningful to the patient and family.

• Discuss the basic facts about the normal conduction system, such as structure and function of the conduction system, normal and abnormal heart rhythms, and symptoms or significance of abnormal heart rhythms. ➤*Rationale:* The patient and family should understand the conduction system and why the procedure is necessary.

• Provide a basic description of the temporary pacemaker insertion procedure. ➤*Rationale:* The patient and family should be informed of the invasive nature of the procedure and any risks associated with it. An understanding of the procedure may reduce anxiety.

• Describe the precautions and restrictions required while the temporary pacemaker is in place, such as limitation of movement, avoidance of handling the pacemaker or touching exposed portions of the electrodes, and when to notify the nurse (e.g., if the dressing becomes wet, if the patient is experiencing dizziness). ➤*Rationale:* Understanding limitations may improve patient cooperation with restrictions and precautions.

PATIENT ASSESSMENT AND PREPARATION

Patient Assessment

• Assess the patient's baseline cardiac rhythm for the presence of the dysrhythmia necessitating temporary cardiac pacing. ➤*Rationale:* This assessment determines the need for invasive cardiac pacing.

• Assess the patient's hemodynamic response to the dysrhythmia. Rhythm disturbances may reduce cardiac output significantly with detrimental effects on perfusion to vital organs. ➤*Rationale:* This assessment determines the urgency of the procedure. It may indicate the need for temporizing measures, such as vasopressors or transcutaneous pacing.

• Review the patient's current medications. ➤*Rationale:* Medications may be a cause of the dysrhythmia that led to the need for pacemaker therapy, or medications may need to be held because of concomitant effect. Other medications, such as antidysrhythmics, may alter the pacing threshold.

• Review the patient's current laboratory studies, including chemistry or electrolyte profile, arterial blood gases, or cardioactive medication levels. ➥*Rationale:* This review assists in determining if the need for pacing was precipitated by metabolic disturbances or medication toxicity and establishes the pacing milieu.

Patient Preparation

• Ensure that the patient and family understand preprocedural teaching. Answer questions as they arise, and reinforce

information as needed. ➥*Rationale:* This communication evaluates and reinforces understanding of previously taught information.

• Validate that informed consent has been obtained. ➥*Rationale:* Obtaining informed consent protects the rights of the patient and makes a competent decision possible for the patient; however, under emergency circumstances, time may not allow the consent form to be signed.

Procedure for Temporary Transvenous and Epicardial Pacing		
Steps	**Rationale**	**Special Considerations**
Initiating Temporary Pacing		
1. Wash hands.	Reduces the transmission of microorganisms; standard precautions.	
2. Connect the patient to the bedside monitoring system and monitor the ECG continuously (see Procedure 54).	Monitors the patient's intrinsic rhythm and the patient's rhythm during and after the procedure to evaluate for adequate pacemaker function.	
3. Assess pacemaker functioning and insert a new battery into the pulse generator, if needed (Figs. 50-8 and 50-9).	Ensures a functional pacemaker pulse generator.	There are different ways to assess battery function, depending on the model and manufacturer; check manufacturer recommendations for specific instructions.
4. Attach the connecting cable to the pulse generator, connecting the "positive" on the cable to the "positive" on the pulse generator and the "negative" on the cable to the "negative" on the pulse generator.	Prepares the pacing system; the pacing stimulus travels from the pulse generator to the negative terminal, and energy returns to the pulse generator via the positive terminal.	

Procedure continues on the following page

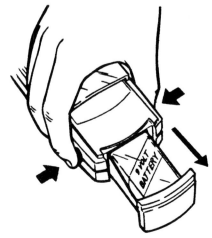

FIGURE 50-8 Replacing the battery. Press both battery drawer buttons to open the battery compartment, and remove the old battery. (*Courtesy Medtronic USA, Inc.*)

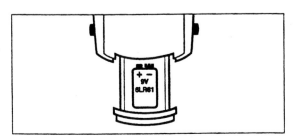

FIGURE 50-9 Placement of the new battery. Insert the new battery, close the compartment, and press the "on" button. (*Courtesy Medtronic USA, Inc.*)

Procedure for Temporary Transvenous and Epicardial Pacing—*Continued*		
Steps	**Rationale**	**Special Considerations**

Assisting With Initiation of Temporary Transvenous Pacing

Steps	Rationale	Special Considerations
1. Follow **Steps 1 through 4** under Initiating Temporary Pacing.		
2. If a central venous catheter is not in place, assist as needed with catheter insertion (see Procedure 81).	A central line is needed for transvenous pacing.	
3. Assist as needed with insertion of the transvenous pacing lead wire.	Provides needed assistance.	
4. All personnel performing and assisting with the procedure should don masks, goggles or face shields, gowns, sterile gloves, and caps.	Prevents infection and maintains standard precautions; maintains sterility.	Gloves should be worn whenever handling the pacing electrodes to prevent microshock.[3]
5. Assist as needed with cleansing the insertion site with antiseptic solution (e.g., 2% chlorhexidine–based preparation).	Prevents infection.	
6. Assist as needed with draping the insertion site.	Provides a sterile field and reduces the transmission of microorganisms.	
7. Assist as needed as the pacing lead is passed through the introducer.	Facilitates the insertion process.	If a balloon-tipped pacing lead is used, balloon inflation occurs when the tip of the pacing lead is in the vena cava. The air-filled balloon allows the blood flow to carry the catheter tip into the desired position in the right ventricle.
8. Verify transvenous pacing lead wire placement via one of the following:	The pacing electrode is positioned in the apex of the right ventricle.	
A. Fluoroscopy	Fluoroscopy allows direct visualization of the pacing electrode.	If fluoroscopy is used, all personnel must be shielded from the radiation with lead aprons or be positioned behind lead shields.

B. Bedside monitoring system or 12-lead ECG machine
   (1) Connect the patient to the limb leads.
   (2) Attach the V lead of the ECG monitoring system or the 12-lead ECG machine to the negative electrode connector pin (distal pin) of the pacing lead wire (an alligator clip or wire with connector pins may be needed).
   (3) Set the monitoring system to record the V lead continuously.
   (4) Observe the ECG for ST-segment elevation in the V lead recording (see Fig. 49-3).
   (5) In addition, a left bundle-branch block pattern and left axis deviation also usually can be identified.
	The ECG is derived directly from the pacing electrode, and the position of the catheter tip is verified by the internal electrical recording, which shows ST-segment elevation when in contact with the myocardium.	

9. After the pacing lead wire is properly positioned, connect the external electrode pins to the pulse	Energy from the pulse generator is directed to the negative electrode.	It is recommended that a connecting cable be used between the pacing wires and the pulse generator.

Procedure for Temporary Transvenous and Epicardial Pacing—*Continued*

Steps	Rationale	Special Considerations
generator via the connecting cable. Ensure that the positive and negative electrode connector pins are connected to the respective positive and negative terminals on the pulse generator via the connecting cable (Figs. 50-10 and 50-11).	The pacing circuit is completed as energy reaches the positive electrode. The lead wires must be connected securely to the pacemaker to ensure appropriate sensing and capture and to prevent inadvertent disconnection.	Some lead wires are labeled *distal* and *proximal*; distal connects to negative, and proximal connects to positive. Some lead wires may not have *negative* and *positive* marked on them. Polarity is established when the wires are placed in the connecting cable. Ensure all connections are secure.
10. *For AV demand pacing when the atrial wires are placed in addition to the ventricular wires,* connect the atrial electrodes to the atrial terminals and the ventricular electrodes to the ventricular terminals. Attach the "positive" on the connecting cable to the "positive" on the pulse generator and the "negative" on the connecting cable to the "negative" on the pulse generator.	Ensures that the atrial electrodes and ventricular electrodes are connected correctly to the pulse generator. Secure connections are essential for proper sensing and conduction of pacemaker energy. The pacing stimulus travels from the pulse generator to the negative terminal, and energy returns to the pulse generator via the positive terminal.	

Procedure continues on the following page

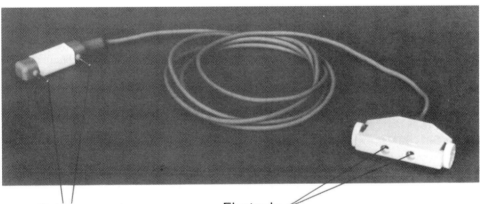

Pulse generator connection sites   Electrode connection sites

FIGURE 50-10 Connecting cable.

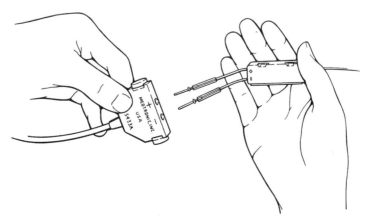

FIGURE 50-11 Inserting the lead wires into the connecting-bridging cable. *(Courtesy Medtronic USA, Inc.)*

Procedure **for Temporary Transvenous and Epicardial Pacing**—*Continued*

Steps	Rationale	Special Considerations
11. *For atrial pacing when atrial wires are placed,* connect the atrial electrodes to the atrial terminals. Attach the "positive" on the connecting cable to the "positive" on the pulse generator, and the "negative" on the connecting cable to the "negative" on the pulse generator.	Secure connections are essential for proper sensing and conduction of pacemaker energy. The pacing stimulus travels from the pulse generator to the negative terminal, and energy returns to the pulse generator via the positive terminal.	

Assisting With Initiating Temporary Pacing via a Pulmonary Artery Catheter

Steps	Rationale	Special Considerations
1. Follow **Steps 1 through 4** under Initiating Temporary Pacing.	Prepares equipment.	
2. Assist the physician or advanced practice nurse with insertion of the PA catheter (see Procedure 72).	Provides assistance as needed.	Pacing electrodes may be inserted at the time of PA catheter insertion, or they may be inserted at a later time, when temporary pacing is required because of a change in patient condition.
3. Obtain the appropriate pacing lead for insertion.	Only probes specifically manufactured for use with the PA catheter should be used; check specific manufacturer's recommendations.	Continuous monitoring of the right ventricular pressure waveform via the pacing lumen is recommended before insertion of the electrode to ensure correct placement of the right ventricular port 1-2 cm distal to the tricuspid valve.
4. Assist the physician or advanced practice nurse with insertion of the pacing lead wire.	Close monitoring of the ECG during insertion of the pacing lead is necessary to detect potentially lethal dysrhythmias.	Follow specific manufacturer's instructions regarding pacing lead insertion and securing the pacing lead in place within the catheter lumen.
5. After the electrodes are properly positioned, connect the positive and negative electrode connector pins to the pulse generator via the connecting cable. Ensure that the positive and negative electrodes are connected to the respective positive and negative terminals on the pulse generator via the connecting cable.	Energy from the pulse generator is directed to the negative electrode. The pacing circuit is completed as energy reaches the positive electrode. The electrodes must be connected securely to the pulse generator to ensure appropriate sensing and capture and to prevent inadvertent disconnection.	Gloves should be worn whenever handling the pacing electrodes to prevent microshock.
6. Check institutional policy or obtain specific physician prescription regarding the purposeful wedging of the PA pacing catheter that is being used actively for pacing therapy.	Intermittent capture has been noted during the wedging procedure as a result of movement of the electrode with catheter migration into the wedge position.[1]	Usually the PA catheter is not wedged during pacing therapy.

Epicardial Pacing

Steps	Rationale	Special Considerations
1. Follow **Steps 1 through 4** under Initiating Temporary Pacing.		
2. Don nonsterile gloves.	Gloves should be worn whenever handling the epicardial wires to prevent microshock.	
3. Expose the epicardial pacing wires, and identify the chamber of origin. Wires exiting to the right of the sternum are atrial in origin. Wires exiting to the left of the sternum are ventricular in origin (see Fig. 43-1).	Identifies the correct chamber for pacing.	

Procedure for Temporary Transvenous and Epicardial Pacing—*Continued*

Steps	Rationale	Special Considerations
4. Connect the epicardial wires to the pulse generator via the connecting cable. Ensure that the positive and negative electrodes are connected to the respective positive and negative terminals on the pulse generator via the connecting cable.	The epicardial wires must be connected securely to the pulse generator to ensure appropriate sensing and capture and to prevent inadvertent disconnection. Use of unipolar or bipolar configuration needs to be established; this depends on where the epicardial wires are located. In a unipolar pacing system, there is only one electrode in contact with the chamber being paced (the negative electrode). The positive, or indifferent, electrode may be sewn to the subcutaneous tissue of the chest wall. With bipolar pacing, both electrodes are in direct contact with the myocardial tissue of the chamber being paced.	The epicardial wire connected to the negative terminal determines where the energy is delivered. The wire connected to the positive terminal determines how the energy returns to the pulse generator. With AV demand pacing, be sure to place both atrial wires in the terminal labeled *atrium* (via cable) and ventricular wires in the terminal labeled *ventricle* (via cable). With bipolar pacing, either wire can be the negative electrode. With unipolar pacing (one electrode in contact with the heart), the epicardial wire must be the negative electrode, and the skin wire must be the positive electrode.
All Methods of Temporary Pacing 1. Determine the mode of pacing desired.	The pacing mode chosen should be the one that best achieves the goal of pacing therapy. Possibilities include atrial, ventricular, or AV asynchronous (fixed rate) pacing or atrial, ventricular, or AV synchronous (demand) pacing.	Asynchronous pacing in the presence of an intrinsic rhythm may result in R-on-T phenomenon, leading to a lethal dysrhythmia, and should be used only in the absence of an intrinsic rhythm.
2. Set the pacemaker mode, pacemaker rate, and level of energy (output or mA) as prescribed or as determined by sensitivity and stimulation threshold testing (see **Steps 3, 4, and 5**).	Determination of pacemaker settings is based on patient response and the capture threshold measured after the wires are connected.	The demand mode is recommended to avoid competition between the pacemaker-initiated beats and the patient's intrinsic rhythm. Output is set to ensure capture of the myocardium. In AV demand pacing, separate output settings are used to ensure capture of the atrium and the ventricle.
3. Depending on the pulse generator, turn all settings to the lowest level, then turn the pulse generator on.	Prepares the equipment.	Some pulse generators perform a self-test when turned on; after the self-test is completed the settings can be adjusted.
4. Determine the sensitivity threshold (for each chamber as appropriate).	*Sensitivity threshold* is the level at which intrinsic myocardial activity is recognized by the sensing electrodes. For demand pacing, the sensitivity must be measured and set.	When determining sensitivity threshold, the mAs should be turned to the lowest level to avoid the possibility of a pacemaker stimulus falling on the T wave (R-on-T phenomenon) and inducing a potentially lethal dysrhythmia. After sensitivity threshold is determined, some physicians prefer to set sensitivity settings all the way to the demand mode (most sensitive), regardless of the sensitivity threshold.
A. Gradually turn the sensitivity dial counterclockwise (or to a higher numerical setting), and observe the pace indicator light for flashing.		

Procedure continues on the following page

Procedure for Temporary Transvenous and Epicardial Pacing—*Continued*

Steps	Rationale	Special Considerations
B. Slowly turn the sensitivity dial clockwise (or to a lower numerical setting) until the sense indicator light flashes with each complex, and the pace indicator light stops. This value is the *sensing threshold.* C. Set the sensitivity dial to the number that was half the sensing threshold to provide a 2:1 safety margin.		If sensitivity is set to the most sensitive, the pacemaker may be inappropriately inhibited because it may detect and interpret extramyocardial activity (e.g., muscle movement, artifact) as actual myocardial activity.
5. Determine the stimulation threshold (for each chamber as necessary): A. Set the pacing rate approximately 10 beats above the patient's intrinsic rate. B. Gradually decrease the output from 20 mA until capture is lost. C. Gradually increase the mA until 1:1 capture is established. This is the stimulation threshold. D. Set the mAs at least two times higher than the stimulation threshold.[4] This output setting is sometimes referred to as the *maintenance threshold.*	The output dial regulates the amount of electrical current (mAs) that is delivered to the myocardium to initiate depolarization. The maintenance threshold is set at least two times above the stimulation threshold to allow for increases in the stimulation threshold without loss of capture.[4]	This step should be performed by a physician in a patient who is pacemaker-dependent for bradyarrhythmia. Individual institutional policies govern when threshold determination should be done and whether a nurse may test the stimulation threshold; thresholds may not be determined if sensitivity is poor or if the patient's inherent heart rate is greater than 90 beats/min. Threshold may increase or decrease within hours of electrode placement due to fibrosis at the tip of the catheter, medication administration (e.g., some antidysrhythmics), alteration of position, or underlying pathology. In the case of dual-chamber pacing, the threshold for each chamber must be assessed.
6. Set the prescribed pacemaker rate.	Ensures adequate cardiac output.	
7. Assess the cardiac rhythm for appropriate pacemaker function:	The ECG tracing should reflect appropriate response to the	

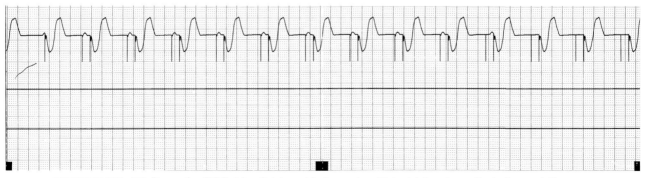

FIGURE 50-12 Pacemaker ECG strip of atrioventricular pacing. Note atrial pacing spike before each P wave and ventricular pacing spike before each QRS complex.

Procedure for Temporary Transvenous and Epicardial Pacing—*Continued*

Steps	Rationale	Special Considerations
A. *Capture:* Is there a QRS complex for every ventricular pacing stimulus? Is there also a P wave for every atrial pacing stimulus? (Fig. 50-12) B. *Rate:* Is the rate at or above the pacemaker rate if in the demand mode? C. *Sensing:* Does the sensitivity light indicate that every QRS complex is sensed?	pacemaker settings if functioning properly. Sometimes, P-wave activity may not be visible due to low-voltage amplitude. If the patient is solely atrially paced, ventricular tracking and response should follow the atrial rate setting.	
8. After the settings are adjusted for optimal patient response, place the protective plastic cover over the pacemaker controls, or place the controls in the locked position.	Pacemaker settings may be inadvertently altered by patient movement or handling if the controls are not covered or locked.	The patient may need to be reminded not to touch the pulse generator.
9. Assess patient response to pacing, including blood pressure, level of consciousness, heart rhythm, and other hemodynamic parameters, if available.	Pacemaker settings are determined by patient response.	When single-chamber ventricular pacing is used, a higher rate may be necessary to compensate for the loss of atrial contribution to cardiac output.
10. Apply a sterile, occlusive dressing over the insertion site.	Prevents infection.	The epicardial electrodes and the insertion sites may be covered by a 4-inch × 4-inch dressing and taped to the chest. The wires may be placed over the dressing and covered with gauze. Finger cots may also be used to cover the wires.
11. Secure the necessary equipment to provide some stability for the pacemaker, such as hanging the pulse generator on an intravenous pole, strapping the pulse generator to the patient's torso, hanging the pulse generator around the patient's neck, or securing the pulse generator under a draw sheet.	The pulse generator should be protected from falling or becoming inadvertently detached by patient movement. Disconnection or tension on the pacing electrodes may lead to pacemaker malfunction.	
12. Discard supplies and wash hands.	Reduces the transmission of microorganisms; standard precautions.	
13. Obtain a chest radiograph as prescribed.	In the absence of fluoroscopy, a radiograph is essential to detect potential complications associated with insertion and to visualize lead position.	Not necessary for epicardial pacing.
14. Selectively restrict patient mobility depending on the insertion site.	Prevents electrode dislodgment.	Check institutional policy regarding ambulation for the patient with a temporary pacemaker.

Expected Outcomes

- ECG shows paced rhythm consistent with parameters set on the pacemaker, as evidenced by appropriate heart rate, proper sensing, and proper capture.
- Patient exhibits hemodynamic stability, as evidenced by a systolic blood pressure greater than 90 mm Hg, a mean arterial blood pressure greater than 60 mm Hg, being alert and oriented, and no syncope or ischemia.
- Pacemaker leads and wires are isolated from other electrical equipment by maintaining secure connections into the pulse generator. If disconnected from the pulse generator, the leads and wires need to be insulated by an insulating material.[3]
- When pacing with a PA catheter, proper pacemaker function is maintained during hemodynamic monitoring procedures.

Unexpected Outcomes

- Failure of the pacemaker to sense, causing competition between the pacemaker-initiated impulses and the patient's intrinsic cardiac rhythm
- Failure of the pacemaker to capture the myocardium
- Pacemaker oversensing causing the pacemaker to be inappropriately inhibited
- Stimulation of the diaphragm causing hiccupping may be related to pacing the phrenic nerve, perforation, wire dislodgment, or excessively high pacemaker mA setting
- Phlebitis, thrombosis, embolism, or bacteremia
- Ventricular dysrhythmias from manipulation within the cardiac chamber
- Pneumothorax or hemothorax from the insertion procedure
- Myocardial perforation and cardiac tamponade from the insertion procedure and electrode placement
- Air embolism
- Lead dislodgment
- Pacemaker syndrome as a result of loss of AV synchrony with ventricular demand pacing
- Intermittent pacing function with PA catheter when obtaining wedge reading

Patient Monitoring and Care

Steps	Rationale	Reportable Conditions
		These conditions should be reported if they persist despite nursing interventions.
1. Monitor vital signs and hemodynamic response to pacing as often as patient condition warrants.	The goal of cardiac pacing is to improve cardiac output by increasing heart rate or by overriding life-threatening dysrhythmias.	• Change in vital signs associated with signs and symptoms of hemodynamic deterioration
2. Evaluate the ECG for the presence of the paced rhythm or resolution of the initiating dysrhythmia.	Proper pacemaker functioning is assessed by observing the ECG for pacemaker activity consistent with the parameters set.	• Inability to obtain a paced rhythm • Oversensing • Undersensing

3. Monitor the patient's level of comfort:
  A. Assess level of comfort.
  B. Administer analgesic or sedative, as needed.
  C. Evaluate patient response to interventions.
	Discomfort may increase patient's anxiety and decrease tolerance of the procedure, causing hemodynamic compromise.	• Continual hiccups (may indicate wire perforation)
		• Unrelieved discomfort

4. Check and document sensitivity and stimulation threshold at least every 24 hours.	Ensures proper pacemaker functioning and prevents unnecessarily high levels of energy delivery to the myocardium.	• Problems with pacemaker function • Threshold may be checked by physicians in high-risk patients
5. Assess pacemaker functioning after the wedge procedure.	Intermittent pacing may occur during or after the wedge procedure, owing to movement of the pacing electrode during wedging.	• Loss of capture after performing the wedge procedure
6. Change the dressing as determined by institutional policy.	Decreases the potential for infection.	• Increased temperature • Increased white blood cell count

Patient Monitoring and Care—*Continued*

Steps	Rationale	Reportable Conditions
A. Cleanse the pacemaker site with antiseptic solution (e.g., 2% chlorhexidine–based preparation). B. Apply dry, sterile dressing and tape. C. Record date of dressing change.		• Drainage at the insertion site • Warmth or pain at the insertion site
7. Monitor for other complications.	Early recognition leads to prompt treatment.	• Any signs or symptoms of complications, such as embolus, thrombosis, perforation of the myocardium, pneumothorax, hemothorax, or phlebitis
8. Monitor electrolytes daily and as needed.	Electrolyte imbalances may precipitate dysrhythmias.	• Abnormal electrolyte values
9. Ensure, that all connections are secure.	Maintenance of tight connections is necessary to ensure proper pacemaker functioning.	• Inability to maintain tight connections with available equipment jeopardizes pacing therapy

Documentation

Documentation should include the following:

- Patient and family education
- Date and time of initiation of pacing
- Description of events warranting intervention
- Vital signs and hemodynamic parameters before, during, and after the procedure
- ECG monitoring strip recording before and after pacemaker insertion
- Type of pacemaker wire inserted and location
- Pacemaker settings: mode, rate, output, sensitivity setting, threshold measurements, and whether the pacemaker is on or off
- Patient response to the procedure
- Complications and interventions
- Medications administered and patient response to the medication
- Date and time pacing was discontinued
- Adjustment to monitoring system settings to ensure detection of paced rhythms

References

1. Atlee, J.L. (1996). *Arrhythmias and Pacemakers*. Philadelphia: W.B. Saunders, 247-329.
2. Baas, L.S., Beery, T.A., and Hickey, C.S. (1997). Care and safety of pacemaker electrodes in intensive care and telemetry nursing units. *Am J Crit Care,* 6, 302-11.
3. Busch, M.M., and Haskin, J.B. (1995). Pacemakers and implantable defibrillators. In: Woods, S.L., et al, editors. *Cardiac Nursing*. 3rd ed. Philadelphia: J.B. Lippincott, 618-61.
4. Moses, H.W., et al. (1995). *A Practical Guide to Cardiac Pacing*. Boston: Little, Brown, 89-112.

Additional Readings

Fitzpatrick, A., and Sutton, R. (1992). A guide to temporary pacing. *BMJ,* 304, 365-9.
Furman, S., Hayes, D.L., and Holmes, D.R. (1993). *A Practice of Cardiac Pacing*. Mount Kisco, NY: Futura Publishing, 231-60.

Futterman, L.G., and Lemberg, L. (1993). Pacemaker update: Part II. atrioventricular synchronous and rate-modulated pacemakers. *Am J Crit Care,* 2, 96-8.
Hickey, C.S., and Baas, L.S. (1991). Temporary cardiac pacing. *AACN Clin Issues Crit Care Nurs,* 2, 107-17.
Lynn-McHale, D.J., Riggs, K.L., and Thurman, L. (1991). Epicardial pacing after cardiac surgery. *Crit Care Nurse,* 11, 62-74.
Manion, P.A. (1993). Temporary epicardial pacing in the postoperative cardiac surgical patient. *Crit Care Nurse,* 13, 30-8.
Morton, P.G. (1997). The pacemaker and defibrillator codes: Implications for critical care nursing. *Crit Care Nurse,* 17, 50-9.
Overbay, D., and Criddle, L. (2004). Mastering temporary invasive cardiac pacing. *Crit Care Nurse,* 24, 25-32.
Schurig, L., Gura, M., and Taibi, B., editors, for the NASPE/CAP: Council of Associated Professionals. (1997). *Educational Guidelines: Pacing and Electrophysiology*. 2nd ed. Armonk, NY: Futura Publishing.
Witherell, C.L. (1994). Cardiac rhythm control devices. *Crit Care Nurs Clin North Am,* 6, 85-101.

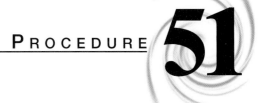
Circulatory Assist Devices

PROCEDURE **51**

Intraaortic Balloon Pump Management

P U R P O S E : Intraaortic balloon pump (IABP) therapy is designed to increase coronary artery perfusion, increase systemic perfusion, decrease myocardial workload, and decrease afterload.

Susan Quaal

PREREQUISITE NURSING KNOWLEDGE

- Knowledge of the anatomy and physiology of the cardiovascular system
- Understanding of the principles of hemodynamic monitoring, electrophysiology, dysrhythmias, and coagulation
- Clinical and technical competence related to the use of the IABP
- Advanced cardiac life support knowledge and skills
- Indications for IABP therapy are as follows:
  - ❖ Cardiogenic shock
  - ❖ Refractory unstable angina
  - ❖ Acute myocardial infarction (MI) complicated by left ventricular failure[18]
  - ❖ Refractory unstable angina
  - ❖ Recurrent ventricular dysrhythmias as a result of ischemia
  - ❖ Support before, during, and/or after coronary artery bypass graft surgery[7]
  - ❖ Support before, during, and/or after coronary artery angioplasty or additional interventional cardiology procedures for high-risk patients[9,13]
  - ❖ Mechanical complications of acute MI, including aortic stenosis, mitral stenosis, mitral valvuloplasty, mitral insufficiency, ventricular septal defect, and left ventricular aneurysm
  - ❖ Intractable ventricular dysrhythmias[20]
  - ❖ Bridge to cardiac transplantation, ventricular assist devices, or total artificial hearts
  - ❖ Cardiac injury, including contusion and coronary artery tears
  - ❖ Septic shock
  - ❖ High-risk patient having noncardiac surgery[20,32]

- Contraindications to IABP therapy are as follows:
  - ❖ Moderate to severe aortic insufficiency
  - ❖ Thoracic and abdominal aortic aneurysms
  - ❖ The relative value of IABP therapy in the presence of severe aortoiliac disease, major coagulopathies, and terminal disease should be evaluated individually.
- IABP therapy is an acute, short-term therapy for patients with reversible left ventricular failure or an adjunct to other therapies for irreversible heart failure. Cardiac assistance with the IABP is performed to improve myocardial oxygen supply and reduce cardiac workload. Intraaortic balloon (IAB) pumping is based on the principles of counterpulsation (Fig. 51-1).

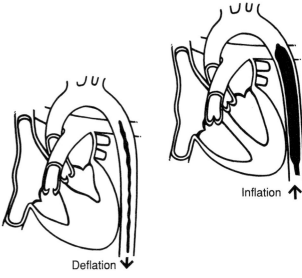

Inflation ↑

Deflation ↓

FIGURE 51-1 Counterpulsation. *(From Datascope Corp., Montvale, New Jersey).*

- The events of the cardiac cycle provide the stimulus for balloon function, and the movement of helium gas between the balloon and the control console gas source produces inflation and deflation of the balloon.
- Recognition of the R wave or the QRS complex on the electrocardiogram (ECG) is the most commonly used trigger source.
- Inflation occurs during ventricular diastole, causing an increase in aortic pressure. This increased pressure displaces blood proximally to the coronary arteries and distally to the rest of the body. The result is an increase in myocardial oxygen supply and subsequent improvement in cardiac output.
- Deflation occurs just before ventricular systole or ejection. This decreases the pressure within the aortic root, reducing afterload and cardiac workload.
- Insertion and placement verification proceed as follows:
  - The IAB catheter is commonly placed in the femoral artery via percutaneous puncture or arteriotomy.
  - Surgical placement via the transthoracic approach also may be used.
  - The IAB catheter lies approximately 2 cm inferior to the subclavian artery and superior to the renal arteries. This position allows for maximum balloon effect without occlusion of other arterial supplies (Fig. 51-2).
  - The IAB should not fully occlude the aorta during inflation. It should be 85% to 90% occlusive.
  - Fluoroscopy may be used to aid in proper IAB catheter positioning, especially for patients with a tortuous aorta.
  - Correct catheter position is verified via radiography if fluoroscopy is not used during catheter insertion.
- The central lumen of many IAB catheters provides a means for monitoring aortic pressure.
- Timing methods of IABP therapy vary slightly from manufacturer to manufacturer. Using the traditional or conventional method, the IAB deflates before isovolumetric contraction. Using the real-time method, the inflation of the IAB extends throughout diastole.[5,6,15,21,24]
- The mechanics of the IABP control console vary from manufacturer to manufacturer.
- Specific information concerning controls, alarms, troubleshooting, and safety features is available from each manufacturer and should be read thoroughly by the nurse before use of the equipment.

EQUIPMENT

- IABP, gas supply
- ECG and arterial pressure monitoring supplies
- IAB catheter (size range 8 to 10 Fr for adults; balloon catheters vary in balloon volumes)
- IAB catheter insertion kit
- Antiseptic solution (e.g., 2% chlorhexidine-based preparation)
- Caps, goggles or face shields, masks, sterile gowns, gloves, and drapes
- Sterile dressing supplies

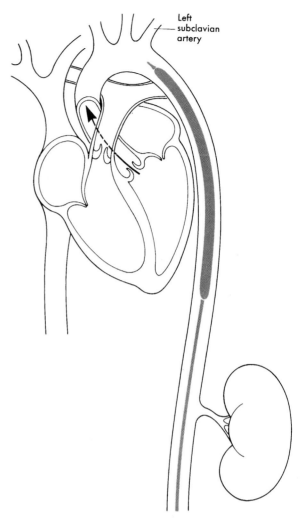

FIGURE 51-2 Intraaortic balloon (IAB) positioned in the descending thoracic aorta, just below the left subclavian artery but above the renal artery. *(From Quaal S.J. [1993]. Comprehensive Intraaortic Balloon Counterpulsation, 2nd ed. St. Louis: Mosby-Year Book.)*

- O-silk suture on a cutting needle, used to suture the catheter to the skin
- Number 11 scalpel, used for skin entry
- 1% lidocaine without epinephrine, one 30-ml vial
- Stopcocks, one 2-way and one 3-way
- One Luer-Lok plug
- 500 ml normal saline with 1000 units of heparin or the flush solution recommended according to institution standards
- Single-pressure transducer system (see Procedure 75)

  Additional equipment to have available depending on patient status includes the following:
- Analgesics and sedatives as prescribed
- Lead apron (needed if procedure is performed using fluoroscopy)
- Prescribed intravenous (IV) solutions
- Emergency medications and resuscitation equipment
- Vasopressors as prescribed
- Antibiotics as prescribed
- Heparin infusion or dextran if prescribed

PATIENT AND FAMILY EDUCATION

- Assess patient and family understanding of IABP therapy and the reason for its use. ➤*Rationale:* Clarification or reinforcement of information is an expressed family need during times of stress and anxiety.
- Explain the standard care to the patient and family, including the insertion procedure, IABP sounds, frequency of assessment, alarms, dressings, need for immobility of the affected extremity, expected length of therapy, and parameters for discontinuation of therapy. ➤*Rationale:* Encourages the patient and family to ask questions and voice specific concerns about the procedure.
- After catheter removal, instruct the patient to report any warm or wet feeling on the leg and any dizziness or lightheadedness. ➤*Rationale:* Indicative of bleeding at the insertion site.

PATIENT ASSESSMENT AND PREPARATION

Patient Assessment

- Assess the patient's medical history, specifically related to competency of the aortic valve, aortic disease, or peripheral vascular disease. ➤*Rationale:* Provides baseline data regarding cardiac functioning and identifies contraindications to IABP therapy.
- Assess the patient's cardiovascular, hemodynamic, peripheral vascular, and neurovascular status. ➤*Rationale:* Provides baseline data.
- Assess the extremity for the intended IAB catheter placement for the quality and strength of the femoral, popliteal, dorsalis pedal, and posterior tibial pulses.
- Assess the ankle/arm index as follows:
  - ❖ Record the brachial systolic pressure with a Doppler signal.
  - ❖ Locate the posterior tibial or dorsalis pedalis pulse with a Doppler signal.
  - ❖ Apply the blood pressure cuff around the ankle, above the maleolus.
  - ❖ Inflate the cuff to 20 mm Hg above the brachial systolic pressure.
  - ❖ Note the reappearance of the Doppler signal as the cuff deflates.
  - ❖ Divide the ankle systolic pressure by the brachial systolic pressure to determine the ankle/arm index (normal is 0.8-1.2).[11] ➤*Rationale:* The IAB catheter will be inserted into the vasculature of the extremity

exhibiting the best perfusion. Provides baseline data related to peripheral blood flow, which may be compromised by the IAB.

- Assess the patient's current laboratory profile, including complete blood count (CBC), platelet count, prothrombin time (PT), partial thromboplastin time (PTT), bleeding time, and International Normalized Ratio (INR). ➤*Rationale:* Baseline coagulation studies are helpful in determining the risk for bleeding. Platelet function may be affected by the mechanical trauma from balloon inflation and deflation.
- Assess for signs and symptoms of cardiac failure requiring IABP therapy, including the following:
  - ❖ Unstable angina
  - ❖ Altered mental status
  - ❖ Heart rate greater than 110 beats per minute
  - ❖ Dysrhythmias
  - ❖ Systolic blood pressure less than 90 mm Hg
  - ❖ Mean arterial pressure (MAP) less than 70 mm Hg with vasopressor support
  - ❖ Cardiac index less than 2.4[1]
  - ❖ Pulmonary artery wedge pressure (PAWP) greater than 18 mm Hg
  - ❖ Decreased mixed venous oxygen saturation (Svo_2)
  - ❖ Inadequate peripheral perfusion
  - ❖ Urine output less than 0.5 ml/kg per hour

  ➤*Rationale:* Physical signs and symptoms result from the heart's inability to adequately contract and from inadequate coronary or systemic perfusion.

Patient Preparation

- Ensure that the patient and family understand preprocedural teaching. Answer questions as they arise, and reinforce information as needed. ➤*Rationale:* Evaluates and reinforces understanding of previously taught information.
- Validate that the informed consent form has been signed. ➤*Rationale:* Protects the rights of the patient and makes a competent decision possible for the patient; however, under emergency circumstances, time may not allow the form to be signed.
- Validate the patency of central and peripheral intravenous access. ➤*Rationale:* Central access is needed for vasopressor administration; peripheral access is needed for fluid administration.
- Place the patient in a supine position and prepare the intended insertion site with an antiseptic solution. ➤*Rationale:* Prepares the intended access site and positions the patient for IAB insertion.

Procedure for Assisting With IAB Catheter Insertion

Steps	Rationale	Special Considerations
1. Wash hands and don caps, goggles or face shields, masks, sterile gowns, and gloves for all health care personnel involved in the procedure.	Reduces the transmission of microorganisms and body secretions; standard precautions.	
2. Turn on the helium gas.	Activates the gas driving the balloon pump.	Follow the manufacturer's recommendations.
3. Sedate the patient as needed; the affected extremity may need to be restrained.	Movement of the lower extremity may inhibit insertion of the catheter or contribute to catheter kinking once the IAB is in place.	A knee immobilizer or a sheet placed over the affected leg and tucked in may minimize movement of the affected leg.
4. Establish ECG input to the IABP console and obtain an ECG configuration with optimal R wave amplitude and absence of artifact. Indirect ECG input can be obtained via "slave" of the bedside ECG to the IABP console.	The R wave is the preferred trigger signal from which the IABP can reference systole and diastole and therefore establish inflation and deflation points.	A secondary ECG source is desirable in the event of lead disconnection or loss of trigger. Review the manufacturer's instructions for selecting the appropriate trigger control. If the patient has a pacemaker, the trigger should be set to reject the pacemaker artifact.
5. Assist with placement of hemodynamic monitoring lines if they are not already present.	Hemodynamic monitoring is necessary for assessment and management of the patient requiring IABP therapy.	A radial arterial line is commonly inserted. The arterial line tracing is used to assess and optimize timing and also may be used as a trigger source.
6. Complete the IABP console preparation. Refer to the instruction manual.	Ensures adequate functioning of the IABP device.	Models of the pump console vary. Review of manufacturer's instructions is recommended.
7. Remove the IAB catheter from the sterile packing and place the catheter and insertion tray on the sterile field.	Makes supplies available while maintaining sterility. Select the most appropriate size of balloon catheter. Most adult balloons are 40 ml in size. However, smaller balloon volumes (30 to 34 ml) are commonly placed in adults 5 ft 4 in and under, whereas larger balloon volumes (50 ml) are commonly placed in adults 6 ft and taller.	Catheters vary in balloon volumes. An adequate volume is necessary to achieve optimal hemodynamic effects from IABP therapy.
8. Administer a heparin bolus before arterial puncture, if prescribed.	Anticoagulation may decrease the incidence of thromboemboli related to the indwelling IAB catheter.	Systemic anticoagulation may not be used in all patients.[33]
9. Attach the supplied one-way valve to the Luer tip of the distal end of the balloon lumen.	Creates a device for air removal from the balloon catheter.	Maintains the wrap of the balloon for insertion.
10. Pull back slowly on the syringe until all the air is aspirated.	Removes air from the balloon, creating a vacuum.	
11. Disconnect the syringe only.	Prevents air entry back into the balloon.	Leave the one-way valve in place.

Procedure continues on the following page

Procedure **for Assisting With IAB Catheter Insertion**—*Continued*

Steps	Rationale	Special Considerations
12. Lubricate the IAB catheter with sterile saline.	Decreases "drag" on the catheter during insertion.	
13. The inner lumen of the IAB catheter should be flushed with heparinized saline before insertion.	Removes air from the central lumen.	If the catheter is not flushed before insertion, allow the backflow of arterial blood before connection to the flush system.
14. Assist with the introducer sheath or dilator assembly and insertion.	Prepares for balloon catheter entry.	Some IABs are inserted without a sheath. If the IAB is inserted via the sheathless method, only the dilator will be used.[10]
15. Assist with balloon catheter insertion.	Catheter placement is a necessary part of IAB setup.	
16. Assist with removal of the one-way valve according to manufacturer's recommendations.	Releases the vacuum and readies the balloon for counterpulsation.	
17. If the inner lumen of a double-lumen catheter is used to monitor arterial pressure, attach a three-way stopcock with a continuous heparinized flush and transducer to the monitor. Set the alarms.	Monitors arterial pressure.	The inner lumen, if used, must be attached to an alarm system because undetected disconnection could result in life-threatening hemorrhage. Refer to your institution's policy in regard to use of a heparinized flush system. Note that the proximal tip of the inner lumen used for arterial pressure monitoring is at the level of the left subclavian artery, NOT at the aortic arch; therefore this is NOT the same location as a "central" line placed at the aortic root.[25,26]
18. Aviod fast flush and blood sampling from the central aortic lumen.	Air may enter the system during fast flush and also during blood sampling, resulting in air emboli.	Some manufacturers and institutions recommend hourly manual flush of central lumen lines. If fast flush is required, ensure that the IABP is on standby (not pumping) during the flush. However, the risk of air embolus entry or dislodging a thrombus at the lumen tip is a major concern. Refer to your institution's policy in regard to fast flush or manual flushing of central lumen catheters.
19. Attach the balloon-lumen tubing to the IABP console.	Attachment is necessary because the console programs and operates balloon counterpulsation.	
20. Follow steps for timing, troubleshooting, and patient monitoring.	Provides for appropriate operation of counterpulsation.	Many IABP consoles have features for automatic timing. Refer to specific manufacturer instructions.
21. Level the air-fluid interface of the stopcock and zero the hemodynamic monitoring system.[23,27]	Ensures accurate arterial pressure measurement.	Refer to specific manufacturer instructions.

Procedure for Assisting With IAB Catheter Insertion—*Continued*

Steps	Rationale	Special Considerations
22. Obtain a portable chest x-ray as soon as possible.	Correct IAB catheter position must be confirmed to prevent complications associated with the interference of the arterial blood supply.	If fluoroscopy is used for insertion of the catheter, an x-ray immediately after placement is not necessary.
23. Apply a sterile dressing to the catheter insertion site.	Allows for aseptic management.	
24. Remove and discard personal protective equipment, and wash hands.	Reduces the transmission of microorganisms; standard precautions.	

Procedure for Timing of the IABP

Steps	Rationale	Special Considerations
1. Select an ECG lead that optimizes the R wave.	The R wave is usually used to trigger the balloon.	An alternate trigger can also be used if necessary.
2. Time the IABP using the arterial waveform.	The arterial waveform assists in identifying accurate IAB inflation and deflation.	Refer to specific manufacturer instructions for automatic timing.
3. Set the IABP frequency to the every-other-beat setting (1:2, or 50%) (Fig. 51-3).	Comparison can be made between the assisted and unassisted arterial waveforms.	
4. Inflation A. Identify the dicrotic notch of the assisted systolic waveform (see Fig. 51-3).	The dicrotic notch represents closure of the aortic valve.	
B. Adjust inflation later to expose the dicrotic notch of the unassisted systolic waveform.	Identifies the landmark for accurate inflation.	
C. Slowly adjust inflation earlier until the dicrotic notch disappears and a sharp V wave forms (see Fig. 51-3).	Balloon augmentation should occur after the aortic valve closes.[24]	A sharp V wave may not be seen in patients with low systemic vascular resistance.

Procedure continues on the following page

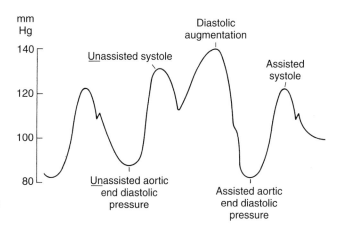

FIGURE 51-3 1:2 Intraaortic balloon pump frequency. *(From Datascope Corp., Montvale, New Jersey.)*

Procedure   for Timing of the IABP—*Continued*

Steps	Rationale	Special Considerations
D. Compare the augmented pressure with the patient's unassisted systolic pressure.	Balloon augmentation should be equal to or greater than the patient's unassisted systolic blood pressure.	If balloon augmentation is less than the patient's systolic pressure, consider the possibility that the balloon is positioned too low, the patient is hypovolemic or tachycardic, or the balloon volume is set too low.[19]
E. Adjust inflation if needed.	Necessary to achieve optimal diastolic augmentation.	Timing of inflation will vary slightly depending on the location of the arterial line. Radial: Inflate 40 to 50 ms before the dicrotic notch. Femoral: Inflate 120 ms before the dicrotic notch (Fig. 51-4). Because of the distance[24] of the radial and femoral arteries from the actual closure of the aortic valve, the arterial waveforms are delayed.[26]

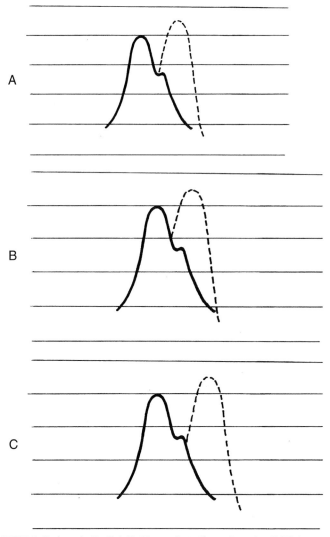

FIGURE 51-4 IABP inflation. **A,** Radial. **B,** Femoral. **C,** Central aortic. *IABP,* intraaortic balloon pump.

Procedure for Timing of the IABP—*Continued*

Steps	Rationale	Special Considerations
5. Deflation A. Identify the assisted and unassisted aortic end-diastolic pressures and the assisted and unassisted systolic pressures. (see Fig. 51-3).[34]	These landmarks are important in determining accurate IAB deflation.	IABP frequency is set at 1:2 (50%).
B. Set the balloon to deflate so that the balloon-assisted aortic end-diastolic pressure is as low as possible (lower than the patient's unassisted diastolic pressure) while still maintaining optimal diastolic augmentation and not impeding on the next systole (the assisted systole).	The assisted systolic pressure will be less than the unassisted systolic pressure as a result of a decrease in afterload, thus reducing the myocardial workload.[15]	Reduction of afterload will decrease the energy required by the heart during systole. It is important to achieve afterload reduction without diminishing diastolic augmentation.
6. Set the IABP frequency to 1:1 (100%) (Fig. 51-5).	Ensures that each heartbeat is assisted.	
7. Assess timing every hour, and whenever the heart rate changes by more than 10 beats per minute and when the rhythm changes.	Inappropriate timing prevents effective IABP therapy.	The computerized IABPs vary in the degree of adjustment to changes in heart rate and rhythm. Refer to the specific manufacturer's guidelines for automatic timing adjustment information.
8. Assess and intervene to correct inappropriate timing. A. Problem: **Early inflation** (Fig. 51-6). Intervention: **Move inflation later.**	Ensures accurate timing and optimal functioning of the IABP. Inflation occurs before closure of the aortic valve, leading to premature aortic valve closure, increased left ventricular volume, and decreased stroke volume.	

Procedure continues on the following page

Timing Errors
Early Inflation

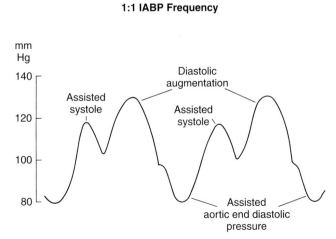

FIGURE 51-5 Correct intraaortic balloon pump timing (1:1). *(From Datascope Corp., Montvale, New Jersey.)*

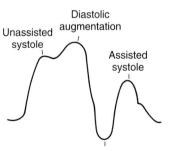

Inflation of the IAB prior to aortic valve closure

Waveform Characteristics:
• Inflation of IAB prior to dicrotic notch
• Diastolic augmentation encroaches onto systole (may be unable to distinguish)

Physiologic Effects:
• Potential premature closure of aortic valve
• Potential increased in LVEDV and LVEDP or PCWP
• Increased left ventricular wall stress or afterload
• Aortic regurgitation
• Increased MVO_2 demand

FIGURE 51-6 Early inflation. *(From Datascope Corp., Montvale, New Jersey.)*

Procedure for Timing of the IABP—*Continued*

Steps	Rationale	Special Considerations
B. Problem: **Late inflation** (Fig. 51-7). Intervention: **Adjust inflation earlier.**	A delay in inflation leads to a decrease in coronary artery perfusion.	
C. Problem: **Early deflation** (Fig. 51-8). Intervention: **Adjust deflation later.**	Deflation occurs before the aortic valve opens, leading to decreased balloon augmentation and less or no afterload reduction; coronary artery perfusion may also be decreased.	Note the sharp diastolic wave after augmentation and the increase in the assisted systolic pressure.
D. Problem: **Late deflation** (Fig. 51-9). Intervention: **Adjust deflation earlier.**	Deflation occurs after the aortic valve has opened, leading to an increase in the aortic end-diastolic pressure and an increase in afterload.	Note the delayed diastolic wave after augmentation and the diminished assisted systole. If using the real-time method of timing, late deflation is not identified by changes in the aortic end-diastolic pressure but is identified by a diminished assisted systolic pressure, an increase in heart rate, an increase in filling pressures, and a decrease in cardiac output and cardiac index.[5,6,10,14,15]

Timing Errors
Late Inflation

Inflation of the IAB markedly after closure of the aortic valve

Waveform Characteristics:
• Inflation of the IAB after the dicrotic notch
• Absence of sharp V
• Sub-optimal diastolic augmentation

Physiologic Effects:
• Sub-optimal coronary artery perfusion

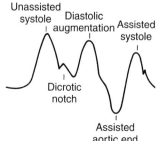

FIGURE 51-7 Late inflation. (*From Datascope Corp., Montvale, New Jersey.*)

Timing Errors
Early Deflation

Premature deflation of the IAB during the diastolic phase

Waveform Characteristics:
• Deflation of IAB is seen as a sharp drop following diastolic augmentation
• Sub-optimal diastolic augmentation
• Assisted aortic end diastolic pressure may be equal to or less than the unassisted aortic end diastolic pressure
• Assisted systolic pressure may rise

Physiologic Effects:
• Sub-optimal coronary perfusion
• Potential for retrograde coronary and carotid blood flow
• Angina may occur as a result of retrograde coronary blood flow
• Sub-optimal afterload reduction
• Increased MVO_2 demand

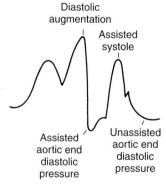

FIGURE 51-8 Early deflation. (*From Datascope Corp., Montvale, New Jersey.*)

Timing Errors
Late Deflation

Deflation of the IAB late in
diastolic phase as aortic valve
is beginning to open

Waveform Characteristics:
• Assisted aortic end-diastolic
  pressure may be equal to
  or greater than the
  unassisted aortic end
  diastolic pressure
• Rate of rise of assisted
  systole is prolonged
• Diastolic augmentation
  may appear widened

Physiologic Effects:
• Afterload reduction is essentially
  absent
• Increased MVO$_2$ consumption due
  to the left ventricle ejecting against
  a greater resistance and a prolonged
  isovolumetric contraction phase
• IAB may impede left ventricular
  ejection and increase the afterload

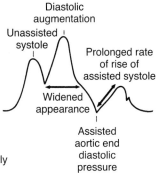

FIGURE 51-9 Late deflation. *(From Datascope Corp., Montvale, New Jersey.)*

Procedure for Balloon Pressure Waveform

Steps	Rationale	Special Considerations
1. Determine whether the IABP console has a balloon pressure waveform.	Helium is shuttled in and out of the IAB catheter, and the balloon pressure waveform represents this movement.	Refer to the specific manufacturer instructions regarding the balloon pressure waveform.
2. Assess the balloon pressure waveform.	Reflects pressure that is in the IAB.	
3. Determine whether the balloon pressure waveform is normal (Fig. 51-10). A normal balloon pressure waveform:	A normal balloon pressure waveform reflects that the IAB is inflating and deflating properly.[22]	
A. Has a fill pressure (baseline pressure)[16] slightly above zero.	Reflects pressure in the tubing between the IAB and the IABP driving mechanism.	

Procedure continues on the following page

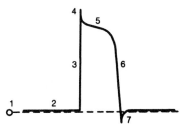

FIGURE 51-10 Normal balloon gas waveform. **1,** zero baseline; **2,** fill pressure; **3,** rapid inflation; **4,** peak inflation artifact; **5,** plateau pressure or inflation plateau pressure; **6,** rapid deflation; **7,** peak deflation pressure and return to fill pressure. *(From Arrow International.)*

Procedure for **Balloon Pressure Waveform**—*Continued*

Steps	Rationale	Special Considerations
B. Has a sharp upstroke.	Occurs as gas inflates the IAB catheter.	
C. Has peak inflation artifact.	This overshoot pressure artifact is caused by gas pressure in the pneumatic line.[2]	
D. Has a pressure plateau.	This plateau is created as the IAB remains inflated during diastole.	The plateau indicates the length of time of inflation as well as whether full inflation (volume) has been delivered to the IAB. If there is no plateau pressure, the IAB may not be fully inflated.
E. Has a rapid deflation.	Gas is quickly shuttled from the IAB.	
F. Has a negative deflection below baseline, then returns to baseline.	Gas returns to the IABP console, then stabilizes within the system.	
4. Compare the balloon pressure waveform with the arterial pressure waveform (Fig. 51-11). Note the similarity in the width of the balloon pressure waveform and the augmented arterial waveform.[16]	Demonstrates the relationship between the balloon pressure waveform and the arterial waveform. Reflects the effect of the balloon on the augmented arterial pressure.	
5. Determine whether the balloon pressure waveform meets the description above.	Abnormal balloon pressure waveforms may indicate problems with the IAB or the IABP console.	Refer to the specific manufacturer instructions regarding troubleshooting abnormal balloon pressure waveforms.

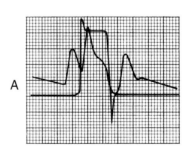

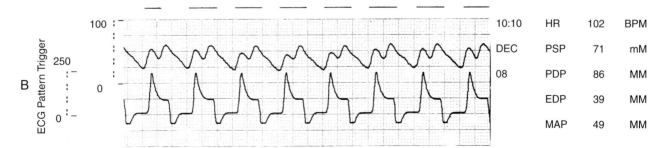

FIGURE 51-11 **A,** Balloon pressure waveform superimposed on the arterial pressure waveform. **B,** Actual recording of an arterial pressure waveform (*top*) and balloon gas waveform (*bottom*) from a balloon-pumped patient. (*From Arrow International.*)

Procedure for Troubleshooting

Steps	Rationale	Special Considerations
1. Atrial Fibrillation A. Set the IABP to inflate and deflate the majority of the patient's beats.	IABP therapy will not be 100% effective during atrial fibrillation (AF) because of the irregular rhythm.	The underlying cause of the AF should be treated. IABPs will automatically deflate the balloon on the R wave. Use the atrial fibrillation trigger mode or the R wave deflation mode. The real-time method of timing may track dysrhythmias better than traditional or conventional IABP timing.[5,15]
2. Tachycardia A. Change the IABP frequency to 1:2.	Because diastole is shortened during tachycardia, the balloon augmentation time is shortened. Pumping every other beat may improve MAP.	The underlying cause of the tachycardia should be treated.
3. Asystole A. Switch the trigger to arterial pressure.	This trigger can be used if there is a rise of at least 15 mm Hg in arterial pressure.	Refer to the manufacturer's manual for this information because the minimum mm Hg needed to use this feature varies.
B. Set inflation to provide diastolic augmentation; set deflation to occur before the upstroke of the next systole. *(Level IV: Limited clinical studies to support recommendations.)*	Programs the machine for appropriate preset timing.	Preliminary research suggests that when used during cardiopulmonary resuscitation, IAB counterpulsation increases cerebral and coronary perfusion.[3]
C. If chest compressions do not provide an adequate trigger: • Turn to internal trigger.	The internal trigger will keep the IAB catheter moving so that clot formation is minimized.	
• Set the rate at 60 to 80 beats per minute.	Maintains consistent movement of IAB catheter.	
• Set the IABP frequency to 1:2.	1:2 frequency is adequate to prevent thrombus formation on the IAB catheter.	
• Turn the balloon augmentation down to 50%.	Slight inflation and deflation of the IAB catheter will prevent clot formation.	
4. Ventricular Tachycardia or Ventricular Fibrillation A. Ensure that personnel are cleared from the patient and equipment before cardioverting or defibrillating.	Prevents the spread of energy to health care personnel. Maintains electrical safety.	
B. Cardiovert or defibrillate as necessary (see Procedures 36 and 37).	Attempts to convert the rhythm.	The IABP console is electrically isolated.
5. Loss of Vacuum or IABP Failure A. Check and tighten the connections on the pneumatic tubing.	A loose connection may contribute to a loss of vacuum.	
B. Check the compressor power source.	Ensures that power is available to drive the helium.	
C. Hand inflate and deflate the balloon every 5 minutes with half the total balloon volume if necessary.	Prevents clot formation along the dormant balloon.	
D. Change the IAB console.	Establishes a power source and effective IABP therapy.	

Procedure continues on the following page

Procedure for Troubleshooting—*Continued*

Steps	Rationale	Special Considerations
6. Suspected Balloon Perforation		
A. Observe for loss of augmentation.	Gas may be gradually leaking from the balloon catheter.	Always set the alarms so the alarm will sound if there is a drop of 10 mm Hg in diastolic augmentation.
B. Check for blood in the catheter tubing.	Blood in the tubing indicates that the balloon has perforated and that arterial blood is present.	It is possible for a balloon leak to be self-sealing as a result of the surface tension between the inside and the outside of the IAB membrane. This may be evidenced by the presence of dried blood in the catheter tubing. The dried blood may appear as a brownish, coffee-ground–like substance.
C. Assess for changes or lack of a normal balloon pressure waveform.	The balloon pressure waveform may be absent if the balloon is unable to retain gas, or the pressure plateau may gradually decrease if the IAB is leaking gas.	
7. Balloon Perforation		
A. Place the IABP on standby.	Prevents further IAB pumping and continued gas exchange.	Some IABP consoles will automatically shut off if a leak is detected. The IAB catheter should be removed within 15 to 30 minutes.
B. Clamp the IAB catheter.	Prevents arterial blood back-up.	
C. Disconnect the IAB catheter from the IABP console.	Prevents blood from backing up into the IABP console.	
D. Notify the physician.	The IAB catheter will need to be removed or replaced immediately.	If the IAB leak has sealed itself off, this may result in entrapment of the IAB in the vasculature. Surgical removal may be required.
E. Prepare for IAB catheter removal or replacement.	The IAB catheter should not lie dormant for longer than 30 minutes.	
F. Discontinue anticoagulation therapy.	Clotting will occur more readily if anticoagulation is stopped (necessary if removing the catheter).	

Procedure for Weaning and IAB Catheter Removal

Steps	Rationale	Special Considerations
1. Wash hands.	Reduces the transmission of microorganisms and body secretions; standard precautions.	
2. Assess clinical readiness for weaning.	Optimal clinical and hemodynamic parameters validate readiness for weaning.	Patient hemodynamic status should be optimal before weaning from IABP therapy. Signs of clinical readiness include the following: no angina, heart rate less than 110 beats per minute, absence of lethal or unstable dysrhythmias, MAP greater than 70 mm Hg with minimal or no

Procedure for Weaning and IAB Catheter Removal—*Continued*

Steps	Rationale	Special Considerations
		vasopressor support, PAWP less than 18 mm Hg, cardiac index greater than 2.4, mixed venous oxygen saturation between 60% and 80%, capillary refill less than 2 seconds, and urine output greater than 0.5 ml/kg/hr.
3. Change the assist ratio to 1:2 (50%), and monitor the patient's response for 1 to 6 hours or as noted per institution's protocol.	The length of time required to wean from IABP therapy depends on the hemodynamic response of the patient and the length of time the patient has received IABP therapy.[12,28]	
4. If hemodynamic parameters remain satisfactory, further change the ratio from 1:3 to 1:8 (depending on the patient and the balloon console assist frequencies, or as prescribed).	IABP consoles vary in assist ratios.	Refer to the institution's policy on weaning procedures.
5. Discontinue heparin or dextran 4 to 6 hours before IAB catheter removal, or reverse heparin with protamine (as prescribed) just before catheter removal.	This will decrease the likelihood of bleeding after balloon removal.	
6. Turn the IABP to standby or off.	Ensures deflation of the IAB catheter.	
7. Assist the physician or advanced practice nurse with removal of the percutaneous balloon.	Facilitates removal.	
8. Ensure that pressure is held on the insertion site for 30 to 45 minutes after the IAB catheter is withdrawn.	Decreases the incidence of bleeding and hematoma formation.	Ensure that hemostasis is obtained.
9. Assess the insertion site for signs of bleeding or hematoma formation before application of a sterile pressure dressing.	Assists in the detection of bleeding.	
10. Apply a pressure dressing to the insertion site for 2 to 4 hours.	Minimizes bleeding from the insertion site.	
11. Monitor vital signs and hemodynamic parameters every 15 minutes × 4, every 30 minutes × 2, then every hour as the patient's condition warrants.	Validates patient stability or identifies hemodynamic compromise.	
12. Assess the quality of perfusion to the decannulated extremity immediately after removal and every 1 hour × 2, then every 2 hours.	Removal of the IAB catheter may dislodge thrombi on the catheter and lead to arterial occlusion.	
13. Maintain immobility of the decannulated extremity and maintain bed rest with the head of the bed no greater than 30 degrees for 8 hours.	Promotes healing and decreases stress at the insertion site.	Follow institution standard.
14. Discard used supplies and wash hands.	Reduces the transmission of microorganisms and body secretions; standard precautions.	

Expected Outcomes

- Increased myocardial oxygen supply
- Decreased myocardial oxygen demands
- Increased cardiac output
- Increased tissue perfusion, including cerebral, renal, and peripheral circulation

Unexpected Outcomes

- Impaired perfusion to the extremity with the IAB catheter in place
- Balloon perforation
- Inappropriate IAB placement
- Pain
- Bleeding or coagulation disorders
- Aortic dissection
- Infection

Patient Monitoring and Care

Steps	Rationale	Reportable Conditions
		These conditions should be reported if they persist despite nursing interventions.
1. Perform systematic cardiovascular, peripheral vascular, and hemodynamic assessments every 15 to 60 minutes as patient status requires.		
A. Level of consciousness	Assesses for adequate cerebral perfusion; thrombi may develop and dislodge during IABP therapy; the IAB may migrate, decreasing blood flow to the carotid arteries.	• Change in level of consciousness
B. Vital signs and pulmonary artery pressures	Demonstrates effectiveness of IABP therapy.	• Unstable vital signs • Significant changes in hemodynamic pressures • Lack of response to IABP therapy
C. Arterial catheter and IAB waveforms	Ensures effectiveness of IABP timing and therapy.	• Difficulty achieving effective IABP therapy
D. Cardiac output, cardiac index, and systemic vascular resistance determinations	Demonstrates effectiveness of IABP therapy.	• Abnormal cardiac output, cardiac index, and systemic vascular resistance values
E. Circulation to extremities	Validates adequate peripheral perfusion. If reportable conditions are found, they may indicate catheter or embolus obstruction of perfusion to the extremity. Specifically, decreased perfusion to the left arm may indicate misplacement of the IAB catheter.[3]	• Capillary refill greater than 2 seconds • Diminished or absent pulses (e.g., antecubital, radial, popliteal, tibial, pedal) • Color pale, mottled, or cyanotic • Diminished or absent sensation • Pain • Diminished or absent movement • Cool or cold to touch
F. Urine output	Validates adequate perfusion to the kidneys.	• Urine output less than 0.5 ml/kg/hr
2. Assess heart and lung sounds every 4 hours and as needed.	Abnormal heart and lung sounds may indicate the need for additional treatment. *Special Note:* When the patient's condition permits, place the IABP on standby to accurately auscultate heart and lung sounds, because IABP therapy creates extraneous sounds and impairs heart and lung sound assessment.	• Abnormal heart and lung sounds
3. Maintain head of bed at less than 45 degrees.	Prevents kinking of the IAB catheter and migration of the catheter.	

Patient Monitoring and Care—*Continued*

Steps	Rationale	Reportable Conditions
4. Monitor for signs of inappropriate IAB placement.	The IAB catheter may be positioned too high or too low, thus occluding the left subclavian, celiac, inferior or superior mesenteric, or renal arteries.	• Diminished or absent antecubital or radial pulse • Color of left arm pale, mottled, cyanotic • Diminished or absent sensation to the left arm • Dampened radial arterial pressure waveform • Diminished or absent movement of the left arm • Diminished or absent bowel sounds • Increased abdominal girth • Abdomen firm to touch • Tympany • Abdominal pain • Decreased urine output, less than 0.5 ml/kg/hr • Increased urine osmolality • Increased blood urea nitrogen or creatinine • Reduced IABP augmentation
5. Monitor for signs of balloon perforation.	In the event of balloon perforation, a very small amount of helium will be released into the aorta, potentially causing an embolic event.	• Blood or brown flecks in tubing • Loss of IABP augmentation • Control console alarm activation (e.g., gas loss)
6. Maintain accurate IABP timing.	If timing is not accurate, cardiac output may decrease rather than increase.	
7. Log-roll patient every 2 hours. Prop pillows to support patient and to maintain alignment. Consider use of pressure-relief devices. *(Level V: Clinical studies in more than one or two different patient populations and situations to support recommendations.)*	Promotes comfort and skin integrity and prevents kinking of the IAB catheter. ***Special Note:*** Log rolling may not be tolerated in severely hemodynamically compromised patients; low-pressure beds are necessary for these patients. Low-pressure beds can decrease the occurrence of pressure ulcers in patients requiring IABP therapy.[4,5]	
8. Immobilize the cannulated extremity with a draw sheet tucked under the mattress or by using a soft ankle restraint or a knee immobilizer.	Prevents dislodgment and migration of the IAB catheter. ***Special Note:*** Assess skin integrity and perfusion distal to the restraint every hour.	
9. Initiate passive and active range-of-motion exercises every 2 hours to extremities that can be mobilized.	Prevents venous stasis and muscle atrophy.	
10. Assess the area around the IAB catheter insertion site every 2 hours and as needed for evidence of hematoma or bleeding.	IAB catheter inflation and deflation traumatize red blood cells and platelets. Anticoagulation therapy may alter hemoglobin and hematocrit and coagulation values.[33]	• Bleeding at insertion site • Hematoma at insertion site

Procedure continues on the following page

Patient Monitoring and Care—*Continued*

Steps	Rationale	Reportable Conditions
11. Maintain anticoagulation as prescribed; monitor coagulation studies.	Prophylactic anticoagulation may be used to prevent thrombi and emboli development.	• Abnormal coagulation studies
12. Monitor patient for systemic evidence of bleeding or coagulation disorders.	Hematologic and coagulation profiles may be altered as a result of blood loss during balloon insertion, anticoagulation, and platelet dysfunction as a result of mechanical trauma by balloon inflation and deflation.[33]	• Bleeding from IAB insertion site • Bleeding from incisions or mucous membranes • Petechiae or ecchymoses • Guaiac-positive nasogastric aspirate or stool • Hematuria • Decreased hemoglobin or hematocrit • Decreased filling pressures • Increased heart rate • Retroperitoneal hematoma • Pain in the lower abdomen, flank, thigh, or lower extremity

13. Change the IAB catheter site dressing every 24 hours.
  A. Cleanse the site with normal saline.
  B. Cleanse the site with an antiseptic solution.
  C. Allow time for the antiseptic solution to dry.
  D. Apply a sterile dressing; label with date, time, and nurse's initials.
	Decreases the incidence of infection and allows an opportunity for site assessment.	• Signs or symptoms of infection

14. Assess for balloon entrapment.[8,29,31]	Entrapment is the inability to remove the IAB because of the presence of a large hardened mass of blood within the IAB. As a result, the IAB is entrapped somewhere in the aortoiliac system or possibly in the abdominal aorta. A pinhole leak or tear in the IAB allows blood to be sucked into the IAB, and a clot forms. Blood dries/becomes dehydrated because of the repeated passage of helium over the IAB.	• Flecks of blood within the catheter or bright red blood
15. Assess for balloon migration.	The IAB should be positioned 2 cm below the left subclavian artery and just above the renal arteries. If the IAB migrates proximally, it may occlude the subclavian or carotid arteries. If the IAB migrates too low, it could occlude the renal or mesenteric arteries.	• Signs of possible subclavian artery occlusion; unequal or absent radial pulse and dampening or loss of the arterial pressure waveform in the ipsilateral radial artery. • Signs of possible carotid artery occlusion include change in level of consciousness and orientation or unilateral neurological deficit. • Signs of renal artery occlusion: oliguria or anuria, back or flank pain, nausea, and anorexia.

Patient Monitoring and Care—*Continued*

Steps	Rationale	Reportable Conditions
		• Signs of mesenteric occlusion: abdominal pain, diarrhea, nausea, and decreased bowel sounds.
16. Identify parameters that demonstrate clinical readiness to wean from IABP therapy.	Close observation of the patient's tolerance to weaning procedures is necessary to ensure that the body's oxygen demands can be met. The presence of these reportable conditions indicates that consideration should be given to weaning the patient from the IABP.	• No angina • Heart rate less than 110 beats per minute • Absence of lethal or unstable dysrhythmias • MAP greater than 70 mm Hg with little or no vasopressor support • PAWP less than 18 mm Hg • Cardiac index greater than 2.4 • SvO_2 between 60% and 80% • Capillary refill less than 2 seconds • Urine output greater than 0.5 ml/kg/hr

Documentation

Documentation should include the following:

- Patient and family education
- Insertion of the IAB catheter (including size of catheter used and balloon volume)
- Peripheral pulses and neurovascular assessment of the affected extremity
- Any difficulties with insertion
- IABP frequency
- Patient response to the procedure and to IABP therapy
- Confirmation of placement (e.g., chest x-ray)
- Insertion site assessment
- Hemodynamic status
- IABP pressures (unassisted end-diastolic pressure, unassisted systolic pressure, balloon augmented pressure, assisted systolic pressure, assisted end-diastolic pressure, and MAP)
- Occurrence of unexpected outcomes
- Additional nursing interventions taken

References

1. Anderson, R.D., et al. (1997). Use of intra-aortic balloon counterpulsation in patients presenting with cardiogenic shock: Observations from the GUSTO-I study. *J Am Coll Cardiol,* 30, 708-15.
2. Arafa, O.E., et al. (2000). Intra-aortic balloon pumping for predominantly right ventricular failure after heart transplantation. *Ann Thoracic Surgery,* 70, 1587-93.
3. Arafa, O.E., et al. (1999). Vascular complications of the intra-aortic balloon pump in patients undergoing open heart operations: 15-year experience. *Ann Thoracic Surgery* 67, 645-51.
4. Brodie, B.R., et al. (1999). Intra-aortic balloon counterpulsation before primary percutaneous transluminal coronary angioplasty reduces catheterization laboratory events in high-risk patients with acute myocardial infarction. *Am J Cardiol,* 84, 18-23.
5. Cadwell, C.A., and Tyson, G. (1993). Real timing. In: Quaal S., ed. *Comprehensive Intraaortic Balloon Counterpulsation.* 2nd ed. St. Louis: Mosby-Yearbook.
6. Cadwell, C.A., Hobson, K.S., and Petis, S. (1996). Clinical observations with real timing. *Crit Care Nurs Clin North Am,* 8, 357-70.
7. Castelli, P., et al. (2001). Intra-aortic balloon counterpulsation outcome in cardiac surgical patients. *J Cardiovas Vasc Anesth,* 15, 700-03.
8. Chaus, N., et al. (2000). *Intra-aortic Balloon Counterpulsation in High-Risk Coronary Angioplasty.* Presented at First World Conference on Intra-Aortic Balloon Counterpulsation. Athens, Greece.
9. Cook, L., et al. (1999). Intra-Aortic balloon pump complications: A five-year retrospective study of 283 patients. *Heart and Lung,* 28, 195-202.
10. Diver, D. (1993). Sheathless balloon insertion. In Quaal S.J., ed. *Comprehensive Intra-Aortic Balloon Counterpulsation.* St. Louis: Mosby-Yearbook.
11. Flewelling-Goran, S. (1989). Vascular complications of the patient undergoing intra-aortic balloon pumping. *Crit Care Nurs Clin N Am,* 459, 459-68.
12. Hanlon-Pena, P.M., Ziegler, J.C., and Stewart, R. (1996). Management of the intra-aortic balloon pump patient. *Crit Care Nurs Clin N Am,* 8, 389-408.
13. Hochman, J.S., et al. (2000). Cardiogenic shock complicating acute myocardial infarction-etiologies. Management and outcome: A report from the SHOCK trial registry. Should we emergently revascularize occluded coronaries for cardiogenic shock? *J Am Coll Cardiol,* 36(3A), 1663-10.
14. Intra-aortic balloon pumps. (1997). *Health Devices,* 26, 184-216.
15. Joseph, D.L., and Spadoni, S.M. (1996). Timing waveform analysis. *Crit Care Nurs Clin N Am,* 8, 349-56.

16. Kalina, J. (1993). Use of the balloon pressure waveform in conjunction with the augmented arterial pressure waveform. In Quaal S.J., ed. *Comprehensive Intra-Aortic Balloon Counterpulsation*. 2nd ed. St. Louis: Mosby-Yearbook.

17. Kang, N., Edwards, M., and Larbalestier, R. (2001). Preoperative intra-aortic balloon pumps in high risk patients undergoing open heart surgery. *Ann Thoracic Surgery*, 72, 54-7.

18. Mouloupolos, S.D. (2001). Intra-aortic balloon counterpulsation in the treatment of cardiogenic shock: hemodynamic effects and clinical challenges. *Cardiology Clinical Updates*. Available at: http://www.medscape.com/viewprogram607/pmt. Accessed May 24, 2001.

19. Pantalos, G.M., et al. (1999). Estimation of timing errors for intra-aortic balloon pump use in pediatric patients. *ASIA OJ*, 45, 166-71.

20. Prunler, F., et al. (2000). *Intra-Aortic Balloon Counterpulsation (IABP) in High-Risk Acute Myocardial Infarction (abstract)*. Presented at First World Conference on Intra-Aortic Balloon Counterpulsation. Athens, Greece.

21. Quaal, S.J. (2000). Conventional timing using the arterial pressure waveform. In Quaal, S.J., ed. *Comprehensive Intra-Aortic Balloon Counterpulsation*. 2nd ed. St. Louis: Mosby-Yearbook.

22. Quaal, S.J. (1996). Caring for the intra-aortic balloon pump patient: Most frequently asked questions. *Crit Care Nurs Clin N Am*, 8, 471-76.

23. Quaal, S.J. (1993). Interactive hemodynamics of IABC. *Comprehensive Intra-Aortic Balloon Counterpulsation*. St. Louis: Mosby-Yearbook, 118-43.

24. Quaal, S.J. (1997). Intra-aortic balloon pumping timing: An overview. *Critical Care Int*, January-February, 12-14.

25. Quaal, S.J. (1999). Nursing care of the intra-aortic balloon catheter's inner lumen. *Prog Cardiovasc Nursing*, Winter, 14, 11-13.

26. Quaal, S.J. (2001). Interpreting the arterial pressure waveform in the intra-aortic balloon pumped patient. *Prog Cardiovas Nursing*, 15, 116-18.

27. Quaal, S.J. (2000). Physiological and clinical analysis of the arterial pressure waveform in the IABP patient. *Can Perfusion Canadienne*, 10, 6-13.

28. Sitzer, V.A., and Atkins, P.J. *Developing and Implementing a Standard of Care for Intra-Aortic Balloon Counterpulsion*. (Unpublished ms.).

29. Stavarski, D.H. (1996). Complications of intra-aortic balloon pumping: Preventable or not preventable? *Crit Care Nurs Clin N Am*, 8, 409-21.

30. Spadoni, S. (2000). Preoperative intra-aortic balloon counterpulsation in high-risk coronary patients. *Can Perfusion Canadienne*, 10, 30-3.

31. Stone, G.W., Ohman, E., and Miller, M. (2003). Contemporary utilization and outcomes of intra-aortic balloon counterpulsation in acute myocardial infarction. *JACC*, 41, 1940-47.

32. Torchiana, D.F., et al. (1997). Intra-aortic balloon pumping for cardiac support; trends in practice and outcome. *J Thoracic & CV Surgery*, 114, 758-64.

33. Vanderheide, R.H., Thadhani, R., and Kufer, D.J. (1998). Association of thrombocytopenia with the use of intra-aortic balloon pumps. *Am J Med*, 105, 27-32.

34. Wojner, A.W. (1994). Assessing the five points of the intra-aortic balloon pump waveform. *Crit Care Nurs*, 14, 45-52.

Additional Readings

Bates, E.R., et al. (1998). The use of intra-aortic balloon counterpulsation as an adjunct to reperfusion therapy in cardiogenic shock. *J Cardiol*, 65(Suppl 1), S37-S42.

Berger, P.B., et al. (1997). Impact of an aggressive invasive catheterization and revascularization strategy on mortality in patients with cardiogenic shock in the Global Utilization of Streptokinase and Tissue Plasminogen Activator for Occluded Coronary Arteries (GUSTO-I) trial. An observational study. *Circulation*, 96, 122-27.

Blusch, T., et al. (1997). Vascular complications related to intra-aortic balloon counterpulsation: An analysis of ten years experience. *Thoracic Cardiovasc Surg*, 45, 55-9.

Christenson, J.T., et al. (1997). Evaluation of preoperative intra-aortic balloon pump support in high risk coronary patients. *Eur J Cardiothoracic Surg*, 11, 1097-1103.

Christenson, J.T., Schmuziber, M., and Simonet, F. (2001). Effective surgical management of high-risk coronary patients using preoperative intra-aortic balloon counterpulsation therapy. *Cardiovasc Surg*, 9, 383-90.

Garrett, K., and Grady, K.L. (2000). Intra-aortic balloon pumping through the common iliac artery: Management of the ambulatory intra-aortic balloon pump patient. *Prog Cardiovasc Nurs*, 15, 14-20.

Kovak, P.J., et al. (1997). Thombolysis plus aortic counterpulsation improved survival of patients who present to the community hospital with cardiogenic shock. *J Am Coll Cardiol*, 29, 454-58.

Low, R. (2003). Intra-aortic balloon counterpulsation in acute myocardial infarction: Too few or too many? *JACC*, 41, 1946-47.

Mertlich, G.B., et al. (1992). Effect of increased intra-aortic balloon pressure on catheter volume: Relationship to changing attitude. *Crit Care Med* 20, 297-303.

Ohman, E., and Hochman, J. (2001). Aortic counterpulsion in acute myocardial infarction: Physiologically important, but does the patient benefit? *Am Heart J*, 141, 889-92.

Talley, J.D., Ohman, E.M., and Mark, O.B. (1997). Economic implications of the prophylactic use of intra-aortic balloon counterpulsation in the setting of acute myocardial infarction. The Randomized IABP Study Group. *AM J Cardiol*, 79, S90-S94.

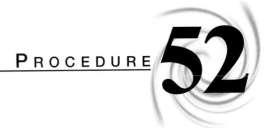

PROCEDURE **52**

External Counterpressure With Pneumatic Antishock Garments

PURPOSE: External counterpressure accomplished with a pneumatic antishock garment (PASG) is designed as a short-term therapy to increase blood pressure, stabilize bleeding, and function as an effective splint for lower extremity or pelvic fractures.

Denise M. Lawrence

PREREQUISITE NURSING KNOWLEDGE

- Knowledge of anatomy and physiology of the cardio-vascular and peripheral vascular systems is needed.
- Advanced cardiac life support knowledge and skills are needed.
- Clinical and technical competence related to use of the PASG is required.
- PASG is a short-term intervention used for patients experiencing acute trauma. PASG is used to control hemorrhage, increase blood pressure, and improve perfusion to the vital organs. PASG also functions as an effective splinting device for preventing blood loss, particularly when transport to definitive care is delayed.
- PASG may be used in the following situations:
  - ❖ Patients with hypotension caused by blood loss or loss of vascular tone
  - ❖ Patients with systolic blood pressure of less than 90 mm Hg
  - ❖ Patients with penetrating injuries of the lower abdomen and lower extremities when transport time exceeds 20 minutes
  - ❖ For compression and splinting of fractures or external wounds of the lower abdomen, pelvis, or lower extremities when transport time exceeds 20 minutes
- Controversy exists in the medical community regarding the clinical efficacy of PASG in decreasing mortality and increasing outcomes.
- Contraindications for PASG include the following:
  - ❖ Pulmonary edema
  - ❖ Congestive heart failure

- ❖ Impaled foreign body of the lower torso
- ❖ Pregnancy
- ❖ Abdominal wounds with evisceration
- ❖ Tension pneumothorax
- ❖ Cardiac tamponade
- ❖ Head injuries with increased intracranial pressure
- ❖ Diaphragmatic rupture
- Application of pneumatic counterpressure to the abdomen and legs causes pneumatic compression to the vessels. This compression increases the pressure outside the vessel wall, increasing the peripheral vascular resistance. In addition, decreasing perfusion of the capillary beds of the lower extremities with pneumatic counterpressure increases the blood pressure.
- PASG has three independently controlled compartments, each with its own high-pressure tubing and pressure control valve. The garment is made of heavy-duty nylon or polyvinyl. PASG is manufactured in sizes appropriate for adults and children older than age 6 years. Velcro fasteners are used to secure the PASG to the abdomen and legs.
- Each compartment is connected to separate tubing for airflow and pressurization. Each individual compartment tube is interconnected to a single connection that is attached to a foot pump. Each tube contains two valves: (1) an on/off flow valve, which allows independent pressurization of the compartment, and (2) a pressure-relief or pop-off valve, which is a safety device to prevent inflation pressure from exceeding 104 mm Hg (Fig. 52-1).
- The abdominal compartment extends from the costal margins to the pubis. Each leg compartment extends from the groin crease to the ankle.

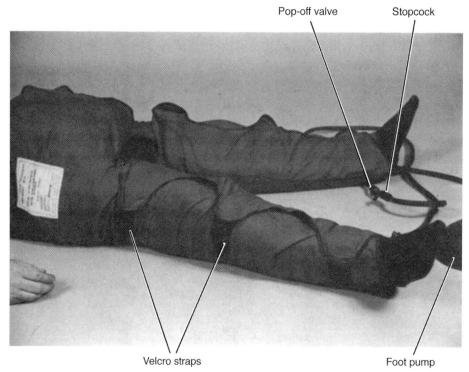

Pop-off valve   Stopcock

Velcro straps   Foot pump

FIGURE 52-1 Complete pneumatic antishock garment. *(From Jastremski, M.S., Dumas, M., and Penalver, L. [1992]. Emergency Procedures. Philadelphia: WB Saunders.)*

EQUIPMENT

- PASG
- Foot pump
- Blood pressure monitoring unit
- Nonsterile gloves

Additional equipment to have available as needed includes the following:

- Intravenous solutions as prescribed
- Emergency medications and resuscitative equipment

PATIENT AND FAMILY EDUCATION

- Explain the purpose of the PASG and its anticipated benefits. ➤*Rationale:* This explanation informs the patient and family about the device. This information prepares the patient and family for what to expect and may decrease anxiety.
- Explain the procedure for PASG to the patient and family. ➤*Rationale:* This explanation encourages patient and family cooperation and understanding of the procedure.

PATIENT ASSESSMENT AND PREPARATION

Patient Assessment

- Assess the patient's cardiovascular, peripheral vascular, respiratory, and neurovascular status. ➤*Rationale:* This

assessment provides baseline information that may aid in determining the need for PASG.

- Assess the patient for signs and symptoms of hemorrhagic shock. ➤*Rationale:* Physical signs and symptoms of shock may result from major blood volume loss and require immediate treatment.
- Assess the patient's skin, including possible sites of hemorrhage, before application of the PASG. ➤*Rationale:* After the PASG is applied, the area beneath the garment is difficult to assess.
- Assess the patient's arterial blood gas and lactate levels. ➤*Rationale:* These levels can be used for comparison because metabolic acidosis can develop as a result of muscle necrosis and tissue ischemia.

Patient Preparation

- Ensure that the patient and family understand preprocedural teaching. Answer questions as they arise, and reinforce information as needed. ➤*Rationale:* This communication evaluates and reinforces understanding of previously taught information.
- Ensure proper immobilization of the patient's spine. ➤*Rationale:* Spine alignment is maintained until spinal injury has been ruled out.
- Ensure that the patient has a patent airway and a decompressed bladder and stomach. ➤*Rationale:* Increased abdominal and intrathoracic pressure can result in compromised airway, aspiration, and bladder rupture.

Procedure for External Counterpressure With Pneumatic Antishock Garments

Steps	Rationale	Special Considerations
Application of PASG		
1. Wash hands, and don nonsterile gloves.	Reduces transmission of microorganisms; standard precautions.	
2. Search for and remove objects that are between the patient and the suit (including clothing).	Removal of objects prevents patient injury.	Thorough assessment and documentation of skin integrity are essential before PASG application.
3. Completely unfold the PASG, and lay it flat; smooth out wrinkles.	Prepares the device for use.	
4. Carefully logroll the patient, and place the PASG under the patient.	Maintains spine immobilization.	
5. Position the PASG so that the abdominal section is positioned below the costal margin, and the leg section ends at the ankle.	Proper placement of the trousers minimizes the risk of respiratory compromise. Diaphragmatic compression interferes with thoracic movement.[1,6]	
6. Fold the trousers around one leg and secure with velcro. Repeat the procedure with the other leg. Secure the PASG around the abdomen.	Prepares the PASG.	Check the dorsalis pedis and posterior tibial pulses before and after PASG application.
7. Attach the foot pump and air tubes to the PASG. Ensure that all stopcocks are open.	Allows for trouser compartment inflation.	
Inflation of PASG		
1. Open the valve(s) of the compartment(s) to be inflated (e.g., leg) and close the valve(s) of the compartment(s) that will not be inflated (e.g., abdomen).	Allows for proper inflation of the device.	*Both extremity compartments must be inflated before inflation of the abdominal compartment.* Leg-compartment inflation is contraindicated if there is an impaled object in the leg.
2. Inflate the leg segments until the velcro crackles or the pressure gauge reads greater than 100 mm Hg. *(Level IV: Limited clinical studies to support recommendations.)*	Inflation should increase peripheral vascular resistance; this allows increased blood flow to the heart, brain, and kidneys.[1,2,4,7]	
3. Inflate the abdominal segment if the patient's hemodynamic status does not improve. *(Level IV: Limited clinical studies to support recommendations.)*	Tamponade of intraabdominal hemorrhage may be achieved by abdominal inflation.[1-3,6]	Abdominal inflation is contraindicated in patients during pregnancy and in patients with impaled objects, evisceration, tension pneumothorax, penetrating chest trauma, or diaphragmatic rupture.
4. Monitor the patient's blood pressure response during inflation.	Monitors hemodynamic status.	PASG is not a substitute for fluid volume replacement. Intravenous fluids should be administered as prescribed.
5. Continue inflation until the desired blood pressure is achieved or maximal suit pressure is reached and the pop-off valve is activated.	Maintains PASG pressure at the lowest level for which the arterial blood pressure is stabilized.[1,6]	As a safety mechanism, release valves are activated when the pressure in the PASG is greater than 104 mm Hg or the suit crackles.
6. When optimal blood pressure is reached, close all valves.	Prevents air leakage from the valves.	

Procedure continues on the following page

Procedure | **for External Counterpressure With Pneumatic Antishock Garments**—*Continued*

Steps	Rationale	Special Considerations
7. Do not remove the PASG suddenly.	Sudden deflation of the PASG without adequate fluid resuscitation may cause the patient's blood pressure to drop precipitously. Sequential release allows for a gradual return of blood flow. Intrasuit pressure is assessed to determine the amount of pressure exerted on the tissues.[1-3,5]	
8. Assess the patient for clinical indicators that hemodynamic stability has been achieved.	Hemodynamic stability must be confirmed before safe deflation of the PASG. Instability may occur before PASG deflation. Additional intravenous fluids may be required.	The PASG should not be used for greater than 24 hours because of the potential for tissue damage.

Deflation of the PASG

Steps	Rationale	Special Considerations
1. Confirm hemodynamic stability before deflation.	PASG weaning should be considered when the patient's condition stabilizes and before 24 hours of therapy.	Suggested parameters: systolic blood pressure, greater than 90 mm Hg; heart rate, 60-120 beats/min; urine output, greater than 0.5 ml/kg/hr; palpable peripheral pulses.
2. Prepare intravenous solutions as prescribed.	Blood pressure serves as a clinical parameter during the deflation process.	When systolic blood pressure drops greater than 5-10 mm Hg, prepare to administer intravenous fluid until the blood pressure returns to baseline.
3. Obtain physician prescription before deflation that includes increments of deflation and parameters for fluid resuscitation.	Guides the deflation process.	Deflation should occur no more quickly than 10 mm Hg/min and should be guided by patient response.
4. Initiate the deflation process with the abdominal wall compartment of the PASG.	Deflation begins with the abdomen first, then leg compartments one at a time.	
5. Deflate the PASG slowly by opening the stopcock.	Allows gradual release of the pressure.	
6. Monitor vital signs at the time of deflation and every 5-10 minutes during deflation.	Compartments should be deflated sequentially to allow for gradual return of blood flow from the central circulation to prevent a sudden drop in circulatory blood volume.[1-4,6]	
7. After the abdominal compartment is deflated and vital signs remain stable, deflate one leg at a time, continuing to assess vital signs.	Validates hemodynamic stability.	When systolic blood pressure drops greater than 5-10 mm Hg, stop deflation and prepare to administer intravenous fluid until the blood pressure returns to baseline.
8. After deflation, continue to monitor vital signs every 15 minutes for 1 hour, then every hour for 24 hours.		
9. Discard used supplies, wash hands.	Reduces transmission of microorganisms; standard precautions.	

Expected Outcomes	Unexpected Outcomes
• Control of hemorrhage • Hemodynamic stability • Proper placement of PASG	• Hemodynamic instability • Respiratory compromise • Continued hemorrhage • Compartment syndrome • Impaired skin integrity • Metabolic acidosis • Increased cerebral edema

Patient Monitoring and Care

Steps	Rationale	Reportable Conditions
		These conditions should be reported if they persist despite nursing interventions.
1. Perform ongoing assessment of the patient's cardiovascular system every 15-60 minutes as patient condition warrants.	Shows effectiveness of PASG therapy; may indicate need for volume replacement.	• Significant changes in vital signs
2. Assess the patient's respiratory status every 15-60 minutes.	Abnormal respiratory status may indicate increased intrathoracic pressure and increased workload of the heart.	• Tachypnea • Cough • Crackles • Hypoxia • Distended neck veins
3. Assess the patient's circulation to the extremities every 15-60 minutes.	Validates adequate peripheral perfusion. Abnormal findings may indicate the development of compartment syndrome.	• Pain • Pallor • Diminished or absent movement, sensation, or pedal pulse • Capillary refill greater than 2 seconds
4. Monitor arterial blood gas and lactate levels as prescribed.	May indicate the development of muscle necrosis, tissue ischemia, and inadequate resuscitation.	• Abnormal arterial blood gas and lactate levels
5. Monitor intake and output.	Assesses fluid status.	• Urine output of less than 0.5 ml/kg/hr
6. Monitor PASG pressures.	Determines the amount of pressure exerted on the tissues beneath the garment.	• PASG pressure of greater than 100 mm Hg
7. Monitor the patient's skin integrity before PASG is inflation and after PASG deflation.	Skin integrity is difficult to assess after the PASG is inflated. When the PASG is removed, vigilant skin assessment is necessary.	• Skin breakdown • Redness • Hematoma • Lacerations

Documentation

Documentation should include the following:

- Patient and family education
- Rationale for institution of PASG
- Vital signs
- Patient response to PASG therapy
- Laboratory results
- Skin integrity assessment
- Time compartment was inflated and deflated
- Intake and output
- Unexpected outcomes
- Additional interventions

References

1. Cardona, V., et al. (2002). *Trauma Nursing: From Resuscitation Through Rehabilitation.* 3rd ed. Philadelphia: W.B. Saunders.
2. Chang, F.C., et al. (1995). PASG: Does it help in the management of traumatic shock? *J Trauma,* 39, 453-6.
3. Dickinson, K.R. (2000). Medical anti-shock trousers (pneumatic anti-shock garment) for circulatory support in patients with trauma. *Cochrane Database Sys Rev,* 1856-60.
4. Hauswald, M.G. (2003). Regional blood flow after pneumatic anti-shock garment inflation. *Prehosp Emerg Care,* April-June, 225-8.
5. Mattox, K.L., et al. (1986). Prospective randomized evaluation of antishock garment in penetrating cardiac wounds. *JAMA,* 266, 2398.
6. Maull, K. (1996). Role of military antishock trousers. In: Ivatury, R.R., and Cayten, C.G., editor. *The Textbook of Penetrating Trauma.* Media, PA: Williams & Wilkins.

Additional Readings

Chank, A.K., et al. (1996). MAST 96. *J Emerg Med,* 4, 419-24.
Salvucci, A., Koenig, K.L., and Stratton, S.J. (1998). The pneumatic anti-shock garment (PASG): Can we really recommend it? *Prehosp Emerg Care,* 2, 86-7.

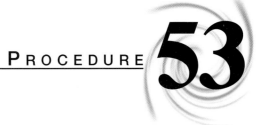

PROCEDURE **53**

Ventricular Assist Devices

P U R P O S E : Ventricular assist devices (VADs) are used in patients for cardiogenic shock and postcardiotomy support to allow for myocardial recovery, for bridge to cardiac transplantation, and for destination therapy (permanent implantation) in patients with New York Heart Association class IV heart failure on optimal medical therapy who are not eligible for cardiac transplantation.[3,5,6]

Desiree A. Fleck
Joelle Hargraves

PREREQUISITE NURSING KNOWLEDGE

- Understanding of the normal anatomy and physiology of the cardiovascular, peripheral vascular, and pulmonary systems is required.
- Understanding of the management of congestive heart failure is required.
- Knowledge of principles of hemodynamic monitoring, cardiopulmonary bypass, electrophysiology and dysrhythmias, and coagulation is needed.
- Clinical and technical competence related to use of VADs is needed.
- Advanced cardiac life support knowledge and skills are needed.
- Complications of VAD therapy include, but are not limited to, bleeding, cardiac tamponade, right ventricular failure with univentricular support, hepatic dysfunction, pulmonary dysfunction, renal dysfunction, infection, cerebral infarcts, and embolism.
- Effective cardiac assistance by the VAD is affected greatly by preload, afterload, right ventricular failure, cardiac tamponade, and cardiac dysrhythmias; the interaction between the patient and the device requires close monitoring.
- The device is implanted surgically in the operating room. Specific information concerning controls, alarms, troubleshooting, and safety features is available from each manufacturer and should be read thoroughly by the nurse before use of the equipment. *Please refer to the operator's manual for all systems for more detail.*

- Indications for VAD therapy include the following:[4,6,7]
  - ❖ Inability to wean from cardiopulmonary bypass
  - ❖ Bridge to cardiac transplantation
  - ❖ New York Heart Association class IV status in a patient not responding to optimal medical therapy and not a transplant candidate
  - ❖ Bridge to myocardial recovery
- Relative contraindications of VAD therapy include the following:
  - ❖ Body surface area (BSA) less than 1.3 m^2 (ABIOMED BVS 5000 or AB 5000 Ventricle)[1-3]
  - ❖ BSA less than 1.5 m^2 (HeartMate LVAD [left ventricular assist device][8,9] and Novacor LVAD)[10]
  - ❖ Renal or liver failure unrelated to cardiac incident
  - ❖ Comorbidity that would limit life expectancy to less than 3 years
  - ❖ Psychosocial and cognitive conditions may limit use of a VAD except in bridge to recovery
- ABIOMED BVS 5000 Circulatory Support System (CSS) (Fig. 53-1)[2]
  - ❖ The ABIOMED BVS 5000 (ABIOMED Inc, Danvers, MA) is an extracorporeal, pneumatically driven pump capable of delivering short-term (less than 3 weeks) left, right, or biventricular support.
  - ❖ The drive console controls systole by delivering air into the lower rigid plastic pumping chamber, displacing blood from the blood sac. Blood drains passively from the patient's atrium into the atrial chamber of the blood pump. When the atrial chamber of the blood pump is full and the pressure inside the atrial chamber exceeds the pressure inside the ventricular chamber,

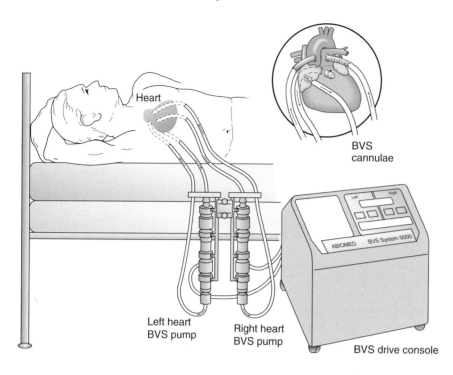

FIGURE 53-1 ABIOMED BVS 5000 System. *(From Dixon, J.F., and Farris, D.D. [1991]. The ABIOMED BVS 5000 System. AACN Clin Issues Crit Care Nurs, 2, 552-61.)*

the trileaflet valve opens, allowing blood to flow into the ventricular chamber of the blood pump. Blood pump diastole is completed as soon as the ventricular chamber is filled with 100 ml. The diastolic filling time is adjusted automatically to changes in the patient's preload to ensure the ventricular chamber is filled to full capacity (100 ml).

❖ The vertically aligned pneumatic blood pumps are adjusted to optimize flow. The blood flow from the patient to the blood pump depends on the console used. The BVS 5000t (transport) console and the AB 5000 console allow for vacuum-assisted filling of the chamber. Filling of the pumps depends solely on gravity when the BVS 5000 or BVS 5000i (high flow) consoles are used. The top of the blood pump should be between 0 and 10 inches below the level of the patient's atria when a 42 Fr atrial cannula is used and 4 to 14 inches when a 32 Fr or 36 Fr atrial cannula is used (see Fig. 53-1). Moving the pump above or below this level can affect flow. Adjusting the height of the blood pump alters filling of the blood chambers. Always allow 2 minutes for the system to adjust before making additional changes.

❖ Outflow from the BVS is used in place of cardiac output for calculations such as systemic vascular resistance, pulmonary vascular resistance, and cardiac index.

❖ External heat is not applied externally to the blood pump, tubing, or cannulas.

❖ Use Abiomed tubing insulators to retain heat in tubing.

❖ Anticoagulation with heparin is required.

• ABIOMED AB 5000 Ventricle[1] (Fig. 53-2)

❖ The AB 5000 Ventricle is a pulsatile, pneumatically driven blood pump approved for short-term (less than

3 weeks) support to allow time for myocardial recovery. It can provide support for one or both ventricles. It must be used in conjunction with the AB 5000 Circulatory Support System Console. The ventricle holds approximately 100 ml of blood. Cannulas exit the skin, and the ventricle lies on the patient's abdomen. Filling of the ventricle is facilitated by a vacuum within the console and is not affected by height. The ventricle is made partially of aluminum and plastic and has inflow and outflow valves to ensure unidirectional blood flow.

❖ The following items must *never* come in contact with the ventricle because they could damage the plastic within the ventricle: ketones such as acetone, aromatic hydrocarbons such as gasoline, halogenated hydrocarbon–based anesthetic agents, other hydrocarbonated hydrocarbons such as chloroform, and highly alkaline chemicals such as sodium hydroxide.

❖ Anticoagulation with heparin initially followed by warfarin (Coumadin) is required.

• HeartMate XVE (Extended Lead Vented Electric) LVAS (left ventricular assist system)[8]

❖ Thoratec Corporation (Pleasanton, CA) offers two implantable VADs used for left ventricular assistance. The implantable pneumatic (IP) is powered pneumatically and served as a predecessor to and currently as a backup for the HeartMate XVE LVAD (Fig. 53-3).

❖ These VADs are for longer term support.

❖ The LVAD may be implanted intraabdominally or preperitoneally in a rectus muscle pocket.

❖ The HeartMate XVE LVAD is made of titanium, holds 83 ml of blood, and weighs approximately 3 pounds. Blood flows through a small tube placed in

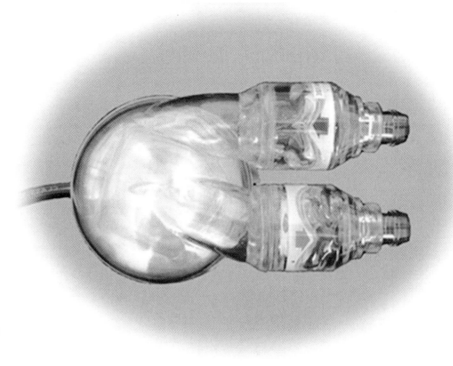

FIGURE 53-2 ABIOMED AB 5000 Ventricle. *(Courtesy ABIOMED, Inc., Danvers, MA.)*

the left ventricular apex through a porcine inflow valve into the pump. When the pump fills with blood, a sensor inside the device starts the electric motor. Blood is pumped through a second porcine outflow valve through a graft into the aorta. The LVAD is placed in the left upper quadrant of the abdomen.

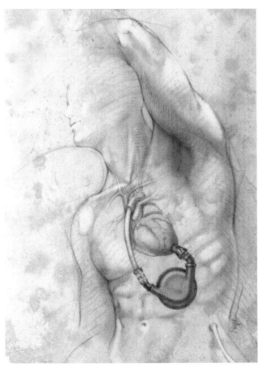

FIGURE 53-3 HeartMate implantable pneumatic VAD. *(Courtesy Thoratec Corporation, Pleasanton, CA.)*

❖ A driveline is passed underneath the skin and exits the right upper quadrant of the abdomen. The driveline connects the LVAD to a controller and a power source (batteries or a power base unit) and vents the electric motor that is within the LVAD. The LVAD can run on the fixed rate mode (set rate) or on the automatic mode, which responds to changes in preload. On the automatic mode, the pump rate varies between 50 and 120 beats/min to meet the physiologic needs of the patients. Anticoagulation with heparin or warfarin (Coumadin) is not necessary with this LVAD. Most patients receive aspirin, 81 mg or 325 mg daily, however.

• HeartMate Pneumatic IP LVAD
 ❖ The HeartMate IP LVAD is made of titanium and is pneumatically driven. A flexible polyurethane diaphragm divides the blood chamber. An influx of pressurized air (through the pneumatic tubing and into the VAD) drives the flexible diaphragm against the blood chamber, pushing blood from the VAD to the patient and controls the duration of systole. Porcine valves provide unidirectional blood flow.
 ❖ The HeartMate IP LVAD is connected via the driveline and a cable to the drive console, which controls pump function. Patients are able to walk around by pushing a rolling cart, which holds the drive console. The console is plugged into an electrical outlet when the patient is not ambulating. This LVAD is primarily for short-term use.

• Thoratec VAD[9]
 ❖ The Thoratec VAD (Thoratec Corporation, Pleasanton, CA) is an extracorporeal system approved for postcardiotomy use and as a bridge to transplantation. It can

provide univentricular or biventricular support. It is the only device approved for long-term (greater than 3 weeks if necessary) biventricular support. It is also the device of choice in patients requiring ventricular support with a BSA less than 1.5 m^2. The three major components of the system are the blood pump, cannulas, and drive console. The smooth, seamless blood sac is enclosed within a rigid case. Two mechanical valves provide unidirectional blood flow. A fill switch with the VAD signals the console to eject the blood when the VAD is filled with blood. Either the dual-drive console or the TLC-II portable driver can operate the VAD (Fig. 53-4).

❖ The Thoratec is driven by a dual-drive console, which contains two independent drive modules for left and right ventricular support. Patients with biventricular assist devices (BiVADs) require both modules, and patients with a right ventricular assist device (RVAD) or a LVAD require one module. When only one module is being used, the other module can serve as a backup if pump failure occurs. The console supplies air pressure to eject blood from the pump into the arterial system and vacuum to assist pump filling. A full 65-ml stroke volume is possible from 20 to 110 beats/min, providing cardiac outputs of 1.2 to 7.2 liters/min.

❖ The recommended control modes for operation include asynchronous/fixed or volume/automatic. A fixed rate allows the operator to choose a VAD rate that is asynchronous with the patient's intrinsic heart rate. The automatic mode also is asynchronous to the patient's intrinsic heart rate, but responds to changes in physiologic conditions.

❖ Anticoagulation with heparin initially followed by warfarin is required.

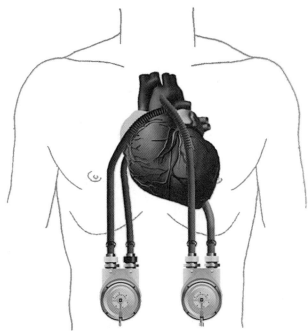

FIGURE 53-4 Thoratec biventricular assist device. *(Courtesy Thoratec Corporation, Pleasanton, CA.)*

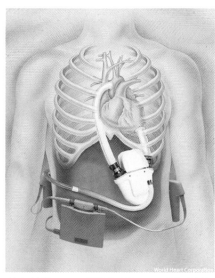

FIGURE 53-5 Novacor LVAS. *(Courtesy World Heart, Inc., Ottawa, Canada.)*

• Novacor LVAS (Fig. 53-5)[10]
   ❖ The Novacor LVAS (World Heart Inc., Ottawa, Canada) provides circulatory support for patients with profound left ventricular failure. The system comprises an implantable electromechanical pump/drive unit, compact controller, wearable power packs, LVAS monitor, and personal monitor.
   ❖ The integrated pulsatile pump and electromechanical driver are implanted in the left anterior abdominal wall. The pump receives blood from the left ventricle via a conduit that cannulates the left ventricular apex. Blood pumped from the device travels through an outflow conduit anastomosed to the ascending aorta.
   ❖ A single percutaneous lead connects the implanted pump/driver to the external compact controller. This lead protects the electrical wires from the pump and vents the pump. The controller is connected to a power source.
   ❖ Anticoagulation with heparin initially followed by warfarin (Coumadin) with or without aspirin is required. Some VAD programs also administer a platelet inhibitor for the first 30 days postoperatively.

EQUIPMENT

• VAD drive console/unit or monitor (Table 53-1)
• Connection cables (specific to device) (see Table 53-1)
• Backup drive console/unit/monitor or batteries (see Table 53-1)
• Emergency pump device (hand crank, foot pump, hand pump or bulb, depending on device) (see Table 53-1)
• Vent filters
• Dressing supplies:
   ❖ Sterile normal saline
   ❖ 4 × 4 sterile gauze pads
   ❖ Tape, 1 and 2 inch
   ❖ 4 × 4 split sterile gauze pads
   ❖ Sterile gloves

TABLE 53-1	Equipment for Various Ventricular Assist (VAD) Devices	
VAD Equipment	**Function**	**Special Consideration**
HeartMate XVE[8]		
Power base unit with cable	Provides electrical power for the LVAD when the patient is attached	Charges batteries
System monitor	Displays the VAD rate, stroke volume, and flow. Used initially in the operating room and early postoperative period to monitor LVAD flow, alarms, change modes, and program fixed rate	
Display module	Displays VAD rate, stroke volume, mode, flow, and alarm status	Used in the hospital and at home
Controller	"Brains" of the system. Computer software programmed to run the LVAD and provide safety alarms is housed in the controller	One controller is connected to the patient, and a backup controller is available in the event of malfunction
Controller cell: one in the controller and a backup	Powers the controller so that in the event of disconnection of all power to the LVAD an alarm sounds	
Vent filter	Filters air that is shuffled back and forth through the driveline during a cycle	
Large batteries	Two batteries are used to power the LVAD to allow for patient ambulation. Batteries are carried in a shoulder holster or fanny pack. Battery life is checked every 30-60 minutes by pushing down the alarm silence button. Batteries are fully charged when 4 green lights appear. Batteries are changed when 2 green lights are lit	Two batteries last approximately 4 hours
Battery clips	Used to hold batteries for portable operation	
Hand pump	Used for a backup emergency	The hand pump always must be with the patient in the event that the pump stops and cannot be started
24-hour emergency battery (outpatient use)	Provides backup energy source	Each patient is given at least a 24-hour battery in the event that electrical power is lost for an extended period
Thoratec Ventricular Assist Device[9]		
Thoratec VAD: The smooth, seamless blood sac is enclosed within a rigid case	Two mechanical valves provide unidirectional blood flow. A fill switch within the VAD signals the console to eject the blood when the VAD is filled with blood	
Dual-drive console:	Contains two independent drive modules for left or right ventricular support	Set rate: 50-60 beats/minute
Asynchronous: rate set by clinician	The console supplies air pressure to eject blood from the pump into the arterial system and supplies vacuum to assist with VAD filling. This should always be kept plugged in except during patient transport/ambulation	
Volume: VAD ejects when electrical lead senses that the VAD is full. The rate and flows change depending on volume status and other physiologic changes		
Set rate: actual rate in asynchronous mode, volume mode: uses backup rate		
Set % of systole: 25-30% (½ of set rate = 300 msec)	% of systole: pump ejection time	
Drive pressure: LVAD: 230-245 mm Hg RVAD: 140-160 mm Hg	Drive pressure: ejects blood from the VAD	
Vacuum: −25 to −40 mm Hg	Vacuum: assists with VAD filling	
Hand pump	Can be used to run a VAD manually in the event of console failure until a backup console can be connected	Always keep hand pumps with the console
Electrical lead	On volume/automatic mode the electrical lead senses when the VAD is full and communicates to the console to empty the VAD	
Pneumatic lead	The console delivers pressurized air through the pneumatic lead to cause collapse of the blood sac and ejection of the blood into the circulation	

Continued

TABLE 53-1	Equipment for Various Ventricular Assist (VAD) Devices—*Continued*	
VAD Equipment	**Function**	**Special Consideration**
TLC-II System Components		
TLC-II driver with carrying case	The portable driver is a lightweight, portable, pneumatic VAD driver powered by batteries or external power	Designed to provide portable pneumatic drive power for ambulatory patients supported with the Thoratec VAD
The carrying case is kept over the driver for protection		
Mobility cart	The driver can be strapped to the cart for easy patient ambulation	
AC adapter	Connects the portable driver to a wall outlet to allow the VAD to be run off of electrical power instead of battery when the patient is not ambulating to conserve battery strength	
Li-ion rechargeable batteries	Provides at least 55 minutes (BiVAD support) to 80 minutes (RVAD or LVAD support)	
TLC-II battery charger	Can fully recharge 1 or 2 batteries in approximately 2 hours	
Docking Station-HeartTouch Computer	Runs an interface-monitoring program that is specially designed to communicate with the TLC-II Driver	Required only for start-up and diagnostic procedures
TLC-II Output Range		
VAD modes: automatic or fixed	Automatic mode allows for more physiologic use of the VAD	
VAD rate: 30-110 beats/minute	Allows for changes in preload	
Ejection time: 230-370 msec		
Peak drive pressure:		
LVAD: 240 mm Hg		
RVAD: 160 mm Hg		
Vacuum: −25 to −40 mm Hg		
Novacor Left Ventricular Assist System[10]		
Compact controller		
Low power	Lights if power is low or power source is not connected	
O.K.	Indicates controller is receiving power and no alarms are present	
Temp check	Lights if internal temperature exceeds limits	
Replace	Indicates out-of-limit condition (i.e., low pump output) or detected fault condition within the controller	
	Indicates a more serious condition requiring urgent attention: check pump connection and replace the controller	
Wearable power pack	Provides power to the compact controller	Primary power pack is the principal source during untethered use. The reserve power pack is the backup
LVAS monitor: connects to the compact controller by a monitor/controller connecting cable	Provides power to the controller via AC power or its internal rechargeable battery	If internal rechargeable battery wears down completely, LVAS fails
	Permits evaluation of LVAS function, setup, and adjustment of parameters	
Personal monitor	Provides information on pump operation and system alarm status	Designed for placement on a table or nightstand for home use

LVAD, left ventricular assist device; *LVAS*, left ventricular assist system; *RVAD*, right ventricular assist device.

❖ Cap
❖ Mask
❖ Sterile gown
❖ Sterile drape
❖ Ace wrap (6 inch)
❖ 6 × 6 bordered gauze
❖ Suture removal kit
Additional equipment as needed includes the following:
• Emergency equipment and medications
• Flashlight
• Intravenous pole

• Four smooth chest clamps
• Blood pump set

PATIENT AND FAMILY EDUCATION

• Assess patient and family understanding of VAD therapy and the reason for its use. ➥*Rationale:* Clarification or reinforcement of information is an expressed patient and family need during times of stress and anxiety.
• Explain the environment and care planned to the patient and family, including frequency of assessment, sounds and

function of equipment, placement of device, explanation of alarms, dressings and therapy, decreased or assisted mobility, and parameters for discontinuation of therapy. Preoperatively, it might be helpful for the patient and family to meet another patient on a VAD if both patients are agreeable. ➻*Rationale:* This communication provides information and encourages the patient and family to ask questions or voice concerns or fears related to the therapy. Meeting another patient with a VAD provides social support.

- If appropriate, begin discharge teaching to include operation of VAD, dressing changes, battery changes, placing self on and off of battery and power base unit or monitor, changing the controller, and appropriate bathing techniques with use of shower equipment. ➻*Rationale:* This teaching provides information and ensures that the patient will be safe at home. It also allows the patient and family to ask questions as needed.

PATIENT ASSESSMENT AND PREPARATION

Patient Assessment

- Assess the patient's past medical history, specifically related to the competency of the aortic/pulmonic valves, competency of the mitral/tricuspid valves, primary pulmonary hypertension, right ventricular failure, left ventricular failure, and peripheral vascular disease. ➻*Rationale:* This assessment provides baseline data regarding cardiac functioning and facilitates decision making regarding insertion of the appropriate device and postoperative management.

- Perform cardiovascular, hemodynamic, peripheral vascular, neurovascular, and psychosocial assessment and assessment of body mass index and BSA. ➻*Rationale:* These assessments provide baseline data and help to determine the type of device to use.

- Assess the current laboratory profile, including complete blood count, platelet count, prothrombin time, partial thromboplastin time (PTT), international normalized ratio (INR), blood chemistry, and liver profile. ➻*Rationale:* This assessment provides baseline data and may indicate end-organ dysfunction related to low-flow state. It also may predict risk of bleeding.

Patient Preparation

- Ensure that the patient and family understand preoperative teaching. Answer questions as they arise, and reinforce information as needed. ➻*Rationale:* This communication evaluates and reinforces understanding of previously taught information.

- Provide emotional support to the patient and family. ➻*Rationale:* The patient and family are under an extreme amount of stress.

- Ensure that informed consent has been obtained (if it is known preoperatively that the VAD will be placed). ➻*Rationale:* Obtaining informed consent protects the rights of the patient and makes a competent decision possible for the patient and family.

Procedure for Ventricular Assist Devices

Steps	Rationale	Special Considerations

ABIOMED BVS 5000 VAD
1. Obtain the needed equipment:
  A. ABIOMED BVS 5000 blood chamber(s)
  B. ABIOMED BVS 5000, 5000i, or 5000t console, ABIOMED AB 5000 console		

2. Ensure that the console is plugged into a three-pronged outlet with emergency generator backup.	The battery life is approximately 1 hour.	
3. Adjust the level of the blood pump(s) between 0 and 10 inches below the level of the patient's atria when a 42 Fr atrial cannula is used and 4 to 14 inches when a 32 Fr or 36 Fr atrial cannula is used, for optimal filling.	The level of the pump is important in assisting with gravity filling of the atrial chamber(s) of the blood pumps, especially when using the BVS 5000 or 5000i console.	

Procedure continues on the following page

Procedure for **Ventricular Assist Devices**—*Continued*

Steps	Rationale	Special Considerations
4. Inspect the blood chambers for complete filling and emptying.	Ensures adequate VAD output.	Optimize blood pump filling by: • Lowering the blood pump • Administering fluids or blood products as prescribed • Assessing for cardiac tamponade. • Administer inotropes (e.g., milrinone, dobutamine) as required to optimize right ventricular function when the patient has only LVAD support.
5. Inspect the valves within the blood pump chamber at least every 2 hours for thrombus formation. Use a flashlight to assist in visualization.	Thrombus formation can lead to pulmonary embolism or stroke.	Administer a heparin infusion to maintain a PTT of 2-2.5 times the laboratory's normal value or an activated coagulation time (ACT) of 180-200 seconds or as prescribed. A heparin bolus is not recommended unless specifically prescribed; heparin is usually started after the mediastinal drainage is less than 50-75 ml/hr × 3 hours. PTT or ACT should be monitored hourly until therapeutic and then every 2 hours. For unresolved atrial or ventricular dysrhythmias, the ACT may be increased to 250-300 seconds, or the PTT may be increased to 2.5-3 times normal.
6. Ensure the connection between the cannula and tubing is secured.	Disconnection of the cannula/tubing can result in exsanguination.	Tie bands should be applied in the operating room. When transporting a patient, a team member (e.g., nurse, perfusionist, and physician) must be responsible for monitoring the tubing and blood chambers.

ABIOMED AB 5000 Ventricle

Steps	Rationale	Special Considerations
1. Obtain the needed equipment: A. AB 5000 ventricle(s) B. AB 5000 console		
2. Ensure that the AB 5000 console is plugged into a three-pronged outlet with emergency generator backup.	The AB 5000 ventricle can be used only with the AB 5000 console; the battery life is approximately 1 hour.	
3. Inspect the valves within the ventricle at least every 8 hours for thrombus formation. Use a flashlight to assist in visualization.	Thrombus formation can lead to pulmonary embolism or stroke.	Administer heparin infusion to maintain a PTT of 2-2.5 times the laboratory's normal value or an ACT of 180-200 seconds or as prescribed by the physician. A heparin bolus is not recommended unless specifically prescribed; heparin is usually started after mediastinal drainage is less than 50 to 75 ml/hr × 3 hours.

Procedure for Ventricular Assist Devices—*Continued*

Steps	Rationale	Special Considerations
		PTT or ACT should be monitored hourly until therapeutic and then every 2 hours.
		For unresolved atrial or ventricular dysrhythmias, the ACT may be increased to 250-300 seconds, or the PTT may be increased to 2.5-3 times normal.
4. Troubleshooting ABIOMED BVS 5000 and AB 5000 console alarms	Alarms must be addressed promptly to prevent complications.	
A. Low flow	Inadequate VAD output and decreased organ perfusion may be due to:	
• Assess for obstruction of lines, and correct the problem if present.	Obstruction of blood lines.	
• Lower the blood pump chamber.	Blood pump placed too high.	
• Administer fluids or blood products as prescribed.	Inadequate blood volume.	
• Provide inotropic support or pulmonary vasodilators or both to improve right ventricular function for patients with only LVAD support.	Right ventricular failure.	
B. High pressure/low flow	Inadequate VAD output and decreased organ perfusion may be due to:	
• Check tubing/cannula for kinks.	Cannula or blood pump tubing kinked or occluded.	
• Decrease systemic vascular resistance; keep systolic blood pressure less than 140 mm Hg or as prescribed.	Increased systemic vascular resistance.	
C. Low pressure/low flow	If tubing disconnects from the console, the VAD stops, which can lead to death.	Check lines; reconnect driveline to resume flow.
• Ensure the tubing is connected to the console	Disconnection of the tubing from the console.	
• Check the tubing for leaks and replace the tubing if needed	Leak in the tubing.	
D. Low battery	Potential for VAD stoppage.	The battery life is approximately 1 hour.
• Ensure that the console is plugged into a three-pronged outlet with emergency generator backup.	The battery has less than 10 minutes of power.	
E. Continuous audible alarm	VAD failure.	Remove the foot pump.
• Use the foot pump (BVS 5000, 5000i, 5000t) or hand pump (AB 5000) to operate the VAD		Move the transfer level to the vertical position.
• Call for help and change the console.		
F. Complete console failure	VAD failure.	Remove the foot pump.
• Use the foot pump (BVS 5000, 5000i, 5000t) or hand pump (AB 5000) to operate theVAD.		
• Call for help to change the console.		

Procedure continues on the following page

Procedure for **Ventricular Assist Devices**—*Continued*

Steps	Rationale	Special Considerations
HeartMate XVE		
1. Changing from the power base unit to batteries.	Ensures that the battery is charged.	Batteries are fully charged when 4 green lights appear.
A. Check the battery life every 30-60 minutes by pushing down the alarm silence button.		Batteries are changed when 2 green lights are lit.
B. Place a battery into each battery clip by lining up the arrow on the large battery and battery clip and inserting until the battery "clicks" securely into the holder.	Allows patients to be ambulatory.	Ensure location of hand pump.
C. Disconnect the white controller cable from the power base unit cable by loosening the white nut and then pulling them apart.	An alarm sounds once per second and a yellow wrench lights indicating disconnection from the power base unit.	Do not disconnect both power cables at the same time, or the VAD loses power and may stop.
D. Connect the white controller cable to the battery clip.	The alarm is resolved.	
E. Disconnect the black controller cable from the power base unit cable by loosening the black nut and then pulling them apart.	An alarm sounds once per second and a yellow wrench lights indicating disconnection from the power base unit. The alarm resolves after the cable is connected properly.	
2. Changing from batteries to power base unit		Patients are attached to the power base unit at night.
A. Disconnect the white controller cable from the battery clip.		An alarm sounds once per second and a yellow wrench lights indicating disconnection from the battery. Do not disconnect both cables at the same time because power failure occurs.
B. Connect the white controller cable to the white power base unit cable connection.	Patient data returns to the personal or display monitor.	The alarm is resolved.
C. Disconnect the black controller cable from the battery clip.	Allows the power to be returned to the power base unit.	An alarm sounds once per second and a yellow wrench lights indicating disconnection from the battery.
D. Connect the black controller cable to the black power base unit cable connection.	Returns the power to the power base unit.	The alarm is resolved.
E. Remove the batteries from clips and place batteries back into the power base unit.	Allows the batteries to recharge.	
3. Changing modes		Some physicians use fixed mode for the initial 24 hours of insertion and on select patients.
A. Touch the mode button (cloud/swirl picture) on the controller.	In the fixed mode, the pump runs at a predetermined set rate; the factory set rate is 50 and is adjusted specific to the patient's needs.	One beep indicates that the mode changed to fixed; two beeps indicate that the mode changed to automatic.
B. Adjust the rate while in the fixed mode as needed or prescribed.	In the automatic mode, the pump rate adjusts between 50 and 120 beats/min based on preload and right ventricular function.	

Procedure for Ventricular Assist Devices—*Continued*

Steps	Rationale	Special Considerations
4. Self-test		
A. Place the patient on the power base unit, then hold down the mode button until all the lights on the controller light and a loud alarm sounds.	A self-test is done each day to check the function of the pump, controller, and controller cell strength.	If the controller cell is low, the red battery light goes on and then off, then flashes for the duration of the self-test; at the end of the self-test a yellow wrench lights, and the display screen reads "controller cell low."
B. Observe the battery picture on the right top corner of the controller to assess battery strength.	A controller cell battery usually lasts 3-6 months.	The patient should be in a sitting or lying position. The pump slows to 40 beats/min during the self-test.
5. Changing the controller		
A. Place the controller cell (small round black) battery in the new controller	Provides power to the controller.	The patient should be in a sitting or lying position.
B. Lay out the new controller next to the old controller.	Eases transition and changing of the controllers.	
C. Ensure the hand pump is available.	The hand pump nearby allows easy use in the event of the inability to connect the new controller.	
D. Disconnect the white cable from the battery or power base cable.	Allows for the controller change.	The controller alarms once a second, and a yellow wrench lights.
E. Disconnect the black cable from the battery or power base cable.	Allows for the controller change.	The controller alarms continuously; the pump stops.
F. Push down the black release button, and disconnect the controller from the driveline.	Allows for the controller change.	The controller stops alarming.
G. Line up the "black triangles," and connect the new controller.	Eases the transition when connecting the new controller.	The controller starts alarming.
H. Connect the new white cable to a battery or power base cable.	Allows the patient data to be displayed and the power to be restored.	The pump starts at a fixed rate of 50; it alarms once per second, and a yellow wrench lights.
I. Connect the new black cable to a battery or power base cable.	Restores power.	The controller stops alarming.
J. Switch the mode to automatic by touching the swirl/cloud mode button on the controller.	The pump turns on in the fixed mode at a rate of 50. The automatic mode is considered to be more physiologic.	The fixed rate can be adjusted at a later time if needed.
6. Hand pumping	Used when the VAD fails.	*Never hand pump if the LVAD is still pumping.* The controller continues to alarm until disconnected or the controller battery cell is removed.
A. Remove the vent filter and connect the hand pump.	Allows for hand pumping.	
B. Push in the white button (purge valve) and hold.	Purges the air.	
C. Push in the black ball and hold.	Provides vacuum.	
D. Let go of the white button.	Allows for reinflation of the ball.	
E. Let go of the black ball.	The ball inflates.	
F. Count to 10 slowly.	Allows for adequate vacuum.	
G. Swing the handles around and pump 60-90 times a minute.	Allows for adequate VAD pumping and flow.	Ensure the black ball is fully depressed during pumping and fills completely.

Procedure continues on the following page

Procedure for **Ventricular Assist Devices**—*Continued*

Steps	Rationale	Special Considerations
7. Switching from hand pumping to the pneumatic console.	Used when the VAD fails.	Hand pumping must be done before changing the patient to the pneumatic console.
A. Ensure that the stroke volume limiter is attached to the pneumatic connection on the back of the console, and ensure that the console is plugged into the AC outlet.	The stroke volume limiter is required to shuttle air back and forth between the VAD and the console.	
B. Turn on the pneumatic console.	Supplies power.	The button is located on the front of the console on the far left.
C. Disconnect the hand pump from the vent port of the driveline and connect it to the stroke volume limiter.	The patient could become unresponsive.	The LVAD is stopped for approximately 1 minute. Ensure the patient is lying down. Maintain a patent airway and proceed.
D. Ensure the vent clip on the stroke volume limiter is open.	Allows for adequate pumping.	
E. Push the vent button.	It reads, "vent cycle activated" when it is venting. When the cycle is complete, it disappears.	The system vents itself; this takes about 10 seconds.
F. Close the vent clip on the stroke volume limiter before the vent cycle is complete.	Allows for the VAD to function.	
G. Push the fixed button. Gradually over the next few minutes, increase the rate to the patient's normal rate.	The pump starts at a rate of 72.	The pump runs only on fixed. Record the rate. Flows will not be displayed.
H. The pump must be vented every 4 hours by opening the vent clip and pushing the vent button. When the cycle is complete, close the vent clip. Pumping resumes.	Assess the stroke volume limiter for movement of the diaphragm and buildup of moisture.	Ensure the patient is lying down throughout the entire procedure.
8. Troubleshooting HeartMate XVE[8] alarms (Alarm Symbol)		
A. Alarm: Red Heart	The VAD may not be functioning adequately.	Emits a steady tone.
Alarm: Red Heart and Yellow Wrench • Check if the LVAD is still pumping by listening for the sound and feeling over the abdomen. • Check that the controller is connected securely to the driveline. • Change the power source. (Change batteries or, if on the power base unit, change to batteries.) • Remove the vent filter. • If the device still fails to operate, disconnect the system controller power connections, and begin manual pumping with the HeartMate hand pump. • Seek additional help.		Can occur if the LVAD flow is less than 1.5 liters/min. Give fluids and treat the dysrhythmias.
B. Alarm: Yellow Wrench • Check the connections. • Check that the batteries are in the battery clips properly. • Prepare to change the controller. • Call the VAD coordinator before changing the controller.	The VAD may not be functioning adequately.	Emits 1 beep per second.

Procedure for Ventricular Assist Devices—*Continued*

Steps	Rationale	Special Considerations
C. Alarm: ½ Yellow Wrench • Call for help. • Replace the system controller.	The VAD may not be functioning adequately.	Emits 1 beep per second.
D. Alarm: Red Battery • Immediately replace the batteries, or change to an alternate power source. The LVAD automatically goes into the Power Saver Mode (50 beats/min)	Less than 5 minutes of battery power remains.	Emits a steady tone.
E. Alarm: Yellow Battery • Change to an alternate power source.	Less than 15 minutes of battery power remains.	Emits 1 beep per second.
F. Alarm: Yellow Battery—flashing • Replace the system controller battery cell. • Perform a system controller self-test to clear the alarm.		Does not emit an audio sound.
G. Power Base Unit Alarm: *AC Fail* • Change the power sources. Switch from the power base unit to batteries. • Ensure that the power base unit is plugged into an outlet with emergency power backup. • If all batteries are used up before electrical power is restored, use the emergency power pack or prepare to hand pump. • Discharge teaching: instruct the patient to place a flashlight on his or her nightstand.	External power to the power base unit is off. The power base unit internal battery powers the pump for 45 minutes.	Emits a steady tone.
H. Power Base Unit Alarm: *Lo Batt*: • Change the power sources. Switch from the power base unit to batteries. • If all batteries are used up before the electrical power is restored, use the emergency power pack or prepare to hand pump.	The power base unit internal battery is almost depleted.	This alarm is a steady tone.
I. Power Base Unit Alarm: *Alarm Reset*: • Press the alarm reset switch. • The AC fail alarm is silenced and does not come back on.	Used to silence the power base unit AC fail alarm.	If the patient is connected to the power base unit, all alarms sound at the power base unit and controller; both need to be silenced.

Thoratec Dual Driver and TLCII

1. Dual driver console: switching to the dual driver console		
A. Open the back door of the console.	Allows access to some of the controls.	
B. Turn on the top and bottom module using the toggle switch.	Allows use in the biventricular mode.	
C. Turn on the top and the bottom compressor by switching the "light" switches on.	Turns on the power to both VADs.	
D. Place the emergency valve on the back inside console door to the center "normal" position.	Allows for emergency protection.	

Procedure continues on the following page

Procedure for Ventricular Assist Devices—*Continued*

Steps	Rationale	Special Considerations
E. Adjust the set rate to the previous setting.	Allows for optimal use of VADs.	
F. Adjust the set % systole to the previous setting.	Allows for optimal emptying and filling.	
G. Adjust the pressure to the previous setting.	Optimal setting is determined in the operating room.	
H. Adjust the vacuum to the previous setting.	Optimal setting is determined in the operating room.	
I. Connect the pneumatic lines; change the LVAD (red) line first, then the RVAD (blue) line.	Allows the VADs to function.	
J. Connect the electric leads.	Provides data input.	
K. Place on the volume mode.	Provides for better cardiac output or VAD flow.	
L. Assess for VAD filling and emptying.	Ensures adequate filling and emptying.	
M. Readjust pressure and the vacuum as needed.	Optimizes filling and emptying.	Do not exceed a pressure of 250 mm Hg or a vacuum of 50 mm Hg.
2. Assessment of VAD filling		
A. Check the green fill light on the console.	The green light flashes with each VAD ejection.	
B. Visually inspect the VAD to ensure that the blood sac is filling completely.	Ensures adequate filling.	

C. Incomplete VAD filling:
• Correct as needed:
  Volume load
  Coagulopathies
  Medications to improve right ventricular output
  Increase pharmacologic support
	Incomplete VAD filling may occur for physiologic reasons, including hypovolemia, bleeding, right ventricular failure (LVAD only), ventricular recovery, cardiac tamponade, or inadequate pharmacologic support.	

D. Incomplete VAD filling:
• Correct as needed:
  Increase vacuum
  Decrease set rate
  Decrease set % systole
	Mechanical reasons for incomplete VAD filling may occur because of a kinked cannula or pneumatic hose, insufficient vacuum, set rate too high, or eject time too long.	

3. Assessment of VAD ejection		
A. Flash test is done by shining the light from a flashlight at an angle through the VAD housing and assessing for a flash of light on the opposite side.	If the flash of light is seen, the blood sac is emptying completely.	If the VAD is not ejecting completely the displayed VAD flows are not accurate.
B. Incomplete VAD emptying: • Increase the drive pressure (should be at least 100 mm Hg higher than the pulmonary artery systolic pressure for a RVAD and 100 mm Hg higher than the systolic blood pressure for a LVAD).	VAD drive pressures too low	
• Lower the systolic blood pressure (goal less than 140 mm Hg)	Systolic pulmonary artery or systemic blood pressure too high	
• Increase the set % systole	Outflow cannula kinked Set % systole too low	
4. Start up procedure for TLC-II		
A. Place the driver in the docking station.		
B. Connect the power, and turn it on.		

Procedure for **Ventricular Assist Devices**—*Continued*

Steps	Rationale	Special Considerations
C. Connect the power cable (yellow) and the computer cable (green).		
D. Place the two charged batteries in the holders.		
E. Use the setup plugs to eliminate pressure alarms during setup.		
F. Turn on the key switch, remove the key, and place it in the pocket of the carrying case on the key chain.	Ensures VAD functioning and maintains key location.	
G. Press the "Silence" button.	Silences the alarm for 30 seconds.	

H. On the HeartTouch computer, touch the VAD settings, press initialize, and confirm the following parameters or adjust to the individual patient:
• VAD configuration: BiVAD or LVAD
• Mode: Automatic or fixed
• Low rate: 50 beats/min
• LVAD beat rate: 80 beats/min (default rate on fixed mode)
• RVAD beat rate: 70 beats/min
• Eject time: 300 msec
• Accumulator pressure:
  BiVAD: 250 mm Hg
  LVAD: 250 mm Hg
  RVAD: 220 mm Hg
	Ensures adequate use and function of the VAD system.	

I. Enter the patient's name and ID number.	Maintains the settings for the patient.	
J. Verify that the patient is connected to the appropriate pneumatic and electric lines.	Ensures adequate VAD function.	The 5-foot section comes from the VAD and the 7-foot section from the console; they connect together to form a 12-foot line. The lines are color coded; red is LVAD and blue is RVAD. Always change the LVAD lead first, then the RVAD.
K. Connect the patient to the TLC-II driver. Connect the pneumatic LVAD line to the console first by separating the 12-foot line. Connect the 5-foot section to the console. Next connect the RVAD pneumatic line.		
L. Connect the "fill" electric cable(s) next. The 5-foot section connects to the console.		
M. Switch to the automatic mode.	Allows for more physiologic use of the VAD.	
N. Adjust the vacuum regulator. Ensure the VADs are filling properly.	Allows for more efficient use of the VAD.	
5. Troubleshooting Thoratec[9] alarms A. Pressure alarm: Drive pressure less than 100 mm Hg or greater than 250 mm Hg • Adjust pressure to recommended settings and assess VAD emptying. • Ensure pneumatic line is connected (low pressure). • Change pneumatic line if leaking. • Change to backup console.	The pressure may be high or low because of VAD rate change, pressure changed by staff, pneumatic leak, transducer failure or calibration incorrect, compressor or uninterruptible power supply failure.	

Procedure continues on the following page

Procedure for Ventricular Assist Devices—*Continued*

Steps	Rationale	Special Considerations
B. Low battery alarm • Plug the console into a wall outlet.	Module batteries have less than 30 minutes power; uninterruptible power supply has less than 5 minutes of power.	Uninterruptible power supply battery time is 40 minutes; the status panel is on the lower front console indicated by 4 green lights, which disappear one at a time; keep the console plugged in at all times except when the patient is ambulating or being transported to another department
C. Synch alarm (-E- instead of VAD output) • Treat the physiologic causes. • Adjust the pressure and the vacuum to the recommended settings, and change the console. • Change the gray electrical lead.	The synch alarm may be due to no fill signal, poor VAD filling, fill cable (gray electric lead) malfunction, drive pressure less than 100 mm Hg or greater than 250 mm Hg, eject time less than 250 msec, set rate too high, set % systole too high, fill cable disconnection, fill switch failure (extremely rare—VAD functions only on asynch mode), module failure.	
6. Troubleshooting TLC-II Alarms A. Low batteries. • Replace the battery packs immediately, replace the indicated battery first: change battery A or B. • Switch to backup driver immediately. • Then change the emergency battery in the initial driver.	The battery needs to be replaced because there is less than 10 minutes of battery life left.	
B. Loss of full signal: No L or R full signal, check the cable. • Check the VAD for filling; fill the cable, pneumatic lead, and all connections. • Change the fill cable if the VAD is filling completely. • Administer volume if not filling completely.	Loss of full signal may be due to poor VAD filling, electric lead malfunction or disconnection, full switch failure in the VAD, pneumatic lead disconnected, or driver malfunction.	
C. High pressure: High L or R pressure. • Check the VAD cannula and the pneumatic leads.	Pneumatic lead occlusion, cannula kinked or occluded, transducer failure.	
D. Low pressure: Low L or R pressure, check, replace. • Check VAD, pneumatic lines, and for system leak. • Replace with backup driver.	Pneumatic line disconnection, compressor failure, system air leak.	
E. High vacuum: High L or R vacuum; replace. • Verify the VAD is working. • Adjust the vacuum regulator to reduce vacuum; if not corrected, replace the driver.	A high vacuum alarm may be due to a transducer error or failure or compressor or vacuum relief valve occlusion.	
F. Low vacuum: Low L or R vacuum; replace. • Check the VAD. • Adjust the vacuum regulator; if not corrected, replace the driver.	A low vacuum alarm may be due to compressor failure, solenoid failure, or a system leak.	

Procedure for Ventricular Assist Devices—*Continued*

Steps	Rationale	Special Considerations
G. Occlusion alarms: RVAD or LVAD occlusion; check lines and VAD. • Check the pneumatic lines, cannula, and VAD. • Call for assistance.	Occlusion alarms may be due to pneumatic line occlusion or cannula occluded or kinked.	
H. High temperature: High temperature; replace. • Check the air vent, clear the air intake filter if necessary, replace.	The high temperature alarm may be due to a blocked air vent.	
I. Low temperature: Low temperature; wait. • Wait until the driver warms up.	The driver may be too cold.	
J. Service interval: Service interval; replace. • Replace with backup; return to Thoratec for service.	Preset at 1500 hours (62 days of continuous use).	
K. Internal alarm: Alarm 18-22; replace. • Replace immediately. • Notify the team.	A problem exists within the driver electronics.	
L. Emergency backup: No message or emergency system on. • Message display off: Check if driver has poser before replacing.	All power sources have been removed, solenoid drive electronics fail, motor electronics fail to deliver sufficient pressure, microprocessor fails.	
Complete Mechanical Failure		
1. Assess the patient; determine need for cardiopulmonary resuscitation (CPR).		
2. Observe the VAD/console/blood pumps and identify the alarm.		
3. If pumps have stopped, connect hand pump(s) to the driveline(s), and squeeze at 60 beats/min.		Do not hand pump RVAD greater than LVAD. Keep the hand pump with the patient at all times.
4. If the patient is on the dual-driver console and only one module fails, the VAD(s) can be driven temporarily by the module that is working by placing the emergency selector valve into the appropriate position.	Provides a source of power.	The emergency selector valve is located on the inside of the console back door; this has three positions. The center position is "normal," and the driver modules operate independently. The "out" position allows the top module to drive both VADs. The "in" position allows the bottom module to drive both VADs.
5. Change to the backup console.		
6. Notify the cardiac transplant VAD surgeon. Consider CPR.	If VAD(s) are not restarted, may result in patient death.	
Novacor Left Ventricular Assist System[10]		
1. Changing from the LVAS monitor to the primary power pack. A. Remove a fully charged primary power pack from the charger. B. Verify the reserve power pack is charged to greater than 80%.	Provides energy source.	

Procedure continues on the following page

Procedure for **Ventricular Assist Devices**—*Continued*

Steps	Rationale	Special Considerations
C. Disconnect the monitor/controller cable from the power input port. D. Connect the primary power pack. E. Silence the LVAS monitor.		

2. Primary power pack replacement or return to tethered operation.
  A. Remove a fully charged battery from the charger, and press the display mute button to verify the charge.
  B. Verify the reserve power pack is charged.
  C. Unplug the primary power pack from the compact controller.
  D. Plug the replacement battery into the vacant power port.
  E. Plug the used power pack into the charger.
	Replace the reserve power pack before changing the primary battery if less than 50% charged (red light and alarm).	

3. Reserve power pack replacement.
  A. Verify the primary power source is connected to the compact controller
  B. Remove the fully charged reserve power pack.
  C. Unplug the reserve power pack from the controller.
  D. Plug the replacement reserve power pack into the vacant power port on the controller.
  E. Plug the removed reserve power pack into the power pack charger.
	Provides a backup power source.	The power pack charger can charge three power packs simultaneously in any combination of types; yellow is charging, green when fully charged.

4. Personal monitor setup.
  A. Place the personal monitor and the standby power source on an appropriate flat surface.
  B. Plug into the grounded power outlet.
  C. Connect the standby power source to the personal monitor using the standby power source cable.
  D. Ensure the monitor controller cable is connected to the rear of the personal monitor.
	Provides stability for the personal monitor.
	
	Decreases the risk of shock.
	Allows for power source.	

5. Changing from the personal monitor to the primary power pack.
  A. Remove a fully charged primary power pack from the charger.
  B. Verify the reserve power pack is charged to greater than 80%.
  C. Push the black button on the front of the personal monitor before changing to battery operation. Change to the battery within 20 seconds of pressing the black button.
  D. Disconnect the monitor/controller cable from the power input port.
  E. Connect the primary power pack.
	Allows for adequate power for the LVAS.
	If this is not done the monitor alarms continuously, necessitating reconnection from the battery to the personal monitor.
	
	Changes the source of power.	

Expected Outcomes

- Increased myocardial oxygen supply and decreased myocardial oxygen demand
- Increased cardiac output
- Increased tissue perfusion
- Safe bridge to heart transplantation or recovery
- Improved exercise tolerance and quality of life

Unexpected Outcomes

- Device failure
- VAD infection
- Systemic infection
- Neurologic dysfunction
- Bleeding and coagulation disorders
- Multisystem organ failure
- Thrombotic event

Patient Monitoring and Care

Steps	Rationale	Reportable Conditions
		These conditions should be reported if they persist despite nursing interventions.
1. Perform systematic cardiovascular, peripheral vascular, and hemodynamic assessment every 60 minutes and as patient status requires.		
A. Level of consciousness	Assesses for adequacy of cerebral perfusion; thrombi may develop and dislodge during VAD therapy.	• Change in level of consciousness
B. Vital signs and pulmonary artery pressures	Shows effectiveness of VAD therapy and evaluates ventricular function.	• Unstable vital signs and significant changes in hemodynamic pressures • Lack of response to VAD therapy
C. VAD flow and mixed venous oxygen saturation	Shows effectiveness of VAD therapy.	• Abnormal values
D. Circulation to extremities	Validates adequate peripheral perfusion. If reportable conditions are found, they may indicate thrombotic or embolic obstruction of perfusion to an extremity.	• Capillary refill greater than 2 seconds • Diminished or absent pulses (radial, popliteal, tibial, pedal) • Color pale, mottled, or cyanotic • Diminished or absent sensation • Pain • Diminished or absent movement • Cool or cold to touch
E. Urine output	Validates adequate perfusion to the kidneys.	• Urine output less than 0.5 ml/kg/hr
2. Assess VAD, heart, and lung sounds every 4 hours and as needed.	Abnormal VAD, heart, and lung sounds may indicate the need for additional treatment.	• Abnormal VAD sounds, such as grinding, sputtering • Diastolic murmur • Crackles or rhonchi
3. Monitor for signs of inadequate filling and emptying.	Adequate VAD function depends on an appropriate volume status. See each section for more detail. *ABIOMED BVS 5000:* Atrial and ventricular chambers expand and collapse completely when adequate filling and emptying occurs. *Thoratec:* Absence of a "flash" indicates incomplete emptying; absence of green fill light indicates incomplete filling. *Novacor:* Monitor peak fill (normal greater than 200) and residual volume (higher volume indicates decreased emptying and increased afterload).	• Inadequate filling or emptying
4. Logroll the patient every 2 hours. Prop pillows to support the patient and to maintain alignment.	Promotes comfort and skin integrity, and prevents kinking of the VAD drivelines.	• Disruption of skin integrity

Procedure continues on the following page

Patient Monitoring and Care—*Continued*

Steps	Rationale	Reportable Conditions
	Note: This step is for hemodynamically stable patients only.	
5. Initiate passive and active range-of-motion exercises every 2 hours.	Prevents venous stasis and muscle atrophy.	• Contractures
6. Assess the area around the VAD cannulas/driveline exit site every 2 hours and as needed for evidence of bleeding.	Anticoagulation therapy increases the risk of bleeding.	• Bleeding at exit/driveline site
7. Assess coagulation studies: A. Monitor complete blood count, platelet, prothrombin time, PTT, and INR as prescribed. B. Anticoagulation guidelines (per hospital policy as prescribed for each individual patient):	All VADs except the *HeartMateXVE* require prophylactic anticoagulation to prevent thrombi and emboli development.	• Abnormal values of complete blood count, platelet, prothrombin time, PTT, INR

ABIOMED BVS 5000 and AB5000 Ventricle[1,2]

A. Initiate heparin as prescribed when mediastinal drainage is 50-75 ml/hr for 3 consecutive hours.
B. Heparin bolus is not recommended.
C. Initiate heparin infusion as prescribed, but usually not greater than 16 hours postoperatively.
D. Initial heparin infusion 10-15 units/kg/hour or as prescribed.
E. Monitor activated PTT or ACT every hour until therapeutic, then every 2 hours.
F. Goal activated PTT: 2-2.5 × laboratory normal value or as prescribed.
G. Goal ACT: 180-200 seconds or as prescribed.
H. ACT: increased to 250-300 seconds or activated PTT 2.5-3 × normal for atrial or ventricular fibrillation or VAD flows less than 3 liters/min or as prescribed.

Thoratec[7]

A. Initiate heparin as prescribed when mediastinal drainage is 50-75 ml/hr for 3 consecutive hours.
B. Initiate heparin infusion as prescribed, but usually not greater than 16 hours postoperatively
C. Heparin bolus is not recommended.
D. Initiate heparin at 10 units/kg/hour or as prescribed.
E. Goal activated PTT: 1.5-2 × control or as prescribed.
F. Monitor activated PTT 2 hours after change and when stable every 4 hours.
G. Start warfarin when stable and take orally as prescribed.
H. INR goal 3-3.5 or as prescribed.

Patient Monitoring and Care—*Continued*

Steps	Rationale	Reportable Conditions

Novacor[10]
  A. Initiate heparin as prescribed when mediastinal drainage is 50-75 ml/hour for 3 consecutive hours.
  B. Initiate heparin infusion as prescribed, but usually not greater than 16 hours postoperatively.
  C. Early postoperative heparin goal: activated PTT 40-51 seconds or as prescribed.
  D. Standard infusion (greater than 24 hours postoperatively): activated PTT goal: 46-62 seconds or as prescribed.
  E. If change in infusion, recheck activated PTT in 4 hours.
  F. Heparin bolus is not recommended.
  G. Some institutions recommend clopidogrel (Plavix) for the first 30 days.
  H. Start warfarin and aspirin when stable, and take orally as prescribed.
  I. INR goal: 2.5-3.5 with aspirin and greater than 3 without aspirin or as prescribed.		

8. Monitor the patient for systemic evidence of bleeding or coagulation disorders.	Hematologic and coagulation profiles may be altered as a result of blood loss during VAD insertion, anticoagulation, platelet dysfunction, and hemolysis.	• Bleeding from the VAD insertion site • Bleeding from incisions or mucous membranes • Petechiae/ecchymosis • Guaiac-positive nasogastric aspirate or stool • Hematuria • Decreased hemoglobin/hematocrit • Decreased filling volumes • Increased heart rate • Decreased VAD flow
9. Change the VAD site dressing every 24 hours and as needed. Do not use prophylactic topical agents because they may increase maceration and increase the risk of resistant microorganisms.[4]	Decreases the incidence of infection and allows an opportunity for site assessment. *Special note:* Most manufacturers do not recommend using povidone-iodine because of degradation of the drivelines. Also, no acetone should be in the patient's room. Patients with an open sternotomy may require a physician at the bedside during dressing changes.	• Signs and symptoms of infection
10. Change the air filter weekly (HeartMate and Novacor LVADs) and as needed.	Decreases the risk of overheating the VAD.	• Any signs of fluid in the driveline or filter
11. Assess and manage the patient's pain.	The patient may experience pain from VAD placement or limited mobility.	• Unrelieved pain

Procedure continues on the following page

Patient Monitoring and Care—*Continued*

Steps	Rationale	Reportable Conditions
12. Early ambulation is essential to patient rehabilitation. When the patient is hemodynamically stable, ambulate the patient progressively. Use of an interdisciplinary rehabilitation team is essential.[4]	Prevents hazards of immobility and begins rehabilitation.	• Postural hypotension • Decrease in VAD flow with position changes • Unrelieved dizziness • Prolonged deconditioning • Signs of transient ischemic attack or cerebrovascular accident
13. Identify parameters that show clinical readiness to wean from VAD therapy (postcardiotomy support—ABIOMED or Thoratec VAD). Most frequently, this is done in the operating room and requires additional anticoagulation. ACT is usually greater than 300 seconds when VAD flow is less than 3 liters/minute. Weaning is done only with the surgeon present. Before weaning: A. Absence of lethal or unstable dysrhythmia B. Mean arterial pressure greater than 70 mm Hg with little or no vasopressor support C. Pulmonary artery wedge pressure less than 18 mm Hg D. Mixed venous oxygen saturation 60-80% E. Capillary refill less than 2 seconds F. Urine output greater than 0.5 ml/kg/hour G. Return of native aortic valve opening and closing on the arterial waveform trace H. Return of heart sounds I. Return of native tricuspid valve opening and closing on the pulmonary artery waveform trace During weaning: A. Ability to maintain normal LVAD flow when the RVAD is weaned off B. Ability to maintain normal blood pressure and pulmonary pressures with the LVAD weaned off	Determines hemodynamic readiness for weaning and stability during weaning; short-term support postcardiotomy or for cardiogenic shock is usually 5-14 days.	• Signs and symptoms of hemodynamic instability
14. Begin patient and family education as early as possible.[4]	Before discharge, patients and families must show adequate knowledge and understanding regarding the mechanics and alarms of the device (HeartMate and Thoratec VADs).	

Documentation

Documentation should include the following:

- Patient and family education
- Patient response to the VAD
- Confirmation of placement
- Hemodynamic status
- Pain level
- Activity level
- Unexpected outcomes
- Additional interventions
- Levels of pumps
- ABIOMED: level of pump (BVS 5000), complete filling and emptying, flow

- Thoratec: mode, set rate, set % systole, LVAD and RVAD drive pressures, complete filling and emptying
- HeartMate: flow, rate and stroke volume, mode
- Novacor: flow, stroke volume and rate, mode, peak fill, residual volume
- Driveline site
- Backup drive console and emergency pump device
- Dressing condition and dressing changes
- Skin integrity
- Patient tolerance
- Complete filling/emptying

References

1. ABIOMED Inc. (2003). *AB 5000 Ventricle Training Guide.* Danvers, MA: Author.
2. ABIOMED Inc. (2003). *Clinical Reference Manual.* Danvers, MA: Author.
3. Chillocott, S., Atkins, P., and Adamson, R. (1998). Left ventricular assist as a viable alternative for cardiac transplantation. *Crit Care Nurs Q, 20,* 64-9.
4. Frazier, O.H. (2003). Prologue: Ventricular assist devices and total artificial hearts: A historical perspective. *Cardiol Clin, 21,* 1-13.
5. Holmes, E.A. (2003) Outpatient management of long-term assist devices. *Cardiol Clin, 21,* 93-9.
6. Kukuy, E.L., et al. (2003). Devices as destination therapy. *Cardiol Clin, 21,* 67-73.
7. Rose, E.A., et al. (2001). Long-term mechanical left ventricular assistance for end stage heart failure. *N Engl J Med, 345,* 1435-43.
8. Thoratec Corporation. (2003). *HeartMate XVE LVAS Operating Manual.* Pleasanton, CA: Author.
9. Thoratec Corporation. (2003). *Thoratec VAD Clinical Operation and Patient Management.* Pleasanton, CA: Author.
10. World Heart Corporation. (2000). *Novacor LVAS Operator's Manual.* Oakland, CA: Author.

Additional Readings

Arabia, F., et al. (1998). Biventricular cannulation for the Thoratec ventricular assist device. *Ann Thorac Surg, 66,* 2119-20.

Bond, A.E., et al. (2003). The left ventricular assist device. *Am J Nurs, 103,* 32-41.

DeRose, J., et al. (1997). Implantable left ventricular assist devices provide an excellent outpatient bridge to transplantation and recovery. *J Am Coll Cardiol, 30,* 1773-7.

Dixon, J.F., and Farris, D.D. (1991). The ABIOMED BVS 5000 System. *AACN Clin Issues Crit Care Nurs, 2,* 552-61.

Goldstein, D.J., and Oz, M.C. (2000). *Cardiac Assist Devices.* New York: Futura Publishing.

Livinston, E., et al. (1996). Increased activation of the coagulation and fibrinolytic systems leads to hemorrhagic complications during left ventricular assist implantation. *Circulation, 94*(Suppl II), II227-34.

McCarthy, P., et al. (1998). One hundred patients with the HeartMate left ventricular assist device: Evolving concepts and technology. *J Thorac Cardiovasc Surg, 115,* 904-12.

Mussivand, T., et al. (1992). Critical anatomic dimensions for intrathoracic circulatory assist devices. *Artif Organs, 16,* 281-5.

Schakenbach, L.H. (2002). Care of the patient with a ventricular assist device. In: *Protocols for Practice.* Aliso Viejo, CA: American Association of Critical-Care Nurses.

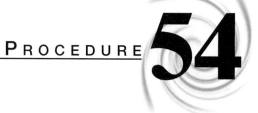
Electrocardiographic
Leads and Cardiac
Monitoring

PROCEDURE 54

Electrophysiologic Monitoring: Hardwire and Telemetry

PURPOSE: Continuous electrophysiologic monitoring is performed routinely for most critically ill patients. A key component of electrophysiologic monitoring is the electrocardiogram (ECG). The ECG provides a continuous graphic picture of cardiac electrical activity. The ECG can be used for diagnostic, documentation, and treatment purposes.

Mary G. McKinley

PREREQUISITE NURSING KNOWLEDGE

- Knowledge of the anatomy and physiology of the cardiovascular system, principles of cardiac conduction, principles of electrophysiology, ECG lead placement, basic dysrhythmia interpretation, and electrical safety is required.
- Advanced cardiac life support knowledge and skills are needed.
- Electrophysiologic monitoring by hardwire and telemetry is indicated for all patients in critical care units and for patients in selected acute care settings, postanesthesia areas, operating rooms, and emergency departments.
- Electrophysiologic monitoring is designed to give a graphic display of the electrical activity in the heart generated by depolarization and repolarization of cardiac tissue.
- Hardwire ECG monitors have electrodes and lead wires that are attached directly to the patient. Impulses are transmitted directly from the patient to the monitor (Fig. 54-1).
- Telemetry systems have electrodes and lead wires that are attached from the patient to a battery pack transmitting impulses to the monitor via radio wave transmission (Fig. 54-2).
- Telemetry is useful in progressive ambulation and to evaluate toleration of activity. A disadvantage to telemetry is

that ambulation and activity can increase distortion of the ECG pattern.
- Specific areas of the chest are used for electrode placement to obtain a view of the electrical activity in a particular area of the heart (commonly called a *lead*).
- ECG monitors use a three-lead or five-lead wire system to provide different views (leads) of the heart's electrical activity.
- Standardized placement of leads is important so that information obtained is assessed within a common frame of reference and so that appropriate judgments can be made on the patient's cardiac status. Alterations of electrode position may distort the appearance of the waveform significantly and can lead to misdiagnosis or mistreatment.
- The two major factors that determine the views of the ECG deflection on the monitor are the location of the electrodes on the body and the direction of the cardiac impulse in relation to the position of the electrode.
- A basic rule of electrocardiography is the rule of electrical flow. This rule notes that if electricity flows toward the positive electrode, an upright pattern is produced on the monitor or graph paper. If the electricity flows away from the positive electrode (or toward the negative electrode), a downward pattern or deflection is produced on the monitor or graph paper. Lead wires attached to the

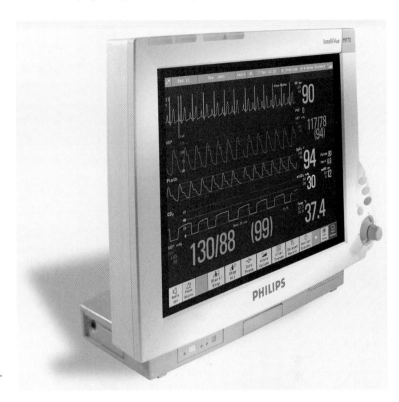

FIGURE 54-1 Bedside monitoring system. *(Courtesy Philips Medical Systems.)*

patient are coded (+, P [positive] or −, N [negative]; RA [right arm]; RL [right leg]; LA [left arm]; LL [left leg]; V or C) in some way for ease in correct placement. Placement of the leads gives different views of the electrical conduction through the heart.

- Information from the bedside via hardwire or telemetry can be transferred to a central monitor, where it can be printed, stored, and analyzed (Fig. 54-3).

- Most five-lead bedside monitoring systems provide a continuous readout of two or more leads simultaneously. This readout provides more information and a comparison of the ECG patterns. Optimal lead selection is based on the goals of monitoring for each patient's clinical situation.

- A more recent application of bedside electrophysiologic monitoring is reduced lead continuous 12-lead ECG

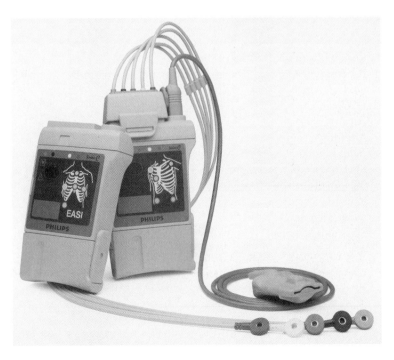

FIGURE 54-2 Telemetry monitoring system. *(Courtesy Philips Medical Systems.)*

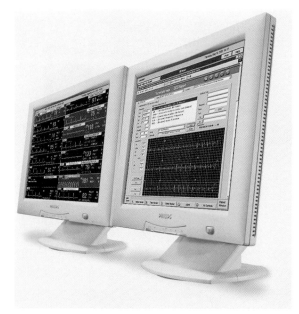

FIGURE 54-3 Central station. *(Courtesy Philips Medical Systems.)*

acquisition (e.g., the EASI lead system). In this application, the reduced lead configuration varies according to the manufacturer and the device, but provides the availability of obtaining a continuous 12-lead ECG, which can be accessed for information over a predetermined time (commonly 24 hours). This application greatly expands the information available from bedside monitors and requires accurate and consistent lead placement based on the manufacturer's requirements.

EQUIPMENT

- ECG monitor (central and bedside monitor) or battery pack (telemetry monitoring only)
- Electrodes, pregelled and disposable
- Gauze pads or terry cloth washcloth
- Cleansing pads or nonemollient soap and water in a basin
- Lead wires (no longer than 18 inches)
- Patient cable (should be compatible with the monitor and the lead wires)
- ECG calipers
- Alcohol pads
  Additional equipment to have available as needed includes the following:
- Skin preparation solution, such as skin barrier wipe or tincture of benzoin, if needed
- Pouch or pocket gown to hold telemetry unit (telemetry monitoring only)
- Scissors to clip hair from the chest as needed

PATIENT AND FAMILY EDUCATION

- Assess the readiness of the patient and family to learn. ➤*Rationale:* Anxiety and concerns the patient and family have may inhibit their ability to learn.
- Provide explanations of the equipment and alarms to the patient and family. ➤*Rationale:* These explanations assist in making the patient and family feel more comfortable with monitoring and may reduce anxiety.
- Reassure the patient and family that monitoring is continuous and that the patient's heart rate and rhythm will be monitored and treated as indicated. ➤*Rationale:* This reassures the patient and family that immediate care is available.
- Emphasize that the patient should feel free to move about in bed. ➤*Rationale:* This encourages movement on the part of the patient and allays fears about disruption of the monitoring system.
- Explain the importance of reporting any symptoms, such as pain, dizziness, palpitations, or chest discomfort. ➤*Rationale:* Reporting of symptoms ensures appropriate and timely assessment and intervention.

PATIENT ASSESSMENT AND PREPARATION

Patient Assessment

- Assess the patient's peripheral pulses, vital signs, heart sounds, level of consciousness, lung sounds, neck vein distention, presence of chest pain or palpitations, and for peripheral circulatory disorders (i.e., clubbing, cyanosis, and dependent edema). ➤*Rationale:* This assessment provides baseline assessment data.
- Assess if the patient has a history of cardiac dysrhythmias or cardiac problems. ➤*Rationale:* The history provides baseline data and may guide selection of monitoring leads.
- Assess landmarks for identification of correct placement of electrodes. ➤*Rationale:* This ensures accurate placement of leads for accurate interpretation.

Patient Preparation

- Ensure that the patient and family understand preprocedural teaching. Answer questions as they arise, and reinforce information as needed. ➤*Rationale:* This communication evaluates and reinforces the understanding of previously taught information.
- Assist the patient to the supine position. ➤*Rationale:* This position enables easy access to the chest for electrode placement.

Procedure for Electrophysiologic Monitoring: Hardwire and Telemetry

Steps	Rationale	Special Considerations
1. Wash hands.	Reduces the transmission of microorganisms; standard precautions.	
2. Turn on the computerized central monitoring system.	When activated, the central monitoring system alarm sounds to notify the nurse of problems with the ECG for interpretation and attention.	The nurse must assess the patient to confirm findings, verify patterns, and evaluate computer interpretations.
3. For telemetry monitoring, insert a battery into the telemetry unit, matching polarity markings on the transmitter.	Batteries can fail if left sitting on the shelf or in the unit. Polarity must match for proper functioning of the unit.	Refer to the manufacturer's recommendations about battery storage and replacement.
4. Ensure that the monitor is plugged into a grounded alternating current (AC) wall outlet.	Maintains electrical safety.	
5. Turn the bedside monitor on.	Provides the power source to the monitor.	The equipment may require self-test and warm-up time.
6. Identify whether a three-lead or a five-lead wire system is available.	Assists in determining possible placement of electrodes and leads that can be viewed.	Optimal lead selection should be based on the type of lead system available and the goals of monitoring for each patient's clinical situation.
7. Check the cable and lead wires for fraying, broken wires, or discoloration.	Detects conditions that may give an inaccurate ECG trace.	Safety must be maintained; if equipment is damaged, obtain alternative equipment and notify the biomedical engineer for repair.
8. Plug the patient cable into the monitoring system.	Hardware systems require a direct connection to the bedside monitoring system.	
9. Check that the lead wires are plugged into the patient cable correctly and securely. A. Three-lead system (Fig. 54-4): • The negative wire plugs into the opening marked *N, −,* or *RA.*	Reduces the chance of disconnection, distortion, or outside interference with the ECG tracing.	Manufacturers code the lead connections so that the correct attachments can be made; often these are color coded, but they may be letter or symbol coded.

Procedure continues on the following page

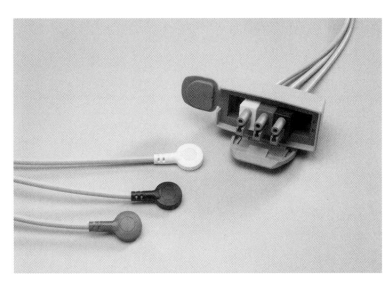

FIGURE 54-4 Three-lead wire system.
(Courtesy Philips Medical Systems.)

Procedure for Electrophysiologic Monitoring: Hardwire and Telemetry—*Continued*

Steps	Rationale	Special Considerations
• The positive wire plugs into the opening marked *P*, *+*, *LL*, or *LA*. • The ground wire plugs into the opening marked *G*, *Neutral*, or *RL*. B. Five-lead system (Fig. 54-5): • The right arm wire plugs into the opening marked *RA*. • The left arm wire plugs into the opening marked *LA*. • The left leg wire plugs into the opening marked *LL*. • The right leg wire plugs into the opening marked *RL*. • The chest wire plugs into the opening marked *C* or *V*.		
10. Connect the electrodes to the lead wires before placing the electrodes on the patient.	Prepares the monitoring system.	Placing electrodes on the chest and then attaching the lead wires can be uncomfortable for the patient and can contribute to the development of air bubbles in the electrode gel, which can decrease conduction.
11. Choose electrode placement. A. Three-lead system: • First choice: MCL_1 • Second choice: MCL_6 B. Five-lead system: • First choice: Single-lead monitoring: V_1; dual-lead monitoring: V_1 and the limb lead appropriate for the clinical situation (see special considerations for tips). • Second choice: Substitute V_6 for V_1 when the patient cannot have an electrode at the sternal	In a three-lead system, MCL_1 or MCL_6 is used because the QRS morphology approximates V_1 or V_6, which is more useful in providing specific information.[1] Choice is based on constraints on chest wall space (dressings or injury sites) and type of information required or desired.	Tips for selection of limb lead appropriate for the clinical situation[3,4]: 1. Atrial flutter: II, III, or AVF. 2. Inferior myocardial infarction (MI) II, III, or AVF select the lead with maximal elevation of ST segment on the 12-lead ECG. 3. Anterior MI: Select the lead with maximal elevation of ST segment on the 12-lead ECG. 4. After angioplasty: Select III or AVF—whichever has the tallest R wave.

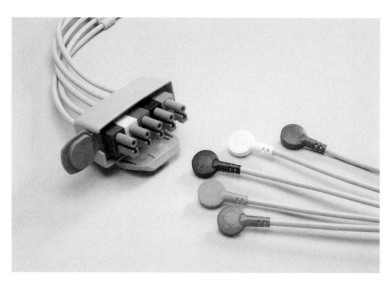

FIGURE 54-5 Five-lead wire system.
(*Courtesy Philips Medical Systems.*)

Procedure for Electrophysiologic Monitoring: Hardwire and Telemetry—*Continued*

Steps	Rationale	Special Considerations
border or when the QRS complex amplitude is not adequate for optimized computerized monitoring.		5. If three channels are available, use $V_1 + I + AVF$.[3] 6. Use lead II if none of these clinical situations apply

12. Identify the sternal notch or angle of Louis.
    A. Palpate the upper sternum to identify where the clavicle joins the sternum (suprasternal notch).
    B. Slide fingers down the center of the sternum to the obvious bony prominence. This is the sternal notch, which identifies the second rib and provides a landmark for noting the fourth ICS.
    C. Locate the fourth ICS.
	The sternal notch identifies the second rib and assists in locating the fourth intercostal space (ICS) so that accurate placement may be achieved.	

13. Clean the area for the application of electrodes with cleansing pads or soap and water and dry thoroughly. *(Level IV: Limited clinical studies to support recommendations.)*	Provides for adequate transmission of electrical impulses. Moist skin is not conducive to electrode adherence.[2]	It may be necessary to clip chest hair to ensure good skin contact with the electrodes.
14. Clean the intended sites with alcohol pads. Consider using skin preparation solutions. *(Level IV: Limited clinical studies to support recommendations.)*	Alcohol or skin preparations may be needed to remove oils to improve impulse transmission.[2]	Skin preparation solutions should not be applied to the area of the skin that will be in direct contact with the electrode gel because transmission of impulses may be decreased.
15. Abrade the skin using a washcloth, scratch pad on electrode pack, or gauze pad.	Removes dead skin cells, promoting impulse transmission.	
16. Remove the backing from the pregelled electrodes and test the center of the pads for moistness.	Gel can dry out in storage; gel should be moist to allow for impulse transmission.	
17. Apply electrodes to the sites, ensuring a seal. Avoid pushing on the gel pads.	Electrodes must be placed tightly to prevent external influences from affecting the ECG. Pressing on the gel pad can cause the gel to leak onto the adhesive surfaces and may interfere with transmission.	

18. Place electrodes as follows:
 	
    A. Three-lead system: MCL$_1$ and MCL$_6$ (Fig. 54-6):
    • Apply right arm (RA) electrode to the patient's left shoulder.
    • Apply left arm (LA) electrode at fourth ICS right sternal border.
    • Apply left leg (LL) electrode to the fifth ICS at midaxillary line.
    • Select lead I to obtain MCL$_1$ and lead II to obtain MCL$_6$.
	Proper positioning is essential to ensure a correct view of the leads.[1,3]	Lead selection is based on chest wall constraints and the clinical situation.

Procedure continues on the following page

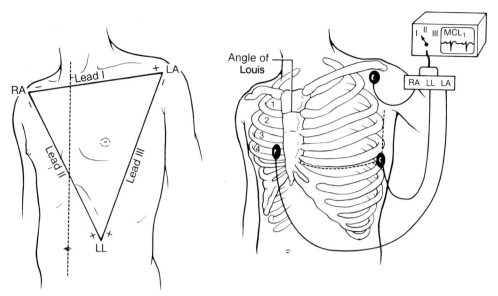

FIGURE 54-6 Three-lead application. *(From Drew, B. [1993]. Bedside electrocardiographic monitoring. AACN Clin Issues Crit Care, 4, 28.)*

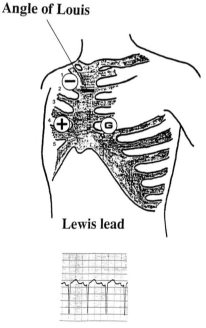

FIGURE 54-7 Three-lead system with Lewis lead.

Procedure	**for Electrophysiologic Monitoring: Hardwire and Telemetry**—*Continued*	
Steps	**Rationale**	**Special Considerations**
B. Lewis lead (Fig. 54-7): • Apply right arm (RA) electrode at first ICS right sternal border. • Apply left arm (LA) electrode to fourth ICS right sternal border. • Apply left leg (LL) electrode to fourth ICS left sternal border • Set the lead selector to lead I.		Lewis lead offers the best visualization of P waves.

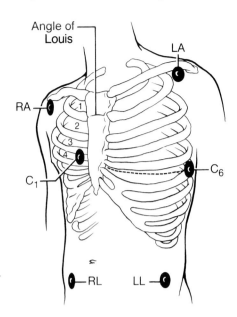

FIGURE 54-8 Five-lead application. *(From Drew, B. [1993]. Bedside electrocardiographic monitoring.* AACN Clin Issues Crit Care, *4, 26.)*

Procedure for Electrophysiologic Monitoring: Hardwire and Telemetry—*Continued*		
Steps	**Rationale**	**Special Considerations**
C. Five-lead system (Fig. 54-8): • Apply right arm (RA) to the right shoulder close to the junction of the right arm and torso. • Apply left arm (LA) to the left shoulder close to the junction of the left arm torso. • Apply right leg (RL) electrode at the level of the lowest rib, on the right abdominal region or on the hip. • Apply left leg (LL) electrode at the level of the lowest rib, on the left abdominal region, or on the hip.	Arm electrodes that are placed under the clavicle or leg electrodes that are placed too high on the ribs can alter the point of view of the leads and result in inaccurate recording.[1,3]	
• Apply the chest lead electrode on the selected site: V_1 fourth ICS right sternal border or V_6 fifth ICS midaxillary line. • Set the lead selector or monitor the appropriate leads.	Only one precordial lead can be displayed—placement of the electrode identifies the lead used.	
19. Reduce tension on the lead wires and cables.	Decreases tension on the lead wires to alleviate undue stress, causing interference or faulty recordings.	
A. For hardwire monitoring, fasten the lead wire and patient cable to the patient's gown, making a stress loop.	Minimizes pulling on the electrodes, which can be uncomfortable for the patient.	
B. For telemetry monitoring, secure the transmitter in a pouch or pocket in the patient's gown.	The transmitter must be secure so that it is not dropped or damaged.	

Procedure continues on the following page

Procedure for Electrophysiologic Monitoring: Hardwire and Telemetry—*Continued*

Steps	Rationale	Special Considerations
20. Examine the ECG tracing on the monitor for the size of the R and T waves.	The R wave should be approximately twice the height of the other components of the ECG to ensure proper detection by the heart rate counter in the equipment. The accuracy of the alarm system often depends on the R wave. If the T wave is nearly equal to the R wave, double counting can occur, resulting in false alarms.	Manufacturers provide for calibration of the ECG to 1 mV, and monitors have size adjustments that can be used to increase or decrease the size of the ECG.
21. Obtain an ECG strip (Fig. 54-9) and interpret it for rhythm, rate, presence and configuration of P waves, length of P-R interval, length of QRS complexes, presence and configuration of T waves, length of Q-T intervals, presence of extra waves (e.g., U waves), and presence of dysrhythmias.	Reviews the normal conduction sequence and identifies abnormalities that may require further evaluation or treatment.	
22. Set the alarms. Upper and lower alarm limits are set on the basis of the patient's current clinical status and heart rate.	Activates the bedside or telemetry monitor alarm system.	Monitoring systems allow for setting alarms at the bedside or the central console. The types of alarms may include rate (high or low), abnormal rhythms or complexes, pacemaker recognition, and others, depending on the manufacturer. *Caution:* Never turn off bedside monitor alarms. Alarms should be adjusted according to the known clinical status of the patient.
23. Discard used supplies and wash hands.	Reduces the transmission of microorganisms; standard precautions.	

Expected Outcomes

- Properly applied electrodes
- A clear ECG monitor tracing displayed (see Fig. 54-9)
- Alarms set appropriate to the patient's clinical status
- Prompt identification and treatment of dysrhythmias

Unexpected Outcomes

- Altered skin integrity
- AC interference, also called 60-cycle interference (Fig. 54-10)
- Wandering baseline (Fig. 54-11)
- False alarms
- Artifact or waveform interference (Fig. 54-12)
- Microshock

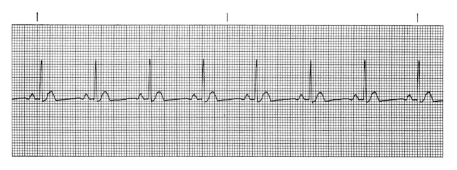

FIGURE 54-9 Monitor strip of clear ECG pattern.

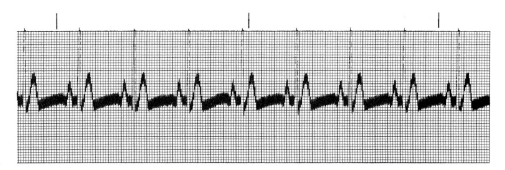

FIGURE 54-10 Monitor strip with 60-cycle interference.

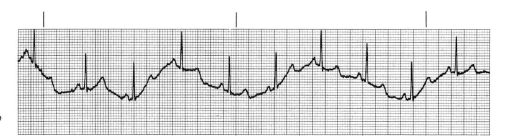

FIGURE 54-11 Monitor strip with erratic baseline.

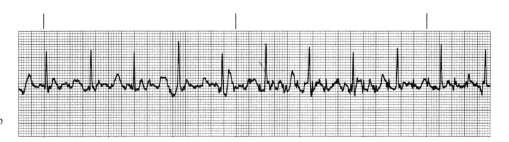

FIGURE 54-12 Monitor strip with interference.

Patient Monitoring and Care

Steps	Rationale	Reportable Conditions
		These conditions should be reported if they persist despite nursing interventions.
1. Evaluate the ECG monitor pattern for the presence of P waves, QRS complexes, a clear baseline, and absence of artifact or distortion. Obtain a rhythm strip on admission, every shift (as per institution protocol), and with rhythm changes.	A clear pattern is required to make accurate judgments about the patient's status and treatment.[5]	• Changes in cardiac ECG complexes, rate, and rhythm
2. Evaluate the ECG pattern continually for dysrhythmias, assess patient tolerance of the change, and provide prompt nursing intervention.	Changes in the ECG pattern may indicate significant problems for the patient and may require immediate intervention or additional diagnostic tests, such as a 12-lead ECG.	• Changes in cardiac rate and rhythm • Hemodynamic instability

Procedure continues on the following page

Patient Monitoring and Care—*Continued*

Steps	Rationale	Reportable Conditions
3. Evaluate skin integrity around the electrodes on a daily basis, and change the electrodes every 48 hours. Rotate sites when changing electrodes. Monitor the skin for any allergic reaction to the adhesive or gel. Change all electrodes if a problem occurs with one.	Skin integrity must be maintained to have a clear picture of the ECG. Replacing electrodes every 48 hours prevents drying of the gel and may prevent skin breakdown. It may be necessary to change to different leads if sites become irritated. Electrode resistance changes as the gel dries, so changing all electrodes at once prevents differences in resistance between electrodes.[2]	• Alteration in skin integrity
4. Check electrode placement every shift.	Accurate interpretation of many dysrhythmias depends on proper placement of the electrodes and knowing which lead is being viewed.	

Documentation

Documentation should include the following:

- Patient and family education
- An initial or baseline ECG strip, noting the lead, interpretation, any dysrhythmias, and treatments
- Routine ECG strips according to institution protocol
- An ECG strip should be recorded whenever there is a change in cardiac rate or rhythm, the patient experiences chest pain, there is a change in lead placement, and when evaluating the effect of antidysrhythmic agents
- Unexpected outcomes
- Additional nursing interventions

References

1. Drew, B.J. (2002). Celebrating the 100th birthday of the electrocardiogram: Lessons learned from research in cardiac monitoring. *Am J Crit Care,* 11, 378-86.
2. Jacobson, C. (1996). Bedside cardiac monitoring. In: *AACN Research Based Practice Protocol, Technology Series.* Aliso Viejo, CA: American Association of Critical Care Publications, 1-32.
3. Jacobson, C. (2000). Optimal bedside cardiac monitoring. *Prog Cardiovasc Nurs,* 15, 134-7.
4. Leeper, B. (2003). Continuous ST-segment monitoring. *AACN Clin Issues,* 14, 145-54.
5. Marquez, M.F., et al. (2002). Common electrocardiographic artifacts mimicking arrhythmias in ambulatory monitoring. *Am Heart J,* 144, 187-97.

Additional Readings

Alspach, J. (1998). *Core Curriculum for Critical Care Nursing.* Philadelphia: W.B. Saunders.

Drew, B.J., et al. (2004). An American Heart Association Scientific Statement from the Councils on Cardiovascular Nursing, Clinical Cardiology, and Cardiovascular Disease in the Young. *Circulation,* 110, 2721-46.
Kadish, A.H., et al. (2001). ACC/AHA clinical competence statement on electrocardiography and ambulatory electrocardiography: A report of the ACC/AHA/ACP-ASIM Task Force on Clinical Competence. *Circulation,* 18, 3169-78.
Reinelt, P., et al. (2001). Incidence and type of cardiac arrhythmias in critically ill patients: A single center experience in medical cardiological ICU. *Intensive Care Med,* 27, 1466-73.
Sole, M., Klein, D., and Moseley, M. (2005). *Introduction to Critical Care Nursing.* 4th ed. Philadelphia: W.B. Saunders.
Tuna, N. (2000). Electrocardiography, In: Willerson, J., and Cohn, J. (2000). *Cardiovascular Medicine.* 2nd ed. New York: Churchill Livingstone.

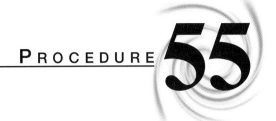

PROCEDURE **55**

Extra Electrocardiographic Leads: Right Precordial and Left Posterior Leads

P U R P O S E : Extra electrocardiographic (ECG) leads are used in conjunction with the standard 12-lead ECG to provide additional diagnostic information.

Shu-Fen Wung
Barbara J. Drew

PREREQUISITE NURSING KNOWLEDGE

- Understanding of the anatomy and physiology of the cardiovascular system, basic rhythm interpretation, and electrical safety is required.
- Advanced cardiac life support knowledge and skills are needed.
- Familiarity with principles of electrophysiology is needed:
  - ❖ The right ventricular (RV) V_{1R} through V_{6R} and left posterior leads V_7 through V_9 are unipolar leads in which the chest electrode serves as the "exploring" electrode or positive pole of the lead. These precordial leads view the heart from the vantage point of their electrode positions on the chest, similar to the standard left precordial leads V_1 through V_6.
  - ❖ To record RV or left posterior leads, the three limb electrodes (right arm [RA], left arm [LA], left leg [LL]) also are required to create a central terminal (negative pole), and one limb electrode (right leg [RL]) is used to stabilize the ECG recording.
- Accuracy in identifying anatomic landmarks to locate electrode sites and knowledge of the importance of accurate electrode placement are required. It is essential for nurses to locate accurately the electrode positions for the standard 12-lead ECG because the same anatomic landmarks are used to locate the RV and left posterior leads. Accurate ECG interpretation is possible only when the recording electrodes are placed in the proper positions. Slight alterations of the electrode positions may distort significantly the appearance of the ECG waveforms and can lead to misdiagnosis.[7] Reliable comparison of

serial (more than two ECGs recorded at different times) ECG recordings relies on accurate and consistent electrode placement. It is recommended that an indelible marker be used to identify clearly the electrode locations to ensure that the same electrode locations are selected when serial ECGs are recorded.

- Nurses should be aware of body positional changes that can alter ECG recordings. Serial ECGs should be recorded with the patient in a supine position to ensure that all recordings are done in a consistent manner. Side-lying positions and elevation of the torso may change the position of the heart within the chest and can change the waveforms on the ECG recording.[8,14] If another position other than supine is clinically required, notation of the altered position should be made on the tracing.
- Right precordial leads are useful in diagnosing a RV myocardial infarction (MI).[1,6,12] These RV leads are important because they enable clinicians to identify MI patients who are at high risk of developing atrioventricular (AV) conduction disturbances,[1] to predict the site of coronary artery occlusion, and to guide appropriate hemodynamic monitoring and interventions.[11] Left posterior leads are used to aid in the detection of true posterior MI[9] or left circumflex coronary artery–related occlusion[15] and to facilitate timely reperfusion treatment. Recording left posterior leads also can help in the differential diagnosis of tall R waves in lead V_1 and V_2.[4]
- Nurses should be able to operate the 12-lead ECG machine used in the unit. Calibration of 1 mV = 10 mm and paper speed of 25 mm/sec are standards used in clinical practice. For ST-segment analysis, filter settings of 0.05 to 100 Hz are recommended by the American Heart Association.[13]

Any variation used for particular clinical purposes should be noted on the tracing. Large QRS amplitudes require the use of a calibration of 5 mm/mV. Specific information regarding configuring the ECG machine, troubleshooting, and safety features is available from the manufacturer and should be read before use of the equipment.

- Nurses should be able to interpret recorded ECGs for the presence or absence of myocardial ischemia, MI, and dysrhythmias so that patients can be treated appropriately. Acute inferior MI patients with RV involvement, determined by ST-segment elevation in the right precordial leads, are at high risk for developing high-degree AV block. Nurses should monitor patients closely for conduction disturbances and anticipate the need for temporary pacing. Patients with RV infarction are prone to developing hypotension and shock that responds to treatment with intravenous fluids.

- Indications for recording a right precordial ECG are as follows:
  - ❖ Patients admitted for evaluation and treatment of suspected acute MI, especially patients with inferior wall MI (ST-segment elevation in leads II, III, and aVF)
  - ❖ To evaluate the risk for developing AV node conduction disturbances and to anticipate treatment plans
  - ❖ To predict the site of coronary artery occlusion (RV infarction occurs with proximal right coronary artery [RCA] occlusion)
  - ❖ To determine the risk of developing "volume-responsive" shock, in which case intravenous fluids are warranted and vasodilators (e.g., intravenous nitroglycerin) are contraindicated

- Indications for recording a left posterior ECG are as follows:
  - ❖ Patients admitted for evaluation and treatment of acute or suspected MI, especially patients with isolated ST-segment depression in the left precordial ECG leads V_1 through V_3 or patients with a nondiagnostic ECG
  - ❖ Presence of chest pain or "anginal equivalent" symptoms (e.g., jaw, left shoulder or arm discomfort, or shortness of breath) or ST-segment depression in the left precordial ECG leads V_1 through V_3 after catheter-based interventions of the left circumflex artery
  - ❖ Patients with any of these ECG characteristics indicative of posterior MI in lead V_1: R waves greater than or equal to 6 mm in height, R wave greater than or equal to 40 msec in duration, R/S ratio* greater than or equal to 1, or S wave less than or equal to 3 mm. In lead V_2: R wave greater than or equal to 15 mm in height, R wave greater than or equal to 50 msec in duration, R/S ratio greater than or equal to 1.5, or S wave less than or equal to 4 mm[10]
  - ❖ To differentiate true posterior MI from other conditions that can cause tall R waves in lead V_1, such as RV hypertrophy, right bundle-branch block, Wolff-Parkinson-White syndrome, and ventricular septal hypertrophy

- In patients with RV infarction who exhibit shock, volume expansion is used to provide adequate RV and left ventricular filling pressures and to restore arterial pressure

and peripheral blood flow. Positive inotropic agents also may be indicated to augment the contractile force of the residual functioning fibers in the damaged RV. Avoid the use of vasodilators (e.g., nitroglycerin). Vasodilators cause venous dilation and reduced preload. Also avoid the use of diuretics (e.g., furosemide [Lasix]). Diuretics reduce preload and left ventricular filling.[5]

EQUIPMENT

- Gauze pads or terry cloth washcloth
- Cleaning tissue or soap and water in basin
- Indelible marker
- 12-lead ECG machine with attached patient cable
- Lead wires (one end connects to the patient cable and one end connects to ECG electrodes on the patient)
- ECG electrodes
  Additional equipment to have available as needed includes the following:
  - ❖ Clipper
  - ❖ Temporary pacing equipment
  - ❖ Alcohol pads
  - ❖ Skin preparation solution, such as skin barrier wipe or tincture of benzoin

PATIENT AND FAMILY EDUCATION

- Describe the procedure and reasons for obtaining extra ECG leads. Reassure the patient that the procedure is painless. ➤*Rationale:* This communication clarifies information, reduces anxiety, and gains cooperation from the patient.
- Explain the patient's role in assisting with the ECG recording, and emphasize actions that improve the quality of the ECG tracing, such as relaxing, avoiding conversation and body movement, and breathing normally. ➤*Rationale:* This explanation ensures the patient's cooperation to improve the quality of the tracing and avoids unnecessarily repeating ECGs because of muscle artifact.

PATIENT ASSESSMENT AND PREPARATION

Patient Assessment

- Interpret previously recorded ECGs. ➤*Rationale:* Each patient has his or her own individual baseline ECG. Previous ECG recordings can help clinicians to determine whether a change is acute or chronic.
- Evaluate the presence of anginal symptoms, such as chest pain, pressure, tightness, heaviness, fullness, or squeezing sensation; radiated pain; or shortness of breath. ➤*Rationale:* This evaluation correlates ECG changes with patient's symptoms.
- Determine the patient's past medical history of cardiac diseases, such as MI, and pervious interventions and medications. ➤*Rationale:* Knowledge about the patient's prior cardiac history and medications can help in interpreting ECG recordings (Fig. 55-1). Digitalis therapy causes chronic ST-segment depression that does not indicate

---

*R wave amplitude in mm over S wave amplitude in mm.

ischemia. A normal-looking isoelectric ST segment in a digitalized patient may indicate acute ischemia. Patients with a prior posterior MI might have abnormal Q waves in the left posterior leads.

- Interpret the patient's standard 12-lead ECG for any signs of myocardial ischemia or MI and dysrhythmias. ➧*Rationale:* Nurses should be able to evaluate the standard 12-lead ECG for the location of ischemia or infarction and assess the possibility of RV and posterior involvement (Fig. 55-2).

Patient Preparation

- Ensure that the patient and family understand preprocedural teaching. Answer questions as they arise, and reinforce information as needed. ➧*Rationale:* This communication evaluates and reinforces the understanding of previously taught information.
- Assist the patient to the supine position. ➧*Rationale:* This position enables easy access to the chest for electrode placement.

FIGURE 55-1 Baseline ST-segment deviation as a result of left bundle-branch block before percutaneous transluminal coronary angioplasty (pre-PTCA, *left panel*). During angioplasty balloon inflation of the proximal left circumflex coronary artery (LC occlusion, *right panel*), the patient developed myocardial ischemia with chest pain radiating to the left arm. ST segments in the left posterior leads (V$_7$, V$_8$, and V$_9$) became elevated compared with the baseline pre-PTCA tracing to produce a normal-looking, isoelectric ST segment. This pseudonormalization of the ST segment during ischemia can be misinterpreted as normal without assessment of the baseline ECG.

Pre-PTCA

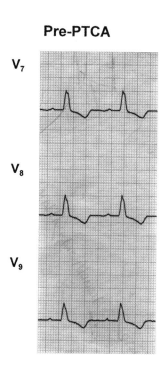

LCX Occlusion

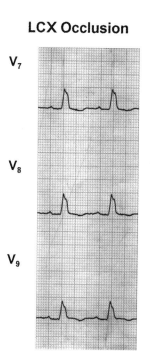

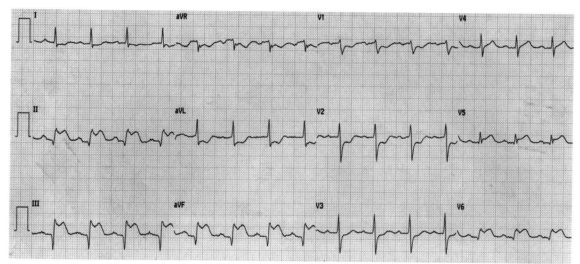

FIGURE 55-2 Initial ECG in a patient admitted to the emergency department with acute inferior MI (elevated ST segments and Q waves in leads II, III, and aVF) with apical involvement (elevated ST segment in leads V$_4$, V$_5$, and V$_6$). ST-segment depression in leads V$_1$, V$_2$, and V$_3$ suggests posterior involvement. Left posterior and right precordial leads should be recorded to assess posterior and RV involvement.

Procedure   for Extra Electrocardiographic Leads

Steps	Rationale	Special Considerations
1. Wash hands.	Reduces the transmission of microorganisms; standard precautions.	
2. Check the patient cable and lead wires for fraying or broken wires.	Detects any condition that might cause the ECG recording to be incomplete or inaccurate.	If the equipment is damaged, obtain alternative equipment and notify a biomedical engineer for repair.
3. Check the lead wires for accurate labels.	Obtains accurate ECG recordings.	
4. Plug the ECG machine into a grounded wall outlet.	Maintains electrical safety.	Follow manufacturer's recommendation and institution's protocol on electrical safety per biomedical department.
5. Turn the ECG machine on, and program the ECG machine: paper speed, 25 mm/sec; calibration, 10 mm/mV; filter settings, 0.05 to 100 Hz. *(Level II: Theory based, no research data to support recommendations; recommendations from expert consensus group may exist.)*	In accordance with clinical practice and recommendation for ST-segment analysis by the American Heart Association (AHA).[13]	Follow the manufacturer's recommendation in configuring the ECG machine.
6. Place the patient in a supine position. *(Level IV: Limited clinical studies to support recommendations.)*	Body position changes can cause ST-segment deviation and QRS waveform alteration.[8,14]	If another position is clinically required, note the altered position on the ECG recording. ECGs should be recorded in the same body position to ensure ECG changes are not caused by a change in body position.
7. Expose the body parts for electrode placement.	Overexposing body parts may cause shivering and lack of privacy.	
8. Identify the electrode sites and mark with an indelible marker.	When multiple ECG recordings are required, it is important to minimize ECG changes caused by altered electrode placement.[7]	After accurately identifying the locations, an indelible marker should be used to mark the electrode sites.
Limb Leads • Right arm (RA): inside right forearm		The limb leads are placed in the same way as when recording a standard 12-lead ECG (see Procedure 57).
• Left arm (LA): inside left forearm		
• Right leg (RL): anywhere on the body; by convention, usually on the right ankle or inner aspect of the calf	RL electrode is a ground electrode that does not contribute to the ECG tracings.	
• Left leg (LL): left ankle or inner aspect of the calf		
Right Precordial Leads (Fig. 55-3) • V_{1R}: fourth intercostal space (ICS) at the left sternal border (same as V_2).	All patients with an acute inferior wall MI should have right precordial leads recorded in addition to left precordial leads V_1 through V_6.	These right precordial leads are placed across the right precordium using the same landmarks that are used for the left precordial leads.[9]
• V_{2R}: fourth ICS at the right sternal border (same as V_1).	Accurate electrode placement is essential for obtaining valid and reliable data for ECG recordings.	V_{1R} is at the same location as V_2, and V_{2R} is at the same location as V_1 in the standard 12-lead ECG (Fig. 55-4).

Right Precordial Leads

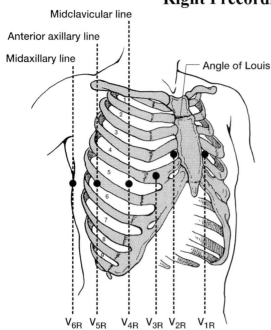

V_{1R}: 4th intercostal space (ICS) at left sternal border (same as V_2)

V_{2R}: 4th ICS at right sternal border (same as V_1)

V_{3R}: halfway between V_{2R} and V_{4R}

V_{4R}: right midclavicular line in the 5th ICS

V_{5R}: right anterior axillary line at the same horizontal level as V_{4R}

V_{6R}: right mid-axillary line at the same horizontal level as V_{4R}

FIGURE 55-3 Electrode locations for recording a right precordial ECG. *(From Drew, B.J., and Ide, B. [1995]. Right ventricular infarction. Prog Cardiovasc Nurs, 10, 46.)*

Conventional 12–Lead ECG   Right Precordial Leads

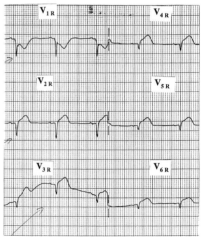

FIGURE 55-4 ST-segment elevation in leads II, III, and aVF indicates acute inferior wall MI. Three characteristics on the standard 12-lead ECG *(left panel)* suggest a RV infarction: **(1)** Diagnosis of inferior MI. **(2)** ST-segment elevation in lead III exceeding that of lead II. **(3)** ST-segment elevation confined to V_1 without elevation in the remaining left precordial leads. Definitive diagnosis of RV infarction is made by observing ST-segment elevation greater than or equal to 1 mm in one or more of the right precordial leads. In the *right panel*, ST-segment elevation is seen in V_{2R} (V_1) through V_{6R}. *(From Drew, B.J., and Ide, B. [1995]. Right ventricular infarction. Prog Cardiovasc Nurs, 10, 46.)*

Procedure for Extra Electrocardiographic Leads—*Continued*

Steps	Rationale	Special Considerations
• V_{3R}: halfway between V_{2R} and V_{4R} • V_{4R}: right midclavicular line in the fifth ICS • V_{5R}: right anterior axillary line at the same horizontal level as V_{4R} • V_{6R}: right midaxillary line at the same horizontal level as V_{4R}	Slight alterations in the position of one precordial electrode may distort significantly the appearance of the cardiac waveforms and can have a significant impact on the diagnosis.[7]	The redundancy of V_1 (or V_{2R}) and V_2 (or V_{1R}) can be used to ensure that the ECGs are recorded accurately. Identify the sternal notch and move downward to locate the angle of Louis; the second ICS is located right below the angle of Louis.
Left Posterior Leads (Fig. 55-5) • V_7: posterior axillary line at the same level as V_4 through V_6 • V_8: halfway between V_7 and V_9 • V_9: left paraspinal line at the same level as V_4 through V_6	Left posterior leads are placed to view the posterior wall of the left ventricle. Left posterior leads should be recorded in patients admitted with a suspected posterior MI or known to have left circumflex artery disease.[3,15]	Help the patient turn to the right side to expose the left side of the back. Ensure the patient is safely turned. Leads V_4 through V_6 are located at the midclavicular line in the fifth ICS; leads V_7 through V_9 are at the same horizontal level as V_4 through V_6.
9. Clean the area for the application of electrodes with cleansing pads or soap and water and dry thoroughly.	Provides the effective contact between electrode and skin.	Poor electrode contact may produce instability of the recording, causing baseline wander.
10. Clean the intended sites with alcohol pads.	Removes body oils.	Clip hair if necessary.
11. Abrade the skin using a washcloth.	Removes dead skin cells and may promote impulse transmission.	
12. Place the electrodes on the marked locations.	Secure the electrodes to obtain quality ECG recordings.	If limb plate electrodes are used, do not overtighten and cause discomfort.

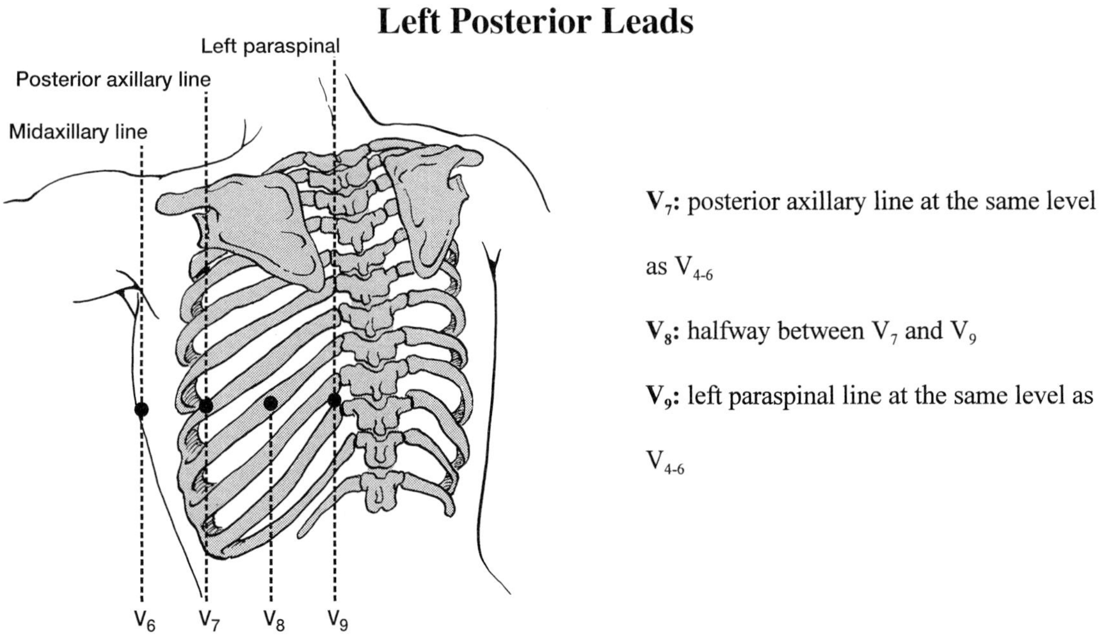

Left Posterior Leads

V_7: posterior axillary line at the same level as V_{4-6}

V_8: halfway between V_7 and V_9

V_9: left paraspinal line at the same level as V_{4-6}

FIGURE 55-5 Electrode locations for recording a left posterior ECG.

Procedure for Extra Electrocardiographic Leads—*Continued*

Steps	Rationale	Special Considerations
13. Identify the number of available ECG channels for simultaneous recording in the ECG machine.	Newer multiple-channel machines can record 16 leads at a time, which would allow simultaneous recording of a standard 12-lead ECG and four channels of RV leads V_{3R} through V_{6R} or three channels of left posterior leads V_7 through V_9.	If the ECG machine can record only 12 leads, record three separate ECGs: (1) standard 12-lead with left precordial leads, (2) RV leads, (3) left posterior leads. Some newer generation ECG machines may allow recording for greater than 12 leads. If the machine can record 16 leads, you could record two ECGs: (1) standard 12-lead plus RV leads (V_{3R} through V_{6R}), then (2) standard 12-lead plus left posterior leads (V_7 through V_9). An institutional protocol for recording these extra leads should be developed so that a consistent method is used to avoid confusion.
14. Connect the lead wires to the electrodes and record the ECG. Correctly label the ECG tracings, noting the extra leads.	Identifies RV and posterior leads.	Make notation on the ECG tracing that these are RV leads.
A. Recording RV leads using a 12-lead ECG machine, connect as follows: V_1 wire to electrode V_{1R} V_2 wire to electrode V_{2R} V_3 wire to electrode V_{3R} V_4 wire to electrode V_{4R} V_5 wire to electrode V_{5R} V_6 wire to electrode V_{6R}	When the unipolar left precordial lead wires V_1 through V_6 are connected to the RV or left posterior electrodes, the ECG machine records signals from where the electrodes are placed.	Change the labels on the ECG printouts from V_1 to V_{1R}, V_2 to V_{2R}, V_3 to V_{3R}, V_4 to V_{4R}, V_5 to V_{5R}, and V_6 to V_{6R}. Labels on the ECG printout depend on the connected lead wire and the location of the electrode.
B. Recording left posterior leads using a 12-lead ECG machine, connect as follows: V_4 wire to electrode V_7 V_5 wire to electrode V_8 V_6 wire to electrode V_9		Make a notation of "left posterior leads" and relabel appropriately on the ECG printouts: Change V_4 to V_7, V_5 to V_8, and V_6 to V_9.
15. Assess the quality of the tracing.	Ensures a clear tracing is obtained and no lead is off.	
16. Discard used supplies, and wash hands.	Reduces the transmission of microorganisms; standard precautions.	

Expected Outcomes

- Clean and accurate recording of ECG tracings allows clinicians to diagnose dysrhythmias and ischemia.
- Institutional protocol should be developed for recording the extra posterior and RV leads according to the availability and type of the ECG machine so that the recording method is consistent.

Unexpected Outcomes

- Inaccurate lead placement: electrode misplacement or incorrect lead connection.
- Failure to identify the recordings as either RV or left posterior ECGs and to change the ECG leads to their correct labels. This could lead to misdiagnosis.
- Poor ECG tracing caused by electrical artifact from external or internal sources.
- External artifact introduced by line current (60-cycle interference) may be minimized by disconnecting nearby electrical devices, unplugging the ECG machine and operating on battery, improving grounding, or replacing lead wires.
- Internal artifact may result from body movement, shivering, muscle tremors, and hiccups.

Patient Monitoring and Care

Steps	Rationale	Reportable Conditions
		These conditions should be reported if they persist despite nursing interventions.
1. Evaluate the ECG recordings for acute RV or posterior myocardial ischemia or infarction (Fig. 55-6). Record whether the patient has chest pain on the ECG tracing. Use 0 to 10 score to quantify pain severity (e.g., "8/10 chest pain").	Promptly initiates appropriate interventions, such as reperfusion treatment or vasodilators.	• Abnormal ST-segment deviation (elevation or depression) may indicate acute myocardial ischemia, injury, or infarction.
2. Assess the presence of chest pain or anginal equivalent symptoms (e.g., jaw, left shoulder or arm discomfort, or shortness of breath).	Ischemia caused by decreased coronary blood flow or increased myocardial oxygen demand may produce anginal symptoms.	• Angina
3. Check the patient's ECG for signs of AV node conduction disturbances in patients with RV infarction (e.g., second-degree or third-degree AV block).	The RCA supplies blood to the AV node in 90% of patients. Occlusion of the RCA proximal to the RV branch decreases the blood supply to the AV nodal artery. The incidence of high-degree AV block in inferior MI patients with RV involvement is significantly higher (48%) than in patients without RV MI (13%).[1]	• Acute MI patients with RV involvement, as evidenced by a QRS pattern or ST-segment elevation greater than or equal to 1 mm in the right precordial leads[2]
4. Assess the patient's hemodynamic status: elevated mean atrial pressure, reduced cardiac output, hypotension, and prominent venous engorgement.	Hypotension and reduced cardiac output in patients with RV infarction could be attributed to inadequate left ventricular filling.[5]	• Cardiovascular and hemodynamic changes associated with RV ischemia, injury, or infarction

Standard 12-Lead ECG   **Left Posterior Leads**

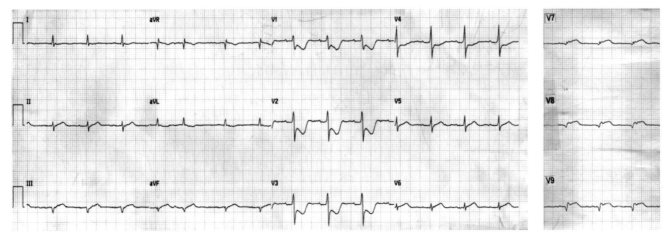

FIGURE 55-6 An ECG recorded in a 76-year-old diabetic patient during occlusion of the left circumflex artery. ST-segment depression is observed in left precordial leads V_{1-4}, which suggests posterior MI *(left panel)*. Left posterior leads V_{7-9} are helpful in recording ST-segment elevation that confirms posterior myocardial ischemia *(right panel)*. Observing ST-segment elevation in the contiguous posterior leads allows patients with acute MI to benefit from thrombolytic therapy, which they would be denied based on analysis of the standard 12-lead ECG alone.

Documentation

Documentation should include the following:

- Patient and family education
- The reason the extra leads are recorded (e.g., suspected RV infarction, posterior MI)
- Description of associated symptoms

- Interpretation of the ECGs recorded
- Interventions as indicated from the recorded ECG
- Occurrence of unexpected outcomes
- Additional interventions

References

1. Braat, S.H., et al. (1984). Value of lead V4R for recognition of the infarct coronary artery in acute inferior myocardial infarction. *Am J Cardiol,* 53, 1538-41.
2. Braat, S.H., et al. (1988). Value of the ST-T segment in lead V4R in inferior wall acute myocardial infarction to predict the site of coronary arterial occlusion. *Am J Cardiol,* 62, 140-2.
3. Brady, W. (1998). Acute posterior wall myocardial infarction: Electrocardiographic manifestations. *Am J Emerg Med,* 16, 409-13.
4. Casas, R.E., Marriott, H.J.L., and Glancy, L. (1997). Value of leads V7-V9 in diagnosing posterior wall acute myocardial infarction and other causes of tall R waves in V1-V2. *Am J Cardiol,* 80, 508-9.
5. Cohn, J.N., et al. (1974). Right ventricular infarction: Clinical and hemodynamic features. *Am J Cardiol,* 33, 209-14.
6. Correale, E., et al. (1999). Electrocardiographic patterns in acute inferior myocardial infarction with and without right ventricle involvement: Classification, diagnostic and prognostic value, masking effect. *Clin Cardiol,* 22, 37-44.
7. Drew, B.J., and Ide, B. (1995). Importance of accurate lead placement. *Prog Cardiovasc Nurs,* 9(2), 44.
8. Drew, B.J., et al. (1998). Bedside diagnosis of myocardial ischemia with ST segment monitoring technology: Measurement issues for real-time clinical decision-making and trial designs. *J Electrocardiol,* 30(Suppl), 157-165.
9. Drew, B.J., and Ide, B. (1995). Right ventricular infarction. *Prog Cardiovasc Nurs,* 10, 45-6.
10. Haisty, W.K., et al. (1992). Performance of the automated complete Selvester QRS scoring system in normal subjects and patients with single and multiple myocardial infarction. *J Am Coll Cardiol,* 19, 341-6.
11. Jacobs, A.K., et al. (2003). Cardiogenic shock caused by right ventricular infarction: A report from the SHOCK registry. *J Am Coll Cardiol,* 41, 1273-9.
12. Madias, J., Mahjoub, M., and Wijetilaka, R. (1997). Standard 12-lead ECG versus special chest leads in the diagnosis of right ventricular myocardial infarction. *Am J Emerg Med,* 15, 89-90.
13. Mirvis, D.M., et al. (1989). Instrumentation and practice standards for electrocardiographic monitoring in special care units. *Circulation,* 79, 464-71.
14. Wung, S.F. (2001). Computer-assisted continuous ST-segment analysis for clinical research: Methodological issues. *Biol Res Nurs,* 3, 65-77.
15. Wung, S.F., and Drew, B.J. (2001). New electrocardiographic criteria for posterior wall acute myocardial ischemia validated by a percutaneous transluminal coronary angioplasty model of acute myocardial infarction. *Am J Cardiol,* 87, 970-4.

Additional Reading

Drew, B.J., et al. (2004). An American Heart Association Scientific Statement from the Councils on Cardiovascular Nursing, Clinical Cardiology, and Cardiovascular Disease in the Young. *Circulation,* 110, 2721-46.

PROCEDURE **56**

Continuous ST-Segment Monitoring

P U R P O S E : Bedside ST-segment monitoring is used to detect myocardial ischemia. This technology can be applied to patients who are diagnosed with acute coronary syndromes (ACS), including acute myocardial infarction (MI) and unstable angina.[6,13,15,16,20] For these patients, continuous ST-segment monitoring is valuable in determining the success of thrombolytic therapy or percutaneous coronary interventions (PCI) or detecting recurrent or transient ischemia with unstable angina. The goal of continuous ST-segment monitoring is to detect acute ischemia, which requires immediate intervention to restore blood flow to the myocardium.

Mary G. Adams
Michele M. Pelter

PREREQUISITE NURSING KNOWLEDGE

- Understanding of the anatomy and physiology of the cardiovascular system, principles of cardiac conduction, electrocardiogram (ECG) lead placement, basic dysrhythmia interpretation, and electrical safety is required.
- Advanced cardiac life support knowledge and skills are necessary.
- Continuous monitoring of the ECG for ischemic ST-segment changes is more reliable than patients' symptoms because more than three quarters of ECG-detected ischemic events are clinically silent.[2,15,17,23,26] Patients who experience transient ischemia detected with continuous ST-segment monitoring are more likely to have unfavorable outcomes, including MI and death, compared with patients without such events.[3,5,11,21,24]
- Because of the dynamic, unpredictable, and silent nature of myocardial ischemia, it is essential to monitor patients continuously for ischemia. Clinicians should monitor the trend of the ST segments over time and evaluate any ST-segment changes (elevation or depression) for possible ischemia (Fig. 56-1). Other causes for a change in the ST-segment trend are (1) movement of the skin electrodes, (2) dysrhythmias, (3) intermittent bundle-branch block pattern, and (4) body position changes.
- The first type of ischemia seen in patients with ACS is occlusion-related ischemia. Coronary occlusion is brought on by disruption of an atherosclerotic plaque followed by cycles of plaque rupture, platelet stimulation, coronary vasospasm, and thrombus formation.[7,18-20] Because this type of ischemia threatens the entire thickness of the myocardium, immediate treatment to reestablish blood flow to the heart is essential. The typical ECG manifestation of total coronary occlusion is ST-segment elevation visible in the ECG leads that lie directly over the ischemic myocardial zone. Occlusion of the right coronary artery (RCA) typically produces ST-segment elevation in leads II, III, and aVF (Fig. 56-2). Occlusion of the left anterior descending (LAD) coronary artery typically produces ST-segment elevation in leads V_2, V_3, and V_4 (Fig. 56-3). Diagnosing total coronary occlusion of the left circumflex coronary artery (LCX) is more complex because placement of the standard ECG electrodes is on the anterior chest, opposite the wall that this coronary artery supplies. Occlusion of the LCX may produce ST-segment depression in leads V_1, V_2, or V_3, which reflects the reciprocal, or mirror image, ST-segment elevation occurring in the posterior wall of the myocardium.

- A second type of ischemia that patients with ACS or stable angina are at risk for is "demand-related" ischemia. This type of ischemia may occur when the demand for oxygen (i.e., exercise, tachycardia, or stress) exceeds the flow capabilities of a coronary artery with a stable atherosclerotic plaque. The ST-segment pattern of demand-related ischemia is depression, often appearing in

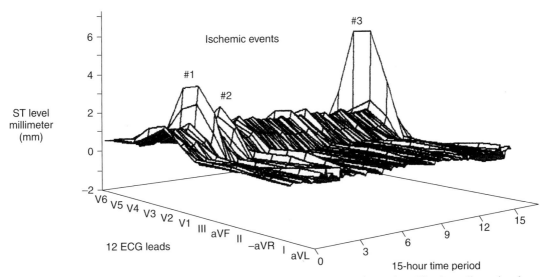

FIGURE 56-1 The importance of assessing the trend of the ST segments over time. The three-dimensional image illustrates ST-segment deviation in millimeters (Y-axis), in all 12 ECG leads (X-axis), over a 15-hour period (Z-axis) in a 78-year-old Cantonese-speaking man admitted to the telemetry unit with unstable angina. Illustrated are three separate ischemic events, characterized by ST-segment elevation, in leads V_3 to V_5. The nurses were unaware of these ischemic events because the patient did not complain of chest pain during any of the events and because there were no ST deviations greater than 1 mm in the routine monitoring leads II and V_1. This patient, who was initially admitted with unstable angina and a normal troponin I level, subsequently "ruled-in" for a MI with a troponin I of 3.5. The patient's angiogram later revealed a nearly 100% occluded LAD coronary artery, which was treated with a stent. *(Adapted from Pelter, M.M., Adams, M.G., and Drew, B.J. [2003]. Transient myocardial ischemia is an independent predictor of adverse in-hospital outcomes in patients with acute coronary syndromes treated in the telemetry unit.* Heart Lung, *32, 71-8.)*

several ECG leads (Fig. 56-4), with maximal ST-segment depression often occurring in lead V_5.[25]

- Accurate diagnosis of myocardial ischemia requires continuous monitoring of all 12 ECG leads because the mechanism of ischemia may vary (i.e., occlusion versus demand-related ischemia), resulting in distinctly different ST-segment patterns (e.g., elevation or depression). If only two ECG leads are available, however, the best two are leads III and V_3. Patient-specific monitoring also may be done if a prior 12-lead ECG was obtained during acute ischemia (i.e., ST-segment elevation MI, PCI, or treadmill test). In this scenario, the ECG lead or leads showing maximal ST-segment deviation should be selected for continuous monitoring to detect recurrent ischemia.

- According to a current consensus statements,[9,14a] multilead ST-segment monitoring should be initiated in hospitalized patients with the following diagnoses:
  - ❖ Acute MI
  - ❖ Unstable angina
  - ❖ Chest pain prompting a visit to the emergency department

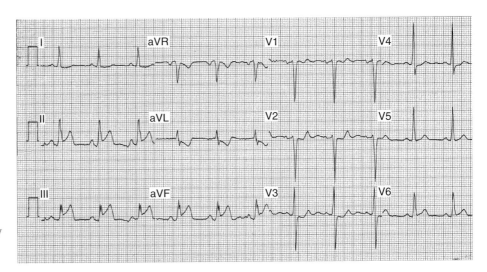

FIGURE 56-2 The typical ST-segment pattern of occlusion-related ischemia in the ECG leads that lie directly over the ischemic myocardial zone. The RCA is likely occluded resulting in ST-segment elevation in leads II, III, and aVF.

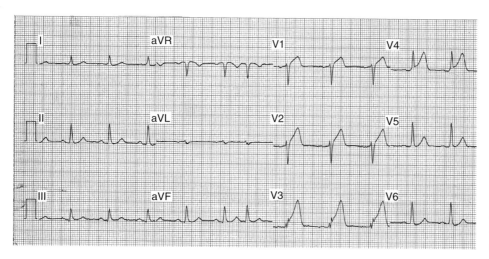

FIGURE 56-3 The typical ST-segment pattern of occlusion-related ischemia in the ECG leads that lie directly over the ischemic myocardial zone. The LAD artery is likely occluded resulting in ST-segment elevation in leads V_1 to V_4.

- After complicated PCI procedures (e.g., coronary angioplasty, stent placement, atherectomy)
  - After cardiac surgery
  - After noncardiac surgery
- According to these same guidelines,[9,14a] ST-segment monitoring may be useful for:
  - Assessing the success of thrombolytic therapy or primary angioplasty in patients with acute MI
  - Detecting reocclusion of the infarct-related artery after thrombolytic therapy or PCI in patients with acute MI
  - Detecting recurrent ischemia in patients with acute MI or transient myocardial ischemia in patients with unstable angina
  - Assessing the efficacy of antiischemic therapies
  - Differentiating ischemic from nonischemic chest pain
  - Detecting silent myocardial ischemia
- ST-segment monitoring may not be appropriate for certain patient groups because current software cannot reliably interpret ST-segment changes resulting from myocardial ischemia.[9,14a] Specifically, patients who may not be suitable for ST-segment monitoring include patients with:
  - Left bundle-branch block
  - Intermittent right or left bundle-branch block

- Patients who have a ventricular paced rhythm
- Patients who are extremely confused or restless causing excessive artifact
- A variety of bedside and telemetry cardiac monitors are currently available for use in clinical practice. Not all monitoring systems are equipped with ST-segment monitoring software, however. Clinicians must determine if their cardiac monitoring system has ST-segment monitoring capabilities.

EQUIPMENT

- Disposable electrodes
- Cardiac monitor with ST-segment monitoring capability and patient cable
- Alcohol pads
- 2 × 2 gauze pads
- ECG calipers

Additional equipment to have available as needed includes the following:

- Skin preparation solution (e.g., skin barrier wipe or tincture of benzoin) if needed
- Scissors
- Indelible marker

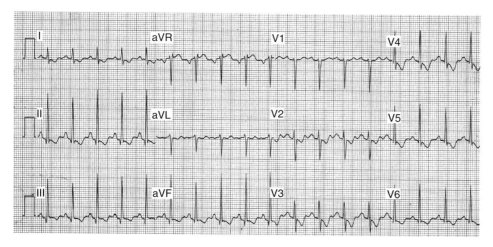

FIGURE 56-4 The typical ST-segment pattern of demand-related ischemia. Note the ST-segment depression appearing in nearly every ECG lead with the exception of V_1 and aVR. Note also that this patient is experiencing tachycardia, a common cause of demand-related ischemia.

PATIENT AND FAMILY EDUCATION

- Explain the purpose of ST-segment monitoring. ➤*Rationale:* This explanation decreases patient and family anxiety.
- Encourage the patient to report any symptoms of chest pain or anginal equivalent (e.g., arm pain, jaw pain, shortness of breath, or nausea). ➤*Rationale:* This heightens the patient's awareness of cardiac sensations and encourages communication of anginal symptoms.

PATIENT ASSESSMENT AND PREPARATION

Patient Assessment

- Identify patients at risk for ischemia (see earlier).[9,14a] ➤*Rationale:* Patients at risk for myocardial ischemia need to be identified.

- Assess the patient's cardiac rate and rhythm. ➤*Rationale:* This assessment provides baseline data and ensures the patient has a cardiac rhythm suitable for ST-segment monitoring.
- Identify the patient's baseline ST-segment levels before initiating ST-segment monitoring. ➤*Rationale:* This identifies the patient's baseline ST-segment level for comparison to subsequent changes.

Patient Preparation

- Ensure that the patient and family understand preprocedural teaching. Answer questions as they arise, and reinforce information as needed. ➤*Rationale:* This communication evaluates and reinforces understanding of previously taught information.
- Place the patient in a resting supine position in bed, and expose the patient's torso while maintaining modesty. ➤*Rationale:* This provides access to the patient's chest for electrode placement and ensures that an artifact-free ECG is obtained.

Procedure for Continuous ST-Segment Monitoring		
Steps	**Rationale**	**Special Considerations**
1. Wash hands.	Reduces the transmission of microorganisms; standard precautions.	
2. Identify accurate electrode placement (Fig. 56-5; see also Procedures 54 and 57).	Ensures accurate ECG data.[10]	Electrodes (V_3 through V_5) should be placed immediately below a pendulous breast so that the breast lies on top of the electrode preventing motion artifact.
3. Cleanse the area for the application of electrodes with cleansing pads or soap and water, and dry thoroughly. (*Level IV: Limited clinical studies to support recommendations.*)	Provides for adequate transmission of electrical impulses.	

Procedure continues on the following page

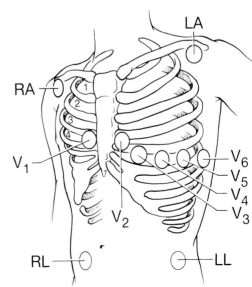

FIGURE 56-5 Correct lead placement for 12-lead ST-segment monitoring. Limb electrodes must be located as close as possible to the junction to the limb and the torso. To diminish the impact of respirations on the tracing, it is especially important that the LL electrode be placed well below the level of the umbilicus. For V_1, the electrode is located at the fourth intercostal space to the right of the sternum. V_2 is in the same fourth intercostal space just to the left of the sternum, and V_4 is in the fifth intercostal space on the midclavicular line. Placement of lead V_3 is halfway on a straight line between leads V_2 and V_4. Leads V_5 and V_6 are positioned on a straight line from V_4, with V_5 in the anterior axillary line and V_6 in the midaxillary line.

Procedure for Continuous ST-Segment Monitoring—*Continued*

Steps	Rationale	Special Considerations
4. Prepare the skin with alcohol pads and dry briskly with gauze pads. *(Level IV: Limited clinical studies to support recommendations.)*	Alcohol or skin preparations may be needed to remove oils, improving impulse transmission.[4,10,22] Removes dead skin cells, promoting impulse transmission. Moist skin is not conducive to electrode adherence.[4,10,22]	It may be necessary to clip chest hair to ensure good skin contact with the electrodes.
5. If possible, mark any precordial location with a black indelible marker.	Prevents inaccurate electrode placement after bathing or inadvertent removal of the electrodes.	Continuous ST-segment monitoring trends depend on stable electrode placement. Sudden changes in ST-segment trends often indicate electrode movement.
6. Connect the ECG leads to the electrodes before placing the electrodes on the patient (see Procedure 54).	Prepares the monitoring system and prevents unnecessary pressure on the patient's chest when connecting the lead wires to the electrodes.	
7. Select the monitoring leads.	Although any ECG lead can be used for ST-segment monitoring, it is desirable to monitor all 12 ECG leads or to select a lead based on the myocardial zone at risk (e.g., inferior or anterior).[12]	If continuous 12-lead ECG monitoring is unavailable, lead-specific ischemia monitoring is encouraged. Lead III is sensitive to inferior ischemia, and V_3 is sensitive to anterior or posterior ischemia.[9,14a]
8. If required by the bedside monitor manufacturer, identify the ECG complex landmarks and select the J point +60 msec landmark.[9,14a]	Prepares the monitoring system and ensures accurate monitoring.	Refer to manufacturer's recommendations.
9. Set the ST-segment alarm threshold according to hospital policy.	Maximizes the sensitivity and specificity of ST-segment monitoring and may reduce unnecessary false alarms.	For bedside cardiac monitoring, the alarm threshold should be set 1 to 2 mm above and below the patient's baseline ST-segment level (Fig. 56-6).[9,14a]

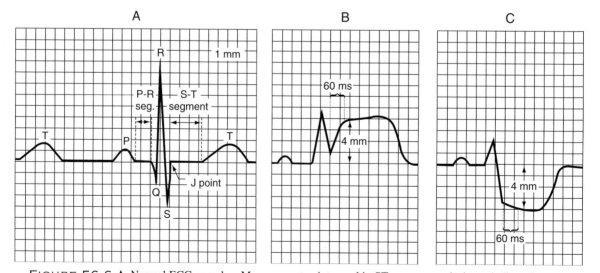

FIGURE 56-6 **A,** Normal ECG complex. Measurement points used in ST-segment analysis are indicated. The P-R segment is used to identify the isoelectric line. The ST segment begins at the J point, which is the end of the QRS complex. The ST-segment measurement point can be measured at 60 or 80 msec past the J point. **B,** ST-segment elevation. The ST segment shown measures +4 mm. **C,** ST-segment depression. The ST segment shown measures –4 mm. *(Adapted from Tisdale, L.A., and Drew, B.J. [1993]. ST segment monitoring for myocardial ischemia. AACN Clin Issues Crit Care Nurs, 4, 36.)*

Procedure for Continuous ST-Segment Monitoring—*Continued*

Steps	Rationale	Special Considerations
		Establishing a patient-specific ST-segment level, rather than an isoelectric ST-segment level is important because the patient's baseline ST-segment level is rarely isoelectric.[4]
10. Discard used supplies, and wash hands.	Reduces the transmission of microorganisms; standard precautions.	
11. Print the baseline ECG tracing to evaluate the quality of the signal and secure for future reference.	Ensures a quality baseline ECG for comparing subsequent changes because ST-segment monitoring is based on continuous trending.	Verify that lead wires are not reversed, especially the limb leads.
12. If possible, obtain an ECG with the patient in right and left side-lying positions and secure these for future reference.	Comparison of side-lying ECGs with ECGs from subsequent alarms may prevent interpreting false-positive ST-segment deviations caused by changes in body position as ischemia.[1,8]	ECGs can also be obtained with the patient in the upright position.

Expected Outcomes

- Accurate ECG monitoring that allows clinicians to interpret ST-segment changes
- Timely detection of myocardial ischemia
- An increase in the number of bedside alarms when the ST-segment software is initiated. These may be caused by the following: (1) actual ischemia, (2) body position changes, (3) transient dysrhythmias, (4) heart rate changes, (5) noisy signal, or (6) lead misplacement[14]

Unexpected Outcomes

- Skin sensitivity to electrodes
- Undetected ST-segment changes
- Inappropriate intervention based on a false ST-segment alarm[8]

Patient Monitoring and Care

Steps	Rationale	Reportable Conditions
		These conditions should be reported if they persist despite nursing interventions.
1. Confirm adequate electrode and lead wire placement every shift.	Enhances the quality of ST-segment monitoring.	
2. Evaluate ST-segment trends routinely while obtaining vital signs.	Ensures that there are no significant deviations in the ST-segment trend.	• Change in ST segment trends
3. Interpret all ST-segment alarms and determine the cause.	Ensures accurate interpretation.	• Clinically significant ST-segment deviation
4. If actual ischemia is noted, obtain a 12-lead ECG, assess the patient for signs and symptoms suggesting acute ischemia, anginal equivalents, hemodynamic changes, or dysrhythmias.	A 12-lead ECG assists with determining the extent of ischemia. Determines the patient response to ischemia.	• New ST-segment changes • New onset of symptoms or anginal equivalent
5. Assess the patient for signs and symptoms suggesting acute ischemia even if no new ST-segment changes are identified, and obtain a 12-lead ECG as needed.	Determines the presence of ischemia. A 12-lead ECG assists with determining the extent of ischemia.	• New ST-segment changes • New onset of symptoms or anginal equivalent

Documentation

Documentation should include the following:

- Patient and family education
- Initiation of ST-segment bedside monitoring
- To determine real versus false ST-segment alarms due to body position changes, print out and have available baseline ECGs with the patient assuming left, right, upright, and supine body positions

- Document any new ST segment changes or any new symptoms suggesting acute ischemia
- Interpret ST-segment trends
- Presence and intensity of chest pain or anginal equivalent
- Unexpected outcomes
- Additional interventions taken

References

1. Adams, M.G., and Drew, B.J. (1997). Body position effects on the ECG: Implication for ischemia monitoring. *J Electrocardiol, 30,* 285-91.
2. Adams, M.G., et al. (1999). Frequency of silent myocardial ischemia with 12-lead ST segment monitoring in the coronary care unit: Are there sex-related differences? *Heart Lung, 28,* 81-6.
3. Bugiardini, R., et al. (1995). Relation of severity of symptoms to transient myocardial ischemia and prognosis in unstable angina. *J Am Coll Cardiol, 25,* 597-604.
4. Clochesy, J.M., Cifani, L., and Howe, K. (1991). Electrode site preparation techniques: A follow-up study. *Heart Lung, 20,* 27-30.
5. Currie, P., and Saltissi, S. (1993). Significance of ST-segment elevation during ambulatory monitoring after acute myocardial infarction. *Am Heart J, 125,* 41-7.
6. Dellborg, M., Topol, E.J., and Swedberg, K. (1991). Dynamic QRS complex and ST segment vectorcardiographic monitoring can identify vessel patency in patients with acute myocardial infarction treated with reperfusion therapy. *Am Heart J, 122,* 943-8.
7. DeWood, M.A., et al. (1980). Prevalence of total coronary occlusion during the early hours of transmural infarction. *N Engl J Med, 303,* 897-902.
8. Drew, B.J., and Adams, M.G. (2001). Clinical consequences of ST-segment changes caused by body position mimicking transient myocardial ischemia: Hazards of ST-segment monitoring? *J Electrocardiol, 34,* 261-4.
9. Drew, B.J., Krucoff, M.W., for the ST-Segment Monitoring Practice Guideline International Working Group. (1999). ST segment monitoring of patients with unstable coronary syndromes: A clinical practice guideline for healthcare professionals. *Am J Crit Care, 8,* 372-88.
10. Drew, B.J., Ide, B., and Sparacino, P. (1991). Accuracy of bedside ECG monitoring: A report on the current practices of critical care nurses. *Heart Lung, 20,* 597-607.
11. Drew, B.J., Pelter, M.M., and Adams, M.G. (2002). Frequency, characteristics, and clinical significance of transient ST segment elevation in patients with acute coronary syndromes. *Eur Heart J, 23,* 941-7.
12. Drew, B.J., and Tisdale, L.A. (1993). ST segment monitoring for coronary artery reocclusion following thrombolytic therapy and coronary angioplasty: Identification of optimal bedside monitoring leads. *Am J Crit Care, 2,* 280-92.
13. Drew, B.J., et al. (1996). ST segment monitoring with a derived 12-lead electrocardiogram is superior to routine cardiac care unit monitoring. *Am J Crit Care, 5,* 198-206.
14. Drew, B.J., et al. (1998). Bedside diagnosis of myocardial ischemia with ST-segment monitoring technology: Measurement issues for real-time clinical decision making and trial design. *J Electrocardiol, 30*(Suppl), 157-65.
14a. Drew, B.J., et al. (2004). An American Heart Association Scientific Statement from the Councils on Cardiovascular Nursing, Clinical Cardiology, and Cardiovascular Disease in the Young. *Circulation, 110,* 2721-46.
15. Gottlieb, S.O., et al. (1986). Silent ischemia as a marker for early unfavorable outcomes in patients with unstable angina. *N Engl J Med, 314,* 1214-8.
16. Klootwijk, P., et al. (1996). Non-invasive prediction of reperfusion and coronary artery patency by continuous ST segment monitoring in the GUSTO-I trial. *Eur Heart J, 17,* 689-98.
17. Klootwijk, P., et al. (1997). Comparison of usefulness of computer assisted continuous 48-h 3-lead with 12-lead ECG ischemia monitoring for detection and quantitation of ischemia in patients with unstable angina. *Eur Heart J, 18,* 931-40.
18. Krucoff, M., et al. (1993). Continuously updated 12-lead ST-segment recovery analysis for myocardial infarct artery patency assessment and its correlation with multiple simultaneous early angiographic observations. *Am J Cardiol, 71,* 145-51.
19. Kwon, K., et al. (1991). The unstable ST segment early after thrombolysis for acute infarction and its usefulness as a marker of recurrent coronary occlusion. *Am J Cardiol, 67,* 109-15.
20. Langer, A., et al. (1995). Noninvasive assessment of speed and stability of infarct-related artery reperfusion: Results of the GUSTO ST segment monitoring study. *J Am Coll Cardiol, 25,* 1552-7.
21. Langer, A., et al. (1992). Pathophysiology and prognostic significance of Holter-detected ST segment depression after myocardial infarction. The Tissue Plasminogen Activator: Toronto (TPAT) Study Group. *J Am Coll Cardiol, 20,* 1313-7.
22. Medina, V., Clochesy, J.M., and Omery, A. (1989). Comparison of electrode site preparation techniques. *Heart Lung, 18,* 456-60.
23. Patel, D., et al. (1996). Early continuous ST segment monitoring in unstable angina: Prognostic value additional to clinical characteristics and the admission electrocardiogram. *Heart, 75,* 222-8.
24. Pelter, M.M., Adams, M.G., and Drew, B.J. (2002). Association of transient myocardial ischemia with adverse in-hospital outcomes for angina patients treated in a telemetry unit or a coronary care unit. *Am J Crit Care, 11,* 318-25.
25. Quyyumi, A., et al. (1986). Value of the bipolar lead CM5 in electrocardiography. *Br Heart J, 56,* 372-6.
26. Romeo, F., et al. (1992). Unstable angina: Role of silent ischemia and total ischemic time (silent plus painful ischemia), a 6-year follow-up. *J Am Coll Cardiol, 19,* 1173-9.

Additional Readings

Adams, M.G., and Pelter, M.M. (2003). In hospital cardiac monitoring. In: Conover, M., editor. *Understanding Electrocardiography*. 8th ed. St. Louis: Mosby, 431-43.

Adams-Hamoda, M.G., et al. (2003). Factors to consider when analyzing 12-lead electrocardiograms for evidence of acute myocardial ischemia. *Am J Crit Care, 12,* 9-18.

Drew, B.J. (2002). Celebrating the 100th birthday of the electrocardiogram: Lessons learned from research in cardiac monitoring. *Am J Crit Care,* 11, 378-88.

Drew, B.J., et al. (2002). Comparison of a new reduced lead set ECG with the standard ECG for diagnosing cardiac arrhythmias and myocardial ischemia. *J Electrocardiol,* 35, 13-21.

Pelter, M.M., Adams, M.G., and Drew, B.J. (2003). Transient myocardial ischemia is an independent predictor of adverse in-hospital outcomes in patients with acute coronary syndromes treated in the telemetry unit. *Heart Lung,* 32, 71-8.

Wagner, G.S. (1994). *Marriott's Practical Electrocardiology.* 9th ed. Baltimore: Williams & Wilkins.

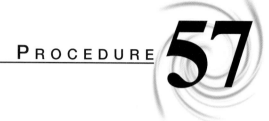

PROCEDURE **57**

Twelve-Lead Electrocardiogram

PURPOSE: A 12-lead electrocardiogram (ECG) provides information about the electrical system of the heart from 12 different views or leads. Common uses of a 12-lead ECG include diagnosis of acute coronary syndromes, identification of dysrhythmias, and determination of the effects of medications or electrolytes on the electrical system of the heart.

Mary G. McKinley

PREREQUISITE NURSING KNOWLEDGE

- Understanding of the anatomy and physiology of the cardiovascular system, principles of cardiac conduction, cardiac cycle, properties of cardiac tissue (automaticity, excitability, conductivity, and refractoriness), principles of electrophysiology, ECG lead placement, basic dysrhythmia interpretation, and electrical safety is required.
- Advanced cardiac life support knowledge and skills are needed.
- Clinical and technical competence in the use of the 12-lead ECG machine and recorder is necessary.
- A 12-lead ECG provides different views or leads of the electrical activity of the heart. The leads are standard limb leads (I, II, III), augmented limb leads (aVR, aVF, and aVL), and six chest leads (V_1 to V_6).
- The standard and augmented leads view the heart from the vertical or frontal plane (Fig. 57-1), and the chest leads view the heart from the horizontal plane (Fig. 57-2).
- The graphic display consists of the P, Q, R, S, and T waves, which represent electrical activity within the heart.
- Serial 12-lead ECGs (more than two ECGs recorded at different times) may be obtained. The accuracy of interpretation relies on consistent electrode placement. Indelible markers can be used to identify the electrode locations to ensure that the same lead placement is used when serial ECGs are recorded.
- Advances in technology have allowed for online or wireless transmission, networking capabilities, and computerized interpretation of the 12-lead ECG (Fig. 57-3). The 12-lead

ECG cable is attached to a processing device that digitizes the 12-lead ECG recording and transfers the information to the wireless laptop device, which transmits the information to the medical record. This increases access to the 12-lead ECG for review and can assist with rapid interpretation and treatment of the patient.

EQUIPMENT

- 12-lead ECG machine and recorder
- Electrodes
- Gauze pads or terrycloth washcloth
- Cleansing tissue or nonemollient soap and water in basin
- Patient cable and lead wires
- Alcohol pads

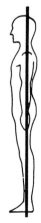

FIGURE 57-1 Vertical plane leads—I, II, III, aVR, aVL, aVF.

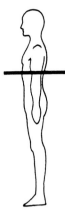

FIGURE 57-2 Horizontal plane leads—V_1 to V_6.

Additional equipment to have available as needed includes the following:
- Skin preparation solution (e.g., skin barrier wipe or tincture of benzoin)
- Indelible marker
- Scissors to clip hair from chest if needed

PATIENT AND FAMILY EDUCATION

- Assess the readiness of the patient and family to learn. **»Rationale:** Anxiety and concerns of the patient and family may inhibit their ability to learn.
- Provide explanations of the equipment and procedure to the patient and family. **»Rationale:** Information may decrease anxiety.
- Emphasize that the patient should not talk, but should relax, lie still, and breathe normally. **»Rationale:** Chest movement can distort the ECG picture.

- Reassure the patient and family that the 12-lead ECG will be reviewed and that any alterations or problems will be addressed. **»Rationale:** Patients and families need to be reassured that immediate care is available if it is needed.

PATIENT ASSESSMENT AND PREPARATION

Patient Assessment

- Assess the patient's peripheral pulses, vital signs, heart sounds, level of consciousness, lung sounds, neck vein distention, presence of chest pain or palpitations, and for peripheral circulatory disorders (e.g., clubbing, cyanosis, and dependent edema). **»Rationale:** Physical signs and symptoms may result from alterations in performance of the cardiovascular system.
- Assess the patient's history of cardiac dysrhythmias or cardiac problems. **»Rationale:** Provides baseline data.
- Assess medications the patient is on. **»Rationale:** Provides baseline data.
- Assess previous 12-lead ECGs. **»Rationale:** Provides baseline data.

Patient Preparation

- Ensure that the patient and family understand preprocedural teaching. Answer questions as they arise, and reinforce information as needed. **»Rationale:** This information evaluates and reinforces understanding of previously taught information.
- Assist the patient to a supine position. **»Rationale:** This position allows easy access to the chest for electrode placement; changes in body position may affect the accuracy of the ECG recording.

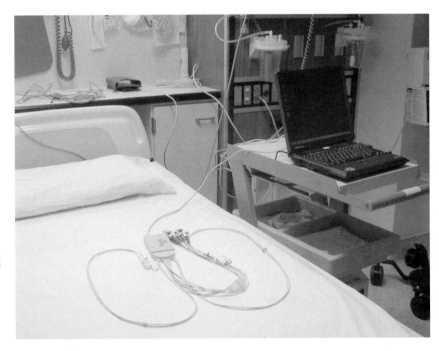

FIGURE 57-3 Example of a wireless ECG device. The 12-lead cable is attached to a processing device that digitizes the 12-lead recording and transfers the information to the wireless laptop device that transmits the information to the medical record.

Procedure for Twelve-Lead Electrocardiogram

Steps	Rationale	Special Considerations
1. Wash hands.	Reduces the transmission of microorganisms; standard precautions.	
2. Check cables and lead wires for fraying, broken wires, or discoloration.	Detects conditions that would give an inaccurate ECG trace.	If equipment is damaged, obtain alternative equipment and notify the biomedical engineer for repair.
3. Plug the ECG machine into a grounded alternating current (AC) wall outlet or ensure functioning if battery operated.	Maintains electrical safety.	
4. Turn the ECG machine on and input the information required.	Equipment may require self-test and warm-up time. Multichannel machines may require input of information to store the ECG appropriately.	Follow the manufacturer's recommendations and requirements regarding input of information and warm-up.
5. Ensure that the patient is in the supine position, not touching the bedrails or footboard.	Provides adequate support for limbs so that muscle activity is minimal. Touching the bedrails or footboard may increase the chance of distortion of the trace. Body position changes can cause alterations in the ECG tracing.	The supine position is best, but Fowler or other positions may be used for comfort. ECGs should be recorded in the same position to ensure that tracing changes are not caused by changes in body position. If another position is clinically required, note the position on the tracing or in the comments of the LCD input.
6. Expose only the necessary parts of the patient's legs, arms, and chest.	Provides privacy and warmth, which reduces shivering.	Ensuring privacy may reduce anxiety, which can alter the ECG reading. Shivering interferes with the recording.
7. Identify lead sites: A. Limb leads (Fig. 57-4).	Ensures the accuracy of the lead placement. Promotes correct positioning of the limb leads. Ensures an accurate tracing of the heart from a view in the vertical and frontal plane.	Mark the sites with an indelible marker if serial ECGs are anticipated. Limb leads should be placed in fleshy areas, and bony prominences should be avoided. The limb leads need to be placed equidistant from the heart and should be positioned in approximately the same place on each limb.
B. Chest leads (Fig. 57-5), as follows: Identify the angle of Louis or the sternal notch: • Palpate the upper sternum to	The angle of Louis or the sternal notch assists with identifying the second rib for correct placement of precordial leads in the	

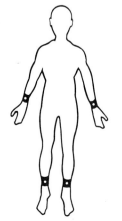

FIGURE 57-4 Limb lead placement in 12-lead ECG.

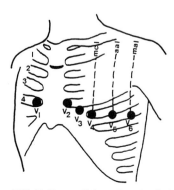

FIGURE 57-5 Precordial or chest lead placement.

Procedure for Twelve-Lead Electrocardiogram—*Continued*

Steps	Rationale	Special Considerations
identify where the clavicle joins the sternum (suprasternal notch). Slide fingers down the center of the sternum to the obvious bony prominence. This is the sternal notch, which identifies the second rib and provides a landmark for noting the fourth ICS. • When the fourth ICS is located, place the V leads: V_1 at the fourth ICS right sternal border; V_2 at the fourth ICS left sternal border; V_3 equidistant between V_2 and V_4; V_4 at the fifth ICS midclavicular line; V_5 horizontal level to V_4 at the anterior axillary line; V_6 horizontal level to V_4 at the midaxillary line.	appropriate intercostal space. Accurate placement ensures correct electrical tracing of the heart from the horizontal plane. Slight alterations in the position of any of the precordial leads may alter the ECG significantly and can have impact on diagnosis and treatment.[1]	
8. Cleanse the area for the application of electrodes with cleansing pads or soap and water, and dry thoroughly. *(Level IV: Limited clinical studies to support recommendations.)*	Provides for adequate transmission of electrical impulses. Moist skin is not conducive to electrode adherence.[2]	It may be necessary to clip chest hair to ensure good skin contact with the electrode.
9. Clean the intended sites with alcohol pads. Consider using skin preparation solutions. *(Level IV: Limited clinical studies to support recommendations.)*	Alcohol or skin preparations may be needed to remove oils, improving impulse transmission.[2]	Skin preparation solutions should not be applied to the area of the skin that will be in direct contact with the electrode gel because transmission of impulses may be decreased.
10. Abrade the skin using a washcloth, scratch pad on electrode pack, or gauze pad.	Removes dead skin cells, promoting impulse transmission.	
11. For pregelled electrodes, remove the backing and test for moistness. For adhesive electrodes, remove the backing and check the adhesive pads—it should be sticky or moist.	Allows for appropriate conduction of impulses.	Gel must be moist. If pregelled electrodes are not moist or adhesive electrodes are not sticky, replace the electrodes.
12. Apply the electrodes securely.	Electrodes must be secure to prevent external influences from affecting the ECG.	
13. Fasten the lead wires to the limb electrodes, avoiding bending or strain on the wires, and use the correct lead-to-electrode connection.	Provides for correct lead-to-limb connection.	
14. Identify the multiple-channel machine recording setting (Fig. 57-6).	Multiple-channel machines run several leads simultaneously and can be set to run leads in different configurations.	Obtain the tracing that is needed for the clinical situation.
15. Check the settings on the ECG machine: paper speed, 25 mm/sec; sensitivity, 1 or 10 mm/sec; baseline at center.	Ensures an accurate trace within standard limits for proper interpretation.	Manufacturers provide a calibration check in the machine to identify the sensitivity setting. Most machines have automatic settings.
16. Obtain a 12-lead ECG recording. Most systems record each lead for	The ECG must be marked accurately and have a clear	

Procedure continues on the following page

Procedure for Twelve-Lead Electrocardiogram—*Continued*

Steps	Rationale	Special Considerations
3 to 6 seconds and automatically mark the correct lead.	baseline without artifact for correct interpretation. Three to six seconds is all that is needed for a permanent record; a longer strip may be obtained if a rhythm strip is needed. A rhythm strip is a long recording of a lead; lead II is commonly used.	
17. Record the chest leads as above. *Note:* A multiple-channel machine runs the limb and chest leads simultaneously.	The chest leads may be set up and done automatically by the machine. The 12-lead ECG tracing should be free of respiratory artifact.	Respiratory artifact can be common in doing the chest leads and may require position changes to ensure a good baseline. If sequential ECGs are to be obtained, chest lead sites should be marked to ensure that the same lead sites are used in subsequent ECGs.
18. Examine the 12-lead ECG tracing to see if it is clear, and repeat the ECG if it is not.	While the patient is still connected to the machine, the nurse should examine the ECG to see if any leads of the entire ECG need to be repeated.	
19. Interpret the recording for rhythm, rate, presence and configuration of P waves, length of P-R intervals, length of QRS complexes, configuration	Reviews the normal conduction sequence and identifies abnormalities that may require further evaluation or treatment.	

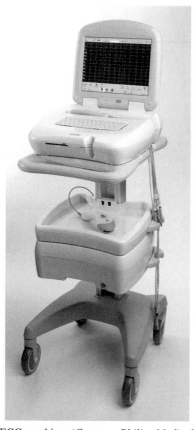

FIGURE 57-6 Multiple-channel ECG machine. (*Courtesy Philips Medical Systems.*)

Procedure for Twelve-Lead Electrocardiogram—*Continued*

Steps	Rationale	Special Considerations
and deviation of the ST segments, presence and configuration of T waves, length of Q-T intervals, presence of extra waves (e.g., U waves), and identification of dysrhythmias.		
20. Evaluate the 12-lead ECG for any signs of ischemia, injury, or infarct and other significant myocardial alterations.	Identifies pathophysiologic processes that may require further evaluation or treatment.	
21. Disconnect the equipment, and clean the gel off the patient (if necessary) and prepare the equipment for future use.	Increases patient comfort.	Some pregelled electrodes can be left in place for repeat ECGs. Follow the manufacturer's directions and hospital policy for electrode use and removal in these cases.
22. Discard used equipment, and wash hands.	Reduces the transmission of microorganisms; standard precautions.	

Expected Outcomes

- A clear 12-lead ECG recording obtained (Fig. 57-7)
- Prompt identification of abnormalities

Unexpected Outcomes

- Altered skin integrity
- Inaccurate lead placement or limb lead reversal (Fig. 57-8)
- AC interference, also called 60-cycle interference (see Fig. 54-10)
- Wandering baseline (see Fig. 54-11)
- Artifact or waveform interference (see Fig. 54-12)

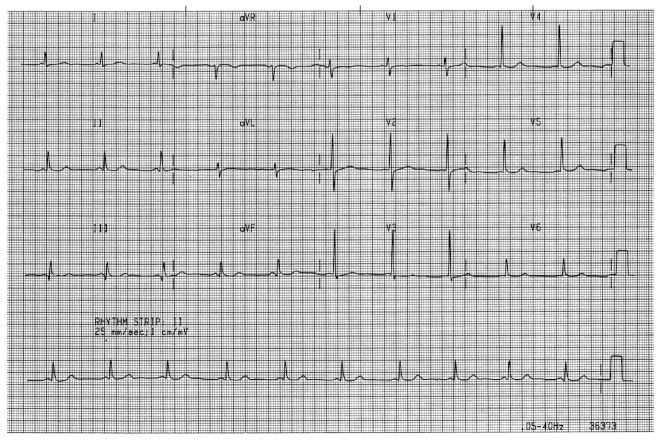

FIGURE 57-7 Clear 12-lead ECG recording.

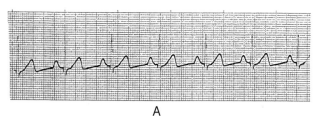

A

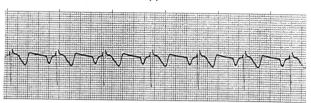

B

FIGURE 57-8 Limb lead reversal on 12-lead ECG in lead I. **A,** Correct placement. **B,** Incorrect placement.

Patient Monitoring and Care

Steps	Rationale	Reportable Conditions
		These conditions should be reported if they persist despite nursing interventions.
1. Obtain a 12-lead ECG as prescribed and as needed (e.g., for angina or dysrhythmias).	Provides determination of myocardial ischemia, injury, and infarction. Aids in diagnosis of dysrhythmias.	• Angina • Dysrhythmias • Abnormal 12-lead ECG
2. Compare the 12-lead ECG with the previous 12-lead ECGs.	Determines normal and abnormal findings.	• Any changes in the 12-lead ECG

Documentation

Documentation should include the following:

• Patient and family education
• The fact that a 12-lead ECG was obtained
• The reason for the 12-lead ECG
• Symptoms that the patient experienced (e.g., chest pain or palpitations)

• Follow-up to the 12-lead ECG, as indicated
• Unexpected outcomes
• Additional nursing interventions

References

1. Drew, B.J. (2002). Celebrating the 100th birthday of the electrocardiogram: Lessons learned from research in cardiac monitoring. *Am J Crit Care,* 11, 378-86.
2. Jacobson, C. (1996). Bedside cardiac monitoring. In: *AACN Research Based Practice Protocol, Technology Series.* Aliso Viejo, CA: American Association of Critical Care Publications, 1-32.

Additional Readings

ACC/AHA clinical competence statement on electrocardiography and ambulatory electrocardiography. A report of the ACC/AHA/ACP-ASIM Task Force on Clinical Competence. (2001). *Circulation,* 18, 3169-78.
Adams-Hamoda, M.G., et al. (2003). Factors to consider when analyzing 12-lead electrocardiograms for evidence of acute myocardial ischemia. *Am J Crit Care,* 12, 9-16.
Adams-Hamoda, M.G., and Pelter, M. (2003). Interpreting a postoperative 12-lead ECG waveform. *Am J Crit Care,* 2003, 12, 267-8.

Crater, S., et al. (2000). Real-time application of continuous 12-lead ST segment monitoring: 3 case studies. *Crit Care Nurse,* 20, 93-9.
Drew, B.J., et al. (2004). An American Heart Association Scientific Statement from the Councils on Cardiovascular Nursing, Clinical Cardiology, and Cardiovascular Disease in the Young. *Circulation,* 110, 2721-46.
Hurst, J.W. (2000). Images in cardiovascular medicine: "Switched" precordial leads. *Circulation,* 101, 2870-1.
Jefferies, P., Woolf, S., and Linde, B. (2003). Technology-based vs. traditional instruction: A comparison of two methods for teaching the skill of performing a 12-lead ECG. *Nurs Educ Perspect,* 24, 70-4.
Kadish, A.H., et al. (2000). Revisiting the question: Will relaxing safe current limits for electromedical equipment increase hazards to patients? *Circulation,* 102, 823-5.
Leeper, B. (2003). Continuous ST-segment monitoring. *AACN Clin Issues,* 14, 145-54.
Tuna, N. (2000). Electrocardiography. In: Willerson, J., and Cohn, J., editors. *Cardiovascular Medicine.* 2nd ed. New York: Churchill Livingstone.

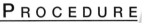
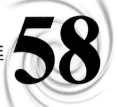

SECTION NINE

Hemodynamic
Monitoring

PROCEDURE **58**

Arterial Catheter Insertion (Perform)

PURPOSE: Arterial catheters are used to continuously monitor blood pressure and for frequent arterial blood gas and laboratory sampling.

Deborah E. Becker

PREREQUISITE NURSING KNOWLEDGE

- Knowledge of anatomy and physiology of the vasculature and adjacent structures
- Nurses must be adequately prepared to insert arterial catheters. This preparation should include specific educational content about arterial catheter insertion and opportunities to demonstrate clinical competency.
- Understanding of the principles of hemodynamic monitoring
- Clinical competence in suturing
- Conditions that warrant the use of arterial pressure monitoring include patients with the following:
  - ❖ Acute hypotension or hypertension (hypertensive crisis)
  - ❖ Hemodynamic instability or circulatory collapse
  - ❖ Cardiac arrest
  - ❖ Hemorrhage
  - ❖ Shock from any cause
  - ❖ Continuous infusion of vasoactive medications
  - ❖ Frequent arterial blood gas measurements
  - ❖ Nonpulsatile blood flow (i.e., those using nonpulsatile ventricular assist devices or receiving extracorporeal membrane oxygenation)
  - ❖ Intraaortic balloon pump therapy
  - ❖ Neurologic injury
  - ❖ Coronary interventional procedures
  - ❖ Major surgical procedures
  - ❖ Multiple trauma
  - ❖ Respiratory failure
  - ❖ Sepsis
  - ❖ Obstetric emergencies
- Noninvasive, indirect blood pressure measurements determined by auscultation of Korotkoff sounds distal to an occluding cuff consistently average 10 to 20 mm Hg lower than simultaneous direct measurement.[6]
- Arterial waveform inspection can help rapidly diagnose the presence of valvular disorders, the effects of dysrhythmias on perfusion, the effects of the respiratory cycle on blood pressure, and the effects of intraaortic balloon pumping or ventricular assist devices on blood pressure.
- The preferred artery for arterial catheter insertion is the radial artery (see Fig. 79-1). Though this artery is smaller than the ulnar artery, it is more superficial and can be more easily stabilized during the procedure.[4] Some research has found that the brachial artery is a safe and reliable alternative site for arterial puncture and line placement.[9]
- At times, the femoral artery may be used for arterial catheter insertion. The use of this artery can be technically difficult because of the proximity of the femoral artery to the femoral vein (see Fig. 79-2).
- The most common complications associated with arterial puncture include pain, vasospasm, hematoma formation, infection, hemorrhage, and neurovascular compromise.[1,3,9]
- Site selection is as follows:
  - ❖ Use the radial artery as the first choice. Perform a modified Allen test to determine the patency of the radial and ulnar arteries before performing the arterial puncture (see Fig. 79-3). Normal palmar blushing is complete before 7 seconds, indicating a positive result; 8 to 14 seconds is considered equivocal; and 15 or

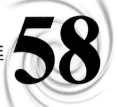

more seconds indicates a negative test. Doppler flow studies or plethysmography can also be performed to ensure the presence of collateral flow. Research shows these studies to be more reliable than the Allen test.[11] Thrombosis of the arterial cannula is a common complication. Ensuring collateral flow distal to the puncture site is important for preventing ischemia.

❖ Use the brachial artery as the second choice, except in the presence of poor pulsation caused by shock, obesity, or a sclerotic vessel (e.g., because of previous cardiac catheterization). The brachial artery is larger than the radial artery. Hemostasis after arterial cannulation is enhanced by its proximity to the bone if the entry point is approximately 1.5 inches above the antecubital fossa.

❖ Use the femoral artery in the case of cardiopulmonary arrest or altered perfusion to the upper extremities. The femoral artery is a large superficial artery located in the groin. It is easily palpated and punctured. Complications related to femoral artery puncture include hemorrhage and hematoma formation (because bleeding can be difficult to control), inadvertent puncture of the femoral vein (because of its close proximity to the artery), infection (because aseptic technique is difficult to maintain in the groin area), and limb ischemia (if the femoral artery is damaged).

EQUIPMENT

- 2-in, 20-G, nontapered Teflon cannula-over-needle; or prepackaged kit that includes a 6-in, 18-G Teflon catheter with appropriate introducer and guide wire
- Single-pressure transducer system (see Procedure 75)
- Monitoring equipment consisting of a connecting cable, monitor, oscilloscope display screen, and recorder
- Nonsterile gloves and goggles
- Sterile gloves
- Antiseptic solution (e.g., 2% chlorhexidine-based preparation)
- Sterile 4 × 4 gauze pads
- Suture material
- 1% lidocaine without epinephrine, 1 ml to 2 ml
- 3-ml syringe with 25-G needle
- Sheet protector
- Sterile towels
- 2-in tape

Additional supplies to have available as needed include the following:
- Bath towel
- Small wrist board

PATIENT AND FAMILY EDUCATION

- Explain the procedure and the purpose of the arterial catheter. ➼*Rationale:* Decreases patient and family anxiety.
- Explain to the patient that the procedure may be uncomfortable but that a local anesthetic will be used first to alleviate most of the discomfort. ➼*Rationale:* Elicits patient cooperation and facilitates insertion.
- Explain the patient's role in assisting with catheter insertion. ➼*Rationale:* Elicits patient cooperation and facilitates insertion.
- Inform the patient about potential complications. ➼*Rationale:* Fully informs the patient of complications as well as alleviates anxiety.

PATIENT ASSESSMENT AND PREPARATION

Patient Assessment

- Obtain the patient's medical history including history of diabetes, hypertension, peripheral vascular disease, vascular grafts, arterial vasospasm, thrombosis, or embolism. Obtain the patient's history of prior coronary artery bypass graft surgery in which radial arteries were removed for use as conduits or presence of A-V fistulas or shunts. ➼*Rationale:* Extremities with any of the above problems should be avoided as sites for cannulation because of the potential for complications. Patients with diabetes mellitus or hypertension are at higher risk for arterial or venous insufficiency. Previously removed radial arteries are a contraindication for ulnar artery cannulation.
- Assess the patient's medical history of coagulopathies, use of anticoagulants, vascular abnormalities, or peripheral neuropathies. ➼*Rationale:* Assists in determining safety of the procedure and aids in site selection.
- Assess the patient's allergy history (e.g., allergy to lidocaine, topical anesthetic cream, antiseptic solutions, or tape). ➼*Rationale:* Decreases the risk for allergic reactions.
- Assess the patient's current anticoagulation therapy, known blood dyscrasias, and pertinent laboratory values (e.g., platelets, PTT, PT/INR) prior to the procedure. ➼*Rationale:* Anticoagulation therapy, blood dyscrasias, or alterations in coagulation studies could increase the risk for hematoma formation or hemorrhage.
- Presence of collateral flow to the area distal to the arterial catheter should be evaluated before cannulating the artery. For radial or ulnar arterial lines, a modified Allen test should be performed. ➼*Rationale:* Ensures presence of collateral flow to the hand to reduce vascular complications.
- Assess the intended insertion site for the presence of a strong pulse. ➼*Rationale:* Identification and localization of the pulse increases the chance of a successful arterial cannulation.

Patient Preparation

- Ensure that the patient and family understand preprocedural teaching. Answer questions as they arise and reinforce information as needed. ➼*Rationale:* Evaluates and reinforces understanding of previously taught information.
- Obtain informed consent. ➼*Rationale:* Protects the rights of the patient and makes a competent decision possible for the patient; however, under emergency circumstances, time may not allow form to be signed.

- Place the patient supine with the head of the bed at a comfortable position. The limb that the arterial catheter will be inserted into should be resting comfortably on the bed. ➥*Rationale:* Provides patient comfort and facilitates insertion.
- Place a towel under the back of the wrist to hyperextend the wrist and tape it in place or have someone hold it (if the radial artery is being used). ➥*Rationale:* Positions the arm and brings the artery closer to the surface.

- Elevate and hyperextend the patient's arm. Support the arm with a pillow (when using the brachial artery). ➥*Rationale:* Increases accessibility of the artery.
- When using the femoral artery, position the patient supine with the head of the bed at a comfortable angle. The patient's leg should be straight with the femoral area easily accessible. ➥*Rationale:* Provides the best position for localizing the femoral artery pulse.

Procedure for Performing Arterial Catheter Insertion

Steps	Rationale	Special Considerations
1. Wash hands.	Reduces the transmission of microorganisms; standard precautions.	
2. Prepare a single pressure transducer system (see Procedure 75).	Prepares equipment.	
3. If the radial artery is to be used, it is recommended to perform the modified Allen test before arterial catheter insertion (see Fig. 79-3). *(Level II: Theory-based, no research data to support recommendations; recommendations from expert consensus group may exist.)*	Although there is evidence in support of and against the use of the Allen's test or the modified Allen's test, it can be performed before a radial artery puncture in an attempt to assess the patency of the ulnar artery and to assess for an intact superficial palmar arch.[1,2,4,10]	
A. With the patient's hand held overhead, instruct the patient to open and close his or her hand several times.	Forces the blood from the hand.	If the patient is unconscious or unable to perform the procedure, clench the fist passively for the patient.
B. With the patient's fist clenched, apply direct pressure on both the radial and ulnar arteries.	Obstructs the flow of blood to the hand.	
C. Instruct the patient to lower and open his or her hand.	Allows observation for pallor.	Performed passively if the patient is unconscious or unable to assist.
D. While maintaining pressure on the radial artery, release the pressure over the ulnar artery and observe the hand for the return of color.[4,9]	Return of color within 7 seconds indicates patency of the ulnar artery and an intact superficial palmar arch; this is interpreted as a normal Allen test. If color returns between 8 and 14 seconds, the test is considered equivocal and the health care provider must consider the risk and benefits of continuing with performing this procedure. If it takes 15 or more seconds for color to return, the test is considered abnormal and another site should be considered.	If the test is abnormal, the modified Allen test should be performed on the opposite hand. If both hands are abnormal, consider using a site other than the radial arteries.
4. Wash hands and don goggles, gown, and nonsterile gloves.	Reduces the transmission of microorganisms; minimizes splash; standard precautions.	

Procedure continues on the following page

Procedure **for Performing Arterial Catheter Insertion**—*Continued*

Steps	Rationale	Special Considerations
5. Prepare the site with the antiseptic solution (e.g., 2% chlorhexidine-based preparation). Starting at the insertion site, cleanse back and forth briskly for 3 seconds.	Limits the introduction of potentially infectious skin flora into the vessel during the puncture. Antiseptic cleansing solution and brisk cleansing enhances cleansing of the area.	Allow time for the solution to dry.
6. Wash hands and change to sterile gloves.	Reduces the transmission of microorganisms; standard precautions.	
7. Drape the area around the site with sterile towels.	Provides a sterile field and minimizes the transmission of organisms.	
8. Locally anesthetize the puncture site. (*Level IV: Limited clinical studies to support recommendations.*)	Provides local anesthesia for the arterial puncture.	It has been reported that most patients experience pain during arterial puncture.[2]
A. Use a 1-ml syringe with a 25-G needle to draw up 0.5 ml of 1% lidocaine without epinephrine.	Minimizes vessel trauma. Absence of epinephrine decreases the risk for peripheral vasoconstriction.	Recent research exploring the efficacy of lidocaine ointment as an alternative to intradermal lidocaine shows promising results.[5,7,8] If this method is used, the manufacturer's recommendations should be followed.
B. Aspirate before injecting the local anesthetic.	Determines whether or not a blood vessel has been inadvertently entered.	
C. Inject intradermally and then with full infiltration around the intended arterial insertion site. Use approximately 0.2 to 0.3 ml for an adult.	Decreases the incidence of localized pain while injecting all skin layers. Patients report reduced pain when a local, intradermal anesthetic agent is used before arterial puncture.[2]	
9. Perform the percutaneous puncture of the selected artery.	Increases the likelihood of correctly locating the artery and decreases the chance of the vessel rolling.	
A. Palpate and stabilize the artery with the index and middle fingers of the nondominant hand.		
B. With the needle bevel-up and the syringe at a 30- to 60-degree angle to the radial or brachial artery, puncture the skin slowly. Adjust the angle to a 60- to 90-degree angle to the femoral artery.	A slow, gradual thrust promotes entry into the artery without inadvertently passing through the posterior wall.	
10. Advance the needle and the cannula until a blood return is noted in the hub; then slowly advance the catheter about 1/4 to 1/2 inch farther to ensure that the cannula is in the artery.	Advancing the cannula farther ensures that the entire cannula is in the artery and not just the tip of the stylet.	
11. If, on initial insertion, a blood return is not noted, a 3-ml syringe may be placed at the end of the cannula. While advancing the catheter, gentle withdrawing of the syringe plunger may be performed in an effort to determine proper placement in the artery.	Some arteries may vasospasm as a result of sudden insertion of the catheter. Taking the time to place a syringe on the catheter and withdrawing slightly during insertion may allow the artery to relax and also help to determine whether proper placement within the artery has been achieved.	

Procedure for Performing Arterial Catheter Insertion—*Continued*

Steps	Rationale	Special Considerations
12. Level the catheter to the skin; then continue to advance the cannula to its hub with a firm, steady rotary action.	The rotary action helps to advance the catheter through the skin.	
13. Correct positioning is confirmed by the presence of pulsatile blood return on the removal of the stylet.	Arterial blood is pulsatile, which confirms intraarterial placement.	
14. Once positioning is confirmed, remove the stylet and connect the catheter to the single-pressure transducer system and flush the system.	Maintains catheter patency and prepares the system for arterial blood pressure monitoring.	
15. Level the air-fluid interface (zeroing stopcock) to the phlebostatic axis, zero the monitoring system, verify the arterial waveform, and activate the alarm system (see Procedure 59).	Prepares the monitoring system; provides notification of abnormal blood pressure parameters and system disconnections.	
16. Suture the arterial catheter in place.	Maintains arterial catheter positioning; reduces the chance of accidental dislodgment.	
17. Apply a dry, occlusive sterile dressing and label the insertion information.	Provides a sterile environment; reduces the risk for infection.	
18. Discard used supplies; dispose of needles and other sharp objects in appropriate containers; remove gloves and wash hands.	Safely removes sharp objects; reduces the transmission of microorganisms; standard precautions.	

Expected Outcomes

- Successful cannulation of the artery
- Ability to obtain blood samples from the arterial line
- Peripheral vascular and neurovascular systems intact
- Alterations in hemodynamic stability identified and treated accordingly

Unexpected Outcomes

- Pain or severe discomfort during the insertion procedure
- Complications of puncture or vasospasm
- Complications after puncture, such as the following: change in color, temperature, or sensation of the extremity used for insertion; or hematoma, hemorrhage, infection, or clot at the insertion site
- Inability to cannulate the artery

Patient Monitoring and Care

Steps	Rationale	Reportable Conditions
		These conditions should be reported if they persist despite nursing interventions.
1. Observe the insertion site for signs of hemostasis after the procedure.	Postinsertion bleeding can occur in any patient but is more likely to occur in patients with coagulopathies or patients receiving anticoagulation therapy.	• Excessive bleeding • Hematoma • Changes in vital signs

Procedure continues on the following page

Patient Monitoring and Care—*Continued*

Steps	Rationale	Reportable Conditions
2. Assess the arterial catheter insertion site and involved extremity for signs of postinsertion complications.[6]	Arterial catheter insertion can result in peripheral vascular and neurovascular compromise of the extremity distal to the puncture site.	• Changes in color, size, temperature, sensation, or movement in the extremity used for the arterial catheter insertion
3. Monitor the arterial catheter insertion site for signs of local infection.	Infection related to the procedure may result from failure to maintain asepsis during insertion. Use of the femoral site for arterial line insertion may be related to an increased incidence of local infection.	• Erythema, warmth, hardness, tenderness, or pain at the arterial line insertion site • Presence of purulent drainage from the arterial line insertion site

Documentation

Documentation should include the following:

- Patient and family education
- Performance of the modified Allen test before insertion and its results (when using the radial artery)
- Signed consent form
- Arterial site used
- Insertion of the arterial catheter (date, time, and initials marked on the dressing itself)
- Size of cannula-over-needle catheter used

- Any difficulties in the insertion
- Patient tolerance
- Appearance of the site
- Appearance of the limb, capillary refill time, and temperature of the extremity after insertion is complete
- Occurrence of unexpected outcomes
- Nursing interventions taken

References

1. Buffington, S. (1996). Specimen collection and testing. In: *Nursing Procedures.* 2nd ed. Springhouse, PA: Springhouse Corp, 145-7.
2. Clarke, S. (1999). Arterial lines: An analysis of good practice. *J Child Healthcare,* 3, 22-27.
3. Cummins, R.O., ed. (1997). *Advanced Cardiac Life Support.* Dallas, TX: American Heart Association, 13.9-13.10.
4. Giner, J., et al. (1996). Pain during arterial puncture. *Chest,* 110, 1443-5.
5. Hussey, V.M., Poulin, M.V., and Fain, J.A. (1997). Effectiveness of lidocaine hydrochloride on venipuncture sites. *AORN J,* 66, 472-5.
6. Imperial-Perez, F., and McRae, M. (1998). *Protocols for Practice: Hemodynamic Monitoring Series. Arterial Pressure Monitoring.* Aliso Viejo, CA: American Association of Critical-Care Nurses.
7. Martin, C., et al. (2001). Long-term arterial cannulation in ICU patients using the radial artery or dorsalis pedis artery. *Chest,* 119, 901-6.
8. Okeson, G.C., and Wulbrecht, P.H. (1998). The safety of brachial artery puncture for arterial blood sampling. *Chest,* 114, 748-51.
9. Qvist, J., Peterfreund, R., and Perlmutter, G. (1996). Transient compartment syndrome of the forearm after attempted radial artery cannulation. *Anesth Analogs,* 83, 183-5.
10. Seneff, M. (1999). Arterial line placement and care. In: Rippe, J.M., et al. *Procedures and Techniques in Intensive Care Medicine.* 3rd ed. Philadelphia: Lippincott Williams & Wilkins, 36-45.
11. Williams, D.J., Ahmed, S.T., and Latto, I.P. (2003). A survey of venous and arterial cannulation techniques used for routine adult coronary artery bypass grafting. *Internet Journal Anesthesiology,* 6, 12p.

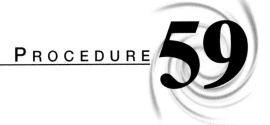

PROCEDURE **59**

Arterial Catheter Insertion (Assist), Care and Removal

P U R P O S E : Arterial catheters are used to continuously monitor blood pressure, to titrate vasoactive agents, and to obtain serial blood gases or other laboratory specimens in critically ill patients.

Rose B. Shaffer

PREREQUISITE NURSING KNOWLEDGE

- Knowledge of the anatomy and physiology of the vasculature and adjacent structures.
- Understanding of principles of hemodynamic monitoring.
- Principles of aseptic technique
- Conditions that warrant the use of arterial pressure monitoring include patients with the following:
  - ❖ Acute hypotension or hypertension (e.g., hypertensive crisis)
  - ❖ Hemodynamic instability or circulatory collapse
  - ❖ Cardiac arrest
  - ❖ Hemorrhage
  - ❖ Shock from any cause
  - ❖ Continuous infusion of vasoactive medications
  - ❖ Frequent arterial blood gas measurements
  - ❖ Nonpulsatile blood flow (e.g., those patients with ventricular assist device therapy or receiving extracorporeal membrane oxygenation therapy)
  - ❖ Intraaortic balloon pump therapy
  - ❖ Neurologic injury
  - ❖ Coronary interventional procedures
  - ❖ Major surgical procedures
  - ❖ Multiple trauma
  - ❖ Respiratory failure
  - ❖ Sepsis
  - ❖ Obstetric emergencies
  - ❖ Continuous renal replacement therapy (CRRT)
- Arterial pressure represents the forcible ejection of blood from the left ventricle into the aorta and out into the arterial system. During ventricular systole, blood is ejected into the aorta, generating a pressure wave. Because of the

intermittent pumping action of the heart, this arterial pressure wave is generated in a pulsatile manner (Fig. 59-1). The ascending limb of the aortic pressure wave (anacrotic limb) represents an increase in pressure because of left ventricular ejection. The peak of this ejection is the peak systolic pressure, which is normally 100 to 140 mm Hg in adults. After reaching this peak, the ventricular pressure declines to a level below aortic pressure and the aortic valve closes, marking the end of ventricular systole. The closure of the aortic valve produces a small rebound wave

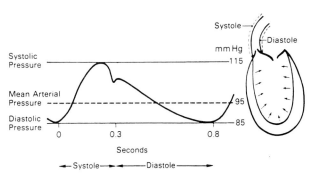

FIGURE 59-1 The generation of a pulsatile waveform. This is an aortic pressure curve. During systole, the ejected volume distends the aorta and aortic pressure rises. The peak pressure is known as the *aortic systolic pressure*. After the peak ejection, the ventricular pressure falls; when it drops below the aortic pressure, the aortic valve closes, which is marked by the dicrotic notch, the end of the systole. During diastole, the pressure continues to decline and the aortic wall recoils, pushing blood toward the periphery. The trough of the pressure wave is the *diastolic pressure*. The difference between the systolic and diastolic pressure is the *pulse pressure*. *(From Smith, J.J., and Kampine, J.P. [1980]. Circulating Physiology. Baltimore, MD: Williams & Wilkins, 55.)*

that creates a notch known as the *dicrotic notch*. The descending limb of the curve (diastolic downslope) represents diastole and is characterized by a long declining pressure wave, during which the aortic wall recoils and propels blood into the arterial network. The diastolic pressure is measured as the lowest point of the diastolic downslope and is normally 60 to 80 mm Hg.

- The difference between the systolic and diastolic pressures is called the *pulse pressure,* with a normal value of 40 mm Hg.
- Arterial pressure is determined by the relationship between blood flow through the vessels (cardiac output) and the resistance of the vessel walls (systemic vascular resistance). The arterial pressure is therefore affected by any factors that change either cardiac output or systemic vascular resistance.
- The average arterial pressure during a cardiac cycle is called the *mean arterial pressure (MAP)*. It is *not* the average of the systolic plus the diastolic pressures, because during the cardiac cycle the pressure remains closer to diastole than to systole for a longer period (at normal heart rates). The MAP is calculated automatically by most patient monitoring systems; however, it can be calculated roughly by using the following formula:

$$MAP = \frac{(\text{systolic pressure}) + (\text{diastolic pressure} \times 2)}{3}$$

- MAP represents the driving force (perfusion pressure) for blood flow through the cardiovascular system. MAP is at its highest point in the aorta. As blood travels through the circulatory system, systolic pressure increases and diastolic pressure decreases, with an overall decline in the MAP (Fig. 59-2).
- The location of the arterial catheter depends on the condition of the arterial vessels and the presence of other catheters (e.g., the presence of a dialysis shunt is a contraindication for placing an arterial catheter in the same extremity). Once inserted, the arterial catheter causes little or no discomfort to the patient and allows continuous blood pressure assessment and intermittent blood sampling. If intraaortic balloon pump therapy is required, arterial pressure may be directly monitored from the tip of the balloon in the aorta.
- When arterial pulse waveforms are recorded from sites distal to the aorta, changes in the arterial waveforms often occur. The anacrotic limb becomes more peaked and narrowed, with increased amplitude; therefore the systolic pressure in distal sites is higher than the systolic pressure recorded from a more central site (see Fig. 59-2). The diastolic downslope may demonstrate a secondary wave, and the dicrotic notch becomes less prominent from distal sites.
- Vasodilators and vasoconstrictors may change the appearance of the waveforms from distal sites. Vasodilators may cause the waveform to take on a more central appearance. Vasoconstrictors may cause the systolic pressure to become more exaggerated because of enhanced resistance in the peripheral arteries.

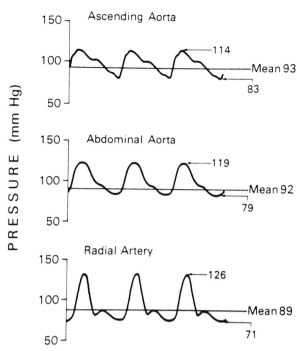

FIGURE 59-2 Arterial pressure from different sites in the arterial tree. The arterial pressure waveform will vary in configuration, depending on the location of the catheter. With transmission of the pressure wave into the distal aorta and large arteries, the systolic pressure increases and the diastolic pressure decreases; with a resulting heightening of the pulse, pressure declines steadily. *(From Smith, J.J., and Kampine, J.P. [1980].* Circulating Physiology. *Baltimore, MD: Williams & Wilkins, 57.)*

- There are several potential complications associated with arterial pressure monitoring. Infection at the insertion site can develop and cause sepsis. Clot formation in the catheter can lead to arterial embolization. The catheter can cause vessel perforation with extravasation of blood and flush solution into the surrounding tissue. Finally, the distal extremity can develop circulatory or neurologic impairment.

EQUIPMENT

- Antiseptic solution (e.g., 2% chlorhexidine-based preparation)
- 1% lidocaine solution without epinephrine
- 3-ml syringe with a 25-G needle
- Disposable pad
- Sterile towels
- 1-in to 2-in (2.5- to 5-cm) over-the-needle catheter (14- to 20-gauge for adults) or prepackaged kit with catheter, introducer, and guide wire
- Sterile 4 × 4 gauze pads
- Tape
- Single-pressure transducer system, including the following: flush solution recommended according to institution standard, a pressure bag or device, pressure tubing with flush device, transducer, and monitor cable (see Procedure 75)
- Nonsterile gloves, sterile gloves, fluid-shield masks, and protective gowns
- IV flush bag with heparin (per institutional protocol)

Additional equipment to have available as needed includes the following:

- Inline blood discard reservoir system
- Arm board
- Transparent dressing
- Suture materials
- Suture removal kit
- Transducer holder, intravenous pole and carpenter or laser level (for pole mounts)
- Bath towel
- Nonvented caps for stopcock
- 70% alcohol

PATIENT AND FAMILY EDUCATION

- Assess patient and family understanding of the reason for arterial line insertion, including how the arterial pressure is displayed on the bedside monitor. ➤*Rationale:* Decreases patient and family anxiety.
- Explain the standard of care to the patient and family, including insertion procedure, alarms, dressings, and length of time the catheter is expected to be in place. ➤*Rationale:* Encourages the patient and family to ask questions and voice concerns about the procedure.
- Explain the patient's expected participation during the procedure. ➤*Rationale:* Encourages patient cooperation during insertion.
- Explain the importance of keeping the affected extremity immobile. ➤*Rationale:* Encourages patient cooperation to prevent catheter dislodgment and ensures a more accurate waveform.
- Instruct the patient to report any warmth, redness, pain, or wet feeling at the insertion site at any time, including after catheter removal. ➤*Rationale:* May indicate infection, bleeding, or disconnection of the tubing or catheter.

PATIENT ASSESSMENT AND PREPARATION

Patient Assessment

- Obtain the patient's medical history, including diabetes, hypertension, peripheral vascular disease, vascular grafts,

AV fistulas or shunts, arterial vasospasm, thrombosis, or embolism. Obtain the patient's history of prior coronary artery bypass graft surgery in which radial arteries were removed for use as conduits. ➤*Rationale:* Extremities with any of these problems should be avoided as sites for cannulation because of their potential for complications. Patients with diabetes mellitus or hypertension are at higher risk for arterial or venous insufficiency.

- Assess the patient's medical history for coagulopathies or a history of heparin-induced thrombocytopenia or recent use of anticoagulants or thrombolytic agents. Assess baseline coagulation studies (prothrombin time [PT], partial thromboplastin time [PTT], international normalized ratio [INR], and platelets). ➤*Rationale:* Assists in determining safety of the procedure.
- Assess the patient's allergy history (e.g., allergy to lidocaine, antiseptic solutions, or tape). ➤*Rationale:* Decreases the risk for allergic reactions.
- Assess the neurovascular and peripheral vascular status of the extremity to be used for the arterial cannulation, including assessment of color, temperature, presence and fullness of pulses, capillary refill, presence of bruit, and motor and sensory function (as compared with the opposite extremity). *Note:* A modified Allen test is performed before cannulation of the radial artery (see Fig. 79-3). ➤*Rationale:* Identifies any circulatory or neurologic impairment before cannulation to avoid potential complications.

Patient Preparation

- Ensure that the patient and family understand preprocedural teaching. Answer questions as they arise and reinforce information as needed. ➤*Rationale:* Evaluates and reinforces understanding of previously taught information.
- Ensure that informed consent is obtained. ➤*Rationale:* Protects the rights of the patient and makes a competent decision possible for the patient; however, in emergency circumstances, time may not allow the form to be signed.
- Place the patient's extremity in the appropriate position with adequate lighting of the insertion site. ➤*Rationale:* Prepares the site for cannulation and facilitates an accurate insertion.

Procedure for Assisting With Insertion of an Arterial Catheter		
Steps	**Rationale**	**Special Considerations**
1. Wash hands.	Reduces the transmission of microorganisms; standard precautions.	
2. If a catheter is to be inserted in the radial artery, perform a modified Allen test (see Fig. 79-3).	Ensures the adequacy of collateral blood flow of the extremity to be cannulated.[2,4-6,13]	

Procedure continues on the following page

Procedure for Assisting With Insertion of an Arterial Catheter—*Continued*

Steps	Rationale	Special Considerations
(Level II: Theory-based, no research data to support recommendations; recommendations from expert consensus group may exist.)		
3. When preparing the flush solution, follow institutional standard for adding heparin to the IV bag, if heparin is not contraindicated. *(Level V: Clinical studies in more than one or two different patient populations and situations to support recommendations.)* Note: Do not use heparinized dextrose solutions. *(Level VI: Clinical studies in a variety of patient populations and situations to support recommendations.)*	Heparinized flush solutions are commonly used to minimize thrombi and fibrin deposits on the catheter. Catheters flushed with heparinized saline are more likely than those flushed with nonheparinized saline to remain patent.[1,7] Dextrose supports the growth of microorganisms. These solutions have been associated with infection.[10,11,16]	The use of heparin is contraindicated in patients with heparin-induced thrombocytopenia or other hematologic disorders. Other factors that promote patency of the arterial line besides heparinized saline include the following: male sex, longer catheters, larger vessels, and short-term use of the catheter.[1]
4. Use a closed tubing system.	May reduce the risk for nosocomial infection.[3]	
5. Consider using tubing with an inline blood discard reservoir. *(Level IV: Limited clinical studies to support recommendations.)*	May reduce the risk for nosocomial anemia.[14,15]	
Assisting with Insertion		
1. Wash hands and don nonsterile gloves, fluid shield masks, and protective gowns.	Reduces the transmission of microorganisms; standard precautions.	
2. Prime or flush the entire pressure transducer system (see Procedure 75).	Removes air bubbles. Air bubbles within the tubing will dampen the waveform. Air bubbles introduced into the patient's circulation can cause an air embolism.	Air is more easily removed from the pressure tubing when the system is not under pressure.
3. Assist with immobilizing the extremity during catheter insertion.	Facilitates insertion; may prevent the needle from lacerating the vessel wall during insertion.	Sedation may be necessary if the patient is restless.
4. Assist with skin preparation and catheter insertion, if needed.	Provides a cooperative effort.	
5. Once the catheter is positioned, connect the primed tubing with the Luer-Lok adapter to the arterial catheter.	Provides a secure attachment and allows the signal to be transmitted to the monitor via the transducer.	The catheter must be held in place while the connections are made.
6. Observe the waveform and perform a dynamic response test (square wave test, Fig. 59-3).	Results indicate whether or not the system is damped.	
7. Assist with securing or suturing the catheter in place.	The catheter is at risk of becoming dislodged until secured.	
8. Once the catheter is secured in place, apply a sterile, occlusive dressing.	Provides a sterile environment; reduces infection.	Refer to the institutional policy. Studies of the efficacy of using antimicrobial ointments at the catheter site to prevent infection are contradictory. The CDC does not

When the fast flush of the continuous flush system is activated and quickly released, a sharp upstroke terminates in a flat line at the maximal indicator on the monitor and hard copy. This is then followed by an immediate rapid downstroke extending below baseline with just 1 or 2 oscillations within 0.12 seconds (minimal ringing) and a quick return to baseline. The patient's pressure waveform is also clearly defined with all components of the waveform, such as the dicrotic notch on an arterial waveform, clearly visible.

Square wave test configuration

A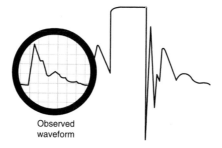

Observed waveform

Intervention

There is no adjustment in the monitoring system required.

The upstroke of the square wave appears somewhat slurred, the waveform does not extend below the baseline after the fast flush and there is no ringing after the flush. The patient's waveform displays a falsely decreased systolic pressure and false high diastolic pressure as well as poorly defined components of the pressure tracing such as a diminished or absent dicrotic notch on arterial waveforms.

Square wave test configuration

B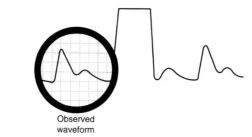

Observed waveform

Intervention

To correct for the problem:
1. Check for the presence of blood clots, blood left in the catheter following blood sampling, or air bubbles at any point from the catheter tip to the transducer diaphragm and eliminate these as necessary.
2. Use low compliance (rigid), short (less than 3 to 4 feet) monitoring tubing.
3. Connect all line components securely.
4. Check for kinks in the line.

The waveform is characterized by numerous amplified oscillations above and below the baseline following the fast flush. The monitored pressure wave displays false high systolic pressures (overshoot), possibly false low diastolic pressures, and "ringing" artifacts on the waveform.

Square wave test configuration

C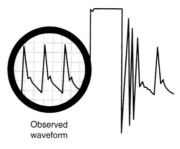

Observed waveform

Intervention

To correct the problem, remove all air bubbles (particularly pinpoint air bubbles) in the fluid system, use large-bore, shorter tubing, or use a damping device.

FIGURE 59-3 Dynamic response test (square wave test) using the fast flush system. **A,** Optimally damped system. **B,** Overdamped system. **C,** Underdamped system. *(From Darovic, G.O., and Zbilut, J.P. [2002]. Fluid-filled monitoring systems. In: Hemodynamic Monitoring. 3rd ed. Philadelphia: W.B. Saunders, 122.)*

Procedure for Assisting With Insertion of an Arterial Catheter—*Continued*

Steps	Rationale	Special Considerations
		recommend the routine application of topical antimicrobial ointment to the insertion site of peripheral intravascular catheters but does not make a specific recommendation for peripheral arterial catheters.[11]
9. Apply an arm board, if necessary.	Ensures the correct position of the extremity for an optimal waveform.	
10. Level the air-fluid interface to the phlebostatic axis and zero the transducer (see Procedure 75).	Prepares the monitoring system. Leveling ensures the air-fluid interface of the monitoring system is level with a reference point on the body. Ideally the reference point is the phlebostatic axis (see Fig. 75-7) because it more accurately reflects central arterial pressure.[9] Using the tip of the catheter as the reference point measures transmural pressure of a specific area in the arterial tree, which may be increased by hydrostatic pressure.[9]	Follow institutional protocol for leveling the air-fluid interface. Use pole mount or patient mount according to institutional protocol (see Procedure 75).
11. Set the alarm parameters according to the patient's current blood pressure.	Alarms should always be on to detect pulseless electrical activity, hypotension, hypertension, accidental disconnection, accidental removal of the catheter, or damping of the waveform.	Follow institution protocol.
12. Discard used supplies and wash hands.	Reduces the transmission of microorganisms; standard precautions.	
13. Run a waveform strip and record baseline pressures.	Obtains baseline data.	Digital values are not used, because they are averaged calculations.
14. Record the manual (noninvasive) blood pressure and compare with the arterial (invasive) blood pressure.	Obtains baseline data.	There is no direct relationship between noninvasive and invasive blood pressures, because noninvasive techniques measure blood flow and invasive techniques measure pressure.

Procedure for Troubleshooting an Overdamped Waveform

Steps	Rationale	Special Considerations
1. Identify the overdamped waveform (Fig. 59-4).	Identifies the problem.	An overdamped waveform results in a falsely low systolic pressure and a falsely high diastolic pressure.
2. Check the patient.	A sudden hypotensive episode can look like an overdamped waveform (Fig. 59-5).	

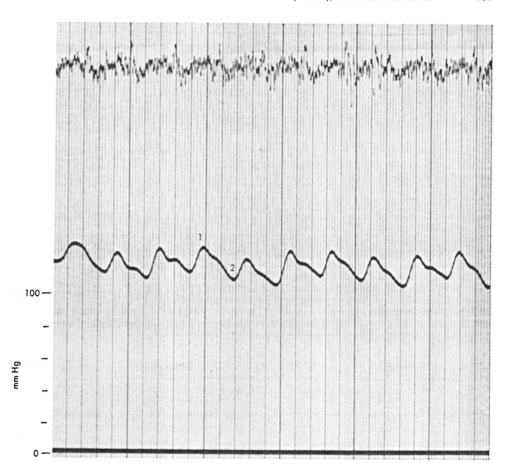

FIGURE 59-4 Overdamped arterial waveform (1 = systole; 2 = diastole). *(From Daily, E.K., and Schroeder, J.S. [1990]. Hemodynamic Waveforms. St. Louis: Mosby-Year Book, 110.)*

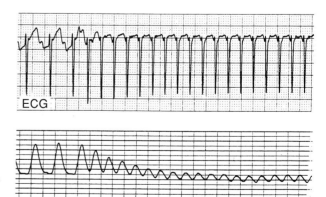

FIGURE 59-5 Patient developed a superventricular tachycardia (SVT) with a fall in arterial pressure. Note how the arterial line appears overdamped but is in fact reflecting a severe hypotensive episode associated with the tachycardia.

Procedure for Troubleshooting an Overdamped Waveform—*Continued*

Steps	Rationale	Special Considerations
3. Perform a dynamic response test if the arterial waveform seems to be overdamped (see Fig. 59-3B).	Overdamping should be assessed immediately to ensure waveform accuracy and to prevent clotting of the catheter.	
4. If the waveform is overdamped, follow these steps: A. Check the arterial line insertion site for catheter positioning.	Wrist movement in the radial site or leg flexion in the femoral site can cause catheter kinking or dislodgment, resulting in an overdamped waveform.	
B. Check the system for air bubbles and eliminate them if they are found.	Air bubbles can be a cause of an overdamped system; air bubbles can also cause emboli.	
C. Check the tubing system for leaks or disconnections and correct the problem if it is found.	Ensures all connections are tight.	
D. Check the flush bag to ensure fluid is present in the bag and that pressure is maintained at 300 mm Hg.	An empty flush bag or a pressure of less than 300 mm Hg may result in an overdamped system.	
E. A catheter with an overdamped waveform should always be aspirated before flushing.	Using the fast-flush device or flushing with a syringe first may force a clot at the catheter tip into the arterial circulation.	
Attempt to aspirate and flush the catheter as follows:	Assists with the withdrawal of air in the tubing or clots that may be at the catheter tip.	
• Wash hands and don nonsterile gloves and a fluid shield mask.	Reduces the transmission of microorganisms; standard precautions.	
• Attach a 5-ml or 10-ml syringe to the blood sampling port of the stopcock closest to the patient.	A 5-ml syringe generates less pressure and may prevent arterial spasm in smaller arteries (e.g., radial artery).	A 10-ml syringe may be needed for larger arteries (e.g., femoral artery).
• Turn the stopcock off to the flush solution (see Fig. 62-3).	Opens the system from the patient to the syringe.	
• Gently attempt to aspirate; if resistance is felt, reposition the extremity and reattempt aspiration. If resistance is still felt, stop and notify the physician or advanced practice nurse.	Assesses catheter patency. Normally, blood should be aspirated into the syringe without difficulty.	
• If blood is aspirated, remove 3 ml, turn the stopcock off to the patient, and discard the 3-ml sample (see Fig. 62-5).	Removes any clotted material within the catheter.	All blood wastes should be disposed of following standard precautions.
• Fast-flush the remaining blood from the stopcock onto a sterile gauze pad or into another syringe and remove the syringe.	Removes blood residue from the stopcock, where it could be a reservoir for bacterial growth. Prevents clotting of blood in the blood sampling port.	

Procedure **for Troubleshooting an Overdamped Waveform**—*Continued*

Steps	Rationale	Special Considerations
• Turn the stopcock off to the blood sampling port (see Fig. 62-1) and replace it with a sterile nonvented cap.	Maintains sterility and a closed system.	
• Use the fast-flush device to clear the line of blood.	Prevents the arterial line from clotting.	
5. Discard used supplies in the appropriate receptacles, and wash hands.	Reduces the transmission of microorganisms; standard precautions.	

Procedure **for Troubleshooting an Underdamped Waveform**

Steps	Rationale	Special Considerations
1. Identify the underdamped waveform and perform a dynamic response test (see Fig. 59-3C).	Identifies the problem.	An underdamped waveform results in a falsely high systolic pressure and a falsely low diastolic pressure.
2. Wash hands and don nonsterile gloves.	Reduces the transmission of microorganisms; standard precautions.	
3. Check the system for air bubbles and eliminate them if they are found.	Air bubbles can contribute to underdamping; air bubbles can also cause emboli.	
4. Check the length of the pressurized tubing system.	Ensures that the tubing length is minimized.	
5. Wash hands.	Reduces the transmission of microorganisms; standard precautions.	

Procedure **for Arterial Line Dressing Change**

Steps	Rationale	Special Considerations
1. The frequency of the dressing change is determined by the type of dressing material used and the institution policy.	Prevents infection at the insertion site.	The CDC recommends replacing the dressing when the catheter is replaced; when the dressing becomes damp, loosened, or soiled; and when inspection of the site is required.[11]
A. Wash hands and don nonsterile gloves.	Reduces the transmission of microorganisms; standard precautions.	
B. Gently remove the old dressing, being careful not to place tension on the arterial catheter.	Prevents the inadvertent dislodgment of the catheter.	Use extreme care to secure the catheter while removing the tape. A second health care provider may be needed to assist with the dressing removal to prevent accidental dislodgment or removal of the arterial catheter.
C. Observe for signs of infection.	Early detection may prevent bacteremia.	An infected catheter is removed. Send the tip for culture if prescribed.

Procedure continues on the following page

Procedure for Arterial Line Dressing Change—*Continued*

Steps	Rationale	Special Considerations
D. Cleanse the insertion site with a 2% chlorhexidine-based preparation.[11]	Decreases the risk for bacterial growth at the insertion site.	Allow time for the solution to dry.
E. Replace the dressing, using aseptic technique.	Maintains asepsis.	
F. Discard used supplies and wash hands.	Reduces the transmission of microorganisms; standard precautions.	

Procedure for Removal of the Arterial Catheter

Steps	Rationale	Special Considerations
1. Assess the patient's coagulation profile (PT, PTT, INR, platelets) prior to removal of the arterial catheter.	Elevated PT, PTT, INR, and/or decreased platelets will affect bleeding times.	If laboratory values are abnormal, pressure will need to be applied for a longer period in order to achieve hemostasis.
2. Wash hands and don nonsterile gloves, a fluid-shield mask, and a protective gown.	Reduces the transmission of microorganisms; standard precautions.	Refer to the institutional policy regarding which arterial catheters nurses can remove.
3. Turn off the monitoring alarms.	Prevents false alarms.	
4. Remove the dressing.	Prepares the catheter for removal.	Clip sutures if present.
5. Attach a 3-ml or 5-ml syringe to the blood sampling port, turn the stopcock off to the flush solution (see Fig. 62-3), and draw blood back through the tubing.	Prepares for removal. A 5-ml syringe generates less pressure and may prevent arterial spasm in smaller arteries (e.g., radial artery).	A 10-ml syringe may be needed for larger arteries (e.g., femoral artery).
6. Apply pressure 1-2 fingerwidths above the insertion site.	The arterial puncture site is above the skin puncture site because the catheter enters the skin at an angle. Prepares for removal.	
7. Pull out the arterial catheter using a sterile 4 × 4 gauze pad to cover the site as the catheter is removed.	Prevents splashing of blood.	
8. Continue to hold proximal pressure and immediately apply firm pressure over the insertion site as the catheter is removed.	Prevents bleeding.	
9. Continue to apply pressure for a minimum of 5 minutes for the radial artery.	Achieves hemostasis.	Longer periods of direct pressure may be needed to achieve hemostasis in patients receiving systemic heparin or thrombolytics or patients with catheters in larger arteries (e.g., in the femoral artery). Follow institutional standard.
10. Apply a pressure dressing to the insertion site.	A pressure dressing will help prevent rebleeding.	The dressing should not encircle the extremity in order to prevent ischemia of the extremity.
11. Discard supplies and wash hands.	Reduces the transmission of microorganisms; standard precautions.	

Expected Outcomes	**Unexpected Outcomes**
• Minimal discomfort from the arterial catheter • Maintenance of baseline hemoglobin and hematocrit levels • Adequate circulation to the involved extremity • Adequate sensory and motor function of the extremity • Remaining euvolemic • Maintenance of catheter site without infection	• Pain or discomfort from the arterial catheter insertion site • Decreased hemoglobin and hematocrit • Catheter disconnection with significant blood loss • Impaired peripheral tissue perfusion (e.g., edema, coolness, pain, paleness, or slow capillary refill of fingers or toes of cannulated extremity) • Presence of a new bruit • Impaired sensory or motor function of the extremity • Fluid volume overload or deficit • Elevated temperature or elevated white blood cell count • Redness, warmth, edema, or drainage at or from the insertion site

Patient Monitoring and Care

Steps	Rationale	Reportable Conditions
		These conditions should be reported if they persist despite nursing interventions.
1. Assess the neurovascular and peripheral vascular status of the cannulated extremity immediately after catheter insertion and every 4 hours or more often if warranted, according to unit policy.	Validates adequate peripheral circulation and neurovascular integrity. Changes in sensation, motor function, pulses, color, temperature, or capillary refill may indicate ischemia, arterial spasm, or neurovascular compromise.	• Diminished or absent pulses • Pale, mottled, or cyanotic appearance of the extremity • Extremity that is cool or cold to the touch • Capillary refill time of more than 2 seconds • Diminished or absent sensation • Diminished or absent motor function
2. Check the arterial line flush system every 4 hours to ensure the following: • Pressure bag or device is inflated to 300 mm Hg. • Fluid is present in the flush solution.	Ensures the accuracy of the pressure waveform and functioning of the system. Ensures accuracy of pressure readings and prevents overdamped waveform. Ensures that approximately 1-3 ml/hour of flush solution is delivered through the catheter, thus maintaining patency and preventing backflow of blood into the catheter and tubing. The catheter will clot off if fluid is not continuously infusing.	
3. Monitor for overdamped or underdamped waveforms. • An overdamped waveform is characterized by a flattened waveform, a diminished or absent dicrotic notch, or a waveform that does not fall to baseline (see Fig. 59-4).	An optimally damped system provides an adequate waveform with appropriate blood pressure readings. With an overdamped waveform, the patient's systolic pressure may be read inaccurately low. Common causes of an overdamped waveform include the following: air bubbles in the system, use of compliant tubing, loose connections in the system, too many stopcocks in the system, cracked tubing or stopcock, arterial cannula	• Overdamped or underdamped waveform that cannot be corrected with troubleshooting procedures

Procedure continues on the following page

Patient Monitoring and Care—*Continued*

Steps	Rationale	Reportable Conditions
• An underdamped waveform is characterized by catheter fling (see Fig. 59-3C).	occlusion, catheter tip against the arterial wall, blood in the transducer, and insufficient pressure of the flush solution. With an underdamped waveform, systolic pressures may be read inaccurately high. Common causes of an underdamped waveform include the following: excessive tubing length, movement of the catheter in the artery, patient movement, and air bubbles in the system.	
4. Perform a dynamic response test every 8-12 hours, when the system is opened to air or when the accuracy of readings is in question (see Fig. 59-3A-C).	An optimally damped system provides an accurate waveform.	• Overdamped or underdamped waveform that cannot be corrected with troubleshooting procedures
5. Zero the transducer during the initial setup and before insertion, if the transducer and the monitoring cable are disconnected, if the monitoring cable and the monitor are disconnected, and when the values obtained do not fit the clinical picture.	Ensures accuracy of the hemodynamic monitoring system; minimizes the risk for contamination of the system.	
6. Observe the insertion site for signs of infection.	Infected catheters must be removed as soon as possible to prevent bacteremia. The CDC does not recommend routinely replacing peripheral arterial catheters to prevent catheter-related infections.[11]	• Purulent drainage • Tenderness or pain at the insertion site • Elevated temperature • Elevated white blood cells
7. Change the pressure tubing, flush solution, and transducer every 96 hours or with each change of the catheter if it is changed more frequently. The flush solution may need to be changed more frequently if it is empty of solution. *(Level VI: Clinical studies in a variety of patient populations and situations to support recommendations.)*	Changing the flush solution and system more often than every 96 hours may cause contamination and increase the risk for infection.[8,11,12]	
8. Run an arterial pressure strip and obtain measurement of the arterial pressures during end-expiration.	Eliminates the effect of the respiratory cycle on the arterial pressure waveform.	
9. Obtain an arterial waveform strip to place on the patient's chart at the start of each shift and whenever there is a change in the waveform.	The printed waveform allows assessment of the adequacy of the waveform, damping, or respiratory variation.	
10. Monitor hemoglobin or hematocrit daily or whenever a significant amount of blood is lost through the catheter (e.g., through accidental disconnection).	Allows assessment of nosocomial anemia.	• Changes in hemoglobin and hematocrit

Documentation

Documentation should include the following:

- Patient and family education
- Peripheral vascular and neurovascular assessment before and after the procedure and after the catheter is removed
- Date and time of insertion with the size of catheter placed and site of placement
- Assessment of insertion site
- Patient response to insertion procedure
- Status of the patient alarms and their parameters

- Type of flush solution used
- Intake of flush solution (e.g., 3 ml/hr) on intake and output sheet
- Initial insertion waveform (recorded), labeled with the date, time, and systolic and diastolic pressures
- Time of arterial catheter removal
- Unexpected outcomes
- Additional nursing interventions

References

1. American Association of Critical-Care Nurses. (1993). Evaluation of the effects of heparinized and nonheparinized flush solutions on the patency of arterial pressure monitoring lines: The AACN Thunder Project. *Am J Crit Care*, 2, 3-15.
2. Buffington, S. (1996). Specimen collection and testing. In: *Nursing Procedures*. 2nd ed. Springhouse, PA: Springhouse Corp.
3. Crow, S., et al. (1989). Microbial contamination of arterial infusions used for hemodynamic monitoring: A randomized trial of contamination with sampling through conventional stopcocks versus a novel closed system. *Infect Control Hosp Epidemiol*, 10, 557-61.
4. Cummins R.O., ed. (1997). *Advanced Cardiac Life Support*. Dallas, TX: American Heart Association.
5. DeGroot, K.D., and Damato, G. (1986). Monitoring intra-arterial pressure. *Crit Care Nurse*, 6, 74-8.
6. Hadaway, L.C. (1995). Anatomy and physiology related to intravenous therapy. In: Terry, J., et al, eds. *Intravenous Therapy: Clinical Principles and Practice*. Philadelphia: W.B. Saunders.
7. Kulkarni, M., et al. (1994). Heparinized saline versus normal saline in maintaining patency of the radial artery catheter. *Can J Surg*, 37, 37-42.
8. Luskin, R.L., et al. (1986). Extended use of disposable pressure transducers. *JAMA*, 255, 916-20.
9. McGhee, B.H., and Bridges, M.E.J. (2002). Monitoring arterial blood pressure: What you may not know. *Crit Care Nurse*, 22, 60-79.
10. Mermel, L.A., and Maki, D.G. (1989). Epidemic bloodstream infections from hemodynamic pressure monitoring: Signs of the times. *Infect Control Hosp Epidemiol*, 10, 47-53.
11. O'Grady, N.P., et al. (2002). Guidelines for the prevention of intravascular catheter-related infections. Centers for Disease Control and Prevention. *Morbidity and Mortality Weekly Report. Recommendations and Reports*, 51(RR-10), 1-29.
12. O'Malley, M.K., et al. (1994). Value of routine pressure monitoring system changes after 72 hours of continuous use. *Crit Care Med*, 22, 1424-30.
13. Perucca, R. (1995). Obtaining vascular access. In: Terry, J., et al, eds. *Intravenous Therapy: Clinical Principles and Practice*. Philadelphia: W.B. Saunders.
14. Peruzzi, W.T., et al. (1993). A clinical evaluation of a blood conservation device in medical intensive care unit patients. *Crit Care Med*, 21(4), 501-6.
15. Silver, M.J., et al. (1993). Evaluation of a new blood-conserving arterial line system for patients in intensive care units. *Crit Care Med*, 21(4), 507-11.
16. Solomon, S.L., et al. (1986). Nosocomial fungemia in neonates associated with intravascular pressure-monitoring devices. *Pediatr Infect Dis*, 5, 680-5.

Additional Readings

Aherns, T.S., and Taylor, L.A. (1992). *Hemodynamic Waveform Analysis*. Philadelphia: W.B. Saunders.

Bridges, E.J., et al. (1997). Ask the experts. *Crit Care Nurse*, 17, 96-7, 101-2.

Chulay, M., and Holland, S. (1996). Ask the experts. Where should the transducer be leveled for radial or femoral arterial pressure monitoring? *Crit Care Nurse*, 16, 103-7.

Clark, C.A., and Harmon, E.M. (1990). Hemodynamic monitoring: Arterial catheters. In: Taylor, R.W., Civetta, J.M., and Kirby, R.R. *Techniques and Procedures in Critical Care*. Philadelphia: J.B. Lippincott.

Clark, V.L., and Kruse, J.A. (1992). Arterial catheterization. *Crit Care Clin*, 8, 687-97.

Daily, E.K., and Schroeder, J.S. (1994). *Techniques in Bedside Hemodynamic Monitoring*. 5th ed. St. Louis: C.V. Mosby.

Darovic, G.O. (2002). Arterial pressure monitoring. In: *Hemodynamic Monitoring: Invasive and Noninvasive Clinical Application*. 3rd ed. Philadelphia: W.B. Saunders.

Dech, Z.F. (1994). Blood conservation in the critically ill. *AACN Clin Issues Crit Care Nurs*, 5, 169-77.

Foster, B. (1997). Continuing discussion on transducer placement ... Ask the experts column of the December 1996 ... zero referencing arterial lines. *Crit Care Nurse*, 17, 18.

Gleason, E., Grossman, S., and Campbell, C. (1992). Minimizing diagnostic blood loss in critically ill patients. *Am J Crit Care*, 1, 85-90.

Gorny, D.A. (1993). Arterial blood pressure measurement technique. *AACN Clin Issues Crit Care Nurs*, 4, 66-80.

Hoffman, K.K., et al. (1992). Transparent polyurethane film as an intravenous catheter dressing: A meta-analysis of the infection risks. *JAMA*, 267, 2072-76.

Imperial-Perez, F., and McRae, M. (2002). Protocols for practice: Applying research at the bedside. Arterial pressure monitoring. *Crit Care Nurse,* 22, 70-72.

Imperial-Perez, F., and McRae, M. (1998). *Protocols for Practice: Hemodynamic Monitoring Series—Arterial Pressure Monitoring.* Aliso Viejo, CA: American Association of Critical-Care Nurses.

O'Grady, N.P., et al. (2003). Patient safety and the science of prevention: The time for implementing the guidelines for the prevention of intravascular catheter-related infections is now. *Crit Care Med,* 31, 291-92.

Pizov, R., et al. (1996). Positive end-expiratory pressure-induced hemodynamic changes are reflected in the arterial pressure waveform. *Crit Care Med,* 24, 1381-7.

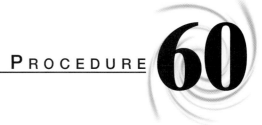

PROCEDURE **60**

Blood Sampling From an Arterial Catheter

PURPOSE: Blood sampling from an arterial catheter is performed to obtain blood specimens for arterial blood gas analysis or for other laboratory testing.

Rose B. Shaffer

PREREQUISITE NURSING KNOWLEDGE

• Knowledge of sterile technique
• Knowledge of the vascular anatomy and physiology
• Understanding of the technique for specimen collection and labeling
• Understanding of the principles of arterial pressure monitoring and stopcock manipulation (see Procedure 59)

EQUIPMENT

• Nonsterile gloves
• Sterile 4 × 4 gauze pads
• Appropriate blood specimen tubes (or arterial blood gas [ABG] kit)
• Labels with the patient's name and appropriate identifying data
• Laboratory forms
• Goggles or fluid shield face mask
  Additional equipment as needed includes the following:
• Alcohol pads or swab sticks
• VACUTAINER®
• "Needleless" VACUTAINER® Luer-Lok adapter needle
• Cup/bag of ice (for ABG specimen)
• Extra blood specimen tube (for discard)
• Syringes, 5 ml and 10 ml
• Sterile nonvented caps

PATIENT AND FAMILY EDUCATION

• Assess patient and family understanding of the reason for blood sampling from the arterial catheter. ➤*Rationale:* Alleviates anxiety and promotes understanding.
• Explain the procedure to the patient and family. ➤*Rationale:* Alleviates anxiety and encourages questions.
• Explain the importance of keeping the affected extremity immobile. ➤*Rationale:* Encourages patient assistance during blood withdrawal.

PATIENT ASSESSMENT AND PREPARATION

Patient Assessment

• Assess the patency of the arterial catheter. ➤*Rationale:* If the arterial catheter is clotted, blood sampling will not be able to be performed.
• Assess the patient's previous laboratory results. ➤*Rationale:* Provides data for comparison.

Patient Preparation

• Ensure that the patient and family understand preprocedural teaching. Answer questions as they arise and reinforce information as needed. ➤*Rationale:* Evaluates and reinforces understanding of previously taught information.
• Expose the stopcock to be used for blood sampling and position the patient's extremity so that the site can easily be accessed. ➤*Rationale:* Prepares the site for blood withdrawal.

Procedure for Blood Sampling From an Arterial Catheter

Steps	Rationale	Special Considerations
1. Wash hands and don nonsterile gloves and goggles or fluid shield face mask.	Reduces the transmission of microorganisms and body fluids; standard precautions.	
2. When obtaining an ABG, open the ABG kit and use the plunger to rid excess heparin and air from the syringe (heparin is usually in powder form).	An excess amount of heparin may alter ABG results.	If prepackaged ABG kits are not available, draw up 0.5 ml of a 1:1000 dilution of heparin in a 3-ml syringe. Pull back on the plunger to coat the inside of the syringe and the needle. Rid the excess heparin and air from the syringe.[1]
3. If using a VACUTAINER,® attach the "needleless" Luer-Lok adapter needle to the VACUTAINER® (Fig. 60-1).	Prepares for blood sampling.	If possible, use a needleless system for obtaining blood samples to prevent needlestick injury. The VACUTAINER® blood sampling system is designed for sampling venous blood. Studies are needed to determine the accuracy of arterial blood for laboratory testing using the VACUTAINER® system.
4. Suspend the arterial alarms.	Prevents the alarm from sounding as the pressure waveform is lost during the blood draw.	
5. Turn the stopcock off to the patient (Fig. 60-2).	Prevents the backflow of arterial blood from the patient when the three-way stopcock blood sampling port is opened.	There will be loss of the arterial pressure waveform and digital display.
6. Remove the nonvented occlusive cap from the blood sampling port of the three-way stopcock closest to the patient.	Prepares for blood sampling.	If using a system where blood samples are obtained through a rubber diaphragm, swab the area with alcohol before entering the system.[6]
7. Place a VACUTAINER® with a "needleless" Luer-Lok adapter needle into the blood sampling port of the three-way stopcock (Fig. 60-3).	Prepares for blood sampling.	A syringe may be used in place of the VACUTAINER.®

"NEEDLELESS" VACUTAINER

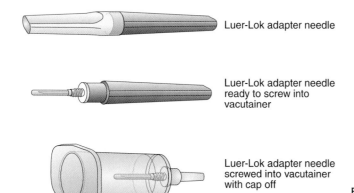

Luer-Lok adapter needle

Luer-Lok adapter needle ready to screw into vacutainer

Luer-Lok adapter needle screwed into vacutainer with cap off

FIGURE 60-1 "Needleless" VACUTAINER® Luer-Lok adapter needle.

Procedure for Blood Sampling From an Arterial Catheter—*Continued*

Steps	Rationale	Special Considerations
8. Turn the stopcock off to the flush solution.	Opens the arterial line to the VACUTAINER® or syringe.	
9. Attach one blood specimen tube (for discard) into the VACUTAINER.®		

Procedure continues on the following page

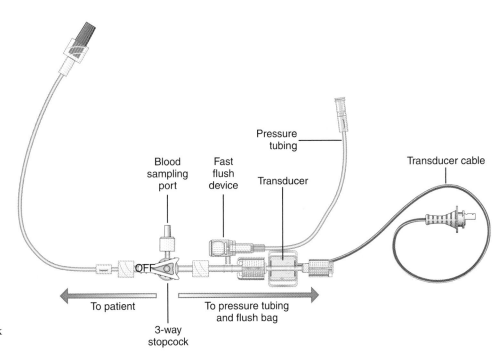

FIGURE 60-2 Disposable transducer with continuous flush device. In this picture, the stopcock is turned "off" to the patient.

Blood sampling port

Fast flush device

Pressure tubing

Transducer

Transducer cable

OFF

To patient

To pressure tubing and flush bag

3-way stopcock

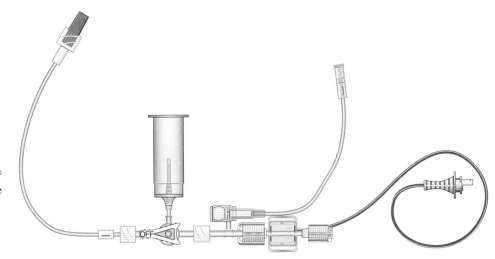

FIGURE 60-3 VACUTAINER® with "needleless" Luer-Lok needle attached to the blood sampling port of the three-way stopcock. The stopcock is "off" to the patient.

OFF

Procedure   for Blood Sampling From an Arterial Catheter—*Continued*

Steps	Rationale	Special Considerations
10. Completely engage the blood specimen tube into the VACUTAINER® to obtain the discard volume (see **Step 11**).	Engages the vacuum to withdraw flush solution and blood from the arterial catheter.	If using a syringe, gently aspirate the discard volume (see **Step 11**).
11. Remove the minimal volume of blood needed for discard.	Clears the arterial line of any flush solution that may affect the laboratory results.	If possible, use a blood-conserving closed system to avoid nosocomial anemia (Fig. 60-4).
A. When obtaining blood for an ABG, use a discard volume of two times the dead-space volume of the catheter and tubing to the sampling site. *(Level V: Clinical studies in more than one or two different patient populations and situations to support recommendations.)*	Use of this discard volume prevents dilution of the ABG sample by saline and excess heparin.[7,8]	
B. When obtaining blood for coagulation studies from a heparinized arterial line, use a discard volume of six times the dead-space volume of the catheter and tubing to the sampling site. *(Level VI: Clinical studies in a variety of patient populations and situations to support recommendations.)*	Use of this discard volume prevents contamination of the specimen with heparin, preventing inaccurate coagulation results.[2,3,4,5]	This recommendation does not apply to patients receiving systemic heparin therapy. More research is needed with these patient populations.
12. Remove the discard specimen tube from the VACUTAINER.®	Discards blood containing flush solution.	Place the discard specimen away from the field so as not to mistake

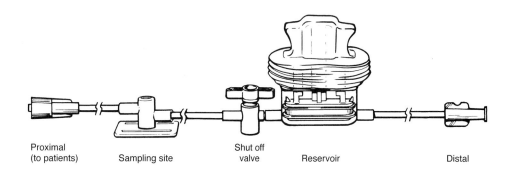

Proximal (to patients)   Sampling site   Shut off valve   Reservoir   Distal

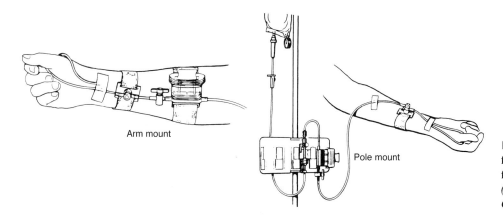

Arm mount

Pole mount

FIGURE 60-4 VAMP system for needleless blood withdrawal from hemodynamic lines. *(Courtesy Edwards Lifesciences Corporation, Irvine, CA.)*

Procedure **for Blood Sampling From an Arterial Catheter**—*Continued*

Steps	Rationale	Special Considerations
If using a syringe for the discard specimen, turn the stopcock off to the patient before removing the syringe (see Fig. 62-5).	Prevents backflow of arterial blood from the patient.	it with the actual blood specimens for laboratory analysis.
13. Engage each blood specimen tube into the VACUTAINER.® A. The stopcock should remain off to the flush solution as each blood specimen tube is engaged (see Fig. 62-4). B. When using syringes to draw blood specimens: • Turn the stopcock off to the patient before changing each syringe (see Fig. 62-5). • After each new syringe is attached to the blood sampling port, turn the stopcock off to the flush solution (see Fig. 62-3). B. When obtaining an ABG with other laboratory studies, turn the stopcock off to the patient, remove the VACUTAINER® or the last syringe, and attach the ABG syringe to the blood sampling port. C. Turn the stopcock off to the flush solution. D. Gently aspirate the ABG sample. E. Turn the stopcock off to the patient before removing the ABG syringe. F. Expel any air bubbles from the ABG syringe and cap the syringe.	Obtains the appropriate blood specimens. The VACUTAINER® is a nonvented system, so there will be no backflow of blood from the patient. Prevents backflow of blood through the open blood sampling port. Opens the arterial line from the patient to the syringe. Prepares for connection of the ABG syringe. Opens the arterial line to the ABG syringe. Obtains the ABG sample while minimizing vessel trauma. Prevents the backflow of arterial blood. Ensures accuracy of the ABG results.	If drawing laboratory specimens in addition to coagulation studies and ABG, draw the routine laboratory studies first; then draw the ABG and coagulation studies. The ABG syringe can also be inserted into the VACUTAINER® system.
14. After the last specimen is obtained, turn the stopcock off to the patient.	Detaches the specimen and ensures no backflow of arterial blood from the patient.	
15. Fast-flush the remaining blood from the blood sampling port of the stopcock onto a sterile gauze pad or into a discard blood specimen tube or syringe and remove the VACUTAINER® or syringe.	Prevents clotting of blood in the blood sampling port so that blood can be drawn at a later time. Also removes blood residue from the stopcock, where it could be a reservoir for bacterial growth.	Follow institution standard.
16. Place a new, sterile nonvented cap on the blood sampling port.	Maintains sterility of the system.	
17. Turn the stopcock open to the patient and the flush solution (off to the blood sampling port) and use the fast-flush device to clear the line of blood.	Prevents the arterial line from clotting.	Blood-conserving closed monitoring systems include an option to reinfuse the blood to the patient after the laboratory sample is obtained (see Fig. 60-4).
18. Turn the alarms back on and ensure that the waveform returns.	Provides accurate waveform and safe blood pressure monitoring.	
19. Discard used supplies and wash hands.	Reduces the transmission of microorganisms; standard precautions.	

Procedure continues on the following page

Procedure **for Blood Sampling From an Arterial Catheter**—*Continued*

Steps	Rationale	Special Considerations
20. Label the specimens and complete the laboratory form per institutional protocol.	Properly identifies the patient and laboratory tests to be performed.	For ABGs, note the time the specimen was drawn and the percentage of oxygen therapy, as well as any other data required by institutional protocol. Expedite the delivery of samples to the laboratory. Follow institutional standard regarding the use of ice for ABG samples.

Expected Outcomes

- Adequate blood sample with minimal blood loss
- No hemolysis of specimens
- No arterial spasm
- Arterial line patency maintained

Unexpected Outcomes

- Inadequate blood sample
- Hemolysis of specimens
- Arterial spasm
- Dilution of specimens, causing inaccurate laboratory results

Patient Monitoring and Care

Steps	Rationale	Reportable Conditions
		These conditions should be reported if they persist despite nursing interventions.
1. Use the minimal volume of blood discard.	Helps prevent nosocomial anemia.	
2. Monitor hemoglobin or hematocrit daily or if a significant amount of blood loss occurs.	Allows early detection of nosocomial anemia.	• Decrease in hemoglobin or hematocrit levels
3. Attempt to group blood draws together whenever possible.	Diminishes the number of times the system is entered to help minimize the risk for infection.	
4. Before and after the blood withdrawal, assess and evaluate the arterial waveform.	Ensures accurate arterial pressure monitoring.	
5. Obtain laboratory specimen results.	Monitors test results.	• Abnormal specimen results

Documentation

Documentation should include the following:

- Patient and family education
- Date, time, and type of specimen drawn
- Results of laboratory tests, when available
- Unexpected outcomes
- Additional nursing interventions

References

1. Darovic, G.O. (2002). Arterial pressure monitoring. In: *Hemodynamic Monitoring: Invasive and Noninvasive Clinical Application.* 3rd ed. Philadelphia: W.B. Saunders.
2. Gregersen, R.A., et al. (1987). Accurate coagulation studies from heparinized radial artery catheters. *Heart Lung,* 16(6), 686-92.
3. Heap, M.J., et al. (1997). Are coagulation studies on blood sampled from arterial lines valid? *Anaesthesia,* 52, 640-5.
4. Kaplow, R. (1988). Comparison of two techniques for obtaining samples for coagulation studies: Venipuncture and intraarterial. *Heart Lung,* 17, 651-3.
5. Molyneaux, R.D., Papciak, B., and Rorem, D.A. (1987). Coagulation studies and the indwelling heparinized catheter. *Heart Lung,* 16, 20-23.
6. O'Grady, N.P., et al. (2002). Guidelines for the prevention of intravascular catheter-related infections. Centers for Disease Control and Prevention. *Morbidity and Mortality Weekly Report. Recommendations and Reports.* 51(RR-10), 1-29.
7. Preusser, B.A., et al. (1989). Quantifying the minimum discard sample required for accurate arterial blood gases. *Nurs Res,* 38, 276-9.

8. Rickard, C.M., et al. (2003). A discard volume of twice the deadspace ensures clinically accurate arterial blood gases and electrolytes and prevents unnecessary blood loss. *Crit Care Med,* 31, 1654-58.

Additional Readings

Cannon, K., Mitchell, K.A., and Fabian, T.C. (1985). Prospective randomized evaluation of two methods of drawing coagulation studies from heparinized arterial lines. *Heart Lung,* 14, 392-5.

Dirks, J.L. (1995). Innovations in technology: Continuous intra-arterial blood gas monitoring. *Crit Care Nurs,* 15, 19-29.

Harper, J. (1988). Use of intraarterial lines to obtain coagulation samples. *Focus Crit Care,* 15, 51-5.

Hoste, E.A.J., et al. (2002). Significant increase of activated partial thromboplastin time by heparinization of the radial artery catheter flush solution with a closed arterial system. *Crit Care Med,* 30, 1030-4.

Imperial-Perez, F., and McRae M. (1998). *Protocols for Practice: Hemodynamic Monitoring Series—Arterial Pressure Monitoring.* Aliso Viejo, CA: American Association of Critical-Care Nurses.

Kajs, M. (1986). Comparison of coagulation values obtained by traditional venipuncture and intra-arterial line methods. *Heart Lung,* 15, 622-7.

Laxson, C.J., and Titler, M.G. (1994). Drawing coagulation studies from arterial lines: An integrative literature review. *Am J Crit Care,* 3, 16-24.

Martinez, J.A., et al. (2002). Clinical utility of blood cultures drawn from central venous or arterial catheters in critically ill surgical patients. *Crit Care Med,* 30, 7-13.

Reinhardt, A.C., et al. (1987). Minimum discard volume from arterial catheters to obtain coagulation studies free from heparin effect. *Heart Lung,* 16, 699-705.

Richiuso, N. (1998). Accuracy of aPTT values drawn from heparinized arterial lines in children. *DCCN,* 17, 14-9.

Rudisill, P.T., and Moore, L.A. (1989). Relationship between arterial and venous activated partial thromboplastin time values in patients after percutaneous transluminal coronary angioplasty. *Heart Lung,* 18, 514-9.

Templin, K., Shively, M., and Riley, J. (1993). Accuracy of drawing coagulation samples from heparinized arterial lines. *Am J Crit Care,* 2, 88-95.

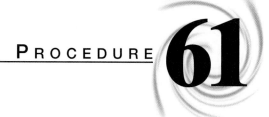

PROCEDURE **61**

Blood Sampling From Central Venous Catheters

P U R P O S E : To obtain blood from the central venous catheter (CVC) for laboratory analysis.

Nancy Munro

PREREQUISITE NURSING KNOWLEDGE

- Knowledge of anatomy and physiology of the cardiovascular system
- Understanding of principles of sterile and aseptic technique and infection control
- Understanding of the technique for specimen collection and labeling
- Signs and symptoms of catheter-related infection and sepsis
- Infection has been identified as a potentially life-threatening complication of central venous catheterization with an associated estimated mortality of 12% for each infection.[4] Appropriate care of the catheter and system is considered to have primary importance in decreasing the risk for catheter-related sepsis.
- Knowledge regarding the care of patients with central venous catheters (see Procedures 66 and 81)
- Understanding of the principles of hemodynamic monitoring
- The effect of heparin and hemolysis on various blood tests and appropriate discard volumes

EQUIPMENT

- Nonsterile gloves
- Goggles or fluid shield face mask
- Syringes, 5 ml and 10 ml
- Sterile 4 × 4 gauze pads
- Blood specimen tubes
- Sterile nonvented caps
- Appropriate laboratory tubes, slips, and labels

Additional equipment to have available as needed includes the following:

- Antiseptic solution
- VACUTAINER®
- Needleless VACUTAINER® Luer-Lok adapter
- Extra blood specimen tube for discard

PATIENT AND FAMILY EDUCATION

- Explain the purpose for blood sampling to the patient and family. ➠*Rationale:* Teaching provides information and decreases anxiety and fear.
- Explain the patient's expected participation during the procedure. ➠*Rationale:* Increases patient cooperation and assistance.
- Explain that the pressure waveform and digital display on the monitor will be absent during the blood sampling procedure. ➠*Rationale:* Alleviates fear and increases knowledge.

PATIENT ASSESSMENT AND PREPARATION

Patient Assessment

- Assess the patency of the central venous catheter. ➠*Rationale:* If the central venous catheter is clotted, blood sampling will not be able to be performed.
- Assess previous laboratory results. ➠*Rationale:* Provides data for comparison.
- Assess the type of fluid infusing through the catheter. ➠*Rationale:* Some fluids/medications may effect the laboratory test result.

Patient Preparation

- Ensure that the patient and family understand preprocedural teaching. Answer questions as they arise and reinforce information as needed. ➤➤*Rationale:* Evaluates and reinforces understanding of previously taught information.

- Position the patient so that the stopcock for blood sampling is exposed. ➤➤*Rationale:* Improves the ease of obtaining the blood sample and minimizes the contamination of the stopcock.

Procedure for Blood Sampling From Central Venous Catheters

Steps	Rationale	Special Considerations
1. Wash hands and don nonsterile gloves and goggles or fluid shield face mask.	Reduces the transmission of microorganisms and body fluids; standard precautions.	
2. If using a VACUTAINER®, attach "needleless" VACUTAINER® Luer-Lok adapter needle to the VACUTAINER® (see Fig. 60-1).	Prepares for blood sampling.	If possible, use a needleless system for obtaining blood samples to prevent needlestick injury.
3. Suspend the CVP monitoring alarms if monitoring is being used and suspend/turn off fluid infusing through the largest lumen.[2]	Prevents the alarm from sounding, because the CVP waveform is lost during the blood draw.	
4. Remove the nonvented cap from the stopcock of the largest lumen of the CVP catheter.	Prepares the line for blood sampling.	If using a system in which blood samples are obtained through a rubber diaphragm, swab the area with an alcohol wipe before entering the system.
5. Place a sterile syringe or VACUTAINER® with needleless Luer-Lok adapter needle into the top port of the stopcock (see Figs. 62-1 and 62-2).	Prepares for blood sampling.	
6. Turn the stopcock off to the monitoring system or flush solution (see Figs. 62-3 and 62-4).	The syringe or VACUTAINER® will now be in contact with central venous blood.	
7. Gently aspirate the discard volume into the syringe or engage a blood specimen tube into the VACUTAINER® to obtain the discard volume.	Clears the catheter of flush solution. The discard volume includes the dead space (from the tip of the lumen to the top port of the stopcock) and the blood diluted by the flush solution.[1,3,5]	Dead space information for a catheter is usually listed in the information that comes with the catheter. If using a blood specimen tube for discard, use one large enough for the appropriate dead space volume. If possible, use a blood-conserving closed system to avoid nosocomial anemia.
8. Turn the stopcock off to the syringe or VACUTAINER® (see Figs. 62-1 and 62-2).	Stops blood flow and closes all ports of the stopcock.	
9. Remove the discard syringe or tube and discard in appropriate receptacle.	Removes discard safely.	

Procedure continues on the following page

Procedure for Blood Sampling From Central Venous Catheters—*Continued*

Steps	Rationale	Special Considerations
10. Insert a new syringe into the stopcock or place a new blood specimen tube into the VACUTAINER® system.	Prepares for removal of the blood sample.	
11. Turn the stopcock off to the hemodynamic flush system/infusing fluid (see Figs. 62-3 and 62-4).	Prepares for blood sampling.	
12. Slowly and gently aspirate blood or engage the blood specimen tube into the VACUTAINER® system.	Obtains the blood specimen.	
13. Turn the stopcock off to the patient (see Figs. 62-5 and 62-6).	Prevents bleeding.	
14. Fast-flush the remaining blood from the stopcock onto a gauze pad or into a discard syringe or blood specimen tube.	Clears blood from the system.	Some monitoring systems may include an option to reinfuse the blood to the patient after the laboratory sample is obtained.
15. Turn the stopcock off to the top port of the stopcock.	This reopens the system for continuous pressure monitoring.	
16. If the system was open, attach a new, sterile nonvented cap to the top port of the stopcock.	Maintains a closed, sterile system.	
17. Flush the remaining blood in the catheter back to the patient.	Promotes patency of the catheter.	
18. Observe the monitor for the return of the CVP waveform if pressure monitoring is being used.	Ensures continuous monitoring of the CVP waveform.	
19. Turn the alarms back on.	Activates the alarm system.	
20. Label the specimen and laboratory form according to institutional procedure.	Properly identifies the patient and the laboratory tests to be performed.	
21. Send the specimen for analysis.		Be aware of the need for timely delivery of coagulation studies that may have distorted results if not delivered promptly.
22. Discard used supplies in the appropriate receptacles and wash hands.	Reduces the transmission of microorganisms; standard precautions.	

Expected Outcomes

- Catheter remains patent with good waveform if monitoring system is used
- Catheter site remains free from infection
- Adequate blood sample with minimal blood loss
- No hemolysis of the specimen

Unexpected Outcomes

- Catheter becomes clotted
- Catheter-related infection
- Inability to obtain blood sample
- Hemolysis of specimens
- Dilution of specimens causing inaccurate laboratory results

Patient Monitoring and Care

Steps	Rationale	Reportable Conditions
		These conditions should be reported if they persist despite nursing interventions.
1. Use minimal volume of blood discard.	Helps prevent nosocomial anemia.	
2. Monitor hemoglobin and hematocrit if a significant amount of blood loss occurs.	Allows early detection of nosocomial anemia.	• Changes in hemoglobin/hematocrit
3. Attempt to group blood draws together when possible.	Diminishes the number of times the system is entered to help minimize the risk of infection.	
4. Before and after the blood withdrawal, assess and evaluate the CVP waveform if used.	Ensures accurate central venous pressure monitoring.	
5. Obtain laboratory specimen results.	Monitor test results.	• Abnormal specimen results

Documentation

Documentation should include the following:

- Patient and family education
- Time and type of specimen drawn
- Results of laboratory tests when available
- Unexpected outcomes
- Additional interventions

References

1. Carlson, K.K., et al. (1990). Obtaining reliable plasma sodium and glucose determinations from pulmonary artery catheters. *Heart Lung,* 19, 613-9.
2. Frey A.M. (2003). Drawing blood samples from vascular access devices: Evidence-based practice. *J Infusion Nursing,* 26, 285-93.
3. Krueger, K.E., et al. (1981). The reliability of laboratory data from blood samples collected through pulmonary artery catheters. *Arch Pathol Lab Med,* 105, 343-4.
4. O'Grady N.P. et al. (2002). Guidelines for the prevention of intravascular catheter-related infections. *Am J Infect Control,* 30, 476-89.
5. Palermo, L.M., Andrews, R.W., and Ellison, N. (1980). Avoidance of heparin contamination in coagulation studies drawn from indwelling lines. *Anesth Analg,* 59, 222-24.

Additional Readings

Infusion Nursing Standards of Practice. (2002). *J Intraven Nurs,* Supplement 1-81.
Centers for Disease Control and Prevention: *www.cdc.gov.*
Infectious Diseases Society of America: *www.idsa.org.*
Intravenous Nursing Society: *www.ins.org.*
National Guidelines Clearinghouse: *www.guidelines.gov.*

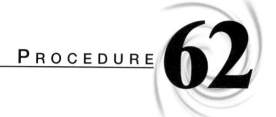

PROCEDURE **62**

Blood Sampling From a Pulmonary Artery Catheter

P U R P O S E :   Blood is removed from the pulmonary artery (PA) catheter to determine mixed venous oxygen saturation (Svo_2).

Teresa Preuss
Debra Lynn-McHale Wiegand

PREREQUISITE NURSING KNOWLEDGE

- Knowledge of sterile technique
- Knowledge of cardiovascular and pulmonary anatomy and physiology
- Understanding of gas exchange and acid-base balance
- Technique for specimen collection and labeling
- Principles of hemodynamic monitoring
- Knowledge about the care of patients with pulmonary artery lines (see Procedure 72) and stopcock manipulation (see Procedure 75)
- The most frequent blood specimen obtained from the pulmonary artery is one for mixed venous oxygen (Svo_2) analysis.
- Svo_2 measures the oxygen saturation of the venous blood in the pulmonary artery (see Procedure 14).
- Svo_2 samples are obtained to calibrate the equipment when continuously monitoring Svo_2 values.
- Routine blood sampling from the pulmonary artery catheter is not recommended because entry into the sterile system may increase the incidence of catheter-related infection.

EQUIPMENT

- Nonsterile gloves
- Goggles or fluid shield face mask
- Syringes, 5 ml and 10 ml
- Sterile 4 × 4 gauze pad
- Blood specimen tube
- Blood gas sampling syringe
- Sterile nonvented cap
- Laboratory form and specimen label
  Additional equipment to have available as needed includes the following:
- Antiseptic solution
- VACUTAINER®
- Needleless VACUTAINER® Luer-Lok adapter
- Bag of ice

PATIENT AND FAMILY EDUCATION

- Explain the purpose for blood sampling. **➤Rationale:** Teaching provides information and may reduce anxiety and fear.
- Explain the patient's expected participation during the procedure. **➤Rationale:** Encourages patient assistance.

PATIENT ASSESSMENT AND PREPARATION

Patient Assessment

- Assess the patient's cardiopulmonary and hemodynamic status, including abnormal lung sounds, respiratory distress, dysrhythmias, decreased mentation, agitation, and skin color changes. **➤Rationale:** These signs and symptoms could necessitate blood sampling for venous oxygenation.
- Assess for a decrease in cardiac output related to changes in preload, afterload, or contractility. **➤Rationale:** Mixed venous blood samples are used to evaluate changes in cardiopulmonary function.

Patient Preparation

- Ensure that the patient understands preprocedural teaching. Answer questions as they arise and reinforce information as needed. ➥*Rationale:* Evaluates and reinforces understanding of previously taught information.

- Position the patient so that the stopcock for blood sampling is exposed. ➥*Rationale:* Improves the ease of obtaining the blood sample and minimizes the contamination of the stopcock.

Procedure	for Blood Sampling From a Pulmonary Artery Catheter	
Steps	**Rationale**	**Special Considerations**
1. Wash hands and don nonsterile gloves and goggles or a fluid shield face mask.	Reduces the transmission of microorganisms and body fluids; standard precautions.	
2. When drawing a mixed venous (Svo$_2$) sample, open the ABG kit and expel the excess air and heparin from the syringe.	Prepares the ABG syringe.	Heparin is usually in powdered form.
3. If using a VACUTAINER®, attach a needleless VACUTAINER® Luer-Lok adapter to the VACUTAINER® (see Fig. 60-1).	Prepares for blood sampling.	If possible, use a needleless system for obtaining blood samples to prevent needlestick injury.
4. Temporarily suspend the pulmonary artery (PA) alarms.	Prevents the alarm from sounding because the PA waveform is lost during the blood draw.	
5. Remove the nonvented cap from the stopcock of the distal lumen of the PA catheter.	Prepares the line for blood sampling.	If using a system where blood samples are obtained through a rubber diaphragm, swab the area with an antiseptic solution before entering the system.[3]
6. Place a sterile syringe or VACUTAINER® with needleless Luer-Lok adapter needle into the top port of the stopcock (Figs. 62-1 and 62-2).	Prepares for blood sampling.	A syringe can be inserted into the Luer-Lok adapter needle for specimen removal.

Procedure continues on the following page

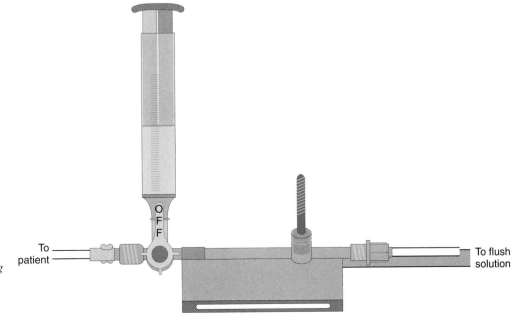

FIGURE 62-1 Sterile syringe placed into the top port of the stopcock. (*Drawing by Paul W. Schiffmacher, Thomas Jefferson University, Philadelphia, PA.*)

To patient

To flush solution

O F F

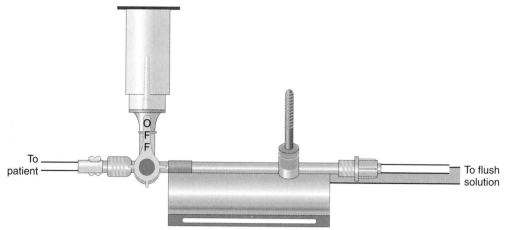

FIGURE 62-2 VACUTAINER® with Luer-Lok adapter needle placed into the top port of the stopcock. *(Drawing by Paul W. Schiffmacher, Thomas Jefferson University, Philadelphia, PA.)*

Procedure for Blood Sampling From a Pulmonary Artery Catheter—*Continued*

Steps	Rationale	Special Considerations
7. Turn the stopcock off to the flush solution (Figs. 62-3 and 62-4).	The syringe or VACUTAINER® will then be in direct contact with the PA.	
8. With a syringe, slowly and gently aspirate the discard volume. If using a VACUTAINER®, engage the blood specimen tube to obtain the discard volume.	Clears the catheter of flush solution. The discard volume includes the dead space (from the tip of the distal lumen to the top port of the stopcock) and the blood diluted by the flush solution (e.g., 2.5 ml).[1,2,4]	If possible, use a blood-conserving closed system to avoid nosocomial anemia (see Fig. 60-4). If additional lab studies are needed, larger discard volumes may be necessary for accurate results.[1,2]
9. Turn the stopcock off to the syringe (see Fig. 62-1).	Stops blood flow and closes all ports of the stopcock.	

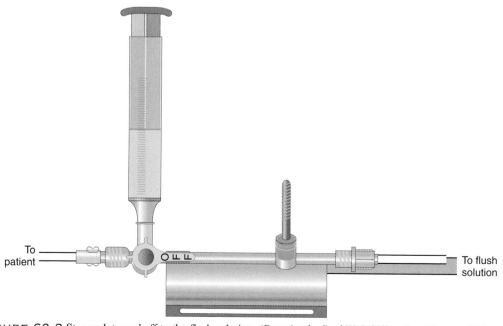

FIGURE 62-3 Stopcock turned off to the flush solution. *(Drawing by Paul W. Schiffmacher, Thomas Jefferson University, Philadelphia, PA.)*

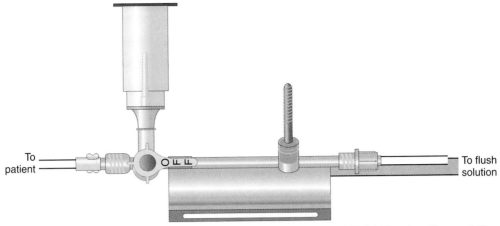

FIGURE 62-4 Stopcock turned off to the flush solution. *(Drawing by Paul W. Schiffmacher, Thomas Jefferson University, Philadelphia, PA.)*

Procedure for Blood Sampling From a Pulmonary Artery Catheter—*Continued*		
Steps	**Rationale**	**Special Considerations**
10. Remove the syringe or the blood specimen tube and discard in the appropriate receptacle.	Removes the discard.	
11. Insert an ABG syringe into the stopcock or insert the ABG syringe into the VACUTAINER® system.	Prepares for removal of a blood sample.	
12. Turn the stopcock off to the flush system (see Figs. 62-3 and 62-4).	Prepares for blood sampling.	
13. Slowly aspirate the SvO₂ sample.	Slow aspiration is important to prevent contamination of the mixed venous sample with arterial blood from the pulmonary capillaries, which will falsely elevate the SvO₂ value.	
14. Turn the stopcock off to the syringe or VACUTAINER® (see Figs. 62-1 and 62-2).	Prevents bleeding.	
15. Remove the ABG syringe.	Detaches the specimen.	
16. Expel any air bubbles from the ABG syringe and cap the syringe.	Ensures the accuracy of the SvO₂ results.	
17. Turn the stopcock off to the patient (Figs. 62-5 and 62-6).		
18. Fast-flush the remaining blood from the top port of the stopcock onto a sterile gauze pad or into a discard syringe or blood specimen tube.	Clears blood from the system.	Some monitoring systems may include an option to reinfuse the blood to the patient after the ABG sample is obtained.
19. Turn the stopcock off to the top port of the stopcock (see Figs. 62-1 and 62-2).	This opens the system up for continuous PA pressure monitoring.	Remove the VACUTAINER® if used.
20. Attach a new, sterile nonvented cap to the top port of the stopcock.	Maintains a closed, sterile system.	

Procedure continues on the following page

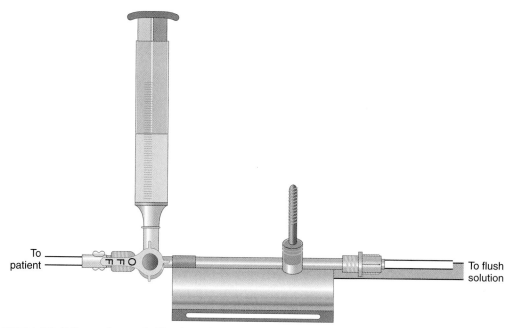

FIGURE 62-5 Stopcock turned off to the patient. *(Drawing by Paul W. Schiffmacher, Thomas Jefferson University, Philadelphia, PA.)*

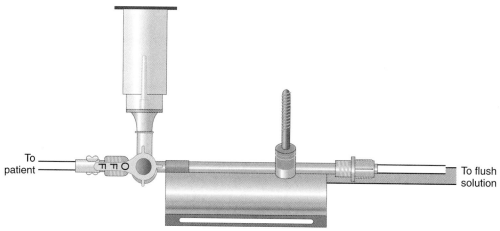

FIGURE 62-6 Stopcock turned off to the patient. *(Drawing by Paul W. Schiffmacher, Thomas Jefferson University, Philadelphia, PA.)*

Procedure **for Blood Sampling From a Pulmonary Artery Catheter**—*Continued*

Steps	Rationale	Special Considerations
21. Flush the remaining blood in the PA catheter back into the patient.	Promotes patency of the PA catheter.	
22. Turn the alarms back on.	Activates the alarm system.	
23. Observe the monitor for return of the PA waveform.	Ensures continuous monitoring of the PA waveform.	
24. Label the specimen and laboratory form.	Properly identifies the patient and laboratory tests to be performed.	

Procedure for Blood Sampling From a Pulmonary Artery Catheter—*Continued*

Steps	Rationale	Special Considerations
25. Send the specimen for analysis.		Label the blood-gas laboratory slip as a mixed venous sample. Follow the hospital policy about using ice for ABG samples.
26. Discard used supplies and wash hands.	Reduces the transmission of microorganisms; standard precautions.	

Expected Outcomes

- Adequate blood sample with minimal blood loss
- PA catheter patency maintained
- Svo_2 value and trends within normal range (60% to 80%)

Unexpected Outcomes

- Inability to obtain Svo_2 sample
- Arterial sample obtained instead of mixed venous oxygen sample for blood-gas analysis

Patient Monitoring and Care

Steps	Rationale	Reportable Conditions
		These conditions should be reported if they persist despite nursing interventions.
1. Before and after the blood withdrawal, assess and evaluate the PA waveform.	Ensures that the PA catheter is properly positioned.	
2. Correlate the Svo_2 results with the measured cardiac output.	Svo_2 is usually decreased when the cardiac output is decreased.	• Abnormal mixed venous oxygen saturation, cardiac output, cardiac index, and afterload
3. Correlate the Svo_2 results with the clinical assessment data.	Svo_2 will decrease with increased O_2 consumption.	• Fever • Shivering • Seizures

Documentation

Documentation should include the following:

- Patient and family education
- Time and date of the Svo_2 sample
- Svo_2 results
- Any difficulties with PA catheter blood sampling
- Nursing interventions performed
- Unexpected outcomes

References

1. Carlson, K.K., et al. (1990). Obtaining reliable plasma sodium and glucose determinations from pulmonary artery catheters. *Heart Lung*, 19, 613-9.
2. Krueger, K.E., et al. (1981). The reliability of laboratory data from blood samples collected through pulmonary artery catheters. *Arch Pathol Lab Med*, 105, 343-4.
3. O'Grady, N.P., et al. (2002). Guidelines for the prevention of intravascular catheter-related infections. *Am J Infect Control*, 30(8), 476-489.
4. Palermo, L.M., Andrews, R.W., and Ellison, N. (1980). Avoidance of heparin contamination in coagulation studies drawn from indwelling lines. *Anesth Analg*, 59, 222-4.

Additional Readings

Ahrens, T.S., and Taylor, L.A. (1992). *Hemodynamic Waveform Analysis.* Philadelphia: W.B. Saunders.
Darovic, G.O. (2002). *Hemodynamic Monitoring: Invasive and Noninvasive Clinical Application.* 3rd ed. Philadelphia: W.B. Saunders.
Schactman, M., et al. (1995). *Hemodynamic Monitoring.* El Paso, TX: Skidmore-Roth Publishing.

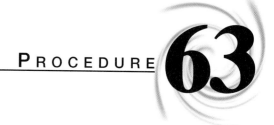
PROCEDURE **63**

Cardiac Output Measurement Techniques (Invasive)

P U R P O S E : Cardiac output (CO) measurements are performed to assess and monitor cardiovascular status. CO measurements are used to evaluate patient responses to clinical interventions, mechanical assist devices, and vasoactive and inotropic medications. When a pulmonary artery catheter is in place, CO measurements provide useful initial and trend data that may augment care for critically ill patients with hemodynamic instability.

Nancy M. Albert

PREREQUISITE NURSING KNOWLEDGE

- Understanding of the normal anatomy and physiology of the cardiovascular system and pulmonary system.
- Understanding of basic dysrhythmia recognition and treatment of life-threatening dysrhythmias.
- Understanding of pathophysiologic changes associated with structural heart disease (e.g., ventricular dysfunction from myocardial infarction, diastolic or systolic changes and valve dysfunction).
- Understanding of the principles of aseptic technique.
- Understanding of the pulmonary artery (PA) catheter (see Fig. 72-1) lumens and ports and the location of the PA catheter in the heart and PA (see Fig. 72-2).
- Understanding multiple pressure transducer systems (see Procedure 75).
- Competence in the use and clinical application of hemodynamic waveforms and values obtained with a PA catheter. Hemodynamic waveform interpretation of right atrial pressure (RAP) or central venous pressure (CVP), PA pressure (PAP), and PA wedge or occlusion pressure (PAWP) provide confirmation of proper catheter placement.
- Knowledge of vasoactive and inotropic medication therapies and their clinical effects on cardiac function, cardiac tissue, ventricular function, coronary vessels, and vascular smooth muscles.

- *Cardiac output* is defined as the amount of blood ejected by the left ventricle per minute and is the product of stroke volume (SV) and heart rate (HR). It is measured in liters per minute.

$$CO = SV \times HR$$

- The normal CO is *4 to 8* L/min. The four physiologic factors that affect CO are preload, afterload, contractility, and heart rate.
- *Stroke volume* is the amount of blood volume ejected from either ventricle during one beat. Left ventricular stroke volume is the difference between left ventricular end-diastolic volume and left ventricular end-systolic volume. Left ventricular stroke volume is normally between 60 and 100 ml/beat. Major factors that influence stroke volume are preload, afterload, and contractility.
- *Right heart preload* refers to the amount of blood in the RV at the end of diastole, measured by the RAP (central venous pressure). Elevations in left heart filling pressures may be accompanied by parallel changes in RAP, especially in patients with systolic left ventricular dysfunction. Other factors that affect RAP are venous return, intravascular volume, vascular capacitance, and pulmonary pressure. Right heart preload is raised in right heart failure, right ventricular infarction, pericardial tamponade, tension pneumothorax, tricuspid regurgitation, and fluid overload and is lowered in hypovolemic states.[29]

- *Left heart preload* refers to the amount of blood in the LV at the end of diastole; it is measured by the PAWP. When LV preload or end-diastolic volume increases, the muscle fibers are stretched. The increased tension or force of cardiac contractions that accompanies an increase in diastolic filling is called the *Frank-Starling law*. The Frank-Starling law allows the heart to adjust its pumping ability to accommodate various levels of venous return.[28] *Note:* In patients with advanced chronic LV dysfunction and remodeled hearts (spherical or globular-shaped LV instead of the normal, elliptical-shaped LV), the Frank-Starling law does not apply; instead, increased tension or force of contraction is associated with a decrease in diastolic filling.

- *Afterload* refers to the force the ventricular myocardium must overcome in order to shorten (contract). It is the force that resists contraction. The amount of force the LV must overcome influences the amount of blood ejected into the systemic circulation. Afterload is assessed through study of peripheral vascular resistance (the force opposing blood flow within the vessels), systolic blood pressure, systolic stress, and systolic impedance. Peripheral resistance is affected by several factors, including length and radius of the blood vessel, arterial blood pressure, and venous constriction or dilation.[1] Change in peripheral resistance has a direct effect on afterload. The myocardium exerts effort (thus, increase in afterload) to maintain SV in conditions such as aortic stenosis, hypertension, other vasoconstrictive states, or hyperviscosity of blood (e.g., polycythemia). The systolic force of the heart is decreased in conditions that cause vasodilation or decrease viscosity of blood (e.g., anemia). Right ventricular afterload is measured as pulmonary vascular resistance.

Left ventricular afterload is measured as systemic vascular resistance.

- *Contractility* is defined as the ability of the myocardium to develop force or the strength of the myocardium independent of loading factors (preload, afterload, and myocardial mass). Contractility is influenced by the sympathetic nervous system. It is increased by the release of calcium and norepinephrine and decreased by parasympathetic neural stimulation, acidosis, and hyperkalemia. Contractility and HR are inherent to the cardiac tissues but can be influenced by neural, humoral, and pharmacologic factors.

- In addition to stroke volume, CO is affected by *heart rate*. Normally, nerves of the parasympathetic and sympathetic nervous system regulate heart rate through specialized cardiac electrical cells. Ultimately, cardiac rate and rhythm is influenced by many factors, including neural, humoral, and pharmacologic factors. A decrease in HR can be the result of increased parasympathetic neural stimulation, decreased sympathetic neural stimulation, or decreased body temperature. An increase in HR can be triggered by exercise, catecholamine release, or hypotension. At HRs greater than 180 beats per minute, there may be inadequate time for diastolic filling, resulting in decreased CO. Because of the interaction of factors that regulate cardiac performance and impact CO, it is essential that factors specific to individual patients be assessed (Fig. 63-1).

- *Cardiac index* is CO per square meter. It is a more precise measurement of cardiac performance than CO since it is calculated by incorporating CO and the patient's body surface area.

- Refer to Table 63-1 for normal hemodynamic values and calculations.

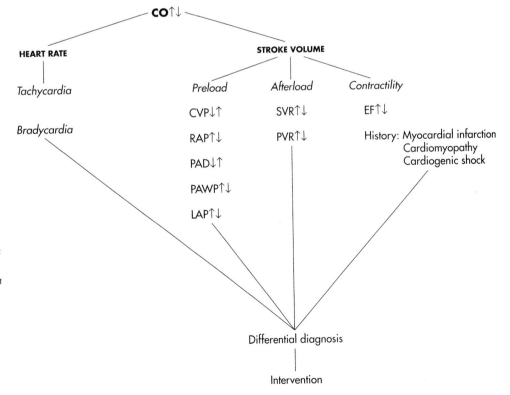

FIGURE 63-1 Systematic assessment of the determinants of cardiac output may assist the clinician in defining the etiologic factors of cardiac output alteration more precisely. *(From Whalen, D.A., and Keller, R. [1998]. Cardiovascular patient assessment. In: Kinney, M.R., et al., eds.* AACN Clinical Reference for Critical Care Nurse. *4th ed. St. Louis: Mosby-Year Book, 227-319.)*

- At the bedside, cardiac measurements are obtained through a PA catheter via the intermittent bolus thermodilution CO method (TDCO) or the continuous CO (CCO) method.
- The TDCO method proceeds as follows:
  - ❖ An injectate (5% dextrose in water) of a known volume (10 ml) and temperature (room or cold temperature) is injected into the right atrium (RA) through the proximal port of the PA catheter. This injectate exits in the RA, where it mixes with blood and flows through the right ventricle to the PA. The computer integrates the temperature change in the PA until the difference between the actual blood temperature and the baseline blood temperature has decreased to a specific percentage (e.g., 30%) of the maximum difference during the injection of the thermal indicator (heat of the injectate).
  - ❖ CO can be calculated from PA catheters with two types of thermistors:
    - ○ A *single thermistor* has one inline temperature sensor near the tip of the catheter (commonly used) that lies in the PA when in proper position.
    - ○ A *dual thermistor* has two inline temperature sensors, one in the right atrium/superior caval vein (immediately above the injectate port opening) and one near the tip of the catheter (same position as

single thermistor). Since there is a temperature sensor in the right atrium, there is no need to enter a "correction factor" or "computation constant" into the computer to account for the loss in thermal indicator from the hub of the RA injectate port to the RA. Investigators found that the second thermistor improved accuracy when compared with Fick CO measurements and also improved precision or repeatability of CO measurements, both cold and room temperature.[4,19] In one study, cold injectate had excellent precision with the standard, single-thermistor PA catheter. Researchers concluded that the dual-thermistor PA catheter provided the greatest benefit in decreasing measurement variability when room temperature injections were used to measure CO.[4]
  - ❖ The change in temperature over time is plotted as a curve and displayed on the computer screen. CO is mathematically calculated from the area under the curve and is displayed digitally and graphically on the oscilloscope (Fig. 63-2). The area under the curve is inversely proportional to the rate of blood flow. Thus a high CO is associated with a small area under the curve, whereas a low CO is associated with a large area under the curve (Fig. 63-3).

TABLE 63-1	Hemodynamic Parameters	
Parameters	**Calculations**	**Normal Value**
Body surface area (BSA)	Weight (kg) × height (cm) × 0.007184	Varies with size Range = 0.58-2.9 m²
CO		4-8 L/min
Stroke volume (SV)	CO = HR × SV	60-100 ml/per beat
Stroke volume index (SVI)	CO × 1000 ÷ HR	35-75 ml/m² per beat
Cardiac index (CI)	SV ÷ BSA	2.8-4.2 L/min/m²
Heart rate (HR)	CO ÷ BSA	60-100 beats/min
Preload		
Central venous pressure (CVP) or RAP		2-6 mm Hg
Left atrial pressure (LAP)		4-12 mm Hg
Pulmonary artery diastolic pressure (PAD)		5-15 mm Hg
PAWP		4-12 mm Hg
RVEDP		0-8 mm Hg
LVEDP		4-10 mm Hg
Afterload		
Systemic vascular resistance (SVR)	MAP − CVP/RAP × 80 ÷ CO	900-1600 dynes sec cm⁻⁵
SVR index (SVRI)	MAP − CVP/RAP × 80 ÷ CI	1970-2390 dynes sec/cm⁻⁵/m²
Pulmonary vascular resistance (PVR)	PAM − PAWP × 80 ÷ CO	155-255 dynes sec/cm⁻⁵
PVR index (PVRI)	PAM − PAWP × 80 ÷ CI	255-285 dynes sec/cm⁻⁵
Systolic blood pressure		100-140 mm Hg
Contractility		
Ejection fraction (EF)—Left	LVEDV × 100 ÷ SV	60%-75%
—Right	RVEDV × 100 ÷ SV	45%-50%
Stroke work index—Left	SVI (MAP − PAWP) × 0.0136	45-65 gm-m/m²/beat
—Right	SVI (MAP − CVP) × 0.0136	5-10 gm-m/m²/beat
Pressures		
MAP	DBP + ⅓ (SBP − DBP)	70-105 mm Hg
Mean PAP	PAD + ⅓ (PASP − PAD)	9-16 mm Hg

Adapted from Whalen, D.A., and Keller, R. (1998). Cardiovascular patient assessment. In: Kinney, M.R., et al., eds. *AACN Clinical Reference for Critical Care Nursing.* 4th ed. St. Louis: Mosby-Yearbook, 299; and Ahrens, T. (1999). Hemodynamic monitoring. *Crit Care Nurs Clin N Am,* 11(1), 19-31.
MAP, mean arterial pressure; *LVEDP,* left ventricular end-diastolic pressure; *RVEDP,* right ventricular end-diastolic pressure; *PAM,* pulmonary artery mean; *PAWP,* pulmonary artery wedge pressure; *LVEDV,* left ventricular end-diastolic volume; *RVEDV,* right ventricular end-diastolic volume; *PASP,* pulmonary artery systolic pressure.

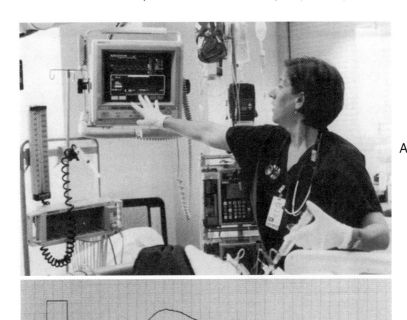

FIGURE 63-2 **A,** Examining cardiac output curves to establish reliability of values. **B,** Normal cardiac output curve with rapid upstroke and smooth progressive decrease in temperature sensing. *(From Ahrens, T. [1999]. Hemodynamic monitoring.* Crit Care Nurs Clin N Am, *11[1], 28.)*

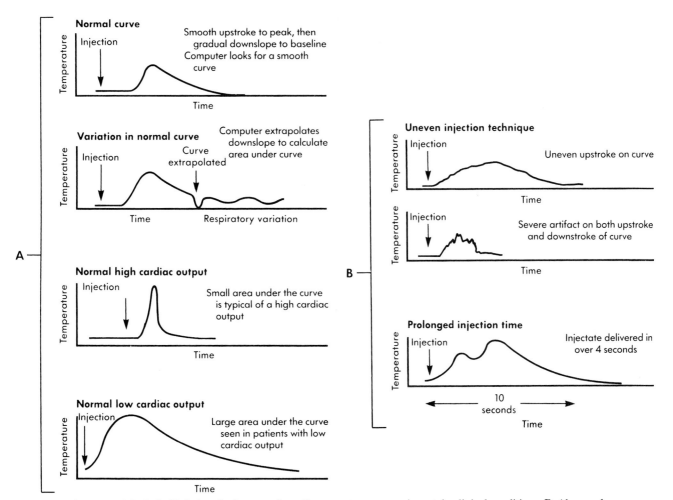

FIGURE 63-3 **A,** Variations in the normal cardiac output curve seen in certain clinical conditions. **B,** Abnormal cardiac output curves that will produce an erroneous cardiac output value. *(From Urden, L.D., Stacy, K.M., and Lough, M.E. [2002].* Thelan's Critical Care Nursing: Diagnosis and Management. *4th ed. St. Louis: Mosby.)*

❖ The thermistor near the distal tip of the catheter detects the temperature change (as stated above) and sends a signal to the CO computer. The computer calculates the CO using the modified Stewart Hamilton equation. A CO number is displayed on the screen. The average result of three to five measurements is used to determine CO.

❖ There are limitations to the use of the TDCO method. For accuracy to be maintained, specific assumptions must be met. These assumptions include adequate mixing of blood and injectate, forward blood flow, steady baseline temperature in the PA, and appropriate procedural technique.[3,13] In addition, loss of thermal indicator, respiratory artifact, and hemodynamic instability can cause variability from one injection to another.[13,22]

❖ Commercially available closed system delivery sets (CO-Set®) can be used with both cold and room temperature injectate (Figs. 63-4 and 63-5).

• The CCO method proceeds as follows:

❖ CO can be obtained using a heat-exchange CO catheter. This catheter has a membrane that allows for heat to exchange with blood in the right atria. Continuous measurement of CO can be performed without the need for injected fluid.

❖ The PA catheter with CCO capability contains a 10-cm thermal filament located close to the injection port (15 to 25 cm from the tip of the catheter; near the proximal lumen port). When a PA catheter is properly placed, the thermal filament section of the catheter is located in the right ventricle. This filament emits a pulsed low heat energy signal in a 30- to 60-second pseudorandom binary (on/off) sequence,[12] allowing blood to be heated and the heat signal to be adequately

processed over time as blood passes through the ventricle. A bedside computer constructs thermodilution curves detected from the pseudorandom heat impulses and measures CO automatically. The computer screen displays digital readings updated every 30 to 60 seconds, reflecting the average CO of the preceding 3 to 6 minutes. The CCO eliminates the need for fluid boluses, reduces contamination risk, and provides a continuous CO trend.[1,12,22]

❖ Because the CCO monitor constantly displays and frequently updates the CO, treatment decisions may be expedited. Derived hemodynamic calculations (e.g., cardiac index and systemic vascular resistance) can be obtained with greater frequency, thereby providing up-to-time information when assessing response to therapies that affect hemodynamics.[1]

❖ CCO has been compared to TDCO, transesophageal Doppler technique, and aortic transpulmonary technique to determine its precision. Study results all demonstrate small bias, limits of agreement, and 95% confidence limits, reflecting that CCO provides accurate measurement of CO and is a reliable method.[1,2,5,16,22,25,27]

❖ Adequate mixing of blood and indicator (heat) is required for accurate CCO measurements. Conditions that prevent appropriate mixing or directional flow of the indicator or blood include intracardiac shunts or tricuspid regurgitation.

❖ The CCO method is based on the same physiologic principle as the TDCO method: the indicator-dilution technique. The TDCO method uses a bolus of injectate as the indicator for measurement of CO. The CCO method uses heat signals produced by the thermal

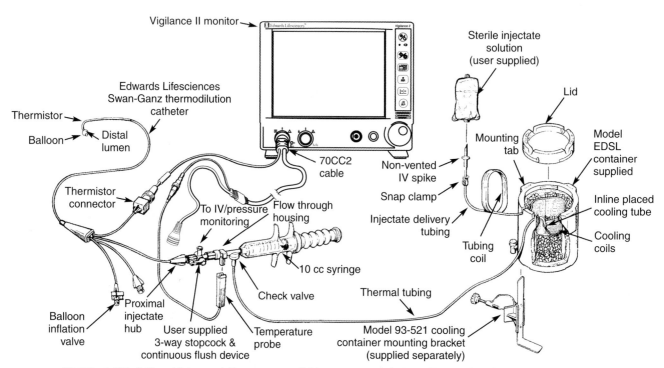

FIGURE 63-4 Closed injectate delivery system. Cold temperature injectate. *(From Edwards Lifesciences, LLC, Irvine, CA.)*

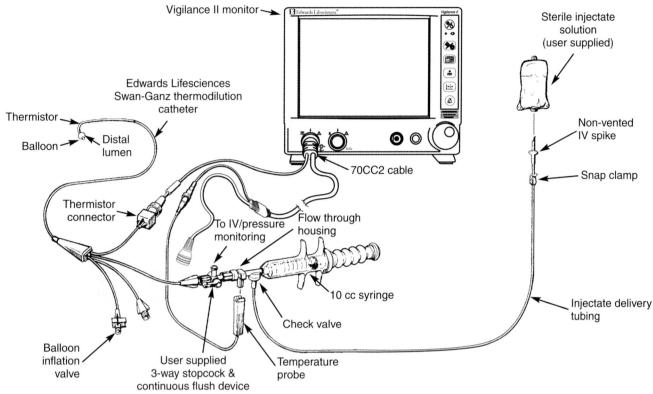

FIGURE 63-5 Closed injectate delivery system. Room temperature injectate. *(From Edwards Lifesciences, LLC, Irvine, CA.)*

filament as the indicator. The CCO computer provides a time-averaged rather than an instantaneous CO reading.[5] CCO values are influenced by the same principles as TDCO.

❖ The CCO computer and catheter may not appreciate body temperatures greater than 40°C to 43°C. The heated thermal filament has a temperature limit to a maximum of 44°C (111.2°F). When calibrated by the manufacturer, CCO computers produce reliable calculations within a temperature range of 30°-40°C (86°-104°F) or 31°-43°C (87.8°-109.4°F). An error message will appear if the temperature in the PA is out of range.

❖ Infusions through proximal lumens should be limited to maintaining patency of the lumen. Concomitant infusions through the proximal lumen can theoretically affect CCO measurements by altering the pulmonary artery temperature. Studies have shown that such infusions can cause variations in TDCO measurements. To date, no published data describing the effect of concurrent central line infusions on the accuracy of CCO measurements are available,[18] but large infusions of fluid are discouraged.[24]

❖ Because bolus injections are not required with the CCO method, the prevalence of user error is theoretically reduced.[8,11]

❖ The CCO catheter can be used to obtain both CCO and TDCO measurements.

❖ The CCO does not reflect acute changes in CO values since the updated value on the monitor display is an average of 3-6 minutes of data. Expect a delay of approximately 10 or more minutes to detect a change of 1 liter/minute in CO. When monitoring an unstable patient that is being aggressively treated with medication or other therapies, be aware of the lag in data displayed.

EQUIPMENT

- Nonsterile gloves
- Cardiac monitor
- Hemodynamic monitoring system (see Procedure 75)
- PA catheter (in place)
- CO computer or module
- Connecting cables
- Injectate temperature probe
- Injectate solution
  Additional equipment as needed includes the following:
- Bolus thermodilution:
  ❖ Four 10-ml syringes (prefilled or empty with cold or room temperature solution)*
  ❖ Injectate solution bag with intravenous (IV) tubing and three-way Luer-Lok stopcock*
  ❖ Ice (for cold injectate only)
  ❖ Nonvented caps for stopcocks
- Setup for CCO
- Printer

---

*CO-Set® may be used in lieu of these items. CO-Set® is a closed system that contains IV tubing with a snap clamp, syringe, and stopcock.

PATIENT AND FAMILY EDUCATION

- Explain the procedure for CO and the reason for its measurement. Include expectations related to sensations during the procedure (the patient should not experience pain or discomfort). ➤➤*Rationale:* Decreases patient and family anxiety. Preparatory information of sensations decreases patient fear of the impending procedure.
- Explain the monitoring equipment involved, the frequency of measurements, and the goals of therapy. ➤➤*Rationale:* Encourages the patient and family to ask questions and voice specific concerns about the procedure.
- Explain any potential variations in temperature the patient may or may not experience if a cold injectate is used. ➤➤*Rationale:* Acknowledges the varying physical responses to the injectate and the possible perception of cold solution. May decrease anxiety associated with the procedure.

PATIENT ASSESSMENT AND PREPARATION

Patient Assessment

- Assess the patient's history of medication therapy, including medication allergies, recent bolus therapies, and current pharmacologic regime. ➤➤*Rationale:* Pharmacologic therapies and changing dosages of therapies can influence the variability of CO measurements. Information may provide the rationale for CO results.

- Assess the patient's past medical history for the presence of coronary artery disease, valvular heart disease, and left or right ventricular dysfunction. ➤➤*Rationale:* Provides baseline information regarding cardiovascular performance.
- Assess current intracardiac pressures and PAP, RAP, and PAWP waveforms. ➤➤*Rationale:* Ensures the PA catheter is positioned properly with a free-floating thermistor sensor. Provides useful information about the presence and severity of mitral and tricuspid regurgitation.
- Assess the patient's vital signs, fluid balance, heart and breath sounds, skin color, temperature, mentation, peripheral pulses, cardiac rate and rhythm, and hemodynamic variables. In patients with advanced systolic heart failure, assess for pulsus alternans (alternating strong and weak pulses). ➤➤*Rationale:* Clinical information provides data regarding blood flow and tissue perfusion. Abnormalities can influence variability of CO measurements.

Patient Preparation

- Ensure that the patient and family understand preprocedural teaching. Answer questions as they arise and reinforce information as needed. ➤➤*Rationale:* Evaluates and reinforces understanding of previously taught information.
- Assist the patient to the supine position. ➤➤*Rationale:* TDCO measurements are most accurate in the supine position, but head elevation angle can be varied slightly for comfort, between 0° and 20°. Lateral recumbent positioning increases variability in CO measurements.[6,20] CCO measurements are most accurate in a supine position, but head of bed angle can be varied for comfort, between 0° and 45°.[10]

Procedure	for Measurement of Cardiac Output Using the Closed or Open Thermodilution Method	
Steps	**Rationale**	**Special Considerations**
1. Select the injectate delivery system—open or closed method. *(Level IV: Limited clinical studies to support recommendations.)*	The closed system has infection control benefits by reducing multiple entries into the system.[25]	A closed system may eliminate cost and time expenditures of individual syringe preparation.
2. Select cold or room temperature injectate. *(Level VI: Clinical studies in a variety of different patient populations and situations to support recommendations.)*	Room temperature injectate may be used for most patients. Cold injectate may improve the accuracy of CO measurement for patients with low or high CO. Research on room temperature versus cold injectate supports the accuracy of either method when 10-ml injectate volume is used.[7,9,17,30,31]	The acceptable temperature range for cold and room temperature injectate varies by system (manufacturer). Generally, room temperature is 18°-25°C and cold is 0°-12°C.
3. Select the injectate bolus amount (generally 10 ml). *(Level VI: Clinical studies in a variety of different patient populations and situations to support recommendations.)*	Common injectate volumes are 5 ml or 10 ml for critically ill adults with low to high CO.[21,30] In hypothermic patients, 10 ml of injectate is recommended	10 ml is the most commonly used volume and is recommended unless fluid restrictions are warranted. 5 ml volumes may necessitate four injections

Procedure	for Measurement of Cardiac Output Using the Closed or Open Thermodilution Method—*Continued*	
Steps	**Rationale**	**Special Considerations**
	since the blood temperature is closer to the injectate temperature (lower signal-to-noise ratio).	(rather than three) due to greater variability of individual measurements[21]; however, when fluid restriction is important, the 5-ml bolus decreases the risk for volume overload.
4. Connect the CO cable to the PA catheter.	Prepares the system.	
5. Select the computation constant consistent with the injectate volume and injectate temperature. Also, confirm the type and size of the PA catheter and confirm the injectate delivery system.	The computation constant is a correction factor determined by the computer manufacturer that corrects for the gain of the indicator (heat) that occurs as the injectate moves through the catheter from the hub of the injectate port to the injection port opening in the RA. The computer manufacturer provides a table to assist with determining the correct computation constant. The computation constant must be accurate for valid and reliable CO measurements.	Carefully select the correct computation constant for catheter size, cold or room temperature injection, and injectate volume. Confirm the setting on the CO computer. Recheck the computation constant before each series of CO measurements.
6. Connect the CO computer to the power source. Turn the CO computer or module on.	Supplies the energy source.	
7. Note the temperature of the injectate (on the computer or monitor screen).	The injectate temperature should be at least 10° less than the patient's core temperature.[8]	
8. Position the patient supine, with the head of the bed not elevated more than 20 degrees. *(Level V: Clinical studies in one or two different patient populations and situations to support recommendations.)*	Studies of patients in the supine position with the head of bed flat or elevated up to 20 degrees have not shown significant differences in TDCO measurements.[6,14] Consistency in patient position may increase stability in consecutive CO readings.	The patient's medical condition and level of instability may determine positioning. Position should be documented and communicated in shift report. Consistent positioning when obtaining CO measurements over time decreases measurement variability. Some patients may be more susceptible to hemodynamic changes with position change. Comparison with CO in the flat position may be warranted.
9. Verify the position of the PA catheter by assessing both the RA and PA waveforms for proper waveform contours.	Proper positioning of the PA catheter ensures that the distal thermistor is located in the pulmonary artery. The distal thermistor sensor calculates the time-temperature data. Excessive coiling of the PA catheter in the RA or right	Improper positioning of the PA catheter tip may result in false values.[9,16,30]

Procedure continues on the following page

Procedure	for Measurement of Cardiac Output Using the Closed or Open Thermodilution Method—*Continued*

Steps	Rationale	Special Considerations
	ventricle can result in poor positioning of the distal thermistor in relation to the injectate port.[17]	
10. Observe the patient's cardiac rate and rhythm.	A rapid heart rate and/or dysrhythmias decrease CO and lead to variability in CO measurements.	
11. If possible, consider restricting infusions delivered through the introducer or other central lines. (*Level IV: Limited clinical studies to support recommendations.*)	TDCO measurements obtained while receiving other infusions can cause variability in CO measurements (by as much as 40% higher).[9]	

Procedure	for Closed Method of Syringe Preparation and Cardiac Output Determination

Steps	Rationale	Special Considerations
Note: Follow Steps 1-11 of the Procedure for Measurement of Cardiac Output Using the Closed or Open Thermodilution Method.		
1. Wash hands and don nonsterile gloves.	Reduces the transmission of microorganisms; standard precautions.	
2. Obtain the injectate solution of 5% dextrose in water (D_5W).	The specific gravity of D_5W is a component in the formula used to derive CO by the TDCO method. The use of saline can result in a 2% decrease in TDCO measurement.[9]	Normal saline may be used if the patient's medical condition requires it.
3. Aseptically connect the IV tubing to the injectate solution.	Prepares the system.	
4. Hang the IV injectate solution on an IV pole; prime the tubing.	Eliminates air from the tubing.	
5. Connect the injectate tubing to the proximal lumen of the PA catheter via a three-way Luer-Lok stopcock (see Figs. 63-4 and 63-5).	Connects the injectate solution to the PA catheter.	
6. Connect the injectate syringe to the three-way stopcock (see Figs. 63-4 and 63-5).	The syringe will be used for solution injection.	Connect the system so that the CO syringe will be in a straight line with the PA catheter to decrease resistance when injecting solution.
7. Connect the inline temperature probe (see Figs. 63-4 and 63-5).	Measures the injectate temperature.	
8. If using cold injectate, set up the cold injectate system (e.g., CO-Set® closed injectate system) (see Fig. 63-4).	If using cold injectate, cool the injectate solution to 0°-12°C (32°-53°F).	Refer to the manufacturer recommendations. Cold injectate may be proarrhythmic in some patients.[31]

Procedure **for Closed Method of Syringe Preparation and Cardiac Output Determination**—*Continued*

Steps	Rationale	Special Considerations
9. Withdraw 10 ml of the injectate solution into the syringe. *(Level IV: Limited clinical studies to support recommendations.)*	Prepares for injection.	
10. Support the stopcock with the palm of the nondominant hand.	Minimal handling (less than 30 seconds) of the syringe is recommended to avoid thermal indicator variation that may introduce error into the CO calculation.	Syringe holders or automatic injector devices are available and can be used to aid in injectate administration.
11. Activate the CO computer, and wait for the "ready" message.	The CO computer or module needs to be ready before injecting solution.	Manufacturer recommendations may vary.
12. Prior to administering the bolus injectate, observe for a steady baseline temperature in the PA (e.g., the line before CO curve begins should be flat without undulations) on the monitor screen. *(Level IV: Limited clinical studies to support recommendations.)*	An abnormal baseline may increase variability in CO measurements and introduce error.	Patients with advanced systolic heart failure (low ejection fraction) are more prone to having a wavering initial baseline due to unstable PA blood temperature. If possible, have the patient lie still and not talk while you are preparing to administer the bolus injection.
13. Observe the patient's respiratory pattern. Prepare to begin administering the injectate at end-expiration to decrease variance in CO measurements due to the respiratory cycle.	Significant variations in transthoracic pressure during respiration can affect CO. End-expiration is defined as the phase of the respiratory cycle preceding the start of inspiration. In patients who are spontaneously breathing, it is easier to find and associated with a relatively constant intra-thoracic pressure waveform.[20,26]	
14. Administer the bolus injectate rapidly and smoothly in 4 seconds or less.	Prolonged injection time may result in false low CO. Rates of 2 to 4 seconds for injection of 5 to 10 ml of injectate yield accurate results.[9,15,17,30] One respiratory cycle generally lasts less than 1-4 seconds. One ventilation cycle on a ventilator is generally 4 seconds.	A prolonged injection time interferes with the time and temperature calculations.
15. Determine the validity of individual CO values by observing the CO on the monitor screen (see Figs. 63-2 and 63-3).	The CO curve needs to be a normal curve. A normal curve starts at baseline (baseline must be a straight, flat, nonwavering line) and has a smooth upstroke and a gradual downstroke. If the CO curve is not normal, the CO measurement obtained from the injection should be discarded. Abnormal contours of the curve may indicate improper catheter position. An abnormal CO curve may represent technical error.	The normal CO is 4 to 8 L/min. Abnormal CO curves may also provide information about the patient's abnormal clinical condition, such as tricuspid valve regurgitation.

Procedure continues on the following page

Procedure	**for Closed Method of Syringe Preparation and Cardiac Output Determination**—*Continued*		
Steps	**Rationale**	**Special Considerations**	
16. Repeat Steps 9 through 15 (generally up to three times total for cold injectate and up to five times total for room temperature injectate).	Discard all CO measurements that do not have normal CO curves or have wandering baselines.	Subsequent injections should be performed after a wait period of 1 to 2 minutes. Consistent volumes and temperatures are necessary for accuracy.	
17. Determine the CO measurement by calculating the average of three measurements within 10% of a middle (median) value. *(Level IV: Limited clinical studies to support recommendations.)*	Determines accurate CO value.[20]		
18. Return the proximal stopcock at the RA lumen to the original position.	Initiates continued hemodynamic monitoring.		
19. Assess the flow of infusions through the RA port to ensure that flow has resumed.	Continues therapy.		
20. Observe the PA and RA waveforms on the monitor.	Continues hemodynamic monitoring.		
21. Discard used supplies and wash hands.	Reduces the transmission of microorganisms; standard precautions.		
22. Determine the hemodynamic calculations. Compare the values to prior values and determine whether the plan of care requires alterations.	Assesses cardiac performance and hemodynamic status.		

Procedure	**for Open Method of Syringe Preparation and Cardiac Output Determination**		
Steps	**Rationale**	**Special Considerations**	
Note: Follow Steps 1-11 of the Procedure for Measurement of Cardiac Output Using the Closed or Open Thermodilution Method.			
1. Wash hands and don nonsterile gloves.	Reduces the transmission of microorganisms; standard precautions.		
2. Prepare syringes or obtain manufactured prefilled syringes for CO determination.	Prepares the injectate for CO determination.	Prefilled syringes decrease variability related to injectate volume.	
A. Clean the injectate port of the D₅W IV bag with an alcohol wipe or apply a dispensing port to the bag's injectate port.	Reduces surface contamination. A dispensing port negates the use of needles or a needleless drawing system and reduces the incidence of accidental needle sticks.	Not necessary if using manufactured prefilled sterile syringes.	
B. Aseptically withdraw the injectate solution from the D₅W IV bag into three to five 10-ml syringes and cap securely.	Prepares the injectate for CO measurements.	Additional syringes may be necessary because syringes may be inadvertently dropped or contaminated.	

Procedure	for Open Method of Syringe Preparation and Cardiac Output Determination—*Continued*	

Steps	Rationale	Special Considerations
C. If not using immediately, label the container or syringes with the date and time they were prepared.	Prefilled syringes at the bedside or in the refrigerator must be labeled (e.g., "for CO injection only").	
3. Cold injectate: Cool the syringes by filling a syringe container with sterile water and ice.	Iced slush is used to cool syringes. Use of water and ice prevents air pockets that can cause variability in the temperature of different injectate syringes.	Not necessary if using room temperature syringes. Handling of a cold syringe will cause warming and hamper validity of CO measurements. Cold injectate may be proarrhythmic.[31]
4. Remove the nonvented cap from the right atrial lumen stopcock of the PA catheter.	Prepares the stopcock.	
5. Aseptically connect one of the sterile CO injectate syringes onto the right atrial lumen stopcock of the PA catheter.	Reduces the risk of introducing microorganisms into the system.	
6. Turn the stopcock so that it is closed to the flush solution and open between the injectate syringe and the patient.	Prepares the system for injectate administration.	
7. Follow Steps 5 and 6 above; then follow Steps 10 through 15 of the closed method.	Obtains CO measurements.	Asepsis is essential as the stopcock is turned and syringes are exchanged between CO measurements.
8. Determine the CO measurement by calculating the average of three measurements within 10% of a middle (median) value. *(Level IV: Limited clinical studies to support recommendations.)*	Determines accurate CO value.[20]	
9. After the last injectate is completed, turn the right atrial lumen stopcock of the PA catheter so that the system is open between the patient and the transducer; aseptically remove the last injectate syringe; and place a new, sterile, nonvented cap on the stopcock port.	Closes the system; maintains the sterility of the system.	
10. Observe the PA and RA waveforms on the monitor.	Continues hemodynamic monitoring.	
11. Discard used supplies and wash hands.	Reduces the transmission of microorganisms; standard precautions.	
12. Determine hemodynamic calculations. Compare values with prior values and determine whether the plan of care requires alterations.	Assesses cardiac performance and hemodynamic status.	

Procedure for Measurement of Cardiac Output Using Continuous Cardiac Output Method

Steps	Rationale	Special Considerations
1. Wash hands and don nonsterile gloves.	Reduces the transmission of microorganisms; standard precautions.	Although there is no exposure of patient body fluids or IV fluids during this procedure, handwashing is a standard precaution.
2. Turn on the CO computer.	Provides energy.	
3. Connect the CO cable to the PA catheter.	Supplies the energy source.	
4. Observe the right atrial waveform. The proximal lumen opening of the PA catheter should be located in the RA.	A right atrial waveform indicates that the thermal filament is properly placed. The thermal filament should be located in the right ventricle between the infusion port and the distal tip of the catheter. Advancement of the thermal filament into the PA will result in erroneous measurements.	The thermal filament should float free in the right ventricle to prevent the loss of indicator (heat) into the cardiac tissue. If the loss of indicator occurs, the CO will be overestimated, giving erroneous readings.
5. Position the patient supine with the head of the bed elevated up to 45 degrees. *(Level IV: Limited clinical studies to support recommendations.)*	CCO measurements are most accurate in a supine position but head of bed angle can be varied for comfort, between 0 and 45 degrees.[10]	Studies are needed to describe the effect of patients' body position on CCO measurements. Document body position at the time of hemodynamic data collection.
6. Check the heat signal indicator on the CO computer.	CCO systems provide the quality of the heat signal by assessing the quality of the measured thermal signal. Relationships are in response to thermal noise or signal-to-noise ratio.	CCO monitors provide messages for troubleshooting signal-to-noise ratio interferences. Refer to the manufacturer recommendations. Technologic advances provide success in suppressing the effects of blood thermal noise.[30]
7. Note that the CCO readings on the monitor reflect an average of the preceding 3 to 6 minutes of data collection. CCO measurements are not timed to the respiratory cycle.	Continuous data collection reflects phasic changes in the respiratory cycle.	
8. When documenting CCO values, also document other hemodynamic findings displayed on the monitor screen.	CCO measurements are averaged over the preceding 3 to 6 minutes and are not individual measurements.	CCO is calculated by a bedside computer displaying graphic trends and by a continuous graphic reading that is updated every 30 to 60 seconds.
9. Validate the CCO with the patient's clinical status and concurrent hemodynamic findings. Review the physical, medication, and other patient findings/changes in the preceding 3- to 6-minute period to determine the significance of a CCO value.	CCO is a global assessment parameter and must be appreciated as part of the patient's total hemodynamic profile at a given time.	CCO method eliminates many of the potential user and technique-related errors associated with intermittent bolus CO. Research demonstrates clinically acceptable correlation between the TDCO technique and the CCO method in the steady state.[1,5,22,23] Future studies are needed to determine efficacy in patients in various phases of acute hemodynamic instability and in specific patient populations. Also, the effects of

Procedure	for Measurement of Cardiac Output Using Continuous Cardiac Output Method—*Continued*	
Steps	**Rationale**	**Special Considerations**
		changes in positioning need to be studied further, especially in patients with structural or functional heart damage.
Note: The CCO catheter system can be used to obtain TDCO. Follow Steps 1-11 of preprocedure for obtaining the CO *before* initiating steps for the open or closed method of syringe preparation and CO measurements and CO determination.		

Expected Outcomes

- Accurate measurement of CO obtained
- Hemodynamic profile and derived parameters obtained with accuracy, whether through the continuous or intermittent method
- PA catheter and lines maintain sterility and patency

Unexpected Outcomes

- Inability to accurately measure CO
- Erroneous readings because of technical, equipment, or operator error
- Contamination of the system
- Occlusion of the proximal PA lumen

Patient Monitoring and Care

Steps	Rationale	Reportable Conditions
		These conditions should be reported if they persist despite nursing interventions.
1. Maintain patency of the PA catheter (see Procedures 72 and 74).	PA catheter patency is essential for accurate monitoring.	• Inability to maintain PA catheter patency
2. Monitor RA and PA waveforms for confirmation of proper catheter position.	Proper placement determines accurate hemodynamics and CO measurement.	• Abnormal RA or PA waveforms and/or values
3. Maintain the sterility of the PA catheter.	Reduces the risk for catheter-related infections.	• Fever, site redness, drainage, or symptoms consistent with infection
4. Calculate cardiac index, systemic vascular resistance, and other parameters as prescribed or indicated.	Determines cardiac performance and current hemodynamic status.	• Abnormal cardiac index, systemic vascular resistance, or other hemodynamic values
5. Monitor vital signs and respiratory status hourly and as required.	Changes in vital signs or respiratory status may indicate hemodynamic compromise.	• Sudden or significant change in the patient's clinical status
6. Calculate the additional fluid volume for the bolus method or the continuous infusion into the patient's total fluid volume intake.	Additional volume added intermittently should be included in the total intake for an accurate fluid volume assessment.	• Signs or symptoms of fluid overload (e.g., respiratory distress, crackles, increased PA diastolic or PAW pressures, elevated jugular venous pressure, new or worsening S_3 gallop, worsening edema).
7. Assess the patient's response to therapies.	Hemodynamic monitoring may expedite treatment decisions.	• Significant worsening or improvement in CO, volume parameters (PAWP, RA pressure), and vascular resistance (PVR and SVR).

Procedure continues on the following page

Patient Monitoring and Care—*Continued*

Steps	Rationale	Reportable Conditions
8. If using a closed system delivery set (CO-Set®), change the system components (tubing, syringe, stopcocks, and IV solution) every 96 hours with the hemodynamic monitoring system (see Procedure 75).	No recommendations exist that are specific to the closed system delivery set.	

Documentation

Documentation should include the following:

- Patient and family education
- CO, cardiac index, systemic vascular resistance, volume indicators (PAWP and RAP)
- Characteristics and reliability of the CO curves and baseline PA blood temperature reflects the reliability of the data obtained
- Continuous or intermittent bolus method
- Volume and temperature of injectate
- Concurrent headrest elevation, vital signs, and hemodynamic measurements
- Titration or administration of pharmacologic agents affecting CO (e.g., dobutamine or milrinone infusions; epinephrine and norepinephrine), vascular resistance (e.g., intravenous nitrates or arterial vasodilator therapy-nitroprusside or nesiritide), and/or intravascular volume (e.g., intravenous loop or thiazide diuretics)
- Significant medical or nursing interventions affecting CO (e.g., intraaortic balloon pump or ventricular assist device therapies, volume expanders, position changes, other clinical factors), vascular resistance, or intravascular volume (e.g., sedation therapy, blood/blood products, headrest elevation, fluid restriction, sodium restriction)
- Unexpected outcomes
- Additional interventions, including psychosocial or emotional/psychiatric interventions that might influence hemodynamic trends

References

1. Albert, N.M., Spear, B., and Hammell, J. (1998). Agreement and clinical utility of two techniques for measuring cardiac output in patients with low cardiac output. *Am J Crit Care,* 8, 464-7.
2. Baillard, C., et al. (1999). Haemodynamic measurements (continuous cardiac output and systemic vascular resistance) in critically ill patients: Transesophageal Doppler versus continuous thermodilution. *Anaesth Intensive Care,* 27, 33-7.
3. Balik, M., Pachl, J., and Hendl, J. (2002). Effect of the degree of tricuspid regurgitation on cardiac output measurements by thermodilution. *Intensive Care Med,* 28, 1117-21.
4. Berthelsen, P.G., et al. (2002). Thermodilution cardiac output. Cold vs. room temperature injectate and the importance of measuring the injectate temperature in the right atrium. *ACTA Anaesthesiologica Scandinavia,* 46, 1103-10.
5. Boldt, J., et al. (1994). Is continuous cardiac output measurement using thermodilution reliable in the critically ill patient? *Crit Care Med,* 22, 1913-8.
6. Evans, D. (1994). The use of position during critical illness: Current practice and review of the literature. *Aust Crit Care,* 7, 16-21.
7. Gardner, P.E., and Bridges, E.J. (1995). Hemodynamic monitoring. In: Woods, S.L., et al., eds. *Cardiac Nursing.* 3rd ed. Philadelphia: J.B. Lippincott, 424-58.
8. Gardner, P., and Woods, S. (1995). Hemodynamic monitoring. In: Woods, S.L., ed. *Cardiac Nursing.* 3rd ed. Philadelphia: J.B. Lippincott, 424-58.
9. Gawlinski, A. (1998). *Protocols for Practice: Hemodynamic Monitoring Series—Cardiac Output Monitoring.* Aliso Viejo, CA: American Association of Critical-Care Nurses.
10. Giuliano, K.K., et al. (2003). Backrest angle and cardiac output measurement in critically ill patients. *Nurs Research,* 52, 242-8.
11. Goede, D.S., and Ackerman, M.A. (1994). We've come a long way: From Fick to continuous cardiac output monitoring. *Am J Nurs,* 94(Suppl), 24-9.
12. Grap, M.J., et al. (1999). Use of backrest elevation in critical care: A pilot study. *Am J Crit Care,* 8, 495-6.
13. Groeneveld, A.B., et al. (2000). Effect of mechanical ventilatory cycle on thermodilution right ventricular volumes and cardiac output. *J Appl Physiol,* 89, 89-96.
14. Grose, B.L., Wood, S.L., and Laurent, D.J. (1981). Effect of backrest position on cardiac output measured by the thermodilution method in acutely ill patients. *Heart Lung,* 10, 661-5.
15. Headley, J.M. (1998). Invasive hemodynamic monitoring: Applying advanced technologies. *Crit Care Nurs,* 21, 73-84.
16. Kalassian, K.G., and Raffin, T.A. (1996). The technique of thermodilution cardiac output measurements. *J Crit Illness,* 11, 249-56.
17. Kerns, M. (1999). Hemodynamic data. In: *The Cardiac Catheterization Handbook.* St. Louis: Mosby-Yearbook, 123-223.
18. Kiely, M., Byers, L.A., and Greenwood, R. (1998). Thermodilution measurement of cardiac output in patients with low output: Room temperature versus iced injectate. *Am J Crit Care,* 7, 436-8.
19. Lehmann, K.G., and Platt, M.S. (1999). Improved accuracy and precision of thermodilution cardiac output measurement using a dual thermistor catheter system. *J Am Coll Cardiol,* 33, 883-91.
20. Loveys, B.J., and Woods, S.L. (1986). Current recommendations for thermodilution cardiac output measurement. *Progress Cardiovasc Nurs,* 1, 24-32.
21. McCloy, K., Leung, S., and Beldon, J. (1999). Effects of injectate volume on thermodilution measurements of cardiac output in patients with low ventricular ejection fraction. *Am J Crit Care,* 8, 86-92.
22. Medin, D.L., et al. (1998). Validation of continuous thermodilution cardiac output in critically ill patients with analysis of systematic errors. *J Crit Care,* 13, 184-9.

23. Mihaljevic, T., et al. (1995). Continuous versus bolus thermodilution cardiac output measurement: A comparative study. *Crit Care Med, 23,* 944-9.

24. Nelson, L.D. (1996). The new pulmonary arterial catheters: Right ventricular ejection fraction and continuous cardiac output. *Crit Care Clin, 124,* 795-818.

25. Rodig, G., et al. (1998). Intraoperative evaluation of a continuous versus intermittent bolus thermodilution technique of cardiac output measurement in cardiac surgical patients. *Eur J Anesthesiology, 15,* 196-201.

26. Riedinger, M.S., Shellock, F.G., and Swan, H.J. (1981). Reading pulmonary artery and pulmonary capillary wedge pressure waveforms with respiratory variations. *Heart Lung, 10,* 675-8.

27. Rocca, G.D., et al. (2002). Continuous and intermittent cardiac output measurement: Pulmonary artery catheter versus aortic transpulmonary technique. *Brit J Anaesth, 88,* 350-6.

28. Stewart, S., and Vitello-Cicciu, J.M. (1998). Cardiovascular clinical physiology. In: Kinney, M.R., eds. *AACN Clinical Reference for Critical Care Nurse.* 4th ed. St. Louis: Mosby-Yearbook, 249-76.

29. Weiniger, C.F., et al. (2001). Arterial and pulmonary artery catheters. In: Parrillo, J.E., and Dellinger, R.P., eds. *Critical Care Medicine.* 2nd ed. St. Louis: Mosby, 3661.

30. Woods, S., and Oshuthorpe, S. (1993). Cardiac output determination. AACN CL issue. *Crit Care Nurs, 4*(1), 81-97.

31. Zellinger, M. (1995). *Advanced Concepts in Hemodynamics—Current Issues in Critical Care Nursing.* New York: Medical Information Services.

Additional Readings

Ahrens, T. (1999). Hemodynamic monitoring. *Crit Care Nurs Clin N Am, 11,* 19-31.

Brandsteller, R.D., et al. (1998). Swan-Ganz catheter: Misconceptions, pitfalls, and incomplete user knowledge—an identified trilogy in need of correction. *Heart Lung: J Acute Crit Care, 27,* 218-22.

Burchell, S.A., et al. (1997). Evaluation of a continuous cardiac output and mixed venous oxygen saturation catheter in critically ill surgical patients. *Crit Care Med, 25,* 388-91.

Cason, C.L., and Lambert, W. (1993). Positioning during hemodynamic monitoring. *DCCN.* 12, 226-33.

Daily, E.K., and Schroeder, J.F. (1994). *Techniques in Bedside Hemodynamic Monitoring.* 5th ed. St. Louis: Mosby-Yearbook.

Ditmyer, C.E., Shively, M., and Burns, C.B. (1995). Comparison of continuous with intermittent bolus thermodilution cardiac output measurement. *Am J Crit Care, 4,* 460-5.

Doering, L., and Dracup, K. (1988). Comparisons of cardiac output in supine and lateral positions. *Nurs Res, 37,* 114-8.

Driscoll, A., et al. (1995). The effect of patient positioning on reproducibility of cardiac output measurements. *Heart Lung, 24,* 38-44.

Elkayam, U., et al. (1983). Cardiac output by thermodilution technique: Effect of injectate's volume and temperature on accuracy and reproducibility in the critically ill patient. *Chest, 84,* 418-22.

Headley, J.M. (1995). Strategies to optimize the cardiorespiratory status of the critically ill. *AACN Clin Issues Crit Care Nurs, 6,* 121-34.

Headley, J. (1996). *Invasive Hemodynamic Monitoring: Physiological Principles and Clinical Application.* Irvine, CA: Baxter Health Care Corp.

Hollenberg, S.M., and Hoyt, J. (1997). Pulmonary artery catheters in cardiovascular disease. *N Horiz, 5,* 207-13.

Jansen, J.R., et al. (2001). Mean cardiac output by thermodilution with a single controlled injection. *Crit Care Med, 29,* 1868-73.

Marcum, J., Liberatone, K., and Willard, G. (1995). A comparison of varying injectate volumes in determining thermodilution cardiac output in critically ill post-surgical patients. *Am J Crit Care, 2,* 262.

Munro, H.M., et al. (1994). Continuous invasive cardiac output monitoring: The Baxter/Edwards Critical Care Swan-Ganz Intelli Cath and Vigilance system. *Clin Intensive Care, 5,* 52-5.

Nadia, S., and Noble, W.H. (1986). Limitations of cardiac output measurements by thermodilution. *Can Anaesth Soc J, 33,* 780-4.

Pesola, G.R., Rostata, H.P., and Carlon, G.C. (1992). Room temperature thermodilution cardiac: Central venous vs. right ventricular port. *Am J Crit Care, 1,* 76-80.

Pulmonary Artery Catheter Consensus Conference Participants. (1997). Pulmonary Artery Catheter Consensus Conference: Consensus statement. *Crit Care Med, 25,* 910-25.

Sandham, J.D., et al. (2003). A randomized, controlled trial of the use of pulmonary-artery catheters in high-risk surgical patients. *N Engl J Med, 348,* 5-14.

Stetz, C.W., et al. (1982). Reliability of the thermodilution method in the determination of cardiac output in clinical practice. *Am Rev Respire Dis, 126,* 1001-4.

Taylor, R.W. (1997). Controversies in pulmonary artery catheterization. *N Horiz, 5,* 1-296.

Whalen, D.A., and Keller, R. (1998). Cardiovascular patient assessment. In: Kinney, M.R., et al., eds. *AACN Clinical Reference for Critical Care Nurse.* 4th ed. St. Louis: Mosby-Yearbook, 227-319.

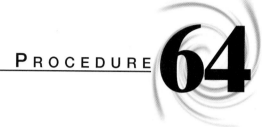

PROCEDURE **64**

Central Venous Catheter Removal

P U R P O S E :   Central venous catheters are removed when therapy is completed, a mechanical malfunction has occurred, the catheter has become occluded or malpositioned, or the patient has developed a catheter-related infection.

Nancy Munro

PREREQUISITE NURSING KNOWLEDGE

- Knowledge of the normal anatomy and physiology of the cardiovascular system
- Knowledge of the anatomy and physiology of the vasculature and adjacent structures of the neck
- Clinical and technical competence in central line removal is necessary. Knowledge of state nurse practice act is necessary since some states do not allow this intervention to be performed by a registered nurse.
- The nurse will need to validate that the catheter has been removed intact. Knowing the catheter design and length will assist the nurse in determining whether the catheter is removed completely.[1]
- The pathogenesis of a nontunneled central venous catheter (CVC) is the extraluminal colonization of the catheter originating from the skin primarily with less common hematogenous seeding of the catheter tip or intraluminal colonization of the hub and lumen.[3,5]
- Air embolism can occur during the removal of the catheter. Air embolism after the removal of the catheter is a result of air drawn in along the subcutaneous tract and into the vein. During inspiration, negative intrathoracic pressure is transmitted to the central veins. Any opening external to the body to one of these veins may result in aspiration of air into the central venous system. The pathologic effects depend on the volume and rate of air aspirated.
- Consider whether a culture tube or agar plate is needed to culture the tip of the catheter, because there is poor evidence to support a recommendation for or against use of this practice.[6]

EQUIPMENT

- Goggles or face shield mask, and nonsterile and sterile gloves
- Antiseptic solution (e.g., 2% chlorhexidine-based preparation)
- Suture removal kit or sterile scissors
- 4 × 4 gauze pads
- 2 × 2 gauze pads
- One roll of 2-inch tape
  Additional equipment to have as needed includes the following:
- Container for culture

PATIENT AND FAMILY EDUCATION

- Explain the procedure for catheter removal to the patient and family. ➥*Rationale:* Enhances patient and family understanding, increases patient cooperation, and reduces anxiety.
- Instruct the patient to report any signs and symptoms of shortness of breath, chest or groin pain, or other changes. ➥*Rationale:* May aid in early recognition of complications.

PATIENT ASSESSMENT AND PREPARATION

Patient Assessment

- Review the patient's laboratory data for platelet count, prothrombin time (PT), activated partial thromboplastin time (aPTT), and international normalized ratio (INR). Review the patient's past medical history or hospital course for coagulopathy issues. ➥*Rationale:* Pressure on the catheter site may be required for a longer period if coagulation studies are abnormal.

- Determine whether the patient is receiving anticoagulant therapy. ➤*Rationale:* Pressure on the catheter site may be required for a longer period.
- Assess the patient's vital signs. ➤*Rationale:* Provides baseline data.
- Observe the catheter site for redness, warmth at the site, tenderness, or presence of drainage. ➤*Rationale:* Assesses for signs and symptoms of infection.

Patient Preparation

- Ensure that the patient and family understand pre-procedural teaching. Answer questions as they arise and reinforce information as needed. ➤*Rationale:* Evaluates and reinforces understanding of previously taught information.
- Position the patient supine in Trendelenburg position or with the head of the bed flat if Trendelenburg position is contraindicated. ➤*Rationale:* A normal pressure gradient exists between atmospheric air and the central venous compartment that promotes air entry if the compartment is open. The lower the site of entry below the heart, the lower the pressure gradient, thus minimizing the risk for venous air embolism.
- Start a new peripheral intravenous (IV) line or ensure that an existing peripheral IV is patent. ➤*Rationale:* Establishes IV access for fluids or medications.

Procedure for Central Venous Catheter Removal

Steps	Rationale	Special Considerations
1. Wash hands.	Reduces the transmission of microorganisms; standard precautions.	
2. Open the suture removal kit or sterile scissors and sterile gauze pads.	Prepares supplies for use.	
3. Turn off the IV infusion.	Prevents saturating the bed, patient, or work area with IV solution on catheter removal.	
4. Don personal protective equipment (goggles, mask, and nonsterile gloves).	Reduces the transmission of microorganisms; standard precautions.	
5. Place the patient supine in slight Trendelenburg position.[2,4,7] Have the patient turn his or her head away from the catheter (if removing an internal jugular or subclavian catheter).	Positions the patient for central line removal; decreases the risk for air entry and reduces the transmission of microorganisms.	Place the patient flat if Trendelenburg is contraindicated or not tolerated by the patient.
6. Remove the catheter dressing and discard.	Exposes the catheter site.	
7. Remove the nonsterile gloves, wash hands, and don a pair of sterile gloves.	Reduces the transmission of microorganisms; standard precautions.	
8. Carefully cut the suture, and pull the suture through the skin.	Allows for removal of the catheter.	Ensure that the entire suture is removed. Retained sutures can form epithelialized tracts that can lead to infection.
9. Instruct the patient to take a deep breath in and hold it (if removing an internal jugular or subclavian catheter).	Minimizes air being accidentally drawn into the systemic venous circulation.	If the patient is mechanically ventilated, withdraw the catheter during the inspiratory phase of the respiratory cycle or while delivering a breath via a bag-valve device.

Procedure continues on the following page

Procedure for Central Venous Catheter Removal—*Continued*

Steps	Rationale	Special Considerations
10. Remove the catheter, following these steps: A. Grasp the catheter with the dominant hand and withdraw the catheter in one continuous motion. B. With the nondominant hand, quickly apply pressure over the puncture site with a sterile 4 × 4 gauze pad.	Withdrawing the catheter with a continuous motion decreases trauma to the vein. The distal end of a multilumen catheter should be removed quickly because the exposed proximal and medial openings could permit the entry of air. Minimizes the risk for air entry and bleeding.	If there are signs of infection, send the catheter tip to the laboratory for culture and sensitivity testing if prescribed.
11. Maintain pressure for 5 minutes until hemostasis has been achieved.	Prevents bleeding and hematoma formation.	Pressure may be needed for a longer period of time if the patient has been receiving anticoagulant therapy or if coagulation studies are abnormal.
12. Once hemostasis has been achieved, apply an occlusive, sterile dressing over the site.	Minimizes the risk for air entry and infection at the site.	
13. Inspect the catheter after it is removed.	Ensures that the entire catheter has been removed.	
14. Reposition the patient after application of the occlusive dressing.		
15. Discard used supplies in appropriate waste containers and wash hands.	Reduces the transmission of microorganisms; standard precautions.	

Expected Outcomes

- The catheter is removed intact.
- Hemostasis is achieved at the catheter site.

Unexpected Outcomes

- Inability to remove the catheter
- Catheter not removed intact
- Air embolism
- Pulmonary embolism
- Catheter site infection
- Difficulty attaining hemostasis at the puncture site; formation of hematoma

Patient Monitoring and Care

Steps	Rationale	Reportable Conditions
		These conditions should be reported if they persist despite nursing interventions.
1. Monitor the patient's vital signs, pulse oximetry, and level of consciousness before and after the central venous catheter is removed.	Changes in mental status, heart rate, blood pressure, and respiratory rate may indicate pulmonary air embolism. If an embolus is suspected, position the patient on the *left* side and in *Trendelenburg position.*	• Changes in vital signs • Persistent shortness of breath or tachypnea • Cyanosis or decreased oxygen saturation • Changes in mental status
2. Assess the dressing for the first 15 minutes after catheter removal, then every 15 minutes for the next hour, for bleeding.	Assesses for hemostasis and early evidence of bleeding.	• Bleeding or hematoma development

Patient Monitoring and Care—*Continued*

Steps	Rationale	Reportable Conditions
3. Assess the catheter integrity.	Catheter debris could cause further complications such as pulmonary embolism.	• Altered catheter integrity • Changes in vital signs • Persistent shortness of breath or tachypnea • Cyanosis • Decreased oxygen saturation
4. Observe the catheter site daily for signs of infection.	Infection of the skin site may occur after the removal of the catheter.	• Redness, tenderness, or drainage at the catheter site • Elevated temperature or white blood cell counts
5. Remove the dressing and assess for site closure 24 hours after removal.	Verifies healing and closure of the site.	• Abnormal healing

Documentation

Documentation should include the following:

- Patient and family education
- Date and time of catheter removal
- Site assessment
- Culture specimen sent (if appropriate)
- Ease of catheter removal
- Inspection of the catheter
- Length of time pressure applied to obtain hemostasis
- Application of occlusive dressing
- Patient tolerance of the procedure
- Unexpected outcomes and interventions

References

1. Andris, D.A., and Krzywda, E.A. (1997). Central venous access: Clinical practice issues. *Nurs Clin North Am,* 32, 719-40.
2. Ely, E.W., et al. (1999). Venous air embolism from central venous catheterization: A need for increased physician awareness. *Crit Care Med,* 27, 2113-7.
3. Hebden, J.N. (2002). Preventing intravascular catheter-related bloodstream infections in the critical care setting. *AACN Clinical Issues: Advanced Practice in Acute and Critical Care,* 13, 373-81.
4. McCarthy, P.M., et al. (1995). Air embolism in single-lung transplant patients after central venous catheter removal. *Chest,* 107, 1178-9.
5. Mermel, L.A., et al. (2001). Guidelines for the management of intravascular catheter-related infections. *J Intraven Nurs,* 24, 180-205.
6. O'Grady, N.P., et al. (1998). Practice guidelines for evaluating new fever in critically ill adult patients. *Crit Care Med,* 2, 392-408.
7. Woodrow, P. (2002). Central venous catheters and central venous pressure. *Nurs Standard,* 16, 45-52, 54.

Additional Readings

O'Grady, N.P., et al. (2002). Guidelines for the prevention of intravascular catheter-related infections. *Am J Infect Control,* 30, 476-89.
Centers for Disease Control and Prevention: *www.cdc.gov.*
Infectious Diseases Society of America: *www.idsa.org.*
Intravenous Nursing Society: *www.ins.org.*
National Guidelines Clearinghouse: *www.guidelines.gov.*

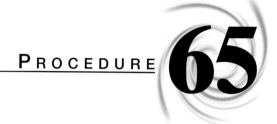
PROCEDURE **65**

Central Venous Catheter Site Care

P U R P O S E : Site care of the central venous catheter (CVC) allows for assessment of the catheter insertion site for signs of infection or catheter dislodgment, skin integrity, and the integrity of the suture. Site care involves cleansing the area around the catheter to minimize the growth of microorganisms.

Nancy Munro

PREREQUISITE NURSING KNOWLEDGE

- Knowledge of the normal anatomy and physiology of the cardiovascular system
- Understanding of the principles of aseptic technique and infection control
- Infection has been identified as a potentially life-threatening complication of central venous catheterization with an associated estimated mortality of 12% for each infection.[1] Appropriate care of the catheter site is considered to have primary importance in decreasing the risk for catheter-related sepsis.
- Migration of skin organisms at the insertion site into the cutaneous catheter tract with colonization of the catheter tip has been designated as the primary mechanism in the pathogenesis of catheter-related infections.[1]
- Knowledge of the signs and symptoms of catheter-related infection and sepsis
- The dressing should be examined for evidence of moisture and evaluated for its ability to provide a protective barrier. The thorax has a greater density of cutaneous flora and a higher skin temperature than other areas.[1] These factors play a major role in the risk for infection with central venous catheters placed in the chest or neck.
- Knowledge of the advantages and disadvantages of transparent dressings and gauze dressings. The advantages of transparent dressings are that they (1) permit continuous visual inspection of the site, (2) may require fewer dressing changes, (3) secure the device, and (4) permit the patients to bathe and shower without saturating the dressing. The disadvantages of transparent dressings are that they (1) are more expensive than gauze, (2) may allow for the accumulation of moisture, which may increase the opportunity of microorganism transmission, and (3) are difficult to apply to diaphoretic patients. Gauze dressings absorb moisture and are less expensive but lack continuous visualization of the insertion site and require more frequent changing of the dressing.

EQUIPMENT

- Nonsterile and sterile gloves
- Transparent dressing or sterile 2 × 2 gauze
- Sterile 4 × 4 gauze
- Roll of 2-in tape
- Prepackaged sterile dressing kit with the above contents can also be used
- Antiseptic solution (e.g., 2% chlorhexidine-based) Additional equipment as needed includes the following:
- 70% alcohol solution, pads, or swabsticks
- 10% povidone-iodine solution, pads, or swabsticks

PATIENT AND FAMILY EDUCATION

- Explain the dressing change procedure. ➥*Rationale:* Prepares the patient and decreases patient anxiety.
- Explain the importance of patient positioning during the dressing change. ➥*Rationale:* Increases patient cooperation and decreases the potential for contamination.

PATIENT ASSESSMENT AND PREPARATION

Patient Assessment

- Assess the patient's arm, shoulder, neck, and chest on the same side as the catheter insertion site for signs of pain, swelling, or tenderness. Assess the patient's leg size and assess for signs of pain, swelling, or tenderness on the same side as the catheter insertion site if placed in the femoral vein. **→*Rationale:*** Evaluates for thrombophlebitis or venous thrombosis.
- Evaluate the patient's clinical status for signs and symptoms of infection or sepsis—that is, fever, chills, change in mental status, hypotension, leukocytosis with left shift (increase in bands), respiratory alkalosis, metabolic acidosis, or glucose intolerance. **→*Rationale:*** Careful assessment of the patient's clinical status and the catheter site is performed to evaluate for catheter-related sepsis.
- Assess the patient's history for sensitivity to antiseptic solutions. **→*Rationale:*** Decreases the risk for allergic reactions.

Patient Preparation

- Ensure that the patient and family understand preprocedural teaching. Answer questions as they arise and reinforce information as needed. **→*Rationale:*** Evaluates and reinforces understanding of previously taught information.
- If the patient is on ventilatory support, assess the patient's need for suctioning before beginning the procedure. Femoral line sites need to be inspected for contamination with urine or stool. **→*Rationale:*** Minimizes the risk for catheter site contamination by secretions/excretions.
- Instruct the patient to turn his or her head, or turn the patient's head, away from the insertion site. **→*Rationale:*** Minimizes contamination of the site with microorganisms from the patient's respiratory tract.

Procedure for Central Venous Catheter Site Care

Steps	Rationale	Special Considerations
1. Wash hands and don nonsterile gloves.	Reduces the transmission of microorganisms; standard precautions.	
2. Remove the central venous line dressing.	Exposes the catheter site for inspection and site care.	
3. Inspect the catheter, insertion site, suture, and surrounding skin.	Assesses for signs of infection, catheter dislodgment, leakage, or loose sutures.	
4. Remove and discard gloves and wash hands.	Reduces the transmission of microorganisms; standard precautions.	
5. Prepare/open kit or supplies needed for site care on a stable surface.	Prepares the equipment.	
6. Don sterile gloves.	Maintains aseptic and sterile technique.	
7. Cleanse the catheter and skin with antiseptic solution (e.g., 2% chlorhexidene-based preparation).	Reduces the rate of recolonization of skin flora.	Allow the solution to dry. If used, povidone-iodine needs to be in contact with the skin for at least 2 minutes.[1]
8. Do not use topical antibiotic ointment or creams on the insertion site.	There is potential to promote fungal infections and antimicrobial resistance with the use of antibiotic ointment or cream.[1]	
9. Apply an occlusive dressing using either of the following: A. A transparent dressing B. A 2 × 2 gauze dressing	Provides a sterile environment. If the patient is diaphoretic or if the site is bleeding or oozing, a gauze dressing is preferred.[1]	Use either a transparent dressing alone or gauze dressing with tape. Do not combine dressing types. A gauze dressing covered with a transparent dressing can harbor moisture and provide an environment for bacterial growth.[1]

Procedure continues on the following page

Procedure for Central Venous Catheter Site Care—*Continued*

Steps	Rationale	Special Considerations
10. If using a gauze dressing, cover the gauze with tape, leaving the catheter hub and tubing connection exposed.	Provides the occlusive seal to prevent site contamination.	
11. Secure the tubing with tape close to the insertion site.	Reduces tension on the catheter caused by patient movement. May prevent accidental dislodgement of the catheter.	Loop the tubing prior to taping it to the skin.
12. Discard used supplies in appropriate receptacle and wash hands.	Reduces the transmission of microorganisms; standard precautions.	

Expected Outcomes

- Dressing remains dry, sterile, and intact
- Catheter site remains free from infection
- Catheter remains in place without dislodgment

Unexpected Outcomes

- Catheter-related infection
- Accidental removal or dislodgement of the catheter or malpositioning of the tip
- Impaired integrity of the skin under the dressing

Patient Monitoring and Care

Steps	Rationale	Reportable Conditions
		These conditions should be reported if they persist despite nursing interventions.
1. Assess the dressing every 2 to 4 hours and as necessary.	Ensures an occlusive, dry sterile dressing.	
2. Replace gauze dressings every 2 days and transparent dressings at least every 7 days.[1] Cleanse the site with an antiseptic solution (e.g., 2% chlorhexidine-based preparation).	Decreases the risk for infection at the catheter site. The CDC recommends replacing the dressing when it becomes damp, loosened, or soiled or when inspection of the site is necessary.[1]	• Signs or symptoms of infection
3. Assess for signs and symptoms of infection.	The catheter should be removed if signs of infection are present.	• Redness, pain, or drainage at the insertion site • Fever without obvious cause • Elevated white blood cell count

Documentation

Documentation should include the following:

- Patient and family education
- Date and time of the procedure
- Condition of the catheter site
- Type of dressing applied

- Date and time of dressing change and initials of the person changing the dressing (documented on the dressing)
- Unexpected outcomes
- Additional interventions

Reference

1. O'Grady, N.P., et al. (2002). Guidelines for the prevention of intravascular catheter-related infections. *Am J Infect Control,* 30, 476-89.

Additional Readings

Infusion Nursing Standards of Practice. (2002). *J Intraven Nurs,* 23(Suppl), 1-81.

Centers for Disease Control and Prevention: *www.cdc.gov.*
Infectious Diseases Society of America: *www.idsa.org.*
Intravenous Nursing Society: *www.ins.org.*
National Guidelines Clearinghouse: *www.guidelines.gov.*

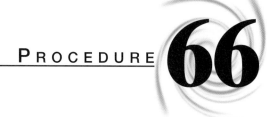

PROCEDURE **66**

Central Venous/Right Atrial Pressure Monitoring

P U R P O S E :   Central venous/right atrial pressure monitoring provides information about the patient's fluid volume status and right ventricular preload. The central venous pressure (CVP) or the right atrial pressure (RAP) allows for evaluation of right-sided heart hemodynamics and evaluation of patient response to therapy. CVP and RAP are used interchangeably.

Nancy Munro

PREREQUISITE NURSING KNOWLEDGE

- Knowledge of the normal anatomy and physiology of the cardiovascular system.
- Understanding of the principles of aseptic technique and infection control.
- Understanding of the principles of hemodynamic monitoring.
- Invasive lines increase susceptibility to infection. Adherence to aseptic technique when handling these lines can decrease the potential for infection.[17]
- The central venous pressure (CVP) or the right atrial pressure (RAP) is the pressure measured at the tip of a catheter placed within a central vein near or in the right atrium (RA).
- CVP influences and is influenced by venous return and cardiac function. Although the CVP is used as a measure of changes in the right ventricle, the relationship is not linear. Because the right ventricle has the ability to expand and alter its compliance, changes in volume can occur with little change in pressure.
- A single reading of a CVP is not significant. Monitoring trends in CVP readings is more meaningful.
- Normal CVP is 2 to 6 mm Hg.
- The CVP represents right-sided heart preload or the volume of blood found in the right ventricle at the end of diastole.
- CVP values can be obtained by using a hemodynamic monitoring system or a fluid manometer system.
- Understanding of *a, c,* and *v* waves is necessary. The *a* wave reflects right atrial contraction. The *c* wave reflects

closure of the tricuspid valve. The *v* wave reflects the right atrial filling during ventricular systole.
- The nurse must be technically and clinically competent in using the monitoring system chosen for obtaining CVP measurements. Hemodynamic monitoring systems allow for analysis of the waveform and measurement of the pressure. Water manometers provide only a numerical value. If changing from one system to the other, it is important to know that the values will be different. Water manometers measure centimeters of water pressure (cm H_2O), whereas transducers measure millimeters of mercury (mm Hg). Water manometer values will be higher than mercury readings. The formula for conversion is as follows:

$$\text{cm } H_2O \div 1.36 = \text{mm Hg}^1$$

- CVP readings can be affected by location of the air-fluid interface of the monitoring system (see Procedure 75).
- CVP values are useful in evaluating volume status, effect of medication therapy (especially medication that decreases preload), and cardiac function (Table 66-1).
- Monitoring parameters from the femoral central line site is not recommended. The catheter is too distant from the right atrium to produce reliable data.

EQUIPMENT

- Hemodynamic monitoring system (see Procedure 75)
- Bedside monitor
- Analog recorder
- Carpenter's level or laser level

TABLE 66-1	Central Venous Pressure

Conditions Causing Increased CVP

Elevated intravascular volume
Depressed right-sided cardiac function (RV infarct, RV failure)
Cardiac tamponade
Constrictive pericarditis
Pulmonary hypertension
Chronic left ventricular failure

Conditions Causing Decreased CVP

Reduced intravascular volume*
Decreased mean arterial pressure (MAP)
Venodilation

---

*Although the measured CVP is low, cardiac function may be depressed, normal, or hyperdynamic when there is reduced vascular volume.

Additional equipment to have available as needed includes the following:
- Water manometer and intravenous (IV) fluid, normal saline
- Indelible marker

PATIENT AND FAMILY EDUCATION

- Discuss the purpose of the CVP catheter and monitoring with both the patient and family. ➵*Rationale:* Reduces anxiety and includes the patient and family in the plan of care.
- Explain the patient's expected participation during the procedure. ➵*Rationale:* Encourages patient assistance.

PATIENT ASSESSMENT AND PREPARATION

Patient Assessment

- Assess for signs and symptoms of fluid volume deficit, including weakness, thirst, decreased urine output, increased urine specific gravity, output that is greater than intake, sudden weight loss or gain, decreased pulmonary artery wedge pressure, hemoconcentration, hypernatremia, postural hypotension, tachycardia, decreased skin turgor, dry mucous membranes, decreased pulse pressure, weak and thready pulse, abnormal paradoxical pulse on the arterial line waveform, and altered mental status. ➵*Rationale:* The patient's clinical picture should correlate with the CVP value. Fluid volume deficit will usually result in a decreased CVP.

- Assess for signs and symptoms of fluid volume excess, including dyspnea, orthopnea, anxiety, sudden weight gain, intake greater than output, pulmonary congestion, abnormal breath sounds (e.g., crackles), S_3 heart sound, dependent edema, pleural effusion, anasarca, tachypnea, dilutional decrease in hemoglobin and hematocrit, tachycardia, dysrhythmias, increased pulmonary artery pressures or pulmonary artery wedge pressure, jugular vein distention, oliguria, decreased urine specific gravity, altered electrolytes, and altered mental status. ➵*Rationale:* The patient's clinical picture should correlate with the CVP values. Fluid volume overload will usually result in an elevated CVP.

- Assess for signs and symptoms of air embolus, including a sucking sound on inspiration, dyspnea, tachypnea, hypoxia, hypercapnia, wheezing, a bell-shaped air bubble in the pulmonary outflow tract on the chest x-ray film, increased pulmonary artery pressures, tachycardia, cyanosis, jugular vein distention, hypotension, increased systemic vascular resistance, substernal chest pain, ST segment changes on electrocardiogram (ECG), cor pulmonale, cardiac arrest, lightheadedness, confusion, anxiety, fear of dying, aphasia, localized neurologic deficits, hemiplegia, unresponsiveness, and seizures.[10] ➵*Rationale:* Air embolus is a rare but potentially fatal complication of CVP catheterization. This may develop during insertion, with an accidental disconnection of the catheter, or during catheter removal.

- Assess for signs and symptoms of infection. Potential for infection can occur with improper catheter care or contamination. Contamination may occur during insertion or any time while the catheter is in place.[17] ➵*Rationale:* Infection is a potential complication of any invasive line.

Patient Preparation

- Ensure that the patient and family understand preprocedural teaching. Answer questions as they arise and reinforce information as needed. ➵*Rationale:* Evaluates and reinforces understanding of previously taught information.
- Place patient in the supine position. ➵*Rationale:* Allows for accurate leveling of the air-fluid interface of the monitoring system with the atria.

Procedure	for Central Venous/Right Atrial Pressure Monitoring	
Steps	**Rationale**	**Special Considerations**
CVP Measurement Using Water Manometer Method		
1. Wash hands.	Reduces the transmission of microorganisms; standard precautions.	
2. Locate the phlebostatic axis (see Procedure 75).	Ensures accuracy of measurement.	Once the phlebostatic axis has been identified, the nurse should mark the patient's skin with an indelible marker at the level. This will ensure that future readings are taken at the same location.

Procedure continues on the following page

Procedure for Central Venous/Right Atrial Pressure Monitoring—*Continued*

Steps	Rationale	Special Considerations
3. Position the patient in the supine position with the head of the bed from 0-45 degrees. *(Level VI: Clinical studies in a variety of patient populations and situations to support recommendations.)*	Studies have determined that the RA and PA pressures are accurate in this position.[4,5,6,7,12,14,16,24,25]	
4. Attach the water manometer to the CVP tubing system and flush the tubing with normal saline while the system is off to the patient.	Prepares the system.	
5. Place the zero level of the water manometer at the level of the phlebostatic axis (Figs. 66-1 and 66-2).	Levels the water manometer for accurate measurements. Ensures accuracy in measurement.	If the water manometer is attached to an IV pole, use a carpenter's level or laser leveling device to ensure that the zero level of the manometer is level with the phlebostatic axis.
6. Turn the water manometer stopcock open to the flush solution (Fig. 66-3, system A).	Permits fluid to fill the water manometer.	
7. Open the IV tubing roller clamp so that fluid flows from the IV fluid solution into the water manometer. A. Fill the manometer two-thirds full or above the level of the expected CVP measurement. B. Ensure that there are no air bubbles in the manometer. C. Close the roller clamp on the IV tubing.	Prepares the water manometer for pressure measurement. If fluid is allowed to overflow the top of the manometer, contamination can result. Underfilling the water manometer will result in an inaccurate measurement.	

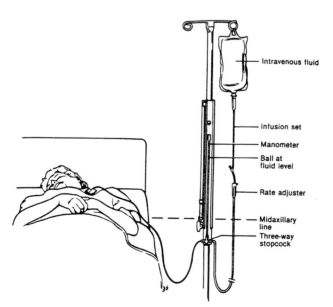

FIGURE 66-1 Central venous pressure water manometer flush system. This manometer is attached to the IV pole, and the height is adjusted to the phlebostatic axis using a carpenter's level or laser leveling device. *(From Hudack, C. [1989].* Critical Care Nursing: A Holistic Approach. *Philadelphia: J.B. Lippincott.)*

Labels: Intravenous fluid / Infusion set / Manometer / Ball at fluid level / Rate adjuster / Midaxillary line / Three-way stopcock

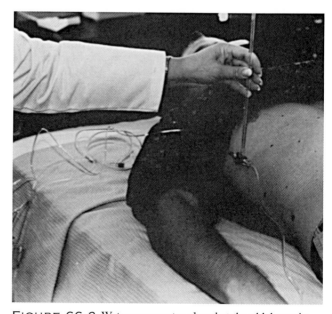

FIGURE 66-2 Water manometer placed at the phlebostatic axis on the patient.

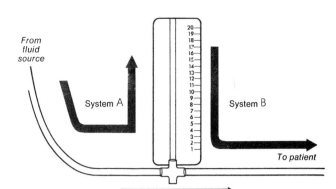

FIGURE 66-3 Central venous pressure measurement. System *A*, Stopcock closed to the patient for filling of the manometer. System *B*, Stopcock closed to the fluid source and open to the patient. System *C*, Stopcock closed to the manometer with the fluid system opened to the patient. *(From Hudack, C. [1989].* Critical Care Nursing: A Holistic Approach. *Philadelphia: J.B. Lippincott.)*

Procedure for Central Venous/Right Atrial Pressure Monitoring—*Continued*		
Steps	Rationale	Special Considerations
8. Turn the water manometer stopcock open to the patient and closed to the IV solution (Fig. 66-3, system B).	Allows fluid to flow into the patient until the fluid column equalizes with the pressure in the right atrium.	
9. Observe the fluid column closely. It should fluctuate with the patient's respiratory cycle.	The fluid column may fall rapidly. Care should be taken not to allow all of the fluid to flow out of the manometer.	If the manometer is allowed to empty, air may enter the patient.
10. The fluid column should fall quickly and then fluctuate gently at the point where the fluid column equalizes with the right atrial pressure. Measure the CVP reading at end expiration.	The pressure within the manometer equalizes with the pressure in the right atrium. The height of the fluid column reflects the right atrial pressure.	The fluid level will fluctuate with the patient's respiratory cycle once the fluid has equalized. The CVP should be measured at end-expiration.
11. Turn the water manometer stopcock open to the flush solution and the patient (Fig. 66-3, system C), and reestablish the IV fluid infusion.	Prevents clotting of the catheter and reestablishes IV flow.	
12. Wash hands.	Reduces the transmission of microorganisms; standard precautions.	
CVP Measurement Using a Hemodynamic Monitoring System		
1. Wash hands.	Reduces the transmission of microorganisms; standard precautions.	
2. Validate the waveform as CVP/RAP on the bedside monitor.	Ensures that the catheter is in proper location.	
3. Position the patient in the supine position with the head of the bed from 0 to 45 degrees. *(Level VI: Clinical studies in a variety of patient populations and situations to support recommendations.)*	Studies have determined that the RA and PA pressures are accurate in this position.[4,5,6,7,12,14,16,24,25]	RA and PA pressures may be accurate for patients in the supine position with the head of the bed elevated up to 60 degrees,[6,16] but additional studies are needed to support this. Only one study[13] supports the accuracy of hemodynamic values for patients in the lateral positions; other studies do not.[4,9,12,18,23] The majority of studies support the accuracy of hemodynamic monitoring

Procedure continues on the following page

Procedure | for Central Venous/Right Atrial Pressure Monitoring—*Continued*

Steps	Rationale	Special Considerations
		for patients in the prone position.[2,3,8,11,15,19,22] Two studies demonstrated that prone positioning caused an increase in hemodynamic values.[20,21]
4. Prepare the hemodynamic monitoring system (see Procedure 75).	Ensures accuracy in measurement.	
5. Level the air-fluid interface of the monitoring system to the phlebostatic axis (see Procedure 75).	Ensures accuracy in measurement.	
6. Run a dual-channel strip of the ECG and right atrial waveform (Fig. 66-4).	Right atrial pressures should be determined from the graphic recording so that end expiration can be properly identified.	Some monitors have the capability of "freeze framing" waveforms. A cursor can be used to determine pressure measurements.
7. Measure the CVP or RAP at end-expiration.	Measurement is most accurate as the effects of intrathoracic pressure changes are minimized.	
8. Using the dual-channel recorded strip, draw a vertical line from the beginning of the *P* wave of one of the ECG complexes down to the RAP waveform. Repeat this with the next ECG complex[1] (see Fig. 72-7).	Compares electrical activity with mechanical activity. Usually three waves will be present on the RAP waveform.	At times, the *c* wave will not be present.
9. Align the PR interval with the RAP waveform (see Fig. 66-4).[1]	The *a* wave correlates with this interval.	
10. Identify the *a* wave (see Fig. 66-4).[1]	The *a* wave is seen approximately 80 to 100 ms after the *P* wave. The *c* wave follows the *a* wave, and the *v* wave follows the *c* wave.	The *a* wave reflects atrial contraction. The *c* wave reflects closure of the tricuspid valve. The *v* wave reflects passive filling of the right atrium.

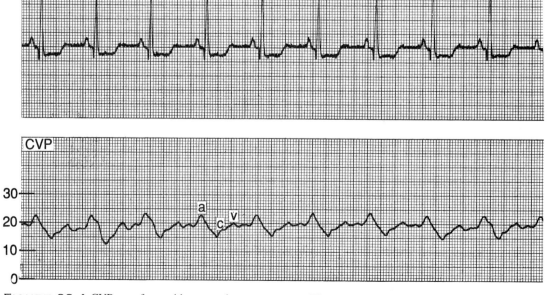

FIGURE 66-4 CVP waveform with *a, c,* and *v* waves present. The *a* wave is usually seen just after the *P* wave of the ECG. The *c* wave appears at the time of the RST junction on the ECG. The *v* wave is seen in the TP interval. *CVP,* central venous pressure; *ECG,* electrocardiogram.

Procedure for Central Venous/Right Atrial Pressure Monitoring—*Continued*

Steps	Rationale	Special Considerations
11. Identify the scale of the RAP tracing.[1]	Aids in determining the pressure measurement.	The RAP scale commonly is set at 20 mm Hg.
12. Measure the mean of the *a* wave to obtain the RAP pressure[1] (Fig. 66-5).	The *a* wave represents atrial contraction and reflects ventricular filling at end-diastole.	
13. Wash hands.	Reduces the transmission of microorganisms; standard precautions.	

Expected Outcomes

- Accurate CVP/RAP measurements
- Adequate and appropriate waveforms
- CVP/RAP readings that correlate with physical findings

Unexpected Outcomes

- Air embolus or other complication
- Inaccurate readings
- CVP readings that do not correlate with physical findings
- Infection/sepsis

Patient Monitoring and Care

Steps	Rationale	Reportable Conditions
		These conditions should be reported if they persist despite nursing interventions.
1. Monitor the patient's vital signs every 2 hours or more frequently if the patient's condition indicates.	Monitoring vital signs will alert the nurse to the beginning signs and symptoms of complications or infections.	• Changes in vital signs

Procedure continues on the following page

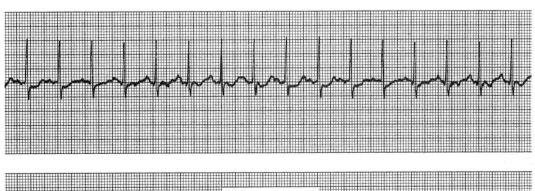

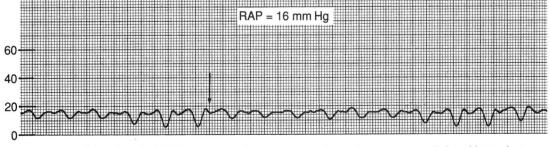

RAP = 16 mm Hg

FIGURE 66-5 Reading the RAP from paper printout at end-expiration in a spontaneously breathing patient. While observing the patient, identify inspiration. The point just before inspiration is end-expiration. Arrow indicates the point of end-expiration. Reading is taken as a mean value. The RAP value for this patient is 16 mm Hg. *RAP*, right atrial pressure.

Patient Monitoring and Care—*Continued*

Steps	Rationale	Reportable Conditions
2. Continuous monitoring of the CVP waveform if using the hemodynamic monitoring system.	Changes in the waveform may indicate a change in catheter position or change in patient condition.	• Abnormal CVP values or waveforms
3. Measure the CVP every 2 hours and as needed if using the water manometer method.	Indicate changes in patient condition.	• Abnormal CVP values

Documentation

Documentation should include the following:

- Patient and family education
- Patient tolerance of the procedure
- Cardiopulmonary assessment
- Assessment and labeled CVP waveform if appropriate
- IV intake, including amount of flush solution
- Assessment of fluid balance
- Confirmation of RA catheter placement using x-ray or waveforms
- Unexpected outcomes
- Additional interventions

References

1. Ahrens, T., and Taylor, L. (1992). *Hemodynamic Waveform Analysis.* Philadelphia: W.B. Saunders.
2. Blanch, L., et al. (1997). Short-term effect of prone position in critically ill patients with acute respiratory distress syndrome. *Intensive Care Med,* 23, 1003-39.
3. Brussel, T., et al. (1993). Mechanical ventilation in the prone position for acute respiratory failure after cardiac surgery. *J Cardiothorac Vasc Anesth,* 7, 541-6.
4. Cason, C.L., et al. (1990). Effects of backrest elevation and position on pulmonary artery pressures. *Cardiovasc Nurs,* 26, 1-5.
5. Chulay, M., and Miller, T. (1984). The effect of backrest elevation on pulmonary artery and pulmonary capillary wedge pressures in patients after cardiac surgery. *Heart Lung,* 13, 138-40.
6. Clochesy, J., Hinshaw, A.D., and Otto, C.W. (1984). Effects of change of position on pulmonary artery and pulmonary capillary wedge pressure in mechanically ventilated patients. *NITA,* 7, 223-5.
7. Dobbin, K., et al. (1992). Pulmonary artery pressure measurement in patients with elevated pressures: Effect of backrest elevation and method of measurement. *Am J Crit Care,* 1, 61-9.
8. Fridrich, P., et al. (1996). The effects of long-term prone positioning in patients with trauma-induced adult respiratory distress syndrome. *Anesth Analg,* 83, 1206-11.
9. Groom, L., Frisch, S.R., and Elliot, M. (1990). Reproducibility and accuracy of pulmonary artery pressure measurement in supine and lateral positions. *Heart Lung,* 19, 147-51.
10. Hadaway, L.C. (2002). Air embolus. *Nursing 2002,* 32, 104.
11. Jolliet, P., Bulpa, P., and Chevrolet, J.C. (1998). Effects of prone position on gas exchange and hemodynamics in severe acute respiratory distress syndrome. *Crit Care Med,* 26, 1977-85.
12. Keating, D., et al. (1986). Effect of sidelying positions on pulmonary artery pressures. *Heart Lung,* 15, 605-10.
13. Kennedy, G.T., Bryant, A., and Crawford, M.H. (1984). The effects of lateral body positioning on measurements of pulmonary artery and pulmonary wedge pressures. *Heart Lung,* 13, 155-8.
14. Lambert C.W., and Cason, C.L. (1990). Backrest elevation and pulmonary artery pressures: research analysis. *Dimensions Crit Care Nurs,* 9, 327-35.
15. Langer, M., et al. (1982). The prone position in ARDS patients. *Chest,* 94, 103-7.
16. Laulive, J.L. (1982). Pulmonary artery pressures and position changes in the critically ill adult. *Dimensions Crit Care Nurs,* 1, 28-34.
17. O'Grady, N.P., et al. (2002). Guidelines for the prevention of intravascular catheter-related infections. *Am J Infect Control,* 30, 476-89.
18. Osida, C. (1989). Measurement of pulmonary artery pressures: Supine verses side-lying head elevated positions. *Heart Lung,* 18, 298-9.
19. Pappert, D., et al. (1994). Influence of positioning on ventilation-perfusion relationships in severe adult respiratory distress syndrome. *Chest,* 106, 1511-6.
20. Pelosi, P., et al. (1998). Effects of the prone position on respiratory mechanics and gas exchange during acute lung injury. *Am J Respir Crit Care Med,* 157, 387-93.
21. Voggenreiter, G., et al. (1999). Intermittent prone positioning in the treatment of severe and moderate posttraumatic lung injury. *Crit Care Med,* 27, 2375-82.
22. Vollman, K.M., and Bander, J.J. (1996). Improved oxygenation utilizing a prone positioner in patients with acute respiratory distress syndrome. *Intensive Care Med,* 22, 1105-11.
23. Wild, L. (1984). Effect of lateral recumbent positions on measurement of pulmonary artery and pulmonary artery wedge pressures in critically ill adults. *Heart Lung,* 13, 305.
24. Wilson, A.E., et al. (1996). Effect of backrest position on hemodynamic and right ventricular measurements in critically ill adults. *Am J Crit Care,* 5, 264-70.
25. Woods, S.L., and Mansfield, L.W. (1976). Effect of body position upon pulmonary artery and pulmonary capillary wedge pressures in noncritically ill patients. *Heart Lung,* 5, 83-90.

Additional Readings

Anonymous. (1997). Pulmonary artery catheter consensus conference: Consensus statement. *Crit Care Med*, 25, 910-25.

Bridges, E.J., and Woods, S.L. (1993). Pulmonary artery pressure measurement: State of art. *Heart Lung*, 22, 99-111.

Darovic, G.O. (2002). *Hemodynamic Monitoring: Invasive and Noninvasive Clinical Application.* 3rd ed. Philadelphia: W.B. Saunders.

Keckeisen M. (1997). *Protocols for Practice: Hemodynamic Monitoring Series—Pulmonary Artery Pressure Monitoring.* Aliso Viejo, CA: American Association of Critical-Care Nurses.

Pulmonary Artery Catheter Education Program: www.pacep.org. This is a website that is the result of a joint effort of the American Association of Critical Care Nurses, the American College of Chest Physicians, the Society of Critical Care Medicine, and other organizations to standardize the education for using the pulmonary artery catheter, which includes CVP monitoring.

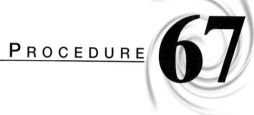

PROCEDURE **67**

Esophageal Doppler Monitoring of Aortic Blood Flow: Probe Insertion

P U R P O S E : Insertion of an esophageal probe for monitoring aortic blood flow is used to assess the hemodynamic condition of critically ill patients. Esophageal Doppler monitoring (EDM) uses Doppler ultrasound technology to provide information regarding left ventricular performance and patient fluid status.

Deborah Lamarr
Maureen Turner

PREREQUISITE NURSING KNOWLEDGE

* Knowledge of cardiovascular anatomy and physiology
* Understanding of the upper gastrointestinal tract anatomy
* Ability to recognize the EDM aortic waveforms by visual display and auditory pitch
* Understanding of normal and associated values aortic waveforms (Fig. 67-1; see Fig. 68-1)
* Understanding of additional waveforms that guide esophageal probe insertion (see Fig. 68-2)
* Clinical and technical competence in esophageal probe insertion and esophageal monitoring
* Indications for the EDM are as follows:
  * Potential status of hypoperfusion (hypovolemia, hemorrhagic shock, septic shock)
  * Hemodynamic monitoring and evaluation of patients with major organ dysfunction (e.g., renal failure, respiratory failure, liver failure)
  * Differential diagnosis of hypotensive states
  * Aid in the diagnosis of heart failure, cardiogenic shock, papillary muscle rupture, mitral regurgitation, ventricular septal rupture, or cardiac rupture with tamponade
  * Management of high-risk cardiac patients undergoing surgical procedures during preoperative, intraoperative, and postoperative periods
* Contraindications to EDM include oral or upper gastrointestinal tract anomalies, coagulopathies, coarctation of the aorta, and intraaortic balloon pump therapy
* Proper positioning of the esophageal probe is essential for accurate data collection
* EDM technology utilizes a thin silicone probe, approximately 6 mm in diameter and 90 cm in length
* Once the patient's age, height, and weight are entered into the monitor, they are burned into a memory chip within the probe. EDM currently has nomogram limits:
  * Age: 16-99 years
  * Weight: 66-330 pounds
  * Height: 59-83 inches
* When nomogram limits are surpassed, calculated data such as systemic vascular resistance (SVR), stroke volume (SV), stroke volume index (SVI), cardiac output (CO), and cardiac index (CI) are not obtainable. Velocity data such as flow time corrected (FTc), peak velocity (PV), stroke distance (SD), and minute distance (MD) will still be measured. (Follow specific manufacturer nomogram limits.)

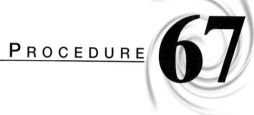

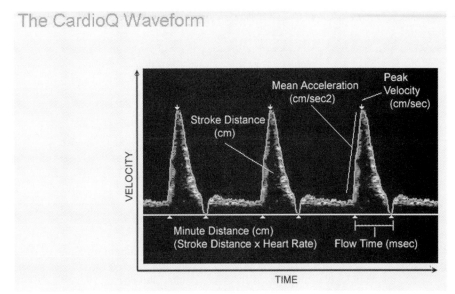

FIGURE 67-1 Normal aortic Doppler waveform. May vary depending on manufacturer's recommendations. *(Adapted from Cardio Q Reference Guide. [2003]. Severna Park, MD: Deltex Medical Inc.)*

EQUIPMENT

- EDM monitor, patient interface cable, power cord
- EDM probe
- Water soluble lubricant
- Nonsterile gloves, gown, mask, and goggles or face shield
- Sedative or analgesic
  Additional equipment to have available if needed:
- Topical lidocaine
- Tongue blade
- Supportive equipment if conscious sedation is necessary (e.g., oxygen, ambu bag, suction, oral airway)

PATIENT AND FAMILY EDUCATION

- Explain the procedure and the reason for the EDM monitoring. ➤*Rationale:* Decreases patient and family anxiety.
- Explain that the procedure may stimulate gagging and that sedation may be given to promote comfort. ➤*Rationale:* Prepares the patient and decreases anxiety.
- Inform the patient and family of the risks and anticipated benefits of the esophageal monitoring probe. ➤*Rationale:* Allows the patient and family to make an informed decision.

PATIENT ASSESSMENT AND PREPARATION

Patient Assessment

- Obtain the patient's past medical history specifically related to oral or upper gastrointestinal anomalies

(e.g., esophageal strictures, varicies, oral surgery, trauma, or ulcers). ➤*Rationale:* Assesses for contraindications to insertion.
- Assess the patient's hemodynamic, cardiovascular, peripheral vascular, and neurovascular status. ➤*Rationale:* Provides baseline data that can be used for comparison with post-insertion data.
- Determine the patient's baseline pulmonary status. If the patient is mechanically ventilated, note the type of support—ventilator-assisted breathing or continuous positive airway breathing. ➤*Rationale:* Sedation and/or local anesthesia may be needed for probe insertion and tolerance.
- If the patient currently has respiratory compromise or could develop respiratory compromise with the adjunct of conscious sedation, consider mechanical ventilation. ➤*Rationale:* Sedation and/or local anesthesia may be needed for probe insertion and tolerance.
- Assess the patient's current laboratory profile, including electrolytes and coagulation studies. ➤*Rationale:* Baseline coagulation studies are helpful in determining the risk for bleeding. Electrolyte abnormalities may contribute to cardiac irritability.

Patient Preparation

- Ensure that the patient and/or family understand the preprocedural teaching. Answer questions as they arise and reinforce information as needed. ➤*Rationale:* Evaluates and reinforces the understanding of previously taught information.
- Obtain informed consent. ➤*Rationale:* Protects the rights of the patients and makes a competent decision possible for the patient; however, under emergency circumstances, time may not allow for this form to be signed.
- Consider administration of sedation or analgesics as needed. ➤*Rationale:* Decreases anxiety and gagging, with enhanced probe tolerance.

Procedure for Esophageal Doppler Monitoring of Aortic Blood Flow: Probe Insertion

Steps	Rationale	Special Considerations
1. Wash hands.	Reduces the transmission of microorganisms; standard precautions.	
2. Plug the esophageal Doppler monitor into the wall outlet and turn it on.	Provides the energy source.	
3. Connect the interface cable to the esophageal Doppler monitor.	Prepares the equipment.	
4. Connect the esophageal probe to the interface cable.	Prepares the equipment.	
5. When prompted, enter the patient's age, weight, and height into the esophageal Doppler monitor. (If the probe has been used previously, the patient information will appear on the screen. Probes are reusable by the same patient.) Confirm that the correct data are on the screen. A. Turn the control knob to change the values. B. Press the control knob to enter the selected values. C. Push the key pad under the words "accept data". D. If any data are incorrect, press "change data" to return to the nomogram screen and change any data that have been incorrectly entered; then repress the "accept data" key pad.	Prepares the monitor. The monitor will confirm data entry and change to the probe focus mode.	Data must be in the following ranges: Age: 16-99 years Weight: 66-330 pounds Height: 59-83 inches If a patient's data are outside the nomogram limits, estimated values cannot be obtained, but velocity data are available. See manufacturer's recommendations for nomograms.
6. Wash hands and don personal protective equipment.	Reduces the transmission of microorganisms.	
7. Administer sedation if necessary.	Promotes patient comfort during esophageal probe insertion.	The esophageal probe may cause gagging. Topical lidocaine may be used to reduce gagging.
8. Apply a water-based lubricant on 6-10 cm of the distal end of the esophageal probe.	Minimizes mucosal injury and irritation during insertion; facilitates insertion and aids in signal acquisition.	It is important that only water-soluble lubricant be used in probe placement. Oil-soluble lubricant cannot be absorbed through the pulmonary mucosa and may cause respiratory complications should the probe be inadvertently placed in the lungs.
9. Insert the probe orally with the bevel edge toward the hard palate.	Begins the insertion process.	Insertion should never be forced. Forceful insertion can cause mucosal damage to the posterior pharynx or the esophagus.
10. Utilize the depth markings on the esophageal probe to facilitate positioning.	Aides in proper probe depth adjustment.	Proper probe depth is essential to obtain optimal aortic signal. Generally the patient's incisors should be between the 35 cm and the 40 cm length markings.

Procedure	**for Esophageal Doppler Monitoring of Aortic Blood Flow: Probe Insertion**—*Continued*	

Steps	Rationale	Special Considerations
11. Look at the esophageal Doppler monitor and listen for an auditory signal to establish the optimal descending aortic waveform while rotating, inserting, and withdrawing the probe until the ideal waveform appears and is heard as the sharpest audible pitch (see Figs. 67-1 and 68-2). If unable to obtain an aortic waveform, consider that the probe may be in the trachea. Remove the probe and attempt reinsertion.	Enhances the accuracy of the probe position.	The ideal waveform has a black center outlined with red and yellow. The sound pitch should be clear and should correspond with the aortic flow pattern noted on the monitor screen.
12. Press the peak velocity display (PVD) button on the monitor to assess for the greatest peak velocity achieved.	The highest peak velocity is usually associated with the best visual and auditory signal.	Use specific manufacturer's recommendation for PVD (e.g., sharp upstroke with moderately crisp peak to the waveform).
13. Press the filter button to activate the 2.5-cm/sec filter when appropriate.	Eliminates visual and auditory low frequency signals (usually due to excess heart valve or wall motion noise).	Use specific manufacturer's recommendations for noise filters.
14. Press the auto gain button for optimal amplification of the signal.	Optimizes amplification of the waveform.	Use specific manufacturer's recommendations for optimal waveform management.
15. Press the scale button to change the waveform scale.	Aids in visualization of the waveform display.	Use specific manufacturer's recommendations for optimal waveform visualization.
16. If activation of auto gain does not provide parameter display, press "run" after an optimal signal is obtained. A green line called the *follower* should hug the contour of the waveform.	Indicates initiation of monitoring.	A white arrow depicts the beginning and end of systole and the peak velocity of each cycle. Use manufacturer's recommendations for beginning the monitoring process.
17. Record the displayed data from the top of the EDM screen.	Peak velocity (PV) and corrected flow time (FTc) are direct measurements. All other data are calculated from these two measurements along with BSA.	Use specific manufacturer's recommendations for obtaining and recording data.
18. Discard used supplies and wash hands.	Reduces the transmission of microorganisms; standard precautions.	
19. Compare FTc and PV values with normal values (see Fig. 68-1).	Determines hemodynamic status.	

Expected Outcomes

- Accurate placement of the esophageal probe
- Adequate and appropriate waveforms
- Ability to obtain accurate information regarding hemodynamic parameters
- Evaluation of information obtained to guide therapeutic interventions

Unexpected Outcomes

- Oral, pharyngeal, or esophageal mucosal tears, ulceration, or infections
- Hematoma
- Hemorrhage
- Probe placed into the trachea or bronchus
- Vagal response during insertion or from gagging
- Vomiting or aspiration
- Esophageal-tracheal fistula formation

Patient Monitoring and Care

Steps	Rationale	Reportable Conditions
		These conditions should be reported if they persist despite nursing interventions.
1. Perform systematic cardiovascular and neurological assessments before, during, and after the insertion of the probe: • Assess level of consciousness • Assess vital signs • Assess hemodynamic parameters	Obtains baseline data and assesses patient status. Assesses for signs of adequate perfusion. Evaluates patient response to the procedure and medications administered.	• Changes in level of consciousness • Changes in vital signs • Abnormal hemodynamic parameters
2. Monitor the patient's mouth for signs of trauma from the probe insertion.	Identifies skin breakdown.	• Redness, ulceration • Swelling, drainage • Foul odor • Bleeding • Skin breakdown
3. Perform oral care every 2 hours and as needed while the probe is in place. The esophageal probe may be left in place if tolerated; the weight of the probe usually maintains placement.	Oral tubes tend to cause mouth dryness and increase the potential for mucosal breakdown.	• Patient unable to tolerate esophageal probe placement (e.g., inability to relieve gagging)
4. Administer sedatives and analgesics as needed and prescribed.	Promotes patient comfort. Additional sedation may be required for probe tolerance.	• Unrelieved patient discomfort • Anxiety
5. Monitor aortic waveforms while the esophageal probe is in place. Waveforms should be assessed when data collection is needed.	Ensures proper probe placement.	• Abnormal waveforms

Documentation

Documentation should include the following:

- Patient and family education
- Signed informed consent form
- Appearance of waveforms
- Sedatives or analgesia administered
- Hemodynamic data obtained
- Unexpected outcomes
- Interventions

Additional Readings

Cardio Q, Cardiac Function Monitor Operating Manual. (2003). Severna Park, MD: Deltex Medical, Inc.

DiCorte, C.J., et al. (2000). Esophageal Doppler monitor determinations of cardiac output and preload during cardiac operations. *Ann Thoracic Surgery,* 69, 1782-6.

Gan T.J., and Arrowsmith, J.E. (1997). The oesophageal Doppler monitor. *Brit Med J,* 315, 893-4.

Iregui, M.G., et al. (2003). Physician estimates of cardiac index and intravascular volume based on clinical assessment versus transesophageal Doppler measurements obtained by critical care nurses. *Am J Crit Care Nurses,* 12, 336-42.

Singer, M., and Bennett, E.D. (1991). Noninvasive optimization of left ventricular filling using esophageal Doppler. *Crit Care Med,* 19, 1132-7.

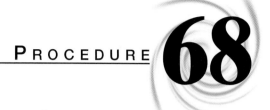
PROCEDURE **68**

Esophageal Doppler Monitoring of Aortic Blood Flow: Care and Removal

P U R P O S E : Esophageal Doppler monitoring of aortic blood flow is used to assess the hemodynamic condition of critically ill patients. Esophageal Doppler monitoring (EDM) uses Doppler ultrasound technology to provide information regarding left ventricular performance and patient fluid status.

Deborah Lamarr
Maureen Turner

PREREQUISITE NURSING KNOWLEDGE

- Knowledge of the cardiovascular anatomy and physiology
- Understanding of the upper gastrointestinal tract anatomy
- Ability to recognize the EDM aortic waveforms by visual display and auditory pitch
- Understanding of normal and associated values aortic waveforms (Fig. 68-1; see Fig. 67-1)

- Understanding of additional waveforms that guide esophageal probe insertion (Fig. 68-2).
- Understanding of the technique and importance of obtaining an optimal signal
- Clinical and technical competence in understanding the esophageal Doppler monitor functions and options
- Corrected flow time (FTc), peak velocity (PV), and minute distance (MD) come directly from the Doppler velocity measurements; stroke volume (SV) and cardiac output (CO)

Normal Ranges*

Corrected Flow Time (FTc)	Peak Velocity (PV)[1,2]	
330-360 milliseconds	**20 years**	**90-120 cm/sec**
* Note: Normal Ranges should not be confused with a Pysiological Target.	30 years	85-115 cm/sec
	40 years	80-110 cm/sec
[1]Singer, M (1993). Esophageal Doppler monitoring of aortic blood flow: beat-by-beat cardiac output monitoring. **Inter Anaesthesia Clin** 31; 99-125. *Normal range values appear in bold.*	**50 years**	**70-100 cm/sec**
	60 years	60-90 cm/sec
[2]Gardin, J.M., Davidson, D.M., Rohan, M.K., et al. Relationship between age, body size, gender, and blood pressure and Doppler flow measurements in the aorta and pulmonary artery, **Am Heart J**, 113; 101-109. *Extrapolated values do not appear in bold.*	**70 years**	**50-80 cm/sec**
	80 years	40-70 cm/sec
	90 years	30-60 cm/sec

FIGURE 68-1 Measured parameters obtained from esophageal Doppler monitoring.

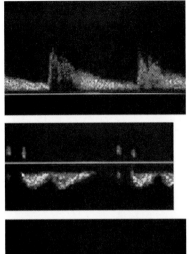

Celiac Axis: Probe too low.

Intracardiac: Correct depth or slightly high. Rotate probe and/or increase depth slightly.

Azygos Vein: Correct depth or slightly low. Rotate probe and/or decrease depth slightly.

FIGURE 68-2 Additional waveforms that guide esophageal probe insertion. *(Adapted from* Cardio Q Reference Guide. *[2003]. Severna Park, MD: Deltex Medical Inc.)*

are derived using an algorithm generated from the patient nomogram information (see Fig. 68-1).

- The base of the waveform is used as a marker of left ventricular preload and displayed as FTc.
- The waveform height is used as a marker of contractility and is displayed as PV.
- MD is the distance (cm) moved by the column of blood through the aorta in 1 minute.
- A narrowed waveform base with decreased FTc may indicate hypovolemia.
- A widened waveform base with increased FTc may indicate euvolemia.
- A reduced waveform height with low PV may indicate left ventricular failure.
- An increased waveform height with increased PV may indicate a hyperdynamic state.
- A reduced waveform height with narrow waveform base may indicate elevation in systemic vascular resistance (SVR).
- Optimal positioning of the probe is essential for accurate data collection (refer to Procedure 67).

EQUIPMENT

- EDM monitor, patient interface cable, power cord
- EDM probe
- Water-soluble lubricant
- Nonsterile gloves, gown, mask, and goggles or face shield
    Additional equipment to have available if needed includes:
- Topical lidocaine
- Sedatives or analgesics as necessary

PATIENT AND FAMILY EDUCATION

- Explain the monitoring and troubleshooting procedures to the patient and family. ➤*Rationale:* Keeps the patient and family informed and reduces anxiety.
- Explain the patients expected participation. ➤*Rationale:* Encourages patient participation.
- Instruct the patient/family of signs and symptoms to report to the critical care nurse and staff, including oral bleeding, sore throat, displacement of the probe. ➤*Rationale:* Encourages patient and families to report changes and problems.

PATIENT ASSESSMENT AND PREPARATION

Patient Assessment

- Assess the patient's current laboratory profile, including coagulation studies. ➤*Rationale:* Coagulation studies are helpful in determining the risk for bleeding.
- Obtain the patient's vital signs and assess cardiovascular status. ➤*Rationale:* Provides baseline data.

Patient Preparation

- Ensure that the patient and/or family understand the pre-procedural teaching. Answer questions as they arise and reinforce information as needed. ➤*Rationale:* Evaluates and reinforces understanding of previously taught information.
- Provide sedation, analgesics, and apply local anesthetics as prescribed. ➤*Rationale:* Decreases anxiety and gagging with probe manipulation.

Procedure	**for Esophageal Doppler Monitoring of Aortic Blood Flow: Care and Removal**

Steps	Rationale	Special Considerations
1. Wash hands and don nonsterile gloves.	Reduces the transmission of microorganisms, standard precautions.	
2. Administer sedation, analgesic, and topical anesthetics as prescribed and as needed.	Promotes patient comfort.	The esophageal monitoring probe can cause gagging.
3. Compare the EDM values to normal values and patient baseline values.	Increases and decreases in both PV or FTc depicts specific hemodynamic physiology.	Follow manufacturer's recommendations for normal values and interpretation. Normal values should not be confused with physiologic targets (see Fig. 68-1).
4. Institute medical therapy (administration of IV fluid or vasoactive agents) as prescribed for the specific values.	Values may show the need for therapy adjustments.	
5. Validate the effectiveness of medical therapy by obtaining values again after the prescribed therapy has been completed.	Values may show the need for therapy adjustments.	It is important the probe is refocused prior to each patient assessment, ensuring an optimal signal.
6. Leave the probe in place throughout therapy adjustments or remove the probe and replace as needed for specific care measurements.	Monitoring can be done on a continuous or intermittent basis.	An advanced practice nurse or a physician may need to adjust the position of the esophageal probe. Follow institution standard.

Finding the Maximum Flow

Steps	Rationale	Special Considerations
1. Adjust the volume control knob on the esophageal Doppler monitor.	Auditory signals are necessary for accurate probe placement.	
2. Grasp the probe gently in one hand.	Manipulates the position of the esophageal probe.	
3. Rotate left and right and then slowly pull back and insert the probe while listening for the sharpest audible pitch associated with the highest peak velocity.	Facilitates locating the appropriate aortic signal.	An advanced practice nurse or a physician may need to adjust the position of the esophageal probe. Follow institution standard. The esophageal probe should be adjusted until the sharpest aortic waveform possible is obtained, in terms of both visual display and audible pitch.

Troubleshooting the Absence of the Aortic Waveform

Steps	Rationale	Special Considerations
1. Check that the probe has not been dislodged by locating the depth markings.	An optimal waveform is obtained when the distance to aortic flow is closest.	
2. Ensure the monitor, cable, and probe are all connected appropriately.	Loose connections will distort values.	
3. Readjust the esophageal probe as needed according to the insertion procedure.	Ensures accurate positioning.	An advanced practice nurse or a physician may need to adjust the position of the esophageal probe. Follow institution standard.

Procedure continues on the following page

Procedure for Esophageal Doppler Monitoring of Aortic Blood Flow: Care and Removal—*Continued*

Steps	Rationale	Special Considerations
Removal of the Esophageal Probe		
1. Wash hands and don nonsterile gloves, gown, mask, and goggles or face shield.	Reduces the transmission of microorganisms; standard precautions.	An advanced practice nurse or a physician may need to remove the esophageal probe. Follow institution standard.
2. Gently pull the esophageal probe from the esophagus and mouth.	The esophageal probe may cause mucosal tears if forcefully removed.	
3. Either discard the probe or place the probe in a clean container or wrap it for future reuse.	Probes may be used on an intermittent or continuous basis.	
4. Discard supplies and wash hands.	Reduces the transmission of organisms; standard precautions.	

Expected Outcomes

- Optimal aortic waveforms
- Absence of oral, pharyngeal, or esophageal injury
- Absence of discomfort from the probe

Unexpected Outcomes

- Presence of aortic waveforms
- Oral, pharyngeal, or esophageal injury
- Probe discomfort and gagging

Patient Monitoring and Care

Steps	Rationale	Reportable Conditions
		These conditions should be reported if they persist despite nursing interventions.
1. Monitor the EDM waveforms while the esophageal probe is in place.	Provides assessment of proper placement of the probe; normal and abnormal waveforms.	• Abnormal waveforms
2. Monitor hemodynamic status as frequently as prescribed and as needed (e.g., SV, CO, CI, SVR, FTc, PV).	Guides appropriate care.	• Changes in hemodynamic monitoring values
3. Assess EDM waveforms and values before and after troubleshooting.	Identifies that troubleshooting has been successful.	• Unsuccessful troubleshooting attempts
4. Perform oral care every 2 hours and as needed while the probe is in place. The esophageal probe may be left in place if tolerated; the weight of the probe usually maintains placement.	Oral tubes tend to cause mouth dryness, which increases the potential for mucosal breakdown.	• Patient unable to tolerate esophageal probe placement (e.g., inability to relieve gagging)
5. Administer sedatives and analgesics as needed and prescribed.	Promotes patient comfort.	• Unrelieved patient discomfort

Documentation

Documentation should include the following:

- Patient and family education
- Appearance of waveforms
- Sedatives or analgesia administered
- Hemodynamic data obtained
- Patient tolerance
- Site assessment
- Occurrences of unexpected outcomes and interventions

Additional Readings

Cardio Q, Cardiac Function Monitor Operating Manual. (2003). Severna Park, MD: Deltex Medical, Inc.

DiCorte, C.J., et al. (2000). Esophageal Doppler monitor determinations of cardiac output and preload during cardiac operations. *Ann Thoracic Surgery,* 69, 1782-6.

Gan Tong, J., and Arrowsmith, J.E. (1997). The oesophageal Doppler monitor. *Brit Med J,* 315, 893-4.

Iregui, M.G., et al. (2003). Physician estimates of cardiac index and intravascular volume based on clinical assessment versus transesophageal Doppler measurements obtained by critical care nurses. *Am J Crit Care Nurses,* 12, 336-42.

Singer, M., and Bennett, E.D. (1991). Noninvasive optimization of left ventricular filling using esophageal Doppler. *Crit Care Med,* 19, 1132-7.

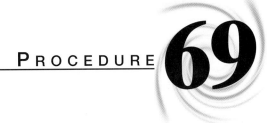
PROCEDURE **69**

Left Atrial Catheter: Care and Assisting With Removal

PURPOSE: The left atrial catheter measures pressure from the left atrium to assess left ventricular function in the postoperative cardiac surgical patient. It also provides information about left-sided intra-cardiac pressure. Hemodynamic information obtained with the left atrial catheter is used to guide therapeutic intervention, including administration of fluids and diuretics and titration of vasoactive and inotropic medications.

Sandra Schlup Woods
Merrie Jackson

PREREQUISITE NURSING KNOWLEDGE

- Knowledge of the cardiovascular anatomy and physiology
- Understanding of basic dysrhythmia recognition and treatment of life-threatening dysrhythmias
- Advanced cardiac life support knowledge and skills
- Understanding of the setup of the hemodynamic monitoring system (see Procedure 75)
- Understanding of hemodynamic monitoring (see Procedure 72)
- Understanding of principles of aseptic technique
- The left atrial pressure (LAP) waveform is configured similarly to that of a pulmonary artery wedge pressure waveform (Fig. 69-1).
- Understanding of *a, c,* and *v* waves is necessary. The *a* wave reflects left atrial contraction. The *c* wave reflects closure of the mitral valve. The *v* wave reflects passive filling of the left atrium during left ventricular systole.
- The LAP is measured with a polyvinyl catheter placed in the left atrium during cardiac surgery. The left atrial catheter can be inserted via a needle puncture of the right superior pulmonary vein, with subsequent threading into the left atrium, or it can be inserted via a direct cannulation of the left atrium through a needle puncture at the intraatrial groove.[7]
- LAP monitoring may be used[2] in the following situations:
  - ❖ For patients with prosthetic tricuspid or pulmonic valves, in whom pulmonary artery catheters are contraindicated

  - ❖ For patients with abnormal heart anatomy (e.g., those with a single ventricle or tricuspid atresia)
  - ❖ For patients with high pulmonary artery pressures, which may interfere with the accuracy of the pulmonary artery wedge pressure
  - ❖ To provide accurate information when vasoconstriction medications are infused in conjunction with pulmonary vasodilator medications
  - ❖ For patient monitoring after cardiac transplantation.

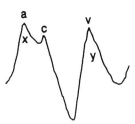

FIGURE 69-1 LAP (left atrial pressure) waveform and its components: *a* wave—the presystolic wave resulting from atrial contraction; *x* descent—the down slope of the *a* wave caused by atrial relaxation; *c* wave—a sharp inflection caused by mitral valve closure; *v* wave—an atrial pressure wave rising to a peak during late ventricular systole caused by filling of the atrium while the mitral valve is closed; *y* descent—the down slope of the *v* wave caused by early diastolic runoff through the mitral valve. Changes in the waveform configuration may indicate valve or myocardial disease. For example, an elevated *a* wave is seen in mitral stenosis and an elevated *v* wave in mitral insufficiency. Both the *a* and *v* waves are elevated in cardiac tamponade.

- The normal LAP is 4 to 12 mm Hg.
- One danger of using this catheter is the potential for air or a blood clot emboli to enter the left atrium and be carried to the brain or other body organs. Close attention to the hemodynamic monitoring system and assessment of the waveform is imperative.

EQUIPMENT

- Left atrial catheter (inserted in the operating room)
- Hemodynamic monitoring system (Refer to Procedure 75)
- Sterile dressing supplies
- Indelible marker
- Nonsterile gloves
- Gown, goggles or face shield
  Additional equipment to have available, if needed, includes the following:
- Air filter (institution-specific) between the left atrial (LA) catheter and the pressure transducer tubing

PATIENT AND FAMILY EDUCATION

- Assess the patient and family understanding of LAP monitoring. ➤➤*Rationale:* Provides information about patient and family knowledge.

- Discuss the purpose of the catheter. ➤➤*Rationale:* Informs the patient and family and may decrease anxiety.
- Discuss with the patient and family the location of the catheter and the importance of not touching this line or putting tension on this line. ➤➤*Rationale:* Prevents line contamination and inadvertent line removal.

PATIENT ASSESSMENT AND PREPARATION

Patient Assessment

- Assess the patient's hemodynamic, cardiovascular, peripheral vascular, and neurovascular status. ➤➤*Rationale:* Provides baseline data that can be used to compare with the LAP.
- Assess the patient's current laboratory values profile, including coagulation studies. ➤➤*Rationale:* Identifies laboratory value abnormalities. Baseline coagulation studies are helpful in determining the risk for bleeding.

Patient Preparation

- Ensure that the patient and family understand teaching. Answer questions as they arise and reinforce information as needed. ➤➤*Rationale:* Evaluates and reinforces understanding of previously taught information.
- Consider sedation. ➤➤*Rationale:* An agitated or restless patient could accidentally pull the LA line out.

Procedure	for Care of the Left Atrial Catheter

Steps	Rationale	Special Considerations
1. Wash hands.	Reduces the transmission of microorganisms; standard precautions.	
2. Check the hemodynamic monitoring system for the following (refer to Procedure 75): A. Flush bag has solution. B. Maintain pressure in the flush bag at 300 mm Hg.	Ensures that the hemodynamic monitoring system is set up appropriately. Maintains catheter patency. At 300 mm Hg, the flush system will deliver 1-3 ml/hr to maintain patency of the system.	The LA hemodynamic monitoring system is set up in the operating room. **Do not use rapid flush technique to ensure patency—this may introduce air into the line/system. The LA line should be flushed only by a physician.**
C. Connections are tight. D. The entire system is air-free.	Maintains enclosed, sterile system. Reduces the risk for air embolization.	
3. Connect the pressure cable from the left atrial transducer to the bedside monitor.	Connects the LA catheter to the bedside monitoring system.	
4. Set the scale on the bedside monitor for LAP monitoring.	Permits waveform analysis.	The scale for LAP is commonly set at 20 mm Hg.
5. Level the left atrial air-fluid interface (zeroing stopcock) to the phlebostatic axis (see Procedure 75).	The phlebostatic axis approximates the level of the atria and should be used as the reference point for patients in the supine position.	The reference point for the atria changes when a patient is in the lateral position (see Procedure 75).

Procedure continues on the following page

Procedure for Care of the Left Atrial Catheter—*Continued*

Steps	Rationale	Special Considerations
6. Secure the system to the IV pole, patient's chest, or arm.	Ensures that the air-fluid interface (zeroing stopcock) is maintained at the level of the phlebostatic axis. If the air-fluid interface is above the phlebostatic axis, the LAP will be falsely low. If the air-fluid interface is below the phlebostatic axis, the LAP will be falsely high.	The point of the phlebostatic axis should be marked with an indelible marker.
7. Zero the left atrial hemodynamic monitoring system (see Procedure 75).	Zeroing negates the effects of atmospheric pressure.	
8. Position the patient in the supine position with the head of the bed from 0 to 45 degrees.	Ensures the accuracy of the LAP.	Refer to Procedure 75: Single and Multiple Pressure Transducer Systems for more information on lateral and prone positioning. Research for positioning has been conducted on PA catheters, not LA lines.
9. Run a dual-channel strip of the ECG and the left atrial waveform.	The LAP should be determined from the graphic strip as the effect of ventilation can be identified.	
10. Measure the LAP at end-expiration.	Measurement is most accurate as the effects of pulmonary pressures are minimized.	
11. Using the dual-channel–recorded strip, draw a vertical line from the beginning of the P wave of one of the ECG complexes down to the LAP waveform. Repeat this with the next ECG complex.	Compares electrical activity with mechanical activity. Three waveforms will be present between the two lines drawn.	
12. Align the end of a QRS complex of the ECG strip with the LAP waveform.	Compares electrical activity with mechanical activity.	
13. Identify the *a* wave.	The *a* wave correlates with the end of the QRS complex. The *c* wave (mitral valve closure) correlates with the ST segment, and the *v* wave (ventricular systole) follows the *c* wave and correlates with the T-P interval.	
14. Measure the mean of the *a* wave to obtain the LAP.	The *a* wave represents left atrial contraction as the left ventricle is filled during diastole.	If the patient's positive end-expiratory pressure (PEEP) is more than 10 ml H_2O, adjustments in determining the pressure may be necessary.
15. Set alarms. Upper and lower alarm limits are set on the basis of the patient's current clinical status and the LAP values.	Activates the bedside and central alarm system.	
16. Continuously monitor the waveform for any changes (overdamping, left ventricular waveform, or absence of a waveform) and correlate with changes in physical findings.	Indicates problems with the LA catheter that require troubleshooting.	Overdamping may be caused by a hypovolemic state, air in the system, or a clot in the catheter. The presence of a left ventricular waveform (Fig. 69-2) indicates that the catheter has migrated into the left ventricle.

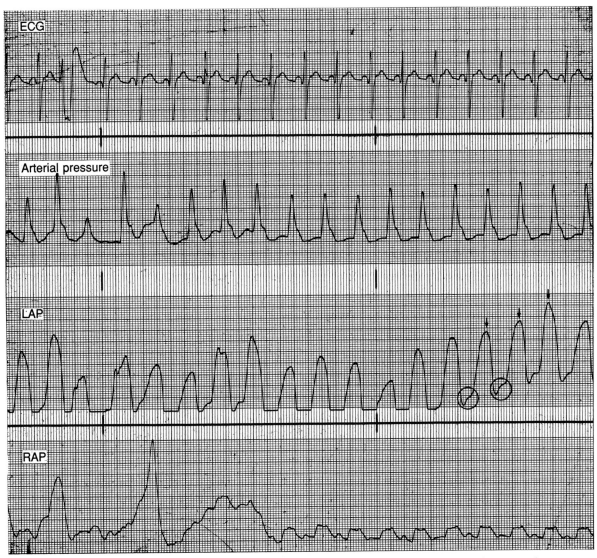

FIGURE 69-2 LAP catheter that has slipped into the left ventricle (LV). Note anacrotic notch on upstroke of LV waveform (*circled*). Note also that paper was not calibrated in this example. *LAP,* left atrial pressure; *ECG,* electrocardiogram; *RAP,* right atrial pressure.

Procedure	**for Care of the Left Atrial Catheter**—*Continued*	
Steps	**Rationale**	**Special Considerations**
		Cardiac arrest, a clotted catheter, a perforated left ventricle, or a problem within the hemodynamic monitoring system may cause an absent waveform. **It is important in all of these situations *not* to irrigate the catheter.**[8]
17. **Do not use the LA catheter for blood withdrawal, administration of medications, or IV therapy. The catheter is for pressure monitoring.**	Each time the left atrial line is entered, there is a significant risk for introducing air emboli or bacteria directly into the heart.	
18. Wash hands.	Reduces the transmission of microorganisms; standard precautions.	

Procedure | for Assisting With Removal of the Left Atrial Catheter

Steps	Rationale	Special Considerations
1. Wash hands and don nonsterile gloves, gown, and goggles or face shield.	Reduces the transmission of microorganisms; standard precautions.	
2. Position the patient in the supine position.	Prepares the patient and provides access to the site.	
3. Turn off the LAP alarm.	Monitoring no longer needed.	
4. Turn the stopcock off to the patient.	Turns off the administration of flush solution and stops hemodynamic monitoring.	
5. Remove the dressing.	Prepares for LA catheter removal.	
6. Clip the sutures if present.	Frees the LA catheter for removal.	
7. Assist the physician or advanced practice nurse as needed with catheter removal and hold firm pressure on the site.	Provides assistance if needed.	
8. Apply a sterile, occlusive dressing to the site.	Decreases the risk for infection until the insertion site has healed.	
9. Dispose of used supplies and wash hands.	Reduces the transmission of microorganisms; standard precautions.	

Expected Outcomes

- Normal cerebral, myocardial, and peripheral perfusion
- LAP readings that correlate with physical findings
- Normal LAP value (4 to 12 mm Hg)
- LAP catheter removed when prescribed

Unexpected Outcomes

- Infection
- Hemorrhage at removal site
- Air embolus
- Cardiac tamponade caused by LA line removal.
- Retention, migration, or embolization of the catheter[4]

Patient Monitoring and Care

Steps	Rationale	Reportable Conditions
		These conditions should be reported if they persist despite nursing interventions.
1. Continuously monitor the LA waveform and obtain pressure measurements every hour and as needed.	Identifies trends in monitoring.	• Abnormal LAP values and waveforms
2. Monitor the LAP hemodynamic monitoring system every 1 to 2 hours for integrity of the system and for presence of air bubbles in the system.	Could result in air embolism. If air is observed, it must be removed immediately.	• Air in the system that requires assistance with removal
3. Zero the system at the time of the patient's admission to the intensive care unit (ICU), if the transducer and the monitoring cable become disconnected, if the monitoring cable and the monitor become disconnected, and when the values obtained do not fit the clinical picture.	Ensures the accuracy of the hemodynamic monitoring system; minimizes the risk for contamination of the system.	

Patient Monitoring and Care—*Continued*

Steps	Rationale	Reportable Conditions
4. Change hemodynamic monitoring system (flush solution, pressure tubing, transducer, and stopcock) every 96 hours. (*Level V: Clinical studies in more than one or two different patient populations and situations to support recommendations.*)	The Centers for Disease Control and Prevention (CDC)[5] and research findings[4,5] recommend that the hemodynamic flush system can be used safely for 96 hours. This recommendation is based on research conducted with disposable pressure monitoring systems used for peripheral and central lines. No studies report this data specific to left atrial catheters.	
5. Follow institution standard for frequency and type of dressing change.	Decreases the risk for infection at the catheter site. The CDC[5] has made no recommendations for the frequency of routine LA catheter dressing changes. For central lines, the CDC recommends replacing transparent dressings when they become damp, loosened, or soiled, when inspection of the site is necessary, and/or every 7 days. Gauze dressings are to be changed every 2 days.	
6. Follow institution standard for application of antimicrobial ointment to the LA catheter site.	Routine use of antimicrobial ointment at central venous catheter insertion sites is not recommended, because of the potential to promote fungal infections and antimicrobial resistance.[1,5] Specific data are not available related to LA catheter sites.	
7. Before removal of the LA catheter, assess the patient's prothrombin time (PT), partial thromboplastin time (PTT), International Normalized Ratio (INR), and platelet levels.	Ensures that the patient will not have any difficulty forming a clot at the LA insertion site after its removal. Failure to form a clot can lead to cardiac tamponade. PT, PTT, and INR values should be normal before the catheter is removed. Platelet count should be at least 60,000/mm^3 before the catheter is removed.	• Abnormal coagulation results
8. After removal of the LA catheter, follow these steps: • Maintain bed rest for 2 hours. • Monitor vital signs, chest tube drainage, and heart sounds every 15 minutes × 4, then every 30 minutes × 2, then again in 1 hour.	Changes in vital signs and bleeding from the chest tube (greater than 100 ml/hr) suggest that the insertion site did not clot and that the patient is hemorrhaging.	• Tachycardia • Hypotension • Increased chest tube bleeding • Cessation of chest tube bleeding • Narrowing of pulse pressure • Muffled heart sounds

Documentation

Documentation should include the following:

- Patient and family education
- Left atrial pressure waveform recording strip (identify the *a* and *v* waves, inspiration and expiration, and the location where the LAP value was determined)
- Amount of intake of flush solution
- Assessment of the dressing or catheter insertion site or both
- Unexpected outcomes
- Additional interventions

References

1. Akl, B.F., et al. (1984). Unusual complication of direct left atrial pressure monitoring line. *J Thorac Cardiovasc Surg,* 88, 1033-35.
2. Bojar, R.M. (1999). *Manual of Perioperative Care in Cardiac and Thoracic Surgery,* 3rd edition, Malden, MA: Blackwell Sciences, 116-118.
3. Ducharme, F.M., et al. (1988). Incidence of infection related to arterial catheterization in children: A prospective study. *Crit Care Med,* 16, 272-76.
4. Luskin, R.L., et al. (1986). Extended use of disposable pressure transducers: A bacteriologic evaluation. *JAMA,* 255, 916-20.
5. O'Grady, N.P., et al. (2002). Guidelines for the prevention of intravascular catheter-related infections. *Am J Infection Control,* 30, 476-89.
6. O'Mailley, M.K., et al. (1994). Value of routine pressure monitoring system changes after 72 hours of use. *Crit Care Med,* 22, 1424-30.
7. Recker, D.H. (1985). Procedure for left atrial catheter insertion. *Crit Care Nurse,* 5, 36-41.
8. Taylor, T. (1986). Monitoring left atrial pressures in the open-heart surgical patient. *Crit Care Nurse,* 6, 62-8.

Additional Readings

Ahrens, T.S., and Taylor, L.A. (1992). *Hemodynamic Waveform Analysis.* Philadelphia: W.B. Saunders.
Leitman, B.S., et al. (1992). The left atrial catheter: Its uses and complications. *Radiology,* 185, 611-12.
Rao, P.S., Sathyanarayana, P.V. (1993). Transseptal insertion of left atrial line: A simple and safe technique. *Ann Thorac Surg,* 55, 785-86.
Santini, F., et al. (1999). Routine left atrial catheterization for the post-operative management of cardiac surgical patients: Is the risk justified? *Eur J Cardiothoracic Surg,* 16, 218-21.
Yeo, T.C., et al. (1998). Retained left atrial catheter: An unusual cardiac source of embolism identified by transesophageal echocardiography. *J Am Soc Echocardiogr* 11, 66-70.

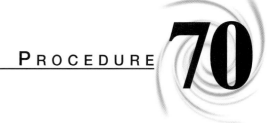

PROCEDURE **70**

Noninvasive Hemodynamic Monitoring: Impedance Cardiography

P U R P O S E : Impedance cardiography is a continuous, non-invasive method to obtain hemodynamic data (cardiac output, afterload, and contractility) and assess thoracic fluid status.

Kathryn T. Von Rueden
Kevin B. Wagner
Paul R. Jansen

PREREQUISITE NURSING KNOWLEDGE

- Knowledge of the normal cardiovascular anatomy and physiology
- Understanding of the principles of hemodynamic monitoring
- Impedance (Z) is resistance to flow of electrical current. Impedance cardiography (ICG) measures electrical resistance changes in the thorax using four sets of external electrodes to input a high-frequency, low-amplitude current (similar to an apnea monitor). Fluids, such as blood and plasma, are good conductors of electricity and result in lower impedance. These electrodes also receive the patient ECG signal.
- Blood volume and flow velocity increases and decreases in the ascending aorta during systole and diastole, respectively. Pulsatile flow generates electrical impedance changes. Impedance to electrical current decreases during systole as a result of increased blood volume, flow velocity, and alignment of red blood cells. Thus the measurement of the magnitude and velocity of impedance changes directly reflect ascending aortic blood flow and left ventricular function.
- The dZ/dt (change in impedance/change in time) waveform depicts the change in impedance related to time and is similar to the aortic blood flow waveform (Fig. 70-1).
- Stable, noise-free ECG and ICG waveforms are requirements for reliable monitoring.
- Z_o is the measurement of the base or average thoracic impedance and reflects all of the fluid in the thorax. Its inverse, thoracic fluid content (TFC) is a clinical

parameter used to describe the overall thoracic fluid status. Greater amounts of fluid in the intravascular, interstitial, or intracellular spaces reduce thoracic electrical impedance and increase the TFC. Because intravascular blood volume is relatively constant, an increase in TFC usually reflects alveolar and interstitial edema; however, bleeding in the chest or pleural effusions also will increase the TFC value. Normal TFC and Z_o ranges may vary slightly by manufacturer. Typically, normal TFC

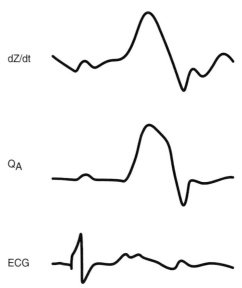

FIGURE 70-1 Relationship of dZ/dt impedance waveform, ascending aortic blood flow tracing (Q_A), and ECG. *(Courtesy Noninvasive Medical Technologies, Inc., formerly Renaissance Technology, Inc.)*

ranges from 30 to 50/k ohms in adult males; women tend to have slightly lower values than men (21 to 37/k ohms).

- Myocardial contractility is assessed by the dZ/dt, velocity index (VI) and acceleration contractility index (ACI) values. Both VI and ACI are measured from the upslope of the dZ/dt waveform during systole and indexed by the base impedance (Z_o). Normal range for VI is 33-65/1000 sec. Normal range of ACI is 70-150/100 sec² for males and 90-170/100 sec² for females.[26] Normal range of dZ/dt is 0.8 to 2.5 ohms/sec. Higher values of all these parameters reflect enhanced left ventricular contractility.
- TFC, VI, mean arterial pressure (MAP), central venous pressure (CVP), and the electrocardiogram (ECG) are used in the calculations of impedance-based hemodynamic parameters.
- Impedance-based cardiac output is calculated from stroke volume and heart rate. Precise determination of the aortic valve opening and closing (ventricular ejection time) and the maximum point of blood flow velocity (dZ/dt$_{max}$) are essential for accurate stroke volume measurement[16,23,24,26] (Fig. 70-2).
- Table 70-1 lists the ICG hemodynamic and thoracic fluid parameters, definitions, and normal values.
- Indications for hemodynamic monitoring using ICG are varied.[12,28] Primary indications include the following:
  - Potential for or signs and symptoms of pulmonary or cardiovascular dysfunction[2,9,22,25]
  - Evaluation of a patient's thoracic fluid and hemodynamic status in locations outside of areas that can provide the close observation required for invasive hemodynamic monitoring[4,5,14,19,22]
  - Evaluation and differentiation of cardiac or pulmonary cause of shortness of breath[14,19,20]
  - Evaluation of etiology and management of hypotension or hypoperfusion[2,14,22]

- Evaluation and titration of pharmacologic therapy[7,14,21]
- Evaluation of myocardial contractility and diagnosis of rejection following cardiac transplantation[29]
- Indication and justification for use of more invasive hemodynamic monitoring, such as a pulmonary artery catheter[22,26,28]
- Hemodynamic monitoring following discontinuation of a pulmonary artery catheter[22,26,28]
- Adjustment of pacemaker rate and atrioventricular delay timing to optimize stroke volume and cardiac output[17,18]
- Contraindication to impedance cardiography monitoring: The ICG monitor should not be used for patients with minute ventilation (impedance-based) pacemakers that regulate heart rate based on respiration rate sensed through changes in impedance. In this situation, the ICG impedance current interferes with the pacemaker impedance current and may cause pacemaker rate acceleration.[1]

EQUIPMENT

- Impedance cardiography monitor
- Impedance cardiography monitor cable
- ICG electrodes (4 dual ICG and ECG electrodes); additional ECG leads required by some manufacturers
- Blood pressure measuring device (to obtain systemic vascular resistance)
- Washcloth, soap, and water or cleansing pads
- Nonsterile gloves

Additional equipment to have available as needed includes the following:
- Slave cable for blood pressure monitor
- Thoracic calipers, as determined and provided by manufacturer
- Skin preparation solution, such as skin barrier or tincture of benzoin
- Scissors to clip hair from neck or chest

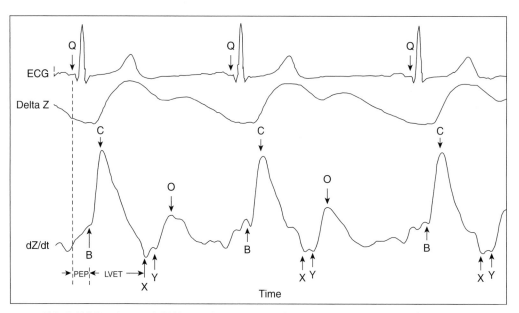

FIGURE 70-2 ECG and normal dZ/dt waveform. *Q*, start of ventricular depolarization; *B*, opening of aortic and pulmonic valves; *C*, maximum deflection of dZ/dt (dZ/dt$_{max}$); *X*, closure of aortic valve; *Y*, closure of pulmonic valve; *O*, mitral opening snap and early ventricular diastolic filling. (*Courtesy Cardiodynamics International, Inc.*)

TABLE 70-1 Impedance Cardiography Hemodynamic and Thoracic Fluid Parameters		
Parameter	**Definition**	**Normal Values**
Cardiac output (CO)	CO: liters of blood flow/min from left ventricle	4-8 L/min
Cardiac index (CI)	CI: CO/body surface area (m^2)	2.8-4.2 L/min/m^2
Stroke volume (SV)	SV: blood volume ejected/beat from left ventricle	60-100 ml/beat
SV index (SVI)	SVI: stroke volume/body surface area	35-75 ml/m^2/beat
Systemic vascular resistance (SVR)	SVR: afterload, resistance to ejection of blood during left ventricular contraction	900-1600 dynes sec/cm^{-5}
SVR index (SVRI)	SVRI: SVR/body surface area	1970-2390 dynes sec/cm^{-5}/m^2
Change in impedance/time (dZ/dt)	Magnitude and rate of impedance change; a direct reflection of force of left ventricular contraction	0.8-2.5 ohms/sec
Velocity index (VI)	Peak velocity of blood flow in the aorta, direct reflection of force of left ventricular contraction $VI = dZ/dt/Z_o/sec$	33-65/1000 sec
Acceleration contractility index (ACI)	Direct reflection of myocardial contractility, initial acceleration of blood flow in the aorta, which occurs within the first 10-20 milliseconds after the opening of the aortic valve (ACI is the second derivative of dZ/dt)	Males: 70-150/100 sec^2 Females: 90-170/100 sec^2
Pre-ejection period (PEP)	Systolic time interval, measuring length of time for isovolumetric contraction, from ECG Q wave to opening of aortic valve, the ICG waveform B point	0.05-0.12 sec; depends on HR, preload, and contractility
Ventricular ejection time (VET)	Systolic time interval, measuring the length of time for left ventricular ejection, from the opening (B point) to closing of aortic valve (ICG × point)	0.25-0.35 sec; depends on HR, preload, and contractility
Left cardiac work (LCW)	An indicator of the amount of work the left ventricle must perform to pump blood each minute	5.4-10 kg m
Left cardiac work index (LCWI)	LCW normalized for body surface area	3.0-5.5 kg m/m^2
Thoracic fluid content status (Z_o)	Base thoracic impedance; the electrical conductivity of the chest cavity, which is primarily determined by the intravascular, intra-alveolar, and interstitial fluids in the thorax; lower Z_o indicates a greater volume of thoracic fluid	Males, 20-30 ohms Females, 25-35 ohms (normal ranges may vary slightly by manufacturer)
Thoracic fluid content (TFC)	The inverse of Z_o ($1/Z_o$ × 1000); the electrical conductivity of the chest cavity, which is primarily determined by the intravascular, intra-alveolar, and interstitial fluids in the thorax; reflects intravascular, interstitial, alveolar, and intracellular fluid. Higher TFC indicates greater thoracic fluid volume.	Males: 30-50/k ohms Females: 21-37/k ohms (normal ranges may vary slightly by manufacturer)

ECG, Electrocardiogram.

PATIENT AND FAMILY EDUCATION

- Explain the purpose of monitoring thoracic fluid and hemodynamic status. ➤*Rationale:* Enhances the understanding of the importance of physiologic assessment and monitoring and may reduce anxiety.
- Explain that four sets of impedance electrodes are placed on the neck and thorax and connected to the leads. ➤*Rationale:* Decreases patient anxiety and elicits cooperation during electrode placement.
- Explain that impedance cardiography monitoring poses no risks or complications and causes no discomfort for the patient. Leads may limit mobility, and electrodes may cause discomfort when removed from the skin. ➤*Rationale:* Decreases patient anxiety.

PATIENT ASSESSMENT AND PREPARATION

Patient Assessment

- Obtain the patient's vital signs and complete a cardiovascular assessment. ➤*Rationale:* Collects baseline data.

- Assess the patient's ability to lie supine with the head of the bed less than 30 degrees for 3 to 5 minutes during placement of the ICG electrodes. ➤*Rationale:* The patient may not tolerate the supine position due to pain, discomfort, or difficulty breathing.

Patient Preparation

- Ensure that the patient understands preprocedural teaching. Answer questions as they arise and reinforce information as needed. ➤*Rationale:* Evaluates and reinforces understanding of previously taught information.
- Place the patient supine with the head of the bed elevated no more than 30 degrees for electrode placement. ➤*Rationale:* Proper electrode placement and hemodynamic assessment is achieved with the patient in a flat supine, or nearly flat supine position. Alternative positions are standing or sitting upright at 90 degrees.
- Prepare the skin for placement of electrodes by cleaning the skin with soap and water or cleaning with an alcohol pad, and using a pad to abrade the skin. If necessary, clip body hair. ➤*Rationale:* Improves ICG electrode adherence required for optimum signal transmission.

Procedure for Noninvasive Hemodynamic Monitoring

Steps	Rationale	Special Considerations
1. Wash hands and don nonsterile gloves.	Reduces the transmission of microorganisms; standard precautions.	
2. Turn on the ICG monitor and enter the patient data: A. Name B. Height and weight C. Gender D. CVP or RAP (or use default CVP value) E. Blood pressure F. If required by the manufacturer, thoracic length, measured using thoracic calipers	Data are used to calculate hemodynamic parameters and indexed values, such as cardiac index and stroke volume index.	A noninvasive blood pressure device may be "slaved" into the ICG monitor for automatic blood pressure and systemic vascular resistance (SVR) updates, thus making manual entry of blood pressure unnecessary. Data entry requirements may vary by manufacturer. Follow instructions from the manufacturer to obtain the thoracic length measurement as required when using some models.
3. Ensure that the patient is in the supine position with the head of the bed elevated no more than 30 degrees.	A flat or near flat position straightens the torso and affords better exposure for accurate electrode placement. Hemodynamic values are position-dependent. Normal hemodynamic values apply only to patients in the supine position.	Options for patients who do not tolerate the nearly supine position include sitting upright at 90 degrees or standing. It is important to document body position when interpreting hemodynamic values so that the proper hemodynamic assessment can be attained.
4. Apply the two sets of upper thoracic ICG electrodes (Fig. 70-3).	The upper ICG electrode sets are placed to define the upper limit	Proper placement of the ICG electrodes above the juncture of the

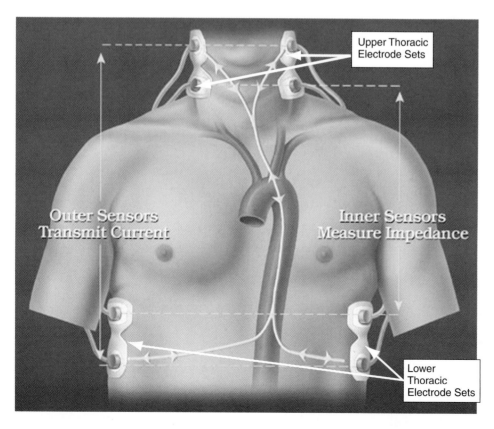

FIGURE 70-3 Placement of thoracic impedance electrodes. *(Courtesy Cardiodynamics International, Inc.)*

Procedure for Noninvasive Hemodynamic Monitoring—*Continued*

Steps	Rationale	Special Considerations
Apply each electrode set on opposite sides of the neck in line with the ears. Ensure that the bottom of the electrode is not lower than the junction of the shoulders at the base of the neck.	of the thorax. Electrodes should be placed 180 degrees opposite from each other to obtain an optimal signal and accurate measurements.	shoulder and neck is critical to accurate data acquisition.[6,8,11,15]
5. Apply the lower two sets of ICG electrodes (see Fig. 70-3). Apply each lower electrode set along the midaxillary line with the top portion of the electrode at the level of xiphoid process.	The lower ICG electrode sets are placed to define the lower limits of the thorax. Electrode sets should be placed 180 degrees opposite from each other to obtain optimal signal and accurate measurements. Proper electrode placement is essential for acquisition of accurate hemodynamic and thoracic fluid status data.[6,8,11,15]	ICG electrodes are typically placed on opposite sides at the base of the neck and lateral from the sternal-xiphoid junction. Dressings or skin tears may necessitate rotating electrode placement to a more anterior to posterior position. If using an alternative electrode placement method, locate the sternal-xiphoid junction and place the second set of lower thoracic electrodes *directly lateral to* that point, 180 degrees opposite the initially placed set.
6. Attach the upper and lower ICG electrode sets to the appropriate leads as noted on the lead array.	Prepares the equipment.	Electrodes may be attached to the leads prior to electrode placement.
7. Observe the ICG and the ECG waveforms displayed on the monitor.	Accurate hemodynamic calculations are dependent on artifact-free ICG and ECG signals.	

Troubleshooting
1. Display screen does not show ECG or ICG waveforms.
   A. Ensure the power source is hospital-grade, grounded outlet.
   B. Ensure all "power" or "on" switches are activated.
   C. Ensure the electrodes are in direct contact with the skin.
   D. Ensure leads are properly connected to the electrodes and ICG monitor.

2. There is excessive noise or 60-cycle interference on the ECG or ICG waveforms.
  A. Ensure the power source is hospital-grade, grounded outlet.
  B. Eliminate nonhospital-grade equipment plugged into the same outlet.
  C. Ensure the electrodes are in direct contact with the skin.
  D. Ensure the leads are properly connected to the electrodes and ICG monitor.
  E. Ask the patient to momentarily hold still to eliminate possible motion artifact as a cause of interference.
	Electrodes need to be in direct contact with skin that is free of hair and not placed over dressings or tape in order to allow ICG signal transmission via the electrode surface.	Skin preparation for ICG electrode placement is based on the same principles that apply to skin preparation for typical ECG monitoring (see Procedure 54).

Procedure continues on the following page

Procedure for Noninvasive Hemodynamic Monitoring—*Continued*

Steps	Rationale	Special Considerations
3. There is a small, damped ICG waveform. A. Verify proper ICG electrode placement and skin contact. B. Assess TFC for extremely high values and VI for extremely low values. C. Options after initial troubleshooting: (1) Continue monitoring; VI will increase as thoracic fluid status improves and TFC decreases with appropriate interventions. (2) Consider invasive means to obtain hemodynamic data.	Extremely high TFC that occurs with a large volume of thoracic fluid may alter the signal to noise ratio and may dampen the ICG waveform.[22]	Inability to obtain ICG hemodynamic data may be considered an indication for invasive hemodynamic monitoring; for example, insertion of a pulmonary artery catheter.[22,26,28]
4. ICG data do not correspond to patient clinical presentation. A. Verify correct electrode placement. B. Ensure good electrode contact with the skin. C. Ensure that the leads are properly connected to all electrodes. D. Validate that the correct patient height, weight, and gender have been entered.	Accurate electrode placement is critical to reliable hemodynamic data acquisition. Since hemodynamic parameters cannot be accurately estimated from physical assessment, rely on ICG hemodynamic values if electrodes and leads are properly applied and the signal quality is good.	
E. Update the blood pressure or mean arterial pressure (MAP) to update the SVR calculation.	The cardiac output and SVR are updated continuously or recalculated by the ICG monitor. The displayed SVR may be erroneous if the blood pressure has changed and the current SVR is calculated based on a blood pressure or MAP that may have been entered several hours before.	Blood pressure should be routinely updated in the monitor if a noninvasive blood pressure monitoring device is not "slaved" into the ICG monitor.
F. Update the CVP pressure in the ICG monitor if large changes (e.g., greater than 10 mm Hg) have occurred in the CVP or the patient has become hypotensive.	Although the CVP has minimal impact on the SVR in most situations, if a patient is hypotensive with a low MAP (e.g., less than 60 mm Hg) and has a high CVP greater than 15 mm Hg, the SVR calculation will be affected and the CVP should be updated.	CVP entered into the monitor may be measured from a CVP catheter or from assessment of the height of the jugular vein pulsation. CVP entered into the ICG monitor must be in mm Hg.

Expected Outcomes

- Generation of reliable, continuous hemodynamic and thoracic fluid status parameters
- Hemodynamic and thoracic fluid data incorporated into patient assessment, diagnosis, prognosis, and therapeutic management

Unexpected Outcome

- Hemodynamic parameters do not reflect clinical presentation.

Patient Monitoring and Care

Steps	Rationale	Reportable Conditions
		These conditions should be reported if they persist despite nursing interventions.

1. Assess baseline and trends in thoracic fluid status (TFC or Z_o) every 1 to 2 hours. Normal values:
    Men: Z_o = 20-30 ohms
          TFC = 30-50/k ohms
    Women: Z_o = 25-35 ohms
            TFC = 21-37/k ohms
(TFC is the inverse of Z_o)
	Men tend to have slightly higher TFC than women due to anthropometric differences.[13] TFC greater than 50/k ohms, in most patients, is indicative of increased thoracic fluid. Rapid TFC increase may be due to intrathoracic bleeding. Gradual increase may be associated with pulmonary edema or pleural or pericardial effusion. Rapid TFC decrease may be due to pneumothorax. Gradual decrease is an expected response to diuretic therapy and reduction of preload, or a reduction in afterload or improved left ventricular contractility, which facilitates forward flow through the pulmonary vasculature and reduce pulmonary congestion. A TFC increase necessitates an evaluation of cardiac output, preload, afterload, and contractility to establish the cause of thoracic fluid accumulation, cardiac or noncardiac origin. Acute pulmonary edema and heart failure exacerbation are associated with higher TFC values.[14,19] A normal TFC (or Z_o) and cardiac index in the presence of respiratory distress may indicate a pulmonary cause of shortness of breath, rather than cardiac origin.	• A TFC increase, indicating increased thoracic fluid accumulation
		• No change in TFC following therapy to relieve pulmonary vascular congestion

2. Assess baseline and trends in continuously displayed cardiac output (CO) or cardiac index (CI) every 1 to 2 hours: Normal CO: 4-8 L/min Normal CI: 2.8-4.2 L/min/m^2 Formula: CO = SV × HR CI = CO/body surface area	Cardiac output and cardiac index are global reflections of cardiac function. Changes in or abnormal CO/CI are related to altered heart rate, preload, afterload, or contractility. Evaluate the determinants of CO/CI to establish the cause of a change and institute appropriate interventions.	• Per institution's standard hemodynamic guidelines; for example, new or continued CO less than 3.5 L/min or CI less than 2.2 L/min/m^2 or sustained cardiac index decrease of 0.5 L/min/m^2 (unrelated to sedation, analgesia, or sleep) assess and report or initiate management protocol • Negligible or absent desired or expected response to therapy
3. Assess baseline and trends in preload by evaluating stroke volume (SV) every 1 to 2 hours: Measure and note SV change.	Preload is ventricular end-diastolic volume. Although direct measurement of preload is not possible with ICG,	• Based on preload assessment, new-onset hypovolemia or left ventricular dysfunction, especially when associated with a reduction in CI

Procedure continues on the following page

Patient Monitoring and Care—*Continued*

Steps	Rationale	Reportable Conditions
Normal SV: 60-100 ml Normal SV index: 35-75 ml/beat/m^2 Formula: SV = VI × LVET × VEPT (Blood velocity × ventricular ejection time × body size factor)	assessment of SV changes can indicate changes in preload, as per the Frank-Starling mechanism. Increases in SV with constant contractility may indicate rising preload levels. Decreases in SV with constant contractility may indicate falling preload levels.[17] Different ICG SV equations may yield different results.[27] Consult with ICG manufacturer for details.	or rise in TFC, should be treated based on institution protocol or reported.
4. Assess baseline and trends in afterload every 1 to 2 hours: Systemic vascular resistance (SVR) Normal SVR: 900–1600 dynes sec/cm^{-5} Normal SVR index: 1970-2390 dynes sec/cm^{-5}/m^2 Formula: $$SVR = \frac{80\,(MAP - CVP)}{CO}$$ $$SVRI = \frac{80\,(MAP - CVP)}{CI}$$	SVR is a measure of resistance to left ventricular emptying. Afterload is inversely related to cardiac output and stroke volume. Ensure SVR is based on current blood pressure or MAP (manually enter or verify that noninvasive blood pressure [NIBP] "slaved" into ICG monitor is functioning) and update default CVP based on measured CVP or jugular venous pressure estimation. Increased SVR often reflects compensatory mechanisms to maintain perfusion. Vasodilation causes SVR to decrease. Monitor SVR to establish response to therapies such as administration of vasodilators or vasoconstricting agents or volume or thermoregulation interventions.	• SVR that has risen above or fallen below normal range or target value • Negligible or absent desired or expected response to therapy
5. Assess baseline and trends in left ventricular contractility every 1 to 2 hours: Acceleration contractility index (ACI) Males: 70-150/100 sec^2 Females: 90-170/100 sec^2 Velocity index (VI): 33-65/1000 sec dZ/dt: 0.8-2.5 ohms/sec	ACI, VI, and dZ/dt are indicators of blood acceleration and velocity in the ascending aorta and directly reflect left ventricular contractility. Impaired contractility is reflected by low dZ/dt, ACI, and VI.[3,10,29] Values increase with improved contractile force. Monitor contractility parameters for an increase to validate appropriate patient response to, for example, positive inotropic agent administration. VI reflects contractility but may be diminished in patients with high TFC.[22]	• Unexpected decrease in dZ/dt, ACI, or VI from baseline values • Negligible or absent desired or expected response to therapy

Documentation

Documentation should include the following:

- Patient and family education
- Initiation of ICG hemodynamic monitoring
- Head-of-bed elevation for initial and subsequent documentation of hemodynamic and thoracic fluid status parameters
- Initial ICG parameters and stroke volume response to physiologic fluid challenge

- Routine every 1 to 2 hours, ICG parameters and trends
- Hemodynamic and TFC (or Z_0) responses to therapeutic interventions
- Printout of dZ/dt waveform or hemodynamic status report at least once per every 12 hours
- Unexpected outcomes
- Additional interventions

References

1. Aldrete, J., et al. (1995). Pacemaker malfunction due to microcurrent injection from a bioimpedance noninvasive cardiac output monitor. *J Clin Monitor,* 11, 131-33.
2. Bishop, M., Shoemaker, W., and Wo, C. (1996). Non-invasive cardiac index monitoring in gunshot wound victims. *Acad Emerg Med,* 7, 682-88.
3. Feng, S., et al. (1988). Detection of impaired left ventricular function in coronary artery disease with acceleration index in the first derivative of the transthoracic impedance change. *Clin Cardiol,* 11, 843-47.
4. Frantz, A. (1996). Home cardiac monitoring and technology. In: Gorski, L., ed. *High-Tech Home Care Manual.* Supplement #2. Rockville, MD: Aspen Publishing.
5. Frantz, A., and Lynn, C. (1999). Cardiac technology in the home. *Home Health Care Management and Practice,* 11, 9-16.
6. Fuller, H. (1992). The validity of cardiac output measurement by thoracic impedance: A meta-analysis. *Clin Invest Med,* 15, 103-12.
7. Hubbard, W., Fish, D., and McBrien, D. (1986). The use of impedance cardiography in heart failure. *Int J Cardiol,* 12, 71-9.
8. Jensen, L., Yakimets, J., and Teo, K.K. (1995). A review of impedance cardiography. *Heart Lung,* 24, 183-93.
9. Jonsson, F., et al. (1995). Thoracic electrical impedance and fluid balance during aortic surgery. *Acta Anaesthesol Scand,* 39, 513-17.
10. Koerner, K., Borzotta, A., and Wilson, J. (1997). Screening for coronary artery disease with impedance cardiography. *Crit Care Med,* 25, A47.
11. Lamberts, R., Visser, K., and Zijlstra, W. (1984). *Impedance Cardiography.* Assen, The Netherlands: Van Gorcum.
12. McFetridge, J., and Sherwood, A. (1999). Impedance cardiography for noninvasive measurement of cardiac output. *Nurs Res,* 48, 109-13.
13. Metry, G., et al. (1997). Gender and age differences in transthoracic bioimpedance. *Acta Physiol Scand,* 161, 171-75.
14. Milzman, D., et al. (1998). Thoracic impedance monitoring of cardiac output in the ED improves heart failure resuscitation. *J Cardiac Failure,* 4, 31.
15. O'Connell, A., Tibballs, J., and Coulthard, M. (1991). Improving agreement between thoracic bioimpedance and dye dilution cardiac output estimation in children. *Anaesth Intens Care,* 19, 434-40.
16. Osypka, M.J., and Bernstein, D.P. (1999). Electrophysiologic principles and theory of stroke volume determination by thoracic electrical bioimpedance. *AACN Clinical Issues,* 10, 385-99.
17. Ovsyshcher, I., and Furman, S. (1993). Impedance cardiography for cardiac output estimation in pacemaker patients: Review of the literature. *PACE,* 16, 1412-22.
18. Ovsyshcher, I., Zimlichman, R., and Katz, A. (1993). Measurements of cardiac output by impedance cardiography in pacemaker patients at rest: Effects of various atrioventricular delays. *J Am Coll Cardiol,* 21, 761-67.
19. Peacock, W.H., et al. (2000). Bioimpedance monitoring: Better than chest x-ray for predicting abnormal pulmonary fluid? *CHF,* 6, 86-9.
20. Pickett, B., and Buell, J. (1993). Usefulness of the impedance cardiogram to reflect left ventricular diastolic function. *Am J Cardiol,* 71, 1099-1103.
21. Scherhag, A., et al. (1997). Continuous measurement of hemodynamic alterations during pharmacologic cardiovascular stress using automated impedance cardiography. *J Clin Pharmacol,* 37, 21S-28S.
22. Shoemaker, W., et al. (1998). Multicenter study for noninvasive monitoring as alternative to invasive monitoring in early management of acutely ill emergency patients. *Chest,* 114, 1643-52.
23. Shoemaker, W., et al. (1994). Multicenter trial of a new thoracic bioimpedance device for cardiac output estimation. *Crit Care Med,* 22, 1907-12.
24. Strobeck, J.E., Silver, M.A., and Ventura, H. (2000). Impedance cardiography: Noninvasive measurement of cardiac stroke volume and thoracic fluid content. *Congestive Heart Failure,* 6, 3-6.
25. Thangathurai, D., et al. (1997). Continuous intraoperative noninvasive cardiac output monitoring using a new thoracic bioimpedance device. *J Cardiothorac Vasc Anesth,* 11, 440-44.
26. Van De Water, J., and Wang, X. (1995). Development of a new impedance cardiograph. *J Clin Engineer,* 20, 218-23.
27. Van De Water, J.M., and Miller, T.W. (2003). Impedance cardiography: The next vital sign technology? *Chest,* 123, 2028-33.
28. Von Rueden, K., and Turner, M. (1999). Advances in continuous, noninvasive hemodynamic surveillance: Impedance cardiography. *Crit Care Nurs Clin North Am,* 11, 63-75.
29. Weinhold, C., et al. (1993). Registration of thoracic electrical bioimpedance for early diagnosis of rejection after heart transplantation. *Heart Lung Transplant,* 12, 832-36.

Additional Readings

Belott, P. (1999). Bioimpedance in the pacemaker clinic. *AACN Clin Issues,* 10, 414-18.

DaMaria, A.N., and Raisinghani, A. (2000). Comparative overview of cardiac output measurement methods: Has impedance cardiography come of age? *CHF,* 6, 60-73.

Drazner, M., et al. (2002). Comparison of impedance cardiography with invasive hemodynamic measurements in patients with heart failure secondary to ischemic or nonischemic cardiomyopathy. *Am J Cardiol,* 89, 993-5.

Lasater, M., and Von Rueden, K. (2003). Outpatient cardiovascular management utilizing impedance cardiography. *AACN Clin Issues,* 14, 240-50.

Peacock, W.H., et al. (2000). Bioimpedance monitoring: Better than chest x-ray for predicting abnormal pulmonary fluid? *CHF,* 6, 86-9.

Pranulis, M. (2000). Impedance cardiography (ICG) noninvasive hemodynamic monitoring provides an opportunity to deliver cost effective quality care for patients with cardiovascular disorders. *J Cardiovasc Management,* 11, 13-8.

Sageman, W.S., Riffenburgh, R.H., and Spiess, B.D. (2002). Equivalence of bioimpedance and thermodilution in measuring cardiac index after cardiac surgery. *J Cardiothorac Vasc Anesth,* Feb. 16, 8-14.

Shoemaker, W.C., et al. (2001). Outcome prediction of emergency patients by noninvasive hemodynamic monitoring. *CHEST,* 120, 528-37.

Summers, R.L., et al. (2003) Bench to bedside: Electrophysiologic and clinical principles of noninvasive hemodynamic monitoring using impedance cardiography. *Acad Emerg Med,* 10, 669-80.

Taler, S.J., Textor, S.C., and Augustine, J.E. (2002). Resistant hypertension: Comparing hemodynamic management to specialist care. *Hypertension,* 39, 982-88.

Tse, H., et al. (2003). Impedance cardiography for atrioventricular interval optimization during permanent left ventricular pacing. *PACE,* 26(Pt. II), 189-91.

Von Rueden, K. (2002). Outpatient hemodynamic monitoring of patients with heart failure. *J Cardiovasc Nurs,* 16, 62-71

Wright, R., and Gilbert, J. (2000). Clinical decision making in patients with congestive heart failure: The role of thoracic electrical bioimpedance. *CHF,* 6, 81-5.

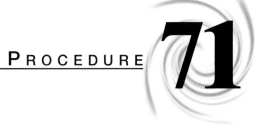

P R O C E D U R E **71**

⊙AP
Pulmonary Artery Catheter Insertion (Perform)

P U R P O S E :   Pulmonary artery (PA) catheters are used to determine hemodynamic status in critically ill patients. PA catheters provide information about right- and left-sided intracardiac pressures and cardiac output. Additional functions available are fiberoptic monitoring of mixed venous oxygen saturation, intracardiac pacing, and assessment of right ventricular volumes and ejection fraction.

Desiree A. Fleck

PREREQUISITE NURSING KNOWLEDGE

- Knowledge of the normal anatomy and physiology of the cardiovascular system
- Knowledge of the normal anatomy and physiology of the vasculature and adjacent structures of the neck
- Understanding of the principles of sterile technique
- Clinical and technical competence in central line insertion and suturing
- Clinical and technical competence in PA catheter insertion[3,6,9-12]
- Competence in chest x-ray interpretation
- Understanding of basic dysrhythmia recognition and treatment of life-threatening dysrhythmias
- Advanced cardiac life support knowledge and skills
- Understanding of pulmonary artery pressure monitoring (see Procedure 72)[3,5,9,10,13]
- Hemodynamic information obtained with a PA catheter is routinely used to guide therapeutic intervention, including administration of fluids and diuretics and titration of vasoactive and inotropic medications.[1,2,8]

- Understanding of *a, c,* and *v* waves: The *a* wave reflects atrial contraction. The *c* wave reflects closure of the atrioventricular valves. The *v* wave reflects passive filling of the atria during ventricular systole.
- Information can be gathered regarding cardiac output (CO), cardiac index (CI), systemic vascular resistance (SVR), pulmonary vascular resistance (PVR), stroke volume/stroke index (SV/SI), mixed venous oxygenation (Svo_2), right heart pressures—pulmonary artery pressure (PAP) and right atrial pressure (RAP)—and a reflection of left ventricular end-diastolic pressure (LVEDP) and volume (LVEDV). Also, information regarding right ventricular ejection fraction (RVEF) and end-diastolic volume (RVEDV) can be determined with certain catheters.
- CO and Svo_2 can be obtained intermittently or continuously.
- There are several types of PA catheters with different functions (e.g., pacing, mixed venous oxygenation saturation monitoring, continuous CO or right ventricular volume monitoring). Catheter selection is based on patient need.
- The PA catheter contains a proximal lumen port, a distal lumen port, a thermistor lumen port, and a balloon inflation lumen port (see Fig. 72-1). Some catheters also have additional infusion ports that can be used for the infusion of medications and intravenous fluids.
- The distal lumen port is used to monitor systolic, diastolic, and mean pressures in the PA. The proximal lumen (or injectate) port is used to monitor the right atrial pressure and to inject the solution used to obtain cardiac

outputs. The balloon inflation lumen port is used to obtain the pulmonary artery wedge pressure (PAWP).

- The standard PA catheter is 7.5 Fr and 110 cm long. The tip of the catheter should reach the PA after being advanced 45 to 55 cm from the internal jugular vein or 70 to 80 cm from a femoral or an antecubital vein. There are black markings every 10 cm to demonstrate where the catheter is positioned.
- Central venous access may be obtained in a variety of places (see Table 80-1).
- The right subclavian vein is a more direct route than the left subclavian vein for placing a PA catheter because the catheter does not cross the midline of the thorax.[1,8]
- Using an internal jugular vein minimizes the risk for a pneumothorax. The preferred site for catheter insertion is the right internal jugular vein. The right internal jugular vein is a "straight shot" to the right atrium.
- Knowledge of West's lung zones helps attain proper placement of the PA catheter (Fig. 71-1). The PA catheter should lie in lung zone 3, below the level of the left atrium in the dependent portion of the lung.[15] In lung zone 3, both arterial and venous pressures exceed alveolar pressure, and PAWP reflects vascular pressures rather than alveolar pressures.[15]
- Common indications for insertion of a PA catheter include the following:
  - ❖ Myocardial infarction (MI) complicated by hemodynamic instability, heart failure, cardiogenic shock, mitral regurgitation, ventral septal rupture, subacute cardiac rupture with tamponade, and postinfarction ischemia, papillary muscle rupture, severe congestive heart failure (e.g., cardiomyopathy, constrictive pericarditis)
  - ❖ Hypotension unresponsive to fluid replacement or with congestive heart failure
  - ❖ Cardiac tamponade, significant dysrhythmias, right ventricular infarct, acute pulmonary embolism, and tricuspid insufficiency
  - ❖ Anesthesia in cardiac surgery with any of the following:
    - ○ Evidence of previous MI
    - ○ Resection of ventricular aneurysm
    - ○ Coronary artery bypass graft (reoperation)
    - ○ Coronary artery bypass graft (left main or complex coronary disease)
    - ○ Complex cardiac surgery (multivalvular surgery)
    - ○ High-risk surgery (e.g., pulmonary hypertension)
  - ❖ General surgery:
    - ○ Vascular procedures (abdominal aneurysm repair, aortobifemoral bypass)
    - ○ High-risk patients
    - ○ Hypotensive anesthesia
  - ❖ Cardiac disorders:
    - ○ Unstable angina requiring vasodilator therapy
    - ○ Congestive heart failure unresponsive to conventional therapy (cardiomyopathy)
    - ○ Pulmonary hypertension during acute drug therapy
    - ○ Distinguishing cardiogenic from noncardiogenic pulmonary edema
    - ○ Constrictive pericarditis or cardiac tamponade
    - ○ Evaluation of pulmonary hypertension for a pre-cardiac transplantation workup
  - ❖ Pulmonary disorders:
    - ○ Acute respiratory failure with chronic obstructive pulmonary diseases

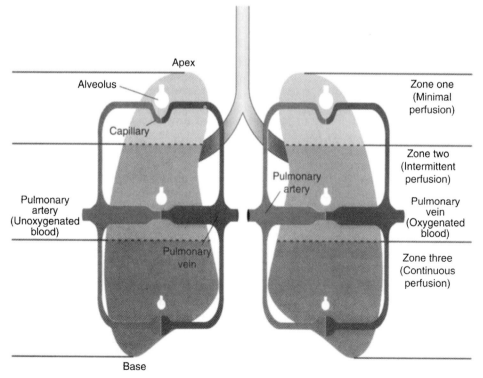

Apex

Alveolus

Capillary

Pulmonary artery (Unoxygenated blood)

Pulmonary vein

Base

Zone one (Minimal perfusion)

Zone two (Intermittent perfusion)

Pulmonary artery

Pulmonary vein (Oxygenated blood)

Zone three (Continuous perfusion)

FIGURE 71-1 West's lung zones. Schema of the heart and lungs demonstrating the relationship between the cardiac chambers and the blood vessels and the physiologic zones of the lungs. *Zone 1* (PA>Pa>Pv): absence of blood flow. *Zone 2* (Pa>PA>Pv): intermittent blood flow. *Zone 3* (Pa>Pv>PA): continuous blood flow, resulting in an open channel between the pulmonary artery catheter and the left atrium. *PA*, pulmonary artery; *Pa*, pressure arterial; *Pv*, pressure venous. (*From Copstead, L.C., and Banasik, J.L. [2000].* Pathophysiology: Biological and Behavioral Perspectives. *2nd ed. Philadelphia: W.B. Saunders.*)

- ○ Cor pulmonale with pneumonia
- ○ Optimization of positive end-expiratory pressure (PEEP) and volume therapy in patients with adult respiratory distress syndrome
  - ❖ Patients requiring intraaortic balloon pump therapy
  - ❖ Critically ill pregnant patients (e.g., severe preeclampsia with unresponsive hypertension, pulmonary edema, persistent oliguria)
  - ❖ Extensive multisystem infection
  - ❖ Severe shock states
  - ❖ Drug overdose
  - ❖ Major trauma or burn
  - ❖ Azotemia
- Relative contraindications to PA catheter insertion include the following:
  - ❖ Preexisting left bundle branch block
  - ❖ Presence of fever (greater than 101°F or 38°C)
  - ❖ Mechanical tricuspid valve
  - ❖ Coagulopathic state
  - ❖ Presence of endocardial pacemaker
  - ❖ History of heparin-induced thrombocytopenia

EQUIPMENT

- Percutaneous equipment tray or introducer kit
- PA catheter (non-heparin-coated catheters are available)
- Sheath introducer
- Sterile catheter sleeve
- Bedside hemodynamic monitoring system with pressure and cardiac output monitoring capability
- Pressure cables for interface with the monitor
- Cardiac output cable with a thermistor/injectate sensor
- Hemodynamic monitoring system, including flush solution recommended according to institution standard, a pressure bag or device, pressure tubing with flush device, and transducers (see Procedure 75)
- Sterile normal saline intravenous fluid for flushing catheter and introducer ports
- Antiseptic solution (e.g., 2% chlorhexidine-based preparation)[12]
- Caps, masks, sterile gowns, sterile gloves, and sterile drapes
- 1% lidocaine without epinephrine
- Sterile basin or cup
- Sterile water or normal saline
- Sterile dressing supplies
- Stopcocks
  Additional equipment to have available as needed includes the following:
- Fluoroscope
- Emergency equipment
- Indelible marker
- Goggles

PATIENT AND FAMILY EDUCATION

- Explain the procedure and the reason for the PA catheter insertion. ➤*Rationale:* Decreases patient and family anxiety; allows for informed consent.
- Explain the need for sterile technique and explain that the patient's face may be covered. ➤*Rationale:* Decreases patient anxiety and elicits cooperation.
- Inform the patient of expected benefits and potential risks. ➤*Rationale:* Allows the patient information to make an informed decision.

PATIENT ASSESSMENT AND PREPARATION

Patient Assessment

- Determine the patient's medical history of cervical disk disease or difficulty obtaining vascular access. ➤*Rationale:* Provides baseline data.
- Determine the patient's medical history of pneumothorax or emphysema. ➤*Rationale:* Patients with emphysematous lungs may be at higher risk for puncture and pneumothorax depending on the approach.
- Determine the patient's medical history of anomalous veins. ➤*Rationale:* Patients may have a history of dextrocardia or transposition of the great vessels, leading to greater difficulty in placing the catheter.
- Assess the intended insertion site. ➤*Rationale:* Scar tissue may impede placement of the catheter.
- Assess the patient's cardiac and pulmonary status. ➤*Rationale:* Some patients may not tolerate a supine or Trendelenburg position for extended periods.
- Assess vital signs and pulse oximetry. ➤*Rationale:* Provides baseline data.
- Assess for electrolyte imbalances (potassium, magnesium, and calcium). ➤*Rationale:* Electrolyte imbalances may increase cardiac irritability.
- Assess the ECG for left bundle branch block. ➤*Rationale:* There are reports of right bundle branch block associated with PA catheter insertion. Caution should be used because complete heart block may ensue.[9]
- Assess for heparin sensitivity or allergy. ➤*Rationale:* PA catheters are heparin-bonded, although non-heparin-bonded catheters are available. If the patient has a heparin allergy or has a history of heparin-induced thrombocytopenia, consider the use of a non-heparin-coated catheter.[14]
- Assess for coagulopathic state and determine whether the patient has recently received anticoagulant or thrombolytic therapy. ➤*Rationale:* These patients are more likely to have complications related to bleeding and may require intervention prior to insertion of the PA catheter.
- Assess for risks and benefits of PA catheter insertion. ➤*Rationale:* Complications do occur with PA catheter insertion, and studies are controversial about the efficacy of PA catheter use.[3,7,8-11]

Patient Preparation

- Ensure that the patient understands preprocedural teaching. Answer questions as they arise and reinforce information as needed. ➤*Rationale:* Evaluates and reinforces understanding of previously taught information. May provide comfort to patient.
- Obtain informed consent. ➤*Rationale:* Protects the rights of a patient and makes a competent decision possible for the patient.
- Place the patient in the supine position and prepare the area with the antiseptic solution (e.g., 2% chlorhexidine-based

preparation).[12] ➤*Rationale:* Prepares site access for PA catheter insertion.
- If the patient is obese or muscular and the preferred site is the internal jugular vein or subclavian vein, place a towel posteriorly between the shoulder blades. ➤*Rationale:* Will help extend the neck and provide better access to subclavian and internal jugular veins.
- If using the arm vein, stabilize the arm on a padded arm board. ➤*Rationale:* Will aid visualization of the arm veins.
- Drape sterile drapes over the prepared area. ➤*Rationale:* Provides an aseptic work area.

Procedure for Performing Pulmonary Artery Catheter Insertion

Steps	Rationale	Special Considerations
1. Wash hands; all health care personnel involved in the procedure should don caps, masks, sterile gowns, and gloves. Goggles or face shields are needed if inserting a new line.	Reduces the transmission of microorganisms and body secretions; standard precautions.	
2. Obtain central venous access with a Teflon introducer (see Procedure 80).	The PA catheter is inserted into a central vein.	
3. Open the PA catheter kit.	Prepares the equipment.	
4. Estimate the length of the catheter needed by holding the catheter over the insertion site to the sternal notch.	Helps ensure proper placement. The catheter should reach the PA after being advanced 45 to 55 cm from the internal jugular vein or 70 to 80 cm from a femoral or an antecubital vein.	Before inserting the catheter, attempt to curl the catheter in the direction it will float.
5. Hand off the ports of the PA catheter to the critical care nurse for connection to the hemodynamic monitoring system (see Procedure 72).	Connects the ports to the flush system; connects the transducer systems to the bedside monitor.	
6. Flush all open lumens.	Removes air from the PA catheter.	
7. Insert the recommended amount of air (1.5 ml) into the balloon and immerse the inflated balloon in sterile water or normal saline.	Checks for integrity of the balloon.	If an air leak is present, air bubbles will be noted.
8. Ensure that the PA catheter thermistor is connected to the cardiac output monitor or module.	Allows the core or blood temperature to be monitored and is needed for cardiac output measurement.	
9. If a PA catheter with the ability to monitor mixed venous oxygenation is being inserted, the fiberoptics are calibrated before removal from the package (see Procedure 14).	Calibrates the system.	Calibrate the catheter according to the manufacturer's guidelines.
10. Ensure that the critical care nurse has zeroed the hemodynamic monitoring system (see Procedure 75).	Prepares the monitoring system so that PA pressures can be obtained during catheter insertion.	

Procedure for Performing Pulmonary Artery Catheter Insertion—*Continued*

Steps	Rationale	Special Considerations
11. Insert the catheter through the sterile catheter sleeve.	Maintains sterility of the PA catheter to allow repositioning of the catheter.	
12. While observing the monitor and the markings on the PA catheter (Fig. 71-2), follow these steps: A. Advance the catheter through the introducer to the superior vena cava into the right atrium.	Waveforms and values change while moving from the superior vena cava to the right atrium to the right ventricle to the pulmonary artery and into the wedge position.	When inserting the PA catheter into the subclavian vein, have the patient bring his or her ear to the shoulder on the side of the insertion site. This creates a sharp angle between the jugular and subclavian veins

Procedure continues on the following page

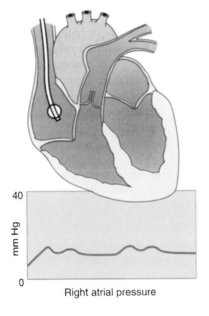

Right atrial pressure

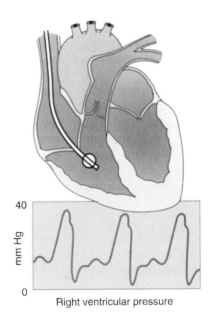

Right ventricular pressure

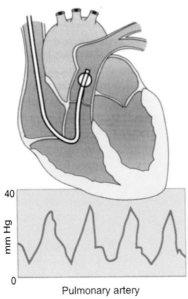

Pulmonary artery

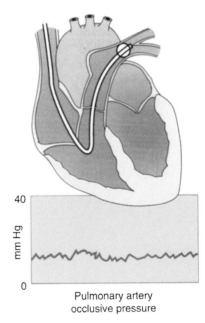

Pulmonary artery
occlusive pressure

FIGURE 71-2 Pulmonary artery catheter advancing through the heart with appropriate waveforms. *(Adapted from Bucher, L., and Melander, S. [1999]. Critical Care Nursing. Philadelphia: W.B. Saunders.)*

Procedure for Performing Pulmonary Artery Catheter Insertion—*Continued*

Steps	Rationale	Special Considerations

B. Inflate the balloon with 1.5 ml of air.
  C. Advance the catheter through the tricuspid valve, into the right ventricle.
  D. Continue to advance the catheter from the right ventricle through the pulmonic valve into the PA.
  E. Advance the catheter to the PA wedge position.
  F. Deflate the balloon.
  G. Observe the PA waveform.
		and may help prevent misdirection of the catheter into the internal jugular vein. During insertion, monitor the ECG tracing for dysrhythmias.

13. Ensure proper placement by rewedging the PA catheter, and confirm placement with a paper tracing.	Ensures proper placement and accurate readings.	
14. Extend the sterile catheter sleeve over the catheter and secure in place.	Maintains catheter sterility for catheter repositioning.[4]	
15. Apply an occlusive, sterile dressing.	Reduces the incidence of infection.	Dressings may be sterile gauze or sterile, transparent, semipermeable dressing.[12]
16. Note the centimeter marking at the introducer site.	Aids in ensuring placement and troubleshooting.	
17. Obtain a chest x-ray.	Confirms catheter placement.	
18. Discard used supplies and wash hands.	Reduces the transmission of microorganisms; standard precautions.	

Expected Outcomes

- Accurate placement of the pulmonary artery catheter
- Adequate and appropriate waveforms
- Ability to obtain accurate information about cardiac pressures
- Evaluation of information to guide therapeutic interventions

Unexpected Outcomes

- Pneumothorax or hemothorax
- Infection
- Ventricular dysrhythmias
- Misplacement (e.g., carotid artery, subclavian artery)
- Valvular damage
- Vessel wall erosion
- Hemorrhage
- Hematoma
- Pericardial or ventricular rupture
- Venous air embolism
- Cardiac tamponade
- Sepsis
- Pulmonary artery infarction
- Pulmonary artery rupture
- Pulmonary artery catheter balloon rupture
- Pulmonary artery catheter knotting
- Heparin-induced thrombocytopenia or thrombosis
- Thromboembolism

Patient Monitoring and Care

Steps	Rationale	Reportable Conditions
		These conditions should be reported if they persist despite nursing interventions.
1. Perform systematic cardiovascular, peripheral vascular, and hemodynamic assessments before and immediately following insertion:		
A. Assess level of consciousness.	Assesses for signs of adequate perfusion; air embolism may present with restlessness; patient may present with decreased level of consciousness if the catheter is advanced into the carotid artery.	• Change in level of consciousness
B. Assess vital signs.	Demonstrates response to procedure and effectiveness of therapies performed.	• Changes in vital signs
C. Assess postinsertion hemodynamic values: pulmonary artery systolic pressure (PASP), pulmonary artery diastolic pressure (PADP), RAP, pulmonary artery wedge pressure, CO, CI, SVR, and other parameters as needed.	Obtains baseline data and assesses patient status.	• Abnormal hemodynamic pressures or cardiac parameters
2. Monitor the site for hematoma or hemorrhage.	If coagulopathies are present, a pressure dressing may be needed.	• Bleeding that does not stop • Hematoma
3. Assess heart and lung sounds.	Abnormal heart or lung sounds may indicate cardiac tamponade, pneumothorax, or hemothorax.	• Diminished or muffled heart sounds • Absent or diminished breath sounds unilaterally
4. Assess the results of the chest x-ray.	Ensures adequate placement in lung zone 3 below the level of the left atrium.	• Abnormal chest x-ray results
5. Monitor for signs of cardiac tamponade and air embolism.	Identifies complications.	• Signs or symptoms of cardiac tamponade or air embolism
6. Monitor the centimeter marking at the introducer site.	Aids in troubleshooting of suspicion that the catheter has moved.	• Change in centimeter marking or PA waveforms

Documentation

Documentation should include the following:

- Patient and family education
- Signed informed consent form
- Insertion of PA catheter and sheath introducer
- Type and size of catheter placed
- Size of introducer sheath
- PA pressure values on insertion (RAP, right ventricular systolic and diastolic pressures, PASP, PADP, PAWP)
- Graphic strip of insertion
- Insertion site of the PA catheter

- Centimeter mark at the edge of the introducer
- Any difficulties encountered during placement (e.g., ventricular ectopy, new bundle branch blocks)
- Patient tolerance
- Confirmation of placement (e.g., chest x-ray)
- Initial values after placement of the catheter (PAPs, PAWP, RAP, CO, CI, SVR, PVR, Svo_2)
- Occurrence of unexpected outcomes
- Additional interventions

References

1. Amin, D.K., Shah, P.K., and Swan, H.J.C. (1993). Deciding when hemodynamic monitoring is appropriate. *J Crit Illness,* 8, 1053-61.
2. Bridges, E.J., and Woods, S.L. (1993). Pulmonary artery measurement: State of the art. *Heart & Lung,* 22, 99-111.
3. Burns, D., Burns, D., and Shively, M. (1996). Critical care nurses' knowledge of pulmonary artery catheters. *Am J Crit Care,* 5, 49-54.
4. Cohen, Y., et al. (1998). The "hands-off" catheter and the prevention of systemic infections associated with pulmonary artery catheter: A prospective study. *Am J Respir Crit Care Med,* 157, 284-87.
5. Darovic, G.O. (2002). Pulmonary artery pressure monitoring. In: *Hemodynamic Monitoring: Invasive and Noninvasive Clinical Application.* Philadelphia: W.B. Saunders.
6. Davis, D., et al. (1999). Impact of formal continuing medical education: Do conferences, workshops, rounds and other traditional continuing education activities change physician behavior or health care outcomes? *JAMA,* 282, 867-74.
7. Eggimann, P., et al. (2000). Impact of a prevention strategy targeted at vascular-access care on incidence of infections acquired in intensive care. *Lancet,* 355, 1864-8.
8. Herbert, K.A., Glancy, D.L. (1994). Indications for Swan-Ganz catheterization. *Heart Dis Stroke,* 3, 196-200.
9. Iberti, T.J., et al. (1990). A Multicenter Study of Physicians' Knowledge of the Pulmonary Artery Catheter. *JAMA,* 22, 2928-33.
10. Iberti, T.J., et al. (1994). Assessment of critical care nurses' knowledge of the pulmonary artery catheter. *Crit Care Med,* 22, 1674-8.
11. Morris, A.H., and Chapman, R.H. (1985). Wedge pressure confirmation by aspiration of pulmonary capillary blood. *Crit Care Med,* 13, 756-9.
12. O'Grady, N.P., et al. (2002). Guidelines for the prevention of intravascular catheter-related infections. *Am J Infect Control,* 30, 476-89.
13. Pulmonary Artery Consensus Conference Participants. (1997). Pulmonary Artery Catheter Consensus Conference: Consensus statement. *Crit Care Med,* 25, 910-25.
14. Silver, D., Kapsch, D.N., and Tsoi, E.K. (1983). Heparin-induced thrombocytopenia, thrombosis, and hemorrhage. *Ann Surg,* 198, 301-6.
15. West, J.B., Dollery, C.T., and Naimark, A. (1964). Distribution of blood flow in isolated lung: Relation to vascular and alveolar pressure. *J Appl Physiol,* 19, 713-24.

Additional Readings

Ahrens, T.S., and Taylor, L.K. (1992). *Hemodynamic Waveform Analysis.* Philadelphia: W.B. Saunders.

American Association of Critical Care Nurses. (1993). Evaluation of the effects of heparinized and nonheparinized flush solutions on the patency of arterial pressure monitoring lines: The AACN Thunder Project. *Am J Crit Care,* 2, 3-15.

Amin, D.K., Shah, P.K., and Swan, H.J.C. (1993). The Swan-Ganz catheter: Techniques for avoiding common errors. *J Crit Illness,* 8, 1263-71.

Amin, D.K., Shah, P.K., and Swan, H.J.C. (1993). The technique of inserting a Swan-Ganz catheter. *J Crit Illness,* 8, 1147-56.

Baxter, J.K., et al. (1997). Effectiveness of right heart catheterization: Time for a randomized trial. *JAMA,* 277, 108.

Chernow, B. (1997). Pulmonary artery flotation catheters: A statement by the American College of Chest Physicians and the American Thoracic Society. *Chest,* 111, 261.

Connors, A.F., et al. (1996). The effectiveness of right heart catheterization in the initial care of critically ill patients. *JAMA,* 276, 889-97.

Daily, E.K., and Schroeder, J.S. (1994). *Techniques in Bedside Hemodynamic Monitoring.* 5th ed. St. Louis: C.V. Mosby.

Darovic, G.O. (2002). *Hemodynamic Monitoring: Invasive and Noninvasive Clinical Application.* Philadelphia: W.B. Saunders.

Friesinger, G.C., Williams, S.V., and ACP/ACC/AHA Task Force on Clinical Privileges in Cardiology. (1990). Clinical competence in hemodynamic monitoring. *J Am Coll Cardiol,* 15, 1460.

Gardner, P.E. (1993). Pulmonary artery pressure monitoring. *AACN Clin Issues Crit Care Nurs,* 4, 98-119.

Gardner, P.E., and Bridges, E.J. (1995). Hemodynamic monitoring. In: Woods, S.L., et al., eds. *Cardiac Nursing,* 3rd ed. Philadelphia: J.B. Lippincott, 424-58.

Ginosar, Y., Pizov, R., and Sprung, C.L. (1995). Arterial and pulmonary artery catheters. In: *Critical Care Medicine.* St. Louis: C.V. Mosby.

Keckeisen, M. (1997). *Protocols for Practice: Hemodynamic Monitoring Series—Pulmonary Artery Pressure Monitoring.* Aliso Viejo, CA: American Association of Critical-Care Nurses.

Leeper, B. (2003). Monitoring right ventricular volumes: A paradigm shift. *AACN Clin Issues: Advanced Practice in Acute and Critical Care,* 14, 208-19.

Marion, P.L. (1991). *The ICU Book.* Philadelphia: Lea & Febiger.

Pulmonary Artery Catheter Consensus Conference Participants. (1997). Pulmonary Artery Catheter Consensus Conference: Consensus statement. *Crit Care Med,* 25, 910-25.

Putterman, C. (1989). The Swan-Ganz catheter: A decade of hemodynamic monitoring. *J Crit Care,* 4, 127-46.

Quail, S.J. (1993). Quality assurance in hemodynamic monitoring. *AACN Clin Issues Crit Care,* 4, 197-205.

Rapoprot, L.J., Teres, D., and Steingrub, J. (2000). Patient characteristics and ICU organizational factors that influencing of frequency of PA catheter. *JAMA,* 283, 2555.

Staudinger, T., et al. (1998). Diagnostic validity of pulmonary artery catheterization for residents at an intensive care unit. *J Trauma,* 44, 902-6.

Steingrub, J.S., Celori, G., and Vickers-Lahti, M. (1991). Therapeutic impact of pulmonary artery catheterization in a medical/surgical ICU. *Chest,* 99, 1451.

Swan, J.H.C. (1993). What role today for hemodynamic monitoring. *J Crit Illness,* 8, 1043-50.

Swan, J.H.C., Ganz, W., and Forrester, J.S. (1970). Catheterization of the heart in a man with the use of a flow-directed balloon-tipped catheter. *N Engl J Med,* 280, 447.

The American Society of Anesthesiologists' Task Force on Pulmonary Artery Catheterization. (1993). Practice guidelines for pulmonary catheterization. *Anesthesiology,* 78, 380-94.

Urban, N. (1990). Hemodynamic clinical profiles. *AACN Clin Issues Crit Care Nurs,* 1, 119-30.

Venus, B., and Mallory, D.L. (1992). Vascular cannulation. In: *Critical Care.* 2nd ed. Philadelphia: J.B. Lippincott.

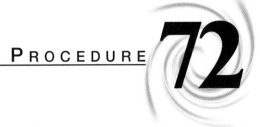
PROCEDURE 72

Pulmonary Artery Catheter Insertion (Assist) and Pressure Monitoring

PURPOSE: Pulmonary artery (PA) catheters are used to determine hemodynamic status in critically ill patients. PA catheters provide information about right- and left-sided intracardiac pressures and cardiac output (CO). Additional functions available are fiberoptic monitoring of mixed venous oxygen saturation, intracardiac pacing, and assessment of right ventricular volumes and ejection fraction. Hemodynamic information obtained with a PA catheter is used to guide therapeutic intervention, including administration of fluids and diuretics and titration of vasoactive and inotropic medications.

Teresa Preuss
Debra Lynn-McHale Wiegand

PREREQUISITE NURSING KNOWLEDGE

- Knowledge of the normal cardiovascular anatomy and physiology
- Knowledge of the normal pulmonary anatomy and physiology
- Knowledge of principles of aseptic technique
- Basic dysrhythmia recognition and treatment of life-threatening dysrhythmias
- Advanced cardiac life support knowledge and skills
- Anatomy of the PA catheter (Fig. 72-1) and the location of the PA catheter in the heart and pulmonary artery (Fig. 72-2)
- The setup of the hemodynamic monitoring system (see Procedure 75).
- Understanding of normal hemodynamic values (see Table 63-1).
- The pulmonary artery catheter contains a proximal injectate lumen port, a PA distal lumen port, a thermistor connector, and a balloon-inflation valve. Some catheters also have two infusion ports, an RA and an RV lumen that can be used for infusion of medications and intravenous fluids.
- The PA distal lumen is used to monitor systolic, diastolic, and mean pressures in the pulmonary artery. This lumen

also allows for sampling of mixed venous blood. The proximal injectate lumen is used to monitor the right atrial pressure and inject the solution used to obtain CO. The balloon-inflation valve is used to obtain the pulmonary artery waveform pressure (PAWP).

- Pulmonary artery wedge pressure may be referred to as *pulmonary artery occlusion pressure.*
- The PA diastolic pressure and the PAWP are indirect measures of left ventricular end-diastolic pressure (LVEDP). Usually, the PAWP is approximately 1 to 4 mm Hg less than the pulmonary artery diastolic pressure (PADP). Because these two pressures are similar, the PADP is commonly followed. This minimizes the frequency of balloon inflation and thus decreases the potential of balloon rupture.
- Differences between the PADP and the PAWP may exist for patients with pulmonary hypertension, chronic obstructive lung disease, acute respiratory distress syndrome (ARDS), pulmonary embolus, and tachycardia.
- Indications for PA catheter therapy (see Procedure 71 for additional indications) are as follows:
  - ❖ Aid in the diagnosis of complications after acute myocardial infarction (MI) that may include heart failure, cardiogenic shock, papillary muscle rupture, mitral regurgitation, ventricular septal rupture, or cardiac rupture with tamponade

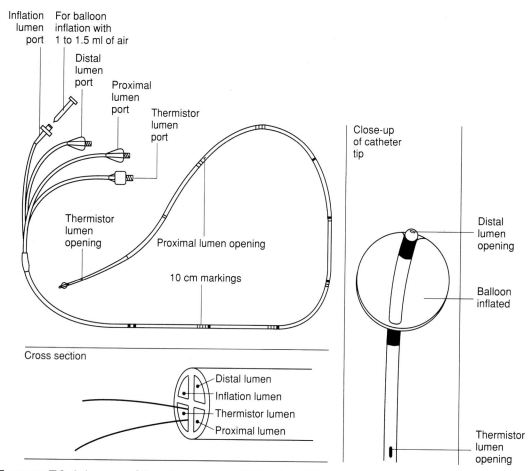

FIGURE 72-1 Anatomy of the pulmonary artery (PA) catheter. The standard No. 7.5-Fr thermodilution PA catheter is 110 cm in length and contains four lumens. It is constructed of radiopaque polyvinyl chloride. In 10-cm increments, there are black markings on the catheter beginning at the distal end. At the distal end of the catheter is a latex rubber balloon of 1.5-ml capacity, which, when inflated, extends slightly beyond the tip of the catheter without obstructing it. Balloon inflation cushions the tip of the catheter and prevents contact with the right ventricular wall during insertion. The balloon also acts to float the catheter into position and allows measurement of the pulmonary artery wedge pressure. The narrow black bands represent 10-cm lengths and the wide black bands indicate 50-cm lengths. *(From Visalli, F., and Evans, P. [1981]. The Swan-Ganz catheter: a program for teaching safe effective use. Nursing, 81[11], 1.)*

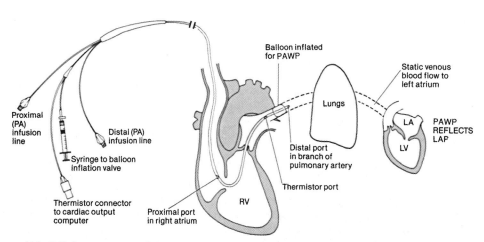

FIGURE 72-2 Pulmonary artery (PA) catheter location within the heart. Pulmonary artery wedge pressure (PAWP) is an indirect measure of left arterial and left ventricular end-diastolic pressure. *(From Kersten, L.D. [1989]. Comprehensive Respiratory Nursing. Philadelphia: W.B. Saunders.)*

- ❖ Assessment of ventricular function in heart failure
- ❖ Management of high-risk cardiac patients undergoing surgical procedures during preoperative, intraoperative, or postoperative periods
- ❖ Differentiation of hypotensive states, such as hypovolemia, sepsis, heart failure, and cardiac tamponade
- ❖ Hemodynamic monitoring and evaluation of patients with major organ dysfunction who require fluid management and infusion of vasoactive medications, such as patients with burns, trauma, acute respiratory distress syndrome (ARDS), or gastrointestinal bleeding

- There are no absolute contraindications to hemodynamic monitoring with a PA catheter, but an assessment of risk versus benefit to the patient should be considered. Relative contraindications to pulmonary artery catheter insertion include presence of fever, presence of a mechanical tricuspid valve, and coagulopathic state. A patient with left bundle branch block may develop a right bundle branch block during PA catheter insertion resulting in complete heart block. In these patients a temporary pacing mode should be readily available.
- Pulmonary artery pressures may be elevated as a result of pulmonary artery hypertension, pulmonary disease, mitral valve disease, left ventricular failure, atrial or ventricular left-to-right shunt, pulmonary emboli, or hypervolemia.
- Pulmonary artery pressures may be decreased due to hypovolemia or vasodilation.
- Waveforms that occur during insertion, including right atrial (RA), right ventricular (RV), PA, and pulmonary artery wedge (PAW) (Fig. 72-3).
- The *a* wave reflects atrial contraction, the *c* wave reflects closure of the atrioventricular valve, and the *v* wave reflects passive filling of the atria during ventricular systole (Figs. 72-4 and 72-5).
- The *a* wave reflects right ventricular filling at end-diastole. The mean of the *a* wave is determined by averaging the top and bottom values of the *a* wave.

- Elevated *a* and *v* waves may be evident in right atrial pressure (RAP/CVP) and in PAWP waveforms. These elevations may occur in patients with cardiac tamponade, constrictive pericardial disease, and hypervolemia.
- Elevated *a* waves in the RAP/CVP waveform may occur in patients with pulmonic or tricuspid stenosis, right ventricular ischemia or infarction, right ventricular failure, pulmonary artery hypertension, and atrioventricular (AV) dissociation.
- Elevated *a* waves in the PAWP waveform may occur in patients with mitral stenosis, acute left ventricular ischemia or infarction, left ventricular failure, and AV dissociation.
- Elevated *v* waves in the RAP/CVP waveform may occur in patients with tricuspid insufficiency.
- Elevated *v* waves in the PAWP waveform may occur in patients with mitral insufficiency or a ruptured papillary muscle.
- Insertion and placement verification should occur as follows:
  - ❖ The PA catheter may be inserted through the subclavian, internal jugular, femoral, external jugular, or antecubital veins. Placement of a central venous catheter in a subclavian site instead of a jugular or femoral site reduces the risk for infection.[20]
  - ❖ The standard 7.5-F PA catheter is 110 cm long and has black markings at 10-cm increments and wide black markings at 50-cm increments to facilitate insertion and positioning (see Fig. 72-1). The catheter should reach the PA after being advanced 45 to 55 cm from the internal jugular vein or 70 to 80 cm from a femoral or an antecubital vein.
  - ❖ Verification of PA catheter placement is validated by waveform analysis. Correct catheter placement demonstrates a PAW tracing when the balloon is inflated and a PA tracing when the balloon is deflated.
- Catheter placement is also verified by chest x-ray.
- The PA catheter contains latex which may cause allergic reactions.

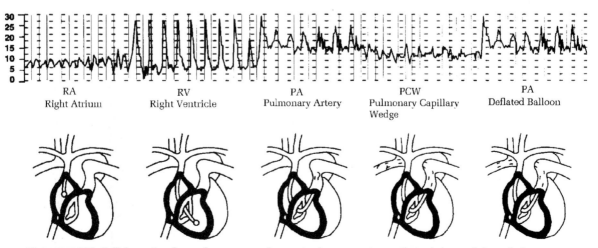

FIGURE 72-3 Schematic of waveform progression as a pulmonary artery catheter is inserted through the various cardiac chambers. *(From Abbott Critical Care Systems, Mountain View, CA.)*

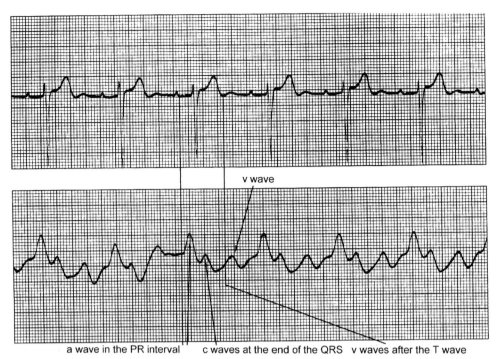

FIGURE 72-4 Identification of *a, c,* and *v* waves in the waveform for right atrial and central venous pressure (RA/CVP). Atrial waveforms are characterized by three components: *a, c,* and *v* waves. The *a* wave reflects atrial cotraction, the *c* wave reflects closure of the tricuspid valve, and the *v* wave reflects passive filling of the atria. *(From Ahrens, T.S., and Taylor, L.K. [1992].* Hemodynamic Waveform Analysis. *Philadelphia: W.B. Saunders.)*

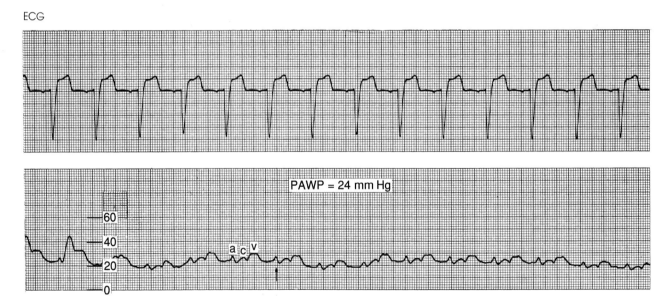

FIGURE 72-5 Normal pulmonary artery wedge pressure (PAWP) waveform and components. Note the delay in the *a, c,* and *v* waves because of the time it takes for the mechanical events to show a pressure change. This waveform is from a spontaneously breathing patient. The arrow indicates end-expiration, where the mean of *a* wave pressure is measured.

EQUIPMENT

- PA catheter (non-heparin-coated PA catheters are available)
- Percutaneous sheath introducer kit and sterile catheter sleeve
- Pressure modules and cables for interface with the monitor
- Cardiac output cable with a thermistor/injectate sensor
- Pressure transducer system, including flush solution recommended according to institution standard, a pressure bag or device, pressure tubing with flush device, and transducers
- Dual-channel recorder
- Sterile normal saline intravenous fluid for flushing the introducer and catheter infusion ports

- Antiseptic solution (e.g., 2% chlorhexidine-based preparation)
- Caps, fluid-shield masks, sterile gowns, sterile gloves, nonsterile gloves and sterile drapes
- 1% lidocaine without epinephrine
- Sterile basin or cup
- Sterile water or normal saline
- Sterile dressing supplies
- Stopcocks (may be included in some pressure tubing systems)
- Nonvented caps for stopcocks
 Additional equipment as needed includes the following:
- Fluoroscope
- Emergency equipment
- Temporary pacing equipment
- Indelible marker
- Transducer holder

PATIENT AND FAMILY EDUCATION

- Provide the patient and family with information about the PA catheter, reason for the PA catheter, and explanation of the equipment. ➤*Rationale:* Assists the patient and family to understand the procedure, why it is needed, and how it will help the patient. Decreases patient and family anxiety.
- Explain the patient's expected participation during the procedure. ➤*Rationale:* Encourages patient assistance.

PATIENT ASSESSMENT AND PREPARATION

Patient Assessment

- Determine baseline hemodynamic, cardiovascular, peripheral vascular, and neurovascular status. ➤*Rationale:* Provides data that can be used for comparison with post-insertion assessment data and hemodynamic values.

- Determine the patient's baseline pulmonary status. If the patient is mechanically ventilated, note the type of support, ventilator mode, and presence or absence of positive end-expiratory pressure (PEEP) or continuous positive airway pressure (CPAP). ➤*Rationale:* The presence of mechanical ventilation alters hemodynamic waveforms and pressures.
- Assess the patient's past medical history specifically related to problems with venous access sites, cardiac anatomy, and pulmonary anatomy. ➤*Rationale:* Identification of obstructions or disease should be made prior to the insertion attempt.
- Assess the patient's current laboratory profile, including electrolyte, coagulation and arterial blood gas studies. ➤*Rationale:* Identifies laboratory abnormalities. Baseline coagulation studies are helpful in determining the risk for bleeding. Electrolyte and arterial blood gas imbalances may increase cardiac irritability.

Patient Preparation

- Ensure that the patient and family understand preprocedural teaching. Answer questions as they arise and reinforce information as needed. ➤*Rationale:* Evaluates and reinforces understanding of previously taught information.
- Ensure that informed consent has been obtained. ➤*Rationale:* Protects the rights of the patient and makes a competent decision possible for the patient.
- Validate the patency of the peripheral IV line. ➤*Rationale:* Access may be needed for administration of emergency medications or fluids.
- Assist the patient to the supine position. ➤*Rationale:* Prepares the patient for skin preparation, catheter insertion, and setup of the sterile field.
- Sedate the patient or provide prescribed analgesics as needed. ➤*Rationale:* Movement of the patient may inhibit insertion of the PA catheter.

Procedure	for Assisting With Pulmonary Artery Catheter Insertion and Pressure Monitoring	
Steps	**Rationale**	**Special Considerations**
Assisting With PA Catheter Insertion		
1. Wash hands.	Reduces the possible transmission of microorganisms and body secretions; standard precautions.	
2. Follow institutional standard for adding heparin to flush solution (see Procedure 75).	Heparinized flush solutions are commonly used to minimize thrombi and fibrin deposits on catheters that might lead to thrombosis or bacterial colonization of the catheter.	Although heparin may prevent thrombosis,[20] it has been associated with thrombocytopenia and other hematologic complications.[4] Further research is needed regarding use of heparin versus normal saline to maintain PA line patency.

Procedure continues on the following page

| **Procedure** | **for Assisting With Pulmonary Artery Catheter Insertion and Pressure Monitoring**—*Continued* |

Steps	Rationale	Special Considerations
3. Prime or flush the entire pressure transducer system (see Procedure 75).	Removes air bubbles. Air bubbles introduced into the patient's circulation can cause air embolism. Air bubbles within the tubing will dampen the waveform.	Air is more easily removed from the hemodynamic tubing when the system is not under pressure.
4. Apply and maintain pressure in the pressure bag or device at 300 mm Hg.	Each flush device delivers 1 to 3 ml/hr to maintain patency of the hemodynamic system.	
5. Wash hands and don caps, fluid shield masks, sterile gowns, and gloves for all health care personnel involved in procedure.	Reduces the transmission of microorganisms and body secretions; standard precautions.	
6. Assist the physician or advanced practice nurse with opening the PA catheter and introducer kits.	Aids in maintaining sterility.	
7. When the sheath introducer is in place, connect a normal saline IV solution to the infusion port.	Maintains the patency of the sheath introducer infusion port.	
8. Connect the pressure transducer/flush system to the PA distal and proximal ports of the PA catheter and flush all lumens.	Removes air from the pulmonary artery catheter.	Flush additional infusion ports prior to insertion.
9. Connect the pressure cables from the PA distal and proximal injectate transducers to the bedside monitor (see Fig. 75-2).	Connects the pulmonary artery catheter to the bedside monitoring system.	
10. Connect the thermistor connector of the PA catheter to the CO monitor or module (see Fig. 75-3).	Allows the core temperature to be monitored and is needed for CO measurement.	
11. If inserting a PA catheter with the ability to monitor mixed venous oxygenation, the fiberoptics are calibrated prior to removal from the package (see Procedure 14).	Calibrates the system.	Follow manufacturer guidelines for catheter calibration.
12. Set the scales for each pressure tracing.	Permits waveform analysis.	The scale for the RA/CVP pressure commonly is set at 20 mm Hg, and the PA scale commonly is set at 40 mm Hg. Scales are adjusted based on patient pressures.
13. Examine the PA catheter for defects in construction and check balloon integrity.	Faulty catheters are replaced.	The inflated balloon can be placed in a container of sterile normal saline or water. No air bubbles should be seen. If air bubbles are seen, there is a defect in the balloon integrity.
14. Level the RA (proximal injectate) air-fluid interface (zeroing stopcock) and the PA (distal) air-fluid interface (zeroing stopcock) to the phlebostatic axis.	The phlebostatic axis approximates the level of the atria and is the reference point for patients in the supine position (see Fig. 75-7).	The reference point for the atria changes when a patient is in the lateral position (see Fig. 75-8).

Procedure **for Assisting With Pulmonary Artery Catheter Insertion and Pressure Monitoring**—*Continued*

Steps	Rationale	Special Considerations
15. Zero the system connected to the PA lumen and RA lumen of the PA catheter by turning the stopcock off to the patient, opening it to air, and zeroing the monitoring system (see Procedure 75).	Prepares the monitoring system so that PA pressures can be obtained during catheter insertion.	
16. The physician or advanced practice nurse places a sterile plastic sleeve over the PA catheter, attaching it to the PA catheter before the catheter is inserted.[20]	A sterile sleeve prevents contamination of the PA catheter, allows repositioning of the catheter after the initial insertion, and reduces blood stream infections.[7]	Research has not yet determined how long the sleeve remains sterile.
17. As insertion begins, continuously run an ECG and PA distal waveform strip.	Provides documentation of RA, RV, and PA pressures during insertion and dysrhythmia occurrence during insertion.	A dual-channel recorder is preferred, because then the ECG and the PA waveform can be simultaneously recorded.
18. After the tip of the PA catheter is in the right atrium, inflate the balloon with no more than 1.25 to 1.5 ml of air and close the gate valve or the stopcock (Fig. 72-6).	The presence of the tip of the catheter in the right atrium is validated by waveform analysis (see Fig. 72-3). Closing the gate valve or the stopcock holds air in the balloon during insertion.	The inflated balloon advances the PA catheter through the right side of the heart and into the PA, minimizing the chance of endocardial damage.
19. Observe for RA, RV, PA, and then PAW waveforms (see Fig. 72-3).	Placement in the PA is validated by waveform analysis.	Monitor the ECG tracing as the PA catheter is inserted, because ventricular dysrhythmias may occur due to right ventricular irritability. Right ventricular pressures are obtained only during insertion.
20. Verify that the catheter is in the proper position. When the balloon is deflated, the monitor shows a PA tracing; when the balloon is inflated, the monitor will show a PAW tracing.	When the balloon is inflated, the catheter floats from the pulmonary artery to a smaller arteriole (see Fig. 72-3).	The catheter usually reaches the PA after being advanced 45 to 55 cm from the internal jugular or subclavian vein or 70 to 80 cm from a femoral or antecubital vein. Placement may vary depending on patient size. A chest x-ray is obtained to verify catheter position.

Procedure continues on the following page

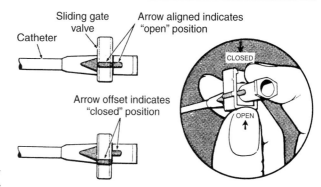

Sliding gate valve

Arrow aligned indicates "open" position

Catheter

CLOSED

OPEN

Arrow offset indicates "closed" position

FIGURE 72-6 Gate valve in the open position on the pulmonary artery (PA) (distal) lumen of the PA catheter. *(From Baxter Edwards Corporation.)*

Gate Valve Operation

Procedure	for Assisting With Pulmonary Artery Catheter Insertion and Pressure Monitoring—*Continued*

Steps	Rationale	Special Considerations
21. After the pulmonary artery catheter is in place, open the balloon inflation gate valve or stopcock and remove the PA syringe.	The gate valve or stopcock is closed during insertion to retain air in the balloon. The air is then released so that continuous monitoring of the PA waveform can be performed.	Air is expelled from the PA syringe, and the empty syringe is reconnected to the end of the balloon inflation valve.
22. Reassess accurate leveling and secure the system to the patient's chest or arm or to a pole mount.	Ensures that the air-filled interface (zeroing stopcock) is maintained at the level of the phlebostatic axis. If the air-fluid interface is above the phlebostatic axis, PA pressures will be falsely low. If the air-fluid interface is below the phlebostatic axis, PA pressures will be falsely high.	Leveling ensures accuracy. The point of the phlebostatic axis should be marked with an indelible marker, especially if using a pole-mount setup.
23. Zero both the RA and PA hemodynamic monitoring systems (see Procedure 75).	Ensures accuracy of the system with the established reference point.	
24. Observe the waveform and perform a dynamic response test (square wave test) (see Fig. 59-3).	Results indicate whether the system is correctly damped.	
25. Place a sterile, occlusive dressing on the insertion site.	Reduces the risk for infection.	
26. Document the external cm marking of the PA catheter at the introducer exit site.	Identifies the length of the PA catheter inserted and allows for evaluation of PA catheter movement.	If the cm marking is not visible at the exit site, measure the distance from the introducer exit site to the nearest visible marking.
27. Set the alarms. Upper and lower alarm limits are set on the basis of the patient's current clinical status and hemodynamic values.	Activates the bedside and central alarm system.	
28. Discard used supplies and wash hands.	Reduces the transmission of microorganisms; standard precautions.	
29. Obtain the chest x-ray.	Verifies catheter placement.	

Obtaining PA Pressure Measurements
RA/CVP

Steps	Rationale	Special Considerations
1. Position the patient in the supine position with the head of the bed from 0 to 45 degrees. (*Level VI: Clinical studies in a variety of patient populations and situations to support recommendations.*)	Studies have determined that the RA and PA pressures are accurate in this position.[3,5,6,9,14,16,18,28,29]	RA and PA pressures may be accurate for patients in the supine position with the head of the bed elevated up to 60 degrees,[6,18] but additional studies are needed to support this. Only one study[15] supports the accuracy of hemodynamic values for patients in the lateral positions; other studies do not.[3,11,14,22,27] The majority of studies support the accuracy of hemodynamic monitoring for patients in the prone position.[1,2,10,13,17,23,26] Two studies demonstrated that prone positioning caused an increase in hemodynamic values.[24,25]

Procedure	**for Assisting With Pulmonary Artery Catheter Insertion and Pressure Monitoring**—*Continued*	
Steps	**Rationale**	**Special Considerations**
2. Run a dual-channel strip of the ECG and RA waveform (Fig. 72-7).	RA pressures should be determined from the graphic strip, because the effect of ventilation can be identified.	Digital data can be used to determine RA pressure if ventilation does not affect the RA pressure waveform. Some monitors have the capability of 'freeze framing' waveforms. A cursor can be used to determine pressure measurements.
3. Measure RA pressure at end-expiration.	Measurement is most accurate as the effects of pulmonary pressures are minimized.	
4. Using the dual-channel recorded strip, draw a vertical line from the beginning of the P wave of one of the ECG complexes down to the RA waveform. Repeat this with the next ECG complex (see Fig. 72-7).	Compares electrical activity to mechanical activity. Usually three waves are present on the RA waveform.	At times, the *c* wave is not present.
5. Align the PR interval with the RA waveform.	The *a* wave correlates with this interval.	
6. Identify the *a* wave.	The *a* wave is seen approximately 80 to 100 milliseconds after the *P* wave. The *c* wave follows the *a* wave, and the *v* wave follows the *c* wave.	The *a* wave reflects atrial contraction. The *c* wave reflects closure of the tricuspid valve. The *v* wave reflects passive filling of the atria (see Fig. 72-4).
7. Identify the scale of the RA tracing (Fig. 72-8).	Aids in determining the pressure measurement.	RA scale commonly is set at 20 mm Hg.
8. Measure the mean of the *a* wave to obtain the RA pressure (RAP) (see Fig. 72-8).	The *a* wave represents atrial contraction and reflects right ventricular filling at end-diastole.	
PA Systolic and Diastolic Pressures		
1. Position the patient in the supine position with the head of the bed from 0 to 45 degrees. *(Level VI: Clinical studies in a variety of patient populations and situations to support recommendations.)*	Studies have determined that the RA and PA pressures are accurate in this position.[3,5,6,9,14,16,18,28,29]	RA and PA pressures may be accurate for patients in the supine position with the head of the bed elevated up to 60 degrees,[6,18] but additional studies are needed to support this. Only one study[15] supports the accuracy of hemodynamic values for patients in the lateral

Procedure continues on the following page

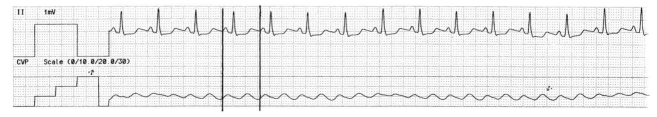

FIGURE 72-7 Note vertical lines drawn from the beginning of the P wave of two of the electrocardiogram (ECG) complexes down to the right atrial (RA) waveform. The first positive deflection of the RA waveform is the *a* wave, the second positive deflection is the *v* wave. The *c* wave, which would lie between the *a* wave and the *v* wave, is not evident in this strip.

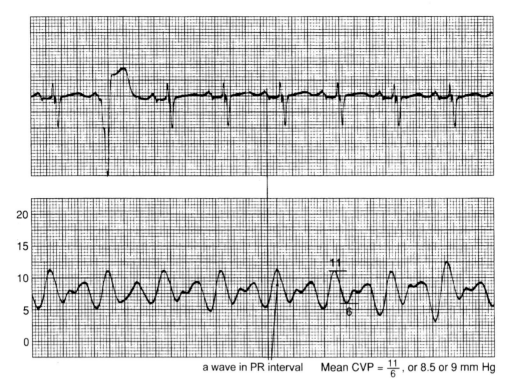

a wave in PR interval   Mean CVP = $\frac{11}{6}$, or 8.5 or 9 mm Hg

FIGURE 72-8 Obtaining measurements of right atrial and central venous pressures (RA/CVP). Aligning the *a* wave on the RA/CVP waveform with the PR interval on the electrocardiogram facilitates accurate measurement of RA/CVP at end-diastole. *(From Ahrens, T.S., and Taylor, L.K. [1992]. Hemodynamic Waveform Analysis. Philadelphia: W.B. Saunders.)*

Procedure	**for Assisting With Pulmonary Artery Catheter Insertion and Pressure Monitoring**—*Continued*	
Steps	**Rationale**	**Special Considerations**
		positions; other studies[3,11,14,22,27] do not. The majority of studies[1,2,10,13,17,23,26] support the accuracy of hemodynamic monitoring for patients in the prone position; yet two studies demonstrated that prone positioning caused an increase in hemodynamic values.[24,25]
2. Run a dual-channel strip of the ECG and PA waveform (Fig. 72-9).	PA pressures are determined from the graphic strip, because the effect of ventilation can be identified.	Some monitors have the capability of "freeze framing" waveforms. A cursor can be used to determine pressure measurements.
3. Measure the PA pressure at end-expiration.	Measurement is most accurate as the effects of pulmonary pressures are minimized.	
4. Identify the QT interval on the ECG strip.	Demonstrates ventricular depolarization.	
5. Align the QT interval with the PA waveform.	Compares electrical activity to mechanical activity.	

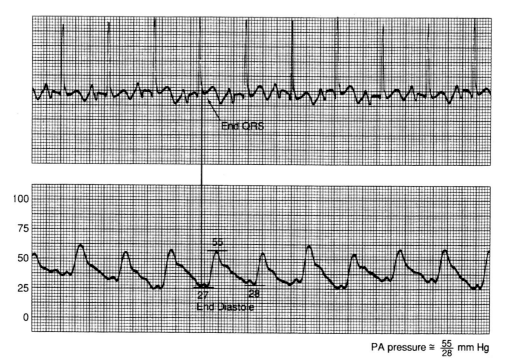

PA pressure ≅ $\frac{55}{28}$ mm Hg

FIGURE 72-9 Obtaining measurements of pressure in the pulmonary artery (PA). For systolic pressure, align the peak of the systolic waveform with the QT interval on the electrocardiogram (ECG). For PA diastolic pressure, use the end of the QRS as a marker to detect the PA diastolic phase. Obtain the reading just before the upstroke of the systolic waveform. *(From Ahrens, T.S., and Taylor, L.K. [1992]. Hemodynamic Waveform Analysis. Philadelphia: W.B. Saunders.)*

Procedure	for Assisting With Pulmonary Artery Catheter Insertion and Pressure Monitoring—*Continued*		
Steps	**Rationale**	**Special Considerations**
6. Identify the scale of the PA tracing.	Aids in determining the pressure measurement.	PA scale is commonly set at 40 mm Hg.
7. Measure the PA systolic pressure at the peak of the systolic waveform on the PA waveform (see Fig. 72-9).	This reflects the highest systolic pressure.	
8. Align the end of the QRS complex with the PA waveform (see Fig. 72-9).	The end of the QRS complex correlates with ventricular end-diastolic pressure.	
9. Measure the PA diastolic pressure at the point of the intersection of this line (see Fig. 72-9).	This point occurs just before the upstroke of the systolic pressure.	
PAWP		
1. Position the patient in the supine position with the head of the bed from 0 to 45 degrees. *(Level VI: Clinical studies in a variety of patient populations and situations to support recommendations.)*	Studies have determined that the RA and PA pressures are accurate in this position.[3,5,6,9,14,16,18,28,29]	RA and PA pressures may be accurate for patients in the supine position with the head of the bed elevated up to 60 degrees,[6,18] but additional studies are needed to support this. Only one study[15] supports the accuracy of hemodynamic values for patients in the lateral

Procedure continues on the following page

Procedure	**for Assisting With Pulmonary Artery Catheter Insertion and Pressure Monitoring**—*Continued*	
Steps	**Rationale**	**Special Considerations**
		positions; other studies[3,11,14,22,27] do not. The majority of studies[1,2,10,13,17,23,26] support the accuracy of hemodynamic monitoring for patients in the prone position, but two studies demonstrated that prone positioning caused an increase in hemodynamic values.[24,25]
2. Fill the PA syringe with 1.5 ml of air.	More than 1.5 ml of air may rupture the PA balloon and the pulmonary arteriole.	
3. Connect the PA syringe to the gate valve or stopcock of the balloon port of the PA catheter (see Fig. 72-6).	This port is designed for PA balloon air inflation.	
4. Run a dual-channel strip of the ECG and PA waveform.	The PAW pressures are determined from the graphic strip, because the effect of ventilation can be identified.	Some monitors have the capability of "freeze framing" waveforms. A cursor can be used to determine pressure measurements.
5. Slowly inflate the balloon with air until the PA waveform changes to a PAW waveform (Fig. 72-10).	A slight resistance is usually felt during inflation of the balloon. Overinflation of the balloon can cause pulmonary arteriole infarction or rupture, resulting in potentially life-threatening hemorrhage.[12]	Only enough air is needed to convert the PA waveform to a PAW waveform. Thus, the entire amount of 1.5 ml of air is not necessarily needed.
6. Inflate the PA balloon for no more than 8 to 15 seconds (two to four respiratory cycles).	Prolonged inflation of the balloon can cause pulmonary arteriole infarction and rupture, with potentially life-threatening hemorrhage.[12]	

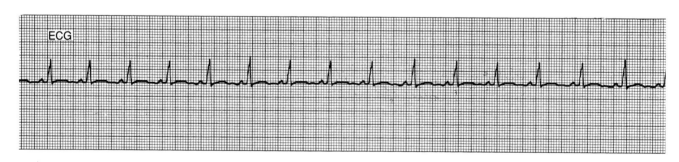

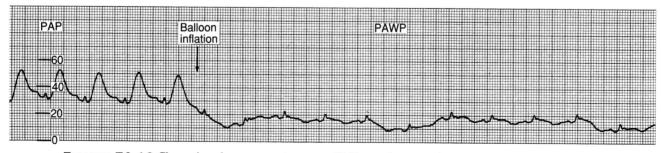

FIGURE 72-10 Change in pulmonary artery pressure (PAP) waveform to pulmonary artery wedge pressure (PAWP) waveform with balloon inflation. The balloon is inflated while observing the bedside monitor for change in the waveform. Balloon inflation *(arrow)* in patient with normal PAWP.

| Procedure | for Assisting With Pulmonary Artery Catheter Insertion and Pressure Monitoring—*Continued* | | |

Steps	Rationale	Special Considerations
7. Disconnect the syringe from the balloon-inflation port.	Allows air to passively escape from the balloon.	Active withdrawal of air from the balloon can weaken the balloon, pull the balloon structure into the inflation lumen, and possibly cause balloon rupture.
8. Observe the monitor as the PAW waveform changes back to the PA waveform.	Ensures adequate balloon deflation.	
9. Expel air from the syringe.	The syringe should remain empty so that accidental balloon inflation does not occur.	
10. Reconnect the syringe to the end of the balloon-inflation valve.	The syringe that is manufactured for the PA catheter should be connected to the PA line so that it is not lost. This syringe can only be filled with 1.5 ml of air, thus serving as a safety feature to minimize the chance of balloon overinflation.	
11. Close the gate valve or stopcock at the end of the balloon-inflation valve.	Prevents accidental use of the balloon-inflation valve.	
12. Using the dual-channel recorded strip, draw a vertical line from the beginning of the P wave of one of the ECG complexes down to the PAW waveform. Repeat this with the next ECG complex.	Compares electrical activity to mechanical activity. Two to three waves will be present on the PAW waveform.	*c* waves commonly are not present on PAW waveforms due to the distance the pressure needs to travel back to the transducer.
13. Align the end of a QRS complex of the ECG strip with the PAW waveform (Fig. 72-11).	Compares electrical activity to mechanical activity.	
14. Identify the *a* wave (see Fig. 72-11).	The *a* wave correlates with the end of the QRS complex. The *c* wave follows the *a* wave, and the *v* wave follows the *c* wave.	If only two waves are present, the first wave is the *a* wave and the second wave is the *v* wave.
15. Identify the scale of the PAW tracing.	Aids in determining pressure measurement.	PA scale commonly is set at 40 mm Hg.
16. Measure the mean of the *a* wave to obtain the PAWP (see Fig. 72-5).	The *a* wave represents atrial contraction and reflects left ventricular filling at end-diastole.	If PEEP is being used and the PEEP is more than 10 cm H_2O, adjustments in determining the pressures may be necessary. Follow institutional standard.
17. Compare the PADP with the PAWP.	The PAWP is commonly 1 to 4 mm Hg less than the PADP. Significant differences between PADP and PAWP may exist for patients with pulmonary hypertension, chronic obstructive lung disease, ARDS, pulmonary embolus, and tachycardia. PADPs that correlate with PAWPs represent left ventricular filling pressures.	

Procedure continues on the following page

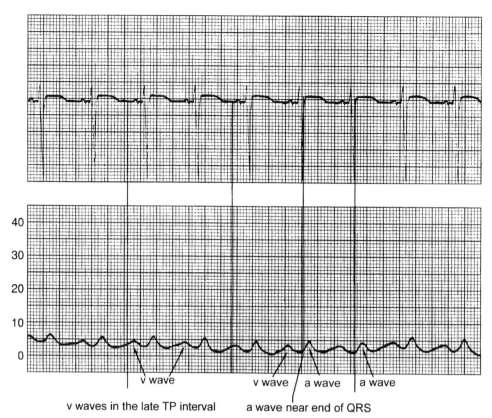

v waves in the late TP interval   a wave near end of QRS

FIGURE 72-11 Obtaining measurement of the pulmonary artery wedge pressure (PAWP). For accurate readings, align the *a* wave from the PAW waveform with the end of the QRS on the electrocardiogram (ECG) at end-diastole. *(From Ahrens, T.S., and Taylor, L.K. [1992]. Hemodynamic Waveform Analysis. Philadelphia: W.B. Saunders.)*

Procedure for Assisting With Pulmonary Artery Catheter Insertion and Pressure Monitoring—*Continued*

Steps	Rationale	Special Considerations
18. Follow PA diastolic pressures if there is a close correlation between PADP and PAWP.	Ensures accuracy of determination of left ventricular filling pressures.	Minimizes the number of times the PA balloon is inflated.
19. Follow the PAWP if there is greater than 4 mm Hg of difference between PAWP and PADP.	Ensures accuracy of measurements.	

Measurement of Hemodynamic Pressures at End-Expiration

1. Measure all hemodynamic pressures at end-expiration to ensure accuracy.	Atmospheric and alveolar pressures are approximately equal at end-expiration. Intrathoracic pressure is closest to zero at end-expiration. Measurement of hemodynamic pressures is most accurate at end-expiration, because pulmonary pressures have minimal effect on intracardiac pressures.	
2. Determine end-expiration by observing the rise and fall of the chest during breathing and use graphic hemodynamic, respiratory, or continuous airway pressure waveforms.	Determines accuracy of end-expiration.	

Procedure	**for Assisting With Pulmonary Artery Catheter Insertion and Pressure Monitoring**—*Continued*	

Steps	Rationale	Special Considerations
Determining End-Expiration for the Patient Breathing Spontaneously		
1. Record a strip of the PA waveform.	A labeled recording aids in determination of accurate hemodynamic pressure values.	In patients who are breathing spontaneously, the normal inspiratory:expiratory ratio is approximately 1:2.
2. Note that the pressure waveform dips down during the inspiratory phase of breathing (Fig. 72-12).	Pleural pressure decreases during spontaneous inspiration, and this decrease is reflected by a fall in the cardiac pressures.	
3. Note that the pressure waveform elevates during the expiratory phase of breathing (see Fig. 72-12).	As pleural pressures equalize, the cardiac pressures reflect a more true normal.	
4. Measure the pressure at the end of the expiratory phase (see Fig. 72-12).	Ensures accurate and consistent pressure measurements.	
Determining End-Expiration for the Patient Receiving Mechanical Ventilation		
1. Record a strip of the PA waveform.	A labeled recording aids in determination of accurate hemodynamic pressure values.	
2. Note that the pressure waveform elevates as a breath is delivered by the ventilator (Fig. 72-13).	As the ventilator delivers a breath to the lungs, an increase in pleural pressure results. This increase in pleural pressure causes an increase in intracardiac pressures.	
3. Note that the pressure waveform dips down as the breath is exhaled (see Fig. 72-13).	As the mechanical breath is exhaled, pulmonary pressures decrease and intracardiac pressures are accurately and consistently measured.	

Procedure continues on the following page

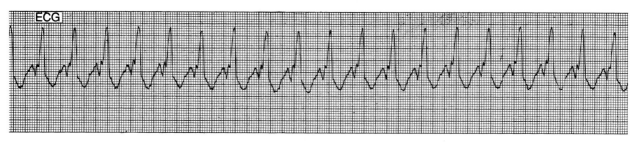

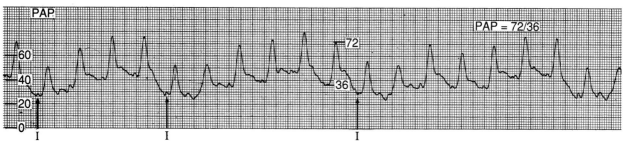

FIGURE 72-12 Respiratory fluctuations of pulmonary artery pressure (PAP) waveform in a spontaneously breathing patient. The location of inspiration (I) is marked on the waveform. The points just before inspiration are end-expiration, where readings will be taken.

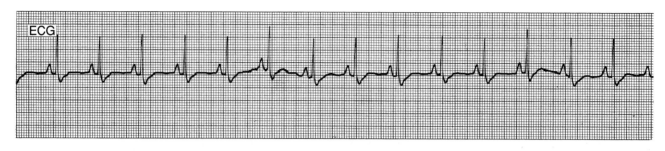

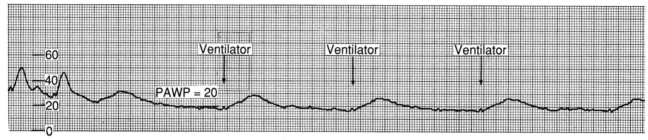

FIGURE 72-13 Mechanically ventilated patient (on pressure support-type ventilator) who had no spontaneous respiration because of neuromuscular blocking agent (vecuronium). The point of end-expiration is located just before the ventilator artifact.

Procedure	for Assisting With Pulmonary Artery Catheter Insertion and Pressure Monitoring—*Continued*	
Steps	**Rationale**	**Special Considerations**

Determining End-Expiration for the Patient Receiving Intermittent Mandatory Mechanical Ventilation

Steps	Rationale	Special Considerations
1. Record a strip of the PA waveform.	A labeled recording aides in determination of accurate hemodynamic pressure monitoring.	
2. If the patient is receiving intermittent mandatory ventilation, measure the pressure during the end-expiration.	Ensures accurate determination of pressure values.	
3. Note that the pressure waveform elevates as a breath is delivered by the ventilator (Fig. 72-14).	As the ventilator delivers a breath to the lungs, an increase in pleural pressure results. This increase in pleural pressure causes an increase in intracardiac pressures.	
4. Note that the pressure waveform dips down as the breath is exhaled (see Fig. 72-14).	As the mechanical breath is exhaled, pulmonary pressures decrease and intracardiac pressures are more accurately reflected.	
5. Identify the patient's spontaneous breath (see Fig. 72-14).	This breath may occur just prior to triggered ventilator breaths.	
6. Determine end-expiration.	Ensures accuracy of measurements.	

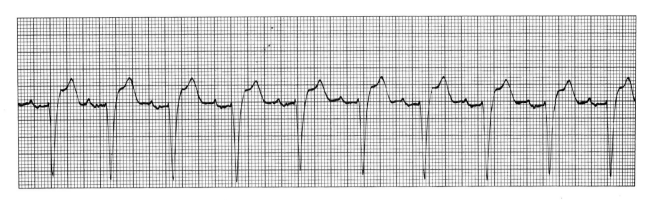

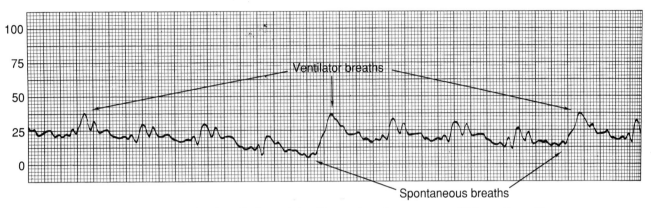

FIGURE 72-14 IMV mode of ventilation and the effect on the pulmonary artery (PA) waveform. *(From Ahrens, T.S., and Taylor, L.K. [1992]. Hemodynamic Waveform Analysis. Philadelphia: W.B. Saunders.)*

Expected Outcomes	Unexpected Outcomes
• Accurate placement of the pulmonary artery catheter • Adequate and appropriate waveforms • Ability to obtain accurate information about cardiac pressures • Evaluation of information obtained to guide therapeutic interventions	• Pneumothorax or hemothorax • Infection • Ventricular dysrhythmias • Heart block • Misplacement (e.g., carotid artery, subclavian artery) • Hemorrhage • Hematoma • Pericardial or ventricular rupture • Venous air embolism • Cardiac tamponade • Sepsis • Pulmonary artery infarction • Pulmonary artery rupture • Pulmonary artery catheter balloon rupture • Pulmonary artery catheter knotting • Heparin-induced thrombocytopenia • Thrombosis • Valvular damage

Patient Monitoring and Care

Steps	Rationale	Reportable Conditions
		These conditions should be reported if they persist despite nursing interventions.
1. Recheck leveling whenever patient position changes.	Ensures accurate reference point for the left atrium.	

Procedure continues on the following page

Patient Monitoring and Care—*Continued*

Steps	Rationale	Reportable Conditions
2. Zero the transducer during initial setup or before insertion, if disconnection occurs between the transducer and the monitoring cable, if disconnection occurs between the monitoring cable and the monitor, and when the values obtained do not fit the clinical picture. Follow manufacturer recommendations for disposable systems.	Ensures accuracy of the hemodynamic monitoring system; minimizes the risk for contamination of the system.	
3. Place sterile nonvented caps on all stopcocks. Replace with new, sterile caps whenever the caps are removed.	Stopcocks can be a source of contamination. Stopcocks that are part of the initial setup are commonly vented. Vented caps need to be replaced with nonvented caps to maintain sterility.	
4. Monitor the pressure transducer system (pressure tubing, transducer, stopcocks, etc.) for air and eliminate air from the system.	Air emboli are potentially fatal.	• Suspected air emboli
5. Continuously monitor hemodynamic waveforms and obtain hemodynamic values (pulmonary artery systolic pressure [PASP], PADP, RAP) hourly and as necessary with condition changes.	Provides for continuous waveform analysis and assessment of patient status.	• Abnormal hemodynamic waveforms and/or pressures
6. Obtain CO, CI, and systemic vascular resistance and additional parameters immediately after catheter insertion and as necessary per patient condition.	Monitors patient status.	• Abnormal hemodynamic parameters or significant changes in hemodynamic parameters
7. Change the hemodynamic monitoring system (flush solution, pressure tubing, transducers, and stopcocks) every 96 hours. *(Level V: Clinical studies in more than one or two different patient populations and situations to support recommendations.)* The flush solution may need to be changed more frequently if near empty of solution.	The Centers for Disease Control and Prevention (CDC)[20] and research findings[19,21] recommend that the hemodynamic flush system can be used safely for 96 hours. This recommendation is based on research conducted with disposable pressure monitoring systems used for peripheral and central lines.	
8. Perform a dynamic response test (square wave test) at the start of each shift, with a change of the waveform, or when the system is opened to air (see Fig. 59-3).	An optimally damped system provides an accurate waveform.	• Overdamped or underdamped waveforms that cannot be corrected with troubleshooting procedures
9. Label the tubing with the date and time the system was prepared.	Identifies when the system needs to be changed.	
10. Maintain the pressure bag or device at 300 mm Hg.	At 300 mm Hg each flush device will deliver approximately 1 to 3 ml/hour to maintain patency of the system.	
11. Do not fast-flush the catheter for longer than 2 seconds.[8]	Pulmonary artery rupture may potentially occur with prolonged flushing of high-pressure fluid.	

Patient Monitoring and Care—*Continued*

Steps	Rationale	Reportable Conditions
12. Never flush the PA catheter when the balloon is wedged in the pulmonary artery.	Excessive PA pressure may cause PA damage and/or rupture.	
13. Use aseptic technique when withdrawing from or flushing the PA catheter.	Prevents bacterial contamination of the system.	
14. Clear the system, including stopcocks, of all traces of blood after blood withdrawal.	Blood can become a medium for bacterial growth.[20] Clots also may be flushed into the catheter if all blood is not eliminated.	
15. Maintain sterility and integrity of the plastic sleeve covering the PA catheter.	Any tear in the sleeve will break the sterile barrier, making catheter repositioning no longer possible.	• Defects in the integrity of plastic sleeve
16. Blood products and albumin should never be infused through the PA catheter.	Viscous blood may occlude the catheter. The accuracy of the PA monitoring system may be adversely affected.	
17. IV fluids are never infused via the distal lumen of the PA catheter and are rarely infused via the proximal lumen of the PA catheter.	PA monitoring is not possible, and a life-threatening situation can occur (e.g., undetected wedged PA catheter).	
18. Replace gauze dressings every 2 days and transparent dressings at least every 7 days.[20] Cleanse the site with an antiseptic solution (e.g., 2% chlorhexidine-based preparation).	Decreases the risk for infection at the catheter site. The CDC recommends replacing the dressing when the dressing becomes damp, loosened, soiled, or when inspection of the site is necessary.[20]	• Signs or symptoms of infection
19. Date, time, and initial the dressing change.	Ensures consistency of dressing change and indicates when the next change will occur.	
20. Follow institutional standard for application of antimicrobial ointment to catheter sites.	Routine use of antimicrobial ointment at central venous catheter sites is not recommended.[20]	
21. Obtain PA waveform strips to place on the patient's chart at the start of each shift and whenever there is a change in the waveform.	The printed waveform allows assessment of the adequacy of the waveform, presence of damping, or respiratory variation.	
22. Consider changing PA catheters every 7 days.	The CDC recommends that PA catheters do not need to be changed more frequently than every 7 days.[20] The CDC makes no specific recommendation regarding routine replacement of PA catheters that need to be in place for greater than 7 days.[20]	• Signs and symptoms of infection.

Documentation

Documentation should include the following:

- Patient and family education
- Insertion of the PA catheter
- External cm marking of PA catheter noted at exit site
- Patient tolerance of procedure
- Confirmation of PA catheter placement (e.g., waveforms, chest x-ray)

- Cardiac rhythm during PA catheter insertion and monitoring
- Site assessment
- PA pressures (RA/CVP, PA systolic, diastolic, mean, and PAWP)
- Waveforms (RA/CVP, PAP, PAWP)
- CO/CI and SVR
- Occurrence of unexpected outcomes and interventions

References

1. Blanch, L., et al. (1997). Short term effects of prone position in critically ill patients with acute respiratory distress syndrome. *Intensive Care Med, 23,* 1033-39.
2. Brussel, T., et al. (1993). Mechanical ventilation in the prone position for acute respiratory failure after cardiac surgery. *J Cardiothorac Vasc Anesth, 7,* 541-46.
3. Cason, C.L., et al. (1990). Effects of backrest elevation and position on pulmonary artery pressures. *Cardiovasc Nurs, 26,* 1-5.
4. Chong, B.H. (1995). Heparin-induced thrombocytopenia. *British J Haematology, 89,* 431-39.
5. Chulay, M., and Miller, T. (1984). The effect of backrest elevation on pulmonary artery and pulmonary capillary wedge pressures in patients after cardiac surgery. *Heart Lung, 13,* 138-40.
6. Clochesy, J., Hinshaw, A.D., and Otto, C.W. (1984). Effects of change of position on pulmonary artery and pulmonary capillary wedge pressure in mechanically ventilated patients. *NITA, 7,* 223-25.
7. Cohen, Y., et al. (1998). The "hands-off" catheter in the prevention of systemic infections associated with pulmonary artery catheter: A prospective study. *Am J Respir Crit Care Med, 157,* 284-87.
8. Daily, E.K., and Schroeder, J.S. (1994). *Techniques in Bedside Hemodynamic Monitoring.* 5th ed. St. Louis: Mosby.
9. Dobbin, K., et al. (1992). Pulmonary artery pressure measurement in patients with elevated pressures: Effect of backrest elevation and method of measurement. *Am J Crit Care, 1,* 61-9.
10. Fridrich, P., et al. (1996). The effects of long-term prone positioning in patients with trauma-induced adult respiratory distress syndrome. *Anesth Analg, 83,* 1206-11.
11. Groom, L., Frisch, S.R., and Elliot, M. (1990). Reproducibility and accuracy of pulmonary artery pressure measurement in supine and lateral positions. *Heart Lung, 19,* 147-51.
12. Hannan, A.T., Brown, M., and Bigman, O. (1984). Pulmonary artery catheter induced hemorrhage. *Chest, 85,* 128-31.
13. Jolliet, P., Bulpa, P., and Chevrolet, J.C. (1998). Effects of prone position on gas exchange and hemodynamics in severe acute respiratory distress syndrome. *Crit Care Med, 26,* 1977-85.
14. Keating, D., et al. (1986). Effect of sidelying positions on pulmonary artery pressures. *Heart Lung, 15,* 605-10.
15. Kennedy, G.T., Bryant, A., and Crawford, M.H. (1984). The effects of lateral body positioning on measurements of pulmonary artery and pulmonary wedge pressures. *Heart Lung, 13,* 155-58.
16. Lambert, C.W., and Cason, C.L. (1990). Backrest elevation and pulmonary artery pressures: Research analysis. *Dimensions Crit Care Nurs, 9,* 327-35.
17. Langer, M., et al. (1988). The prone position in ARDS patients. *Chest, 94,* 103-7.
18. Laulive, J.L. (1982). Pulmonary artery pressures and position changes in the critically ill adult. *Dimensions Crit Care Nurs, 1,* 28-34.
19. Luskin, R.L., et al. (1986). Extended use of disposable pressure transducers: A bacteriologic evaluation. *JAMA, 255,* 916-20.
20. O'Grady, N.P., et al. (2002). Guidelines for the prevention of intravascular catheter-related infections. *Am J Infect Control, 30,* 476-89.
21. O'Malley, M.K., et al. (1994). Value of routine pressure monitoring system changes after 72 hours of use. *Crit Care Med, 22,* 1424-30.
22. Osika, C. (1989). Measurement of pulmonary artery pressures: Supine verses side-lying head-elevated positions. *Heart Lung, 18,* 298-9.
23. Pappert, D., et al. (1994). Influence of positioning on ventilation-perfusion relationships in severe adult respiratory distress syndrome. *Chest, 106,* 1511-16.
24. Pelosi, P., et al. (1998). Effects of the prone position on respiratory mechanics and gas exchange during acute lung injury. *Am J Respir Crit Care Med, 157,* 387-93.
25. Voggenreiter, G., et al. (1999). Intermittent prone positioning in the treatment of severe and moderate posttraumatic lung injury. *Crit Care Med, 27,* 2375-82.
26. Vollman, K.M., and Bander, J.J. (1996). Improved oxygenation utilizing a prone positioner in patients with acute respiratory distress syndrome. *Intensive Care Med, 22,* 1105-11.
27. Wild, L. (1984). Effect of lateral recumbent positions on measurement of pulmonary artery and pulmonary artery wedge pressures in critically ill adults. *Heart Lung, 13,* 305.
28. Wilson, A.E., et al. (1996). Effect of backrest position on hemodynamic and right ventricular measurements in critically ill adults. *Am J Crit Care, 5,* 264-70.
29. Woods, S.L., and Mansfield, L.W. (1976). Effect of body position upon pulmonary artery and pulmonary capillary wedge pressures in noncritically ill patients. *Heart Lung, 5,* 83-90.

Additional Readings

Anonymous. (1997). Pulmonary artery catheter consensus conference: Consensus statement. *Crit Care Med, 25,* 910-25.

Ahrens, T.S., and Taylor, L.A. (1992). *Hemodynamic Waveform Analysis.* Philadelphia: W.B. Saunders.

Bridges, E.J., and Woods, S.L. (1993). Pulmonary artery pressure measurement: State of art. *Heart Lung, 22,* 99-111.

Campbell, M.L., and Greenberg, C.A. (1988). Pulmonary artery wedge pressure at end-expiration. *Focus Crit Care, 15,* 60-3.

Cason, C.L., and Lambert, C.W. (1993). Positioning during hemodynamic monitoring: Evaluating the research. *Dimensions Crit Care Nurs, 12,* 226-33.

Daily, E.K. (2001). Hemodynamic waveform analysis. *J Cardiovasc Nurs, 15,* 6-22, 87-8.

Darovic, G.O. (2002). *Hemodynamic Monitoring: Invasive and Noninvasive Clinical Application.* 3rd ed. Philadelphia: W.B. Saunders.

Ducharme, F.M., et al. (1988). Incidence of infection related to arterial catheterization in children: A prospective study. *Crit Care Med, 16,* 272-76.

Grap, M.J., Pettrey, L., and Thornby, D. (1997). Hemodynamic monitoring: A comparison of research and practice. *Am J Crit Care, 6,* 452-56.

Houghton, D., et al. (2002). Routine daily chest radiography in patients with pulmonary artery catheters. *Am J Crit Care, 11,* 261-65.

Keckeisen, M. (1997). *Protocols for Practice: Hemodynamic Monitoring Series—Pulmonary Artery Pressure Monitoring.* Aliso Viejo, Ca: American Association of Critical-Care Nurses.

Kee, L.L., et al. (1993). Echocardiographic determination of valid zero reference levels in supine and lateral positions. *Am J Crit Care, 2,* 72-80.

Liu, C., and Webb, C. (2000). From the Food and Drug Administration. Pulmonary artery rupture: Serious complication associated with pulmonary artery catheters. *Internat J Trauma Nurs, 6,* 19-26.

Mermel, L.A., et al. (1991). The pathogenesis and epidemiology of catheter-related infection with pulmonary artery Swan-Ganz catheters: A prospective study utilizing molecular subtyping. *Am J Med, 91,* 197S-205S.

Ott, K., Johnson, K., and Ahrens, T. (2001). New technologies in the assessment of hemodynamic parameters. *J Cardiovasc Nurs, 15,* 41-55.

Pearson, M.L. (1996). Hospital Infection Control Practices Advisory Committee: Guideline for prevention of intravascular device-related infections. *Infect Control Hosp Epidemiol,* 17, 438-73.

Quaal, S.J. (2001). Improving the accuracy of pulmonary artery catheter measurement. *J Cardiovasc Nurs,* 15, 71-82.

Quaal, S.J. (1995). Is it necessary to perform a square wave test routinely to test for accuracy in hemodynamic monitoring? Or is it recommended only if there is a problem? *Crit Care Nurse,* 15, 92-3.

Schactman, M., et al. (1995). *Hemodynamic Monitoring.* El Paso, Tex: Skidmore-Roth Publishing.

Vollman, K.M. (2001). What are the practice guidelines for prone positioning of acutely ill patients? Specifically, what are the recommendations related to hemodynamic monitoring and tube feeding? *Crit Care Nurse,* 21, 84-6.

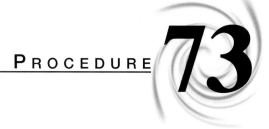

PROCEDURE **73**

Pulmonary Artery Catheter Removal

PURPOSE: The pulmonary artery (PA) catheter is removed when the patient's condition is improved sufficiently that hemodynamic monitoring is no longer necessary, when there is risk for complications from the presence of the catheter (e.g., dysrhythmias, pulmonary infarction), or when there is risk for infection associated with the prolonged use of intravascular lines.

Teresa Preuss
Debra Lynn-McHale Wiegand

PREREQUISITE NURSING KNOWLEDGE

- Knowledge of the normal cardiovascular anatomy and physiology
- Knowledge of normal values for intracardiac pressures
- Knowledge of normal coagulation values
- Knowledge of normal waveform configurations for right atrial pressure (RAP), right ventricular pressure (RVP), pulmonary artery pressure (PAP), and pulmonary artery wedge pressure (PAWP)
- Venous access routes
- Principles of aseptic technique
- Advanced cardiac life support knowledge and skills
- Potential complications associated with removal of the PA catheter
- In collaboration with the physician, determine when the PA catheter should be discontinued
- Indications for the removal of the PA catheter include the following:
  - ❖ The patient's condition no longer requires hemodynamic monitoring.
  - ❖ Complications occurred because of the presence of the PA catheter.
  - ❖ The patient shows evidence of a catheter-related infection that may be associated with the PA catheter.
- Contraindications to percutaneous removal of the PA catheter or introducer include the following:
  - ❖ The patient's coagulation values are prolonged.

- ❖ The PA catheter is knotted (observed on chest x-ray).
- ❖ A permanent pacemaker, temporary transvenous pacemaker, or implantable cardioverter defibrillator (ICD) is present (catheter should be removed by an advanced practice nurse or a physician).

EQUIPMENT

- 1.5-ml syringe
- Sterile and nonsterile gloves
- Gown
- Fluid shield face mask
- 4 × 4 sterile gauze pads
- Central line dressing kit
- Two moisture-proof absorbent pads
  Additional equipment to have available as needed includes the following:
- Obturator/cap for hemostasis valve
- Suture removal kit
- Sterile specimen container (needed if culture of catheter tip will be obtained)
- Emergency equipment

PATIENT AND FAMILY EDUCATION

- Explain the procedure and the reason for catheter removal. ➤*Rationale:* Provides information and decreases anxiety.
- Explain the importance of lying still during the catheter removal. ➤*Rationale:* Ensures patient cooperation and facilitates safe removal of the catheter.

- Instruct the patient and family to report any bleeding or discomfort at the insertion site during or after catheter removal. ➤*Rationale:* Identifies patient discomfort and assists with identification and prompt treatment of bleeding.

PATIENT ASSESSMENT AND PREPARATION

Patient Assessment

- Assess ECG, vital signs, and neurovascular status of the extremity distal to the catheter insertion site. ➤*Rationale:* Serves as baseline data.
- If the introducer will also be removed, assess the current coagulation values of the patient. ➤*Rationale:* If the patient has abnormal coagulation study results, hemostasis may be difficult to obtain after the introducer catheter is removed.
- Verify catheter position by waveform analysis or chest x-ray. ➤*Rationale:* Ensures accuracy of catheter position.
- Determine whether the patient has a permanent pacemaker, temporary transvenous pacemaker or ICD. ➤*Rationale:* PA catheter removal by a critical care nurse

is usually contraindicated in the presence of a permanent pacemaker, temporary transvenous pacemaker, or ICD. Entanglement of the PA catheter and the pacemaker electrodes can occur.

- Assess the integrity of the PA catheter. ➤*Rationale:* The PA catheter should be removed by a physician if the catheter or introducer is not intact (e.g., visible cracks are noted).

Patient Preparation

- Ensure that the patient understands preprocedural teaching. Answer questions as they arise and reinforce information as needed. ➤*Rationale:* Evaluates and reinforces understanding of previously taught information.
- Place the patient in a supine position with the head of the bed in a slight Trendelenburg position (or flat if Trendelenburg is contraindicated or not tolerated by the patient).[2,3,5] ➤*Rationale:* A normal pressure gradient exists between atmospheric air and the central venous compartment that promotes air entry if the compartment is open. The lower the site of entry below the heart, the lower the pressure gradient, thus minimizing the risk of venous air embolism.

Procedure for Pulmonary Artery Catheter Removal		
Steps	**Rationale**	**Special Considerations**
1. Wash hands and don fluid shield face mask, gown, and nonsterile gloves.	Reduces the transmission of microorganisms; standard precautions. Protects against splashing of body fluids during the procedure.	
2. Place a moisture-proof absorbent pad under the patient's upper torso and another under the PA catheter.	Collects blood and body fluids associated with removal; serves as a receptacle for the contaminated catheter.	
3. Place the patient supine in slight Trendelenburg position.[2,3,5] (*Level II: Theory-based, no research data to support recommendations; recommendations from expert consensus group may exist.*)	Minimizes the risk for venous air embolus.	Place the patient flat if Trendelenburg is contraindicated or not tolerated by the patient. If the PA catheter is in the femoral vein, extend the patient's leg and ensure the groin area is adequately exposed.
4. Turn the patient's head away from insertion site so that the PA catheter and introducer sheath are readily visible.	Decreases the risk for infection.	
5. Transfer or discontinue intravenous (IV) solution and flush solutions.	Prepares the catheter for removal.	
6. Open supplies.	Prepares for removal.	

Procedure continues on the following page

Procedure for Pulmonary Artery Catheter Removal—*Continued*

Steps	Rationale	Special Considerations
7. Remove the syringe from balloon inflation port, ensure that the gate valve or stopcock is in the open position, and observe the PA waveform (see Fig. 72-6).	Allows air to passively escape from the balloon and ensures adequate balloon deflation.	Myocardial or valvular tissues can be damaged if PA catheter is removed with the balloon inflated.
8. Turn all stopcocks off to the patient.	Prepares for removal.	
9. Unlock the sheath from the introducer catheter.	Prepares for removal.	
10. Remove the old dressing.	Prepares for removal.	Signs of local or systemic infection may determine the need to send a culture of the catheter tip.
11. Discard gloves, wash hands, and don sterile gloves.	Reduces the transmission of microorganisms; standard precautions ensure asepsis.	
12. If present, clip the sutures securing the PA catheter.	Frees the PA catheter for removal.	
13. Ask the patient to take a deep breath in and hold it. *(Level II: Theory based, no research data to support recommendations; recommendations from expert consensus group may exist.)*	Minimizes the risk for venous air embolus.	If a patient is mechanically ventilated, withdraw the catheter during the inspiratory phase of the respiratory cycle or while delivering a breath via a bag-valve device.
14. While stabilizing the introducer catheter, gently withdraw the PA catheter using a constant, steady motion (Fig. 73-1).	Ensures the removal of an intact catheter.	Observe ECG tracing during removal. Dysrhythmias may occur during removal but are usually self-limiting.[1] If resistance is met, do not continue to remove catheter and notify advanced practice nurse or physician immediately. Resistance may be caused by catheter knotting, kinking, or wedging.

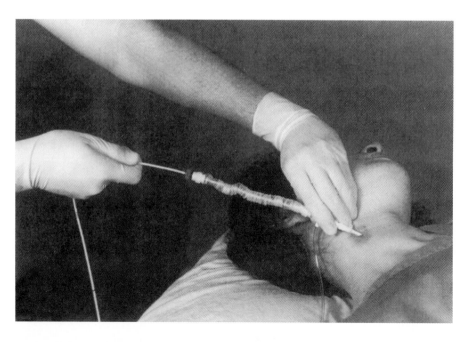

FIGURE 73-1 While stabilizing the introducer, gently withdraw the PA catheter using a constant, steady motion. *(From Wadas, T.M. [1994]. Pulmonary artery catheter removal. Crit Care Nurse, 14, 63.)*

Procedure for Pulmonary Artery Catheter Removal—*Continued*

Steps	Rationale	Special Considerations
15. Temporarily cover the hemostasis valve with a sterile-gloved finger until the obturator/cap is secured.	The hemostasis valve must be occluded to minimize the risk for air embolus and hemorrhage.	
16. Have the patient exhale once the PA catheter is removed.		
17. Place the PA catheter on the moisture-proof absorbent pad and check to be sure that the entire catheter was removed.	Allows for assessment of the catheter.	
18. Send the tip of the PA catheter, if needed, to the laboratory for analysis.	Determines the presence of bacterial colonization of the catheter.	
19. If the introducer remains in place, perform site care and apply a sterile dressing to the site.	Decreases the risk for infection at the insertion site.	
20. If the introducer is to be removed, clip sutures securing the introducer.	Frees the introducer for removal.	
21. Ask the patient to take a deep breath in and hold it.[2,3,5] (*Level II: Theory-based, no research data to support recommendations; recommendations from expert consensus group may exist.*)	Minimizes the risk for venous air embolus. Cases have been reported of venous air embolus occurring after removal of central venous catheters while patients were in the semi-Fowler's position.	If a patient is mechanically ventilated, withdraw the catheter during the inspiratory phase of the respiratory cycle or while delivering a breath via a bag-valve device.
22. Withdraw the introducer, pulling parallel to the skin and using a steady motion.	Minimizes trauma.	If resistance is met, do not continue to remove the introducer. Notify advanced practice nurse or physician immediately. Resistance may be caused by kinks or cracks.
23. As the introducer exits the site, apply pressure with a gauze pad.	Minimizes the risk for venous air embolus and promotes hemostasis.	
24. Have the patient exhale once the introducer is removed.		
25. Lay the introducer on the moisture-proof absorbent pad. Check to be sure that all of the introducer was removed.	Ensures the removal of the entire introducer.	
26. Continue applying firm, direct pressure over the insertion site with the gauze pad until bleeding has stopped.	Ensures hemostasis.	Because a large vein was used for insertion, it may take up to 10 minutes for hemostasis to occur.
27. Apply a sterile occlusive dressing to the insertion site.	Decreases the risk for infection at the insertion site and minimizes the risk for venous air embolus.	
28. Elevate the head of bed to patient comfort.		
29. Dispose of used supplies and wash hands.	Reduces the transmission of microorganisms; standard precautions.	

Expected Outcomes

- The PA catheter is removed.
- The introducer may or may not be removed.

Unexpected Outcomes

- Dysrhythmias
- Valvular damage
- PA rupture
- Thrombosis
- Venous air emboli
- Uncontrolled bleeding
- Infection
- Unable to percutaneously remove the PA catheter because of knotting or kinking
- Hematoma

Patient Monitoring and Care

Steps	Rationale	Reportable Conditions
		These conditions should be reported if they persist despite nursing interventions. • Signs and symptoms of infection
1. Consider changing the PA catheter every 7 days.	The CDC recommends that PA catheters do not need to be changed more frequently than every 7 days.[4] The CDC makes no specific recommendation regarding routine replacement of PA catheters that need to be in longer than 7 days.[4]	
2. Monitor the patient's cardiac rate and rhythm during catheter withdrawal.	Ventricular dysrhythmias may occur as the PA catheter passes through the right ventricle.	• Ventricular dysrhythmias occurring after the PA catheter is removed
3. Monitor for signs and symptoms of venous air embolus and, if present, immediately place the patient in the left lateral Trendelenburg position.	Venous air embolus is a potentially life-threatening complication. The left lateral Trendelenburg position prevents air from passing into the left side of the heart and traveling into the arterial circulation.	• Respiratory distress, cyanosis, gasp reflex, sucking sound, hypotension, petechiae, cardiac dysrhythmias, altered mental status
4. After removal of the PA catheter and introducer, assess the PA catheter site for signs of bleeding every 15 minutes × 2, every 30 minutes × 2, and then 1 hour later.	Bleeding or a hematoma can develop if there is still bleeding from the vessel.	• Abnormal vital signs or signs of bleeding
5. Mark the dressing with the date, time, and your initials.	Indicates when dressing was placed.	

Documentation

Documentation should include the following:

- Patient and family education
- Patient assessment before and after removal of the PA catheter
- Patient's response to the procedure
- Date and time of removal
- Occurrence of unexpected outcomes
- Nursing interventions taken

References

1. Baldwin, I.C., and Heland, M. (2000). Incidence of cardiac dysrhythmias in patients during pulmonary artery catheter removal after cardiac surgery. *Heart Lung*, 29, 155-60.
2. Ely, E.W., et al. (1999). Venous air embolism from central venous catheterization: A need for increased physician awareness. *Crit Care Med*, 27, 2113-7.
3. McCarthy, P.M., et al. (1995). Air embolism in single-lung transplant patients after central venous catheter removal. *Chest*, 107, 1178-9.
4. O'Grady, N.P., et al. (2002). Guidelines for the prevention of intravascular catheter-related infections. *Am J Infect Control*, 30, 476-89.
5. Woodrow, P. (2002). Central venous catheters and central venous pressure. *Nursing Standard*, 16, 45-52, 54.

Additional Readings

Ahrens, T.S., and Taylor, L.A. (1992). *Hemodynamic Waveform Analysis*. Philadelphia: W.B. Saunders.

Arnaout, S., et al. (2001). Rupture of the chordae of the tricuspid valve after knotting of the pulmonary artery catheter. *Chest*, 120, 1742-4.

Darovic, G.O. (2002). *Hemodynamic Monitoring: Invasive and Noninvasive Clinical Application,* 3rd ed. Philadelphia: W.B. Saunders.

Dumont, C.P. (2001). Procedures nurses use to remove central venous catheters and complications they observe: A pilot study. *Am J Crit Care*, 10, 151-5.

Henderson, N. (1997). Central venous lines. *Nursing Standard*, 11, 49-56.

Peter, D.A., and Saxman, C. (2003). Preventing air embolism when removing CVCs: An evidence-based approach to changing practice. *Medsurg Nursing*, 12, 223-9.

Rountree, W.D. (1991). Removal of pulmonary artery catheters by registered nurses: A study in safety and complications. *Focus Crit Care*, 18, 313-8.

Schactman, M., et al. (1995). *Hemodynamic Monitoring*. El Paso, Tex: Skidmore-Roth Publishing.

Wadas, T.M. (1994). Pulmonary artery catheter removal. *Crit Care Nurse,* 14, 62-72.

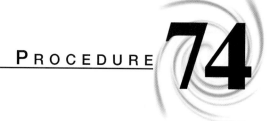

PROCEDURE **74**

Pulmonary Artery Catheter and Pressure Lines, Troubleshooting

P U R P O S E : Troubleshooting of the pulmonary artery (PA) catheter is important to maintain catheter patency, to ensure that data from the PA catheter are accurate, and to prevent the development of catheter-related and patient-related complications.

Teresa Preuss
Debra Lynn-McHale Wiegand

PREREQUISITE NURSING KNOWLEDGE

- Knowledge of cardiovascular anatomy and physiology
- Knowledge of pulmonary anatomy and physiology
- Basic dysrhythmia recognition and treatment of life-threatening dysrhythmias
- Advanced cardiac life support knowledge and skills
- Knowledge of principles of aseptic technique
- Understanding of the set-up of the hemodynamic monitoring system (see Procedure 75)
- Anatomy of the PA catheter (see Fig. 72-1) and the location of the PA catheter in the heart and pulmonary artery (see Fig. 72-2)
- Pulmonary artery wedge pressure may be referred to as *pulmonary artery occlusion pressure.*
- After wedging the PA catheter, air is passively removed by disconnecting the syringe from the balloon-inflation port. Active withdrawal of air from the balloon is avoided because it can weaken the balloon, pull the balloon structure into the inflation lumen, and possibly cause balloon rupture.
- The pulmonary artery diastolic pressure (PADP) and the pulmonary artery wedge pressure (PAWP) are indirect measures of left ventricular end-diastolic pressure (LVEDP). Usually, the PAWP is approximately 1 to 4 mm Hg less than the PADP. Because these two pressures are similar, the PADP is commonly followed. This minimizes the frequency of balloon inflation, thus decreasing the potential of balloon rupture.
- Differences between the PADP and the PAWP may exist for patients with pulmonary hypertension, chronic obstructive lung disease, adult respiratory distress syndrome, pulmonary embolus, and tachycardia.
- Pulmonary artery pressures (PAPs) may be elevated because of pulmonary artery hypertension, pulmonary disease, mitral valve disease, left ventricular failure, atrial or ventricular left-to-right shunt, pulmonary emboli, or hypervolemia.
- PAPs may be decreased because of hypovolemia or vasodilation.
- The waveforms that occur during insertion should be recognized, including right atrial (RA), right ventricular (RV), pulmonary artery (PA), and pulmonary artery wedge (PAW) (see Fig. 72-3).
- The *a* wave reflects atrial contraction. The *c* wave reflects closure of the atrioventricular valves. The *v* wave reflects passive filling of the atria during ventricular systole (see Figs. 72-4 and 72-5).
- Knowledge of normal hemodynamic values (see Table 63-1)
- Elevated *a* and *v* waves may be evident in RA or central venous pressure (CVP) and in PAW waveforms. These elevations may occur in patients with cardiac tamponade, constrictive pericardial disease, and hypervolemia.
- Elevated *a* waves in the RA or CVP waveform may occur in patients with pulmonic or tricuspid stenosis, right ventricular ischemia or infarction, right ventricular failure, pulmonary artery hypertension, and atrioventricular (AV) dissociation.
- Elevated *a* waves in the PAW waveform may occur in patients with mitral stenosis, acute left ventricular ischemia or infarction, left ventricular failure, and AV dissociation.
- Elevated *v* waves in the RA or CVP waveform may occur in patients with tricuspid insufficiency.

- Elevated *v* waves in the PAW waveform may occur in patients with mitral insufficiency or ruptured papillary muscle.

EQUIPMENT

- Nonsterile gloves
- Syringes (5-ml or 10-ml)
- Sterile nonvented caps
- Sterile gauze 4 × 4
- Stopcocks
- Pressure monitoring cable(s)
- Disposable pressure tubing with transducer(s)
- 500-ml bag of normal saline intravenous (IV) solution
- Pressure bag or device
- Dual channel recorder

Additional equipment to have available as needed includes the following:

- Emergency equipment

PATIENT AND FAMILY EDUCATION

- Explain the troubleshooting procedures to the patient. ➤*Rationale:* Keeps the patient and family informed and reduces anxiety.
- Explain the patient's expected participation during the procedure. ➤*Rationale:* Encourages patient assistance.
- Inform the patient and family of signs and symptoms to report to the critical care nurse, including chest pain, palpitations, new cough, tenderness at the insertion site, and chills. ➤*Rationale:* Encourages the patient to report signs of discomfort and potential PA catheter complications.

PATIENT ASSESSMENT AND PREPARATION

Patient Assessment

- Monitor PA waveforms continuously. ➤*Rationale:* The PA catheter may migrate forward into a wedged position or may loop around and move back into the right ventricle.
- Assess the configuration of the PA catheter waveforms. ➤*Rationale:* Thrombus formation at the tip of the catheter lumen may be evidenced by an overdamped waveform.
- Assess the patient's hemodynamic and cardiovascular status. ➤*Rationale:* The patient's clinical assessment should correlate with the PA catheter readings.
- Assess the patient and the PA catheter site for signs of infection. ➤*Rationale:* Infection can develop because of the invasive nature of the PA catheter.

Patient Preparation

- Ensure that the patient understands preprocedural teaching. Answer questions as they arise and reinforce information as needed. ➤*Rationale:* Evaluates and reinforces understanding of previously taught information.
- Validate the patency of the patient's intravenous lines. ➤*Rationale:* Access may be needed for administration of emergency medication or fluids.

Procedure	**for Pulmonary Artery Catheter and Pressure Lines, Troubleshooting**		
Steps	Rationale	Special Considerations	

Troubleshooting an Overwedged Balloon

Steps	Rationale	Special Considerations
1. Wash hands.	Reduces the transmission of microorganisms; standard precautions.	
2. Identify an overwedged balloon (Fig. 74-1).	Determines the need for troubleshooting.	Overinflation of the balloon can cause pulmonary arteriole infarction or rupture, resulting in life-threatening hemorrhage.[9]
3. Remove the syringe from the gate valve or the stopcock of the PA balloon inflation port.	Passively removes air from the PA balloon.	Ensure that the gate-valve or stopcock is in the open position (see Fig. 72-6).
4. Note the change in PA waveform from the overinflated waveform to the PA waveform.	As the balloon deflates, the PA waveform returns.	
5. Note and record the external cm marking of the PA catheter at the introducer exit site.	Identifies whether the PA catheter has migrated forward from the previously documented measurement.	The advanced practice nurse or the physician may need to reposition the catheter.

Procedure continues on the following page

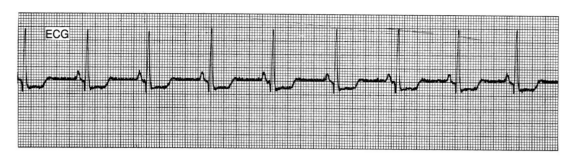

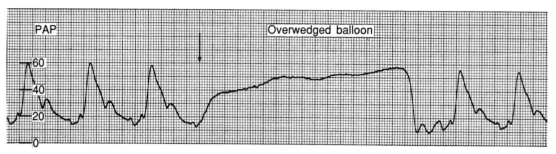

FIGURE 74-1 Balloon inflation (*arrow*). Overwedging of balloon (balloon has been overinflated). The danger of overinflating the balloon is that the pulmonary artery (PA) vessel may rupture from the pressure of the balloon. *PAP*, pulmonary artery pressure; *ECG*, electrocardiogram.

Procedure	**for Pulmonary Artery Catheter and Pressure Lines, Troubleshooting**—*Continued*	
Steps	**Rationale**	**Special Considerations**
6. Note and record the amount of air needed to wedge the PA catheter.	Prevents overwedging of the PA catheter balloon.	
Preventing an Overwedged Balloon		
1. Fill the syringe with 1.5 ml of air.	More than 1.5 ml of air may rupture the PA balloon and the pulmonary arteriole.	
2. Connect the PA syringe to the gate valve or stopcock of the balloon inflation port of the PA catheter.	This port is designed for PA balloon air inflation.	
3. Slowly inflate the balloon with air until the PA waveform changes to a PAW waveform (see Fig. 72-10).	Only enough air is needed to convert the PA waveform to a PAW waveform.	
4. Inflate the PA balloon for no more than 8 to 15 seconds.	Avoids prolonged pressure on the pulmonary arteriole.	
5. Disconnect the syringe from the balloon inflation port.	Allows air to passively escape from the balloon.	
6. Observe the monitor as the PAW waveform changes back to the PA waveform.	Ensures adequate balloon deflation.	
7. Expel air from the syringe.	The syringe should remain empty so that accidental balloon inflation does not occur.	
8. Reconnect the empty syringe to the end of the balloon inflation port.	Retains the safety syringe.	
9. Close the gate valve or the stopcock at the end of the balloon-inflation port (see Fig. 72-6).	Prevents accidental use of the balloon-inflation port.	

Procedure	for Pulmonary Artery Catheter and Pressure Lines, Troubleshooting—*Continued*	
Steps	**Rationale**	**Special Considerations**
10. Wash hands.	Reduces the transmission of microorganisms; standard precautions.	
Troubleshooting an Absent Waveform 1. Wash hands and don nonsterile gloves.	Reduces the transmission of microorganisms; standard precautions.	
2. Check to see whether there is a kink in the pulmonary artery catheter.	Kinks may inhibit waveform transmission.	
3. Ensure that all connections are tight.	Loose connections will allow air into the system and can overdamp or eliminate the waveform.	
4. Ensure that the stopcock is open to transducer (Fig. 74-2).	The stopcocks open to the system allow waveform transmission from the vascular system to the monitor; stopcocks closed to transducer will prevent waveform transmission to the monitor and oscilloscope.	
5. Check that the cables are in the appropriate pressure module.	Necessary for signal transmission.	
6. Ensure that the pressure cable is securely plugged into the monitor.	No waveform will be transmitted without proper connection.	
7. Ensure that the correct monitor parameters are turned on.	Required for specific parameter monitoring.	
8. Ensure the correct scale has been chosen for pressure being monitored; for example, 40 mm Hg scale is used for PA monitoring.	A larger scale (e.g., 100 mm Hg) will cause the waveform to be smaller and possibly to not be visible on the oscilloscope.	

Procedure continues on the following page

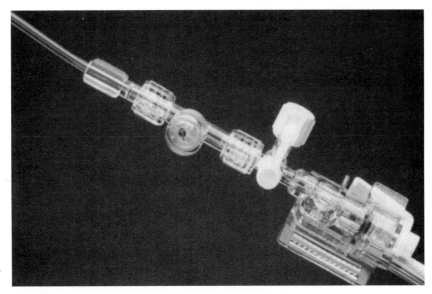

FIGURE 74-2 The stopcock is open to the transducer. *(From Ahrens, T.S., and Taylor, L.K. [1993]. Hemodynamic Waveform Recognition. Philadelphia: W.B. Saunders.)*

Procedure	**for Pulmonary Artery Catheter and Pressure Lines, Troubleshooting**—*Continued*	

Steps	Rationale	Special Considerations
9. Level and zero the monitoring system (see Procedure 75).	Ensures accurate functioning of the monitoring system.	
10. Aspirate through the stopcock that is closest to the catheter to check for blood return (see Fig. 62-3).	Ensures patency of the PA catheter.	A clotted catheter will have no waveform and no blood return when aspirated.
11. Replace the monitoring cable.	A faulty cable can result in an absent waveform.	
12. Replace the disposable pressure tubing with transducer.	A faulty transducer can result in an absent waveform.	
13. Notify the advanced practice nurse or the physician if troubleshooting is unsuccessful.	The catheter will need to be removed or replaced.	
14. Discard used supplies and wash hands.	Reduces the transmission of microorganisms; standard precautions.	
Troubleshooting an Overdamped Waveform		
1. Wash hands and don nonsterile gloves.	Reduces the transmission of microorganisms; standard precautions.	
2. Obtain a monitor strip of the overdamped waveform (Fig. 74-3).	The waveform can be compared with the previous waveforms.	
3. Ensure that all connections are tight.	Loose connections will allow air into the system and can overdamp the waveform.	
4. Ensure that there is fluid in the flush bag and that the pressure on the flush bag or device is delivering 300 mm Hg.	Low counterpressure from the IV flush bag will result in an overdamped waveform.	

5. Check all tubing for air bubbles. If air exists within the transducer, follow these steps:
  A. Remove the nonvented cap from the top port of the stopcock.
  B. Place a sterile syringe or VACUTAINER® with a needleless Luer-Lok adapter needle into the top of the stopcock (see Figs. 62-1 and 62-2).
  C. Turn the stopcock off to the patient (see Figs. 62-5 and 62-6).
  D. Fast-flush the air from the transducer and system into the syringe or insert a blood specimen tube into the VACUTAINER®.
  E. Open the system to the transducer (see Figs. 62-1 and 62-2).
  F. Remove the syringe or VACUTAINER® from the stopcock.
  G. Place a new sterile nonvented cap on the top port of the stopcock.
  H. Evaluate and then monitor the waveform.
	Removes air from the system, prevents the air from entering the patient, and ensures accurate monitoring of waveforms.	

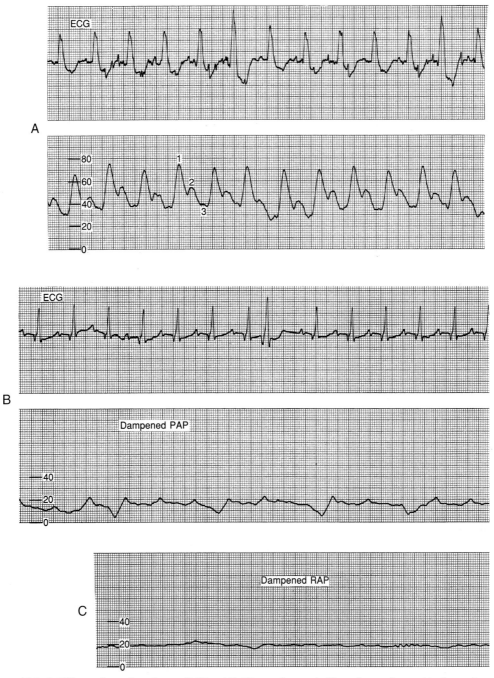

FIGURE 74-3 Effects of overdamping on PAP and RAP waveforms. **A,** Normal waveform with elevated pulmonary artery (PA) pressures (1 = systole; 2 = dicrotic notch; 3 = diastole). **B,** Overdamped PAP waveform. **C,** Overdamping of RAP waveform. Overdamping of the waveform may be due to clots at the catheter tip, catheter against vessel or heart wall, air in lines, stopcock partially closed, or deflated pressure bag. *PAP,* pulmonary artery pressure; *RAP,* right atrial pressure; *ECG,* electrocardiogram.

Procedure	for Pulmonary Artery Catheter and Pressure Lines, Troubleshooting—*Continued*	
Steps	**Rationale**	**Special Considerations**

If air exists between the pressure bag and a stopcock, follow these steps:

A. Remove the nonvented cap from the top port of the stopcock.

B. Place a sterile syringe or VACUTAINER® with a needleless Luer-Lok adapter needle into the top of the stopcock (see Figs. 62-1 and 62-2).

C. Turn the stopcock off to the patient (see Figs. 62-5 and 62-6).

D. Fast-flush the air from the system into the syringe or insert a blood specimen tube into the VACUTAINER®.

E. Open the system to the transducer (see Figs. 62-1 and 62-2).

F. Remove the syringe or VACUTAINER® from the stopcock.

G. Place a new sterile nonvented cap on the top port of the stopcock.

H. Evaluate and then monitor the waveform.

If the air is between the patient and a stopcock (Fig. 74-4), follow these steps:

A. Remove the nonvented cap from the top port of the stopcock.

B. Place a sterile syringe or VACUTAINER® with a needleless Luer-Lok adapter needle into the top port of the stopcock (see Figs. 62-1 and 62-2).

C. Turn the stopcock off to the flush solution (see Figs. 62-3 and 62-4).

D. Gently pull the air back into the syringe or insert a blood specimen tube into the VACUTAINER®.

E. When all the air is removed, turn the stopcock off to the patient (see Figs. 62-5 and 62-6).

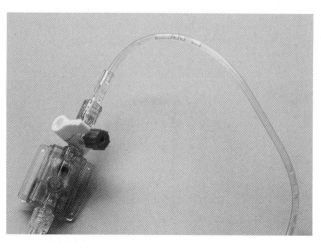

FIGURE 74-4 Air between the patient and stopcock. *(Courtesy Edwards Lifesciences, Irvine, CA)*

Procedure	for Pulmonary Artery Catheter and Pressure Lines, Troubleshooting—*Continued*		
Steps		**Rationale**	**Special Considerations**

Steps	Rationale	Special Considerations
F. Fast-flush the blood from the top port of the stopcock. G. Open the system to the transducer (see Figs. 62-1 and 62-2). H. Remove the syringe or VACUTAINER® from the stopcock. I. Place a new sterile nonvented cap on the top of the stopcock. J. Fast-flush the system. K. Evaluate and then monitor the waveform.	Clears the tubing of blood.	
6. Aspirate through the stopcock of the catheter to check for adequate blood return. A. Remove the nonvented cap from the top port of the stopcock. B. Connect a 5- to 10-ml syringe to the stopcock. C. Turn the stopcock off to the flush solution (see Fig. 62-3). D. Gently aspirate until blood enters the syringe. E. Turn the stopcock open to the transducer (see Fig. 62-1). F. Fast-flush the blood back into the patient. G. Turn the stopcock off to the patient (see Fig. 62-5). H. Fast-flush the blood from the top port of the stopcock. I. Open the stopcock to the transducer (see Fig. 62-1). J. Remove the syringe from the top port of the stopcock. K. Place a new sterile nonvented cap on the top of the stopcock.	Ensures that blood flows easily within the catheter and assesses for the presence of clots.	
7. Check the transducer for the presence of blood. If blood is present, follow these steps: A. Remove the nonvented cap from the top port of the stopcock. B. Turn the stopcock off to the patient (see Fig. 75-4). C. Fast-flush the blood from the transducer into a sterile 4 × 4. D. Turn the stopcock open to the transducer (see Fig. 75-5). E. Place a new sterile nonvented cap on the top port of the stopcock. F. Evaluate and monitor the waveform.	Ensures accurate monitoring of waveforms.	
8. Perform a dynamic response test (square wave test; see Fig. 59-3A and B).	Overdamped waveforms do not accurately represent pulmonary artery pressure waveforms.	

Procedure continues on the following page

Procedure for Pulmonary Artery Catheter and Pressure Lines, Troubleshooting—*Continued*

Steps	Rationale	Special Considerations
9. Notify the advanced practice nurse or physician if troubleshooting is unsuccessful.	The catheter will need to be removed or replaced.	
10. Discard used supplies and wash hands.	Reduces the transmission of microorganisms; standard precautions.	

Troubleshooting a Continuously Wedged Waveform

1. Wash hands.	Reduces the transmission of microorganisms; standard precautions.	
2. Identify the wedged waveform (see Fig. 72-5).	Confirms the need for troubleshooting.	Continuous monitoring of the PA waveform is necessary to assess for the presence of the PA waveform. PA catheters should be wedged for only 10 to 15 seconds to obtain a PAWP measurement.
3. Remove the PA balloon inflation syringe and ensure that the gate valve or stopcock is open (see Fig. 72-6) and that the balloon is deflated.	Ensures that air is not trapped within the PA balloon.	
4. Assist the patient in changing position, or if possible, ask the patient to cough.	This may help the catheter float out of the wedge position.	Monitor the PA waveform for a change from a PAW waveform to a PA waveform.
5. If troubleshooting is unsuccessful, notify the advanced practice nurse or physician.	Immediate repositioning of the catheter is necessary as prolonged wedging can lead to PA infarction.	The critical care nurse may withdraw the PA catheter according to institution policy.
6. Never flush a wedged PA catheter.	Flushing the catheter in the wedged position may lead to PA rupture and hemorrhage.	
7. Wash hands.	Reduces the transmission of microorganisms; standard precautions.	

Troubleshooting a Catheter in the Right Ventricle (RV)

1. Wash hands.	Reduces the transmission of microorganisms; standard precautions.	
2. Identify the RV waveform (Fig. 74-5).	The RV waveform resembles the PA waveform. The RV waveform, however, does not have a dicrotic notch. In addition, the diastolic pressure of the RV waveform is lower than the PADP. The normal PADP is 8 to 15 mm Hg; the normal RV diastolic pressure is 0 to 8 mm Hg.	Note the external cm marking.
3. Inflate the PA balloon with 1.5 ml of air.	The inflated PA balloon may readily float into position in the PA.	

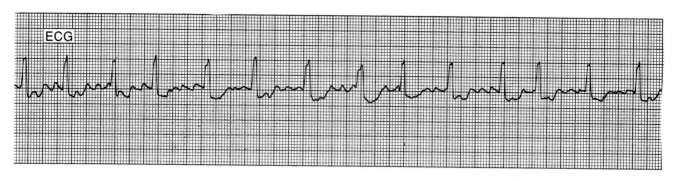

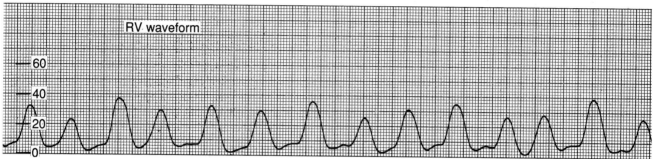

FIGURE 74-5 RVP waveform. This was seen coming from the PA (distal) lumen of a PA catheter. The catheter had become coiled in the RV. *PA,* pulmonary artery; *RV,* right ventricle; *RVP,* right ventricular pressure; *ECG,* electrocardiogram.

Procedure	for Pulmonary Artery Catheter and Pressure Lines, Troubleshooting—*Continued*	
Steps	**Rationale**	**Special Considerations**
4. Observe for change in the waveform from RV to PA to PAW (see Fig. 72-3).	Waveform analysis aids in identification of PA catheter position.	The catheter may not advance to the PAW waveform.
5. Remove the syringe from the PA inflation balloon port.	Air will be released passively from the PA balloon.	
6. Observe the waveform.	The waveform should change from the PAW waveform to a PA waveform.	
7. If the RV pressure waveform is still present, inflate the PA balloon port with 1.5 ml of air.	An inflated PA balloon cushions the catheter tip and prevents endocardial irritation.	The PA catheter tip may cause ventricular dysrhythmias. If the PA balloon is inflated, the ventricular dysrhythmias may decrease because the inflated balloon may cause less irritation of the endocardium.
8. Assist the patient with a change of position.	The inflated PA catheter may float into the PA after a position change.	
9. Observe for change in waveform from RV to PA to PAW (see Fig. 72-3).	Waveform analysis aids identification of the PA catheter position.	
10. Remove the syringe from the PA balloon port.	Deflates the PA balloon.	

Procedure continues on the following page

Procedure **for Pulmonary Artery Catheter and Pressure Lines, Troubleshooting**—*Continued*

Steps	Rationale	Special Considerations
11. If troubleshooting is unsuccessful, notify the advanced practice nurse or physician.	The PA catheter cannot remain in the right ventricle because it may trigger life-threatening ventricular dysrhythmias. Immediate repositioning is necessary.	If ventricular dysrhythmias are present, consider temporarily leaving the balloon inflated until the catheter is repositioned in the PA. If the balloon remains inflated, continuous visual monitoring is necessary in case the catheter floats into the wedge position. The critical care nurse may advance or remove the catheter according to institution policy.
12. Wash hands.	Reduces the transmission of microorganisms; standard precautions.	

Troubleshooting an Inability to Wedge the PA Catheter

1. Wash hands.	Reduces the transmission of microorganisms; standard precautions.	
2. Note the external cm marking of the PA catheter at the introducer exit site and compare to this with the most recent documented marking.	Determines whether the catheter has moved from its previous location. Most PA catheters are in the correct position if the external markings of the catheter are between 45 and 55 cm. The PA catheter tip may not be distal enough in the PA to float into the wedge position.	The advanced practice nurse or physician may need to reposition the catheter.
3. Ensure that the PA balloon is inflated with the maximum 1.5 ml of air.	The full 1.5 ml of air may be necessary to wedge some PA catheters. An insufficient amount of air can prevent wedging.	Repositioning the patient may aid in changing the position of the catheter and may facilitate successful wedging of the PA catheter.
4. Resistance should be felt when inflating the PA balloon.	Resistance is present when the PA balloon is intact.	The balloon may rupture because of overinflation, frequent inflations, or repeated aspiration of air from the balloon rather than allowing it to passively deflate.
5. If no resistance is felt or if blood is aspirated from the balloon lumen, follow these steps: A. Immediately discontinue balloon inflation attempts. B. Tape the balloon inflation port closed. C. Label the tape that the balloon should not be used.	If the balloon is ruptured, no resistance will be felt during an inflation attempt. Blood may also come back through the balloon lumen.	
6. If the balloon is ruptured or troubleshooting is unsuccessful, notify the advanced practice nurse or physician.	A new PA catheter may be placed, or PADP may be followed if the PADPs correlated with the PAWPs.	
7. Wash hands.	Reduces the transmission of microorganisms; standard precautions.	

Procedure	for Pulmonary Artery Catheter and Pressure Lines, Troubleshooting—*Continued*	
Steps	**Rationale**	**Special Considerations**

Troubleshooting Unexpected Changes in PAP

1. Wash hands.	Reduces the transmission of microorganisms; standard precautions.	
2. Ensure that the patient is in the supine position with the head of bed from 0 to 45 degrees. *(Level VI: Clinical studies in a variety of patient populations and situations to support recommendations.)*	Studies have determined that the RA and the PA pressures are accurate in this position.[3,4,5,6,11,13,15,23,24]	RA and PA pressures may be accurate for patients in the supine position with the head of the bed elevated up to 60 degrees,[5,15] but additional studies are needed to support this. Only one study[12] supports the accuracy of hemodynamic values for patients in lateral positions; other studies do not.[3,8,11,17,22] The majority of studies support the accuracy of hemodynamic monitoring for patients in the prone position.[1,2,7,10,14,18,21] Two studies demonstrated that prone positioning caused an increase in hemodynamic values.[19,20]
3. Ensure that the air-fluid interface (zeroing stopcock) is level with phlebostatic axis (see Procedure 75).	Ensures accurate pressure values. If the transducer is higher or lower than the phlebostatic axis, pressures will be inaccurate.	
4. Zero the hemodynamic monitoring system (see Procedure 75).	Ensures accuracy of the monitoring system.	
5. Check for air bubbles in the pressure monitoring system and eliminate bubbles if present (see Troubleshooting an Overdamped Waveform earlier in this procedure).	Air will overdamp the waveform (see Fig. 74-3), resulting in lower readings.	
6. Obtain hemodynamic parameters and correlate with patient assessment data.	Hemodynamic and assessment data should correlate.	
7. If PAP changes are accurate, titrate fluids or vasoactive agents as prescribed and/or notify advanced practice nurse or physician.	Hemodynamic data guide therapeutic intervention.	
8. Wash hands.	Reduces the transmission of microorganisms; standard precautions.	

Troubleshooting Blood Backup into a PA Catheter or Pressure Transducer System

1. Wash hands and don nonsterile gloves.	Reduces the transmission of microorganisms; standard precautions.	
2. Turn the stopcock off to the patient. (see Fig. 75-4)	Prevents blood from going into the transducer.	If blood reaches the transducer, it may have to be replaced.
3. Ensure that all connections are tight and that all stopcocks are closed to air and have nonvented caps.	Loose connections or open stopcocks will cause a decrease in pressure within the fluid-filled system and blood may exert a back pressure into the pressure tubing.	A crack in the system would necessitate replacing the entire monitoring system.

Procedure continues on the following page

Procedure	for Pulmonary Artery Catheter and Pressure Lines, Troubleshooting—*Continued*	

Steps	Rationale	Special Considerations
4. Ensure that there is fluid in the flush bag and that the pressure on the flush bag or device is delivering 300 mm Hg.	Low pressure from the bag will result in blood back-up.	
5. Once the source of the problem is located and corrected, flush the entire line to remove blood from the system.	Prevents clot formation within the monitoring system. Blood can become a medium for bacterial growth.[16]	
6. Zero the hemodynamic monitoring system (see Procedure 75).	Ensures accuracy of the monitoring system.	
7. Evaluate and monitor the PA waveform.	Ensures presence of the correct waveform and system functioning.	
8. Discard gloves and wash hands.	Reduces the transmission of microorganisms; standard precautions.	

Troubleshooting When Patient Develops Hemoptysis or Bloody Secretions from the Endotracheal Tube During PA Catheter Monitoring

Steps	Rationale	Special Considerations
1. Wash hands and don nonsterile gloves.	Reduces the transmission of microorganisms; standard precautions.	
2. Notify the physician immediately.	PA perforation with hemorrhage is a potentially lethal complication of a PA catheter.	
3. Maintain patency of the airway.	Prevents hypoxemia and respiratory arrest.	Prepare for intubation as needed.
4. Remain with the patient for monitoring and reassurance.	Reduces anxiety and fear; provides essential assessment.	
5. Be prepared to follow these steps: A. Send blood specimens for coagulation studies and type and crossmatch. B. Obtain a chest x-ray. C. Prepare the patient for the operating room.	Blood loss from the PA can be fatal. Immediate surgical repair of the PA is necessary.	

Expected Outcomes

- Normal pulmonary tissue perfusion
- Absence of PA catheter-related dysrhythmias
- Absence of signs of PA catheter-related infection
- Absence of discomfort associated with PA catheter
- Accurate pulmonary artery waveforms and pressures

Unexpected Outcomes

- PA balloon rupture
- Pulmonary infarction and rupture
- PA catheter-related infection resulting in sepsis
- Discomfort at PA catheter insertion site
- Ventricular tachycardia unresponsive to antidysrhythmic medications

Patient Monitoring and Care

Steps	Rationale	Reportable Conditions
		These conditions should be reported if they persist despite nursing interventions.
1. The PA waveforms should be continuously monitored.	Provides assessment of proper placement of the PA catheter and abnormal waveforms such as PAW or RV waveforms.	• Abnormal waveforms (e.g., continued PAW tracing and RV tracings)
2. Pressure alarms should be set and remain on at all times.	Alerts the critical care nurse to pressure changes and to disconnections in the pressure monitoring system.	• Abnormal hemodynamic values
3. Evaluate the hemodynamic monitoring system and waveform configurations.	Ensures that the system is intact and functioning appropriately.	• Abnormal waveforms
4. Monitor hemodynamic status (PA, PAW, RA, cardiac output or cardiac index, systemic vascular resistance, etc.).	Guides appropriate therapy.	• Abnormal hemodynamic monitoring values
5. Monitor the patient for catheter-related infections.	The PA catheter should be removed or replaced at the first sign of site infection or catheter-related sepsis.	• Signs and symptoms of infection
6. Assess the hemodynamic waveforms and pressure values before and after troubleshooting.	Identifies that troubleshooting has been successful.	• Unsuccessful troubleshooting attempts

Documentation

Documentation should include the following:

- Patient and family education
- Troubleshooting intervention and outcome
- Occurrence of unexpected outcomes and interventions
- Patient tolerance of procedure
- Site assessment

References

1. Blanch, L., et al. (1997). Short term effects of prone position in critically ill patients with acute respiratory distress syndrome. *Intensive Care Med,* 23, 1033-9.
2. Brussel, T., et al. (1993). Mechanical ventilation in the prone position for acute respiratory failure after cardiac surgery. *J Cardiothorac Vasc Anesth,* 7, 541-6.
3. Cason, C.L., et al. (1990). Effects of backrest elevation and position on pulmonary artery pressures. *Cardiovasc Nurs,* 26, 1-5.
4. Chulay, M., and Miller, T. (1984). The effect of backrest elevation on pulmonary artery and pulmonary capillary wedge pressures in patients after cardiac surgery. *Heart Lung,* 13, 138-40.
5. Clochesy, J., Hinshaw, A.D., and Otto, C.W. (1984). Effects of change of position on pulmonary artery and pulmonary capillary wedge pressure in mechanically ventilated patients. *NITA,* 7, 223-5.
6. Dobbin, K., et al. (1992). Pulmonary artery pressure measurement in patients with elevated pressures: Effect of backrest elevation and method of measurement. *Am J Crit Care,* 1, 61-9.
7. Fridrich, P., et al. (1996). The effects of long-term prone positioning in patients with trauma-induced adult respiratory distress syndrome. *Anesth Analg,* 83, 1206-11.
8. Groom, L., Frisch, S.R., and Elliot, M. (1990). Reproducibility and accuracy of pulmonary artery pressure measurement in supine and lateral positions. *Heart Lung,* 19, 147-51.
9. Hannan, A.T., Brown, M., and Bigman, O. (1984). Pulmonary artery catheter induced hemorrhage. *Chest,* 85, 128-31.
10. Jolliet, P., Bulpa, P., and Chevrolet, J.C. (1998). Effects of prone position on gas exchange and hemodynamics in severe acute respiratory distress syndrome. *Crit Care Med,* 26, 1977-85.
11. Keating, D., et al. (1986). Effect of sidelying positions on pulmonary artery pressures. *Heart Lung,* 15, 605-10.
12. Kennedy, G.T., Bryant, A., and Crawford, M.H. (1984). The effects of lateral body positioning on measurements of pulmonary artery and pulmonary wedge pressures. *Heart Lung,* 13, 155-8.
13. Lambert, C.W., and Cason, C.L. (1990). Backrest elevation and pulmonary artery pressures: Research analysis. *Dimensions Crit Care Nurs,* 9, 327-35.
14. Langer, M., et al. (1988). The prone position in ARDS patients. *Chest,* 94, 103-7.
15. Laulive, J.L. (1982). Pulmonary artery pressures and position changes in the critically ill adult. *Dimensions Crit Care Nurs,* 1, 28-34.
16. O'Grady, N.P., et al. (2002). Guidelines for the prevention of intravascular catheter-related infections. *Am J Infect Control,* 30, 476-89.

17. Osika, C. (1989). Measurement of pulmonary artery pressures: Supine verses side-lying head-elevated positions. *Heart Lung*, 18, 298-9.

18. Pappert, D., et al. (1994). Influence of positioning on ventilation-perfusion relationships in severe adult respiratory distress syndrome. *Chest*, 106, 1511-6.

19. Pelosi, P., et al. (1998). Effects of the prone position on respiratory mechanics and gas exchange during acute lung injury. *Am J Respir Crit Care Med,* 157, 387-93.

20. Voggenreiter, G., et al. (1999). Intermittent prone positioning in the treatment of severe and moderate posttraumatic lung injury. *Crit Care Med*, 27, 2375-82.

21. Vollman, K.M., and Bander, J.J. (1996). Improved oxygenation utilizing a prone positioner in patients with acute respiratory distress syndrome. *Intensive Care Med,* 22, 1105-11.

22. Wild, L. (1984). Effect of lateral recumbent positions on measurement of pulmonary artery and pulmonary artery wedge pressures in critically ill adults. *Heart Lung*, 13, 305.

23. Wilson, A.E., et al. (1996). Effect of backrest position on hemodynamic and right ventricular measurements in critically ill adults. *Am J Crit Care,* 5, 264-70.

24. Woods, S.L., and Mansfield, L.W. (1976). Effect of body position upon pulmonary artery and pulmonary capillary wedge pressures in noncritically ill patients. *Heart Lung,* 5, 83-90.

Additional Readings

Ahrens, T.S., and Taylor, L.A. (1992). *Hemodynamic Waveform Analysis.* Philadelphia: W.B. Saunders.

Darovic, G.O. (2002). *Hemodynamic Monitoring: Invasive and Noninvasive Clinical Application.* 3rd ed. Philadelphia: W.B. Saunders.

Kearney, T.J., and Shabot, M.M. (1995). Pulmonary artery rupture associated with the Swan-Ganz catheter. *Chest,* 108, 1349-52.

Keckeisen, M. (1997). *Protocols for Practice: Hemodynamic Monitoring Series—Pulmonary Artery Pressure Monitoring.* Aliso Viejo, CA: American Association of Critical-Care Nurses.

Schactman, M., et al. (1995). *Hemodynamic Monitoring.* El Paso, TX: Skidmore-Roth Publishing.

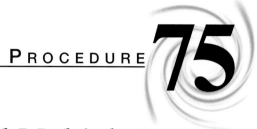

PROCEDURE **75**

Single- and Multiple-Pressure Transducer Systems

PURPOSE: To provide a catheter-to-monitor interface so that intravascular and intracardiac pressures can be measured. The transducer detects a biophysical event and converts it to an electronic signal.

Teresa Preuss
Debra Lynn-McHale Wiegand

PREREQUISITE NURSING KNOWLEDGE

- Knowledge of the anatomy and physiology of the cardiovascular system
- Knowledge of principles of aseptic technique
- Fluid-filled pressure monitoring systems used for bedside hemodynamic pressure monitoring are based on the principle that a change in pressure at any point in an unobstructed system results in similar pressure changes at all other points of the system.
- Pressure transducers detect the pressure waveform generated by ventricular ejection and convert that pressure wave into an electrical signal, which is transmitted to the monitoring equipment for representation as a waveform on the oscilloscope.
- Invasive measurement of intravascular (arterial) pressure requires insertion of a catheter into an artery.
- Invasive measurement of intracardiac (right atrial and pulmonary artery) pressures requires insertion of a catheter into the heart and pulmonary artery.
- A single-pressure transducer system is used to measure pressure from a single catheter (e.g., arterial catheter, central venous) (Fig. 75-1).
- A double-pressure transducer system is used to measure pressure from two catheters (e.g., arterial and central venous) or two ports (e.g., pulmonary artery and right atrial) from a single catheter (e.g., pulmonary artery catheter) (Fig. 75-2).
- A triple-pressure transducer system is commonly used to measure pressures from the arterial and pulmonary artery catheters. Using this system, arterial pressures, pulmonary

artery pressures, and right atrial pressures can be obtained (Fig. 75-3).
- To ensure accuracy of the hemodynamic values obtained from any transducer system, leveling and zeroing are essential.
- All hemodynamic values (pulmonary artery, right atrial, and arterial) are referenced to the level of the atria. The external reference point of the atria is the phlebostatic axis.

EQUIPMENT

- Invasive catheter (e.g., arterial, pulmonary artery)
- Disposable pressure tubing with transducer(s)
- Pressure bag or device
- Monitoring system (central and bedside monitor)
- Pressure monitoring cable(s)
- Analog recorder
- 500-ml bag of normal saline intravenous (IV) solution
- Indelible marker
- Nonvented caps
- Low-intensity laser leveling device
  Additional equipment as needed includes the following:
- Pressure modules for the monitor
- Heparin
- 3-ml syringe
- Vial of sterile water
- Carpenter level
- Transducer holder and IV pole
- Stopcocks
- 4 × 4 gauze pads
- Tape
- Non-sterile gloves

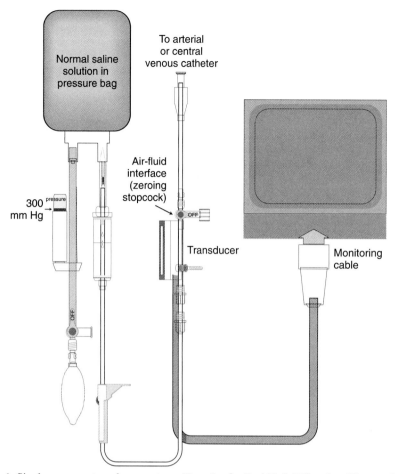

FIGURE 75-1 Single-pressure transducer system. *(Drawing by Paul W. Schiffmacher, Thomas Jefferson University, Philadelphia, PA.)*

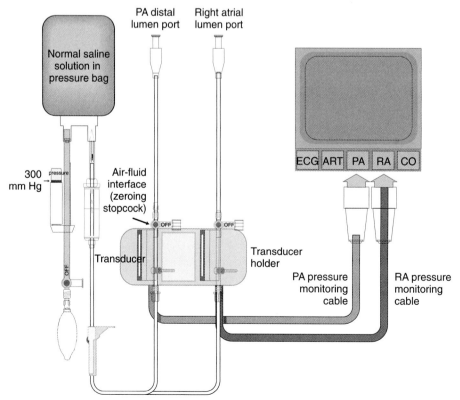

FIGURE 75-2 Double-pressure transducer system. *(Drawing by Paul W. Schiffmacher, Thomas Jefferson University, Philadelphia, PA.)*

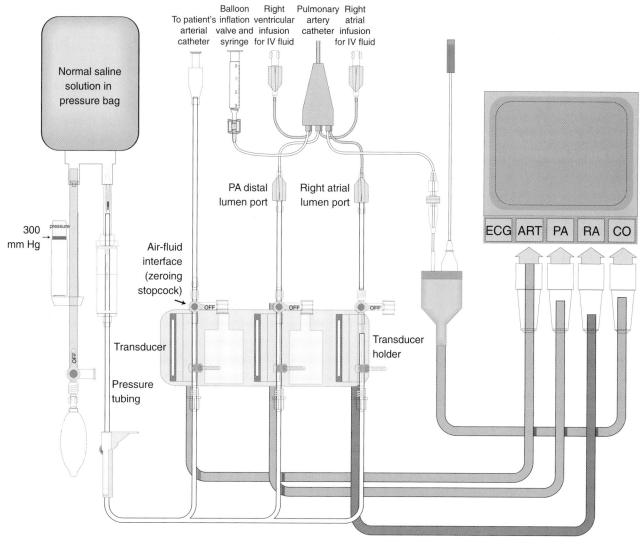

FIGURE 75-3 Triple-pressure transducer system. *(Drawing by Paul W. Schiffmacher, Thomas Jefferson University, Philadelphia, PA.)*

PATIENT AND FAMILY EDUCATION

- Assess patient and family understanding of hemodynamic monitoring and the reason for its use. ➼*Rationale:* Clarification or reinforcement of information is an expressed patient and family need.
- Explain the procedure for hemodynamic monitoring. ➼*Rationale:* Prepares the patient and the family for what to expect; may decrease anxiety.

PATIENT ASSESSMENT AND PREPARATION

Patient Assessment

- Assess the patient for conditions that may warrant the use of a hemodynamic monitoring system, including hypotension or hypertension, cardiac failure, cardiac arrest, hemorrhage, respiratory failure, fluid imbalances, oliguria, anuria, and sepsis. ➼*Rationale:* Provides data regarding signs and symptoms of hemodynamic instability.
- Obtain the patient's medical history of coagulopathies, use of anticoagulants, vascular abnormalities, and peripheral neuropathies. ➼*Rationale:* Assists in determining the safety of the procedure and aids in site selection.

Patient Preparation

- Ensure that the patient and the family understand preprocedural teaching. Answer questions as they arise, and reinforce information as needed. ➼*Rationale:* Evaluates and reinforces understanding of previously taught information.
- Position the patient in the supine position with the head of bed flat or elevated up to 45 degrees. ➼*Rationale:* Prepares the patient for hemodynamic monitoring.

Procedure for Single- and Multiple-Pressure Transducer Systems

Steps	Rationale	Special Considerations

Disposable Pressure Transducer System Setup

Steps	Rationale	Special Considerations
1. Wash hands.	Reduces the transmission of microorganisms; standard precautions.	
2. Use a 500-ml IV bag of normal saline. *(Level VI: Clinical studies in a variety of patient populations and situations to support recommendations.)*	Normal saline is preferred. Solutions containing dextrose increase the incidence of infection.[7,25,27,37]	Follow institution standard.
3. Follow institutional standard for adding heparin to the flush solution. *(Level V: Clinical studies in more than one or two different patient populations and situations to support recommendations.)*	Heparinized flush solutions are commonly used to minimize thrombi and fibrin deposits on catheters that might lead to thrombosis or bacterial colonization of the catheter.	Although heparin may prevent thrombosis[27,34], it has been associated with thrombocytopenia and other hematologic complications.[9] Arterial catheters flushed with heparinized saline are more likely than those flushed with nonheparinized saline to remain patent for up to 72 hours.[1,20] Further research is needed regarding use of heparin versus normal saline to maintain pulmonary artery line patency.
4. Label the IV bag, indicating the date and time the solution was hung, the dose of heparin (if used), and your initials.	Identifies the contents of the IV flush bag and identifies when the IV bag needs to be changed.	
5. Open the prepackaged pressure transducer kit(s) using aseptic technique. A. A single-pressure tubing kit can be used for right atrial or arterial monitoring (see Fig. 75-1). B. A double-pressure tubing kit can be used for pulmonary artery and right atrial monitoring (see Fig. 75-2). C. A triple-pressure tubing kit can be used for arterial, pulmonary artery, and right atrial monitoring (see Fig. 75-3).	Provides the correct pressure tubing.	Assemble the pressure transducers, pressure tubing, and stopcocks if not preassembled by the manufacturer. Use the minimal number of stopcocks and tubing length.
6. Tighten all connections.	Prepares the system.	
7. Spike the outlet port of the IV solution with the pressure tubing.	Allows access to the IV flush solution.	Separate flush systems are needed if invasive catheters are inserted at different times.
8. Open the roller clamp and squeeze the drip chambers to fill the chamber half full.	Primes the drip chamber.	It is important to fill the drip chamber halfway to prevent air bubbles from entering the tubing. Filling halfway will allow the nurse to see that the solution is flowing when performing a manual flush of the invasive line.
9. Insert the IV bag into the pressure bag or device on the IV pole. Do not inflate the pressure bag.	Priming the tubing under pressure increases turbulence and may cause air bubbles to enter the tubing.	Air should never be allowed to develop in a hemodynamic system. Micro or macro air

Procedure for Single- and Multiple-Pressure Transducer Systems—*Continued*

Steps	Rationale	Special Considerations
		emboli can migrate to major organs and present a potentially life-threatening complication.
10. Flush the entire system, including transducer, stopcock, and pressure tubing with the flush solution. A. Using the flush device, flush solution from the IV bag through to the tip of the pressure tubing. B. Turn the stopcock off to the patient end of the tubing (Fig. 75-4). C. Using the flush device, flush solution from the IV bag through the stopcock. D. Replace the vented cap on the stopcock with a nonvented cap. E. Open the stopcock to the transducer (Fig. 75-5).	Eliminates air from the system.	Vented caps are placed by the manufacturer and permit sterilization of the entire system. These vented caps need to be replaced with sterile nonvented caps to prevent bacteria and air from entering the system.
11. If using a double- or triple-pressure tubing kit, repeat step 10 with each of the pressure transducer systems.	Eliminates air from the system(s).	
12. Inflate the pressure bag or device to 300 mm Hg.	Inflating the pressure bag to 300 mm Hg allows approximately 1 to 3 ml per hour of flush solution to be delivered through the catheter, thus maintaining catheter patency and minimizing clot formation.	
13. If using a pole mount, insert the transducer(s) into the pole mount holder (Fig. 75-6).	Secures the transducer(s).	
Monitor Setup		
1. Turn on the bedside monitor.	Prepares the monitor.	
2. Plug the pressure cables into the appropriate pressure modules/jack in the bedside monitor (see Fig. 75-3).	Necessary for signal transmission to the monitor.	Some monitors are preprogrammed to display the waveform that corresponds to the module/jack for cable insertion (e.g., first position arterial, second position pulmonary artery, third position right atrial).
3. Turn the parameters on (e.g., PA, RA).	Visualizes the correct waveforms.	
4. Set the appropriate scale for the pressure being measured.	Necessary for visualization of the complete waveform and to obtain accurate readings. Waveforms vary in amplitude depending on the pressure within the system.	The scale for right atrial pressure is commonly set at 20 mm Hg. The scale for pulmonary artery pressure is commonly set at 40 mm Hg. The scale for arterial blood pressure is commonly set at 180 mm Hg. Scales may vary based on monitoring equipment. Adjustments to the scales may be required.

Procedure continues on the following page

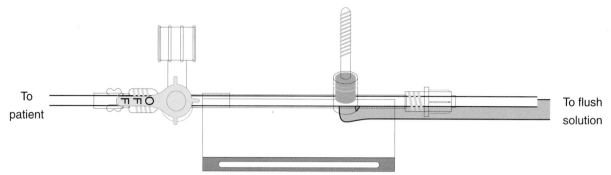

FIGURE 75-4 Stopcock off to the patient. *(Drawing by Paul W. Schiffmacher, Thomas Jefferson University, Philadelphia, PA.)*

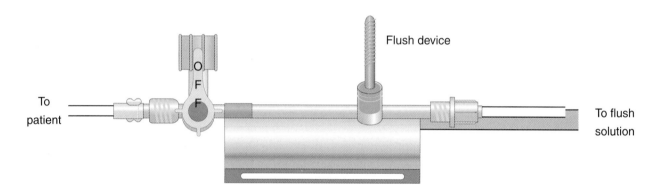

Transducer

FIGURE 75-5 Stopcock open to the transducer. *(Drawing by Paul W. Schiffmacher, Thomas Jefferson University, Philadelphia, PA.)*

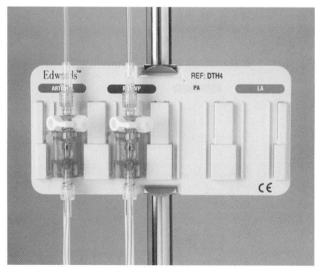

FIGURE 75-6 Transducers in pole mount. *(Courtesy Edwards Lifesciences, Irvine, CA.)*

Procedure for Single- and Multiple-Pressure Transducer Systems—*Continued*

Steps	Rationale	Special Considerations
Leveling the Transducer		
1. Wash hands.	Reduces the transmission of microorganisms; standard precautions.	
2. Position the patient in the supine position with the head of the bed from 0 to 45 degrees. *(Level VI: Clinical studies in a variety of patient populations and situations to support recommendations.)*	Studies have determined that the RA and the PA pressures are accurate in this position.[8,10,11,12,16,21,23,41,42]	RA and PA pressures may be accurate for patients in the supine position with the head of the bed elevated up to 60 degrees,[11,23] but additional studies are needed to support this. Only one study[18] supports the accuracy of hemodynamic values for patients in lateral positions; other studies do not.[4,8,14,16,29,36,40] The majority of studies support the accuracy of hemodynamic monitoring for patients in the prone position.[3,6,13,15,22,31,39] Two studies demonstrated that prone positioning caused an increase in hemodynamic values.[33,38]
3. Locate the phlebostatic axis for the supine position (Fig. 75-7). A. Identify the fourth ICS on the edge of the sternum. B. Draw an imaginary line along the fourth ICS laterally, along the chest wall. C. Draw a second imaginary line from the axilla downward, midway between the anterior and posterior chest walls. D. Where these two lines cross is the level of the phlebostatic axis. E. Mark the point of the phlebostatic axis with an indelible marker.	The phlebostatic axis is at approximately the level of the atria and should be used as the reference point for the air-fluid interface.	The reference point for the left lateral decubitus position is the fourth intercostal space at the left parasternal border (Fig. 75-8).[17,30] The reference point for the right lateral decubitus position is the fourth intercostal space (ICS) at the midsternum (see Fig. 75-8).[17,30]
4. Using pole mount[2,35]: A. Place the low-intensity laser leveling device parallel to the air-fluid interface(s) (zeroing stopcock[s]). B. Point the laser light at the phlebostatic axis. C. Move the pole mount holder up or down until the interface is level with the phlebostatic axis. *(Level V: Clinical studies in more than one or two different patient populations and situations to support recommendations.)*	Ensures that the air-fluid interface is level with the phlebostatic axis.	

Procedure continues on the following page

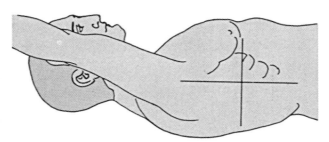

FIGURE **75-7** Phlebostatic axis in the supine position.

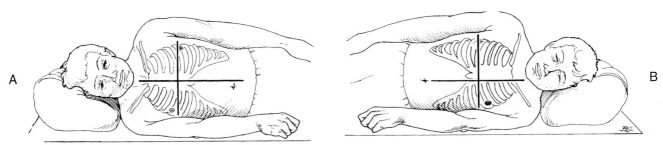

A

B

FIGURE **75-8** Reference points for the hemodynamic monitoring system for patients in lateral positions. **A,** For the right lateral position, the reference point is the intersection of the fourth intercostal space and the midsternum. **B,** For the left lateral position, the reference point is the intersection of the fourth intercostal space and the left parasternal border. *(From Keckelsen M. [1997].* Protocols for Practice: Hemodynamic Monitoring Series—Pulmonary Artery Monitoring. *Aliso Viejo, CA: American Association of Critical-Care Nurses.)*

Procedure for Single- and Multiple-Pressure Transducer Systems—*Continued*		
Steps	**Rationale**	**Special Considerations**
5. Using patient mount: A. Place the pulmonary artery distal/PA air-fluid interface (zeroing stopcock) at the phlebostatic axis. B. Place the pulmonary artery proximal (RA) and arterial air-fluid interfaces (zeroing stopcocks) directly next to the pulmonary artery distal/PA air-fluid interface. C. Place a 4 × 4 gauze pad between each of the transducers and the patient's skin. D. Secure each of the systems in place with tape.	Ensures that the air-fluid interface is level with the phlebostatic axis. Leveling to the phlebostatic axis reflects accurate central arterial pressure values.	Leveling the arterial interface to the tip of an arterial catheter reflects the transmural pressure of a particular point in the arterial tree (e.g., radial artery) and not central arterial pressure.[5,19,26,32]
Zeroing the Transducer 1. Wash hands.	Reduces the transmission of microorganisms; standard precautions.	
2. Turn the stopcock off to the patient end of the tubing (see Fig. 75-4).	Prepares the system for the zeroing procedure.	
3. Remove the nonvented cap from the stopcock, opening the stopcock to air.	Allows the monitor to use atmospheric pressure as a reference for zero.	

Procedure for Single- and Multiple-Pressure Transducer Systems—*Continued*

Steps	Rationale	Special Considerations
4. Push and release the zeroing button on the bedside monitor. Observe the digital reading until it displays a value of zero.	The monitor will automatically adjust itself to zero. Zeroing negates the effects of atmospheric pressure.	Some monitors require that the zero be turned and adjusted manually. Some systems also may require calibration. Refer to manufacturer guidelines for specific information.
5. Place a new, sterile nonvented cap on the stopcock.	Maintains sterility.	
6. Turn the stopcock so that it is open to the transducer (see Fig. 75-5).	Permits pressure monitoring and maintains catheter patency.	
7. Discard used supplies and wash hands.	Reduces the transmission of microorganisms; standard precautions.	

Expected Outcomes

- The pressure monitoring system is prepared aseptically.
- The hemodynamic monitoring system remains intact with secure connections.
- The phlebostatic axis is accurately identified.
- The air-fluid interface of the transducer is leveled to the phlebostatic axis.
- The pressure monitoring system is zeroed.

Unexpected Outcomes

- Loose connections within the hemodynamic monitoring system
- Stopcocks left open to air without nonvented caps
- Air bubbles within the system
- Pressure bag inflated to less than 300 mm Hg

Patient Monitoring and Care

Steps	Rationale	Reportable Conditions
		These conditions should be reported if they persist despite nursing interventions.
1. Check the IV flush bag every 4 hours and as needed.	Ensures that the IV flush bag contains solution to maintain catheter patency.	
2. Check that the IV flush bag is maintained at 300 mm Hg every 4 hours and as needed.	Maintains catheter patency.	
3. **Arterial lines.** Change the flush bag and hemodynamic monitoring system (pressure tubing, transducer, and stopcocks) every 96 hours or with each change of the catheter if it is changed more frequently than every 96 hours. The flush bag may need to be changed more frequently if empty of solution. *(Level VI: Clinical studies in a variety of patient populations and situations to support recommendations.)*	The Centers for Disease Control and Prevention (CDC)[27] and research findings[24,28] indicate that the hemodynamic flush system can be used safely for 96 hours.	
4. **Pulmonary artery lines.** Change the flush bag and hemodynamic monitoring system (pressure tubing, transducer, and stopcocks) every 96 hours or with each change of the catheter if it is changed more	The Centers for Disease Control and Prevention (CDC)[27] and research findings[24,28] indicate that the hemodynamic flush system can be used safely for 96 hours.	

Procedure continues on the following page

Patient Monitoring and Care—*Continued*

Steps	Rationale	Reportable Conditions
frequently than every 96 hours. The flush bag may need to be changed more frequently if empty of solution. *(Level VI: Clinical studies in a variety of patient populations and situations to support recommendations.)*		
5. Zero the hemodynamic monitoring system during initial setup or before insertion, after insertion, if disconnection occurs between the transducer and the monitoring cable, if disconnection occurs between the monitoring cable and the monitor, and when the values obtained do not fit the clinical picture. Follow manufacturer recommendations for disposable systems.	Ensures the accuracy of the hemodynamic monitoring system.	
6. Check the hemodynamic monitoring system every 4 hours and as needed.	Ensures that all connections are tightly secured and that there are no cracks in the system. Ensures that the system is closed with nonvented caps on all stopcocks. Ensures that the system is free of air bubbles.	
7. Set the hemodynamic monitoring system alarms.	Provides immediate alarm for high and low pressures.	

Documentation

Documentation should include the following:

- Patient and family education
- Date and time of hemodynamic monitoring system preparation
- Hemodynamic monitoring system leveling and zeroing
- Type of flush solution
- Unexpected outcomes
- Additional nursing interventions

References

1. American Association of Critical-Care Nurses. (1993). Evaluation of the effects of heparinized and nonheparinized flush solutions on the patency of arterial pressure monitoring lines: The AACN Thunder Project. *Am J Crit Care,* 2, 3-15.
2. Bisnaire, D., and Robinson, L. (1999). Accuracy of leveling hemodynamic transducer systems. *CACCN,* 10, 16-9.
3. Blanch, L., et al. (1997). Short term effects of prone position in critically ill patients with acute respiratory distress syndrome. *Intensive Care Med,* 23, 1033-9.
4. Bridges, E.J., et al. (2000). Effect of 30 degree lateral recumbent position on pulmonary artery and pulmonary artery wedge pressures in critically ill adult cardiac surgery patients. *Am J Crit Care,* 9, 262-75.
5. Bridges, E.J., et al. (1997). Direct arterial vs. oscillometric monitoring of blood pressure: Stop comparing and pick one. (comment). *Crit Care Nurse,* 17, 96-7, 101-2.
6. Brussel, T., et al. (1993). Mechanical ventilation in the prone position for acute respiratory failure after cardiac surgery. *J Cardiothorac Vasc Anesth,* 7, 541-6.
7. Buxton, A.E., et al. (1978). Failure of disposable domes to prevent septicemia acquired from contaminated pressure transducers. *Chest,* 74, 508-13.
8. Cason, C.L., et al. (1990). Effects of backrest elevation and position on pulmonary artery pressures. *Cardiovasc Nurs,* 26, 1-5.
9. Chong, B.H. (1995). Heparin-induced thrombocytopenia. *British J Haematol,* 89, 431-9.
10. Chulay, M., and Miller T. (1984). The effect of backrest elevation on pulmonary artery and pulmonary capillary wedge pressures in patients after cardiac surgery. *Heart Lung,* 13, 138-40.
11. Clochesy, J., Hinshaw, A.D., and Otto, C.W. (1984). Effects of change of position on pulmonary artery and pulmonary capillary wedge pressure in mechanically ventilated patients. *NITA,* 7, 223-5.
12. Dobbin, K., et al. (1992). Pulmonary artery pressure measurement in patients with elevated pressures: Effect of backrest elevation and method of measurement. *Am J Crit Care,* 1, 61-9.
13. Fridrich, P., et al. (1996). The effects of long-term prone positioning in patients with trauma-induced adult respiratory distress syndrome. *Anesth Analg,* 83, 1206-11.
14. Groom, L., Frisch, S.R., and Elliot, M. (1990). Reproducibility and accuracy of pulmonary artery pressure measurement in supine and lateral positions. *Heart Lung,* 19, 147-51.
15. Jolliet, P., Bulpa, P., and Chevrolet, J.C. (1998). Effects of prone position on gas exchange and hemodynamics in severe acute respiratory distress syndrome. *Crit Care Med,* 26, 1977-85.
16. Keating, D., et al. (1986). Effect of sidelying positions on pulmonary artery pressures. *Heart Lung,* 15, 605-10.

17. Keckeisen, M. (1997). *Protocols for Practice: Hemodynamic Monitoring Series—Pulmonary Artery Pressure Monitoring.* Aliso Viejo, CA: American Association of Critical-Care Nurses.

18. Kennedy, G.T., Bryant, A., and Crawford, M.H. (1984). The effects of lateral body positioning on measurements of pulmonary artery and pulmonary wedge pressures. *Heart Lung, 13,* 155-8.

19. Kirkhoff, K.T., and Rebenson-Piano, M. (1984). Mean arterial pressure readings: Variations with positions and transducer level. *Nurs Res, 33,* 343-5.

20. Kulkarni, M., et al. (1994). Heparinized saline versus normal saline in maintaining patency of the radial artery catheter. *Can J Surg, 37,* 37-42.

21. Lambert, C.W., and Cason, C.L. (1990). Backrest elevation and pulmonary artery pressures: Research analysis. *Dimensions Crit Care Nurs, 9,* 327-35.

22. Langer, M., et al. (1988). The prone position in ARDS patients. *Chest, 94,* 103-7.

23. Laulive, J.L. (1982). Pulmonary artery pressures and position changes in the critically ill adult. *Dimensions Crit Care Nurs, 1,* 28-34.

24. Luskin, R.L., et al. (1986). Extended use of disposable pressure transducers: A bacteriologic evaluation. *JAMA, 255,* 916-20.

25. Maki, D.G., and Martin, W.T. (1975). Nationwide epidemic of septicemia caused by contaminated infusion products. IV. Growth of microbial pathogens in fluids for intravenous infusion. *J Infect Dis, 131,* 267-72.

26. McGhee, B.H., and Bridges, M.E.J. (2002). Monitoring arterial blood pressure: What you may not know. *Crit Care Nurse, 22,* 60-79.

27. O'Grady, N.P., et al. (2002). Guidelines for the prevention of intravascular catheter-related infections. *Am J Infect Control, 30,* 476-89.

28. O'Malley, M.K., et al. (1994). Value of routine pressure monitoring system changes after 72 hours of use. *Crit Care Med, 22,* 1424-30.

29. Osika, C. (1989). Measurement of pulmonary artery pressures: Supine verses side-lying head-elevated positions. *Heart Lung, 18,* 298-9.

30. Paolella, L.P., et al. (1988). Topographic location of the left atrium by computed tomography: Reducing pulmonary artery catheter calibration error. *Crit Care Med, 16,* 1154-56.

31. Pappert, D., et al. (1994). Influence of positioning on ventilation-perfusion relationships in severe adult respiratory distress syndrome. *Chest, 106,* 1511-16.

32. Pauca, A.L., et al. (1992). Does radial artery pressure accurately reflect aortic pressure? *Chest, 102,* 1193-8.

33. Pelosi, P., et al. (1998). Effects of the prone position on respiratory mechanics and gas exchange during acute lung injury. *Am J Respir Crit Care Med, 157,* 387-93.

34. Randolph, A.G., et al. (1998). Benefit of heparin in central venous and pulmonary artery catheters. *Chest, 113,* 165-71.

35. Rice, W.P., et al. (2000). A comparison of hydrostatic leveling methods in invasive pressure monitoring. *Crit Care Nurse, 20, 20,* 22-30.

36. Ross, C.J., and Jones, R. (1995). Comparisons of pulmonary artery pressure measurements in supine and 30 degree lateral positions. *Can J Cardiovasc Nurs, 6,* 4-8.

37. Solomon, S.L., et al. (1986). Nosocomial fungemia in neonates associated with intravascular pressure-monitoring devices. *Pediatr Infect Dis, 5,* 680-5.

38. Voggenreiter, G., et al. (1999). Intermittent prone positioning in the treatment of severe and moderate posttraumatic lung injury. *Crit Care Med, 27,* 2375-82.

39. Vollman, K.M., and Bander, J.J. (1996). Improved oxygenation utilizing a prone positioner in patients with acute respiratory distress syndrome. *Intensive Care Med, 22,* 1105-11.

40. Wild, L. (1984). Effect of lateral recumbent positions on measurement of pulmonary artery and pulmonary artery wedge pressures in critically ill adults. *Heart Lung, 13,* 305.

41. Wilson, A.E., et al. (1996). Effect of backrest position on hemodynamic and right ventricular measurements in critically ill adults. *Am J Crit Care, 5,* 264-70.

42. Woods, S.L., and Mansfield, L.W. (1976). Effect of body position upon pulmonary artery and pulmonary capillary wedge pressures in noncritically ill patients. *Heart Lung, 5,* 83-90.

Additional Readings

Bridges, E.J., and Woods, S.L. (1993). Pulmonary artery pressure measurement: State of art. *Heart Lung, 22,* 99-111.

Cason, C.L., and Lambert, C.W. (1993). Positioning during hemodynamic monitoring: Evaluating the research. *Dimensions Crit Care Nurs, 12,* 226-33.

Cason, C.L., and Lambert, C.W. (1987). Backrest position and reference level in pulmonary artery pressure measurement. *Clin Nurse Spec, 1,* 159-65.

Darovic, G.O. (2002). *Hemodynamic Monitoring: Invasive and Noninvasive Clinical Application.* 3rd ed. Philadelphia: W.B. Saunders.

Ducharme, F.M., et al. (1988). Incidence of infection related to arterial catheterization in children: A prospective study. *Crit Care Med, 16,* 272-6.

Gardner, P.E., and Bridges, E.J. (1995). Hemodynamic monitoring. In: Woods, S.I., et al., eds. *Cardiac Nursing.* 3rd ed. Philadelphia: JB Lippincott.

Gardner, R.M., and Hollingsworth, K.W. (1988). Technologic advances in invasive pressure monitoring. *J Cardiovasc Nurs, 2,* 52-5.

Grap, M.J., Pettrey, L., and Thornby, D. (1997). Hemodynamic monitoring: A comparison of research and practice. *Am J Crit Care, 6,* 452-6.

Imperial-Perez, F., and McRae, M. (1998). *Protocols for Practice: Hemodynamic Monitoring Series—Arterial Pressure Monitoring.* Aliso Viejo, CA: American Association of Critical-Care Nurses.

Kee, L.L., et al. (1993). Echocardiographic determination of valid zero reference levels in supine and lateral positions. *Am J Crit Care, 2,* 72-80.

McLane, C., Morris, L., and Holm, K. (1998). A comparison of intravascular pressure monitoring system contamination and patient bacteremia with use of 48- and 72-hour system change intervals. *Heart Lung, 27,* 200-8.

Mermel, L.A., and Maki, D.G. (1989). Epidemic bloodstream infections from hemodynamic pressure monitoring: Signs of the times. *Infect Control Hosp Epidemiol, 10,* 47-53.

Pearson, M.L. (1996). Hospital infection control practices advisory committee: Guideline for prevention of intravascular device-related infections. *Infect Control Hosp Epidemiol, 17,* 438-73.

Quaal, S.J., and Weir, C. (1995). Effect of head of bed position on pulmonary artery pressure measurements: A review of the literature. *The Online Journal of Knowledge Synthesis for Nursing, 2,* 1-10.

Shih, F. (1999). Patient positioning and the accuracy of pulmonary artery pressure measurements. *Int J Nurs Studies, 36,* 497-505.

Vollman, K.M. (2001). What are the practice guidelines for prone positioning of acutely ill patients? Specifically, what are the recommendations related to hemodynamic monitoring and tube feeding? *Crit Care Nurse, 21,* 84-86.

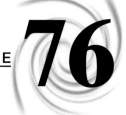

P R O C E D U R E **76**

SECTION TEN

Special Cardiac
Procedures

Arterial and Venous Sheath Removal

P U R P O S E : Arterial and venous sheaths are placed during cardiac catheterization and interventional cardiac procedures. Achieving and maintaining hemostasis after their removal is essential.

Rose B. Shaffer

PREREQUISITE NURSING KNOWLEDGE

- Knowledge of femoral artery and vein anatomy
- Understanding of the technique for percutaneous approach to the insertion of the arterial and venous sheaths
- Technical and clinical competence in removing arterial and venous sheaths
- Understanding of anticoagulation and antiplatelet therapy used during interventional procedures and the appropriate tests used to determine the timing of sheath removal
- Knowledge about the variety of hemostasis options available, including the following:
  ❖ Manual compression alone or in combination with noninvasive hemostasis pads—e.g., Syvek Patch (Marine Polymer Technologies, Inc., Danvers, MA), Clo-Sur Pad (Scion Cardio-Vascular, Inc., Miami, FL).
  ❖ Mechanical compression devices—e.g., C-clamp, FemoStop (Radi Medical Systems, Wilmington, MA) (Fig. 76-1).
  ❖ Collagen plug devices—e.g., VasoSeal (Datascope Corporation, Montvale, NJ), Angioseal (St. Jude Medical, St. Paul, MN).
  ❖ Percutaneous suture-mediated closure devices—e.g., Perclose (Abbott Laboratories, Abbott Park, IL).
- Percutaneous suture-mediated closure devices and collagen plug devices are usually deployed into the artery by the physician at the end of the catheterization or interventional procedure.
- Sheath removal can be associated with many complications, including the following:
  ❖ External bleeding at the site
  ❖ Internal bleeding (e.g., retroperitoneal bleeding)
  ❖ Vascular complications (e.g., hematoma, pseudoaneurysm, arteriovenous [AV] fistula, thrombus, or embolus)
  ❖ Neurovascular complications (sensory or motor changes in the affected extremity)
  ❖ Vasovagal complications
- Prior to vascular access, a baseline assessment of the site should be documented, including the quality and strength of the pulse and assessment for the presence or absence of a bruit.

EQUIPMENT

- Cardiac monitoring system
- Noninvasive automatic blood pressure cuff
- Antiseptic solution (e.g., 2% chlorhexidine-based preparation)
- Nonsterile gloves
- Sterile gloves
- Protective eyewear
- Dressing supplies
- Suture removal kit
  Additional equipment as needed includes the following:
- Readily available emergency medications, additional intravenous fluids, and resuscitation equipment
- Selected hemostasis option (mechanical compression device or noninvasive hemostasis pad)

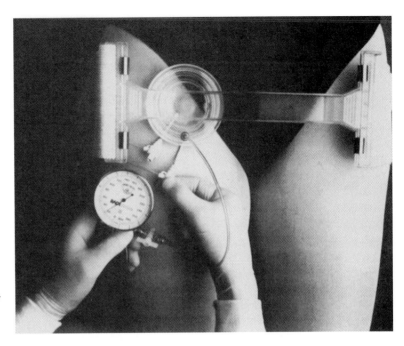

FIGURE 76-1 FemoStop in the correct position. *(From Barbiere C. [1995]. A new device for control of bleeding after transfemoral catheterization.* Crit Care Nurse, *15[1], 52.)*

- Activated clotting time (ACT) machine
- Alcohol pad or swabsticks
- Indelible marker
- 1% lidocaine (without epinephrine)
- 5 ml and 10 ml syringes and needles ($\frac{1}{2}$ inch to $1\frac{1}{2}$ inch)
- Doppler

PATIENT AND FAMILY EDUCATION

- Explain the procedure to the patient and the family. ➤➤*Rationale:* Teaching provides information and may help decrease anxiety and fear. It encourages the patient to ask questions and voice concerns about the procedure.
- Explain the importance of bed rest, of not lifting the head off the pillow, of maintaining the head of the bed at no higher than 30 degrees, and of keeping the affected extremity straight for a specified time to maintain hemostasis after the procedure. ➤➤*Rationale:* Elicits patient cooperation and decreases the risk for bleeding, hematoma, or other vascular complications.
- Explain that the procedure may produce discomfort and that pressure will be felt at the site until hemostasis is achieved. Encourage the patient to report discomfort. ➤➤*Rationale:* Prepares the patient for what to expect.
- After sheath removal, instruct the patient to report any warm, wet feeling or pain at the puncture site. Also instruct the patient to report any sensory or motor changes in the affected extremity. ➤➤*Rationale:* Aids in the early recognition of complications.

PATIENT ASSESSMENT AND PREPARATION

Patient Assessment

- Assess the patient's medical history of bleeding disorders. ➤➤*Rationale:* May increase the risk for bleeding or vascular complications.
- Assess the patient's platelet count, prothrombin time (PT) with international normalized ratio (INR), and partial thromboplastin time (PTT) before sheath removal. ➤➤*Rationale:* Laboratory results should be within acceptable limits to decrease the risk for bleeding after sheath removal.
- Assess the patient's complete blood count (CBC). ➤➤*Rationale:* Establishes baseline assessment.
- Assess the patient's activated clotting time (ACT) before sheath removal. ➤➤*Rationale:* Results should be within acceptable limits to decrease the risk for bleeding after sheath removal.
- Assess the patient's electrocardiogram (ECG) rhythm and vital signs. ➤➤*Rationale:* Establishes baseline data. Consider lowering the patient's blood pressure if the systolic blood pressure is greater than 150 mm Hg in order to achieve and maintain hemostasis.
- Review the documented baseline assessment of the access site before vascular access, including assessment for presence or absence of bruit. ➤➤*Rationale:* Establishes baseline assessment.
- Assess the extremity distal to the sheath for quality and strength of pulses, color, temperature, sensation, and movement. ➤➤*Rationale:* Establishes baseline assessment before sheath removal.
- Assess for patency of intravenous access and ensure that more than 500 ml of fluid remains in the IV solution. ➤➤*Rationale:* Allows for emergency medication or fluids to be administered if necessary (e.g., vasovagal reaction).

Patient Preparation

- Ensure that the patient and the family understand preprocedural teaching. Answer questions as they arise, and reinforce information as needed. ➤*Rationale:* Evaluates and reinforces understanding of previously taught information.
- Administer analgesia before removal of sheaths. ➤*Rationale:* Facilitates pain management.
- Place the patient with the head of the bed flat. ➤*Rationale:* Improves ability to achieve hemostasis.
- Mark the distal pulses with an indelible marker, especially if pulses are confirmed with Doppler. ➤*Rationale:* Facilitates the ability to locate pulses after the procedure.
- If using a mechanical device to maintain pressure, position the device as indicated under the patient. ➤*Rationale:* The device is positioned before sheath removal because patient movement must be minimized after sheath removal.

Procedure for Arterial and Venous Sheath Removal

Steps	Rationale	Special Considerations
1. Wash hands.	Reduces the transmission of organisms; standard precautions.	
2. Place a noninvasive blood pressure cuff on the patient's arm.	Establishes a baseline noninvasive blood pressure before sheath removal and ensures ongoing assessment of the patient's blood pressure during and after sheath removal.	Monitor the patient's blood pressure every 5 minutes during arterial sheath removed until hemostasis is achieved.
3. Place the patient's head of bed flat.	Improves ability to achieve hemostasis.	
4. Don nonsterile gloves and protective eyewear.	Reduces the risk for transmission of microorganisms; standard precautions.	
5. Turn off the arterial catheter alarm.	Monitoring no longer needed; prevents alarm sounding.	
6. Open the suture removal kit if sheaths are sutured in place.	Prepares for sheath removal.	
7. Remove the arterial and venous sheath dressing.	Prepares for sheath removal.	
8. Clean the arterial and venous sites with antiseptic solution before removal.	May decrease the risk for infection.	Follow institutional standard.
9. Consider subcutaneously infiltrating the area around the catheter sites with 1% lidocaine.	May reduce the discomfort experienced during sheath removal.	The benefit of lidocaine infiltration has not been proven to reduce the discomfort associated with sheath removal.[3,14]
10. If using a noninvasive hemostasis pad, in conjunction with manual compression, open the pad using sterile technique.	Prepares for sheath removal and ensures sterility.	
11. Attach a 10-ml syringe to the blood sampling port of the stopcock, turn the stopcock off to the flush bag, and gently draw back 5 to 10 ml of blood into the syringe.	Ensures there is no clot in the catheter.	
12. Discard nonsterile gloves, wash hands, and don sterile gloves.	Maintains asepsis.	
13. Remove sutures, if present.	Prepares for removal of sheath.	

Procedure for Arterial and Venous Sheath Removal—*Continued*

Steps	Rationale	Special Considerations
14. Palpate the femoral pulse.	Allows for more accurate positioning of the hemostasis option (manual or mechanical).	
15. Position the hemostasis option (manual or mechanical) 1 to 2 cm above the site where the arterial sheath enters the skin. (*If using a noninvasive hemostasis pad in conjunction with manual pressure, see step 18.*)	The arterial puncture site (arteriotomy) is superior and medial to the skin puncture site. The arterial sheath is inserted at a 45-degree angle to the artery.	Studies vary on the benefits of manual versus mechanical compression to achieve hemostasis of the femoral artery.[2,10,11,15] If the patient is obese or has a large abdomen, a second person may be needed to assist with sheath removal.
16. Simultaneously depress the hemostasis option (manual or mechanical), gently remove the arterial sheath from the femoral artery during exhalation.	Prevents external bleeding. Pulling the arterial sheath during the exhalation phase of the respiratory cycle may prevent the patient from "bearing down" during arterial sheath removal.	Never withdraw the sheath if resistance is met. Notify the physician or advanced practice nurse.
17. Continue to apply pressure. A. Maintain manual pressure above the arterial puncture site for approximately 20 minutes. B. Maintain mechanical compression device.	Pressure is needed to achieve hemostasis.	The length of time required to achieve hemostasis depends on several factors, including the size of sheath used, the type of procedure, the use of heparin and antiplatelet medications during the procedure, the ACT level at the time of sheath removal, and the patient's anatomy at the femoral insertion site. Additionally, patients who are hypertensive or obese may require longer application of pressure. If using a mechanical device, set the pressure of the device according to the manufacturer's recommendation and institutional standard. Tissue damage may occur if prolonged pressure is maintained (e.g., 2 to 3 hours).[1]
18. If using a noninvasive hemostasis pad in conjunction with manual compression: A. Moisten the pad or insertion site with sterile saline. B. Apply manual pressure 1-2 cm proximal to the skin insertion site (see step 15). C. Place the moistened noninvasive hemostasis pad directly over the puncture site covered with a sterile gauze pad, before pulling the sheath.	Noninvasive hemostasis pads must be moistened before application to activate the hemostatic mechanism.	Check with manufacturer for specific guidelines. Total time of compression depends on the same factors listed for manual compression (see step 17). The noninvasive hemostasis pad is left in place for 24 hours.

Procedure continues on the following page

Procedure for Arterial and Venous Sheath Removal—*Continued*

Steps	Rationale	Special Considerations
D. Continue holding firm pressure proximal to the skin insertion site and apply firm pressure over the gauze pad at the puncture site. E. Remove the sheath. F. Gradually release proximal pressure after 3-4 minutes; however, pressure should be maintained over the puncture site for at least 10 minutes. G. Place a new sterile gauze over the hemostasis pad and cover with a transparent dressing. *(Level I: Manufacturer's recommendations only.)*		
19. Assess the circulation to the extremity distal to the site of the arterial sheath removal.	Verifies adequate circulation while achieving hemostasis.	The pulse may decrease during application of full pressure but should not be obliterated completely. If manual compression is being performed, another person is needed to assess distal perfusion.
20. Palpate the area around the arterial site.	Determines whether any bleeding has occurred around the arterial site.	
21. If using manual compression or mechanical compression, discontinue pressure once hemostasis is achieved.		If using a mechanical device, follow the manufacturer's recommendations, institutional standard, or physician prescription regarding the gradual reduction of pressure from the device. Notify the physician or advanced practice nurse if unable to achieve hemostasis.
22. If there is a venous sheath, remove the venous sheath 10 minutes after the arterial sheath is removed and maintain manual pressure over both sites for approximately 10 additional minutes or until hemostasis is achieved.	Achieves both arterial and venous hemostasis. The arterial sheath is removed first because pressure needs to be applied to the arterial site longer than the venous site to achieve hemostasis.	Collagen plug devices and percutaneous suture-mediated closure devices are not used for venous punctures. Noninvasive hemostasis pads may be used to achieve hemostasis for venous punctures.
23. Apply a sterile bandage to the arterial and venous sites (if both are used).	Maintains asepsis.	If a collagen plug device or a percutaneous suture-mediated closure device is deployed in the arteriotomy immediately after the procedure, the venous sheath must still be removed with manual pressure applied for approximately 10 minutes.
24. Discard used supplies and wash hands.	Reduces the transmission of microorganisms; standard precautions.	

Expected Outcomes	Unexpected Outcomes
• Arterial and venous sheaths removed with hemostasis achieved • Adequate peripheral vascular and neurovascular integrity of the extremity distal to the site of sheath removal (positive sensation, movement, capillary refill, color, temperature, pulse) • No evidence of peripheral vascular or neurovascular complications • Cardiovascular and hemodynamic stability	• Inability to remove the arterial or venous sheaths • Inability to achieve hemostasis • Impaired perfusion to the extremity distal to the site of sheath removal • Impaired motor/sensory status of the extremity distal to the site of sheath removal • Development of a hematoma or new bruit • Development of a retroperitoneal bleed • Development of a pseudoaneurysm or arteriovenous fistula • Vagal response during removal of arterial sheath (ensure patent IV, with IV fluids and emergency medications/equipment available) • Hemodynamic instability • Angina or shortness of breath • Drop in hemoglobin greater than 2 grams compared to preprocedure

Patient Monitoring and Care

Steps	Rationale	Reportable Conditions
		These conditions should be reported if they persist despite nursing interventions.
1. Assess the peripheral vascular and neurovascular status of the affected extremity after arterial sheath removal: q 15 min × 4, q 30 min × 2, q 60 min × 4.	A thrombus or embolus may precipitate changes in peripheral or neurovascular status, requiring early intervention.	• Decrease or change in strength of pulses in the affected extremity (diminished or absent) • Coldness or coolness of the distal extremity • Paresthesia in the affected extremity • Pallor, cyanosis of the affected extremity • Pain in the affected extremity • Decrease in mobility of the affected extremity
2. Obtain vital signs after removal of the arterial sheath: q 15 min × 4, q 30 min × 2, q 60 min × 4.	Changes in vital signs may occur because of a vasovagal response or blood loss.	• Changes in vital signs
3. Assess the puncture site: q 15 min × 4, q 30 min × 2, q 60 min × 4, including assessment of presence or absence of bruit.	Detects presence of bleeding, hematoma, or bruit.	• Bleeding at arterial or venous sites • Hematoma development • New bruit
4. Monitor the ECG during and after sheath removal.	Detects the presence of dysrhythmias.	• Dysrhythmias
5. After hemostasis is achieved, the patient's head of bed can be elevated up to 30 degrees. *(Level VI: Clinical studies in a variety of patient populations and situations to support recommendations.)*	Minimizes back discomfort and does not increase vascular complications.[4,5,12]	• Back pain not relieved with position changes or analgesics.

Procedure continues on the following page

Patient Monitoring and Care—*Continued*

Steps	Rationale	Reportable Conditions
6. Maintain bed rest for 2 to 6 hours after arterial sheath removal when using manual or mechanical pressure. *(Level VI: Clinical studies in a variety of patient populations and situations to support recommendations.)* With collagen plugs, percutaneous suture-mediated closure devices and noninvasive hemostasis pads, the bed rest time is decreased to between 1-4 hours, depending on the manufacturer recommendations and institutional protocol. Maintain bed rest for a maximum of 4 hours after venous sheath removal.	Minimizes back discomfort, minimizes complications of bed rest, and does not increase vascular complications.[4,6,7,8,9,13] Venous punctures require less time in bed than arterial punctures because the chance of complications is decreased.	• Occurrence of bleeding • Hematoma development • Changes in vital signs

Documentation

Documentation should include the following:

- Patient and family education
- Date and time of sheath removal
- Site of arterial and venous sheath removal
- Quality of arterial and venous sheaths that are removed (e.g., intact, cracked)
- Any difficulties with removal
- Patient tolerance of the procedure
- Any medications used

- Time to hemostasis
- Method of hemostasis
- Site assessment
- Vital signs—heart rate, blood pressure, respiratory rate, rhythm
- Peripheral and neurovascular checks to the affected extremity
- Occurrence of unexpected outcomes
- Nursing interventions required
- Evaluation of any nursing intervention required

References

1. Barbiere, C.C. (1995). A new device for control of bleeding after transfemoral catheterization: The FemoStop system. *Crit Care Nurse,* 15, 51-3.
2. Bogart, M.A. (1995). Time to hemostasis: A comparison of manual versus mechanical compression of the femoral artery. *Am J Crit Care,* 4, 149-56.
3. Bowden, S.M., and Worrey, J.A. (1995). Assessing patient comfort: Local infiltration of lidocaine during femoral sheath removal. *Am J Crit Care,* 4, 368-9.
4. Coyne, C., et al. (1994). Controlled trial of backrest elevation after coronary angiography. *Am J Crit Care,* 3, 282-8.
5. Juran, N.B., et al. (1999). Nursing interventions to decrease bleeding at the femoral access site after percutaneous coronary intervention. *Am J Crit Care,* 8, 303-13.
6. Keeling, A.W., et al. (2000). Reducing time in bed after percutaneous transluminal coronary angioplasty (TIBS III). *Am J Crit Care,* 9, 185-7.
7. Keeling, A.W., et al. (1994). Postcardiac catheterization time-in-bed study: Enhancing patient comfort through nursing research. *Appl Nurs Res,* 7, 14-7.
8. Lau, K.W., et al. (1993). Early ambulation following diagnostic 7 French cardiac catheterization: A prospective randomized trial. *Cath Cardiovasc Diag,* 28, 34-8.
9. Logemann, T., et al. (1999). Two versus six hours of bed rest following left-sided cardiac catheterization and a meta-analysis of early ambulation trials. *Am J Cardiol,* 84, 486-8.
10. Rudisill, P.T., et al. (1997). Study of mechanical versus manual-mechanical compression following various interventional cardiology procedures. *J Cardiovasc Nurs,* 11, 15-21.
11. Simon, A., et al. (1998). Manual versus mechanical compression for femoral artery hemostasis after cardiac catheterization. *Am J Crit Care,* 7, 308-13.
12. Sulzbach, L.M., Munro, B.H., and Hirshfeld, J.W. (1995). A randomized clinical trial of the effect of bed position after PTCA. *Am J Crit Care.* 4, 221-6.
13. Vlasic, W., Almond, D., and Massel, D. (2001). Reducing bedrest following arterial puncture for coronary interventional procedures-impact on vascular complications: The BAC Trial. *J Invasive Cardiol,* 13, 788-92.
14. Wadas, T.M., and Hill, J. (1998). Is lidocaine infiltration during femoral sheath removal really necessary? *Heart Lung,* 27, 31-6.
15. Walker, S.B., Cleary, S., and Higgins, M. (2001). Comparison of the FemoStop device and manual pressure in reducing groin puncture site complications following coronary angioplasty and coronary stent placement. *Int J Nurs Pract,* 7, 366-75.

Additional Readings

Baim, D.S., et al. (2000). Suture-mediated closure of the femoral access site after cardiac catheterization: Results of the Suture To Ambulate aNd Discharge (STAND I and STAND II) trials. *Am J Cardiol,* 85, 864-9.
Botti, M., Williamson, B., and Steen, K. (2001). Coronary angiography observations: Evidence-based or ritualistic practice? *Heart Lung,* 30, 138-45.
Bowden, S.M., Matsco, M., and Worrey, J.A. (1998). Time of removal of femoral sheaths after interventional procedures: Comparison of hemoglobin and hematocrit values. *Am J Crit Care,* 7, 197-9.

Christensen, B.V., et al. (1998). Vascular complications after angiography with and without the use of sandbags. *Nurs Res,* 47, 51-3.

Cura, F.A., et al. (2000). Safety of femoral closure devices after percutaneous coronary interventions in the era of glycoprotein IIb/IIIa platelet blockade. *Am J Cardiol,* 86, 780-2.

Davis, C., et al. (1997). Vascular complications of coronary interventions. *Heart Lung,* 26, 118-27.

Homes, L.M., and Hollabaugh, S.K. (1997). Using the continuous quality improvement process to improve the care of patients after angioplasty. *Crit Care Nurse,* 17, 56-65.

Kapadia, S.R., et al. (2001). The 6Fr Angio-Seal arterial closure device: Results from a multimember prospective registry. *Am J Cardiol,* 87, 789-91.

Nickolaus, M.J., Gilchrist, I.C., and Ettinger, S.M. (2001). The way to the heart is all in the wrist: Transradial catheterization and interventions. *AACN Clin Issues,* 12, 62-71.

O'Brien, C., and Recker, D. (1992). How to remove a femoral sheath. *Am J Nurs,* 92, 34-7.

Schickel, S., et al. (1996). Removal of femoral sheaths by registered nurses: Issues and outcomes. *Crit Care Nurse,* 16, 32-6.

Shrake, K. (2000). Comparison of major complication rates associated with four methods of arterial closure. *Am J Cardiol,* 85, 1024-5.

Smith, T.T., and Labriola, R. (2001). Developing best practice in arterial sheath removal for registered nurses. *J Nurs Care Qual,* 16, 61-7.

Zhang, Z., et al. (2001). Impact of the Duett sealing device on quality of life and hospitalization costs for coronary diagnostic and interventional procedures: Results from the Study of Economic and Quality of Life Substudy of the SEAL trial. *Am Heart J,* 142, 982-8.

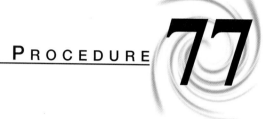

PROCEDURE **77**

Pericardial Catheter Management

PURPOSE: An indwelling pericardial catheter allows for the slow and complete evacuation of a pericardial effusion. The catheter also allows for the infusion of medications such as antibiotics or chemotherapeutic agents into the pericardial space.

Mary Ellen Kern
Kathy McCloy

PREREQUISITE NURSING KNOWLEDGE

- Understanding of the anatomy and physiology of the cardiovascular system, principles of cardiac conduction, electrocardiogram (ECG) lead placement, basic dysrhythmia interpretation, and electrical safety
- Understanding of sterile technique
- Advanced cardiac life support knowledge and skills
- Pericardial effusion is a collection of fluid in the pericardial space.
- The pericardial space normally contains 15 to 50 ml of fluid.[1,3] Injury of the pericardium causes increased production of pericardial fluid, formation of fibrin, and cellular proliferation.[1]
- Causes of pericardial effusion are numerous and include infection, malignant neoplasms, autoimmune disorders, kidney failure, heart failure, acute myocardial infarction, trauma, radiation exposure, inflammatory disorders, and myxedema.[1,7] Pericardial effusion may also be medication-induced, idiopathic, or a complication of invasive procedures.
- Pericardiocentesis is an effective treatment for pericardial effusion (refer to Procedures 41 and 42). An indwelling pericardial catheter may be left in place following pericardiocentesis to drain excess pericardial fluid.
- The pericardial catheter may be connected to a closed drainage system (Fig. 77-1).
- The pericardial catheter may also be left in place to allow instillation of certain medications, (i.e., nonabsorbable corticosteroid or antineoplastic agents) depending on the patient's underlying disease state.[5,7]

- The indwelling pericardial catheter is usually removed within 72 hours after placement to avoid the risk for infection and iatrogenic pericarditis.[4,5] However, the indwelling pericardial catheter may be left in place for longer periods of time to ensure resolution of a pericardial effusion and cardiac tamponade.[6,7] Pericardial catheters are usually removed when the total amount of

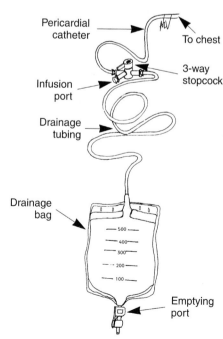

FIGURE 77-1 Indwelling pericardial catheter system. *(From Hammel, W.J. [1998]. Care of patients with an indwelling pericardial catheter. Crit Care Nurse. 18[5], 40-5.)*

drainage has decreased to less than 25 to 30 ml over the preceding 24 hours.[4,5,6,7]

• Extended catheter drainage is associated with a reduction of the reoccurrence of cardiac tamponade compared with a single pericardiocentesis in patients with pericardial effusion related to malignancy.[5,6,7]

EQUIPMENT

• Pericardial catheter
• Sterile and nonsterile gloves, gowns, masks, protective eyewear
• Sterile isotonic normal saline for irrigation
• Syringes: 30 ml or 60 ml Luer-Lok
• Antiseptic solution (e.g., 2% chlorhexidine-based preparation)
• Sterile 4 × 4 gauze
• Transparent occlusive dressing
• Tape
• Three-way stopcock with nonvented caps
  Additional equipment as needed includes the following:
• Drainage tubing (applicable to management with a drainage system)
• Pericardial drainage bag (applicable to management with a drainage system)
• Cytotoxic disposal receptacle (if applicable, for use of chemotherapeutic or cytotoxic agents)

PATIENT AND FAMILY EDUCATION

• Explain the need for the indwelling pericardial catheter and the reason for its insertion. ➥*Rationale:* Teaching decreases patient and family anxiety; meets patient and family need for information.
• Explain the need for frequent monitoring while the pericardial catheter remains in place. ➥*Rationale:* Decreases patient and family anxiety; meets patient and family need for information.
• Explain that the catheter may be uncomfortable and cause some discomfort at the insertion site, possibly with inspiration, and that pain medication will be administered to promote comfort. ➥*Rationale:* Facilitates effective pain management; decreases patient and family anxiety.

• Describe the possible signs and symptoms of cardiac tamponade to the patient and family. ➥*Rationale:* Teaching the patient and family will help them to recognize a possible reoccurrence of pericardial effusion and assist them as they prepare for discharge.

PATIENT ASSESSMENT AND PREPARATION

Patient Assessment

• Assess the patient's cardiovascular and hemodynamic status: heart rate, blood pressure (BP), respiratory rate, heart sounds, peripheral pulses, and if available, pulmonary artery pressures (PAPs), pulmonary artery wedge pressure (PAWP), right atrial pressure (RAP), cardiac output (CO), and cardiac index (CI). ➥*Rationale:* Establishes the patient's baseline for future comparison.
• Assess the patient for dyspnea, tachypnea, tachycardia, muffled heart sounds, precordial dullness to percussion, impaired consciousness; hypotension (systolic BP less than 100 mm Hg or decreased from the patient's baseline); increased jugular venous pressure; pulsus paradoxus (inspiratory fall in systolic BP) greater than 12 to 15 mm Hg or, if auscultated, a disappearance of BP sounds (as the manometer is falling) during inspiration of greater than 12-15 mm Hg; equalization of RAP, PAWP, and pulmonary artery diastolic pressure, low CO/CI.[8] ➥*Rationale:* Assesses for signs and symptoms of cardiac tamponade.

Patient Preparation

• Ensure that the patient and family understand preprocedure teaching. Answer questions as they arise and reinforce information as needed. ➥*Rationale:* Evaluates and reinforces understanding of previously taught information.
• Administer analgesia and/or anxiolytic before pericardial catheter insertion. ➥*Rationale:* Facilitates pain management and reduces anxiety.
• Ensure that in nonemergent situations, an informed consent has been obtained. ➥*Rationale:* Protects the rights of the patient and includes the patient in health care team decision making. It also allows for a competent decision by the patient.

Procedure	for the Pericardial Catheter Management	
Steps	Rationale	Special Considerations
General Management of the Patient With a Pericardial Catheter Without a Drainage System		
1. Wash hands, don nonsterile gloves, mask with protective eyewear, and gown if needed for postinsertion care.	Reduces the transmission of microorganisms; standard precautions.	
2. Assist the physician or advanced practice nurse with the	Provides assistance as needed.	The pericardial catheter may be inserted in the operating room or

Procedure continues on the following page

Procedure for the Pericardial Catheter Management—*Continued*

Steps	Rationale	Special Considerations
pericardiocentesis (see Procedures 41 and 42) as the pericardial catheter is inserted over a guidewire and is positioned in the pericardial sac.		in a special procedure environment (e.g., cardiac catheterization laboratory or interventional laboratory).
3. Determine that the connections between the pericardial catheter and stopcock are tight.	Ensures that the integrity of the system is intact.	At the completion of the pericardial tap, the stopcock is turned off to the patient and a nonvented cap is placed on the stopcock port.
4. Observe the drainage of pericardial fluid for color, amount, and consistency.	Ensures pericardial catheter patency. The presence of fibrin matrix in the drainage can result in obstruction of the catheter and be problematic for future manual taps.	Pericardial fluid is commonly straw-colored, serous drainage. A two-dimensional (2-D) or Doppler echocardiogram is usually performed after the pericardiocentesis to assess for reaccumulation of pericardial fluid.[7]
5. Perform catheter site care:	Prevents infection and avoids dislodgment of the catheter.	
A. Wash hands, don nonsterile gloves, mask, and protective eyewear.	Reduces the transmission of microorganisms; standard precautions.	
B. Remove the dressing.	Prepares for site care.	
C. Assess the catheter, insertion site, suture, and surrounding skin.	Assess for signs of infection, catheter dislodgment, leakage, or loose sutures.	
D. Remove and discard the nonsterile gloves, wash hands, and put on sterile gloves.	Maintains aseptic technique.	
E. Beginning at the insertion site, cleanse the catheter and skin around the insertion site thoroughly with antiseptic solution (e.g., 2% chlorhexidine-based preparation) and allow to dry.	Reduces the rate of recolonization of skin microflora.	Failure to allow the antiseptic solution to dry before applying an occlusive dressing can result in a chemical interaction with the adhesive of the dressing and may cause skin irritation.
F. Ensure that the catheter and stopcock are securely anchored to the chest.	Minimizes the risk for dislodgment.	
G. Apply a sterile occlusive dressing.	Provides a sterile environment.	
H. Label the dressing with the date, time, and initials.	Identifies the last dressing change.	
I. Discard used supplies and wash hands.	Reduces the transmission of microorganisms; standard precautions.	
6. *If pericardial fluid removal is desired,* aspirate the pericardial fluid every 4 to 6 hours or as clinically indicated through a three-way stopcock using sterile technique.[1]	Removes excess pericardial fluid and relieves symptoms of cardiac tamponade; ensures catheter patency.	Follow institutional standards regarding personnel permitted to aspirate and flush pericardial catheters (e.g., registered nurse, advanced practice nurse, physician).
A. Wash hands, and don sterile gloves, mask, and protective eyewear. In some cases a gown may also be indicated.	Reduces the transmission of microorganisms; standard precautions. Prepares for aseptic technique.	
B. Remove the cap from the infusion port (stopcock is turned off to the patient) of the three-way stopcock.		
C. Clean the infusion port of the three-way stopcock with an alcohol swab and allow to dry.	Decreases the risk for infection. Allowing the alcohol to dry before going further ensures its antiseptic property.	

Procedure for the Pericardial Catheter Management—*Continued*

Steps	Rationale	Special Considerations
D. Attach a sterile, 60-ml Luer-Lok syringe to the three-way stopcock.	Connects to the port for pericardial fluid removal without the danger of disconnection.	
E. Turn the stopcock open to the syringe and patient.	Permits the removal of pericardial fluid.	
F. *Gently* aspirate pericardial fluid.	Gentle removal is necessary to avoid pericardial injury.	Pericardial fluid samples may be collected for selected diagnostic tests (e.g., protein, glucose; hematocrit, white blood cell count; bacterial or fungal culture).
G. After completion of the fluid withdrawal, temporarily turn the stopcock off to the patient and disconnect the specimen syringe. Connect the flush syringe, turn the stopcock open to the syringe, and flush the pericardial catheter with 2 to 5 ml of sterile normal saline (NS) or heparinized NS as prescribed.[1]	Clears the pericardial catheter and maintains catheter patency.	Monitor vital signs and the ECG while flushing the pericardial catheter.
H. Return the three-way stopcock off to the patient and disconnect the flush syringe.	Maintains a closed system; prevents pneumopericardium.	
I. Place a new sterile nonvented cap on the infusion port.	Maintains asepsis.	
J. Measure the amount of drainage.	Needed for assessing and recording output.	
K. Discard the drainage and used supplies and wash hands.	Reduces the transmission of microorganisms; standard precautions.	
7. *If the pericardial catheter is blocked or obstructed to flow:*		
A. Assess whether there is an external mechanical cause of the pericardial catheter blockage and, if present, correct. Consider the following measures: (1) Correct tubing kinks. (2) Remove tubing that may be compressed under the patient. (3) Turn or reposition the patient.	Relieves mechanical obstruction to flow of pericardial fluid.	
B. Assess for loose tubing connection and, if loosened, tighten the connection.	Ensures an intact pericardial drainage system.	
C. Determine whether the stopcock is in the correct position and, if needed, correct the position.	Facilitates pericardial fluid collection.	
D. If the above steps do not relieve the catheter blockage, do the following:	Attempts to relieve the blockage.	Follow institutional standards regarding personnel permitted to aspirate and flush pericardial catheters (e.g., registered nurse, advanced practice nurse, or physician).
(1) Wash hands and apply sterile gloves and mask with eye protection and gown if needed.	Reduces the transmission of microorganisms; standard precautions. Prepares for aseptic technique.	

Procedure continues on the following page

Procedure for the Pericardial Catheter Management—*Continued*

Steps	Rationale	Special Considerations
(2) Turn the stopcock off to the patient and remove the cap from the infusion port of the stopcock.	Decreases the risk for infection.	
(3) Clean the infusion port of the stopcock with an alcohol swab and allow to dry.		
(4) Attach the syringe for the flush and turn the stopcock open to the patient.		
(5) Flush the pericardial catheter with 2 to 5 ml of heparinized normal saline, *as prescribed* (e.g., 30 units of heparin per ml of NS) or sterile NS if the patient is sensitive to heparin.[1]	Attempts to improve pericardial catheter patency. Heparinized saline may be used if the drainage is serous or fibrous in consistency.[4]	Monitor vital signs and the ECG while flushing the pericardial catheter.
(6) Gently attempt to aspirate the flush.	Allows drainage of flush solution and pericardial fluid.	Deduct flush solution from the measurement of pericardial drainage.
(7) Determine whether the pericardial catheter is draining and patent.		
(8) If measures do not remove the catheter blockage, notify the physician or advanced practice nurse immediately.		Obtain vital signs and cardiac parameters.
8. *If medications are prescribed for infusion into the pericardium:*		
A. Wash hands and don protective attire for this procedure, including protective eyewear, mask, and sterile gloves and gown if necessary.	Double-gloving, eyewear/mask and gown may be indicated for antineoplastic medication administration.[7] Reduces the transmission of microorganisms and potential for infection.	Follow institutional standards regarding personnel permitted to instill medications into the pericardial sac.
B. Review the prescribed medication, dose, method of delivery, amount, and time for dwell. Assemble the medication, tubing/pump or syringe and two flush syringes of NS (2 to 5 ml each).[1]	Prepares the equipment.	**Caution:** Infusion of medications into the pericardial sac may cause iatrogenic cardiac tamponade.[1]
C. Ensure that the stopcock is off to the patient and remove the cap from the infusion port.		
D. Clean the infusion port with an alcohol wipe and allow to dry.		
E. Attach a flush syringe and turn the stopcock open to the patient. Establish the patency of the catheter by gentle infusion and withdrawal of NS.		
F. Turn the stopcock off to the patient and disconnect the flush syringe.		
G. Attach the prescribed medication (either infusion or syringe). If using a syringe for delivery, gently instill the medication.	Infusion of the medication may activate signs and symptoms of cardiac tamponade.	Monitor vital signs, patient presentation, and cardiac parameters if available in order to identify patient distress and decompensation. If the patient presents with these symptoms, stop the infusion and notify the advanced practice nurse or the physician.

Procedure for the Pericardial Catheter Management—*Continued*

Steps	Rationale	Special Considerations
H. Turn the stopcock off to the patient when the medication delivery is complete. (1) Disconnect the syringe or tubing. (2) Attach a flush syringe of NS. (3) Turn the stopcock open to the patient and instill the flush.	Ensures that the medication is fully in the pericardium and not in the catheter.	
I. Turn the stopcock off to the patient and allow the medication to dwell for the prescribed time. Apply a sterile nonvented cap to the infusion port.		
J. When the dwell time is completed, remove the infusion port cap and attach a syringe large enough to retrieve the medication plus pericardial fluid accumulation.	Retrieval of the medication should be equivalent in amount to what was instilled, plus flush and additional pericardial fluid accumulated during the dwell time.	
K. Gently withdraw the medication and pericardial drainage.		
L. Turn the stopcock off to the patient and disconnect the syringe of the processed medication. Attach a flush syringe of 2-5 ml of NS or heparin flush if prescribed.		
M. Turn the stopcock open to the patient and instill an NS flush or heparin flush. Turn the stopcock off to the patient.		
N. Remove the flush syringe and apply a sterile nonvented cap to the infusion port.		
O. Discard used supplies and wash hands.	Reduces the transmission of microorganisms; standard precautions.	Discard any chemotherapeutic agent and flush including antineoplastics in the designated cytotoxic receptacle.

General Management of the Patient With a Pericardial Catheter Closed Drainage System

1. Wash hands, don nonsterile gloves, mask with protective eyewear, and gown if needed for postinsertion care.	Reduces the transmission of microorganisms; standard precautions.	
2. Assist the physician or the advanced practice nurse with the pericardiocentesis (see Procedures 41 and 42) as the pericardial catheter is inserted over a guidewire and placed in the pericardial sac.	Provides assistance as needed.	The pericardial catheter may be inserted in the operating room or in a special procedure environment (e.g., cardiac catheterization laboratory or interventional laboratory).
3. Determine that connections between the pericardial catheter, stopcock, tubing, and drainage bag are tight.	Ensures that the integrity of the system is intact.	At the completion of the pericardial tap, a nonvented sterile cap is placed on the stopcock port and the stopcock is turned off to the patient or open to drainage as prescribed.

Procedure continues on the following page

Procedure for the Pericardial Catheter Management—*Continued*

Steps	Rationale	Special Considerations
4. Position the drainage bag lower than the catheter insertion point, and observe the drainage of pericardial fluid for color, amount, and consistency.	Promotes drainage and is preventative for catheter blockage. The presence of fibrin matrix in the drainage can result in obstruction of the catheter and be problematic for future manual taps and intermittent or continuous drainage.	Pericardial fluid is commonly straw-colored, serous drainage. A 2-D or Doppler echocardiogram is performed after the pericardiocentesis to assess for reaccumulation of pericardial fluid.[7]
5. Perform catheter site care.	Prevents infection and avoids dislodgment of the catheter.	
A. Wash hands and don nonsterile gloves, mask with protective eyewear, and gown if necessary.	Reduces the transmission of microorganisms; standard precautions.	
B. Remove the dressing.	Prepares for site care.	
C. Assess the catheter, insertion site, suture, and surrounding skin.	Assess for signs of infection, catheter dislodgment, leakage, or loose sutures.	
D. Remove and discard the gloves, wash hands, and put on a sterile pair of gloves.	Maintains aseptic technique.	
E. Beginning at the insertion site, cleanse the catheter and skin around the insertion site thoroughly with antiseptic solution (e.g., 2% chlorhexidine-based preparation) and allow to dry.	Reduces the rate of recolonization of skin microflora.	Failure to allow the antiseptic solution to dry before applying an occlusive dressing can result in a chemical interaction with the adhesive of the dressing and may cause skin irritation.
F. Ensure that the catheter and the stopcock are securely anchored to the chest.		
G. Apply a sterile, occlusive dressing.	Provides a sterile environment.	Observe the site for any evidence of drainage and notify the physician or advanced practice nurse of this finding.
H. Label the dressing with the date, time, and initials.	Identifies the last dressing change.	
I. Discard used supplies and wash hands.	Reduces the transmission of microorganisms; standard precautions.	
6. *If pericardial fluid removal is desired,* intermittently or continuously drain the pericardial fluid as prescribed by turning the stopcock off to the infusion port and open between the patient and drainage bag (see Fig. 77-1). In the case of *intermittent drainage,* the stopcock is usually off to the patient and opened every 4-6 hours to drainage or as clinically indicated by Doppler or 2-D echocardiogram and patient presentation until the accumulation of fluid is resolved (follow prescribed regimen). In *continuous drainage* the stopcock is open between the patient and the drainage bag and off to the infusion port with a nonvented sterile cap on the stopcock port (follow prescribed regimen).	Removes excess pericardial fluid and relieves symptoms of cardiac tamponade; ensures catheter patency.	Follow institutional standards regarding personnel permitted to drain pericardial catheters (e.g., registered nurse, advanced practice nurse, or physician).

Procedure for the Pericardial Catheter Management—*Continued*

Steps	Rationale	Special Considerations
A. Empty the pericardial drainage bag at least every 8 hours.	Reduces the possibility of colonization in the bag and potential reflux of fluid to the patient.	Pericardial fluid samples may be collected for selected diagnostic tests (e.g., protein, glucose; hematocrit, white blood cell count; bacterial or fungal culture).
(1) Wash hands and wear protective eyewear, mask, and nonsterile gloves.	Reduces the chance of organism transmission.	
(2) Turn the stopcock off to the patient.	Decreases the risk for pneumopericardium.	
(3) Open the emptying port of the drainage bag and drain the pericardial fluid into a receptacle for measurement and waste disposal.		
(4) Close the port and secure the drainage bag.		
(5) Resume the prescribed drainage mode.		
B. After completion of intermittent fluid drainage, temporarily turn the stopcock off to the patient for the flush procedure.	Clears the pericardial catheter and maintains catheter patency.	Monitor vital signs and the ECG while flushing the pericardial catheter.
(1) Remove the infusion port cap and clean the port with alcohol and allow to dry.		
(2) Connect the flush syringe, open the stopcock to the patient, and flush the pericardial catheter with 2 to 5 ml of sterile normal saline or the prescribed heparinized solution or as prescribed.[1]		
(3) Turn the three-way stopcock off to the patient and disconnect the flush syringe.	Maintains a closed system; prevents pneumopericardium.	
(4) Place a new sterile nonvented cap on the infusion port.	Maintains asepsis.	
7. *If the pericardial catheter is blocked or obstructed to flow:*		Follow institutional standards regarding personnel permitted to aspirate and flush pericardial catheters (e.g., registered nurse, advanced practice nurse, or physician).
A. Determine whether the drainage system is lower than the insertion point and reposition if needed.	Facilitates drainage.	
B. Assess whether there is an external mechanical cause of pericardial catheter blockage and, if present, correct. Consider the following measures:	Relieves mechanical obstruction to flow of pericardial fluid.	
(1) Correct tubing kinks.		
(2) Remove tubing that may be compressed under the patient.		
(3) Turn or reposition the patient.		

Procedure continues on the following page

Procedure for the Pericardial Catheter Management—*Continued*

Steps	Rationale	Special Considerations
C. Assess for loose tubing connection and, if loosened, tighten the connection.	Ensures an intact pericardial drainage system.	
D. Determine whether the stopcock is in the correct position and, if needed, correct the position.	Facilitates pericardial fluid collection.	
E. If the above steps do not relieve the catheter blockage, do the following:	Attempts to relieve blockage.	Follow institutional standards regarding personnel permitted to aspirate pericardial catheters (e.g., registered nurse, advanced practice nurse, or physician).
(1) Wash hands and apply sterile gloves and mask with eye protection and gown if needed.	Reduces the transmission of microorganisms; standard precautions. Prepares for aseptic technique.	
(2) Remove the cap from the stopcock.	Decreases the risk for infection.	
(3) Clean the infusion port of the stopcock with an alcohol swab and allow to dry.		
(4) Attach the flush syringe and turn the stopcock open to the patient.		
(5) Flush the pericardial catheter with 2 to 5 ml of heparinized normal saline, *as prescribed* (e.g., 30 units of heparin per ml of normal saline) or sterile normal saline if the patient is sensitive to heparin.[1]	Attempts to improve pericardial catheter patency. Heparinized saline may be used if the drainage is serous or fibrous in consistency.[4]	Monitor vital signs and the ECG while flushing the pericardial catheter.
(6) Turn the stopcock off to the infusion port and allow the fluid to passively drain or gently attempt to aspirate the flush with the attached syringe with the stopcock turned open to the patient.	Allows drainage of the flush solution and pericardial fluid.	Deduct the flush solution from measurement of pericardial drainage.
(7) Determine whether the pericardial catheter is draining and patent.		
(8) If the above measures are ineffective for drainage, but the catheter itself is patent, consider changing the tubing and the drainage bag system with the stopcock turned off to the patient at the time of the change.		
(9) After the tubing/bag change, assess the patency of the system.		
(10) If measures do not remove the catheter blockage, notify the advanced practice nurse or the physician immediately.		Obtain vital signs and cardiac parameters.
8. *If infusion of medication into the pericardium is desired:*		Follow institutional standards regarding personnel permitted to aspirate and flush pericardial catheters (e.g., registered nurse, advanced practice nurse, or physician).
A. Wash hands and don protective attire for this procedure, including protective eyewear, mask, sterile and nonsterile gloves and gown if necessary.	Reduces the transmission of microorganisms; standard precautions. Prepares for aseptic technique.	

Procedure for the Pericardial Catheter Management—*Continued*

Steps	Rationale	Special Considerations
	Double-gloving, eyewear/mask and gown may be indicated for antineoplastic medication administration as well as a cytotoxic disposal receptacle for retrieved drainage and flush postinstillation.[7]	
B. Review the prescribed medication, dose, amount, rate of infusion, and length of dwell time.	Ensures the accuracy of medication administration.	
C. Turn the stopcock off to the patient, remove the infusion port cap, clean the infusion port of the stopcock with an alcohol pad or swabstick, and allow to dry.	Decreases the risk for infection.	
D. Connect the medication syringe or IV medication solution to the infusion port of the stopcock. (Patency of the catheter is established by virtue of evident drainage. If there is a question about catheter patency, follow the flush procedure listed in the medication infusion section of *Management of the Patient with a Pericardial Catheter Without a Drainage System* [above], step 8, C-F.)		Infusion of medication into the pericardial sac may cause iatrogenic cardiac tamponade.
E. Turn the stopcock off to the drainage bag.	Prevents inadvertent instillation of medication into the drainage bag.	
F. Infuse the medication or solution slowly as prescribed.	Provides treatment of underlying pathology without compromising hemodynamic stability.	Assess the patient closely for signs and symptoms of tamponade and chest pain. Stop the infusion if chest pain similar to angina develops or if the patient demonstrates tamponade.[1]
G. If the medication is to dwell in the pericardial space before reestablishment of pericardial drainage: (1) Turn the stopcock off to the patient at the completion of the infusion. (2) Disconnect the medication syringe or tubing. (3) Attach a syringe with 2-5 ml of NS flush and turn the stopcock off to the drainage bag. (4) Flush the catheter and turn the stopcock off to the patient for the completion of the dwell time as prescribed. (5) Disconnect the syringe and apply a sterile nonvented cap. (6) After the dwell time is complete, turn the stopcock off to the infusion port and open to drainage. (7) Measure the amount of the solution infused and the drainage collected.	Ensures that the medication is instilled in the pericardial space and does not lie in the catheter. Allows pericardial drainage to resume. Ensure that the volume of drainage collected is equal to or greater than the volume of solution instilled.	

Procedure continues on the following page

Procedure for the Pericardial Catheter Management—*Continued*

Steps	Rationale	Special Considerations
(8) Resume the prescribed drainage mode: continuous or intermittent. If intermittent, follow the prescription for the drain time postinfusion.	The drain time should allow for all of the medication in the concentrated form to exit the pericardium.	
(a) Once the drain time is completed as prescribed, clean the infusion port of the stopcock with alcohol with the stopcock turned off to the patient.		
(b) Attach a flush syringe of 2-5 ml of NS or heparinized NS as prescribed and flush the pericardial catheter.		
(c) Turn the stopcock off to the patient until the next time the patient is due for intermittent drainage.		
(d) Discard supplies and wash hands.	Reduces the transmission of microorganisms; standard precautions.	Discard any chemotherapeutic agent and flush, including antineoplastics in the designated cytotoxic receptacle.

Expected Outcomes

- Patent pericardial drainage system
- Resolution of pericardial effusion
- Hemodynamic stability
- Free of infection
- Free of pain and anxiety
- Medications administered as prescribed

Unexpected Outcomes

- Infection
- Pain
- Catheter blockage
- Reaccumulation of pericardial fluid
- Cardiac tamponade
- Dysrhythmias

Patient Monitoring and Care

Steps	Rationale	Reportable Conditions
		These conditions must be reported if they persist despite nursing interventions.
1. Perform systematic cardiovascular and hemodynamic assessments every 60 minutes and as patient status requires or as prescribed.	Monitors for cardiac tamponade and pericardial catheter-related problems.	• Signs of cardiac tamponade[7]; dyspnea, tachypnea, tachycardia, hypotension, increased jugular venous pressure, pulsus paradoxus, muffled heart sounds, precordial dullness to percussion, altered level of consciousness; equalization of RAP, PA diastolic, PAWP; CI less than 2.5 L per minute/m^2; dysrhythmias
2. Assess the patency of the pericardial catheter: A. Without a closed drainage system: every 4-6 hours and as needed B. With a closed drainage system: every hour and as needed.	Pericardial catheter blockage may predispose the patient to excessive accumulation of pericardial fluid that may lead to cardiac tamponade.	• Inability to obtain pericardial drainage or cessation of pericardial drainage • Signs and symptoms of cardiac tamponade • Evidence of accumulation of pericardial fluid on Doppler or 2-D echocardiography
3. Assess the amount and type of fluid draining from the pericardial catheter.	Monitors the type and amount of pericardial fluid drainage.	• Change in the amount or color of pericardial drainage from the patient's baseline

Patient Monitoring and Care—*Continued*

Steps	Rationale	Reportable Conditions
4. Change the pericardial dressing every 24 hours and when the dressing becomes damp, loosened, or soiled.	Provides an opportunity to assess for signs and symptoms of infection. Infective pericarditis is associated with high mortality and morbidity rates.[7]	• Elevated WBCs • Elevated temperature, greater than 38.5°C • Signs and symptoms of infection at the insertion site (e.g., pain, erythema, drainage)
5. If in use, change the pericardial tubing and drainage bag every 72 hours.[1]	Reduces the incidence of infection.	
6. Assess and manage patient pain and anxiety.	The patient may experience chest pain or pleuritic type pain while the pericardial catheter is in place and anxiety due to the critical nature of this condition.	• Inadequate pain relief with analgesics • Inadequate relief of anxiety
7. Identify parameters that demonstrate clinical readiness for removal of the indwelling pericardial catheter.	Facilitates early removal of the pericardial catheter; decreases infection risk.	• Pericardial drainage less than 25 to 30 ml over the previous 24 hours.[6] • Hemodynamic stability as evidenced by systolic BP greater than 100 mm Hg, CI greater than 2.5 L/minute/m^2, no pulsus paradoxus, no equalization of RAP, PA diastolic, PAWP[1,6] • Absence of pericardial effusion demonstrated on 2-D echocardiography or Doppler echocardiography

Documentation

Documentation should include the following:

• Patient and family education
• Patient toleration of the indwelling pericardial catheter
• Pericardial catheter insertion site assessment
• Dressing changes, tubing changes, drainage bag changes
• Amount of pericardial drainage each shift, including net volumes when the catheter is flushed or medications infused
• Volumes of injectate or aspirate

• Characteristics of pericardial drainage: color, consistency, and any changes
• Hemodynamic status
• Pain and anxiety associated with the indwelling pericardial catheter and interventions
• Occurrence of unexpected outcomes
• Nursing interventions

References

1. Hamel, W.J. (1998). Care of patients with an indwelling pericardial catheter. *Crit Care Nurse*, 18, 40-5.
2. Mayo Clinic. (2004). *Pericarditis and Pericardial Effusion: Patient Education Booklet.* Available at: www.mayoclinic.org. Rochester, Minn.
3. Strimel, W.J. (2002). *Pericardial Effusion.* Available at: www.emedicine.com. Item #1786.
4. Tsang, T.S.M., et al. (1999). Clinical and echocardiographic characteristics of significant pericardial effusions following cardiothoracic surgery and outcomes of echo-guided pericardiocentesis for management: Mayo Clinic experience, 1979-1998. *Chest* 116, 322-31.
5. Tsang, T.S.M., et al. (2000). Outcomes of primary and secondary treatment of pericardial effusion in patients with malignancy. *Mayo Clinic Proceedings,* 75, 248-53.
6. Tsang, T.S.M., et al. (2002). Consecutive 1127 therapeutic echocardiographically guided pericardiocenteses: Clinical profile, practice patterns and outcomes spanning 21 years. *Mayo Clinic Proceedings,* 77, 429-36.
7. Venugopalan, P. (2003). *Pericardial Effusion, Malignant.* Available at: www.emedicine.com. Accessed July. Topic #1764.

Additional Readings

Cummins, R.O., ed. (2001). *ACLS Provider Manual,* Dallas: American Heart Association, 97-109.
Seifert, P.C. (2002). *Cardiac Surgery.* Philadelphia: Mosby, 568-9.

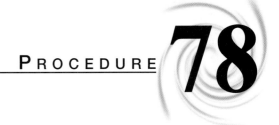

PROCEDURE 78

Transesophageal Echocardiography (Assist)

PURPOSE: Transesophageal echocardiography (TEE) offers an alternative approach for obtaining high-quality images of the heart structure that are not well visualized by conventional transthoracic approach. A TEE obtains images of the heart from a transducer inside the esophagus. The esophagus lies immediately behind the heart, and with this technology, very clear images of the heart can be obtained.

Linda M. Hoke
Janice Y. Dawson

PREREQUISITE NURSING KNOWLEDGE

- Knowledge of cardiovascular anatomy and physiology
- Knowledge of basic dysrhythmia recognition and treatment of life-threatening dysrhythmias
- Advance cardiac life support knowledge and skills
- A topical anesthetic is used in the oropharyngeal area; thus the patient's gag reflex may be diminished or absent, putting the patient at risk for aspiration.[17]
- Implementation of a conscious sedation guideline per institution standard. Sedation that is used can put the patient at risk for respiratory depression.[5,6,11,14]
- A fiberoptic probe with an ultrasound transducer is inserted through the mouth and into the esophagus just behind the heart (Fig. 78-1). The transducer located at the tip of the probe sends high-frequency sound waves toward the heart, which return as echoes. The echoes are converted, by computer, into moving images of the heart. The image is displayed on a screen and can be recorded digitally on videotape and/or printed on paper. This test is used to visualize structures of the heart and aorta that may not be seen by a standard echocardiogram as well as clarify structures, which may be otherwise poorly seen. The test may be performed as an outpatient or inpatient procedure or in the operating room.[1,11,17]
- Various modes of echocardiography are used to examine the heart, blood vessels, valve function, and blood flow. The three techniques are as follows:
    - ❖ Motion-mode (M-mode) echocardiography: This is a one-dimensional echocardiogram, which visualizes

time, depth, and intensity. It looks like a tracing instead of a picture of the heart. It is used to measure the exact size of the heart chambers.
- ❖ Two-dimensional (2-D) echocardiography: This shows the actual shape and motion of the different heart

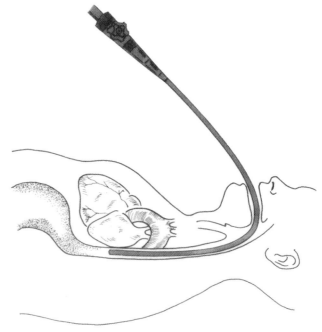

FIGURE 78-1 TEE probe inserted through the mouth and into the esophagus just behind the heart. (*From Brown, L.M., and Brown, A.S. [1994]. Transesophageal echocardiography: implications for the critical care nurse.* Crit Care Nurs, *14, 56.*)

structures. These images represent "slices" of the heart in motion.

- ❖ Doppler echocardiography: This assesses the flow of blood through the heart. The signals that represent blood flow are displayed as a series of black-and-white tracings or color images on the screen.
- TEE imaging is more risky than transthoracic imaging because of the insertion of the probe in the esophagus and the need for conscious sedation.[11]
- Indications for TEE are as follows:
  - ❖ Evaluation of (pre) clot formation in the heart, especially in the atria and appendages, in patients with an atrial dysrhythmia.
  - ❖ Evaluation of spontaneous echocardiographic contrast or "smoke" presenting as dynamic echoes within the left atrium and appendage which resembles swirling smoke in 2-D images. It is manifested by erythrocyte and platelet aggregates in regions of low blood flow. It has a significant correlation with previous embolic events and may serve as a marker for increased risk for embolism.[1,15]
  - ❖ TEE prior to cardioversion is advocated in patients in whom early cardioversion would be clinically beneficial. Patients with atrial fibrillation undergoing electrical cardioversion with short-term anticoagulation have lower hemorrhagic complications. Cardioversion may be performed more safely, after only a short period of anticoagulant therapy, in patients without atrial cavity or appendage thrombus by TEE. Cardioversion is delayed in high-risk patients with thrombus detected by TEE. Conventional treatment has been to give patients undergoing elective cardioversion therapeutic anticoagulation for 3 weeks before and 4 weeks after cardioversion, to decrease the risk for thromboembolism.[2,9]
  - ❖ Transient ischemic attack or stroke evaluation to rule out cardiac source of emboli and structure abnormalities (e.g., patent foramen ovale) or others abnormalities not identified prior to a neurologic event.[11]
  - ❖ Multiple factors may obstruct the penetration of the ultrasound beams from the transthoracic approach. Poor quality transthoracic echocardiogram images can be found in patients with obesity, chronic obstructive lung disease, chest wall deformities, multiple chest trauma, and thick surgical chest dressings.[1,3,17]
  - ❖ Assessment of native cardiac valve defects particularly of the mitral valve[11]
  - ❖ Assessment of prosthetic cardiac valve function
  - ❖ Assessment of intracardiac foreign bodies, tumors or masses
  - ❖ Assessment of vegetative endocarditis and abscess
  - ❖ Assessment of congenital heart defects
  - ❖ The superior sensitivity and specificity of TEE for aortic disease, including aneurysm, dissection, atherosclerosis, mobile plaque, congenital aortic disease, pseudoaneurysm, and traumatic aortic disruption make it the test of choice in many clinical situations.[1,16]
  - ❖ Disease in the ascending and transverse aorta often requires a TEE for complete evaluation; however,

a short portion of the distal ascending aorta and proximal transverse arch is usually not visible. This is a blind area because of the carina passing between the aorta and the esophagus.[16]

- ❖ TEE used in combination with stress test for the evaluation of patients with coronary artery disease. Transesophageal echocardiography-dobutamine stress echocardiography (TEE-DSE) has been reported to be highly accurate for detecting ischemia in patients with suspected coronary artery disease.[8,10,12]
- ❖ Transesophageal atrial pacing stress echocardiography (TAPSE) is an efficient alternative to DSE for the detection of coronary artery disease. The heart rate can be rapidly increased, resulting in myocardial ischemia in regions supplied by stenosed coronary arteries. By contrast to TEE-DSE, termination of pacing results in nearly instantaneous restoration of the patient's intrinsic heart rate.[1,13]
- ❖ Intraoperative guide to left ventricular function and intracardiac blood flow and evaluation of cardiac surgical repair[7]
- ❖ Detection of intracardiac air at the end of cardiac surgery before discontinuing cardiopulmonary bypass[3]
- ❖ Assessing a donor heart for transplantation following a motor vehicle accident for myocardial contusion[1,17]
- ❖ Contrast for TEE is an intravenous injection of microbubbles formed by agitating a saline solution. This results in a marked increase in echogenicity of the right-sided cardiac chambers. Right-sided echocardiography contrast studies are performed to document an atrial septal defect, a patent foramen ovale, and to increase the signal strength of the tricuspid regurgitant jet to allow a more accurate estimate of pulmonary artery pressures. Commercially available contrast agents provide smaller microbubbles that are injected intravenously by traversing the pulmonary capillary bed. This enhances the left ventricular chamber.[11]

- Contraindications to TEE can be divided into absolute and relative.
  - ❖ Absolute contraindications:[1,11]
    - ○ Tumor of the upper gastrointestinal (GI) tract
    - ○ Esophageal obstruction, stenosis, fistulae, or varices
    - ○ A history of esophageal radiation or unresolved esophageal dilation
    - ○ GI bleeding
    - ○ Gastric volvus or perforation
    - ○ Perforated viscus
    - ○ Patient who ate within 8 hours of the study
    - ○ Unwilling patient
    - ○ Inability to obtain intravenous access
  - ❖ Relative contraindications:[1,11]
    - ○ Upper GI surgery
    - ○ Severe thrombocytopenia (platelets 20,000 to 50,000/cubic millimeter[4])
    - ○ Oropharyngeal distortion
    - ○ Prior esophageal surgery
    - ○ Esophagitis
    - ○ Loose teeth

- Antibiotics are no longer administered prior to the procedure in patients with a prosthetic valve. Echocardiography does not pose a risk for infection.[1,11]

EQUIPMENT

- Omniplane or biplane transesophageal probe
- Echocardiography machine (compatible with the probe)
- Contrast
- Constant low wall suction with connecting tubing and rigid pharyngeal suction tip catheter
- Protective mask/goggles
- Nonsterile gloves
- Barrier gowns
- Water-soluble lubricant
- Oxygen with both nasal prongs and mask available
- Topical anesthetic such as an aerosol lidocaine solution, viscous lidocaine, or tetracaine
- Premedications for sedation and their appropriate reversal agent (as prescribed by the physician)
- Syringes for sedation medications (at least 1-5 ml and 1-10 ml)
- Alcohol prep pads
- Intravenous setup with solution (usually 0.9% NSS)
- Tongue depressor
- Emesis basin
- Tonsillar forceps and cotton balls
- Flashlight (to assess the oropharyngeal area, especially in the case of trauma)
- Disposable bite guard (may use the type with or without a strap to hold it in place)
- Thermometer
- Continuous cardiac monitor
- Continuous pulse oximeter
- Automatic blood pressure cuff (with manual blood pressure cuff available for backup use)
- Pillow (to support/position neck when the patient lies on the left side during the procedure)

Additional equipment as needed includes the following:

- Emergency equipment
- Emergency intubation equipment

PATIENT AND FAMILY EDUCATION

- Explain the procedure and the indication for therapy as well as the patient's role in the procedure. ➤*Rationale:* Information about the procedure increases patient cooperation and decreases both anxiety and apprehension.
- Ensure that the patient understands the preparation for the procedure, which includes nothing by mouth (NPO) after midnight, or a minimum of 8 hours. Prior to the test, the patient may take daily medications, with a sip of water, as directed by his or her physician.[17] ➤*Rationale:* Undigested material in the stomach increases the risk for aspiration. Missing a daily medication dose may not be advisable.

- Explain to the patient that the local anesthetic may make the tongue and throat feel swollen and that they may feel unable to swallow. The gag reflex will be inhibited by the local anesthetic. The patient may experience gagging or retching during the numbing process and/or the initial passage of the probe. ➤*Rationale:* Assists in decreasing patient anxiety during the procedure.
- Explain that the patient will be sedated for comfort and for ease in passing the probe. ➤*Rationale:* Assists in decreasing patient and family anxiety.
- Explain that the patient will be monitored closely during and after the procedure. ➤*Rationale:* Assists in decreasing the patient and family anxiety.

PATIENT ASSESSMENT AND PREPARATION

Patient Assessment

- Confirm medications the patient has taken within the last four hours. ➤*Rationale:* Recent sedative, analgesic, and vasoactive medications may effect the patient's tolerance and response to the medications given during the procedure.
- Assess the patient's baseline cardiac rhythm. ➤*Rationale:* The patient's rhythm may have converted if the indication for the procedure was a dysrhythmia. Passage of a large-bore tube may cause vagal stimulation and bradydysrhythmias.
- Assess the patient's baseline respiratory, hemodynamic, and neurologic assessment before anesthetizing the posterior pharynx and administering any sedative agent(s). ➤*Rationale:* Baseline assessment data provides information to use as a comparison for further assessment once medications have been administered.
- Assess the patient's baseline vital signs and pulse oximeter reading. ➤*Rationale:* Close monitoring of vital signs during the procedure and comparison with baseline are essential to assess the patient's tolerance of the procedure.
- Assess the patient's baseline pain characteristic, site, and severity. ➤*Rationale:* Baseline assessment data provides information to use as a comparison during and following the procedure.
- Assess the patient for a history of substance use. ➤*Rationale:* It may affect the patient's tolerance and response to the medications given during the procedure.

Patient Preparation

- Ensure that the patient understands preprocedural teaching. Answer questions as they arise and reinforce information as needed. ➤*Rationale:* Evaluates and reinforces understanding of previously taught information. Assists in decreasing patient anxiety.
- Validate that the informed consent has been signed. ➤*Rationale:* Informed consent is necessary before invasive procedures and the administration of conscious sedation. Protects the rights of the patient and makes a competent decision possible for the patient; however,

under emergency circumstances, time may not allow the form to be signed.

- Ensure that the patient has not eaten for at least 8 hours before the procedure. ➥*Rationale:* Undigested material in the stomach increases the risk for aspiration.
- Instruct the patient to void prior to the procedure. ➥*Rationale:* Minimizes disruption of the exam.
- Place the patient on a cardiac monitor and apply the automatic blood pressure cuff and pulse oximeter. ➥*Rationale:* Allows for close cardiovascular and respiratory monitoring during the procedure.
- Ensure the intravenous (IV) access is in place. ➥*Rationale:* IV access is needed to administer premedications and for emergency medications.
- Maintain IV access at a keep open rate during the procedure. ➥*Rationale:* Ensures the IV is functioning and available should an emergency situation arise.
- Have the patient remove any dentures or dental prostheses. ➥*Rationale:* Dentures may interfere with the safe passage of the transesophageal probe.

- Set up the suction system with the connecting tubing and a rigid pharyngeal suction tip attached and ready for use. ➥*Rationale:* Necessary for suctioning the patient's oral secretions during the procedure.
- Administer a small amount of supplemental oxygen. ➥*Rationale:* Assists the patient's oxygenation during the procedure.
- Have a sedative or analgesic (may include midazolam, diazepam, morphine sulfate, and fentanyl) available (as prescribed) and administer when requested. Naloxone and Romazicon must be available for narcotic or sedative reversal. ➥*Rationale:* Reduces patient anxiety, promotes comfort, facilitates cooperation during the procedure, and decreases myocardial workload.
- Have atropine available at the bedside. ➥*Rationale:* Necessary if a vagal reaction occurs with the insertion and passage of the transesophageal probe.
- Have the contrast agent available if prescribed. ➥*Rationale:* Enhances the ability to evaluate cardiac structures and function.

Procedure for Transesophageal Echocardiography (Assist)

Steps	Rationale	Special Considerations
1. Wash hands and don barrier gown, nonsterile gloves, and protective mask/goggles.	Reduces the transmission of microorganisms; standard precautions. Provides protection against accidental exposure to body fluids.	
2. Assist with anesthetizing the posterior pharynx with the topical agent.	Decreases discomfort caused by passage of the probe.	If possible, allow the patient to sit up to increase comfort and decrease anxiety or the feeling of choking.
A. Position the patient in the left lateral position. Use pillows to ensure correct alignment of the spine with the head and body.[17]	This position allows secretions to collect in the dependent areas of the mouth for ease of suctioning and is the position of choice to prevent aspiration in case the patient vomits.	Endotracheal-intubated patients can be examined in the supine position.[3]
B. Reassess vital signs, pulse oximeter, neurologic status and pain before administration of conscious sedation.	Reconfirms any change in patient condition.	
3. Administer conscious sedation as prescribed.[5,6,11,14]	Allows the patient to cooperate in facilitating passage of the probe during the procedure.	Ensure that the appropriate antagonists are readily available. The patient may need additional medication throughout the procedure.
4. Assist the physician with the insertion of the probe.[3,17]		
A. Insert the bite guard.	Prevents the patient from biting the probe or the inserter's fingers.	Gag and cough reflexes may be compromised by topical

Procedure continues on the following page

Procedure for Transesophageal Echocardiography (Assist)—*Continued*

Steps	Rationale	Special Considerations
	Prevents damage to the teeth and mouth.	anesthetics and the patient may vomit as the probe is passed, increasing the risk for aspiration.
B. Assist with lubrication of the distal end of the probe with lubricant as prescribed.	Minimizes mucosal injury and irritation and facilitates ease of passage of the probe.	
C. Slightly bend the patient's head in a forward flex.	Eases insertion of the probe into the esophagus.	
D. Encourage the patient to simulate swallowing while the probe is being passed as directed by the physician.	The swallowing maneuver causes the epiglottis to close the trachea and directs the probe into the esophagus.	
E. Suction the oral secretions as needed to ensure patency of the airway.[11]	Because of the diminished gag reflex and the presence of the probe in the patient's pharynx, it may not be possible to swallow oral secretions. Manipulation of the probe in the esophagus and stomach may cause stimulation of gastric secretions, which will require additional suctioning.	
F. Provide the patient with reassurance and encouragement to keep the bite guard in place, maintain left lateral position, hold still without attempts to speak, and focus on his or her breathing pattern.	Decreases patient anxiety and promotes patient cooperation.	
5. Assist with the administration of the contrast agent as prescribed.	Enhances the view of the cardiac structures and function.	
6. Assist with the removal of the probe from the patient. Place the probe in an appropriate receptacle for cleaning.	Reduces the transmission of microorganisms; standard precautions.	
7. Discard used supplies and wash hands.	Reduces the transmission of microorganisms; standard precautions.	

Expected Outcomes

- Clear visualization of cardiac structures and function
- Immediate preliminary diagnosis
- (Note: Negative studies are helpful in excluding cardiac sources of compromise.[1])

Unexpected Outcomes

- Esophageal or gastric perforation
- Vasovagal hypotension from esophageal manipulation
- Substernal chest pain
- Temporary dysphagia
- Aspiration
- Respiratory depression
- Hematoma in the oropharynx
- Hypotension
- Hypertension
- Dysrhythmias
- Laryngospasm
- Bronchospasm
- Change in neurologic status
- Air embolism in patients with right-to-left shunt when using saline contrast
- Congestive heart failure

Patient Monitoring and Care

Steps	Rationale	Reportable Conditions
		These conditions should be reported if they persist despite nursing interventions.
1. Monitor cardiovascular, respiratory, and neurologic (level of consciousness) status. Document at a minimum of 5-minute intervals during, and 15-minute intervals after the TEE procedure, until the patient returns to baseline for at least 30 minutes.	Changes in vital signs, heart rhythm, and oximetry may indicate complications related to the procedure.	• Alterations of the following: ❖ Neurologic status ❖ Oximetry reading ❖ Heart rate ❖ Blood pressure
2. Maintain IV access at a keep open rate during the procedure and until the patient returns to baseline status postprocedure.	Ensures IV patency for emergency medications.	
3. Monitor the patient's sedation score (follow institution's preference for tool) based on blood pressure, pulse oxygen saturation, level of consciousness, and respiratory status.	Using a scoring system standardizes assessment of the patient's tolerance of conscious sedation.	• Abnormal sedation scale
4. Assess the patient's pain status at a minimum of 15-minute intervals during and after the TEE procedure until the patient returns to baseline for at least 30 minutes.	May indicate a complication of the procedure and/or a need for increased analgesia.	• New onset of pain • Increased discomfort • Unresolved discomfort not relieved after probe removal
5. Monitor for signs and symptoms of esophageal perforation.[17] A. Esophageal perforation in the cervical area B. Thoracic perforation C. Abdominal esophageal perforation D. A severe perforation can include hemothorax or pneumothorax.	Identifies complications.	 • Pain at the base of the neck • Dysphagia • Crepitus • Deep back pain • Dysphagia • Tachycardia • Dysphagia in the upper epigastric region that is more retrosternal in nature • Chest pain • Respiratory distress • Tachypnea • Dyspnea • Hypotension • Tachycardia
6. Monitor for intraprocedure complications or reasons to terminate the test early.[1,3,11]	Identifies complications.	• Patient becomes agitated, unable to cooperate, or has a significant change in neurologic status • Dental or oropharyngeal trauma • Hypoxemia • New dysrhythmia • New hypotension or hypertension • Perforation or subcutaneous emphysema • GI or other bleeding • Severe chest pain
7. Assess for the return of normal pharyngeal function. Keep the patient on the left side with slight head	Topical anesthesia decreases the gag reflex and increases the risk for aspiration. The left	• Prolonged absence of gag, swallow, or cough reflexes

Procedure continues on the following page

Patient Monitoring and Care—*Continued*

Steps	Rationale	Reportable Conditions
elevation until the gag, swallow, and cough reflexes are intact.	lateral position is the position of choice to prevent aspiration in case the patient is not be able to control secretions or vomit.	
8. Provide clear liquids when prescribed after return of pharyngeal function. Diet should be progressed to solid food as tolerated.	Topical anesthesia decreases the gag reflex and increases the risk for aspiration. Mild throat discomfort is common as the topical anesthetic wears off.	• Nausea • Vomiting • Unusual throat or stomach discomfort • Increase in throat discomfort after 24 hours, possibly indicating a hematoma

Documentation

Documentation should include the following:

- Date and time of procedure
- Initial patient assessment
- Pre- and postprocedure patient and family education
- Signed informed consent form
- Vital signs, pulse oximetry, neurologic status, and pain evaluation immediately prior to sedation, during the procedure and postprocedure

- Medications administered and their effectiveness
- Assessments of gag, swallow, and cough reflexes
- Time of probe insertion and removal
- Characteristics of any secretions obtained when suctioned
- Postprocedure totals for medications and fluid given
- Occurrence of unexpected outcomes
- Nursing interventions

References

1. Allen, M.N. (1999). Transesophageal echocardiography, 2nd ed. In: *Diagnostic Medical Sonography.* Philadelphia: J.B. Lippincott.
2. Asher, C.R., and Klein, A.L. (2000). The ACUTE trial. Transesophageal echocardiography to guide electrical cardioversion in atrial fibrillation. Assessment of cardioversion using transesophageal echocardiography. *Cleve Clin J Med,* 69, 713-8.
3. Brown, L.M., and Brown, A.S. (1994). Transesophageal echocardiography: Implications for the critical care nurse. *Crit Care Nurs,* 14, 55-9.
4. Drews, R.E., and Weinberger, S.E. (2000). Thrombocytopenic disorders in critically ill patients. *Respir Crit Care Med,* 162, 347-51.
5. Gare, M., et al. (2001). Conscious sedation with midazolam or propofol does not alter left ventricular diastolic performance in patients with preexisting diastolic dysfunction: A transmitral and tissue Doppler transthoracic echocardiography study. *Anesth Analg,* 93, 865-71.
6. Goodwin, S.A. (2001). Pharmacology consult. Pharmacological management of patients undergoing conscious sedation. *Clin Nurse Spec,* 15, 269-71.
7. Kallmeyer, I.J., et al. (2001). The safety of intraoperative transesophageal echocardiography: A case series of 7200 cardiac surgical patients. *Anesth Analg,* 92, 1126-30.
8. Kamalesh, M., Matorin, R., and Sawada, S. (2002). Comparative prognostic significance of transesophageal versus transthoracic stress echocardiography. *Echocardiography,* 19, 313-8.
9. Klein, A.L., Murray, D.R., and Grimm, R.A. (2001). Role of transesophageal echocardiography-guided cardioversion of patients with atrial fibrillation. *J Am Coll Cardiol,* 37, 691-704.
10. Loperfido, F., et al. (1999). Echocardiographic imaging in coronary artery disease: New techniques. *Rays,* 24, 60-72.
11. Otto, C.M. (2000). *Textbook of Clinical Echocardiography.* 2nd ed. Philadelphia: W.B. Saunders.
12. Panza, J.A. (1999). Transesophageal echocardiography with stress for the evaluation of patients with coronary artery disease. *Cardiol Clin,* 17, 501-20.
13. Rainbird, A.J., et al. (2000). A rapid stress-testing protocol for the detection of coronary artery disease: Comparison of two-stage transesophageal atrial pacing stress echocardiography with dobutamine stress echocardiography. *J Am Coll Cardiol,* 36, 1659-63.
14. Raipancholia, R., Sentinella, L., and Lynch, M. (2001). Role of conscious sedation for external cardioversion. *Heart,* 86, 571-2.
15. Stockdale, C.Y., and Robinson, J. (2002). TEE: Detecting left atrial thrombi: Using transesophageal echocardiography to detect left atrial thrombi in patients with atrial fibrillation. *AJN,* 102, 24CC, 24EE-FF (Critical Care Extra).
16. Silvestry, F.E. (2001). Aortic disease-descending and abdominal aortic aneurysm. In: Wiegers, S.E., Plappert, T., and St. John Sutton, M., eds. *Echocardiography in Practice: A Case-Oriented Approach.* London: Martin Dunitz.
17. Thompson, E.J. (1993). Transesophageal echocardiography: A new window on the heart and great vessels. *Crit Care Nurs,* 13, 55-66.

Additional Readings

Transesophageal Echocardiography

Eltzschig, H.K., et al. (2002). Transesophageal echocardiography: Perioperative evaluation of valvular function. *Anaesthesist,* 51, 81-102.

Kamalesh, M., et al. (2000). Prognostic value of negative transesophageal dobutamine stress echocardiography in men at high risk for coronary artery disease. *Am J Cardiol,* 85, 41-4.

Madu, E.C. (2000). Transesophageal dobutamine stress echocardiography in the evaluation of myocardial ischemia in morbidly obese subjects. *Chest,* 117, 657-61.

Quinones, M.A., et al. (2003). ACC/AHA clinical competence statement on echocardiography: A report of the American College of Cardiology/American Heart Association/American College of Physicians-American Society of Internal Medicine

Task Force on Clinical Competence. *J Am Coll Cardiol*, 41, 687-708.

Conscious Sedation
Hayes, A., and Buffum, M. (2001). Educating patients after conscious sedation for gastrointestinal procedures. *Gastroenterol Nurs*, 24, 54-7.

Pachulski, R.T., Adkins, D.C., and Mirza, H. (2001). Conscious sedation with intermittent midazolam and fentanyl in electrophysiology procedures. *J Intervent Cardiol,* 14, 143-6.

Waring, J.P., et al. (2003). Guidelines for conscious sedation and monitoring during gastrointestinal endoscopy. *Gastrointest Endosc,* 58, 317-22.

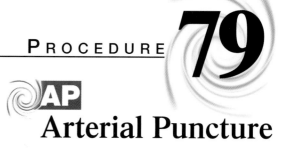

AP
Arterial Puncture

PURPOSE: Arterial puncture is performed to obtain a sample of blood for arterial blood gas (ABG) analysis.

Linda Bucher

SECTION ELEVEN
Vascular Access

PREREQUISITE NURSING KNOWLEDGE

• An arterial blood gas analysis measures the pH and the partial pressure of oxygen (PaO_2) and carbon dioxide ($PaCO_2$). ABG samples are also analyzed for oxygen saturation (SaO_2) and for bicarbonate (HCO_3^-) values. These analyses are done primarily to evaluate a patient's oxygenation status, acid-base balance, and ventilation.[1] Additional laboratory tests (e.g., ammonia and lactate levels) can be performed on arterial blood samples.

• Knowledge of principles of aseptic technique

• Knowledge of the anatomy and physiology of the vasculature and adjacent structures

• The brachial artery, a continuation of the axillary artery in the upper extremity, bifurcates just below the elbow (Fig. 79-1). From the bifurcation, the ulnar artery moves down the forearm on the medial side and the radial artery on the lateral side.[7]

• The preferred artery for arterial puncture is the radial artery. Although this artery is smaller than the ulnar artery, it is more superficial and can be more easily stabilized during the procedure.[7] Some research has found that the use of the brachial artery is a safe and reliable alternative site for arterial puncture.[16]

• At times, the femoral artery is used for arterial puncture. The use of this artery can be technically difficult because of the proximity of the artery to the femoral vein (Fig. 79-2).

• Patient indications for ABGs vary and include patients with chronic obstructive pulmonary disease (COPD), acute respiratory distress syndrome (ARDS), and pneumonia. ABG analysis frequently is performed on patients experiencing shock, cardiopulmonary resuscitation (CPR), and changes in respiratory therapy or status.[1]

• Arterial cannulation is considered for patients who require frequent arterial blood samples, continuous arterial pressure monitoring, or evaluation of vasoactive medication therapy (see Procedures 58 and 59).[17]

• The most common complications associated with arterial puncture include pain, vasospasm, hematoma formation, infection, hemorrhage, and neurovascular compromise.[1,6,16]

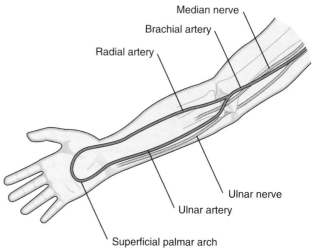

FIGURE 79-1 Anatomic landmarks for locating the radial and brachial arteries.

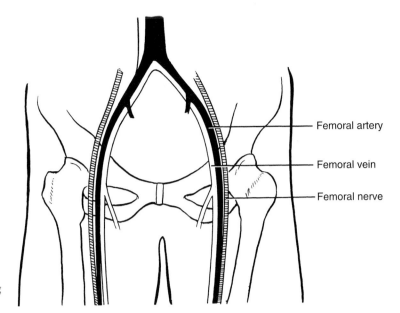

FIGURE 79-2 Anatomic landmarks for locating the femoral artery.

Femoral artery

Femoral vein

Femoral nerve

- Site selection proceeds as follows:
  - ❖ Use the radial artery as first choice. The radial artery is small and easily stabilized as it passes over a bony groove located at the wrist (see Fig. 79-1).
  - ❖ Use the brachial artery as second choice, except in the presence of poor pulsation due to shock, obesity, or sclerotic vessel (e.g., because of previous cardiac catheterization). The brachial artery is larger than the radial artery. Hemostasis after arterial puncture is enhanced by its proximity to bone if the entry point is approximately 1½ inches above the antecubital fossa (see Fig. 79-1).
  - ❖ Use the femoral artery in the case of cardiopulmonary arrest or altered perfusion to the upper extremities. The femoral artery is a large superficial artery located in the groin (see Fig. 79-2). It is easily palpated and punctured. Complications related to femoral artery puncture include hemorrhage and hematoma, because bleeding can be difficult to control; inadvertent puncture of the femoral vein, because of the close proximity of the vein to the artery; infection, because aseptic technique in the groin area is difficult to maintain; and limb ischemia if the femoral artery is damaged.

EQUIPMENT

- One prepackaged ABG kit that contains the following:
  - ❖ One 20- to 25-G, 1- to 1½-in-long hypodermic needle (Note: Longer needles are required for brachial and femoral artery puncture.)

  - ❖ One 1- to 5-ml preheparinized (if available) glass or plastic syringe with a rubber stopper or cap
  - ❖ One 1-ml ampule of sodium heparin, 1:1000 concentration (if preheparinized syringe is not available)
  - ❖ Two 2 × 2 gauze pads
  - ❖ 2% chlorhexidine-based antiseptic solution[2]
- One plastic bag (for transport of sample to laboratory)
- One adhesive bandage
- Appropriate laboratory form, specimen label
- One pair of nonsterile examination gloves and goggles
- 1% lidocaine (without epinephrine), 1 to 2 ml, or eutectic mixture of local anesthetics (EMLA) cream

  Additional supplies as needed include the following:
- Small rolled towel (to support patient's wrist)
- Sterile gloves
- Ice

PATIENT AND FAMILY EDUCATION

- Explain the reason for the arterial puncture to the patient and family. ➤*Rationale:* Clarification of information is an expressed patient and family need and helps to diminish anxiety, enhance acceptance, and encourage questions.
- Describe the overall steps of the procedure, including the patient's role in the procedure. ➤*Rationale:* Decreases patient anxiety, enhances cooperation, and provides an opportunity for the patient to voice concerns; prevents accidental movement during the procedure.

PATIENT ASSESSMENT AND PREPARATION

Patient Assessment

- Assess for factors that influence ABG measurements, including anxiety, endotracheal suctioning, nebulizer treatment, change in oxygen therapy, patient positioning, body temperature, metabolic rate, and respiratory rate. ➤➤*Rationale:* Stated conditions or therapies can alter blood gas analysis.

- Assess the patient's current anticoagulation therapy, known blood dyscrasias, and pertinent laboratory values (e.g., platelets, PTT, PT/INR) before the procedure. ➤➤*Rationale:* Anticoagulation therapy, blood dyscrasias, or alterations in coagulation studies could prolong hemostasis at the puncture site and increase risk for hematoma formation or hemorrhage.
- Assess the patient's allergy history (e.g., lidocaine, antiseptic solutions, tape). ➤➤*Rationale:* Decreases the risk for allergic reactions.
- Determine history of any surgeries (e.g., use of radial artery for coronary artery bypass surgery, fistulas, or shunts). ➤➤*Rationale:* Arterial puncture should be avoided in extremities affected by these conditions.
- Determine the need for arterial cannulation versus puncture. ➤➤*Rationale:* Repeated arterial punctures increase patient discomfort and the risk for complications.
- Ascertain the patient's nondominant hand, if able. ➤➤*Rationale:* A complication to the nondominant hand may have fewer consequences.

Patient Preparation

- Ensure that the patient and family understand preprocedural teaching. Answer questions as they arise and reinforce information as needed. ➤➤*Rationale:* Evaluates and reinforces understanding of previously taught information.
- If the patient is receiving oxygen, check that the current therapy has been underway for at least 20 minutes before

obtaining ABGs.[1,8,11,14,18] ➤➤*Rationale:* Achieves accurate laboratory results. This is most important in patients with an abnormal ventilation/perfusion ratio.[14]

- Position the patient appropriately. ➤➤*Rationale:* Enhances the accessibility to the insertion site and promotes patient comfort.
- Radial artery puncture: (1) Assist the patient to a semirecumbent position. ➤➤*Rationale:* Position of comfort decreases anxiety and may facilitate respiratory effort. (2) Elevate and hyperextend the wrist. A small, rolled towel may be placed under the wrist for support. ➤➤*Rationale:* Moves the artery closer to the skin surface making the artery easier to palpate. (3) Palpate for the presence of a strong radial pulse. ➤➤*Rationale:* Identification and localization of the pulse increases the chance of a successful arterial puncture.
- Brachial artery puncture: (1) Assist the patient to a semirecumbent position. ➤➤*Rationale:* Position of comfort decreases anxiety and may facilitate respiratory effort. (2) Elevate and hyperextend the patient's arm. A small pillow may be placed under the arm for support. ➤➤*Rationale:* Increases accessibility for puncture. (3) Rotate the patient's arm and palpate for the presence of a strong brachial pulse. ➤➤*Rationale:* Identification and localization of the pulse increases the chance of a successful arterial puncture.
- Femoral artery puncture: (1) Assist the patient to a supine, straight-leg position. ➤➤*Rationale:* Provides the best position for localizing the femoral artery pulse. (2) Palpate for the presence of a strong femoral pulse. ➤➤*Rationale:* Identification and localization of the pulse increases the chance of a successful arterial puncture.

Procedure for Arterial Puncture

Steps	Rationale	Special Considerations
1. Wash hands.	Reduces the transmission of microorganisms; standard precautions.	Ensure that hospital policy permits RNs to perform radial, brachial, and femoral arterial punctures.
2. If the radial artery is to be used, perform the modified Allen test prior to the puncture (Fig. 79-3). *(Level IV: Limited clinical studies to support recommendations.)*	The modified Allen test has been recommended before a radial artery puncture to assess the patency of the ulnar artery and an intact superficial palmar arch.[1,3,5,7,10,11,13,14,17]	
A. With the patient's hand held overhead, instruct the patient to open and close the hand several times.	Forces the blood from the hand.	If the patient is unconscious or unable to perform the procedure, clench the fist passively for the patient.
B. With the patient's fist clenched, apply direct pressure on the radial and ulnar arteries.	Obstructs the flow of blood to the hand.	
C. Instruct the patient to lower and open the hand.	Observe for pallor.	Perform passively if the patient is unconscious or unable to assist.
D. Release the pressure over the ulnar artery and observe	Return of color within 7 seconds indicates patency of the ulnar	If the test is *negative* or equivocal, the radial artery should not be

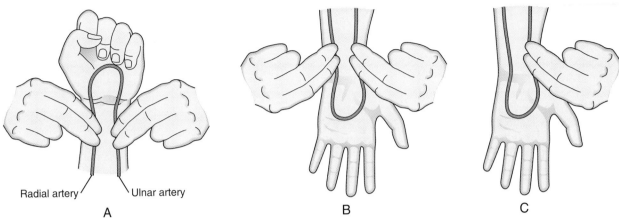

Radial artery   Ulnar artery

A   B   C

FIGURE 79-3 Modified Allen test. Elevate patient's hand and instruct the patient to open and close his or her fist several times. **A,** With patient's fist clenched, simultaneously occlude the radial and ulnar arteries. **B,** Instruct the patient to lower and open his or her fist. Observe for pallor in the patient's hand. **C,** Release the pressure over the ulnar artery and observe the hand for the return of color. *(From Bucher, L., Melander, S.D. [1999].* Critical Care Nursing. *Philadelphia: W.B. Saunders.)*

Procedure for Arterial Puncture—*Continued*

Steps	Rationale	Special Considerations
the hand for return of color.[1,3,11,13,14]	artery and an intact superficial palmar arch and is interpreted as a *positive* Allen test. If color returns between 8 to 14 seconds, the test is considered equivocal. If it takes 15 or more seconds for color to return, the test is considered a negative test.	used and the modified Allen test should be performed on the opposite hand.
3. If a preheparinized syringe is not available, heparinize the syringe and needle. A. Assemble a 22-G needle on the syringe and prime the entire syringe barrel and needle with 1 ml of heparin. Once done, expel the heparin from the syringe.	Prevents specimen coagulation. Excess heparin in the syringe can lower the pH and Pa_{CO_2}.	A small-bore needle is less likely to cause vasospasm of the artery during the procedure.
B. Eliminate any visible air bubbles from the syringe.	Maintains the accuracy of ABG values.	
4. Don goggles and nonsterile gloves.	Reduces the transmission of microorganisms and body secretions; standard precautions.	
5. Prepare the site using a 2% chlorhexidine-based antiseptic solution. Cleanse the site using a back and forth motion while applying friction for 30 seconds. Allow the antiseptic solution to dry.	Limits the introduction of potentially infectious skin flora into the vessel during the puncture.	

Procedure continues on the following page

Procedure **for Arterial Puncture**—*Continued*

Steps	Rationale	Special Considerations
6. Locally anesthetize the puncture site. *(Level IV: Limited clinical studies to support recommendations.)* A. Use a 1-ml syringe with a 25-G needle to draw up 0.5 ml of 1% lidocaine without epinephrine. B. Aspirate before injecting the local anesthetic. C. Inject intradermally and then with full infiltration around the artery puncture site. Use approximately 0.2 to 0.3 ml for an adult.	Provides local anesthesia for arterial puncture. Minimizes vessel trauma. Absence of epinephrine decreases the risk for peripheral vasoconstriction. Determines whether or not a blood vessel has been inadvertently entered. Decreases the incidence of localized pain while injecting all skin layers. Patients have reported reduced pain when a local, intradermal anesthetic agent is used prior to the arterial puncture.[6]	It has been reported that most patients experience pain during arterial puncture.[6] Research exploring the efficacy of lidocaine ointment, amethocaine gel, and EMLA cream as alternatives to intradermal lidocaine for managing the pain associated with arterial puncture has shown mixed results.[9,12,15,19] If these are used, the manufacturer's recommendations should be followed.
7. Perform the percutaneous puncture of the selected artery. A. Palpate and stabilize the artery with the index and middle fingers of the nondominant hand. B. With the needle bevel up and the syringe at a 30- to 60-degree angle to the radial or brachial artery, puncture the skin slowly (Figs. 79-4 and 79-5). For a femoral artery puncture, a 60- to 90-degree angle is used (Fig. 79-6). C. Observe the syringe for a flashback of blood. D. If the puncture is unsuccessful, withdraw the needle to the skin level, angle slightly toward the	Increases the likelihood of correctly locating the artery and decreases the chance of vessel rolling. A slow, gradual thrust will promote entry into the artery without inadvertently passing through the posterior wall. Pulsation of blood into the syringe verifies that the artery has been punctured. Prevents the necessity of a second puncture and changes the needle angle	Use sterile gloves if the site of artery puncture is palpated after it is antiseptically prepared. Enter at an angle that is comfortable for your hand. Certainty of position is more important than angle entry. If too much force is used, the needle may touch the periosteum of the bone and cause considerable pain. Flashback occurs more easily with a glass syringe than a plastic syringe. Gentle aspiration may be necessary with a plastic syringe. Excessive probing of the artery may cause injury to it, as well as to the nerve.

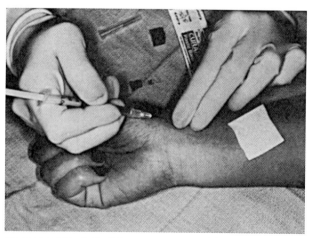

FIGURE 79-4 Radial cardiery puncture with the syringe at a 30-degree angle to the artery.

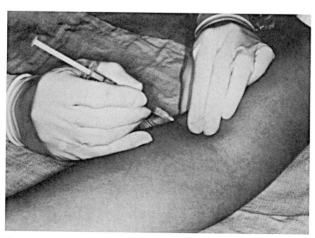

FIGURE 79-5 Brachial artery puncture with the syringe at a 45-degree angle to the artery.

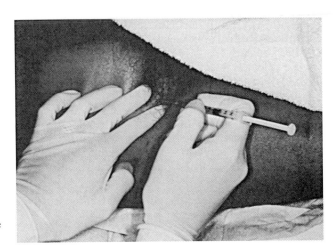

FIGURE 79-6 Femoral artery puncture with the syringe at a 60-degree angle to the artery.

Procedure for Arterial Puncture—*Continued*

Steps	Rationale	Special Considerations
artery, and readvance. Do not withdraw the needle.	to facilitate the location of the artery.	
8. Obtain 1 ml of blood.	Obtain more than 1 ml of blood for rechecking and additional studies, as necessary. An accurate ABG can be done on as little as 1 ml of blood.	Sample volumes may vary with equipment used.
9. Withdraw the needle while stabilizing the barrel of the syringe.	Prevents inadvertent aspiration of air during withdrawal.	Equipment may vary. Should a safety guard be available, it should be snapped onto the needle using a one-handed technique by gently pressing the device against a hard surface.
10. Press a gauze pad firmly over the puncture site for at least 5 minutes or until hemostasis is established.[1] Never ask the patient to assist in applying the pressure. Cover the puncture site with an adhesive bandage once hemostasis is achieved.[1,4]	Hematomas and hemorrhage can occur if pressure is not applied and maintained correctly. Hematomas can cause circulatory impedance and pain and can predispose to infection. The patient's status can be unpredictable, and he or she should not be involved in this aspect of the procedure. If the patient were to fail to apply and maintain pressure correctly, the risk for hematoma and hemorrhage would increase.	If the patient is receiving anticoagulation therapy or has a bleeding dyscrasia, pressure may need to be applied for as long as 15 minutes. If bleeding persists, an ice pack can be placed over the site while maintaining firm pressure.

Procedure continues on the following page

AP This procedure should be performed only by physicians, advanced practice nurses, and other health care professionals (including critical care nurses) with additional knowledge, skills, and demonstrated competence per professional licensure or institutional standard.

Procedure   for Arterial Puncture—*Continued*

Steps	Rationale	Special Considerations
11. Check the syringe for air bubbles and express any air bubbles by slowly ejecting some of the blood onto a 2 × 2 gauze pad.	Air bubbles can alter the Pao_2 results.	If a safety guard is present, it should be removed and a blood/air filter should be placed on the syringe. Excess air should be evacuated through the blood/air filter.
12. Seal the needle or tip of the syringe immediately using a rubber stopper or cap, respectively. Gently roll the syringe for 30 seconds.	Prevents leakage of blood and air from entering the sample. Mixes blood and heparin, thus preventing clot formation.	
13. Immerse the sample into a slurry of ice and water in a plastic bag and prepare to transport to the laboratory.[1,4,11,14]	Ice decreases the temperature of the sample to approximately 4°C. This slows oxygen metabolism and may enhance accuracy of the results.	Follow hospital policy regarding necessity of the use of ice for ABG samples.
14. Label the specimen and complete the laboratory form per institutional protocol. Note the percentage of oxygen therapy, respiratory rate, and ventilator settings, if appropriate, as well as the patient's temperature and time the specimen was drawn.	Helps the laboratory to perform the analysis accurately.	Policies may vary regarding the type of patient information required for laboratory analysis.
15. Expedite the delivery of the sample to the laboratory.	Ideally, the blood gas analysis should be performed within 10 minutes of collection to ensure the accuracy of results.[4,11,14]	
16. Dispose of used supplies properly and wash hands.	Reduces the transmission of microorganisms; standard precautions.	

Expected Outcomes

- The ABG sample is collected correctly such that the accuracy of the results is enhanced.
- The puncture site remains free of hematoma, hemorrhage, and infection.
- The peripheral vascular and neurovascular systems remain intact (free of complications).
- Alterations in the ABGs are identified and treated accordingly.

Unexpected Outcomes

- Pain/severe discomfort during the procedure
- Complications during the puncture or vasospasm
- Complications following the puncture: changes in the color, size, temperature, sensation, or pulse of the extremity used for the arterial puncture; hematoma, hemorrhage, or infection at the puncture site

Patient Monitoring and Care

Steps	Rationale	Reportable Conditions
		These conditions should be reported if they persist despite nursing interventions.
1. Observe the puncture site for signs of hemostasis postprocedure.	Postpuncture bleeding can occur in any patient but is more likely to occur in patients with coagulopathies or patients who are receiving anticoagulation therapy.	• Excessive bleeding • Hematoma • Changes in vital signs
2. Assess the puncture site and involved extremity for signs of postpuncture complications.	Arterial puncture can result in peripheral vascular and neurovascular compromise of	• Changes in color, size, temperature, sensation, movement, or pulse in the extremity used for arterial puncture

Patient Monitoring and Care—*Continued*

Steps	Rationale	Reportable Conditions
	the extremity distal to the puncture site.	
3. Monitor the puncture site for signs of local infection.	Infection related to the procedure may result from failure to maintain asepsis during puncture. Use of the femoral site for puncture may be related to increased incidence of local infection.	• Erythema, warmth, hardness, tenderness, or pain at the puncture site • Presence of purulent drainage from the puncture site

Documentation

Documentation should include the following:

- Patient and family education
- Results of the modified Allen test, if done
- Arterial site used
- Local anesthetic used (if applicable)
- Patient's tolerance of the procedure

- Patient's temperature and amount and type of oxygen therapy
- Postpuncture site assessment and care
- Sample results
- Unexpected outcomes
- Additional nursing interventions

References

1. Buffington, S. (1996). Specimen collection and testing. In: *Nursing Procedures.* 2nd ed. Springhouse, PA: Springhouse Corp, 145-7.
2. Centers for Disease Control and Prevention. (2002). Guidelines for the prevention of intravascular catheter-related infections. *MMWR, 51*(RR-10), 1-31.
3. Cummins, R.O., ed. (1997). *Advanced Cardiac Life Support.* Dallas, TX: American Heart Association.
4. Flynn, J.C. (1999). Special collection procedures. In: Flynn, J.C., ed. *Procedures in Phlebotomy.* 2nd ed. Philadelphia: W.B. Saunders, 124-5.
5. Fuhrman, T.M., Reilly, T.E., and Pippin, W.D. (1992). Comparison of digital blood pressure, plethysmography, and the modified Allen's test as a means of evaluating the collateral circulation to the hand. *Anaesthesia, 47,* 959-61.
6. Giner, J., et al. (1996). Pain during arterial puncture. *Chest,* 110, 1443-5.
7. Hadaway, L.C. (2001). Anatomy and physiology related to intravenous therapy. In: Hankins, J., et al., eds. *Infusion Therapy in Clinical Practice.* 2nd ed. Philadelphia: W.B. Saunders, 65-97.
8. Hess, D., et al. (1985). The validity of assessing arterial blood gases 10 minutes after an F_{IO_2} change in mechanically ventilated patients without chronic pulmonary disease. *Respir Care,* 30, 1037-41.
9. Hussey, V.M., Poulin, M.V., and Fain, J.A. (1997). Effectiveness of lidocaine hydrochloride on venipuncture sites. *AORN J,* 66, 472-5.
10. Intravenous Nurses Society. (2000). Infusion nursing standards of practice. *J Intraven Nurs,* 23, S1-S78.
11. Jacobs, D.S., Oxley, D.K., and DeMott, W.R. (2001). *Jacobs and DeMott Laboratory Test Handbook.* 5th ed. Hudson, OH: Lexi-Comp.
12. Lander, J., et al. (1996). Evaluation of a new topical anesthetic agent: A pilot study. *Nurs Res,* 45, 50-2.
13. Mark, J.B., Slaughter, T.F., and Reves, J.G. (2000). Cardiovascular monitoring. In: Miller, R.D., ed. *Anesthesia.* 5th ed. Philadelphia: Churchill Livingstone, 1125.
14. National Committee for Clinical Laboratory Standards. (1999). *Procedures for the Collection of Arterial Blood Specimens: Approved Standard H11-A3.* 3rd ed. Wayne, PA: NCCLS.
15. Nott, M., and Peacock, J. (1990). Relief of injection pain in adults: EMLA cream for 5 minutes before venipuncture. *Anaesthesia,* 45, 772-4.
16. Okeson, G.C., and Wulbrecht, P.H. (1998). The safety of brachial artery puncture for arterial blood sampling. *Chest,* 14, 748-51.
17. Perucca, R. (2001). Obtaining vascular access. In: Hankins, J., et al., eds. *Infusion Therapy in Clinical Practice.* 2nd ed. Philadelphia: W.B. Saunders, 375-88.
18. Sherter, C.B., et al. (1975). Prolonged rate of decay of arterial P_{O_2} following oxygen breathing in chronic airway obstruction. *Chest,* 67, 259.
19. Tran, N.Q., Pretto, J.J., and Worsnop, C.J. (2002). A randomized controlled trial of the effectiveness of topical amethocaine in reducing pain during arterial puncture. *Chest,* 122, 1357-60.

Additional Readings

Flynn, J.C. (1999). *Procedures in Phlebotomy.* 2nd ed. Philadelphia: W.B. Saunders.
Hankins, J., et al., eds. (2001). *Infusion Therapy in Clinical Practice.* 2nd ed. Philadelphia: W.B. Saunders.
Infusion Nurse Society. (2002). *Policies and Procedures for Infusion Nurses.* 2nd ed. Norwood, MA: Infusion Nurses Society.
Potter, P.A., and Perry, A.G., eds. (1999). *Basic Nursing: A Critical Thinking Approach.* 4th ed. St. Louis: Mosby.

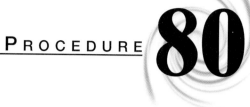

AP
Central Venous Catheter Insertion (Perform)

PURPOSE: Central venous catheters are inserted to measure and obtain right atrial pressure (RAP) and central venous pressure (CVP) with jugular or subclavian catheter placement. Clinically useful information can be obtained about right ventricular preload, cardiovascular status, and fluid balance in patients who do not require pulmonary artery pressure monitoring. Central venous catheters also are placed for infusion of vasoactive medications, total parenteral nutrition, and hemodialysis access.[3,6] In addition, central venous catheters are used to administer medication and intravenous (IV) products to patients with limited peripheral IV access, as well as to provide access for pulmonary artery catheters and transvenous pacemakers.

Desiree A. Fleck

PREREQUISITE NURSING KNOWLEDGE

- Knowledge of the normal anatomy and physiology of the cardiovascular system
- Clinical and technical competence in central line insertion and suturing[4]
- Understanding of principles of sterile technique
- Knowledge of the anatomy and physiology of the vasculature and adjacent structures of the neck, groin, and arm
- Competence in chest x-ray interpretation
- Advanced cardiac life support knowledge and skills
- Indications for a central venous catheter (CVC) include the following:[8]
  - ❖ Blood loss
  - ❖ Hypotension following major surgery
  - ❖ Right ventricular ischemia or infarction
  - ❖ Hemodialysis access
  - ❖ Administration of total parenteral nutrition
  - ❖ Lack of peripheral venous access

- ❖ Assessment of hypovolemia or hypervolemia
- ❖ Monitoring CVC pressures
- ❖ Long-term infusions of medications
- ❖ For the placement of pulmonary artery catheters
- ❖ Transvenous pacemakers[10]
- The CVP can be particularly helpful after major surgery and during active bleeding.
- The CVP can be helpful in differentiating right ventricular failure from left ventricular failure. The CVP is commonly elevated during or following right ventricular failure, ischemia, or infarction because of decreased compliance of the right ventricle while the pulmonary artery wedge pressure is normal.[3,6,10]
- The CVP can be helpful in determining hypovolemia. The CVP value is low if the patient is hypovolemic. Venodilation also decreases CVP.
- Relative contraindications of CVC insertion include the following:
  - ❖ Fever
  - ❖ Coagulopathies
  - ❖ Presence of a permanent pacemaker
  - ❖ Persistent shock
  - ❖ Obstruction of the superior or inferior vena cava, innominate vein, subclavian veins, or internal jugular veins
  - ❖ Respiratory distress

TABLE 80-1	Sites, Complications, and Success Rates[11]	
Access Site	**Complications[4,9]**	**Success Rates (%)**
Internal jugular vein	Carotid artery puncture Carotid artery cannulation	60-90
Right subclavian vein	Pneumothorax Tension pneumothorax Thoracic duct puncture Decreased success rate with inexperience	70-98
Left subclavian vein	Pneumothorax Tension pneumothorax Thoracic duct puncture Decreased success rate with inexperience	70-98

Femoral vein	Infection
	Arterial puncture
	Failure rate during
	  hypotension and shock
	Inability to thread central
	  catheters
		75-99

- The CVP provides information regarding right heart filling pressures and right ventricular function and volume.
- The CVP can be measured using a water manometer system (see Procedure 66) or via a hemodynamic monitoring system (see Procedures 66 and 75).
- The CVP waveform is identical to the right atrial pressure (RAP) waveform.
- The normal CVP value is *2 to 6* mm Hg.
- ECG monitoring is essential in determining accurate interpretation of the CVP value.
- Understanding of *a*, *c*, and *v* waves: the *a* wave reflects right atrial contraction; the *c* wave reflects closure of the tricuspid valve; and the *v* wave reflects right atrial filling during ventricular systole (see Figure 66-4 and 72-7).
- Dysrhythmias may alter CVP or RA pressure waveforms.
- Central venous access may be obtained in a variety of sites (Table 80-1).[9,11]
- The risk for a pneumothorax is minimized by using an internal jugular vein. The preferred site for catheter insertion is the right internal jugular vein. The right internal jugular vein is a "straight shot" to the right atrium.
- The right or left subclavian veins are also sites for central catheter placement. Placement of a central catheter through the right subclavian vein is a shorter and more direct route than the left subclavian vein, because it does not cross the midline of the thorax.[6]
- Femoral veins may be accessed but have the strong disadvantage of forcing the patient to be on bed rest with immobilization of that leg, and there is an increased risk for infection with placement in the groin.
- The presence of a pacemaker may alter choices in placement of CVP lines, because there is a risk for dislodging pacemaker leads when inserting CVP lines.

- Complications may occur during or after insertion of a central venous catheter (see Tables 80-1 and 81-1).

EQUIPMENT

- CVC insertion kit
- Teflon®-coated or antimicrobial/antiseptic impregnated catheter of choice[9] (single, dual, or triple lumen) usually supplied with insertion needle, dilator, syringe, and guidewire
- Large sterile drapes or towels
- 1% lidocaine without epinephrine
- One 25-G 5/8 needle
- Large package of 4 × 4 gauze sponges
- Suture kit (hemostat, scissors, needle holder)
- 3-0 or 4-0 nylon suture with curved needle
- Three-way stopcock
- Syringes: one 10- to 12-ml syringe, two 3- to 5-ml syringes, two 22-G, 11/2-in needles
- Masks, caps, goggles (shield and mask combination may be used), sterile gloves, and sterile gowns
- Number 11 scalpel
- Skin protectant pad or swabstick
- Roll of 2-inch tape
- Dressing supplies
- Moistureproof underpad
- Antiseptic solution (such as 2% chlorhexidine-based preparation)
- Nonsterile gloves
- 0.9% sodium chloride, 10-30 ml
  Additional equipment as needed includes the following:
- Hemodynamic monitoring system (see Procedure 75)
- IV solution with Luer-Lok administration set for IV infusion
- Luer-Lok extension tubing
- Bedside monitor and oscilloscope with pulse oximetry
- Supplemental oxygen supplies
- Emergency equipment
- Package of alcohol pads or swabsticks
- Package of povidone-iodine pads or swabsticks
- Heparin flushes
- Needleless caps
- Arm board

PATIENT AND FAMILY EDUCATION

- Explain the need for the CVC insertion and assess patient and family understanding of CVP. ➥*Rationale:* Clarification and understanding of information decreases patient and family anxiety levels.
- Explain the procedure and the time involved. ➥*Rationale:* Increases patient's cooperation and decreases patient and family anxiety levels.
- Explain the need for sterile technique and that the patient's face may be covered. ➥*Rationale:* Decreases patient anxiety and elicits cooperation.
- Explain the benefits and potential risks for the procedure. ➥*Rationale:* Offers information so that the patient can make an informed decision.

PATIENT ASSESSMENT AND PREPARATION

Patient Assessment

- Determine the patient's past medical history of pneumothorax/emphysema. ➻*Rationale:* Emphysematous lungs may be at increased risk for puncture and pneumothorax, depending on the approach.
- Determine the patient's past medical history of anomalous veins. ➻*Rationale:* Patients may have a history of dextracardia or transposition of the great vessels, leading to greater difficulty in placing the catheter.
- Assess the intended insertion site. ➻*Rationale:* Scar tissue may impede placement of the catheter. Permanent pacemakers or implantable cardioverter defibrillators may preclude placement. Previous surgery and previous placement of a CVC may cause a thrombus to be present.
- Assess the patient's cardiac and pulmonary status. ➻*Rationale:* Some patients may not tolerate a supine or Trendelenburg position for extended periods of time.
- Assess vital signs and pulse oximetry. ➻*Rationale:* Provides baseline data.
- Assess electrolyte levels. ➻*Rationale:* Electrolyte abnormalities may increase cardiac irritability.
- Assess the patient for heparin sensitivity or allergy.[4] ➻*Rationale:* Central venous catheters may be heparin-bonded, although nonheparin-bonded catheters are available. If the patient has a heparin allergy or has a history of heparin-induced thrombocytopenia, use a nonheparin-coated catheter.
- Assess coagulopathic status or whether the patient has recently received anticoagulant or thrombolytic therapy. ➻*Rationale:* These patients are more likely to have complications related to bleeding.

Patient Preparation

- Ensure that the patient and family understand preprocedural teaching. Answer questions as they arise and reinforce information as needed. ➻*Rationale:* Evaluates and reinforces understanding of previously taught information.
- Obtain informed consent. ➻*Rationale:* Protects the rights of the patient and makes a competent decision possible for the patient; however, under emergency circumstances, time may not allow for this form to be signed.
- Prescribe sedation if needed. ➻*Rationale:* The patient may need sedation to ensure adequate cooperation and appropriate placement. During the procedure, restlessness and an altered level of consciousness may represent a pneumothorax, hypoxia, or placement in the carotid artery.
- Place the patient in a supine position and prep the area with an antiseptic solution (e.g., 2% chlorhexidine-based solution)[9] (see Fig. 81-1). ➻*Rationale:* Prepares the access sites for central venous catheter insertion. Decreases the risk for infection.
- If the patient is obese or muscular and the preferred site is the internal jugular vein or subclavian vein, place a towel posteriorly between the shoulder blades. ➻*Rationale:* Helps extend the neck and provide better access to the subclavian and internal jugular veins.
- Place sterile drapes over the prepped area. ➻*Rationale:* Provides an aseptic work area.

Procedure for Performing Central Venous Catheter Insertion

Steps	Rationale	Special Considerations
1. Determine the anatomy of the access site.	Helps ensure proper placement of the catheter.	Catheter placement on the right side is preferred to avoid cannulation of the thoracic duct.
2. Wash hands and don caps, masks, sterile gowns, goggles or face shields, and gloves for all health care personnel involved with the procedure.	Reduces the transmission of microorganisms and body secretions. Prepares for sterile technique.	
3. Check landmarks again for the intended catheter insertion site.	Ensures proper placement of the catheter.	
4. Estimate the length of the catheter needed. This can be done by holding the catheter from the insertion site to the sternal notch.	Helps ensure proper placement.	
Internal Jugular Vein (Fig. 80-1)		
1. Locate the carotid artery by palpation.	Helps prevent placing the introducer in the carotid artery.	
2. Identify the jugular vein and mark it if necessary.	Identifies the intended insertion site.	

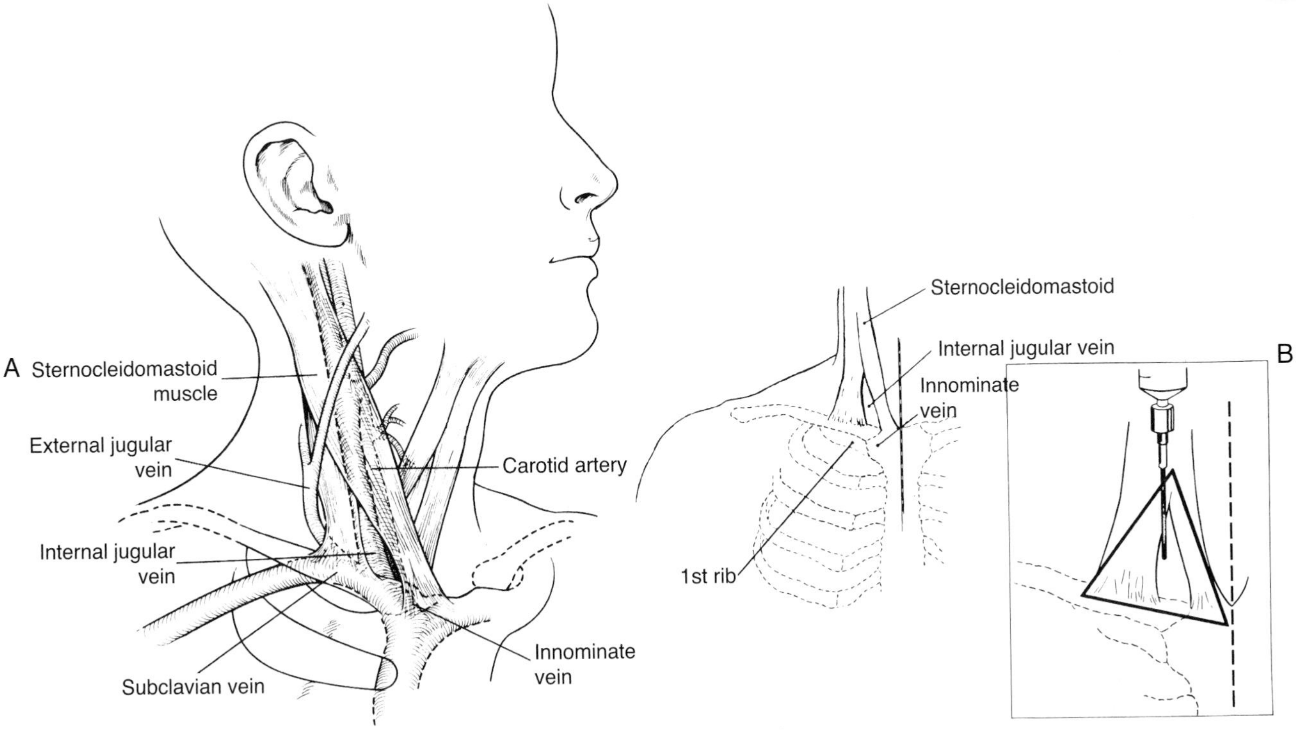

FIGURE 80-1 Anatomy of the jugular vein. **A,** Anatomy of the internal jugular vein showing its lower location within the triangle formed by the sternocleidomastoid muscle and the clavicle. **B,** Triangle drawn over clavicle and sternal and clavicular portions of the sternocleidomastoid muscle is centered over internal jugular vein (*inset*). (*From Dailey, E.K., and Schroeder, J.S. [1994]. Techniques in bedside hemodynamic monitoring. St. Louis: Mosby; and Daily, P.O., Griepp, R.B., and Shumway, N.E. [1970]. Percutaneous internal jugular vein cannulation. Arch Surg, 101, 534-6. Copyright 1970, American Medical Association.*)

Procedure for Performing Central Venous Catheter Insertion—*Continued*

Steps	Rationale	Special Considerations
3. Instruct the patient to turn his or her head away from the insertion site.	Helps identify the landmarks.	Turn the patient's head if the patient is unable to.
4. Place the patient in a 15- to 25-degree Trendelenburg position.	Helps to decrease the risk for air embolism. Helps engorge the veins to help identify the correct site.	
5. Identify the internal jugular vein from the triangle between the medial aspect of the clavicle, the medial aspect of the sternal head, and the lateral head of the sternocleidomastoid muscle (see Fig. 80-1).	A high entry can be made from a posterior approach, a lateral approach, an anterior approach, or a central approach.	The midanterior approach may be preferred in an obese patient. The posterior approach may present a slightly higher risk.

Procedure continues on the following page

Procedure for **Performing Central Venous Catheter Insertion**—*Continued*

Steps	Rationale	Special Considerations
6. Administer a local anesthetic and locate the internal jugular vein with a small needle 3 to 4 cm above the medial clavicle and 1 to 2 cm within the lateral border of the sternocleidomastoid muscle.	Provides patient comfort and aids in insertion.	
7. Attach a 3- or 5-ml syringe with 2 or 3 ml of 1% lidocaine (without epinephrine) to the 18-G needle. Align the needle with the syringe parallel to the medial border of the clavicular head of the sternocleidomastoid muscle. Aim at a 30-degree angle to the frontal plane over the internal jugular vein, toward the ipsilateral nipple.	Helps to anesthetize below the subcutaneous tissue. If the needle bevel is directed medially, the bevel aids in directing the guidewire medially.	
8. Use the Seldinger technique for placement of the catheter (Fig. 80-2).	This technique is the preferred method of central venous catheter placement. This technique uses a dilator and guidewire.	

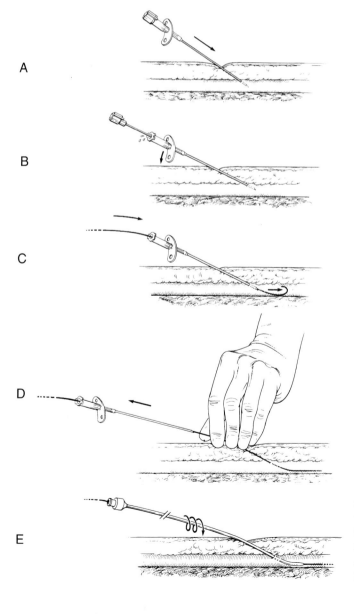

A

B

C

D

E

FIGURE 80-2 Basic procedure for Seldinger technique. **A,** The vessel is punctured with the needle at a 30- to 40-degree angle. **B,** The stylet is removed, and free blood flow is observed; the angle of the needle is then reduced. **C,** The flexible tip of the guidewire is passed through the needle into the vessel. **D,** The needle is removed over the wire while firm pressure is applied at the site. **E,** The tip of the catheter or sheath is passed over the wire and advanced into the vessel with a rotating motion. *(From Dailey, E.K., and Schroeder, J.S. [1994]. Techniques in Bedside Hemodynamic Monitoring. St. Louis: Mosby.)*

Procedure for Performing Central Venous Catheter Insertion—*Continued*

Steps	Rationale	Special Considerations
9. Puncture the skin and advance the needle while maintaining slight negative pressure until a free flow of blood is obtained.	Slight negative pressure helps to ensure placement into the vein and decreases the risk for air embolism and pneumothorax.	If a free flow of blood is not obtained, remove and redirect the needle 5 to 10 degrees more laterally.
10. After a free flow of blood is obtained, have the patient hold his or her breath or hum while the syringe is detached and insert the soft-tipped guidewire 10 to 15 cm through the needle. Remove the needle, wipe the guidewire with the sterile 4 × 4 gauze, and instruct the patient to breathe normally.	A free flow of blood indicates the needle is in the vessel. Holding the breath or humming decreases the risk for air embolus. Wiping the guidewire dry eases manipulation.	
11. With a number 11 blade, knife edge up, make a small (2- to 3-mm) stab wound at the insertion site.	Eases the insertion of the dilator through the skin.	
12. Insert the dilator through the skin, over the guidewire, until 10 to 15 cm of wire extends beyond the dilator. Remove the dilator.	The dilator enlarges the vessel and skin opening, easing the insertion of the catheter.	
13. Insert the catheter over the guidewire until 10 to 15 cm of wire extends beyond the catheter. Remove the guidewire. Advance the catheter. Note the catheter length at the insertion site.	Helps identify the location.	
14. Aspirate and flush the ports with normal saline.	Prevents clotting of the catheter.	
15. Connect to the hemodynamic monitoring system (see Procedure 75) or intravenous fluid.	Necessary for pressure monitoring and maintaining catheter patency.	
16. Suture the catheter in place.	Secures the catheter.	Some institutions use stat locks or a sutureless mechanism for securing the catheter.
17. Apply an occlusive, sterile dressing.	Decreases the risk for infection.	May be gauze or transparent semipermeable dressing.
18. Return the patient to a neutral or head-up position.	Provides comfort.	
19. If monitoring, identify the appropriate waveforms (see Procedure 66).	Ensures accurate monitoring of values.[1,2]	
20. Assess lung sounds and obtain a chest x-ray.	Confirms placement and assesses for pneumothorax.	The x-ray needs to be read before administration of total parenteral nutrition or chemotherapeutic agents.
21. Discard supplies and wash hands.	Decreases the risk for transmission of microorganisms, standard precautions.	

Procedure continues on the following page

Procedure for Performing Central Venous Catheter Insertion—*Continued*

Steps	Rationale	Special Considerations
Subclavian Vein (Fig. 80-3)		
1. Identify the junction of the middle and medial thirds of the clavicle. The needle insertion should be 1 to 2 cm laterally.	Identifies landmarks for catheter placement.	Access from the right side is preferred to avoid inadvertent puncture of the thoracic duct.
2. Depress the area 1 to 2 cm beneath the junction with the thumb of the nondominant hand and the index finger 2 cm above the sternal notch.		To avoid the subclavian artery, select a puncture site away from the most lateral course of the vein and do not aim too posteriorly.
3. Administer a local anesthetic and locate the vein with a 21- to 25-G needle directed to the index finger at a 20- to 30-degree angle.	Provides patient comfort and assists patient cooperation and ease of insertion. Extends the vein to ease the location.	
4. Instruct the patient to turn his or her head away from the insertion site.	Helps identify the landmarks.	Turn the patient's head if he or she is unable to.
5. Place the patient in a 15- to 25-degree Trendelenburg position.	Helps to decrease the risk for air embolism. Helps engorge the veins to help identify the correct site.	
6. Insert the needle under the clavicle and "walk down" until it slips below the clavicle into the vein while maintaining negative pressure within the syringe until free-flowing blood is returned (Fig. 80-4).	Decreases the risk for pneumothorax. Slight negative pressure helps to ensure placement into the vein and decreases the risk for air embolism and pneumothorax.	Insert at a 45-degree angle to prevent pneumothorax. If it is difficult to depress the needle down, the needle may be bent to form an arc. For the elderly: the subclavian vein may be more inferior. Avoiding a too lateral or too deep a needle insertion can reduce the risk for pneumothorax.

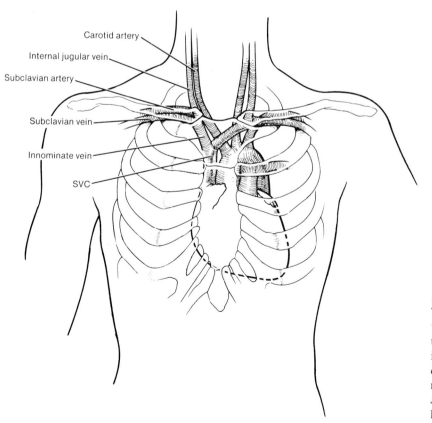

Carotid artery
Internal jugular vein
Subclavian artery
Subclavian vein
Innominate vein
SVC

FIGURE 80-3 Anatomic location of the subclavian vein and surrounding structures. The subclavian vein joins the internal jugular vein to become the innominate vein at about the manubrioclavicular junction. The innominate vein becomes the superior vena cava (SVC) at about the level of the midmanubrium. *(From Dailey, E.K., and Schroeder, J.S. [1994]. Techniques in Bedside Hemodynamic Monitoring. St. Louis: Mosby.)*

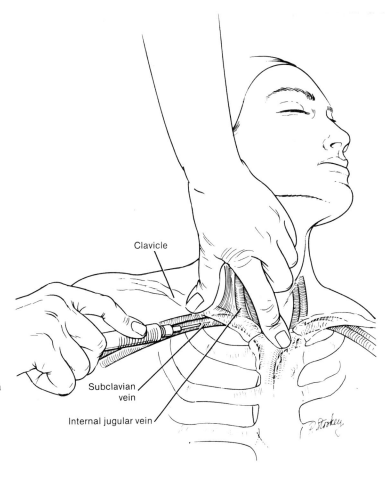

FIGURE 80-4 Puncture of the subclavian vein with the needle inserted beneath the middle third of the clavicle at a 20- to 30-degree angle aiming medially. *(From Dailey, E.K., and Schroeder, J.S. [1994]. Techniques in Bedside Hemodynamic Monitoring. St. Louis: Mosby.)*

Labels: Clavicle; Subclavian vein; Internal jugular vein

Procedure for Performing Central Venous Catheter Insertion—*Continued*

Steps	Rationale	Special Considerations
7. When a free flow of blood is returned, turn the bevel to the 3 o'clock position. Once in the vein, remove the syringe and insert the flexible guidewire after asking the patient to hum or hold his or her breath.	A free flow of blood indicates a vein is entered. Turning the bevel helps the guidewire advance to the correct position. Holding the breath or humming decreases the risk for air embolus.	
8. Insert the guidewire 10 to 15 cm through the needle. Remove the needle and wipe the guidewire with a sterile 4 × 4 gauze.	Wiping the guidewire eases the manipulation of the guidewire.	If the guidewire insertion is not smooth, it may be in the internal jugular vein.
9. Advance the dilator over the guidewire into the vein, using a light twisting motion.	This aids dilation of the subcutaneous tissue to ease insertion and prevents the formation of a false channel.	
10. Remove the dilator from the wire.		
11. Insert the catheter of choice over the guidewire; then remove the guidewire.		

Procedure continues on the following page

Procedure for Performing Central Venous Catheter Insertion—*Continued*

Steps	Rationale	Special Considerations
12. Aspirate and flush the ports with normal saline.	Ensures blood return and maintains catheter patency.	
13. Suture the line in place.	Secures the catheter.	
14. Connect the catheter to the hemodynamic monitoring system (see Procedure 75) or to intravenous fluid.	Necessary for pressure monitoring and catheter patency.	
15. Apply an occlusive, sterile dressing to the site.	Decreases the risk for infection.	
16. If monitoring, identify appropriate waveforms (see Procedure 66).	Ensures accurate monitoring of values.[1,2]	
17. Assess lung sounds and obtain a chest x-ray.	Confirms placement and assesses for pneumothorax.[7]	The x-ray must be read before administration of total parenteral nutrition or chemotherapeutic agents.
18. Discard supplies and wash hands.	Decreases the risk for transmission of microorganisms; standard precautions.	
Femoral Vein (see Fig. 79-2)		
1. Identify the anatomy, including the femoral artery (remember "NAVEL").	NAVEL is an acronym for remembering the anatomy (*N*erve, *A*rtery, *V*ein, *E*mpty space, *L*igament; from lateral to medial).	
2. Administer a local anesthetic and locate the vein with a 21- to 25-G needle lateral to the femoral artery. Aim the needle at a 20- to 30-degree angle.	Anesthetizes the area to provide patient comfort.	
3. Attach a 3- or 5-ml syringe with 2 or 3 ml 1% lidocaine without epinephrine to the 18-G needle.	Anesthetizes the area to provide patient comfort.	
4. Use the Seldinger technique for placement of the catheter (see Fig. 80-2).	This technique is the preferred method of central venous catheter placement. This technique uses a dilator and guidewire.	
5. Puncture the skin and advance the needle while maintaining slight negative pressure until a free flow of blood is obtained.	Negative pressure helps to identify a free flow of blood and ensures proper placement into the vein.	If a free flow of blood is not obtained, remove and redirect the needle 5 to 10 degrees more laterally.
6. After a free flow of blood is obtained, detach the syringe and insert a soft-tipped guidewire through the needle 10 to 15 cm. Remove the needle and wipe the guidewire with a sterile 4 × 4 gauze.	A free flow of blood indicates that the vessel has been accessed. Wiping the guidewire eases the manipulation of the guidewire.	
7. With a number 11 blade, knife edge up, make a small (2- to 3-mm) stab wound at the insertion site.	Eases insertion of the introducer through the skin.	
8. Insert the dilator over the guidewire until 10 to 15 cm of wire extends beyond the sheath. Advance the dilator through the skin.	The dilator dilates the vessel and skin to assist in the ease of the catheter insertion.	

Procedure for Performing Central Venous Catheter Insertion—*Continued*

Steps	Rationale	Special Considerations
9. Remove the dilator.		
10. Insert the catheter of choice over the guidewire and into the vein; then remove the guidewire.		
11. Aspirate and flush the ports with normal saline.	Ensures blood return and maintains catheter patency.	
12. Suture the catheter in place.	Secures the catheter.	Some institutions use sutureless systems.
13. Connect to the hemodynamic monitoring system (see Procedure 75) or to intravenous fluid.	Necessary for pressure monitoring and catheter patency.	
14. Apply an occlusive, sterile dressing.	Decreases the risk for infection.	May be gauze or transparent, semipermeable sterile dressing.
15. Identify the appropriate waveforms (see Procedure 66).	Ensures the accurate monitoring of values.[1,2]	
16. Discard supplies and wash hands.	Decreases the risk for transmission of microorganisms, standard precautions.	
Arm Vein (Fig. 80-5)		
1. Identify the median basilic vein.	Identifies the site for catheter placement.	The basilic vein is deeper and ascends along the ulnar surface of the forearm, joined by the median cubital vein in front of the elbow.
2. Further patient preparation includes applying a tourniquet to locate the vein. Abduct the selected arm 30 to 45 degrees and secure it on a flat, paddedarm board resting on a flat surface.	Aids preparation and allows for engorgement of the vessel.	
3. Use the Seldinger technique for placement of the catheter (see Fig. 80-2).	This technique is the preferred method of central venous catheter placement. This technique uses a dilator and guidewire.	
4. Apply a venous tourniquet to the upper arm. Maintain traction on the skin distal to the insertion with one hand; puncture the vein with the needle bevel up at a 15- to 20-degree angle.	Allows for better visualization of veins. Helps with insertion and prevents the needle from penetrating too deeply.	Do not attempt to place a central venous catheter in a vein that cannot be seen or palpated.
5. When blood appears in the needle, insert the guidewire into the vein approximately 2 to 4 cm beyond the tip.	Ensures appropriate placement of the catheter.	If resistance is met, do not force the catheter to advance. Withdraw the catheter 2 to 3 cm, rotate it, and readvance it.

Procedure continues on the following page

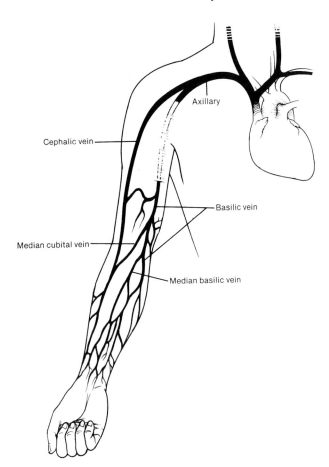

Cephalic vein

Axillary

Basilic vein

Median cubital vein

Median basilic vein

FIGURE 80-5 Anatomy of the arm veins. *(From Dailey, E.K., and Schroeder, J.S. [1994]. Techniques in Bedside Hemodynamic Monitoring. St. Louis: Mosby.)*

Procedure **for Performing Central Venous Catheter Insertion**—*Continued*

Steps	Rationale	Special Considerations
6. Release the tourniquet and advance the guidewire several centimeters. Remove the needle; wipe the guidewire with a sterile 4 × 4 gauze.	Eases manipulation of the guidewire.	
7. Insert the catheter of choice over the guidewire. Remove the guidewire. Note the centimeter marking at the skin.		
8. Aspirate and flush the ports with normal saline.	Maintains line patency.	
9. Suture in place.	Secures the line.	
10. Connect to intravenous fluid.	Maintains line patency.	
11. Apply an occlusive, sterile dressing to the insertion site.	Reduces the incidence of infection.	
12. Immobilize on an arm board.	Ensures that minimal movement of the catheter and sheath occurs.	
13. Discard supplies and wash hands.	Reduces the transmission of microorganisms; standard precautions.	

Expected Outcomes	Unexpected Outcomes
• Successful placement of the central venous catheter • If infusing IV solution, the solution infuses without problems • The *a, c,* and *v* waves identified if hemodynamic monitoring • CVP measurement determined	• Pain or discomfort during the insertion procedure • Pneumothorax, tension pneumothorax, hemothorax, or chylothorax • Nerve injury • Sterile thrombophlebitis • Infection • Cardiac dysrhythmias • Misplacement (e.g., carotid artery, subclavian artery) • Inadvertent lymphatic or thoracic duct perforation • Hemorrhage • Hematoma • Venous air embolism • Pulmonary embolus • Cardiac tamponade • Sepsis • Heparin-induced thrombocytopenia or thrombosis

Patient Monitoring and Care

Steps	Rationale	Reportable Conditions
		These conditions should be reported if they persist despite nursing interventions. • Change in level of consciousness • Changes in vital signs • Abnormal waveforms or pressures

1. Perform cardiovascular, peripheral vascular, and hemodynamic assessments immediately before and after the procedure and as the patient's condition necessitates. This includes:
  A. Level of consciousness
  B. Vital signs, central venous waveform, central venous pressure
	Assess for signs of adequate perfusion; air embolism may present with restlessness; patient may present with decreased level of consciousness if the catheter is advanced into the carotid artery.
	Changes in pressures may indicate change in volume status.
	Changes in the waveform may indicate change in right ventricular function or catheter migration.	

2. Monitor the site for hematoma and hemorrhage.	If the patient is coagulopathic, a pressure dressing may be required.	• Bleeding that does not stop • Hematoma and/or expanding hematoma
3. Assess heart and lung sounds before and after the procedure.	Abnormal heart or lung sounds may indicate cardiac tamponade, pneumothorax, chylothorax, or hemothorax.	• Diminished or muffled heart sounds • Absent or diminished breath sounds unilaterally
4. Assess results of chest x-ray.	Ensures adequate placement and identification of pneumothorax, if present.[7]	• Abnormal x-ray results
5. Monitor for signs of complications.	May decrease mortality and morbidity if recognized early.	• Signs and symptoms of complications
6. Follow institution guidelines for changing CVC.	CVCs are changed according to CDC guidelines when an infection is suspected or the CVC is placed in the femoral vein or is placed emergently.[5,9]	• Signs or symptoms of catheter infection.

Documentation

Documentation should include the following:

- Patient and family education
- Signature on informed consent form
- Insertion of central venous catheter
- Insertion site of central venous catheter
- Vein selected and type and size of catheter placed
- Right atrial pressure and CVP waveform

- Central venous pressure values after insertion
- Centimeter marking at the skin
- Patient response to the procedure
- Confirmation of placement (e.g., chest x-ray)
- Occurrence of unexpected outcomes
- Additional nursing interventions

References

1. Ahrens, T.S., and Taylor, L.K. (1992). *Hemodynamic Waveform Analysis.* Philadelphia: W.B. Saunders.
2. Ahrens, T.S. (1999). Hemodynamic monitoring. *Crit Care Nurs Clin NA,* 11, 19-31.
3. Dailey, E.K., and Schroeder, J.S. (1994). *Techniques in Bedside Hemodynamic Monitoring.* 5th ed. St. Louis: Mosby.
4. Davis, D., et al. (1999). Impact of a formal continuing medical education: do conferences, workshops, rounds and other traditional continuing education activities change physician behavior or health care outcomes? *JAMA,* 282, 867-74.
5. Eggimann, P., et al. (2000). Impact of a prevention strategy targeted at vascular-access care on incidence of infections acquired in intensive care. *Lancet,* 355, 1864-8.
6. Hurford, W.E., and Zapol, W.M. (1988). The right ventricle and critical illness: A review of anatomy, physiology, and clinical evaluation of its function. *Intensive Care Med,* 14, 448-57.
7. Koplef, M.H. (1994). Fallibility of persistent blood return for confirmation of intravascular catheter placement in patients with hemorrhagic thoracic effusion. *Chest,* 106, 1906-8.
8. Kumar, A., and Darovic, G.O. (2000). Establishment of cardiovascular access. In: *Hemodynamic Monitoring Invasive and Noninvasive Clinical Application.* Philadelphia: W.B. Saunders.
9. O'Grady, N.P., et al. (2002). Guidelines for the prevention of intravascular catheter-related infections. *Am J Infect Control,* 30, 476-89.
10. Sibbald, W.J., and Driedger, A.A. (1983). Right ventricular function in acute disease states: Pathophysiologic consideration. *Crit Care Med,* 11, 339-45.
11. Silver, D., Kapsch, D.N., and Tsoi, E.K. (1983). Heparin-induced thrombocytopenia, thrombosis, and hemorrhage. *Ann Surg,* 198, 301-6.

Additional Readings

American Association of Critical Care Nurses. (1993). Evaluation of the effects of heparinized and nonheparinized flush solutions on the patency of arterial pressure monitoring lines: The AACN Thunder Project. *Am J Crit Care,* 2, 3-15.
Darovic, G.O. (2000). *Hemodynamic Monitoring Invasive and Noninvasive Clinical Application.* Philadelphia: W.B. Saunders.
Friesinger, G.C., Williams, S.V., and the ACP/AHA Task Force on Clinical Privileges in Cardiology. (1990). Clinical competence in hemodynamic monitoring. *J Am Coll Cardiol,* 15, 1460.
Hilton, E. (1988). Central catheter infections: Single- versus triple-lumen catheters. *Am J Med,* 84, 667-72.
Marion, P.L. (1991). *The ICU Book.* Philadelphia: Lea & Febiger.
Parsa, M.H., Parsa, C.J., and Sampath, A.C. Intravenous and intra-arterial access. In: *Textbook of Critical Care,* 4th ed. Philadelphia: W.B. Saunders.
Parsa, M.H., Tabora, F., and Al Sawwaf, M. (1989). Vascular access techniques. In: *Textbook of Critical Care,* 2nd ed. Philadelphia: W.B. Saunders.
Roberts, J.R., and Hedges, J.R. (2004). *Clinical Procedures In Emergency Medicine.* 4th ed. Philadelphia: W.B. Saunders.
Venus, B., and Mallory, D.L. (1992). Vascular cannulation. In: *Critical Care.* 2nd ed. Philadelphia: J.B. Lippincott.

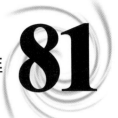

PROCEDURE **81**

Central Venous Catheter Insertion (Assist)

P U R P O S E :   Central venous catheters are inserted to measure and obtain right atrial pressure (RAP) and central venous pressure (CVP) with jugular or subclavian catheter placement. Clinically useful information can be obtained about right ventricular preload, cardiovascular status, and fluid balance in patients who do not require pulmonary artery pressure monitoring. Central venous catheters also are placed for infusion of vasoactive medications, total parenteral nutrition, and hemodialysis access.[1,3] In addition, central venous catheters are used to administer medication and intravenous (IV) products to patients with limited peripheral IV access.

Nancy Munro

PREREQUISITE NURSING KNOWLEDGE

- Knowledge of the normal anatomy and physiology of the cardiovascular system
- Knowledge of the anatomy and physiology of the vasculature and adjacent structures of the neck and groin
- Understanding of basic dysrhythmia interpretation
- Advanced cardiac life support knowledge and skills
- Indications for a central venous catheter include the following:[2]
  - ❖ Blood loss
  - ❖ Hypotension
  - ❖ Hemodialysis access
  - ❖ Administration of total parenteral nutrition or other hyperosmolar solutions
  - ❖ Lack of peripheral venous access
  - ❖ Assessment of hypovolemia or hypervolemia
  - ❖ Right ventricular ischemia or infarction
  - ❖ Monitoring CVC pressures
  - ❖ Long-term infusion of medications
  - ❖ Placement of pulmonary artery catheters
  - ❖ Placement of transvenous pacemakers[10]
- Relative contraindications of CVP line insertion include the following:
  - ❖ Fever
  - ❖ Coagulopathies
  - ❖ Presence of a pacemaker

- ❖ Shock
- ❖ Respiratory distress
- ❖ Vein obstructions
- Site selection is based on the vasculature of the patient. The most common sites include the internal jugular veins, subclavian veins, and the femoral veins.[1,5]
- The type of catheter inserted and purpose of insertion should be considered. Catheters may be single lumen or multiple lumen. Central venous catheters may be inserted for monitoring, infusion of medications, or parenteral nutrition.
- Principles of aseptic technique should be understood. Prevention of infection is a significant concern for patients with indwelling catheters.
- CVP can be measured using a water manometer system (see Procedure 66) or via a hemodynamic monitoring system (see Procedure 75).
- The CVP provides information regarding right heart filling pressures and volume.
- The normal CVP value is 2 to 6 mm Hg.
- ECG monitoring is essential in determining an accurate interpretation of the CVP.
- Understanding of *a, c,* and *v* waves: the *a* wave reflects right atrial contraction; the *c* wave reflects closure of the tricuspid valve; the *v* wave reflects right atrial filling during ventricular systole (see Fig. 66-4).
- Dysrhythmias may alter CVP or RAP waveforms.
- Complications may occur during or after insertion of a central venous catheter (Table 81-1).

TABLE 81-1	**Complications of Central Venous Catheter Insertion**		
Complication	**Clinical Manifestation**	**Treatment**	**Prevention**
Pneumothorax	Sudden respiratory distress Chest pain Hypoxia/cyanosis Decreased breath sounds Resonance to percussion	Confirmation by chest x-ray Symptomatic treatment Small pneumothorax: Bed rest O$_2$ Pneumothorax greater than 25%: Chest tube Cardiopulmonary support	Proper patient preparation Sedation as necessary Proper patient positioning Adequate hydration status Technique and angle of the needle/ catheter on insertion Avoid multiple passes with the needle Clinician skilled and experienced in insertion technique
Tension pneumothorax	Most likely to occur in patients on ventilatory support Respiratory distress Rapid clinical deterioration: Cyanosis Jugular venous distension (may not be present with severe hypovolemia) Hypotension Decreased cardiac output	Treatment must be rapid and aggressive *Immediate* air aspiration followed by chest tube Cardiopulmonary support	Proper patient preparation Sedation as necessary Proper patient positioning Adequate hydration status Reduction of PEEP to less than or equal to 5 cm H$_2$O at the time of venipuncture Technique and angle of the needle/ catheter on insertion Avoid multiple passes with the needle Clinician skilled and experienced in insertion technique Use of peripherally inserted central venous catheter
Delayed pneumothorax	Slow onset of respiratory symptoms Subcutaneous emphysema Persistent pleuritic chest or back pain	Confirmation by chest x-ray Chest tube Cardiopulmonary support	Proper patient preparation Sedation as necessary Proper patient positioning Adequate hydration status Technique and angle of the needle/ catheter on insertion Avoid multiple passes with the needle Clinician skilled and experienced in insertion technique Use of peripherally inserted central venous catheter
Hydrothorax hydromediastinum	Dyspnea Chest pain Muffled breath sounds High glucose level of chest drainage Low-grade fever	Stop infusion Confirmation by chest x-ray; contrast injection may be helpful Cardiopulmonary support	Proper patient preparation Sedation as necessary Proper patient positioning Adequate hydration status Technique and angle of the needle/ catheter on insertion Avoid multiple passes with the needle Clinician skilled and experienced in insertion technique Use of peripherally inserted central venous catheter Placement of catheter tip in lower superior vena cava Aspiration of blood prior to catheter use to confirm vascular placement
Hemothorax	Respiratory distress Hypovolemic shock Hematoma in the neck with jugular insertions	Confirmation by chest x-ray Chest tube Thoracotomy for arterial repair if indicated	Correct coagulopathies before insertion Adequate hydration status Avoid multiple passes with the needle Evaluation by Doppler studies or venogram of suspected thrombosis from prior cannulation before insertion
Arterial puncture/ laceration	Return of bright red blood in the syringe under high pressure Pulsatile blood flow on disconnection of the syringe Arterial waveform/pressures when catheter is connected to transducer system Arterial saturation of sample sent for blood gas analysis Deterioration of clinical status: Hemorrhagic shock Respiratory distress Bleeding from catheter site may or may not be observed	Application of pressure for 3-5 minutes or as needed to promote hemostasis following removal of the needle Elevate head of bed if hemodynamically stable Chest tube as indicated Thoracotomy for arterial repair if indicated	Correct coagulopathies before insertion Adequate hydration status Avoid multiple passes with the needle Evaluation by Doppler studies or venogram of suspected thrombosis from prior cannulation before insertion Use of small-gauge needle to first locate the vein

TABLE 81-1	Complications of Central Venous Catheter Insertion—*Continued*		
Complication	**Clinical Manifestation**	**Treatment**	**Prevention**
Bleeding/hematoma; venous or arterial bleeding	Deviation of trachea with large hematoma in the neck Hemothorax may be detected on chest x-ray Bleeding from insertion site Hematoma formation not likely to be seen with subclavian approach Bleeding may occur internally without visible evidence Tracheal compression Respiratory distress Carotid compression	Application of pressure to the insertion site Thoracotomy for arterial repair Tracheostomy for tracheal deviation from hematoma With the femoral approach, manual pressure slightly above the inadvertent arterial puncture site (see procedure 76 for femoral sheath removal)	Correct coagulopathies before insertion Adequate hydration status Avoid multiple passes with the needle at venipuncture Use of small-gauge needle to first locate the vein Controlling femoral bleeding immediately may prevent large blood loss or hematoma formation
Cardiac dysrhythmias	Cardiac dysrhythmias: Premature atrial contractions Atrial fibrillation or flutter Premature ventricular contractions Supraventricular tachycardia Ventricular tachycardia Sudden cardiovascular collapse	Withdraw the guidewire or catheter from the heart; dysrhythmias should stop if the cause was mechanical in nature Pharmacologic treatment of persistent dysrhythmias	Avoid entry into the heart with the guidewire Observe cardiac monitor; tall peaked P waves can be identified as the catheter tip enters the right atrium
Air embolism	Symptoms depend on amount of air drawn in, especially with spontaneously breathing patients Sudden cardiovascular collapse Tachypnea, apnea, tachycardia Hypotension, cyanosis, anxiety Diffuse pulmonary wheezes "Mill wheel" churning heart murmur Neurologic deficits, paresis, stroke, coma Cardiac arrest	Stop airflow Position patient on left side in Trendelenburg position Oxygen administration Air aspiration; transthoracic needle or intracardiac catheter Cardiopulmonary support	Adequate hydration status Head-down tilt or Trendelenburg position during catheter insertion Use of small-bore needle for insertion Application of thumb over needle or catheter hub during disconnection; needle or hub should not be exposed longer than 1 second Advancement of catheter during positive-pressure cycle in patients on ventilatory support Avoid nicking of catheter with careful suturing technique Avoid catheter exchange from large-bore catheter (pulmonary artery) to smaller catheter Use of Luer-Lok connections Minimal risk with peripherally inserted central venous catheter
Catheter malposition	Pain in ear or neck Swishing sound in ear with infusion Sharp anterior chest pain Pain in ipsilateral shoulder blade Cardiac dysrhythmia Observation on chest x-ray Signs or symptoms may be absent No blood return on aspiration	Make sure bevel of insertion needle is positioned downward (towards feet of patient) prior to placing guide wire Repositioning of catheter with guidewire or new venipuncture Catheter removal	Proper patient positioning Anthropometric measurement for accurate intravascular catheter length Avoid use of force when advancing the catheter Use of a guidewire or blunt-tipped stylet
Catheter embolism	Cardiac dysrhythmias Chest pain Dyspnea Hypotension Tachycardia May be clinically silent	Location of fragment on x-ray Transvenous retrieval of catheter fragment Thoracotomy	Use of "over a guidewire" (Seldinger) insertion technique Extreme caution with use of through-the-needle catheter designs; *never* withdraw a catheter through the needle Use of guidewire or stylet within a catheter that is inserted through a needle
Cardiac tamponade	Retrosternal or epigastric pain Dyspnea Venous engorgement of face and neck Restlessness, confusion Hypotension, paradoxical pulse Muffled heart sounds Mediastinal widening Pleural effusion Cardiac arrest	Treatment must be rapid and aggressive Discontinuation of infusions through the central line Aspiration through the catheter Emergency pericardiocentesis Emergency thoracotomy	Catheter tip position: Parallel to the walls of the superior vena cava 1 to 2 cm above the junction of the superior vena cava and right atrium Use of soft, flexible catheters Minimal risk with peripherally inserted central venous catheter
Tracheal injury	Subcutaneous emphysema Pneumomediastinum Air trapping between the chest wall and the pleura Respiratory distress with puncture of endotracheal tube cuff	Emergency reintubation (for punctured endotracheal tube cuff) Aspiration of air in mediastinum	Clinician skilled and experienced in insertion techniques Use of peripherally inserted central venous catheter

Continued

TABLE 81-1	Complications of Central Venous Catheter Insertion—*Continued*		
Complication	**Clinical Manifestation**	**Treatment**	**Prevention**
Nerve injury	Patient complaints of tingling/numbness in arm or fingers Shooting pain down the arm Paralysis Diaphragmatic paralysis (phrenic nerve injury)	Remove catheter if suspected brachial plexus injury	Clinician skilled and experienced in insertion technique Minimal risk with peripherally inserted central venous catheter
Sterile thrombophlebitis	Potential complication of the peripherally inserted central venous catheter Redness, tenderness, swelling along the course of the vein Pain in the upper extremity or shoulder	Application of heat for 48 to 72 hours Removal of catheter	Strict aseptic technique during catheter insertion Adequate skin preparation Atraumatic insertion
Pulmonary embolism	Potential complication of catheter exchange Often clinically silent Chest pain, dyspnea, coughing, tachycardia, anxiety, fever	Spiral chest tomogram (CT) Lung perfusion scan Cardiopulmonary support with large pulmonary embolism	Avoid catheter exchange in veins with thrombosis

EQUIPMENT

- CVP insertion kit
- Face masks, surgical caps, goggles (shield and mask combination may be used), sterile gloves, and sterile gowns
- Moistureproof underpad
- Antiseptic solution (e.g., chlorhexidine-based preparation)
- Nonsterile gloves
- Sterile large drapes and/or towels
- Catheter of choice (single, dual, or triple lumen), usually supplied with insertion needle, dilator, syringe, and guidewire
- 1% lidocaine vial without epinephrine
- One 25-G $\frac{5}{8}$-inch needle
- 0.9% sodium chloride, 10 to 30 ml
- Number 11 scalpel
- Syringes: one 10- to 12-ml syringe, two 3- to 5-ml syringes, two 22-G, 1½-inch needles
- Large package of 4 × 4 gauze sponges
- Three-way stopcock
- Suture kit (hemostat, scissors, needle holder)
- 3-0 or 4-0 nylon suture with curved needle
- Skin protectant pads or swabsticks
- Roll of 2-inch tape
- 2 × 2 gauze pad or transparent dressing
  Additional equipment as needed includes the following:
- Hemodynamic monitoring system (see Procedure 75)
- IV solution with Luer-Lok administration set for IV infusion
- Luer-Lok extension tubing
- Rolled towel
- Bedside monitor and oscilloscope including pulse oximeter for continuous monitoring
- Supplemental oxygen supplies
- Emergency resuscitation cart readily accessible with airway and cardiac equipment

PATIENT AND FAMILY EDUCATION

- Explain the procedure to the patient and family, and reinforce information given. ➟*Rationale:* Prepares the patient and family and reduces anxiety.

- Explain the required positioning for the procedure and the importance of not moving during the insertion. ➟*Rationale:* Encourages cooperation and reduces anxiety.
- Explain the need for sterile technique and that the patient's face may be covered. ➟*Rationale:* Decreases patient anxiety and elicits cooperation.

PATIENT ASSESSMENT AND PREPARATION

Patient Assessment

- Assess the patient's vital signs and pulse oximetry. ➟*Rationale:* Provides baseline data.
- Assess the patient's cardiac and pulmonary status. ➟*Rationale:* Some patients may not tolerate a supine or Trendelenburg position for extended periods.
- Assess the patient's coagulopathic status or recent anticoagulant or thrombolytic therapy. ➟*Rationale:* Patients are more likely to have complications related to bleeding.

Patient Preparation

- Ensure that the patient and family understand preprocedural teaching. Answer questions as they arise and reinforce information as needed. ➟*Rationale:* Evaluates and reinforces understanding of previously taught information.
- Ensure that informed consent was obtained. ➟*Rationale:* Protects the rights of the patient and makes a competent decision possible for the patient; however, under emergency circumstances, time may not allow for this form to be signed.
- If needed, perform endotracheal or tracheostomy suctioning on ventilated patients before the procedure. ➟*Rationale:* Minimizes the risk for contamination of the sterile field and the need to interrupt the procedure for suctioning.
- Place a rolled towel vertically between the scapulae if the subclavian approach is going to be used. ➟*Rationale:* May improve access to the subclavian vein.[5]
- The patient's legs may need to be positioned slightly apart if the femoral approach is going to be used. ➟*Rationale:* May improve access to the femoral vein.[5]

Procedure for Assisting With Central Venous Catheter Insertion

Steps	Rationale	Special Considerations
1. Wash hands.	Reduces the transmission of microorganisms; standard precautions.	
2. Prepare the IV solution or flush solution.	Prepares the infusion system.	
3. The prime IV tubing and/or the hemodynamic monitoring system (see Procedure 75).	Prepares the infusion system and/or the monitoring system.	
4. Place a moistureproof pad under the selected site of insertion.	Avoids soiling of the bed.	
5. Don sterile gloves, surgical caps, face masks, caps, and goggles or face shields.	Reduces the transmission of microorganisms; standard precautions.	
6. Assist, if needed, with cleansing of the intended insertion site with antiseptic solution (e.g., 2% chlorhexidine-based preparation).[3] A. Subclavian insertion: scrub shoulder to contralateral nipple line and from neck to nipple line (Fig. 81-1A).	Mechanical friction physically removes microbes. Antiseptics chemically destroy microbes.	The patient's skin should be physically clean before the application of an antiseptic solution. Organic material may inactivate antiseptic agents.

Procedure continues on the following page

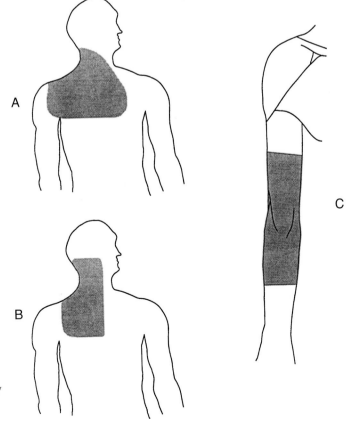

FIGURE 81-1 Area of skin preparation for central venous catheter insertions. **A,** Subclavian insertion: scrub from shoulder to contralateral nipple line and neck to nipple line. **B,** Jugular insertions: scrub midclavicle to opposite border of the sternum and from the ear to a few inches above the nipple. **C,** Peripherally inserted central venous catheters (PICC): scrub the entire arm. *(Courtesy Suredesign.)*

Procedure for Assisting With Central Venous Catheter Insertion—*Continued*

Steps	Rationale	Special Considerations
B. Jugular vein insertion: scrub midclavicle to opposite border of the sternum and ear to a few inches above the nipple line (Fig. 81-1B). C. Femoral vein insertion: scrub femoral area in a 4- to 6-in area.		
7. Allow the area to dry; then cover with a sterile towel.	Protects the cleansed area from contamination until the insertion procedure begins.	
8. Ensure that all individuals in the immediate area of the bedside wear a face mask.[3]	Prevents the transmission of microorganisms.	
9. Turn or instruct the patient to turn his or her head away from the insertion site.	Prevents the transmission of microorganisms.	
10. Remove the sterile towel from the insertion site.	Exposes the area for the sterile preparation.	
11. While the physician or advanced practice nurse completes the skin preparation, ensure patient comfort by explaining what is happening at the time. A. Application of the antiseptic solution will be cold and wet. B. Injection of the local anesthetic may burn or sting as the tissue is being infiltrated.	Reduces anxiety and encourages cooperation.	Continue providing support and comfort throughout the procedure.
12. Place the bed in a 15- to 25-degree Trendelenburg position.	Provides venous dilatation and increases central venous pressure to reduce the risk for air embolism.	May be contraindicated in certain patients (e.g., those with increased intracranial pressure, elevated venous pressure, respiratory or cardiac compromise).
13. Monitor the heart rate, respiratory rate and rhythm, pulse oximetry and any patient response to the procedure.	Assessment may indicate occurrence of complications (see Table 81-1) or inadequate pain control.	
14. During insertion, again ensure that the patient's head is turned away from the side where the guidewire and the catheter are being advanced.	Reduces contamination and may avoid malpositioning of the catheter.	
15. Observe the cardiac monitor while the guidewire and catheter are advanced, and inform the physician or advanced practice nurse immediately if a dysrhythmia occurs.	Advancement of the guidewire or catheter into the heart may induce cardiac dysrhythmias.	Tall, peaked P waves may be identified as the catheter tip enters the right atrium or if the guidewire has been advanced too far into the right atrium. Dysrhythmias may resolve with withdrawal of the guidewire or catheter. If the dysrhythmia continues, antidysrhythmic medications may be required.
16. A scalpel is used to increase the skin access; the vessel is then dilated using a wider diameter tool (dilator),	Prepares the patient for what to expect during the procedure.	Adequate sedation and local anesthetic agent use may also assist with patient comfort and position.

Procedure for Assisting with Central Venous Catheter Insertion—*Continued*

Steps	Rationale	Special Considerations
which is placed over the wire and burrowed into the skin to allow easy access for the catheter into the vessel. Instruct the patient that there may be a sensation of pressure as the dilator is inserted.		
17. Once the catheter is placed and blood return ensured, assist with flushing the lumens with normal saline and connecting the IV or hemodynamic monitoring tubing to the catheter.	Maintains aseptic technique. Immediate connection of the IV or monitoring system to the catheter prevents air embolism.	Ensure a tight connection to prevent accidental disconnection. Luer-Lok devices prevent an accidental disconnection.
18. If monitoring: A. Level the air-fluid interface and zero the system (see Procedure 75). B. Observe the waveform (see Fig. 66-4). C. Obtain a waveform strip. D. Measure the pressure.	Prepares the hemodynamic monitoring system and assesses the central venous pressure waveform.	
19. Apply an occlusive dressing.	Prevents catheter-related infections.	
20. Reposition the patient in a comfortable position.	Head-tilt position is no longer necessary.	Remove the towel roll, if used.
21. Obtain a chest x-ray.	Ensures that the catheter is placed and that there is no pneumothorax present.	Infusions (especially total parenteral nutrition and chemotherapeutic agents) should not be initiated until catheter placement is confirmed.
22. Discard used supplies in appropriate waste containers and wash hands.	Reduces the transmission of microorganisms; standard precautions.	The physician or advanced practice nurse who inserted the catheter should dispose of all sharp objects into the sharps container.

Expected Outcomes

- The placement of the central venous catheter is successful.
- If infusing IV solution, the solution infuses without problems.
- The *a, c,* and *v* waves are identified if hemodynamic monitoring is used.
- CVP measurement is determined if hemodynamic monitoring is used.

Unexpected Outcomes

- Pain or discomfort during/after the insertion procedure
- Pneumothorax, tension pneumothorax, hemothorax, or hydrothorax
- Right ventricular placement of the catheter
- Sterile thrombophlebitis
- Nerve injury
- Infection
- Cardiac dysrhythmias
- Misplacement of the catheter (e.g., carotid artery, subclavian artery)
- Hemorrhage; arterial puncture or laceration
- Hematoma
- Venous air embolism
- Catheter embolism
- Pulmonary embolus
- Cardiac tamponade
- Sepsis
- Heparin-induced thrombocytopenia or thrombosis

Patient Monitoring and Care

Steps	Rationale	Reportable Conditions
		These conditions should be reported if they persist despite nursing interventions.
1. Monitor the patient's vital signs and pulse oximetry and assess level of consciousness before the procedure, after the procedure, and as needed during the procedure.	Identifies signs and symptoms of complications and allows for immediate interventions.	• Abnormal vital signs or low pulse oximetry value • Changes in level of consciousness • Airway compromise
2. If the catheter was placed for obtaining CVP measurement, assess the waveform.	Ensures that the catheter is in the proper location for monitoring. Allows assessment of *a, c,* and *v* waves and measurement of pressure.	• Abrupt and sustained changes in pressure • Abnormal waveforms
3. Observe the catheter site for bleeding or hematoma every 15 to 30 minutes for the first 2 hours after insertion.	Postinsertion bleeding may occur in a patient with coagulopathies or arterial punctures, multiple attempts at vein access, or with the use of through-the-needle introducer designs for insertion.	• Bleeding or hematoma especially with the internal jugular or femoral approach. Subclavian bleeding is more difficult to detect
4. Assess heart and lung sounds before and after the procedure.	Abnormal heart or lung sounds may indicate cardiac tamponade, pneumothorax, or hemothorax.	• Decreased blood pressure, increased CVP and/or pulsus paradoxus • Diminished or muffled heart sounds • Absent or diminished breath sounds unilaterally
5. Monitor for signs and symptoms of complications (see Table 81-1).	May decrease mortality if recognized early.	• Signs and symptoms of complications

Documentation

Documentation should include the following:

- Patient and family education
- Vital signs
- Catheter location
- Medications administered
- Date and time of procedure
- Catheter type
- Lumen size
- Length of catheter inserted and length remaining outside the insertion site

- Nursing interventions
- Fluids administered
- Hard copy of the waveform with analysis, if possible
- Patient tolerance of procedure
- Type of dressing applied
- Any unexpected outcomes encountered and the interventions taken
- Placement confirmed by chest x-ray

References

1. Andris, D.A., and Krzywda, E.A. (1997). Central venous access: Clinical practice issues. *Nurs Clin North Am,* 32, 719-40.
2. Kumar, A., and Darovic, G.O. (2000). Establishment of cardiovascular access. In: *Hemodynamic Monitoring Invasive and Noninvasive Clinical Application.* Philadelphia: W.B. Saunders.
3. O'Grady, N.P., et al. (2002). Guidelines for the prevention of intravascular catheter-related infections. *Am J Infect Control,* 30, 476-89.
4. Sibbald, W.J. and Driedger, A.A. (1983). Right ventricular function in acute disease states: Pathophysiologic consideration. *Crit Care Med,* 11, 339-45.
5. Zimmerman, J.L, et al. (2001). *Fundamental Critical Care Support (FCCS).* Chicago: Society of Critical Care Medicine.

Additional Readings

Centers for Disease Control and Prevention: www.cdc.gov
National Guidelines: www.guidelines.gov
Society of Critical Care Medicine: www.sccm.org

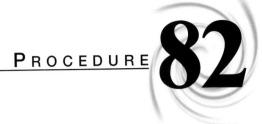
PROCEDURE 82

Implantable Venous Access Device: Access, Deaccess, and Care

PURPOSE: Implantable venous access devices or ports are used to deliver medications, parenteral solutions, blood products, and cytotoxic agents and for blood sampling for patients requiring long term venous access.

Anne C. Muller

PREREQUISITE NURSING KNOWLEDGE

- Understanding of the implantable venous access device, including the septum and outer borders
- Knowledge of the anatomy of the venous system
- Understanding of the principles of medication delivery. Intermittent use requires flushing with normal saline (NS) after each use and instillation of heparin as prescribed.
- Understanding of the principles of aseptic and sterile technique
- Understanding of the properties of chemotherapeutic or cytotoxic agents and preferred delivery techniques
- Understanding of the consequences of infiltration of vesicant substances
- Implanted venous access devices are surgically placed, totally implanted in a cutaneous pocket (usually in the chest wall), and designed to provide venous access for intermittent or continuous infusions while maintaining a patient's intact body image when not accessed.
- Implanted devices consist of a slim tube or catheter connected to a reservoir, which is covered by a disc 2 to 3 cm in width (Fig. 82-1). The disc is made of silicone and is referred to as the *septum*. The septum is capable of resealing when deaccessed. The internal catheter is connected to the patient's venous system.
- The implanted venous access device is percutaneously accessed with a noncoring needle.

- The use of a noncoring needle allows for repeated accessing of the venous device without damage to the silicone core.
- The noncoring needle chosen should be of optimal length with the most common length for adults being 1½ or 1¾ cm in length. Patients with increased subcutaneous tissue may require a longer needle for accessing. Too short a needle may cause the flanges to press against the skin surrounding the portal chamber, leading to patient discomfort and possibly resulting in damage to the skin overlying the venous access device. Too long a needle many result in a rocking motion that can cause discomfort, possible migration out of the portal septum, or damage to the integrity of the septum, impairing it for further use.

EQUIPMENT

- Nonsterile gloves
- Sterile gloves
- 90-degree-angled winged noncoring needle with extension tubing (available in ¾-, 1-, 1¼, and 1½-inch lengths)
- Dressing supplies
- Skin antiseptic solution (e.g., 2% chlorhexidine-based solution)
- Two 10-ml syringes
- Luer-Lok vial access device
- Prepierced needleless injection cap
- Single-use 30-ml vial NS
- ½-inch steri-strips
- Heparin flush, 100 unit/ml concentration
- Central venous catheter dressing change kit
  Additional equipment as needed includes the following:
- 10% betadine solution and 70% alcohol solution site prep swabs
- Supplies for obtaining blood for laboratory analysis

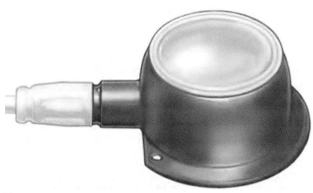

FIGURE 82-1 Vaxcel Port with PASV valve. (*Courtesy Boston Scientific Corporation. Copyright 2003. All rights reserved.*)

PATIENT AND FAMILY EDUCATION

- Assess patient and family readiness to learn and identify factors that will affect learning. ➥*Rationale:* Allows the nurse to individualize teaching and maximize understanding.
- Provide information about the implantable venous access device and the methods used for accessing it. ➥*Rationale:* Assists the patient and family to understand the procedure. Decreases patient and family anxiety.
- Explain the patient's role during the procedure and expected outcomes. ➥*Rationale:* Enables the patient to participate in care and encourages cooperation.
- Explain the anticipated sensations during the accessing procedure. ➥*Rationale:* Allows the patient to alert the clinician of unusual or unexpected sensations during the procedure.

- Explain site care and signs and symptoms of infection and infiltration. ➥*Rationale:* Enables the patient and family to participate in care. Encourages the patient to report untoward events to care providers.

PATIENT ASSESSMENT AND PREPARATION

Patient Assessment

- Review the patient's medical history specifically related to problems with device implantation, complications with previous accesses and allergies to antiseptic solutions. ➥*Rationale:* Provides baseline data.
- Obtain the patient's vital signs. ➥*Rationale:* Provides baseline data.
- Review the patient's current laboratory status, including coagulation results. ➥*Rationale:* Baseline coagulation studies are helpful in determining the risk for bleeding. If abnormal, consult with the primary care provider before accessing the device.[2]

Patient Preparation

- Ensure that the patient and family understand preprocedural teaching. Answer questions as they arise and reinforce information as needed. ➥*Rationale:* Evaluates and reinforces understanding of previously taught information.
- Assist the patient to a supine position with the head of the bed elevated up to a 30-degree angle. ➥*Rationale:* Prepares the patient and allows optimal access to the implanted venous access device.

Procedure for Implantable Venous Access Device: Access, Deaccess, and Care

Steps	Rationale	Special Considerations
Accessing an Implantable Venous Access Device		
1. Wash hands and don nonsterile gloves.	Reduces the transmission of microorganisms; standard precautions.	Both conventional antiseptic containing soap and water or waterless alcohol-based gels or foams are considered acceptable by the Centers for Disease Control and Prevention.[1]
2. Remove patient gown away from the venous access device. Palpate the subcutaneous tissue to determine the borders of access device.[2,3]	Optimizes the viewing area.	
3. Palpate the venous access device borders and locate the septum and the center of the septum.	Allows for palpation of the venous access device borders and identification of the septal center.	
4. Assess the site for signs and symptoms of infection (e.g., erythema, induration, pain, or tenderness at the site).	Minimizes the risk for accessing an infected area.	Erythema, swelling, or tenderness may indicate system leakage. An x-ray is recommended if leakage is suspected.[3]
5. Discard gloves and wash hands.	Reduces the transmission of microorganisms; standard precautions.	

Procedure	**for Implantable Venous Access Device: Access, Deaccess, and Care**—*Continued*	
Steps	**Rationale**	**Special Considerations**
6. Open the central venous catheter dressing kit using the sterile inner surface of the wrap to create a sterile field.	Maintains asepsis and prepares supplies. Creates a sterile field.	Disinfect the table as needed. Venous access devices have the lowest risk for catheter-related blood system infections, provided that aseptic and sterile techniques are used throughout care delivery.[1]
7. Prepare supplies: A. Using sterile technique, remove the wrapper from two 10-ml syringes and place them on the sterile field. B. Remove the packaging and place the winged or safety noncoring needle with extension tubing, needleless injection cap, Luer-Lok vial adapter, and steri-strips on the sterile field.	Places equipment within reach during procedure. Maintains sterility of procedure. Protects the clinician from potential needle injury. Maintains sterile technique.	
8. Aseptically connect the vial adapter device to the vial.	Prepares supplies.	
9. Remove the cap from the NS vial. Wipe off top of the NS vial with an alcohol wipe and allow to dry.	Reduces microorganisms.	
10. Prepare supplies: A. Put a sterile glove on your nondominant hand. B. With the sterile hand, pick up a 10-ml syringe. C. Using the nonsterile, dominant hand, pick up the NS vial with the Luer-Lok adapter while using the sterile, gloved hand to access the NS vial and withdraw 10 ml of NS.	Prepares supplies for procedure.	
11. Repeat step 10 with the second 10-ml syringe; then discard the NS vial.		
12. Don the remaining sterile glove.	Maintains asepsis.	
13. Using sterile technique: A. Attach the needleless injection cap to the extension tubing on the noncoring needle. B. Attach the 10-ml NS syringe to the needleless valve. C. Prime the tubing with NS away from the sterile field.	Prepares the equipment. Removes air from the extension tubing, preventing possible air embolism.	
14. Retain the priming syringe on the needleless cap and return the primed equipment to the sterile field.		

Procedure continues on the following page

Procedure for Implantable Venous Access Device: Access, Deaccess, and Care—*Continued*

Steps	Rationale	Special Considerations
15. Cleanse the implanted venous access device or port with antiseptic solution (e.g., 2% chlorhexidine-based preparation).[1]	Reduces infection.	
16. Use the nondominant hand to stabilize the borders of the venous access device and use the dominant hand to pick up the noncoring needle with the NS syringe attached.		
17. Triangulate the venous access device between the thumb and first two fingers of the nondominant hand and aim the needle for the center point of these three fingers. With the dominant hand, firmly grasp the protective cap or wings of the noncoring needle and insert it firmly into the center of the port septum using a 90-degree angle perpendicular to the skin surface. (Fig. 82-2)	Stabilizes the venous access device within the chest wall and prevents slippage. Protects the clinician from a potential needle injury.	
18. Advance the needle through the skin and septum until reaching the base of the portal reservoir.		If using a noncoring safety needle, grasp the vertical fin between the thumb and middle finger and press downward with the index finger[3,7,8] (Fig. 82-3).
19. Note that resistance will be felt as the needle reaches the base of the reservoir.		Once the septum is punctured, avoid tilting or rocking the needle, which may cause fluid leakage or damage to the system.[2]

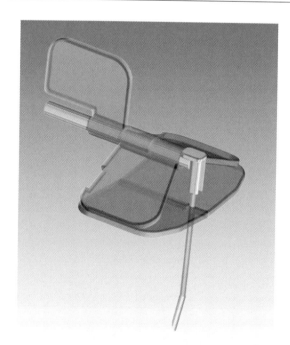

FIGURE 82-2 HuberPlus© noncoring implanted device needle. *(Courtesy NOW Medical Corporation.)*

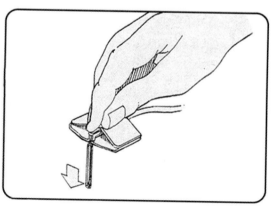

FIGURE 82-3 Accessing venous infusion device. Position of dominant hand with noncoring needle as downward pressure is exerted. *(Courtesy NOW Medical Corporation.)*

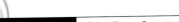

Procedure	**for Implantable Venous Access Device: Access, Deaccess, and Care**—*Continued*	

Steps	Rationale	Special Considerations
20. Flush the venous access device with 5 ml of NS.	Determines the patency of the venous access device.	Avoid using syringes with less than a 10-ml volume for flushing or administering infusate. Smaller syringes exert pressure exceeding 40 psi per square inch and may cause catheter rupture or fragmentation with possible embolization.[2,3]
21. Observe the skin surrounding the noncoring needle for leakage of fluid or infiltration at the access site.	Assesses for potential access problems.	
22. Gently aspirate blood; then flush with the remaining 5 ml of NS.	Verifies placement.	If blood return is not evident, gently flush using push-pull method and reposition patient. If continued lack of aspirate, continue the accessing procedure and apply a dressing to minimize the risk of infection. Confer with care provider and consider administration of lytic agent and radiographic or dye shadow studies to confirm placement.[3]
23. Remove the protective cap from the winged needle. Position the wings flush with the patient's skin.	Anchoring minimizes muscular discomfort for the patient.	
24. Stabilize the needle by attaching steri-strips in a cross or star pattern over the wings of the noncoring needle.	Stabilizes the needle inserted in the septal core and minimizes rocking of the needle, which can cause damage to the septum and patient discomfort. Minimizes needle movement in the septum, thereby ensuring integrity of the septal core for future use.	
25. Apply a dressing according to institution protocol.	May aid in stabilizing the device and maintaining asepsis.	A gauze dressing is preferred if oozing or blood seepage occurs at the insertion site.
26. Label the dressing with the date, time of cannulation, needle gauge/length, and your initials.	Provides important clinical information.	If the accessed device is not to be used immediately, flush with heparin as prescribed.
27. Initiate continuous or intermittent infusion.	Begins therapy.	
28. Discard used supplies and wash hands.	Reduces the transmission of microorganisms; standard precautions.	

Deaccessing an Implantable Venous Access Device

1. Wash hands and don nonsterile gloves.	Reduces the transmission of microorganisms; standard precautions.	
2. Flush the venous access device with 10 ml of NS, followed by heparin as prescribed (e.g., 5 ml of 100 units per ml heparin).[2]	Prepares and optimizes catheter patency while not in use.	

Procedure continues on the following page

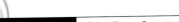

Procedure | **for Implantable Venous Access Device: Access, Deaccess, and Care**—*Continued*

Steps	Rationale	Special Considerations
3. Loosen the transparent or gauze dressing and steri-strips from the site.	Facilitates removal.	
4. Use the thumb and forefinger of the dominant hand to grasp the dressing and steri-strips along with the winged flanges of the needle (Fig. 82-4).	Prepares for needle removal.	
5. With the nondominant hand, apply gentle stabilizing pressure to the venous access device while removing the needle by pulling straight up and out in a firm, continuous motion.	Minimizes patient discomfort and ensures controlled withdrawal of a sharp object.	If using a noncoring safety needle, grasp the horizontal flanges securely, pull up, and squeeze the flanges together. The flanges will fold together, forcing the needle inside the locked wings and covering the needle. The clinician will see and feel the wings lock in place (Fig. 82-5).
6. Assess the site for redness or drainage.	Identifies possible complications.	
7. Discard the noncoring needle in a designated container.	Standard precautions.	
8. Apply a dressing to the site if oozing occurs.	Provides absorption.	
9. Discard supplies and wash hands.	Reduces the transmission of micro-organisms; standard precautions.	

Obtaining a Blood Specimen From an Implantable Venous Access Device

1. Wash hands and don nonsterile gloves.	Reduces the transmission of micro-organisms; standard precautions.	
2. If present, shut off the IV infusion and disconnect the IV tubing from the extension tubing on the noncoring needle.	Maintains asepsis.	
3. Place a sterile cap on the end of the IV tubing.	Maintains asepsis.	
4. Thoroughly cleanse the injection cap with an alcohol wipe and allow it to dry. Do not remove cap.[5,6,9]	Minimizes infection and clinician exposure to blood/body fluids.[3]	

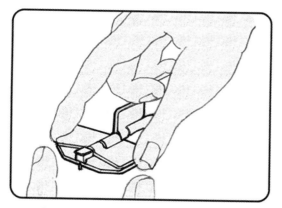

FIGURE 82-4 Position of hands while removing venous access device needle. Nondominant hand secures base of device while dominant hand exerts steady upward pressure while squeezing wings together. (*Courtesy NOW Medical Corporation.*)

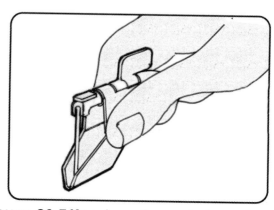

FIGURE 82-5 Noncoring needle secure in sharps safety feature of HuberPlus needle after removal from implanted venous device (*Courtesy NOW Medical Corporation.*)

Procedure for Implantable Venous Access Device: Access, Deaccess, and Care—*Continued*

Steps	Rationale	Special Considerations
5. Attach a 10-ml syringe with NS and flush the venous access device.	Clears the catheter of medication or IV fluid.	
6. Attach a new sterile 10-ml syringe or a VACUTAINER® with a needle-less Luer-Lok adapter needle.	Prepares supplies.	
7. Gently aspirate the discard volume into the syringe or engage a blood specimen tube into the VACUTAINER® to obtain the discard volume and allow the tube to passively fill.[5,6,9]	Discard method recommended for obtaining laboratory samples.[4]	VACUTAINER® system is the current natural standard. Minimizes needle stick injury, exposure to blood, and decreases infection risk to the patient by reducing incidence of opening the catheter system.[5,7]
8. Remove the discard syringe or tube and discard in the appropriate receptacle.	Removes discard safely.	Research shows 95% reliability of laboratory samples using a minimum discard volume of 3 times the dead space volume of the indwelling catheter system.[5,6] Portal reservoirs average 0.5 ml volume; catheters average 0.6 ml for single lumen systems.[2]
9. Insert a new syringe into the injection cap or place a new blood specimen tube into the VACUTAINER® system.	Prepares for removal of the blood sample.	
10. Slowly and gently aspirate blood or engage the blood specimen tube into the VACUTAINER® system.	Obtains the blood specimen.	
11. After the blood specimen is obtained, flush with 10 ml of NS.	Clears blood from the system.	Flush with an additional 10-20 ml of NS if the blood does not clear completely from the extension tubing.
12. Clamp the extension tubing.		
13. Apply a new injection cap using strict aseptic technique.	Reduces infection.	
14. Reconnect the IV and continue infusion.	Resumes therapy.	If the IV is completed, administer heparin as prescribed.
15. Discard used supplies and wash hands.	Reduces the transmission of microorganisms; standard precautions.	
16. Send laboratory specimens for analysis.	Expedites determination of laboratory results.	

Expected Outcomes

- Site without redness, pain, or tenderness
- Venous access device stable
- Venous access device is accessed without difficulty
- Venous access device flushes easily without evidence of resistance or infiltration
- No evidence or leakage at septal site
- Blood specimens are obtained as prescribed
- Venous access device is deaccessed without difficulty

Unexpected Outcomes

- Port reddened, tender, or painful on palpation
- Implanted device unstable in chest wall with palpation
- Patient describes burning sensation in subcutaneous tissue with flushing or infusion
- Sluggish or no blood return with aspiration
- Evidence of leakage of flushing solution at septal site
- Patient describes pain at site, chest, ear or shoulder with flushing
- Signs or symptoms of local or systemic infection
- Swollen neck and/or arm

Patient Monitoring and Care

Steps	Rationale	Reportable Conditions
		These conditions should be reported if they persist despite nursing interventions.
1. During IV infusions assess the venous access device for patency and signs of infiltration every 4 hours and as needed.	Determines adequate functioning of the venous access device.	• Signs or symptoms of infiltration at the venous access site
2. Follow institution standard for frequency and type of dressing change.	The dressing should be changed if it becomes damp, loosened, or soiled or when inspection of the site is necessary.[1]	• Signs or symptoms of infection
3. Replace gauze dressing every 2 days, transparent dressing every 7 days. Change either dressing if soiled, dampened, or loosened.[1,8]	Prevents infection.	
4. Change access device every 7 days.[1]	Maintains patency.	
5. Follow-up care for deaccessed device includes flushing monthly with 5-ml 100 units heparin.[2,7,8]		
6. Assess for signs and symptoms of infection.	Determines the presence of infection.	• Redness, pain, or drainage at the site; fever, elevated white blood cell count

Documentation

Documentation should include the following:

- Location and cannulation of the device
- Needle length and gauge
- Appearance of blood return
- Access of the site
- Deaccess of the site

- Specimens obtained and sent for analysis
- Laboratory results
- Unexpected outcomes
- Additional interventions

References

1. CDC (2002). Guidelines for the prevention of intravascular catheter related bloodstream infection. *Morbidity and Mortality Weekly Report,* 5, 1-26.
2. Beck, S.L., et al. (1990). *Standards of Care for the Patient With a Venous Access Device.* Salt Lake City: American Cancer Society, Utah Division.
3. Deltec Incorporated. (2002). Clinician Information Port-A-Cath®, Port-A-Cath II® and P.A.S. Port® Systems. St. Paul, MN: Deltec, Inc., 1-24.
4. Dougherty, L. (2000). Central venous access devices. *Nursing Standard,* 14, 45-50.
5. Frey, A.M. (2003). Drawing blood from vascular access devices. *J Infusion Nurs,* 26, 285-93.
6. Himberger, J., and Himberger, L. (2001). Accuracy of drawing blood through infusing intravenous lines. *Heart Lung,* 30, 66-73.
7. Intravenous Nurses Society. (2000). Infusion nursing standards of practice, *J Intraven Nurs,* 23.
8. Oncology Nurses Society. (2001). *Chemotherapy and Biotherapy Guidelines and Recommendations for Practice.* Pittsburgh: Oncology Nursing Press, Inc.

9. Yucha, C., and DeAngelo, E. (1996). The minimum discard volume. *J Intraven Nurs,* 19, 141-46.

Additional Readings

Camp-Sorrell, D. (1992). Implantable ports: Everything you always wanted to know. *J Intraven Nurs,* 15, September/October, 262-73.
Rosenthal, K. (2003). Pinpointing intravascular device complications. *Nurs Manage,* June, 37-42.
Sabel, M., and Smith, J. (1988). Principles of chronic venous access: Recommendations based on the Roswell Park experience. *Surg Oncol,* 6, 171-77.
Seemann, S., and Reinhardt, A. (2000). Blood sample collection from a peripheral catheter system compared with phlebotomy. *J Intraven Nurs,* 23, 290-97.
Sterba, K. (2001). Controversial issues in the care and maintenance of vascular access devices in the long-term/subacute care client. *J Infusion Nurs,* 24, July/August, 249-54.

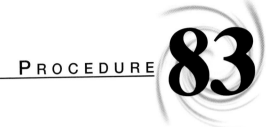
PROCEDURE **83**

Peripheral Intravenous Catheter Insertion

PURPOSE: A peripheral intravenous (IV) catheter is inserted for a variety of purposes: to provide a route for the administration of IV fluids, medications, and blood products; to maintain a patent venous route for use during emergency situations; to obtain venous blood samples for laboratory tests; and to provide nutritional supplements and hydration for patients unable to obtain them by other means.

Linda Bucher

PREREQUISITE NURSING KNOWLEDGE

- Nurses must be adequately prepared to insert a peripheral IV catheter. This preparation should include specific educational content regarding the indications for and the complications and maintenance of IV therapy. Opportunities to demonstrate clinical competency in the insertion of a peripheral IV catheter should also be included.
- Understanding of the principles of aseptic technique
- Knowledge of the anatomy and physiology of the vasculature and adjacent structures in the upper extremities. The most commonly used veins are located on the forearm; specifically the cephalic, basilic, and median veins in the lower arm, and the metacarpal veins in the dorsum of the hand (see Figs. 85-1 and 85-2).[15,22,25]
- Superficial veins lie in loose connective tissue under the skin and are best suited for venous cannulation. Peripheral IV therapy can be maintained longer by selecting the most distal site on the extremity; by using the smallest gauge catheter appropriate to the vein size and the prescribed therapy; by avoiding areas of flexion such as the antecubital fossa and the wrist; by using the nondominant hand, if possible; and by choosing sites that are located above previous insertion sites and sites that are phlebitic, infiltrated, or bruised.[22,25]
- Indications for the insertion of a peripheral IV catheter will vary and can include patients experiencing fluid and electrolyte imbalances, malnutrition, shock, trauma, sepsis, surgery, endocrine disorders, cardiovascular disease, and cancer.

- Complications associated with the insertion of a peripheral IV catheter can be local or systemic. Common local complications include phlebitis, thrombophlebitis, infiltration, and catheter occlusion. Systemic complications occur less frequently than local complications and include septicemia, thromboembolism, and embolism (air, catheter). Circulatory overload, speed shock, and allergic/anaphylactic reactions are systemic complications that are related directly to intravenous therapy. Systemic complications, when they occur, are often life-threatening.[20,21]
- The most common type of IV catheter used for short-term intravenous therapy (7 days or less) is the over-the-needle, plastic catheter (Fig. 83-1).[13] The winged infusion set, or "butterfly," is recommended for use in patients who require IV therapy for less than 24 hours (Fig. 83-2).[19] Through-the-needle peripheral catheters are usually restricted to long-term IV use.
- The length and gauge of catheters used for peripheral IV therapy vary. Over-the-needle plastic catheters range from ⅝ inch to 2 inches in length and from 27 G to 12 G in size. The most common adult sizes are 22 G, 20 G, and 18 G.[13]
- A variety of safety IV devices are available and should be used to reduce the risk for needlestick injury.[9,10,17]

EQUIPMENT

- IV catheter of appropriate type, size, and length
- IV fluid as prescribed with IV administration set and short extension tubing attached and primed for continuous IV infusion (an intermittent infusion cap/adapter may be attached per institutional policy)

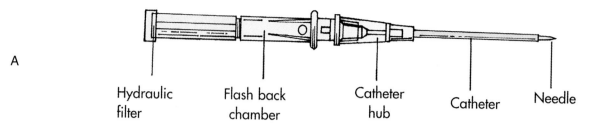

A

Hydraulic   Flash back   Catheter   Catheter   Needle
filter   chamber   hub

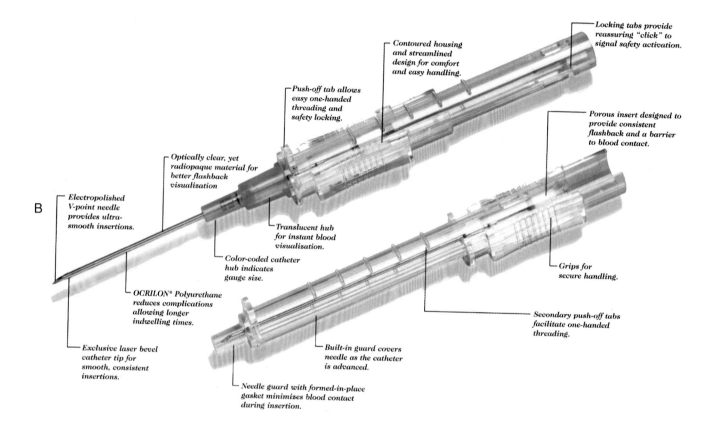

B

Locking tabs provide
reassuring "click" to
signal safety activation.

Contoured housing
and streamlined
design for comfort
and easy handling.

Push-off tab allows
easy one-handed
threading and
safety locking.

Porous insert designed to
provide consistent
flashback and a barrier
to blood contact.

Optically clear, yet
radiopaque material for
better flashback
visualisation

Electropolished
V-point needle
provides ultra-
smooth insertions.

Translucent hub
for instant blood
visualisation.

Color-coded catheter
hub indicates
gauge sise.

Grips for
secure handling.

OCRILON* Polyurethane
reduces complications
allowing longer
indwelling times.

Secondary push-off tabs
facilitate one-handed
threading.

Exclusive laser bevel
catheter tip for
smooth, consistent
insertions.

Built-in guard covers
needle as the catheter
is advanced.

Needle guard with formed-in-place
gasket minimises blood contact
during insertion.

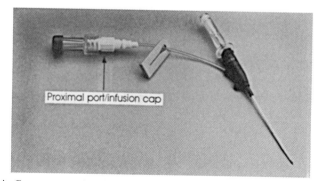

C

Proximal port/infusion cap

FIGURE 83-1 **A,** Components of the over-the-needle catheter. **B,** PROTECTIV* Plus IV Catheter Safety
System. **C,** Multilumen peripheral (over-the-needle) catheter. *(**A,** From Potter, P.A., and Perry, A.G., eds. [2003].
Basic Nursing: A Critical Thinking Approach. 5th ed. St. Louis: Mosby, 863; **B,** courtesy Johnson & Johnson;
C, courtesy Arrow International, Inc.)*

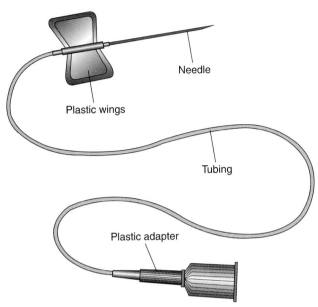

FIGURE 83-2 Components of winged infusion (butterfly) set.

- Short-extension tubing with an intermittent infusion cap/adapter attached and primed with normal saline (NS) for intermittent infusion device (IID)
- Single-use tourniquet
- Antiseptic solution (e.g., 2% chlorhexidine-based preparation)
- 2 × 2 sterile gauze pad or alcohol prep pad
- One roll of 1-inch, nonallergenic tape
- Transparent semipermeable dressing (small)
- One pair of nonsterile gloves
- Biohazard container
  Additional equipment as needed includes the following:
- 3 to 5 ml of NS (flush for IID)
- Scissors or clippers for hair removal
- IV pole
- VACUTAINER® with Luer-Lok adapter and collecting tubes, if venous sampling is needed (a 10-ml syringe may be used in place of the VACUTAINER® system)
- Lidocaine or eutectic mixture of local anesthetics (EMLA) cream (optional)
- 10% povidone-iodine or 70% alcohol

PATIENT AND FAMILY EDUCATION

- Explain the purpose of the peripheral IV catheter and include the patient in the selection of the site (if possible). **➻Rationale:** Clarification of information is an expressed patient and family need and helps to diminish anxiety, enhance acceptance, and encourage questions. Patients often request that their nondominant hand or arm be used for IV catheter placement.
- Explain the overall steps of the procedure, including the patient's role during the procedure. **➻Rationale:** Decreases patient anxiety, enhances cooperation, and

provides an opportunity for the patient to voice concerns; limits the risk for accidental movement during the procedure.
- Instruct the patient and family on the signs and symptoms that should be reported to the nurse (e.g., discomfort, burning, swelling, wetness). **➻Rationale:** Enables the patient and family to recognize possible complications related to the IV catheter and includes them in the plan of care.

PATIENT ASSESSMENT AND PREPARATION

Patient Assessment

- Assess the patient's current anticoagulation therapy, thrombolytic therapy, or known blood dyscrasias. **➻Rationale:** Anticoagulation and thrombolytic therapies or blood dyscrasias could increase the risk for hematoma formation or excessive bleeding at the insertion site. Patients who are receiving thrombolytic therapy should have adequate peripheral access established prior to initiation of therapy.
- Assess the patient's allergy history (e.g., lidocaine, EMLA cream, antiseptic solutions, adhesives, latex). **➻Rationale:** Reduces the risk for allergic reactions by avoiding known allergenic products.
- Assess the patient for a history of mastectomy, fistula, shunt, neurovascular injury, cellulitis, thrombosis, radial artery surgery. **➻Rationale:** These conditions predispose patients to IV-related complications. Insertion of a peripheral IV catheter should be avoided in extremities affected by these conditions.
- Assess the patient's age, general size, skin condition, and anatomy of the venous system. **➻Rationale:** Assists in the determination of the most appropriate catheter size and insertion site. Small-gauge catheters (e.g., 24 to 22 G) are less traumatizing to veins. If large-gauge catheters are required (e.g., 20 to 14 G), the selected vein should be able to accommodate the catheter. Edematous areas or sites of previous hematoma or infection and veins that are very small, sclerosed, scarred, or tortuous should be avoided, because these conditions can inhibit successful insertion of an IV catheter and can contribute to complications.
- Determine whether or not venous sampling is needed. **➻Rationale:** Accurate laboratory samples can be obtained during the process of initiating a peripheral IV catheter.[9,14] Concurrent collection of venous blood for laboratory testing during this procedure limits the number of venipunctures required by the patient.

Patient Preparation

- Ensure that the patient and family understand preprocedural teaching. Answer questions as they arise and reinforce information as needed. **➻Rationale:** Evaluates and reinforces understanding of previously taught information.
- Position the patient in a supine position with the head of the bed slightly elevated and the patient's arms at

the side. **➤➤Rationale:** Proper positioning of the patient enhances accessibility to the venipuncture site and promotes patient comfort.

- Extend the patient's upper extremity to form a straight line from the shoulder to the wrist. A pillow can be placed under the arm for support, if needed. **➤➤Rationale:** Proper positioning of the extremity enhances accessibility to the venipuncture site and reduces the risk for patient movement during the procedure.

Procedure for Peripheral Intravenous Catheter Insertion

Steps	Rationale	Special Considerations
1. Wash hands.	Reduces the transmission of microorganisms; standard precautions.	
2. Prepare the IV infusion and prime the tubing or the intermittent infusion cap or adapter, as indicated. If a multilumen peripheral catheter is used, flush the proximal port through the infusion cap with NS. (see Fig. 83-1C).	Allows the procedure to be completed expeditiously and reduces the risk for occlusion once the IV catheter is established. Avoids infusion of air into the patient.	A short-extension tubing attached to the administration set or intermittent infusion cap/adapter facilitates access to the IV catheter and limits manipulation at the catheter hub.
3. Wash hands and don nonsterile gloves.	Reduces the transmission of microorganisms; standard precautions.	
4. Apply the tourniquet proximal to the proposed puncture site. Tie in a manner such that the tourniquet can be released by pulling on one end (see Fig. 85-5). If the veins are not prominent, instruct the patient to open and close his or her hand (make a fist) several times.	Impedes venous return to the heart and produces venous distention. Proper application of the tourniquet allows for the quick, one-handed release of the tourniquet.	Arterial blood flow should not be impeded. Arterial perfusion should be verified by palpating for the radial pulse. For patients with large, prominent veins, a tourniquet is not recommended. Alternative approaches to facilitating venous distention include gentle tapping of the skin over the venipuncture area with the index and second fingers and permitting the arm to hang dependent below the level of the heart. Warm compresses can also be applied to facilitate venous distention.
5. Select the appropriate venipuncture site and use the most distal branch of the vein selected.	Multiple factors determine the success of securing and maintaining a patent venous access site.	Vein size, elasticity, and distance below the skin should be considered. Shorter and smaller catheters may be needed in the elderly and very young patients. Excessive hair at the selected site should be removed with scissors or clippers to facilitate site preparation, catheter insertion, and adherence of dressings. The site should not be shaved as microabrasions increase the potential introduction of microorganisms into the vascular system.[9,10]
6. Release the tourniquet.	Prolonged vein distension causes undue patient discomfort and impairs circulation to the extremity. In addition, a tourniquet left on for more than 1 to 2 minutes may result in hemoconcentration or a variation in blood test values if blood is to be collected during the procedure.	In some cases (e.g., tortuous or sclerosed veins), a tourniquet may increase venous pressure such that the vein may rupture when punctured.

Procedure for Peripheral Intravenous Catheter Insertion—*Continued*

Steps	Rationale	Special Considerations
7. If lidocaine or EMLA cream is to be used, apply to the site selected for insertion of the IV catheter. *(Level VI: Clinical studies in a variety of patient populations and situations to support recommendations.)*	Provides relief from pain associated with venipuncture and may reduce or eliminate anxiety associated with the procedure.[4,8,9,10,16,18]	Research on the length of time from application of lidocaine or EMLA to the procedure has produced mixed results.[4,8,9,10,16,18] If these products are used, the manufacturer's recommendations should be followed. The time from application to procedure varies from 5 to 280 minutes.
8. Prepare the site using a 2% chlorhexidine-based antiseptic solution.[1,2] Cleanse the site using a back-and-forth motion while applying friction for 30 seconds. Allow the antiseptic to remain on the insertion site and to air-dry completely before catheter insertion.[1,10]	Limits the introduction of potentially infectious skin flora into the vessel during the puncture.	If using alcohol and povidone-iodine, apply alcohol first. Never remove the povidone-iodine solution with alcohol because alcohol cancels the effect of the povidone-iodine.[1,10,15] If you must palpate the area once cleansing has been performed, use sterile gloves or recleanse the area.
9. Reapply the tourniquet.	Produces venous distention.	
10. Draw the skin taut just below the insertion site, using the thumb of the nondominant hand.	Immobilizes the vein for insertion of the IV catheter.	
11. Puncture the skin parallel to the path of the vein with the bevel up and the needle at a 30- to 45-degree angle.	Causes the least amount of discomfort.	Before puncturing the patient's skin, inform the patient that you are about to insert the device.
12. Advance the needle until resistance is met. Next, reduce the angle of the needle and slowly pierce the vein. Observe for dark red blood in the catheter hub (flashback chamber) or tubing of the winged infusion set. Continue to insert the needle approximately ¼ inch into the vein.	Limits the risk for puncturing the posterior wall of the vein. Establishes entry into the vein. Ensures full entry of the catheter into the vein, because the catheter is slightly shorter than the stylet (needle).	A "pop" may or may not be felt when the needle enters the vein. Winged infusion sets can be used to collect venous samples for laboratory testing. When this is the case, the tubing of the infusion set is *not* primed, and retrograde blood flow will be observed on entry of the needle into the vein.
13. Release the tourniquet.	Reduces the risk for rupturing the vein.	Keep the tourniquet in place if blood for laboratory testing is to be collected. If blood flow is found to be sluggish during the collection process, the tourniquet should be kept in place until collection of the blood is completed and then removed.
14. Advance the device, following the appropriate procedure for the needle type: A. Catheter-over-needle (Figs. 83-3 and 83-4): (1) Holding the device stable, advance the catheter into the vein until the hub rests at the insertion site.	Stabilization of the device reduces the risk for puncturing the posterior wall of the vein.	Procedures for advancing the catheter vary according to the device used. It is recommended that safety devices be used to reduce the risk for needlestick injuries.[10,11,12,17]
(2) Place a 2 × 2 gauze or alcohol prep pad under the catheter hub and remove the stylet (or needle guard) while holding the hub securely.	Provides absorption of any blood that may escape when the stylet is removed. Prevents dislodgment of the catheter.	Never reinsert the needle into the catheter, because the needle could cut the catheter, resulting in catheter embolus. The application of digital pressure to the vein just above the tip of the catheter limits the escape of blood.

Procedure continues on the following page

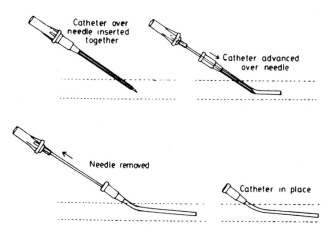

FIGURE 83-3 Schematic for insertion of catheter-over-needle. *(Courtesy Johnson & Johnson.)*

One-handed technique

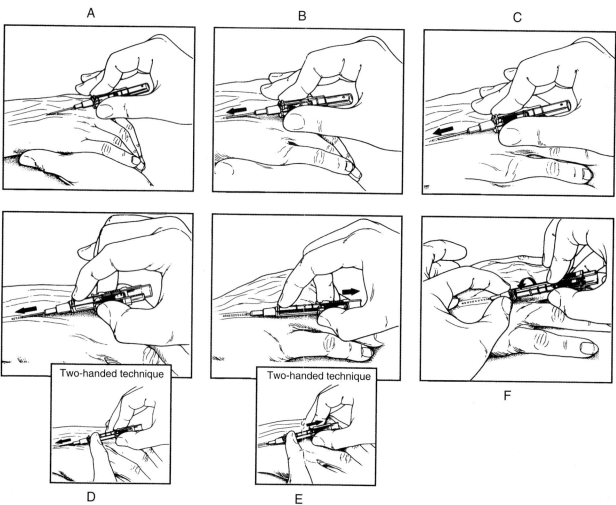

FIGURE 83-4 Insertion of PROTECTIV® Plus IV Catheter System. **A,** One- or two-handed technique: hold the device by the ribbed needle housing with thumb and fingers on opposite sides. **B,** With the bevel and push-off tabs in the "up" position, insert the needle through the skin into the vein. Observe for blood in the flashback chamber. **C,** Slightly advance the catheter and needle together to assume full catheter entry into the vein lumen. **D,** One-handed technique: holding the device stable, place a finger on the primary push-off tab and thread the catheter to the desired length. Two-handed technique: holding the device stable with one hand, place the thumb of the other hand behind the primary push-off tab and thread the catheter to desired length. As you thread the catheter, the needle guard begins to cover the needle. **E,** One-handed technique: using a finger to stabilize the device at the push-off tab, draw the needle into the needle guard by retracting the ribbed needle housing until it locks securely in place. Two-handed technique: with the thumb behind the primary push-off tab to stabilize the device, retract the ribbed needle housing with the other hand until it locks securely in place. Listen for a "click" indicating that the needle is locked. **F,** Secure the hub and remove the needle guard by twisting slightly and pulling it out of the catheter hub.

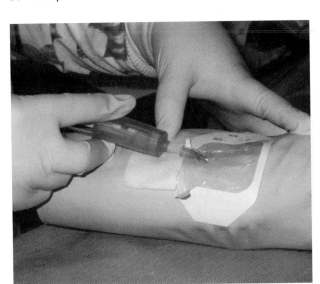

FIGURE 83-5 Collection of blood specimens during the insertion of a peripheral IV using the VACUTAINER® system. *(Courtesy Becton Dickinson.)*

Procedure for Peripheral Intravenous Catheter Insertion—*Continued*

Steps	Rationale	Special Considerations
(3) Properly dispose of sharps.	Limits the risk for a needlestick injury and exposure to bloodborne pathogens.	If blood for laboratory testing is required, attach the VACUTAINER® and collect the appropriate blood samples before connecting the IV or IID (Fig. 83-5). A 10-ml syringe can be used in lieu of the VACUTAINER® system (see Procedure 85).
(4) Connect the primed IV administration set or IID to the catheter hub.	Prompt connection maintains the patency of the vein and sterility. Provides direct entrance for IV fluids or access for the intermittent administration of IV fluids and medications.	Limited data exist on blood sample collection from an infusing IV or IID; thus this is not recommended.[7,10,24]
(5) Initiate the proper IV flow rate or flush the port of the IID with 3 ml of NS flush. *(Level VI: Clinical studies in a variety of patient populations and situations to support recommendations.)*	Use of a NS flush is recommended over heparin flush for maintaining the patency of peripheral IV catheters in adults.[5,6,26]	
(6) Assess for signs of infiltration.	If the stylet has punctured the posterior wall of the vein, fluid or blood will infuse into the surrounding tissue, as evidenced by local edema or hematoma formation.	If infiltration is observed, the catheter must be removed and the procedure must be restarted at a location above the site of the infiltration or on the opposite extremity.[9,10]
(7) Secure the catheter with a transparent semipermeable dressing, sterile gauze and tape, or adhesive bandage. If a transparent semipermeable dressing is used, do not cover the connection between the tubing and catheter hub and do not place tape under the transparent dressing (Fig. 83-6).	Prevents early access of microorganisms to the bloodstream and stabilizes the catheter, thereby reducing irritation of the intimal lining of the vein by the catheter. Facilitates changing of the IV tubing if necessary before the catheter is changed and helps to maintain asepsis of the puncture site.	Procedures for covering peripheral IV sites vary. Antimicrobial ointment at the catheter insertion site is not recommended.[1,9,28] Research is mixed regarding the efficacy of transparent semipermeable dressing, sterile gauze and tape, or adhesive bandages as IV site dressings.[1,3,23,27]

Procedure continues on the following page

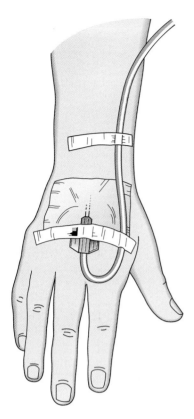

FIGURE 83-6 Transparent semipermeable dressing over the catheter insertion site. An additional ½ inch tape is placed over the connection between the catheter hub and the tubing. Note the intravenous tubing is looped in a "J" loop and secured with additional tape. It is not recommended that tape be placed under the transparent dressing. *(From Farley, K.L. Taping and Dressing Suggestions and Tips for Use With Non-Winged IV Catheters. Courtesy Johnson & Johnson.)*

Procedure for Peripheral Intravenous Catheter Insertion—*Continued*

Steps	Rationale	Special Considerations
B. Winged infusion set (or "butterfly"):		
(1) Prime the device with NS if an IV line or IID is to be established.	Avoids the entrance of air into the vein	If blood for laboratory testing is required, the device should *not* be primed.
(2) Advance the needle fully, if possible, into the vein.	Increases the stabilization of the device in the vein.	If the device is primed, retrograde blood flow usually will *not* be observed in the tubing.
(3) Release the tourniquet and connect the IV tubing or the injection port to the end of the tubing.	Prompt connection maintains patency of the vein and sterility. Provides direct entrance for IV fluids or access for the intermittent administration of IV fluids and medications.	If blood for laboratory testing is required, attach a VACUTAINER® (or a 10-ml syringe) and collect the appropriate blood samples before connecting the IV line or injection port (see Procedure 85). Limited data exist on blood sample collection from an infusing IV or IID; this is not recommended.[7,10,24]
(4) Initiate the proper IV flow rate or flush the port of the IID with 3 ml of NS flush. *(Level VI: Clinical studies in a variety of patient populations and situations to support recommendations.)*	Use of a NS flush is recommended over heparin flush for maintaining the patency of peripheral IV catheters in adults.[5,6,26]	
(5) Assess for signs of infiltration.	If the needle has punctured the posterior wall of the vein, fluid or blood will infuse into the surrounding tissue, as evidenced by local edema or hematoma formation.	If observed, the device must be removed and the procedure must be restarted at a location above the site of the infiltration or on the opposite extremity.[9,10]

Procedure for Peripheral Intravenous Catheter Insertion—*Continued*

Steps	Rationale	Special Considerations
(6) Secure the catheter with a transparent semipermeable dressing, sterile gauze and tape, or adhesive bandage.	Prevents early access of microorganisms to the bloodstream and stabilizes the catheter, thereby reducing irritation of the intimal lining of the vein by the catheter.	Procedures for covering peripheral IV sites vary. Antimicrobial ointment at the catheter insertion site is not recommended.[1,9,28] Research is mixed regarding the efficacy of transparent semipermeable dressings, sterile gauze and tape, or adhesive bandages as IV site dressings.[1,3,23,27]
15. Label the dressing with the date, time, catheter gauge and length, and your initials.	Provides information related to the catheter insertion.	
16. Discard supplies in appropriate containers and wash hands.	Reduces the transmission of microorganisms; standard precautions.	Expedite the delivery of blood specimens to the laboratory, if collected.

Expected Outcomes

- Patent venous access
- Insertion site free of local complications (e.g., pain, edema, tenderness, erythema, blanching, catheter occlusion)
- Patient free of systemic complications (e.g., fever, chills, malaise, tachycardia, respiratory distress, hemoptysis, hypotension, cyanosis)

Unexpected Outcomes

- Pain/severe discomfort during the procedure
- Local complications during or after the procedure (e.g., hematoma, phlebitis, thrombophlebitis, infiltration, catheter occlusion)
- Systemic complications following the procedure (e.g., septicemia, thromboembolus, catheter embolus)

Patient Monitoring and Care

Steps	Rationale	Reportable Conditions
1. Observe the peripheral IV site for signs and symptoms of local complications every hour (continuous infusion) or every 4 hours (IID). Remove the catheter if any of these conditions develop.	Local complications occur more frequently than systemic complications. The catheter (or needle) can become dislodged and can cause infiltration of the infusing substances or blood into the surrounding tissues. Causative factors related to phlebitis can be chemical (related to the infusing solutions), bacterial (related to contamination), or mechanical (related to the catheter).[20] Thrombophlebitis can result from trauma to the vein and venous stasis. Catheter occlusion usually results from inadequate flushing procedures (IID), obstruction to free-flowing infusion (e.g., positional catheter, flexion of extremity), dry solution containers, or precipitate from incompatible solutions or medications.	*These conditions should be reported if they persist despite nursing interventions.* • Edema around the IV site • Pain, tenderness, erythema, blanching • Hardness along the path of the vein when palpated • Drainage from the insertion site

Procedure continues on the following page

Patient Monitoring and Care—*Continued*

Steps	Rationale	Reportable Conditions
2. For IID, assess the catheter for venous blood return and patency before initiating infusions.	Verifies the position of the catheter in the vascular space and patency before initiating infusions.	
3. Assess the patient for signs and symptoms of systemic infection.	Insertion of a peripheral IV catheter causes trauma to the surrounding tissues and the intimal layer of the vessel wall. Proper insertion technique and surveillance will minimize the risk for septicemia. The incidence of infection related to the catheter may result from failure to maintain asepsis during insertion, failure to comply with the dressing change protocols, immunosuppression, frequent access to the catheter, and long-term use of a single peripheral IV access site.	• Fever, chills, malaise, headache (early signs of septicemia)[20] • Tachycardia, hypotension, nausea or vomiting, backache (late signs of septicemia)[20]
4. Assess for signs or symptoms of an emboli. If suspected, place the patient in the left lateral Trendelenburg recumbent position (to trap air in the right heart) and notify the physician immediately.[20]	Emboli can result from the release of a preexisting thrombus, from a portion of the IV catheter, and from the inadvertent introduction of air into the venous system.	• Pulmonary embolus: sudden onset of dyspnea, apprehension, unexplained hemoptysis, tachycardia, shock, cardiac arrest[20] • Catheter embolus: cyanosis, hypotension, tachycardia, jugular venous distension (JVD), loss of consciousness, shock, cardiac arrest • Air embolus: chest pain, shortness of breath, shoulder or back pain, cyanosis, shock, cardiac arrest[20]
5. Follow the institution standard for the frequency and type of dressing change.	Decreases the risk for infection at the catheter site. The CDC has made no recommendation for the frequency of routine peripheral catheter dressing changes, but recommends replacing the dressing when it becomes damp, loosened, or soiled or when inspection of the site is necessary.[1]	
6. Rotate the IV site every 72-96 hours.	The CDC recommends rotating the IV site every 72-96 hours to minimize the risk for phlebitis.[1] IIDs should also be replaced at least every 72-96 hours.[1]	

Documentation

Documentation should include the following:

- Patient and family education
- Known allergies
- Date and time of the procedure
- Catheter type, gauge, and length
- Type and amount of local anesthetic (if used)
- Location of the peripheral IV insertion site and the vein accessed

- Problems encountered during or after the procedure and nursing interventions
- Patient tolerance of the procedure
- Assessment of the insertion site
- Disposition of specimens, if appropriate

References

1. Centers for Disease Control and Prevention. (2002). Guidelines for the prevention of intravascular catheter-related infections. *MMWR,* 51(RR-10), 2-29.
2. Chaiyakunapruk, N., et al. (2002). Chlorhexidine compared with povidone-iodine solution for vascular catheter site care: A meta-analysis. *Ann Intern Med,* 136, 792-801.
3. Craven, D.E., et al. (1985). A randomized study comparing a transparent polyurethane dressing to a gauze dressing for peripheral intravenous catheter sites. *Infect Control,* 6, 361-6.
4. Fetzer, S.J. (2002). Reducing venipuncture and intravenous insertion pain with eutectic mixture of local anesthetic: A meta-analysis. *Nurs Res,* 51, 119-24.
5. Goode, C.J., et al. (1991). A meta-analysis of effects of heparin flush and saline flush: Quality and cost implications. *Nurs Res,* 40, 324-30.
6. Hamilton, R.A., et al. (1988). Heparin sodium versus 0.9% sodium chloride for maintaining patency of indwelling intermittent infusion devices. *Clin Pharm,* 7, 439-443.
7. Himberger, J.R., and Himberger, L.C. (2001). Accuracy of drawing blood through infusing intravenous lines. *Heart Lung,* 30, 66-73.
8. Hussey, V.M., Poulin, M.V., and Fain, J.A. (1997). Effectiveness of lidocaine hydrochloride on venipuncture sites. *AORN J,* 66, 472-5.
9. Infusion Nurses Society. (2002). *Policies and Procedures for Infusion Nursing.* 2nd ed. Philadelphia: Lippincott Williams & Wilkins.
10. Intravenous Nurses Society. (2000). Infusion nursing standards of practice. *J Intraven Nurs,* 23, S1-S78.
11. Jagger, J. (1996). Reducing occupational exposure to bloodborne pathogens: Where do we stand a decade later? *Infect Control Hosp Epidemiol,* 17, 573-5.
12. Jagger, J., et al. (1988). Rates of needle-stick injury caused by various devices in a university hospital. *N Engl J Med,* 319, 284-8.
13. Jensen, B.L. (2001). Infusion therapy equipment: Types of infusion therapy equipment. In: Hankins, J., et al., eds. *Infusion Therapy in Clinical Practice.* 2nd ed. Philadelphia: W.B. Saunders, 300-33.
14. Kennedy, C., et al. (1996). A comparison of hemolysis rates using intravenous catheters versus venipuncture tubes for obtaining blood samples. *J Emerg Nurs,* 22, 566-9.
15. Krozek, C., et al. (1996). Intravascular therapy. In: *Nursing Procedures.* 2nd ed. Springhouse, PA: Springhouse Corp., 380-95.
16. Lander, J., et al. (1996). Evaluation of a new topical anesthetic agent: A pilot study. *Nurs Res,* 45, 50-2.
17. National Committee on Safer Needle Devices. (1997). *Using Safer Needle Devices: The Time Is Now.* Washington, DC: Author.
18. Nott, M., and Peacock, J. (1990). Relief of injection pain in adults: EMLA cream for 5 minutes before venipuncture. *Anaesthesia,* 45, 772-4.
19. Olson, K.L., and Gomes V. (1996). Intravenous therapy needle choices in ambulatory cancer patients. *Clin Nurs Res,* 5, 543-61.
20. Perdue, M. (2001). Intravenous complications. In: Hankins, J., et al., eds. *Infusion Therapy in Clinical Practice.* 2nd ed. Philadelphia: W.B. Saunders, 418-45.
21. Perucca, R. (2001). Infusion monitoring and catheter care. In: Hankins, J., et al., eds. *Infusion Therapy in Clinical Practice.* 2nd ed. Philadelphia: W.B. Saunders, 389-97.
22. Perucca, R. (2001). Obtaining vascular access. In: Hankins, J., et al., eds. *Infusion Therapy in Clinical Practice.* 2nd ed. Philadelphia: W.B. Saunders, 375-88.
23. Pettit, D.M., and Kraus, V. (1995). The use of gauze versus transparent dressings for peripheral intravenous catheter sites. *Nurs Clin North Am,* 30, 495-506.
24. Seeman, S., and Reinhardt, A. (2000). Blood sample collection from a peripheral catheter system compared with phlebotomy. *J IV Nurs,* 23, 290-7.
25. Speakman, E. (1999). Fluid, electrolyte, and acid-base balances. In: Potter, P.A., and Perry, A.G., eds. *Basic Nursing: A Critical Thinking Approach.* 4th ed. St. Louis: Mosby, 857-90.
26. Taylor, N., et al. (1989). Comparison of normal versus heparinized saline for flushing infusion devices. *J Nurs Qual Assur,* 3, 49-55.
27. VandenBosch, T.M., Cooch, J., and Treston-Aurand, J. (1997). Research utilization: Adhesive bandage dressing regimen for peripheral venous catheters. *Am J Infect Control,* 25, 513-9.
28. Zinner, S.H., et al. (1996). Risk of infection with intravenous indwelling catheters: Effect of application of antibiotic ointment. *J Infect Dis,* 120, 616-9.

Additional Readings

Hankins, J., et al., eds. (2001). *Infusion therapy in clinical practice.* 2nd ed. Philadelphia: W.B. Saunders.

Potter, P.A., and Perry, A.G., eds. (2003). *Basic Nursing: A Critical Thinking Approach.* 5th ed. St. Louis: Mosby.

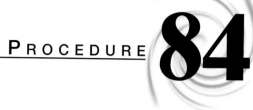
PROCEDURE **84**

Peripherally Inserted Central Catheter

PURPOSE: Peripherally inserted central catheters (PICCs) are used to deliver central venous therapy for 2 weeks to 12 months and to provide venous access for patients who require multiple venipunctures. PICCs are used to administer long-term antibiotic therapy, chemotherapy, total parenteral nutrition, analgesia, blood products, intermittent inotropic (e.g., dobutamine) therapy, and fluids.

Linda Bucher

PREREQUISITE NURSING KNOWLEDGE

- Successful completion of specialized education in PICC insertion and demonstrated competency are required.[5] In addition, opportunities to demonstrate clinical competency on a regular basis (e.g., yearly) may be required.
- Clinical and technical competence in suturing PICC lines in place (if permitted by RN in state of practice)
- Understanding of sterile technique
- Knowledge of the anatomy and physiology of the vasculature and adjacent structures in the upper extremity, neck, and chest. Ideally, the patient receiving a PICC should have a peripheral vein that can accommodate a 14-G or 16-G introducer needle. If necessary, a 22-G microintroducer can be used to dilate a vein to accommodate an introducer sheath. The basilic and cephalic antecubital fossa veins are the preferred veins for cannulation with a PICC (Fig. 84-1). The basilic vein is the larger of the two veins and is the vein of choice for insertion of a PICC. Once inserted, the PICC is advanced to the superior vena cava.[4,5]
- Patient indications for the insertion of a PICC vary. A PICC is used increasingly for patients receiving IV therapy in the home setting for chronic heart failure, cancer treatment, chronic pain management, nutritional support, and fluid replacement (e.g., hyperemesis gravidarum).

- PICCs may be preferred over percutaneously inserted central venous catheters for patients suffering from trauma (e.g., burns) of the chest or from certain pulmonary disorders (e.g., chronic obstructive pulmonary disease, cystic fibrosis).[6]
- PICCs are contraindicated in patients with sclerotic veins and in extremities affected by a mastectomy, an arteriovenous graft, a fistula, or radial artery surgery.
- IV therapy via the PICC poses fewer and less severe complications (including infections) compared with percutaneously inserted central venous catheters. The most common complications associated with the PICC are phlebitis and catheter occlusion.[1,6]
- A variety of PICCs are available for use. PICCs are flexible catheters that are made of silicone or polyurethane. Catheter diameters range from 23 G to 16 G, and catheter length ranges from 40 cm (16 in) to 60 cm (24 in). For adults, 18-G or 20-G catheters that are 60 cm in length are the standard. PICCs are available as single- or double-lumen catheters and can be inserted with or without the use of a guide wire.
- A PICC can be inserted using a guide wire. When a guide wire is used, venous access is achieved with a small gauge (20 or 22 G) peripheral IV catheter (see Procedure 83). Once the IV catheter is inserted, the stylet is removed and the guide wire is threaded through the IV catheter. The IV catheter is then removed, and the dilator/introducer is inserted over the guide wire. The dilator and guide wire are removed, leaving the introducer in the vein to allow for passage of the PICC into the vein. Once the PICC is in place, the introducer is removed. This approach is

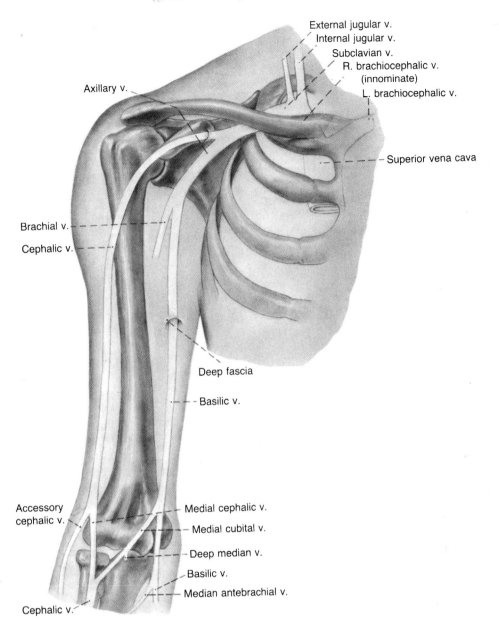

FIGURE 84-1 Location of the veins of the right shoulder and upper arm. *(From Jacob, S.W., and Francone, C.A. [1989]. Elements of Anatomy and Physiology. 2nd ed. Philadelphia: W.B. Saunders.)*

referred to as the modified Seldinger method.[12] Care must be taken with the use of a guide wire. Although advancement of the introducer is enhanced by the firmness provided by the guide wire, the guide wire can inadvertently traumatize the vessel.[6]

- A PICC can also be inserted through a cannula. This involves a venipuncture with a short peripheral IV catheter. The stylet is removed, and the PICC is threaded into the vein. The short peripheral IV catheter is removed by pulling it over the end of the PICC.[12]
- A variety of safety engineered introducers are available and should be used to reduce the risk for blood exposure and needlestick injury.[4,5,8]

EQUIPMENT

- Catheter insertion kit
- PICC catheter of choice
- Single-use tourniquet or blood pressure cuff
- Sterile and nonsterile measuring tape
- Waterproof underpad/linen saver
- Sterile gown and cap
- Mask
- Goggles
- Two pairs of nonpowdered, sterile gloves
- Sterile drapes and towels, including one fenestrated drape
- Antiseptic solution (e.g., 2% chlorhexidine-based preparation)[1]
- 10-ml vial of heparin (concentration and use per institutional policy)
- 30-ml vial of normal saline (NS)
- Luer-Lok injection port (cap) with short extension tubing

- One 10-ml, 20-G, 1-inch needle syringe (blunt needle recommended)
- One 3-ml, 20-G, 1-inch needle syringe or one 5-ml, 20-G, 1-inch needle syringe if inserting a double-lumen catheter (blunt needle recommended)
- Three to four sterile 4 × 4 gauze pads or sponges
- 1% lidocaine without epinephrine, or 1 to 2 ml of eutectic mixture of local anesthetics (EMLA) cream (optional)
- Two sterile 2 × 2 gauze pads or sponges
- Sterile, transparent, semipermeable dressing
  Additional equipment as needed includes the following:
- One 1-ml, 25-G, 5/8-inch needle syringe (if using intradermal lidocaine)
- One 3-0 or 4-0 nylon suture on a small, curved cutting needle (if suturing)
- Alternative catheter securement device (e.g., sterile wound closure strips) if not suturing.

PATIENT AND FAMILY EDUCATION

- Explain the reason for the PICC, as well as the benefits and risks associated with the catheter and the alternatives to PICC placement. ➥*Rationale:* Clarification of information is an expressed patient need and helps to diminish anxiety, enhance acceptance, and encourage questions.
- Describe the major steps of the procedure, including the patient's role in the procedure. ➥*Rationale:* Decreases patient anxiety, enhances cooperation, provides an opportunity for the patient to voice concerns, and prevents accidental contamination of the sterile field and equipment.
- Instruct the patient and family to refuse injections, venipunctures, and blood pressure measurements on the arm with the PICC. ➥*Rationale:* Minimizes the risk for catheter-related complications and catheter damage.
- Provide appropriate patient and family discharge education regarding the care and maintenance of the PICC. ➥*Rationale:* Reduces the risk for catheter-related complications due to lack of knowledge and skills needed to care for the PICC after discharge.

PATIENT ASSESSMENT AND PREPARATION

Patient Assessment

- Assess the patient's past medical history for mastectomy, fistula, shunt, or radial artery surgery. ➥*Rationale:* PICC insertion should be avoided in extremities affected by these conditions, because the risk for complications is increased.
- Obtain the patient's baseline vital signs and cardiac rhythm. ➥*Rationale:* Cardiac dysrhythmias can occur if the catheter is advanced into the heart. Baseline data facilitate the identification of clinical problems and the efficacy of interventions.
- Assess the vasculature of the antecubital space of both arms, focusing on the basilic and cephalic veins (see Fig. 84-1). A tourniquet or blood pressure cuff should be applied on the mid-upper arm for vein assessment and then removed. ➥*Rationale:* Proper vein selection increases the success of insertion and decreases the incidence of postinsertion complications.
- Determine the patient's allergy history (e.g., lidocaine, heparin, EMLA cream, antiseptic solutions, tape, latex). ➥*Rationale:* Decreases the risk for allergic reactions by avoiding known, allergenic products.

Patient Preparation

- Ensure that the patient and family understand preprocedural teaching. Answer questions as they arise and reinforce information as needed. ➥*Rationale:* Evaluates and reinforces understanding of previously taught information.
- Ensure that informed consent has been obtained. ➥*Rationale:* Protects the rights of the patient and allows the patient to make a competent decision.
- Assist the patient to a semi-Fowler's or dorsal recumbent position, depending on the patient's clinical condition and level of comfort. ➥*Rationale:* The upright position allows gravity to assist in directing the catheter downward when advancing the catheter into the innominate vein and superior vena cava. It also may help avoid inadvertent placement of the catheter into the jugular vein.
- Position the selected arm at 45 degrees of extension from the body for anthropometric measurement. For catheter placement in the superior vena cava, use the nonsterile measuring tape to measure the distance from the selected insertion site to the shoulder (Fig. 84-2A) and from the shoulder to the sternal notch (Fig. 84-2B). Add 3 inches (7.5 cm) (or the measured distance from the sternal notch to the third intercostal space) to this number for catheter placement in the superior vena cava. ➥*Rationale:* Extending the extremity allows for displacement of the catheter with arm movement. Accurate measurement ensures proper tip position in the superior vena cava and determines the length of the catheter to be inserted.
- Measure the mid-upper arm circumference of the selected extremity. ➥*Rationale:* Provides a baseline for evaluation of suspected thrombosis. Increases greater than 2 cm over baseline are supportive of venous occlusion.
- Stabilize the position of the arm with a towel or pillow. ➥*Rationale:* Increases patient comfort, secures the work area, and facilitates access to the selected vein.
- Instruct the patient on proper head positioning. The head is positioned to the contralateral side (away from the insertion site) throughout the procedure, except when advancing the catheter from the axillary vein to the superior vena cava. At this point, the patient is instructed to position his or her head toward the ipsilateral side (toward the insertion site) with the chin dropped to the shoulder. ➥*Rationale:* Limits the risk for inadvertently directing the catheter into the jugular vein.

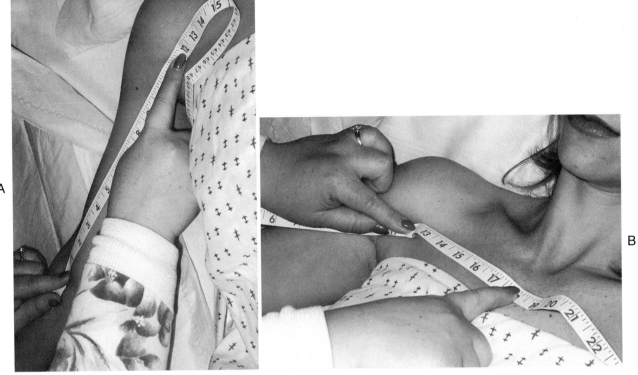

FIGURE 84-2 Measurement of the catheter length for placement in the superior vena cava. **A,** First, measure the distance from the selected insertion site to the shoulder. **B,** Continue measuring from the shoulder to the sternal notch, and add 3 inches (7.5 cm) to this number.

Procedure for Peripherally Inserted Central Catheter

Steps	Rationale	Special Considerations
1. Wash hands.	Reduces the transmission of microorganisms; standard precautions.	
2. Place a waterproof pad under the selected arm.	Avoids soiling bed linens.	
3. Position the tourniquet high on the upper extremity, near the axilla, but do not constrict venous blood flow at this time.	Placement high on the extremity avoids contamination of the sterile field.	A blood pressure cuff may be used in place of a tourniquet.
4. Open the PICC insertion tray and drop the remaining sterile items onto the sterile field.	Maintains aseptic technique; prepares the work area, including procurement of all necessary equipment; avoids interruption of the procedure and contamination of the work area.	
5. Don cap, mask, goggles, sterile gown, and sterile gloves.	Standard precautions; PICC insertion is a sterile procedure.	Blood splashing may occur with the use of guide wires, stylets, and breakaway or peel-away introducers.

Procedure continues on the following page

Procedure for **Peripherally Inserted Central Catheter**—*Continued*

Steps	Rationale	Special Considerations
6. Using the sterile measuring tape, cut the catheter to the predetermined length. A. Add 1 inch (2.5 cm) to the premeasured length to be left outside the insertion site. B. Remove the guide wire and cut the tip of the catheter straight across with the sterile scissors (Fig. 84-3).	Catheters are provided at various lengths. Prevents the catheter tip from lying flush against the vessel wall, which can increase the incidence of clot formation.	A catheter with a guide wire or stylet is recommended to reduce the risk of the catheter coiling or knotting in the vein and for ease in insertion.
7. Reinsert the guide wire so that the tip of the wire is covered by approximately 0.5 to 1 cm of the catheter.	Facilitates the removal of the guide wire; provides softness and flexibility at the catheter tip, thus preventing perforation of the vein during insertion.	
8. Fill the 10-ml syringe with NS. Add the injection port (cap) to the short-extension tubing and prime it with NS. Leave the syringe attached.	Avoids inadvertently introducing air into the system.	If inserting a double-lumen catheter, prime the additional lumen of the catheter with NS.
9. Prepare the site using a 2% chlorhexidine-based antiseptic solution.[1,4,5] Cleanse the site using a back-and-forth motion while applying friction for 30 seconds. Allow the antiseptic to remain on the insertion site and to air-dry completely before catheter insertion.[1,4,5]	Limits the introduction of potentially infectious skin flora into the vessel during the puncture.	
10. Remove gloves, wash hands, and apply the tourniquet (or blood pressure cuff) snugly, approximately 6 inches (15 cm) above the antecubital fossa.	Provides vasodilatation of the vein for venipuncture.	Constriction should effectively cause venous distention without arterial occlusion. A blood pressure cuff may be used and may be more effective, especially with obese patients. After the cuff is inflated, palpate the radial artery to assess for arterial blood flow.

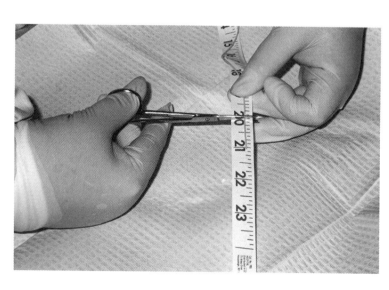

FIGURE 84-3 Measuring and cutting the catheter tip to the premeasured length.

Procedure for Peripherally Inserted Central Catheter—*Continued*

Steps	Rationale	Special Considerations
11. Don a new pair of sterile gloves. Instruct the patient to lift his or her arm, and place a sterile drape underneath and the fenestrated drape over the prepared area, leaving the venipuncture site exposed. Place a sterile 4 × 4 gauze pad over the tourniquet. Instruct the patient to turn his or her head away from the insertion site.	Maintains the sterile field and facilitates aseptic technique. Prevents contamination of the field by organisms from the patient's respiratory tract.	
12. Inject a skin weal of approximately 0.5 ml of 1% lidocaine without epinephrine at or adjacent to the venipuncture site. *(Level V: Clinical studies in more than one or two different patient populations and situations to support recommendations.)*	Provides local anesthesia for venipuncture with large-gauge needles and introducers. Research suggests that local anesthesia should be considered when inserting a PICC.[2,3,4,5,7,9]	Most patients report less pain when a local anesthetic agent is used before venipuncture.[2,3] Lidocaine may produce stinging, burning, obliteration of the vein, or venospasm. The use of EMLA (a topical anesthetic cream) before venipuncture has been researched.[2,7,9] If it is used, the manufacturer's recommendations should be followed.
13. Perform the venipuncture according to catheter design and manufacturer's instructions.	Catheters vary according to design and introducing techniques.	
14. Perform the modified Seldinger technique (Fig. 84-4): A. Insert a peripheral IV and observe for blood return in the flashback chamber (Fig. 84-4[1 and 2]). B. Remove the stylet and advance the guide wire 2 to 4 inches (5-10 cm) through the IV catheter (Fig. 84-4[3]).[6] C. Remove the IV catheter and insert the dilator/introducer over the guide wire (Fig. 84-4[4]). D. Gently advance the dilator/introducer until the tip is well within the vein (Fig. 84-4[5]). E. Remove the dilator and guide wire, leaving the introducer in place (Fig. 84-4[6]).[6] F. Insert the catheter approximately 6 to 8 inches (15 to 20 cm) (Fig. 84-4[7]).	Verifies venous access. Use of a guide wire enhances the advancement of the dilator/introducer. Establishes venous access.	Place a finger over the orifice of the catheter to limit blood loss and risk for air embolism. (Fig. 84-4[2]). If there is no blood return, the procedure should be terminated and an alternate access site selected. A small skin nick may be performed at the venipuncture site to facilitate the advancement of the dilator/introducer (Fig. 84-4[3]). If a scalpel is not provided in the PICC insertion kit, a #11 blade should be used. Place a finger over the orifice of the introducer to limit blood loss and the risk for air embolism (Fig. 84-4[6]). Sterile forceps may be used to insert the catheter into the introducer and advance the catheter into the vein.
15. Release the tourniquet using the sterile 4 × 4 gauze pad.	Continued vasodilatation may not be required for catheter advancement.	If a blood pressure cuff is used, it may remain inflated throughout the advancement of the catheter. Leaving the tourniquet in place (or the blood pressure cuff inflated) may facilitate catheter advancement if vascular insufficiency is evident.

Procedure continues on the following page

Modified Seldinger Technique

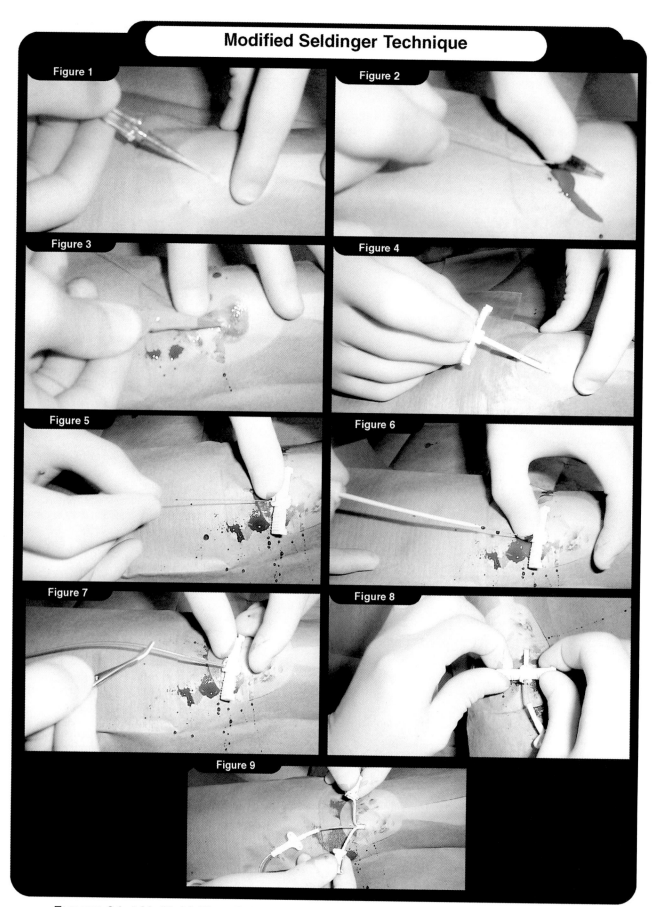

FIGURE 84-4 Modified Seldinger Technique. **1,** Insertion of peripheral intravenous catheter. **2,** Advancement of guide wire through the catheter. **3,** Small skin nick to facilitate advancement of dilator/introducer. **4,** Insertion of dilator/introducer over guide wire. **5,** Advancement of dilator/introducer. **6,** Removal of dilator and guide wire. **7,** Insertion of catheter using sterile forceps. **8,** Removal of introducer. **9,** Introducer peeled apart and removed. *(Courtesy Bard Access Systems, Salt Lake City, UT.)*

Procedure for Peripherally Inserted Central Catheter—*Continued*

Steps	Rationale	Special Considerations
16. Instruct the patient to turn his or her head toward the cannulated arm and to drop his or her chin to the chest.	Changes the angle of the jugular vein and decreases the potential for malpositioning of the catheter in the jugular vein.	
17. Advance the remainder of the catheter until approximately 4 inches (10 cm) remain. Observe (or palpate) the heart rate and rhythm.	Cardiac dysrhythmias may occur if the catheter is advanced into the heart.	Never advance the catheter if resistance is felt. Excessive pushing could lead to perforation of the vein or myocardium.
18. Instruct the patient to return his or her head to the contralateral side (away from the insertion site).	Prevents contamination of the field by organisms from the patient's respiratory tract.	
19. Pull the introducer out of the vein and away from the insertion site and remove (Fig. 84-4[8 and 9]).	The introducer sheath is not needed once the catheter is in place.	Methods of removing the introducer vary according to the manufacturer.
20. Measure the length of the catheter remaining outside the skin and reposition, if necessary, to the predetermined length. Approximately 1 inch (2.5 cm) of the catheter should remain externally.	Ensures proper catheter tip position.	
21. Attach the primed extension tubing (with injection port) to the catheter; aspirate for evidence of blood, and flush with NS using a push/pause technique.	Use of extension tubing provides easier access to the catheter and reduces local trauma at the insertion site. Aspiration affirms patency of the catheter. The push/pause technique while flushing optimizes catheter long-term patency.[4,5]	
22. Inject the recommended amount and concentration of heparin into the catheter, clamp the extension tubing, and remove the syringe. Repeat the procedure if using a double-lumen catheter.	Maintains catheter patency and prevents backflow of blood in the catheter.	Recommendations vary regarding the use, amount, and concentration of heparin to maintain catheter patency.[10,11] Contraindicated in persons with known allergies to heparin. Institutional policies should be followed.
23. Secure the catheter at the insertion site by suturing or by applying an alternate catheter securement device (Fig. 84-5).	Prevents inward or outward migration of the catheter.	A nylon suture is recommended.[10] The procedure should follow institutional guidelines.
24. Cover the insertion site with a sterile, 2 × 2 gauze pad(s). Cover the site with a sterile, transparent, semipermeable dressing (Fig. 84-6).[6]	Decreases catheter-related infections.	2 × 2 gauze can be folded and placed immediately below the insertion site to act as a "wick" for any drainage in the first 24 hours. It is not needed after the first dressing change.

Procedure continues on the following page

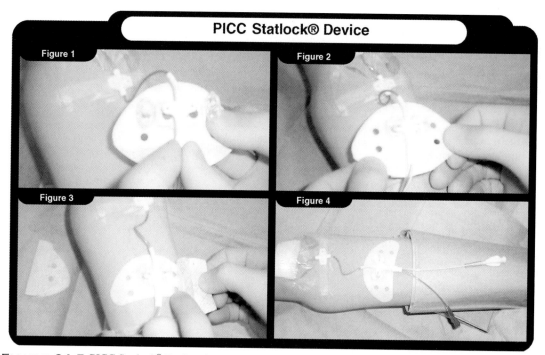

FIGURE 84-5 PICC Statlock® Device. **1,** Insertion of the wings of the PICC onto device. **2,** Placement of device on forearm. **3,** Application of sterile, transparent, semipermeable dressing over device. **4,** Device properly secured. *(Courtesy Bard Access Systems, Salt Lake City, UT.)*

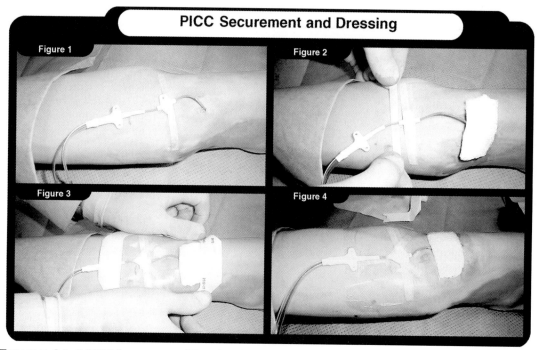

FIGURE 84-6 PICC Securement and Dressing. **1,** Securement of the wings of the PICC with a sterile wound closure strip (if sutures are not used). **2,** Placement of a sterile wound closure strip, using a chevron. Placement of a sterile 2 × 2 gauze pad over the insertion site, if initial dressing. **3,** Application of sterile, transparent, semipermeable dressing. **4,** PICC properly secured and dressed. *(Courtesy Bard Access Systems, Salt Lake City, UT.)*

Procedure for Peripherally Inserted Central Catheter—*Continued*

Steps	Rationale	Special Considerations
25. Discard used supplies and wash hands.	Reduces the transmission of microorganisms and body secretions; standard precautions.	
26. Prepare the patient for a chest x-ray.	Confirms placement of the catheter tip and detects any complications.	Some PICCs require contrast media for good visualization. Infusions should not be initiated until the catheter tip placement is confirmed.

Expected Outcomes

- The PICC tip is positioned in the superior vena cava.
- The PICC remains patent.
- The insertion site and upper extremity remain free of phlebitis and thrombophlebitis.
- The insertion site, catheter, and systemic circulation remain free of infection.

Unexpected Outcomes

- Pain or severe discomfort during the procedure
- Complications on insertion, such as cardiac dysrhythmias, pericardial tamponade, air embolism, catheter embolism, arterial puncture, nerve (brachial plexus) injury
- Complications following insertion, such as phlebitis, thrombophlebitis, catheter occlusion, infection (e.g., insertion site, catheter, systemic), infiltration

Patient Monitoring and Care

Steps	Rationale	Reportable Conditions
		These conditions should be reported if they persist despite nursing interventions.
1. Observe the patient for signs or symptoms of cardiac dysrhythmias and pericardial tamponade during the procedure. If cardiac dysrhythmias occur, pull the catheter back and reassess the patient.	Cardiac dysrhythmias may occur if the catheter is advanced into the heart. Pericardial tamponade may occur if the catheter penetrates the atrium.	- Cardiac dysrhythmias - Hemodynamic instability (changes in vital signs, level of consciousness, peripheral pulses, narrow pulse pressure, jugular venous distention)
2. Assess the patient and obtain the chest x-ray report confirming proper catheter tip placement before initiating any intravenous solutions.	Ensures accurate catheter tip placement and aids in identifying potentially life-threatening complications.	- Abnormal chest x-ray report - Change in lung sounds - Chest pain - Respiratory distress
3. Observe the dressing and insertion site every 30 minutes for the first 4 hours after insertion.	Postinsertion bleeding may occur in patients with coagulopathies or with arterial punctures, multiple attempts at venipuncture, or use of the through-the-needle introducer design for insertion.	- Excessive bleeding, hematoma - Changes in vital signs

Procedure continues on the following page

Patient Monitoring and Care—*Continued*

Steps	Rationale	Reportable Conditions
4. Assess the insertion site and upper extremity every shift for signs and symptoms of phlebitis, thrombophlebitis, or infiltration.	Mechanical phlebitis is the most common complication within the first 72 hours postinsertion. Thrombophlebitis may occur within 0 to 10 days of catheter insertion.	• Pain along the vein • Edema at the puncture site • Erythema • Ipsilateral swelling of the arm, neck, face • Venous occlusion (changes in arm circumference greater than 2 cm from baseline) • Infiltration (infusion continues in spite of restriction to venous blood flow by tourniquet)
5. Assess the catheter for venous blood return and patency before initiating infusions. Connect a 10-ml syringe filled with 10 ml of NS to the extension tubing. Release the clamp and aspirate slowly to verify blood return. Flush with 10 ml of NS (using a push/pause technique) and then administer the infusion.	Verifies position of the catheter in the vascular space and patency before initiating infusions.	• Catheter occlusion (failure to obtain blood return on aspiration or resistance to irrigation)
6. Assess the catheter for dislodgment or migration by measuring the length of the external catheter.	The catheter may no longer be properly positioned if the length of the external catheter is longer or shorter than the length measured at the time of insertion.	• Change in external catheter length • Catheter occlusion • Cardiac dysrhythmias • Pain or burning during infusions • Palpation of the catheter in the internal jugular vein • Palpation of a coiled catheter • Infiltration
7. The initial dressing should be left in place for 24 hours. After this, assess the insertion site and upper forearm while performing a sterile dressing change. Transparent, semipermeable dressings should be changed at least weekly.[1] Sterile gauze dressings should be changed every 48 hours.[4,5] Dressings should be changed if they become damp, loosened, or visibly soiled.[1]	Policies may vary regarding the type of dressing and frequency of dressing changes after the initial dressing change.	• Redness, warmth, hardness, tenderness or pain, swelling at the insertion site • Presence of purulent drainage from the insertion site • Local rash or pustules
8. Monitor the insertion site and patient for signs and symptoms of local or systemic infection.	The incidence of infection related to the catheter may result from failure to maintain asepsis during insertion, failure to comply with dressing change protocols, immunosuppression, frequent access to the catheter, and long-term use of a single IV access site.	• Redness, warmth, hardness, tenderness or pain, swelling at the insertion site • Presence of purulent drainage from the insertion site • Local rash or pustules • Fever, chills, elevated white blood cell count • Nausea and vomiting
9. Avoid measuring blood pressure, performing venipunctures, or administering injections in the extremity with a PICC.	Minimizes the risk for catheter-related complications and catheter damage.	

Documentation

Documentation should include the following:

- Patient and family education
- Signature on the informed consent form
- Known allergies
- Mid-upper arm circumference
- Date and time of the procedure
- Catheter type, size, and length, including the length of catheter remaining outside the insertion site
- Type and amount of local anesthetic (if used)

- The location of the PICC insertion site and the vein accessed
- The method of securing catheter (suture, Steri-Strips)
- Confirmation of the catheter tip placement
- Problems encountered during or after the procedure or nursing interventions
- Patient tolerance of the procedure
- Vital signs and cardiac rhythm
- Assessment of the insertion site

References

1. Centers for Disease Control and Prevention. (2002). Guidelines for the prevention of intravascular catheter-related infections. *MMWR, 51*(RR-10), 2-29.
2. Fetzer, S.J. (2002). Reducing venipuncture and intravenous insertion pain with eutectic mixture of local anesthetic: A meta-analysis. *Nurs Res, 51,* 119-24.
3. Hussey, V.M., Poulin, M.V., and Fain, J.A. (1997). Effectiveness of lidocaine hydrochloride on venipuncture sites. *AORN J, 66,* 472-5.
4. Infusion Nurses Society. (2002). *Policies and Procedures for Infusion Nursing.* 2nd ed. Philadelphia: Lippincott Williams & Wilkins.
5. Intravenous Nurses Society. (2000). Infusion nursing standards of practice. *J Intraven Nurs, 23,* S1-S78.
6. Josephson, D.L. (2004). *Intravenous Infusion Therapy for Nurses.* 2nd ed. Clifton Park, NY: Thomson Delmar Learning.
7. Lander, J., et al. (1996). Evaluation of a new topical anesthetic agent: A pilot study. *Nurs Res, 45,* 50-2.
8. National Committee on Safer Needle Devices. (1997). *Using Safer Needle Devices: The Time Is Now.* Washington, DC: Author.
9. Nott, M., and Peacock, J. (1990). Relief of injection pain in adults: EMLA cream for 5 minutes before venipuncture. *Anaesthesia, 45,* 772-4.
10. Perdue, M. (2001). Intravenous complications. In: Hankins, J., eds. *Infusion Therapy in Clinical Practice.* 2nd ed. Philadelphia: W.B. Saunders, 418-45.
11. Perucca, R. (2001). Infusion monitoring and catheter care. In: Hankins, J., et al., eds. *Infusion Therapy in Clinical Practice.* 2nd ed. Philadelphia: W.B. Saunders, 389-97.
12. Perucca, R. (2001). Obtaining vascular access. In: Hankins, J., et al., eds. *Infusion Therapy in Clinical Practice.* 2nd ed. Philadelphia: W.B. Saunders, 375-88.

Additional Readings

Corrigan, A., Pelletier, G., and Alexander, M. (2000). *Core Curriculum for Intravenous Nursing.* Philadelphia: Lippincott Williams & Wilkins.

Hankins, J., et al., eds. (2001). *Infusion Therapy in Clinical Practice.* 2nd ed. Philadelphia: W.B. Saunders.

Potter, P.A., and Perry A.G., eds. (2003). *Basic Nursing: A Critical Thinking Approach.* 5th ed. St. Louis: Mosby.

Weinstein, S.M. (2000). *Plumer's Principles and Practice of Intravenous Therapy.* 7th ed. Philadelphia: Lippincott Williams & Wilkins.

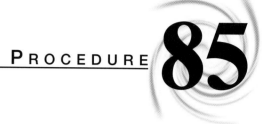

PROCEDURE **85**

Venipuncture

P U R P O S E : Venipuncture is performed to obtain a sample of venous blood suitable for a variety of laboratory tests (e.g., measurement of serum electrolytes, blood urea nitrogen, creatinine, prothrombin time, partial thromboplastin time, cardiac enzymes, complete blood count, amylase). Proper specimen collection and handling are integral to the accuracy of the results; the likelihood of introducing error is greater in these areas than during the actual laboratory analysis.

Linda Bucher

PREREQUISITE NURSING KNOWLEDGE

- Nurses must be adequately prepared to perform venipuncture. This preparation should include specific educational content regarding venipuncture and opportunities to demonstrate clinical competency.
- Understanding of the principles of aseptic technique.
- Knowledge of the anatomy and physiology of the vasculature and adjacent structures in the upper extremity. The most commonly used veins are located on the forearm (e.g., cephalic, median cubital veins), followed by those on the dorsum of the hand (e.g., dorsal venous arch, metacarpal plexus) (Figs. 85-1 and 85-2).[4]
- Superficial veins lie in loose connective tissue under the skin and are best suited for venipuncture.[6] Typically, venipuncture is performed using a vein in the antecubital fossa.[4]
- Patient indications for venipuncture vary and can include patients with suspected electrolyte imbalances, bleeding disorders, infections, and myocardial infarctions.
- For patients who require frequent venous sampling and who have limited peripheral access, cannulation of a central vein should be considered.
- The most common complication associated with venipuncture is hematoma. Less common complications include excessive pain, excessive bleeding, thrombosis, phlebitis, nerve damage and cellulitis.[2]

- Modifications to the specimen collection procedure are related to specific laboratory tests. These can include not using a tourniquet and requesting the patient not to clench his or her fist during the venipuncture (e.g., lactate levels), placing the specimen on ice immediately after collection (e.g., ammonia levels), and avoiding use of alcohol to prep the skin before collection (e.g., blood alcohol levels).[5]
- A variety of safety devices are available and should be used to reduce the risk for needlestick injury.[9,13]

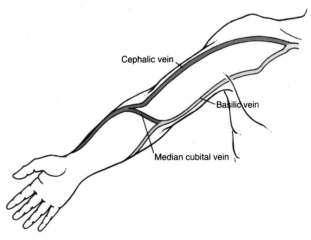

FIGURE 85-1 Superficial veins of the upper extremity. *(From Flynn JC. [1999]. Procedures in Phlebotomy. 2nd ed. Philadelphia: W.B. Saunders.)*

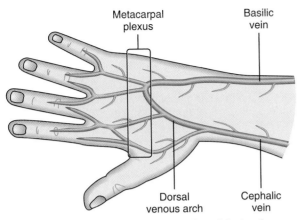

FIGURE 85-2 Superficial veins of the hand.

EQUIPMENT

- One pair of nonsterile gloves
- Single-use tourniquet
- VACUTAINER® adapter
- VACUTAINER® needle (20-, 21-, or 22-G) or 23-G butterfly blood collection set
- Antiseptic solution (e.g., 2% chlorhexidine-based preparation)[1]
- One 2 × 2 gauze pad
- One adhesive bandage
- Biohazard box for discarding used needles
- Appropriate color-coded collection tubes (including extras)
- Appropriate specimen labels and laboratory forms
  Additional equipment as needed includes the following:
- 10-20 ml syringe with a 20-G or 21-G needle (if VACUTAINER® or similar system is not available)
- Additional antiseptic solution (if drawing blood for blood cultures)
- Plastic bag with ice
- Lidocaine or eutectic mixture of local anesthetics (EMLA) cream (optional)

PATIENT AND FAMILY EDUCATION

- Explain the reason for the venipuncture to the patient and family. ➳*Rationale:* Clarification of information is an expressed patient and family need and helps to diminish anxiety, enhance acceptance, and encourage questions.
- Describe the overall steps of the procedure, including the patient's role in the procedure. ➳*Rationale:* Decreases patient anxiety, enhances cooperation, and provides an opportunity for the patient to voice concerns; prevents accidental movement during the procedure.

PATIENT ASSESSMENT AND PREPARATION

Patient Assessment

- Assess the patient's current anticoagulation therapy or blood dyscrasias. ➳*Rationale:* Anticoagulation therapy or blood dyscrasias could prolong hemostasis at the puncture site and increase the risk for hematoma formation or excessive bleeding.
- Assess the patient's allergy history (e.g., lidocaine, EMLA cream, antiseptic solutions, latex, adhesives). ➳*Rationale:* Reduces the risk for allergic reactions.
- Determine whether the patient has a history of mastectomy, fistula, shunt, vascular injury, or radial artery surgery. ➳*Rationale:* Venipuncture should be avoided in extremities affected by these conditions.
- Determine the current intravenous (IV) therapy or blood administration. ➳*Rationale:* Venipuncture should be avoided in extremities with these therapies, because they may alter the accuracy of the test results.[4] If the patient is receiving IV therapy in both arms, venipuncture should be performed below the site of the IV line.
- Determine the best venipuncture site on the patient's arms. ➳*Rationale:* Lower extremities should be avoided in adults. Hand veins should be avoided, because they lie just beneath the surface of the skin and tend to roll. Avoid edematous areas or sites of previous hematoma, infection, or vascular injury and veins that are very small, sclerosed, scarred, or tortuous, because these conditions inhibit successful venipuncture and can contribute to complications.
- Determine whether IV access (peripheral or central) is to be initiated in addition to venipuncture. ➳*Rationale:* Accurate laboratory samples can be collected during the initiation of IV access, thereby limiting the number of venipunctures required.[10,15]

Patient Preparation

- Ensure that the patient and family understand preprocedural teaching. Answer questions as they arise and reinforce information as needed. ➳*Rationale:* Evaluates and reinforces understanding of previously taught information.
- Position the patient in a supine position with the head of the bed slightly elevated and his or her arms at the side. ➳*Rationale:* Proper positioning of the patient enhances accessibility to the venipuncture site and promotes patient comfort.
- Extend the patient's upper extremity to form a straight line from the shoulder to the wrist. A pillow can be placed under the arm for support, if needed. ➳*Rationale:* Proper positioning of the extremity enhances accessibility to the venipuncture site and reduces the risk for patient movement during the procedure.

Procedure for Venipuncture

Steps	Rationale	Special Considerations
1. Gather the supplies, including extra tubes, and attach the VACUTAINER® needle (20-G, 21-G, or 22-G) to the adapter (Fig. 85-3).	Extra tubes avoid interruption of the procedure. Proper needle size minimizes trauma to the vein and the risk for hemolysis.[10]	If using a butterfly (23-G), attach a syringe or a VACUTAINER® adapter to the butterfly blood collection set (Fig. 85-4A). A 10-20 ml syringe with a 20-G or 21-G needle can also be used to perform venipuncture.
2. Wash hands and don nonsterile gloves.	Reduces the transmission of microorganisms; standard precautions.	

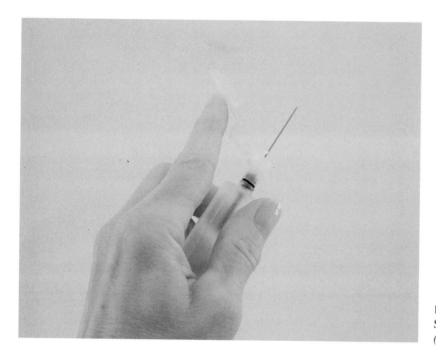

FIGURE 85-3 VACUTAINER® SAFETY-LOK™ needle attached to adapter. *(Courtesy Becton Dickinson.)*

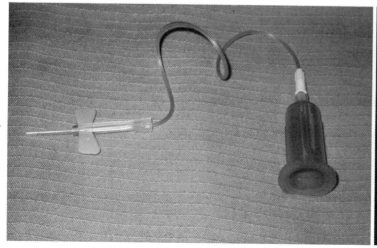
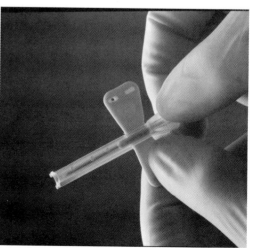

A   B

FIGURE 85-4 VACUTAINER® SAFETY-LOK™ Blood Collection Set. **A,** SAFETY-LOK™ blood collection set before use. **B,** SAFETY-LOK™ blood collection set after use and with needle guard activated. *(Courtesy Becton Dickinson.)*

Procedure for Venipuncture—*Continued*

Steps	Rationale	Special Considerations
3. Apply the tourniquet 2 inches above the area chosen for venipuncture. Tie in a manner so that the tourniquet can be released by pulling on one end (Fig. 85-5).	Impedes venous return to the heart and produces venous dilation. Proper application of the tourniquet allows for the quick, one-handed release of the tourniquet when desired.	Arterial blood flow should not be impeded. Arterial perfusion should be verified by palpating for the radial pulse. For patients with large, prominent veins, a tourniquet is not recommended.[1]
4. Use the tip of the index or second finger to palpate the area across the arm at the elbow. If veins are not prominent, instruct the patient to open and close his or her hand (make a fist) several times, ending with a clenched fist. If a vein still cannot be palpated, remove the tourniquet and apply it to the alternate arm.	Veins should be palpated before venipuncture to improve the chance of success. The milking action of opening and closing the hand causes blood to flow into the veins.	Alternative approaches to facilitating venous distention include gentle tapping of the skin over the venipuncture area with the index and second fingers and permitting the arm to hang dependent below the level of the heart. Warm compresses also can be applied to facilitate venous dilation. The tourniquet should not be left on for more than 2 minutes because it may result in hemoconcentration or variation in blood test values.[4]
5. If lidocaine or EMLA cream is to be used, remove the tourniquet and apply it to the site selected for	Provides relief from pain associated with venipuncture and may reduce or eliminate	Research on the length of time from the application of lidocaine or EMLA cream to the procedure has

Procedure continues on the following page

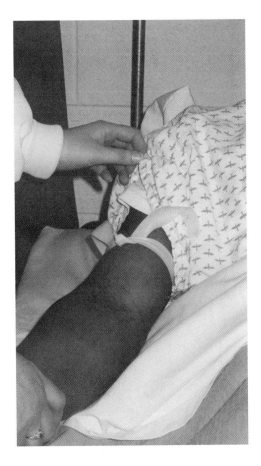

FIGURE 85-5 Proper application of the tourniquet.

Procedure for Venipuncture—*Continued*

Steps	Rationale	Special Considerations
venipuncture. *(Level VI: Clinical studies in a variety of patient populations and situations to support recommendations.)*	anxiety associated with the procedure.[3,7,11,14]	produced mixed results.[3,7,11,14] If used, the manufacturer's recommendations for application should be followed. The time from application to procedure varies from 5 to 170 minutes.
6. Prepare the intended site using a 2% chlorhexidine-based antiseptic solution. Cleanse the site using a back-and-forth motion while applying friction for 30 seconds. Allow the antiseptic to remain on the insertion site and to air-dry completely before catheter insertion.[1,8,9]	Limits the introduction of potentially infectious skin flora into the vessel during the puncture.	If you must palpate the area once cleansing has been performed, use sterile gloves or recleanse the area.[4]
7. Draw the skin taut just below the venipuncture site using the thumb of the nondominant hand.	Immobilizes the vein for venipuncture.	
8. Push the stopper of the collecting tube into the needle up to the guideline on the VACUTAINER® adapter.	Prepares the VACUTAINER® system for blood collection and limits the need for manipulation of equipment once the venipuncture is made.	
9. Collecting tubes are filled in the following order: A. Blood culture tubes B. Empty tubes, generally plain, red-top tubes, or tubes with gel separators without clot enhancers C. Tubes with additives, generally light blue, then lavender, and gray[4]	Minimizes the risk for bacterial contamination.[4] Tissue fluids may interfere with coagulation studies.[4] Additives from the tubes may interfere with the accuracy of the laboratory results if there is any carryover between collection tubes.[4]	Consult the manufacturer's recommendations and protocols within your institution. If a coagulation tube is the only tube requested, a plain, red-top tube should be collected first and discarded.[4] Recent research has suggested that a discard tube may not be necessary.[12]
10. Position the needle with the bevel up and the shaft parallel to (along side of) the path of the vein.	Provides the least traumatic entry through the skin.	
11. Insert the needle through the skin at a 15- to 30-degree angle and ¼ to ½ inches below the intended entry into the vein (Fig. 85-6).	Provides the least traumatic entry of the needle into the vein and limits the risk for hematoma.	As the needle pierces the vein, a sensation of resistance may be felt, followed by ease of penetration.

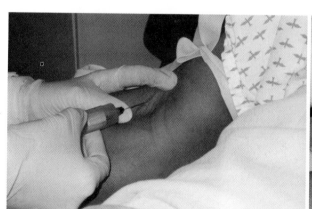
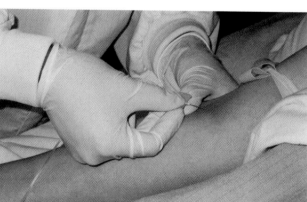

A   B

FIGURE 85-6 Venipuncture. **A,** VACUTAINER® system. **B,** VACUTAINER® butterfly blood collection system. *(Courtesy Becton Dickinson.)*

Procedure for Venipuncture—*Continued*

Steps	Rationale	Special Considerations
12. Grasp the flange of the needle adapter and push the collecting tube forward until the needle punctures the stopper. Observe for the flow of blood into the collecting tube.	Stabilizes the needle in the vein and activates the vacuum within the collecting tube, thereby facilitating the flow of blood into the tube.	If blood does not flow, move the needle slightly in and out. Change the collecting tube to ascertain whether or not the first tube had vacuum. If blood still does not flow, release the tourniquet, remove the needle, apply pressure with the gauze, and attempt a second venipuncture at a new location and with a new needle.
13. If a butterfly is being used, blood flow will first be observed in the tubing (Fig. 85-7A). Once blood flow is established, grasp the flange of the butterfly needle adapter and push the collecting tube forward until the needle punctures the stopper. Observe for the flow of blood into the collecting tube (Fig. 85-7B).	Activates the vacuum within the collecting tube, thereby facilitatingthe flow of blood into the tube.	
14. If a syringe is being used, observe for blood in the hub. Withdraw blood slowly by pulling gently on the plunger of the syringe until the required sample is obtained.		Safety devices should be used to transfer blood from syringe to collecting tubes (Fig. 85-8).
15. Release the tourniquet as soon as blood flow is established. Allow blood to fill the collecting tube until the vacuum is exhausted.	Prevents stasis and hemoconcentration, which can impair the accuracy of test results.[4]	If blood flow is sluggish, the tourniquet may be kept in place. Once blood flow is established, have the patient release his or her clenched fist, if appropriate.
16. While holding the adapter steady, remove the collecting tube and replace it with a new tube. Repeat until all required tubes are filled.	Prevents the inadvertent dislodgment of the needle.	For tubes containing an additive (e.g., anticoagulant), gently rotate five to ten times by inversion. Do not mix tubes that contain no additive.

Procedure continues on the following page

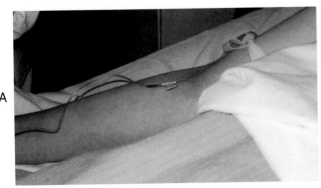
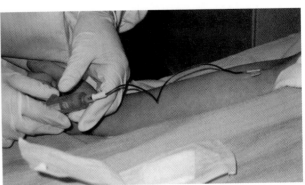

A   B

FIGURE 85-7 Venipuncture using the VACUTAINER® butterfly blood collection system. **A,** Flow of blood into the tubing of the butterfly establishes successful venipuncture. **B,** Flow of blood into the collecting tube once the vacuum is activated. *(Courtesy Becton Dickinson.)*

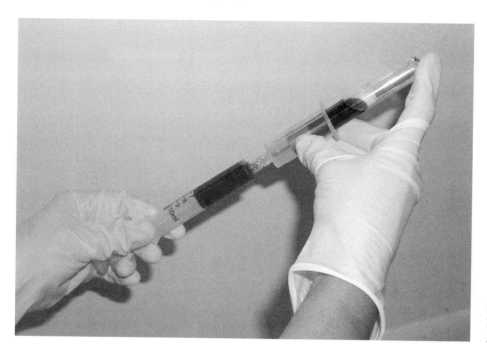

FIGURE 85-8 VACUTAINER®
Blood Transfer Device. *(Courtesy
Becton Dickinson.)*

Procedure for Venipuncture—*Continued*

Steps	Rationale	Special Considerations
17. To remove the needle, release the tourniquet, if not already done. Place a gauze pad over the puncture site and gently remove the needle.	Limits the risk for the development of a hematoma.	The last collecting tube must be removed from the adapter to release the vacuum before removing the needle.
18. Activate the safety device and place the needle and adapter directly into the biohazard container.	Limits the risk for accidental puncture by a contaminated needle.	Equipment varies and should be designed to provide protection from needlesticks on removal of the needle (see Fig. 85-4B).[13]
19. Apply continuous pressure to the gauze pad over the puncture site for 2 to 3 minutes.	Prevents extravasation of blood into the surrounding tissues and limits the development of a hematoma.	Continued pressure may be necessary for patients with a history of blood dyscrasias or receiving anticoagulation therapy. If bleeding persists, the extremity may be elevated above the level of the heart while maintaining pressure to the site. Avoid flexing the extremity because this enhances hematoma formation.
20. Once hemostasis has been established, apply an adhesive bandage to the venipuncture site.	Limits the risk for infection at the venipuncture site.	
21. Label the specimens and complete the laboratory requisitions per protocol.	Ensures accuracy of the results (e.g., right patient, right specimen, right test).	
22. Expedite the delivery of the specimens to the laboratory.	Ensures the timeliness of the laboratory analyses.	
23. Dispose of gloves and equipment properly; wash hands.	Reduces the transmission of microorganisms; standard precautions.	

Expected Outcomes

- Venous sample collected in a way that maintains accuracy of the results
- Puncture site free of complications (e.g., hematoma, pain, excessive bleeding, thrombosis, phlebitis, and cellulitis)
- Alterations in laboratory values identified and treated accordingly

Unexpected Outcomes

- Excessive pain or severe discomfort during the procedure
- Hemolyzed specimens
- Complications following venipuncture: hematoma, excessive bleeding, thrombosis, phlebitis, and cellulitis

Patient Monitoring and Care

Steps	Rationale	Reportable Conditions
		These conditions should be reported if they persist despite nursing interventions.
1. Observe the venipuncture site for signs of hemostasis after the procedure.	A postpuncture hematoma can occur if the needle passes through both walls of the vein, if the needle bevel is not fully seated in the vein, if the extremity is flexed after needle removal, or if insufficient time is spent applying pressure to the venipuncture site. Postpuncture bleeding is more likely to occur in patients with coagulopathies or in patients receiving anticoagulation therapy.	• Excessive bleeding • Large hematoma • Changes in vital signs
2. Assess the venipuncture site and the involved extremity for signs of postprocedure complications (e.g., thrombosis, phlebitis, cellulitis).	All venipunctures cause trauma to the surrounding tissues and the intimal layer of the vessel wall. This trauma causes cells and platelets to aggregate. The greater the trauma, the greater the risk for complications. Proper technique minimizes these risks.	• Erythema, warmth, hardness, tenderness, or pain at the venipuncture site or along the path of the vein • Presence of purulent drainage from the puncture site

Documentation

Documentation should include the following:

- Patient and family education
- Date, time, and laboratory tests requested
- Venipuncture site used
- Local anesthetic used (if applicable)
- Patient's tolerance of the procedure
- Postvenipuncture site care
- Disposition of specimen(s), results, and analysis
- Unexpected outcomes
- Additional interventions

References

1. Centers for Disease Control and Prevention. (2002). Guidelines for the prevention of intravascular catheter-related infections. *MMWR,* 51(RR-10), 2-29.
2. Chukhraev, A.M., Grekov, I.G., and Aivazyan, M. (2000). Local complications of nursing interventions on peripheral veins. *J IV Nurs,* 23, 167-9.
3. Fetzer, S.J. (2002). Reducing venipuncture and intravenous insertion pain with eutectic mixture of local anesthetic: A meta-analysis. *Nurs Res,* 51, 119-24.
4. Flynn, J.C. (1999). Proper procedures for venipuncture. In: *Procedures in Phlebotomy.* 2nd ed. Philadelphia: W.B. Saunders, 87-113.
5. Flynn, J.C. (1999). Special collection procedures. In: *Procedures in Phlebotomy.* 2nd ed. Philadelphia: W.B. Saunders, 115-34.
6. Hadaway, L.C. (2001). Anatomy and physiology related to intravenous therapy. In: Hankins, J., et al., eds. *Infusion Therapy in Clinical Practice.* 2nd ed. Philadelphia: W.B. Saunders, 65-97.

7. Hussey, V.M., Poulin, M.V., and Fain, J.A. (1997). Effectiveness of lidocaine hydrochloride on venipuncture sites. *AORN J, 66*, 472-5.

8. Infusion Nurses Society. (2002). *Policies and Procedure for Infusion Nursing.* 2nd ed. Philadelphia: Lippincott Williams & Wilkins.

9. Intravenous Nurses Society. (2000). Infusion nursing standards of practice. *J Intraven Nurs, 23*, S1-S78.

10. Kennedy, C., et al. (1996). A comparison of hemolysis rates using intravenous catheters versus venipuncture tubes for obtaining blood samples. *J Emerg Nurs, 22*, 566-569.

11. Lander, J., et al. (1996). Evaluation of a new topical anesthetic agent: A pilot study. *Nurs Res, 45*, 50-2.

12. McClasson, D.L., et al. (1999). Clinical practice: hemostasis. Drawing specimens for coagulation testing: Is a second tube necessary? *Clin Lab Sci, 12*, 137-9.

13. Mendelson, M.H., et al. (2003). Evaluation of a safety resheathable winged steel needle for prevention of percutaneous injuries associated with intravascular-access

procedures among healthcare workers. *Infect Control Hosp Epidem, 24*, 105-12.

14. Nott, M., and Peacock, J. (1990). Relief of injection pain in adults: EMLA cream for 5 minutes before venipuncture. *Anaesthesia, 45*, 772-4.

15. Perucca, R. (2001). Obtaining vascular access. In: Hankins, et al., eds. *Infusion Therapy in Clinical Practice.* 2nd ed. Philadelphia: W.B. Saunders, 375-88.

Additional Readings

Flynn, J.C., ed. (1999). *Procedures in phlebotomy.* 2nd ed. Philadelphia: W.B. Saunders.

Hankins, J., et al., eds. (2001). *Infusion Therapy in Clinical Practice.* 2nd ed. Philadelphia: W.B. Saunders.

Potter, P.A., and Perry A.G., eds. (2003). *Basic Nursing: A Critical Thinking Approach.* 5th ed. St. Louis: Mosby.

Wendler, M.C. (2002). Tellington touch before venipuncture: An exploratory descriptive study. *Holistic Nurs Prac, 16*, 51-64.

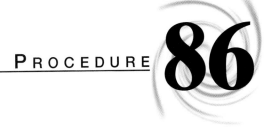

PROCEDURE **86**

Bispectral Index Monitoring

PURPOSE: The bispectral index is a processed EEG-based parameter utilized in critically ill adults to assess patient level of consciousness and responses to sedative/hypnotic/anesthetic agents.[1,2,3,5,17,20] The bispectral index also may indicate an arousal response to painful stimulation.[2] Information derived from bispectral index monitoring may be utilized to guide sedative/hypnotic and analgesic therapy.[1]

Richard B. Arbour

PREREQUISITE NURSING KNOWLEDGE

- Understanding of cerebral physiology
- Sedative, hypnotic, anesthetic, and analgesic agents produce clinical effects as a result of binding, in a dose-related manner, with specific receptors in the brain modulating cerebral physiology.
  - Understanding of the interrelationship between EEG activity and cerebral metabolism
  - EEG tracings are obtained and recorded through the application of scalp electrodes and detect electrical activity in the brain.
  - Examination of EEG waveforms provides a complement to central nervous system (CNS) evaluation obtained through clinical neurologic assessment.
  - On its basic level, EEG activity requires multiple energy-utilizing steps, which need to occur in succession. These steps include electrical impulse discharge at the thalamus and impulse conduction to the cerebral cortex with associated presynaptic release of neurotransmitters.
  - Any clinical state or therapy affecting cerebral metabolism may also affect the EEG.
- Understanding of the close relationship between bispectral index (BIS) and EEG activity
  - When BIS monitoring is initiated, a sensor is placed across the patient's forehead per manufacturer's recommendations to detect one channel of EEG activity.
  - EEG activity is then subjected to multiple processing steps.

- The EEG signal is filtered and digitized within the amplifier headbox near the patient's head.
- Artifacts (low- and high-frequency) are eliminated.
- Multiple processing steps are applied to calculate a specific EEG state (frequency/amplitude) associated with the level of sedation, arousal or anesthesia.
- The level of EEG suppression and near-suppression is determined.
- The EEG features are combined to form the bispectral index, a single value correlating with the level of consciousness and the specific EEG state.[3,17]
- The BIS value is a single number based on the previous 15 seconds of EEG data and is updated frequently. Given this, changes in BIS value may lag behind clinical changes.
- The BIS monitor provides a single channel of an EEG tracing from the right or left frontal-temporal montage electrode placement.
- Understanding factors affecting cerebral metabolism and EEG activity
  - Sedation (dose-related): related to the modulation of the EEG state and level of consciousness from medication administration
  - Analgesic agents (dose-related): related to attenuation of the arousal response or sedation as a side effect of opioid analgesia in higher doses
  - Anesthetic agents (dose-related)
  - Cerebral injury/hypoperfusion (hemodynamic stability, global neurologic injury, severe hypoxemia): related to direct alterations in cerebral metabolic stability

TABLE 86-1 **BIS Values, Corresponding Level of Sedation, and EEG State**[3,13,17,20]

BIS Value	Corresponding Level of Sedation	Descriptors
100	Awake state; patient able to respond appropriately to verbal stimulation	Baseline state presedation
		Anxiolysis
80	Patient able to respond to loud verbal, limited tactile stimulation such as mild prodding/shaking	High-frequency EEG activity (Beta augmentation)
		Moderate sedation
60	Low probability of explicit recall, patient unresponsive to verbal stimulation	Low-frequency EEG activity
		Deep sedation
40	Patient unresponsive to verbal stimulation, less responsive to physical stimulation	Deep hypnotic state
		Drug-induced coma; burst-suppression EEG pattern
20	Minimal responsiveness	Isoelectric or completely suppressed EEG
0	No responsiveness mediated by brain function; spinal reflexes may be present	

Note: Levels of sedation and responsiveness, as well as corresponding BIS value and EEG state, occur on a continuum.
Adapted from Arbour, R. (2003). Continuous nervous system monitoring: EEG, the bispectral index and neuromuscular transmission. *AACN Clin Issues*, 14(2), 192.

- Potential indications for BIS monitoring
  - Use of neuromuscular blockade: BIS monitoring may help to identify patients at risk for awareness, recall, and pain while paralyzed.[3]
  - Use of BIS values to guide sedation and analgesia[1,2,3]
  - Titrating sedation/analgesia in patients receiving controlled ventilation
  - Avoiding extremes of under- and over-sedation
  - Titration of medications for medication-induced coma[19]
  - Procedural sedation
  - Determining the dosage of sedation/analgesia during end-of-life care[3,7]
- Table 86-1 provides BIS values and correlation with clinical endpoints/level of sedation.
- Fig. 86-1 illustrates placement of the BIS sensor.
- Knowledge of factors affecting the BIS value
  - Sedation: decrease in BIS value[1,2,3]
  - Analgesia: decrease in BIS value from attenuation of cerebral arousal or sedation occurring as a side effect of high-dose opioid analgesia[1,2,3]
  - Neuromuscular blocking agents: decrease in BIS value related to attenuation of high-frequency muscle activity across the patient's forehead[6]
  - Painful (noxious) stimulation: if analgesia inadequate, arousal response may be produced within cerebral cortex[2]
  - Sleep: BIS range is lower (20-70) during deep sleep, and BIS range is higher (75-92) during REM (rapid eye movement) sleep.[21]

- Hypothermia: decrease in BIS value[16,23]
- Cerebral ischemia: decrease in BIS value[3,16]
- Neurologic injury: decrease in BIS value[3,8,16] depending on location of injury and degree to which overall cerebral metabolism is affected
- Encephalopathic states: severe anoxic/ischemic encephalopathy (decrease in BIS value)[3,16]
- Electromyographic (EMG) activity (high-frequency activity from muscle activity across forehead)[3,6] may cause increase in BIS value independent of hypnotic state.[3,6]
- High-frequency electrical artifact from patient care equipment, such as pacemaker or muscle activity; rapid head or eye movement (increase in BIS value).
- Knowledge of BIS display screen, monitor controls, and information array available on BIS monitor (Fig. 86-2).
- Knowledge of data obtained from bispectral index monitoring.
  - The BIS value is a single number on a linear (0-100) scale that reflects the level of sedation/cerebral arousal. BIS values correspond with specific clinical endpoints, indicating arousal and consciousness. A BIS value at or near 100 typically corresponds with an awake state. A BIS value at or near 0 corresponds with an isoelectric or near-isoelectric EEG and a deeply comatose patient.[3,4]
  - The suppression ratio (SR) represents the percentage of suppressed EEG over the last 63 seconds of

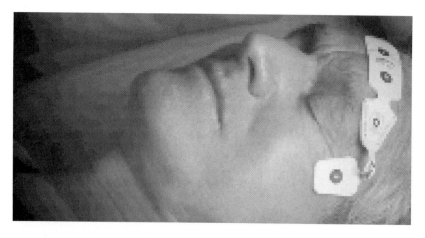

FIGURE 86-1 BIS sensor in place illustrating anatomic landmarks for optimal sensor placement. BIS Extend sensor in place. Sensor may be placed on right or left side. (*Courtesy Aspect Medical Systems, Newton, MA.*)

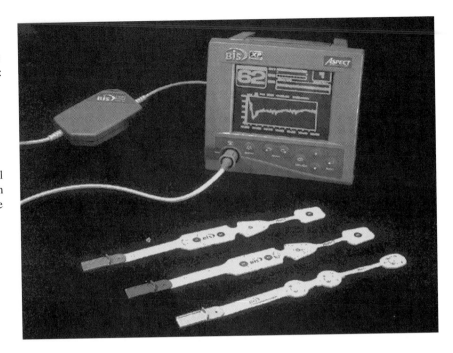

FIGURE 86-2 Equipment and accessories for use of bispectral index monitoring system: BIS monitor, patient cable, patient interface cable, digital signal converter, and available sensors (Extend sensor, Quatro sensor, and pediatric sensors shown). BIS Extend sensor automatically defaults to a 30-second smoothing rate, which may be preferable when patients are lightly sedated and minimal changes in drug delivery or patient stimulation exist, conditions that may apply to an intensive care setting. The BIS Quatro sensor automatically defaults to a 15-second smoothing rate and may be preferable when rapid changes in hypnotic level are anticipated or when maximum sensitivity in assessing arousal response is desired, which may be helpful in an operating room setting. (*Courtesy Aspect Medical Systems, Newton, MA.*)

collected data within the EEG data sample. This parameter may be elevated in patients receiving high-dose propofol or barbiturates. The SR may also be elevated in a patient with severe cerebral injury such as encephalopathy or catastrophic brain trauma. An SR of 15 indicates that the EEG signal was isoelectric over an interval of 15% of the previous 63 seconds of collected data.[3,4]

- The electromyograph (EMG) displays the power (in decibels) within the range of 70-110 Hz (cycles per second). This frequency range includes electrical activity from muscle artifact as well as patient care devices.[3,4]

- Interpretation of BIS value
  - BIS is interpreted over time, in response to stimulation and within the context of whether therapeutic endpoints and overall goals of therapy are met.
  - Decisions to increase or decrease titration of sedative or analgesic therapy should be based on clinical assessment/judgment, goals of therapy, and the BIS value.
  - Relying on the BIS alone for sedation/analgesia management is not recommended.
  - Movement such as in response to painful stimulation may occur with low BIS values.
  - BIS values should be interpreted with caution in patients with brain injury or disease and those receiving psychoactive medications.
  - BIS monitoring is not intended for regional cerebral ischemia monitoring. When using BIS in the presence of known CNS injury, obtaining a baseline BIS value prior to administration of sedative/analgesic or anesthetic agents is recommended.[3,13]

- Elevation in BIS value:
  - Assess for sources of noxious stimuli (arousal response and potential increase in EMG activity).
  - Decrease in level of neuromuscular blockade (affecting EMG activity)[6]
  - Interruption in sedative therapy, development of tolerance
  - Interruption in analgesic therapy, development of tolerance
  - REM sleep
  - Seizure activity (potentially)
  - Environmental noise: cerebral arousal from excessive auditory stimulation

- Decrease in BIS value:
  - Attenuation of arousal response or EMG activity following opioid administration[1,2,3]
  - Administration of neuromuscular blocking agents
  - Attenuation of EMG activity[6]
  - Excessive sedative dose
  - Excessive analgesic dosing
  - Hypothermia (patient cooling)[13,23]
  - Progression to deeper stages of sleep
  - Hemodynamic instability
  - Cerebral hypoperfusion[17]
  - Onset/evolution of neurologic injury[8]

- Knowledge of sedative and analgesic therapy
  - Specific medication therapies (e.g., opioids, benzodiazepines, propofol)[1,12,18]
  - Indications/contraindications of specific medication classes
  - Goals of care
  - Clinical assessment for establishing goals and endpoints of therapy[1,12,18]

- Knowledge of medication effects on BIS value
  - Opioids: may decrease in a dose-related manner (with side effect of sedation at higher doses) and decrease BIS value related to attenuation of arousal response from pain
  - Benzodiazepines: decrease BIS value in dose-related manner
  - Propofol: decrease in BIS value in dose-related manner
  - Single-agent therapy with ketamine may not result in dose-related decrease in BIS value.[3] Ketamine results in increased cerebral blood flow and activation of EEG, specifically in higher frequencies.[13] Higher EEG frequencies are associated with lighter levels of sedation.[3] The BIS value may remain elevated in the presence of deeper sedation as determined by clinical assessment.[13]
- Knowledge of neuromuscular blockade and monitoring issues:
  - Differentiating between monitoring level of sedation/cortical arousal and monitoring level of neuromuscular blockade
    - Monitoring level of sedation/cortical arousal is a phenomenon mediated by the CNS and is evaluated by clinical assessment of level of consciousness/arousal, as well as by a processed EEG parameter such as the bispectral index. Medication effects evaluated include CNS depressants such as propofol, barbiturates, benzodiazepines, and opioids at higher doses.
    - Monitoring level of neuromuscular blockade is a phenomenon mediated by the peripheral nervous system (PNS) and measures the effects of neuromuscular blocking agents at producing varying degrees of skeletal muscle relaxation. The degree of neuromuscular blockade is evaluated two ways. First, clinical assessment of ventilator synchrony, resolution of life-threatening agitation, and the degree to which clinical goals and endpoints are met. Second, peripheral nerve stimulation and assessment of the evoked response are done. Peripheral nerve stimulation is most commonly performed at the ulnar nerve in the wrist. Following nerve localization and electrode placement, an electrical stimulus is applied and the localized response of the target muscle is assessed (see Procedure 104).
  - Risk of awareness and pain while paralyzed
  - Clinical goals for aggressive sedation and analgesia while paralyzed
  - Monitoring parameters
    - Hemodynamic changes (marginal value and affected by multiple factors)
    - Diaphoresis (affected by multiple factors)
    - EEG-based monitoring (bispectral index)
- Initial monitoring and set-up of sensor and equipment:
  - Signal quality index (SQI) is displayed on the monitor screen. The SQI bar extending to right side of the SQI bar graph display indicates optimal (100%) EEG signal quality. The BIS value on the numeric region of monitor display will be shown as a solid number. SQI below 50% (SQI below middle range of display) is indicated by a BIS value shown as an outlined number. If SQI is inadequate to calculate a BIS value, no data will be displayed.[4,13]

EQUIPMENT

- BIS monitor
- Digital signal converter
- Patient interface cable
- BIS sensor
- Detachable power cord
- Alcohol pads
- Gauze pads
- Nonsterile gloves
  Additional equipment includes the following:
- Soap and water
- Emergency equipment

PATIENT AND FAMILY EDUCATION

- Assess factors affecting family readiness to learn. ➤*Rationale:* Individualizes teaching to specific family needs.
- Explain the purpose of BIS monitoring, including content regarding specific information obtained, how it may be used, and an explanation of the equipment. ➤*Rationale:* Patient (if still awake) and family will experience less anxiety and have increased understanding of the patient equipment at the bedside.
- Explain to the patient (if appropriate) and family what will happen with the initiation of BIS monitoring (skin prep, placement of electrodes, moderate pressure for electrode contact). ➤*Rationale:* Prepares the patient and family for events associated with initiating BIS monitoring. This also provides an opportunity to reinforce pre-procedure teaching and assess level of understanding.
- Although rare, some patients may develop mild skin irritation in the area in contact with the sensor. This typically resolves within 1 hour following sensor removal. ➤*Rationale:* Prepares family for possible minor issue with sensor application and possible need for removal or repositioning of the sensor.
- Explain that BIS monitoring and electrode placement pose no risk to the patient beyond that of mild skin irritation (in rare instances) and that the patient experiences no discomfort as part of monitoring procedure. ➤*Rationale:* Decreases anxiety.

PATIENT ASSESSMENT AND PREPARATION

Patient Assessment

- Clinical assessment of level of sedation, responsiveness, and arousal. ➤*Rationale:* Provides baseline data.

- In collaboration with other health care providers, establish overall goals and endpoints of sedative and analgesic therapy. ➤**Rationale:** Establishes coordinated plan with integration of BIS data into decision making regarding sedation/analgesia.
- Assess skin condition at the proposed sites for sensor placement. ➤**Rationale:** Establishes whether skin is intact prior to sensor placement.
- Assess the patient's neurologic status. ➤**Rationale:** Provides baseline data. BIS values may be decreased with significant neurologic injury, and this needs to be determined prior to initiating BIS monitoring. If possible, obtain a baseline BIS value before initiating therapy with sedative, analgesic, or anesthetic agents.

Patient Preparation

- Determine the adequacy of intravenous (IV) access, replace if necessary. Have at least two patent IV accesses. ➤**Rationale:** Ensures reliable IV access for administration and titration of sedative, analgesic, and/or neuromuscular blocking agents. Also ensures vascular access for rapid administration of fluids/medications to treat possible side effects of therapy.
- Determine anatomic landmarks for the BIS sensor placement. ➤**Rationale:** Provides for accurate placement of the sensor.

Procedure for Bispectral Index Monitoring

Steps	Rationale	Special Considerations
1. Connect the power cord to the monitor and plug it into the electrical wall outlet.	Prepares the equipment.	Equipment may vary because a stand-alone monitor may be used or a module may be used that is incorporated into the bedside monitoring system.
2. Connect the digital signal converter (DSC) and the patient interface cable to the monitor.	Prepares the equipment.	
3. Turn the monitor on and observe as a system check is run.	The system initiates a self-test to ensure that the equipment and connections are operating effectively.	If a hardware problem exists such as DSC failure, a message will appear on the display, indicating the need for a hardware part replacement or service. If a problem exists, an error message will appear. Refer to the operator's manual.[4]
4. Wash hands and don nonsterile gloves.	Reduces the transmission of microorganisms; standard precautions.	
5. Cleanse the intended sensor area with alcohol pads and dry with gauze.	A thorough skin prep removes debris and oily residue from the skin and facilitates optimal electrical contact for EEG data acquisition.	Mild soap and water is an acceptable alternative. Ensure that the skin is dry before applying the sensors.
6. Attach the BIS sensor to the patient's forehead (Figs. 86-1 and 86-3): A. Position circle 1 electrode at the center of the forehead, approximately 2 inches above the patient's nose. B. Position circle 4 electrode directly above and parallel to the eyebrow. C. Position circle 3 electrode on the temple area between the hairline and the outer canthus of the eye.	Ensures consistency of the anatomic location for sensor placement and optimizes the electrical contact between the monitoring system and the skin for facilitation of EEG data acquisition. EEG data acquisition begins shortly after optimal connection is established between the patient and the monitoring system.	The conductive parts of the electrodes, sensor, or connectors should not contact other conductive parts of the monitoring system. The patient interface cable should be carefully placed and secured. Data acquisition begins when impedances are acceptable. Electrodes showing high impedance will be highlighted on the sensor check display seen at start-up. For electrodes identified as having high impedance, repeat

Procedure continues on the following page

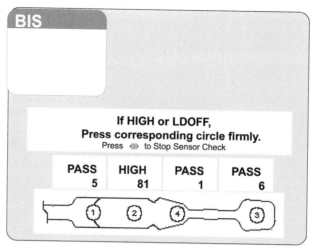

FIGURE 86-3 BIS sensor check at start of monitoring.[4] *Circle 1* is positioned at center of forehead approximately 2 inches (5 cm) above nose. *Circle 4* is placed directly above and parallel to the eyebrow. *Circle 3* is placed on the temple area between the hairline and the outer canthus of the eye. *Circle 2* is placed between *Circles 1* and *4* on the patient's forehead. *(Courtesy Aspect Medical Systems, Newton, MA.)*

Procedure for Bispectral Index Monitoring—*Continued*

Steps	Rationale	Special Considerations
D. Position circle 2 electrode between the first and fourth sensor on the patient's forehead. E. Press the edges of the sensor to ensure adhesion and seal in the conductive gel. F. Press each of the electrodes with continuous direct pressure for 5 seconds to ensure optimal skin contact.		pressing of electrodes to optimize electrical contact. If significant artifact is present, the DSC should be moved away from sources of external electrical or mechanical artifact. Sources of artifact include fluid or forced-air warming systems, ventricular assist devices, high frequency ventilation, suction, pacemakers and oscillating mattresses.[13] Sensor check will be initiated automatically. In the event of an error message such as high impedance or sensor removal, re-prep and replacement of sensor may be necessary.
7. Insert the sensor tab into the patient interface cable until it is engaged.	Connects the BIS sensor and the patient interface cable.	
8. Secure the digital signal converter to an accessible location near the patient's head (e.g., patient's pillow or sheet) avoiding close proximity to sources of mechanical or electrical interference.	The digital signal converter amplifies, filters, and digitizes the patient's EEG signals. It is located close to the patient's head to minimize the vulnerability of the EEG signal to interference from other electronic equipment or patient care devices.[4]	
9. Access the setup menu by pressing "MENU/EXIT" on the monitor to select the specific monitor settings, including BIS smoothing rate, event markers, and display type. This also provides access to the advanced setup menu (Fig. 86-4).	Settings such as display type and BIS smoothing rate (in seconds) may be chosen.	A 15-second smoothing rate provides increased sensitivity and expedited feedback to altered hypnotic or arousal states. A 30-second smoothing rate generates a smoother trend with less variability, is less sensitive to artifact and is often chosen for long-term monitoring.[4]

Procedure for Bispectral Index Monitoring—*Continued*

Steps	Rationale	Special Considerations
10. As noted above, access the advanced setup menu by initially pressing "MENU/EXIT" and then highlighting "Advanced Setup" by using the up or down arrows. Press select when "Advanced Setup" is highlighted (Fig. 86-5).	This is utilized to select secondary parameters displayed with BIS trend such as EMG (electromyography) activity, SR (suppression ratio), and SQI (signal quality index), as well as to alter settings that may be changed less frequently. SQI of 100% indicates an optimal EEG signal. SR is the percentage of suppressed (isoelectric) EEG over the previous 63 seconds within the EEG data sample.[3,13]	If BIS is utilized to monitor a patient's sedation level during neuromuscular blockade, selecting electromyograph as a secondary parameter may provide early information regarding "lightening" of the blockade (electromyograph activity may increase). If used during deep sedation for controlled ventilation, EMG may indicate a pain/arousal response and indicate the need for analgesia.[3] Increased electromyograph activity may also indicate a lighter state of sedation or increased muscle activity. If BIS is used to monitor a patient in a drug-induced coma, suppression ratio (SR) may be monitored as a secondary parameter for continuous evaluation of the degree of EEG suppression.
11. Select additional settings as needed, including: A. Intervals for collection of data in the BIS log B. Accessing "Advanced Setup" as outlined earlier to change the alarm limits and the display type.	The settings, such as the interval for recording of the BIS log values, log displays, alarm limits, and alternative displays such as EEG, density spectral array may be changed based on clinical or other needs for data collection.	The density spectral array display shows changes/trends in the power spectrum of the EEG over time. The BIS log display shows BIS numeric values averaged over the previous minute and can be displayed at varying intervals such as 1, 5, 15, or 60 minutes. Up to 400 hours of data can be stored. The EEG display provides a single channel of raw EEG from a frontal montage.

Procedure continues on the following page

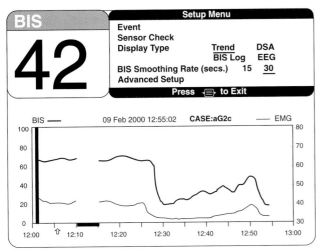

FIGURE 86-4 Set-up menu for selecting monitor settings optimal to specific patient needs.[4] Display of specific monitoring parameters such as BIS trend and smoothing rate may be adjusted on this display. *(Courtesy Aspect Medical Systems, Newton, MA.)*

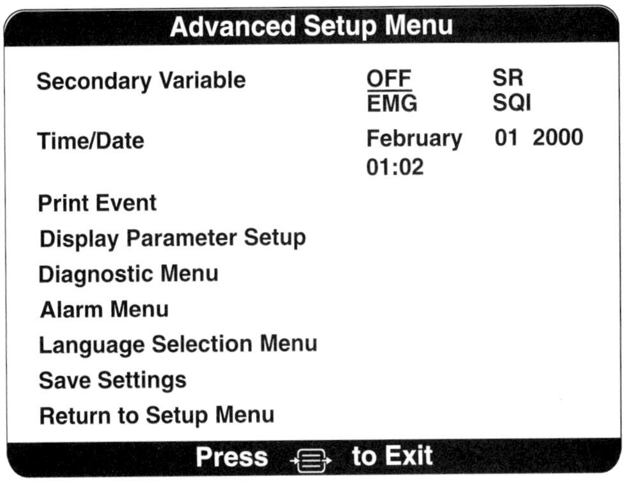

FIGURE 86-5 Advanced set-up menu enabling the operator to select secondary monitoring parameters to be displayed with BIS trend, as well as other, less frequently changed settings. Secondary parameters that may be selected include electromyography (EMG), suppression ratio (SR), and signal quality index (SQI).[4] *(Courtesy Aspect Medical Systems, Newton, MA.)*

Procedure **for Bispectral Index Monitoring**—*Continued*

Steps	Rationale	Special Considerations
12. When the monitor settings have been adjusted to a specific patient, BIS data collection can begin.	BIS data collection can proceed after all preparatory steps and monitor settings are completed appropriately. This ensures optimal electrical contact between the patient and the monitoring system, as well as optimal electrical safety. In addition, confirming display settings and secondary parameters at the outset of monitoring effectively tailors the monitor display and data acquisition to the specific patient.	
13. Observe the monitor display for: A. High impedance alarm (it will be highlighted on the sensor check display at start-up). If displayed, press each electrode again to optimize electrical contact. Remove the sensor, cleanse the skin, and place on new sensor if necessary. B. Lead off alarm (it will be displayed as "LDOFF.") If present, check to see whether the sensor has loosened. Remove the sensor, cleanse the skin, and apply another sensor. C. Artifact. If artifact is present, move the digital signal converter away from sources of external electrical or mechanical artifact.	Data acquisition begins when impedances are acceptable. Artifact may be due to use of fluid or forced-air warming systems, ventricular assist devices, high-frequency ventilation, suction, pacemakers, and oscillating mattresses.[13]	A sensor check is initiated automatically during the system start up (see Fig. 86-3).
14. For a patient receiving neuromuscular blockade, sedation, analgesia therapy, the medication should be titrated for a BIS value between 45 and 60.	A BIS value below 60 is associated with a low probability of explicit recall. A patient with a BIS value less than 45 is approaching a deep hypnotic state.[3,20]	If the BIS value exceeds 60 in a patient receiving neuromuscular blockade in association with stimulation such as airway suctioning or chest physiotherapy, additional analgesics are indicated. If the BIS value decreases below 40-45, downward titration of sedative therapy may be indicated. In addition, the patient should be evaluated for additional clinical changes such as hypotension, hypothermia, or cerebral ischemia, which may cause a decrease in the BIS value.
15. For a patient receiving deep sedation for controlled ventilation, correlate the goal for the BIS value with specific clinical endpoints of therapy.	Correlation of the BIS value with clinical goals of therapy identifies patients who may be progressing to deeper levels of sedation and those who may be at risk for impending breakthrough agitation.	With increased agitation and a BIS value less than 60, movement may be related to pain or reflex responses to noxious stimulation. Additional analgesia should be considered.
16. Discard supplies and wash hands.	Reduces the transmission of microorganisms; standard precautions.	

Expected Outcomes

- Optimal placement of the BIS sensor consistent with anatomic landmarks and consistent with manufacturer's recommendations
- Skin remaining intact in the area of the BIS sensor placement
- Data acquisition and display proceeding after monitor setup and completion of self-test
- SQI above 50, indicating effective EEG data acquisition
- Clear EEG waveform visible on the monitor display
- BIS decrease in response to sedative administration in dose-related manner
- BIS decrease following analgesia administration
- BIS value increase following significant noxious stimulation
- BIS values equal between right and left frontal-temporal montage EEG sensor placement
- BIS data effective in providing feedback on the state of the brain in response to sedative/analgesic/hypnotic administration that can be used to direct therapy

Unexpected Outcomes

- Skin irritation in the area of the BIS sensor placement
- SQI significantly below 50, indicating suboptimal EEG signal acquisition
- A sudden decrease in the BIS value independent of changes in sedative or analgesic therapy (may indicate hemodynamic compromise, cerebral ischemia, or the onset or progression of significant neurologic injury)
- A sudden rise in the BIS independent of stimulation, increased EMG activity, or an outward change in the patient's condition (may indicate seizure activity)
- BIS completely unresponsive to noxious stimulation such as endotracheal suctioning or invasive procedures
- BIS values significantly unequal between the right and left frontal-temporal montage sensor placement (may indicate unilateral cerebral injury/ischemia)
- BIS values not correlating with clinical assessment of sedation level and respond inconsistently to administration of sedative, hypnotic, or analgesic agents

Patient Monitoring and Care

Steps	Rationale	Reportable Conditions
		These conditions should be reported if they persist despite nursing interventions.
1. Assess the skin condition in the area of the sensor placement.	Ensures that the skin is intact.	• Altered skin integrity/irritation following sensor placement
2. Maintain the digital signal converter in close proximity to the patient's head.	Decreases the vulnerability of the EEG signals to electrical interference from other sources.	
3. Monitor the BIS values and secondary parameters, including SQI, EMG, and SR as determined by goals of care, clinical status, and response to interventions. For example, during rapid administration of sedative/analgesic agents prior to the anticipated use of neuromuscular blockade therapy, it may be appropriate to monitor and record the BIS value multiple times per hour. As therapy is stabilized, BIS can be monitored hourly.	Identifies trends in BIS and secondary parameters. Decrease in SQI below 50% may indicate suboptimal EEG data acquisition.	• Increase in EMG activity without a change in medication therapy (may indicate increased arousal response [pain], lightening of neuromuscular blockade, and result in increase in BIS independent of hypnotic state, or decreasing level of sedation or analgesia) • Significant difference in BIS value between right and left frontal montage EEG (may indicate unilateral cerebral injury) • BIS value absolutely invariant to significant noxious stimulation (may indicate significant cerebral injury) • Increased suppression ratio (may indicate onset or evolution of cerebral injury, hemodynamic compromise, ischemia, or excessively deep hypnotic state[3])
4. Identify goals or endpoints of therapy at the beginning of BIS monitoring.	Patient outcomes are improved with an organized, research-based approach to care.[3,12]	• Not progressing toward achievement of goals/end point of therapy

Procedure continues on the following page

Patient Monitoring and Care—*Continued*

Steps	Rationale	Reportable Conditions
5. Observe BIS values at least hourly and in response to titration of medication therapy.	Determines changes in BIS values in response to medication therapy and interventions. This also provides the ability to use "event marker" to closely correlate changes in BIS and secondary parameters for later review.	• Abnormal BIS values or trends: BIS value not decreasing in response to upward titration of sedative or hypnotic therapy; BIS value not increasing following downward titration of sedative or hypnotic therapy
6. Change the BIS sensor at least every 24 hours or more frequently as needed (e.g., diaphoresis, loose electrodes).	Maintains optimal electrical contact between the patient and the monitoring system.	
7. Observe the EEG channel at least every 2 hours and as determined by the patient's clinical state and therapeutic interventions.	The EEG amplitude and frequency will change based on the patient's clinical state, evolving injury, and medication therapy. The EEG will also (under normal conditions), change in response to varying levels and types of stimulation.[10,11,14,20] Under most conditions, ECG artifact is not visible in an EEG waveform.[3] ECG artifact visible in the EEG channel may indicate significant EEG suppression.	• A decrease in EEG frequency or amplitude (e.g., if this occurs with a decrease in the BIS value may indicate neurologic injury) • A significant decrease in the BIS value that is inconsistent with the medication therapy may indicate critical pathology and warrant further evaluation by neuroimaging diagnostic EEG and/or clinical examination • BIS value alone should not be relied on to diagnose neurologic injury
8. Observe the BIS value in response to stimulation	The BIS value should, in most patients, rise in response to stimulation. The EEG, upon which the BIS is based, normally responds to external stimulation. An EEG unresponsive to stimulation may indicate significant neurologic injury and possibly poor prognosis.[9,14,22,24]	• Significant ECG artifact in the EEG channel • A BIS value that is unresponsive to noxious stimulation • A significant difference in BIS values or SR between the right and left frontal-temporal montage (may indicate unilateral cerebral injury)

Documentation

Documentation should include the following:

- Goals and endpoints of sedative, analgesic therapy
- Family education regarding BIS monitoring
- Clinical assessment (if appropriate) of level of sedation
- BIS value at start of monitoring and with changes/titration of therapy
- BIS value recording on flowsheet at least hourly and more frequently as indicated (Fig. 86-6)
- Occurrence of skin irritation at the site of the BIS sensor placement with action taken
- Unexpected outcomes and interventions
- Sudden changes in BIS value (increase or decrease) independent of obvious clinical changes or alterations of medication therapy

- Suppression ratio (as appropriate) for BIS use in medication-induced coma
- Documentation of left versus right frontal montage (location of the BIS sensor on the right or the left side)
- BIS value before and after noxious stimulation and the difference between these two values
- Change in the BIS value in response to noxious/painful stimulation
- For case reviews to track, BIS values/trends and response to stimulation/therapeutic interventions over time; printout/strip of BIS trend data can be obtained if printer is available (Fig. 86-7)

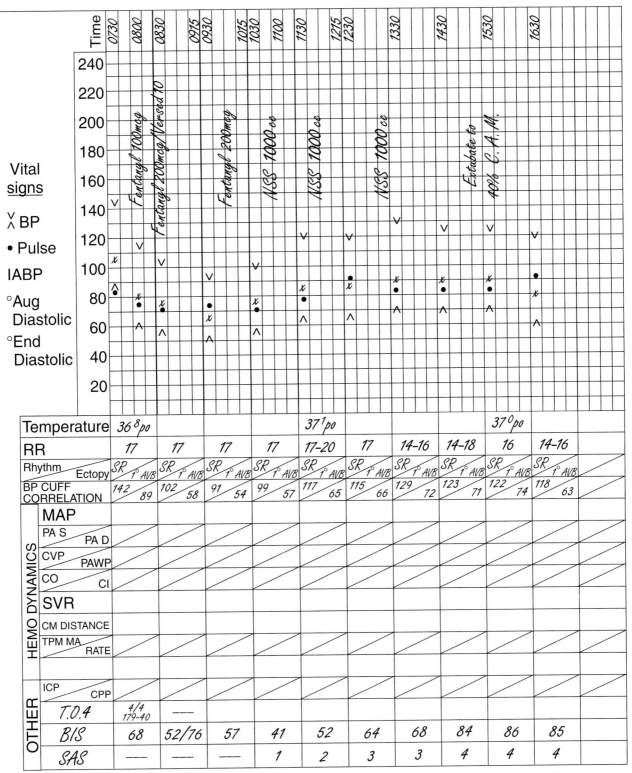

FIGURE 86-6 Documentation of BIS values over time and following medication administration in critically ill patient. At 7:30 a.m., the patient was still receiving neuromuscular blockade with a BIS value of 68. Additional sedation/analgesia was administered (fentanyl and midazolam), with resulting BIS decline to 52. Following stimulation, BIS value elevated to 76, requiring supplemental dosing with analgesics (fentanyl). BIS value remained below 60 and neuromuscular blockade was discontinued. The upward trend in the BIS value tracked recovery of consciousness to baseline mental status. *(Courtesy Aspect Medical Systems, Newton, MA.)*

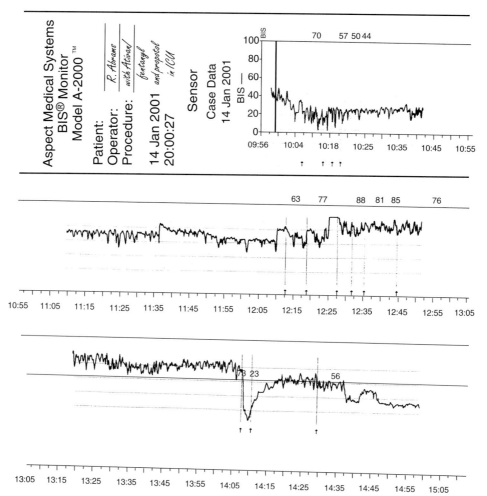

FIGURE 86-7 An illustration of BIS trend recording of sedation/analgesia management in critically ill patient. BIS monitoring was initiated at approximately 10:00 a.m. Sedation was managed initially with fentanyl and lorazepam. Decline in BIS from 90-97 to 55-65 occurred over 25-30 minutes in response to therapy. Decline in BIS value matched clinical assessment of increased level of sedation. The patient had periods of breakthrough agitation and ventilator dyssynchrony beginning at 12:15 p.m. Agitation was refractory to current therapy despite upward titration of sedation and analgesia. The sedation management was changed to propofol at approximately 14:05 p.m. The precipitous drop in BIS value indicated increased sedation. Propofol was titrated back in a controlled, incremental manner. Sedation was more closely and optimally managed with application of BIS monitoring and avoiding, in a controlled manner, extremes of excessive sedation and inadequate sedation/risk of agitation and ventilator dyssychrony. This tracing has been utilized in electronic format beginning in June, 2003 for educational purposes on behalf of Aspect Medical Systems. *(Courtesy Aspect Medical Systems, Newton, MA.)*

References

1. Arbour, R.B. (2000). Sedation and pain management in critically ill adults. *Crit Care Nurs,* 20, 39-56.
2. Arbour, R.B. (2000). Using the bispectral index to assess arousal response in a patient with neuromuscular blockade. *Amer J Crit Care,* 9, 383-7.
3. Arbour, R.B. (2003). Continuous nervous system monitoring, EEG, the bispectral index and neuromuscular transmission. *AACN Clin Iss,* 14, 185-207.
4. Aspect Medical Systems (2001). *A-2000™ Operating Manual.* Newton, MA: Aspect Medical Systems, Inc.
5. Aspect Medical Systems. (1997). *Technology Overview: Bispectral Index.* Newton, MA: Aspect Medical Systems Inc. White Paper.
6. Aspect Medical Systems. (2000). *Overview: The Effects of Electromyography (EMG) and Other High-Frequency Signals*

on the Bispectral Index (BIS). Newton, MA: Aspect Medical Systems Inc. White Paper.
7. Barbato, M. (2001). Bispectral index monitoring in unconscious palliative care patients. *J Pall Care,* 17, 102-8.
8. Gilbert, T.T., et al. (2001). Use of bispectral electroencephalogram monitoring to assess neurologic status in unsedated, critically ill patients. *Crit Care Med,* 29, 1996-2000.
9. Grissom, T.E., and Grissom, J. (2000). Neurologic monitoring in the ICU. *Anesthesiology Online.* Available at: http://www.anesthesiologyonline.com/articles/onepage.cfm?chapter_id=34. Accessed Dec. 19, 2001.
10. Guerit, J.M. (1999). Medical technology assessment: EEG and evoked potentials in the intensive care unit. *Neurophysiol Clin,* 29, 301-17.

11. Huszar, L. (2001). Clinical utility of evoked potentials. *E-Medicine.* Available at: http://www.emedicine.com/neuro/topic69.htm. Accessed Feb., 19, 2001.

12. Jacobi, J., et al. (2002). Clinical practice guidelines for the sustained use of sedatives and analgesics in the critically ill adult. *Crit Care Med,* 30, 119-41.

13. Kelly, S.D. (2003). *Monitoring Level of Consciousness During Anesthesia and Sedation. A Clinician's Guide to the Bispectral Index.* Aspect Medical Systems. Available at: http://www.aspectmedical.com/resources/handbook/default.mspx. Accessed June 4, 2004.

14. Leim, L.K. (2001). Intraoperative neurophysiological monitoring from neurology/electroencephalography and evoked potentials. *E-Medicine.* Accessed 5-14-01 at http://emedicine.com/neuro/topic102.htm.

15. Mathew, J.P., et al. (2001). Bispectral analysis during cardiopulmonary bypass: the effect of hypothermia on the hypnotic state. *J Clin Anesth,* 13: 301-5.

16. Merat, S., et al. (2001). BIS monitoring may allow detection of severe cerebral ischemia. *Can J Anesth,* 48, 1066-9.

17. Rampil, I.J. (1998). A primer for EEG signal processing in anesthesia. *Anesth,* 89, 980-1002.

18. Rhoney, D.H., and Parker, D. (2001). Use of sedative and analgesic agents in neurotrauma patients: effects on cerebral physiology. *Neurol Res,* 23, 237-59.

19. Riker, R.R., Fraser, G.L., and Wilkins, M.L. (2003). Comparing the bispectral index and suppression ratio with burst suppression of the electroencephalogram during pentobarbital infusions in adult intensive care patients. From *Pharmacotherapy.* Available at: http://www.medscape.com/viewarticle/461380. Accessed Sept. 23, 2003.

20. Rosow, C., and Manberg, P.J. (1998). Bispectral index monitoring. *Anesth Clin North Am,* 2, 89-107.

21. Schwartz, G. (2000). Evoked potentials for coma diagnosis and prognosis. *Euroanesthesia.* Available at: http://www.euroanesthesia.org/pages/education/rc_vienna/07rc3.HTM. Accessed May 14, 2001.

22. Sleigh, J.W., Andrezejowski, J., and Steyn-Ross, M. (1999). The bispectral index: a measure of depth of sleep. *Anesthesia & Analgesia,* 88, 659-61.

23. Stecker, M.M., et al. (2001). Deep hypothermic circulatory arrest: I. Effects of cooling on electroencephalogram and evoked potentials. *Ann Thor Surg,* 71, 14-21.

24. Young, G.B. (2000). The EEG in coma. *J Clin Neurophys,* 17, 473-85.

Additional Readings

Arbour, R. (1998). Aggressive management of intracranial dynamics. *Crit Care Nurs,* 18, 30-40.

Arbour, R. (2000). Mastering neuromuscular blockade. *Dimens Crit Care Nurs,* 19, 4-20.

Arbour, R. (2002). Using bispectral index monitoring to detect potential breakthrough awareness and limit duration of neuromuscular blockade. *Am J Crit Care* 13, 66-73.

Bower, A.L., et al. (2000). Bispectral index monitoring of sedation during endoscopy. *Gastrointest Endos,* 52, 192-6.

Crippen, D.W. (1997). Using bedside EEGs to monitor sedation during neuromuscular blockade. *J Crit Ill,* 12, 519-24.

DeDeyne, C., et al. (1998). Use of continuous bispectral EEG monitoring to assess depth of sedation in ICU patients. *Intens Care Med,* 24, 1294-8.

Del Castillo, M.A. (2001). Monitoring neurologic patients in intensive care. *Curr Opin Crit Care,* 7, 49-60.

Ely, E.W., Siegel, M.D., and Inouye S.K. (2001). Delirium in the intensive care unit: an under-recognized syndrome of organ dysfunction. *Sem Resp Crit Care Med,* 22, 115-26.

Epstein, J., and Breslow, M.J. (1999). The stress response of critical illness. *Crit Care Clin,* 15, 17-34.

Frenzel, D., et al. (2002). Is the bispectral index appropriate for monitoring the sedation level of mechanically ventilated surgical ICU patients? *Intens Care Med,* 28, 178-83.

Halliburton, J.R., and McCarthy, E.J. (2000). Perioperative monitoring with the electroencephalogram and bispectral index monitor. *AANA J,* 68, 333-40.

Hatlestad, D. (2001). Assessment of neuromuscular blockade. *J Resp Care Pract,* 14, 37-38, 40.

Hilbish C. (2003). Bispectral index monitoring in the neurointensive care unit. *J Neurosci Nurs,* 35, 336-8.

Jordan, K.G. (1999). Continuous EEG monitoring in the neuroscience intensive care unit and emergency department. *J Clin Neurophys,* 16, 14-39.

Luginbuhl, M., and Schnider, T.W. (2002). Detection of awareness with the bispectral index: Two case reports. *Anesth,* 96, 241-243.

Misulis, K.E. (1997). *Essentials of Clinical Neurophysiology.* Newton, MA: Butterworth-Heinemann.

Nasraway, S.A. (2001). Use of sedative medications in the intensive care unit. *Sem Resp Crit Care Med,* 22, 165-74.

Nasraway, S.A., et al. (2002). How reliable is the bispectral index in critically ill patients? A prospective, comparative, single-blinded observer study. *Crit Care Med,* 30, 1483-7.

Prielipp, R.C., et al. (1995). Complications associated with sedative and neuromuscular blocking drugs in critically ill patients. *Crit Care Clin,* 11, 983-1002.

Primak, L.K., and Lowrie, L. (2001). Paralyzation and sedation of the ventilated trauma patient. *Resp Care Clin N Amer,* 7, 97-126.

Riker, R.R., et al. (2001). Validating the sedation-agitation scale with the bispectral index and visual analog scale in adult ICU patients after cardiac surgery. *Intens Care Med,* 27, 853-8.

Riker, R.R., and Fraser, G.L. (2002). Sedation in the intensive care unit: refining the models and defining the questions. *Crit Care Med,* 30, 1661-3.

Rowlee, S.C. (1999). Monitoring neuromuscular blockade in the intensive care unit: the peripheral nerve stimulator. *Heart Lung,* 28, 352-62.

Rutkove, S.B. (2001). Effects of temperature on neuromuscular electrophysiology. *Muscle Nerve,* 24, 867-82.

Sandler, N.A., Hodges, J., and Sabino, M. (2001). Assessment of recovery in patients undergoing intravenous conscious sedation using bispectral analysis. *J Oral Maxillofac Surg,* 59, 603-611.

Schneider, G., and Sebel, P.S. (1997). Monitoring depth of anesthesia. *Euro J Anaesth,* 14(Suppl 15), 21-28.

Simmons L.E., et al. (1999). Assessing sedation during intensive care unit mechanical ventilation with the bispectral index and the sedation-agitation scale. *Crit Care Med,* 27, 1499-1504.

Stewart-Amidei, C. (1998). Neurologic monitoring in the ICU. *Crit Care Nurs Q,* 21, 47-60.

Venn, R., et al. (1999). Monitoring of the depth of sedation in the intensive care unit. *Clin Intens Care,* 10, 81-90.

Vivien, B., et al. (2002). Detection of brain death onset using the bispectral index in severely comatose patients. *Intens Care Med,* 28, 419-25.

Wagner, B.K.T., et al. (1998). Patient recall of therapeutic paralysis in a surgical critical care unit. *Pharmacotherapy,* 18, 358-63.

Wallace, B.E., et al. (2001). A history and review of quantitative electroencephalography in traumatic brain injury. *J Head Trauma Rehab,* 16, 165-90.

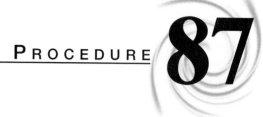

Brain Tissue Oxygen Monitoring: Insertion (Assist), Care, and Troubleshooting

P U R P O S E : Brain tissue oxygen (also abbreviated as $p_{bt}O_2$, $p_{br}O_2$, tiO_2) monitoring is performed in the severely brain-injured patient to measure and continuously monitor intracranial tissue oxygen. Monitoring brain tissue oxygen provides important information relative to the delivery of oxygen to cerebral tissue and the cellular metabolism (oxygen consumption and demand) of the injured brain.

Eileen Maloney-Wilensky
Stephanie Bloom

PREREQUISITE NURSING KNOWLEDGE

- Incorporated as an adjunct monitor of trends in concert with current neurologic multimodality monitoring parameters (ICP, CPP, $Sjvo_2$), $p_{bt}O_2$ monitoring reflects the oxygenation of cerebral tissue local to the sensor placement.
- It is important to note the difference between $Sjvo_2$ measurements and $p_{bt}O_2$ values. Systemic jugular venous oxygen ($Sjvo_2$) is a measure of the oxygen contained in the blood draining from the cerebral venous sinuses into the jugular bulb (a measure of global oxygenation), whereas $p_{bt}O_2$ measures regional (local to the catheter placement in the cerebral white matter) brain tissue oxygenation.
- Understanding of neuroanatomy and physiology, specifically intracranial dynamics
- Knowledge of sterile and aseptic technique
- Brain tissue oxygen probes are available in bolt systems and tunnellable oxygen probes.
- $p_{bt}O_2$ monitoring provides information that reflects brain tissue oxygen levels associated with cerebral oxygen demand and systemic oxygen delivery. $p_{bt}O_2$ monitoring provides data additional to that obtained by current clinical practice in cases where cerebral hypoxia and/or ischemia are a concern.
- $p_{bt}O_2$ values are relative within an individual. Establishing and following the patient's cerebral oxygen trends provides the bedside practitioner information to diagnose cerebral hypoxia as well as determine the effectiveness of therapeutic interventions instituted to respond to brain tissue hypoxia and affecting outcome.
- Indications for $p_{bt}O_2$ monitoring include patients at risk for secondary injury associated with severe traumatic brain injury, aneurysmal and traumatic subarachnoid hemorrhage, brain tumor, and malignant stroke.
- Contraindications for $p_{bt}O_2$ monitoring include patients with a coagulopathy, those receiving anticoagulation therapy, and those having an insertion-site infection.
- $p_{bt}O_2$ probes are MRI-safe as long as the ICP fiberoptic is not in place.
- $p_{bt}O_2$ probes are safe with CT.
- Cerebral oxygen data is accurate and reliable when the $p_{bt}O_2$ probe is located in the deep white matter of the brain, the location where oxygen consumption is most stable.
- Depending on the probe inserted, parameters such as ICP and brain tissue temperature can be measured immediately at the time of probe placement.
- Monitoring of $p_{bt}O_2$ values may be delayed as long as 2 hours as time is required for the brain tissue to settle after the microtrauma caused by probe placement.
- The normal range for brain tissue oxygen values is between 20 and 35 mm Hg.[2,3] Treatment goals usually aim to keep the $p_{bt}O_2$ greater than 20 mm Hg.
- A $p_{bt}O_2$ of less than 15 mm Hg is a critical threshold associated with a greater chance of functional disability and mortality related to cerebral ischemia.[4]

- $p_{bt}O_2$ values of less than 10 mm Hg are directly associated with severe disability, poor outcomes at discharge, and death.[1]
- $p_{bt}O_2$ values of less than 5 mm Hg are indicative of cerebral cell death and approximately 90% mortality.[4]
- $p_{bt}O_2$ values can be used to manage potential cerebral hypoxia by initiating clinical interventions aimed at increasing oxygen delivery and/or decreasing cerebral oxygen demand.
- Decreases in $p_{bt}O_2$ values occur when cerebral blood flow and/or cerebral oxygen delivery are inadequate and/or states of increased metabolic demands exist, indicating the potential for secondary brain injury.
- Increases in $p_{bt}O_2$ values denote decreased oxygen uptake by cerebral cells, indicating a state of "luxury perfusion" (hyperemia) and provide the practitioner with options in the face of intractable intracranial hypertension (e.g., controlled hyperventilation).
- Table 87-1 outlines treatment options for patients with a decrease or increase in $p_{bt}O_2$ values.
- $p_{bt}O_2$ probe placement: The physician placing the probe device will determine the catheter placement location after review of the CT scan and will ascertain the most appropriate monitoring area based on diagnosis and pathology, avoiding areas of infarct or hematoma.
  - ❖ Placement is typically in the area of potential tissue compromise (the ischemic penumbra), but with potentially viable tissue.
  - ❖ Placement may be in or near a lesion when the clinical goal is to monitor oxygen availability to damaged tissue.
  - ❖ Placement may be away from a lesion when the goal of therapy is monitoring oxygen in healthy tissue at risk for secondary injury.
  - ❖ The catheter is usually placed in the nondominant hemisphere (e.g., right frontal region). This is a safer location for catheter placement than the left hemisphere because speech function is located in the left hemisphere in 95% of right-handed individuals and 60% to 70% of left-handed persons.

- ❖ If a patient has a subarachnoid hemorrhage, the probe is placed in the area of the brain expected to develop vasospasm. This is determined by the distribution of subarachnoid blood on CT scan and by aneurysm location.
- ❖ If a patient has a traumatic brain injury, the probe is placed toward the area of greatest injury as indicated on the CT scan.
- ❖ If the patient has diffuse axonal injury with no asymmetry seen on CT, the probe is placed on the patient's right side.
- ❖ If the patient has asymmetry on CT the probe is placed on the same side as the pathology (e.g., edema, contusion, subdural hematoma)
- ❖ If the patient has a subdural, extradural, or intracerebral hematoma, the probe is placed on the same side as the pathology.

EQUIPMENT

- Sterile gowns, sterile drapes, sterile gloves, nonsterile gloves, hair caps, goggles, and facemasks
- Shave prep kit
- Antiseptic solution (e.g., 2% chlorhexidine-based preparation)
- $p_{bt}O_2$ monitor (Fig. 87-1) or module
- Connecting cables
- Cranial access tray
- $p_{bt}O_2$ probe
- # 11 blade
- Dressing supplies, including 4 × 4 gauze and tape
- Sterile dry gauze to be placed at the insertion point in a conical shape
- IV arm board to stabilize monitor probe(s) and cable(s) Additional equipment, as needed, includes the following:
- Intracranial bolt system
- Central line dressing change kit
- Extra transparent and soft cloth adhesive dressing or any appropriate dry, sterile occlusive dressing

TABLE 87-1	Managing Increased or Decreased $p_{bt}O_2$ Values	
Decreased $P_{bt}O_2$ Values		
Increased Demand	Increased ICP	Treat the increased ICP with diuretics, CSF drainage, sedation (e.g., barbiturates, propofol), craniotomy.
	Pain	Administer analgesics.
	Shivering	Rewarm, if needed, or administer agents to stop (e.g., Demerol, Thorazine, paralytic agents).
	Agitation	Administer sedation.
	Seizures	Administer benzodiazepines and adjunct anticonvulsants
	Fever	Treat the underlying cause of the fever, initiate a cooling device, if needed, and administer antipyretics.
Decreased Delivery	Hypotension	Administer isotonic fluids (normal saline or hypertonic saline) or vasopressors.
	Hypovolemia	Administer isotonic fluids (normal saline or hypertonic saline), blood replacement.
	Anemia	Administer blood replacement products.
	Hypoxia	Increase F_{IO_2}, PEEP, and pulmonary toilet.
Increased $P_{bt}O_2$ Values		
Increased Delivery Decreased Demand	Hyperdynamic (hyperemic)	Consider hyperventilation.
	Hypothermia	Rewarm to achieve normothermia.
	Sedatives	Decrease sedation, anesthesia, or paralysis as needed.
	Anesthesia	
	Paralysis	

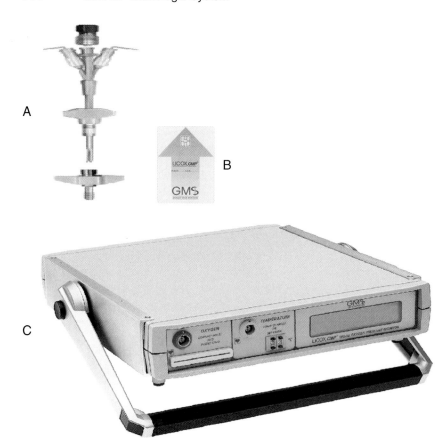

A, Model IM3 Triple Lumen Introducer.

B, Smart Card where calibration data for the oxygen probe is electronically stored.

C, Licox CMP monitor

FIGURE 87-1 **A,** Model IM3 Triple Lumen Introducer. **B,** Smart Card where calibration data for the oxygen probe is electronically stored. **C,** Licox CMP monitor, AC 3.1. *(Courtesy Integra Neurosciences, Plainsboro, NJ.)*

PATIENT AND FAMILY EDUCATION

- Assess patient or family understanding of the purpose of $p_{bt}O_2$ monitoring. ➼*Rationale:* Reduces anxiety and stress, stimulates requests for clarification or additional information, and increases awareness of the goals, duration, and expectations of the monitoring system.
- Explain the standards of insertion, patient monitoring, and care involving the $p_{bt}O_2$ monitoring system. ➼*Rationale:* Alleviates anxiety and stress, stimulates requests for clarification or additional information.
- Explain expected outcomes of the $p_{bt}O_2$ system. ➼*Rationale:* Decreases patient and family anxiety and stress by increasing awareness of $p_{bt}O_2$ monitoring duration and therapy goals.

PATIENT ASSESSMENT AND PREPARATION

Patient Assessment

- Assess the patient's neurologic status. ➼*Rationale:* Data obtained at baseline assessment will provide information necessary to recognize any change that occurs during or as a result of $p_{bt}O_2$ probe insertion.
- Assess the patient for signs or symptoms of local infection at the intended insertion location. ➼*Rationale:* Evidence

of local infection is a contraindication to brain tissue oxygen catheter placement.
- Obtain and review coagulation laboratory parameters (e.g., complete blood count, platelet count, prothrombin time, partial thromboplastin time, bleeding time, and international normalized ratio). ➼*Rationale:* Identifies the patient's risk for bleeding.

Patient Preparation

- Ensure that the patient and family understands the procedure. Answer questions as they arise and reinforce information as needed. The majority of patients who require brain tissue oxygen monitoring are in an altered state of consciousness with a Glasgow Coma Scale score of less than 8. ➼*Rationale:* Evaluates and reinforces information previously taught.
- Administer sedation and/or analgesia as indicated prior to beginning the insertion procedure. ➼*Rationale:* Facilitates the insertion process.
- Assist the patient to the semi-Fowler's position with his or her head in the neutral position and the head of bed elevated 30 to 45 degrees. ➼*Rationale:* Patients who are candidates for brain tissue oxygen monitoring may be experiencing increased intracranial pressure (ICP). Elevating the head of the bed and placing the head in the neutral position acts to decrease intracranial pressure by enhancing jugular venous outflow and also provides for optimal insertion accessibility.

| Procedure | for Brain Tissue Oxygen Monitoring: Insertion (Assist), Care, and Troubleshooting |

Steps	Rationale	Special Considerations
1. Wash hands.	Reduces the possible transmission of microorganisms and body secretions; standard precautions.	
2. Ensure that the patient is in a semi-Fowler's position with his or her head in the neutral position and the head of bed elevated 30 to 45 degrees.	Prepares the patient for probe insertion.	
3. Plug the $p_{bt}O_2$ monitor power cord into an AC wall outlet.	Provides energy.	
4. Attach the cables (e.g., oxygen cable, temperature cable) to the $p_{bt}O_2$ monitor.	Prepares the equipment.	Refer to manufacturer guidelines a needed. Some monitors and cables are color-coded.
5. Wash hands again and assist personnel as needed with donning of goggles or masks with face shields, caps, gowns, and sterile gloves.	Prepares for sterile procedure.	
6. Assist the physician as needed with site preparation (e.g., shave preparation and cleansing with antiseptic solution).	Prepares for sterile procedure.	
7. Assist the physician as needed in draping the head, neck, and chest of the patient in sterile sheets.	Prepares a sterile environment for the insertion process.	
8. Assist the physician as needed with opening of the sterile trays and probes.	Facilitates efficiency of the insertion process.	
9. Turn on the $p_{bt}O_2$ monitor.	Prepares the monitor.	Follow the manufacturer guidelines. The Licox monitor requires confirmation that a card referred to as the smart card has numbers that match those on the oxygen probe that is being inserted. This card is placed into a card slot located on the front of the monitor (see Fig. 87-1B).
10. Assist the physician as needed with insertion of an intracranial bolt (see Procedure 88).	May be inserted prior to $p_{bt}O_2$ probe insertion.	
11. Assist the physician as needed with insertion of the oxygen probe and temperature probe.	Facilitates the insertion process.	
12. Connect the oxygen and temperature probes to the monitor cables.	Prepares for monitoring.	
13. Observe the temperature and $p_{bt}O_2$ values.	Initiates monitoring. The temperature values should be accurate; however, time is required for the brain tissue to settle after the microtrauma caused by catheter placement.	Monitoring and recording of $p_{bt}O_2$ values can be delayed from 10 minutes to 2 hours.

Procedure continues on the following page

Procedure	**for Brain Tissue Oxygen Monitoring: Insertion (Assist), Care, and Troubleshooting**—*Continued*	

Steps	Rationale	Special Considerations
14. If possible, use a cable to pull or "slave" the values from the $p_{bt}O_2$ monitor to the bedside monitor.	Allows integration of the monitoring systems.	Refer to monitor guidelines for specific information.
15. After the system has been placed, apply sterile dry gauze at the insertion point in a conical shape.	Prevents contamination of the insertion site by microorganisms and protects the site.	A conical dressing (formed with dry sterile gauze) provides a base to secure the device to an arm board or other securing method.
16. Secure the $p_{bt}O_2$ monitor cables (Fig. 87-2).		
A. Place an IV arm board or stability anchor to the dressing cone where the device and cables can be secured.	The monitoring cables need to be secured so that there is no tension or disruption of the device at the insertion site.	
B. Anchor the cables from the patient's head to his or her shoulder in place with a transparent or soft cloth adhesive dressing.	The first tension point is directly on the patient's head where the dressing is anchored to the skin at the point of insertion. The second tension point is at the patient's shoulder.	Allow enough slack to accommodate for patient movement and turning.
C. Place rolled towels under the secured system.	Supports the entire mechanism.	
D. Secure the cables so they are not touching the ground.	Prevents gravity drag and tension on the cables and the device.	
17. Discard used supplies and wash hands.	Reduces the transmission of microorganisms and body secretions; standard precautions.	

Troubleshooting the $p_{bt}O_2$ Monitoring System

1. Perform an oxygen challenge test as prescribed.	After the brain tissue has had time to settle from the initial insertion, an oxygen challenge is performed particularly if the $p_{bt}O_2$ reading is unexpectedly low or there is a question of probe accuracy.	Follow manufacturer's guidelines for error codes that are specific to each $p_{bt}O_2$ monitoring system.
A. Place the ventilator F_IO_2 on 100% for 2 to 5 minutes.		
B. Observe, because an accurate probe will demonstrate an increase in $p_{bt}O_2$.		

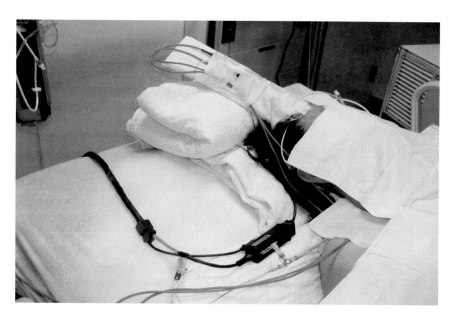

FIGURE 87-2 Demonstration of securing the IM3 Triple Lumen System (oxygen probe, temperature probe, and ICP catheter). *(Courtesy University of Pennsylavania Brain Oxygen Monitor Clinical Practice Guidelines.)*

Steps	Rationale	Special Considerations
C. If there is no response to the increased FIO$_2$, inform the physician as a head CT should be obtained to confirm correct probe placement.		
2. Note whether an electrical disturbance has occurred.	Strong electromagnetic disturbances can result in p$_{bt}$O$_2$ measurement errors. Errors can continue for a few seconds after the disturbance.	These disturbances may occur when a high-frequency scalpel or cauterization is used or during cardioversion.
3. Note whether a cable is damaged; if so, replace the cable.	If the probe cable or the extension cable is damaged, measured values can be incorrect or the measurement can be interrupted.	
4. Avoid changes in temperature of the temperature probe connector:	The temperature measurement may be inaccurate if the connector of the temperature probe is subjected to significant changes in temperature or if the temperature of the connector is beyond the defined range of 18° to 30°C.	
A. Avoid holding the temperature probe connector.	If the probe connector is held with a warm hand, the temperature measurement may be inaccurate until it is released.	
B. Protect the temperature probe connector from direct sunlight or warming devices.	Warming of the connector can cause inaccurate temperature readings.	

Removal of the p$_{bt}$O$_2$ Monitoring System

Steps	Rationale	Special Considerations
1. Wash hands and don goggles or masks with face shields, caps, gowns and sterile gloves. Assist personnel, as needed, with donning of above.	Prepares for removal.	
2. Position the patient in a semi-Fowler's position.	Prepares for removal.	
3. Assist the physician, as needed, with removal of the dressing.	Facilitates the removal process.	
4. Turn off the p$_{bt}$O$_2$ monitor.	Monitoring no longer necessary.	
5. Assist, as needed, with removal of the monitoring probes.	Facilitates the removal process.	
6. Apply a dry sterile dressing to the site.	Reduces the risk for infection.	Assess for bleeding, CSF leak, and signs/symptoms of infection.
7. Discard used supplies and wash hands.	Reduces the transmission of microorganisms and body secretions; standard precautions.	

Expected Outcomes

- p$_{bt}$O$_2$ probe placed in the correct position; monitoring able to begin after brain tissue has had time to settle (10 minutes to 2 hours)
- p$_{bt}$O$_2$ value between 25 and 35 mm Hg, or as prescribed, as an acceptable value for the individual patient
- Accurate and reliable p$_{bt}$O$_2$ monitoring
- Early detection of cerebral hypoxia
- Immediate intervention and management of compromised cerebral oxygenation hypoxia

Unexpected Outcomes

- Brain tissue oxygen reading low, with no response to oxygen challenge
- Infection (less than 2%)
- Hematoma from placement (4.95%)

Patient Monitoring and Care

Steps	Rationale	Reportable Conditions
		These conditions should be reported if they persist despite nursing interventions. • Changes in neurologic status • Changes in vital signs • Changes in ICP
1. Assess the patient's baseline neurologic status, vital signs, and ICP immediately prior to insertion and throughout the procedure.	Provides assessment of patient status before and during the procedure.	
2. Perform an oxygen challenge test as prescribed. A. Place the ventilator FIO_2 on 100% for 2 to 5 minutes. B. An accurate probe will demonstrate an increase in $p_{bt}O_2$.	After the brain tissue has had time to settle from the initial insertion, perform an oxygen challenge, particularly if the $p_{bt}O_2$ reading is unexpectedly low or there is a question of probe accuracy, reliability, or validity.	• Response to oxygen challenge test
3. Obtain the patient's temperature every 1-2 hours or as prescribed.	Provides a comparison of cerebral and body temperatures. Although the temperature measurements do not correlate exactly, there should be a parallel trend.	• Abnormal temperatures
4. Maintain the $p_{bt}O_2$ value between 25-35 mm Hg or as prescribed.	This represents normal values.	• Elevated $p_{bt}O_2$ values • Decreased $p_{bt}O_2$ values

Documentation

Documentation should include the following:

- Patient and family education
- Insertion of the $p_{bt}O_2$ probe
- Patient tolerance of the procedure
- Site assessment
- Neurologic assessments

- Hourly values, including $p_{bt}O_2$, brain tissue temperature, and other hemodynamic (e.g., vital signs, cardiac parameters: CO, CI, SVR) and neurologic multimodality monitoring in use (e.g., ICP, CPP, $SjvO_2$)
- Occurrence of unexpected outcomes and interventions

References

1. Bardt, T.F., et al. (1998). Monitoring of brain tissue Po_2 in traumatic brain injury: Effect of cerebral hypoxia on outcome. *Acta Neurochirurgica (Wien)* 71(Suppl), 153-6.
2. Maas, A.I.R., et al. (1993). Monitoring cerebral oxygenation: experimental studies and preliminary clinical results of continuous monitoring of cerebrospinal fluid and brain tissue oxygen tension. *Acta Neurochirugica,* 59(Suppl), 50-7.
3. Sarrafzadeh, A.S., et al. (1998). Cerebral oxygenation in contusioned vs. nonlesioned brain tissue: Monitoring of $Ptio_2$ with Licox and Paratrend. *Acta Neurochirurgica (Wien)* 71(Suppl), 186-9.
4. Valadka, A.B., et al. (2002). Brain tissue Po_2: correlation with cerebral blood flow. *Acta Neurochirurgica* 81(Suppl), 299-301.

Additional Readings

American College of Surgeons: Committee on Trauma (1977). *Advanced Trauma Life Support for Doctors Faculty Manual.* 6th ed. Chicago, American College of Surgeons, 219-46.
Bader, M.K., Littlejohns, L.R., and March, K. (2003). Brain tissue oxygen monitoring II: Implications for critical care teams and case study. *Critical Care Nurse,* 23, 29-4.
Bruder, N., et al. (1998). Influence of body temperature, with or without sedation, on energy expenditure in severe head injured patients. *Crit Care Med,* 26, 568-72.

Charbel, F.T., et al. (2000). Brain tissue Po_2, Pco_2, and pH during cerebral vasospasm. *Surg Neurology,* 54, 432-8.
Charbel, F.T., et al. (1999). What does measurement of brain tissue Po_2, Pco_2, and pH add to neuromonitoring? *Acta Neurochirurgica,* 75(Suppl), 41-3.
Chestnut, R.M. (1998). Implications of the guidelines for the management of severe head injury for the practicing neurosurgeon. *Surg Neurology,* 50, 187-93.
Dings, J., et al. (1996). Brain tissue Po_2 in relation to cerebral perfusion pressure, TCD findings and TCD-CO_2 reactivity after severe head injury. *Acta Neurochirurgica,* 138, 425-34.
Dings, J., Meixenberger, J., and Roosen, K. (1997). Brain tissue PO_2 monitoring: Catheter stability and complications. *J Neurologic Res,* 19, 1-4.
Fitch W. (2001). Brain metabolism. In: Cottrell, J., and Smith, D., eds. *Anesthesia and Neurosurgery.* St. Louis: Mosby, 1-17.
Ginsberg, M., et al. (1992). Therapeutic modulation of brain temperature: Relevance to ischemia brain injury. *Cerebrovasc & Brain Metab Rev,* 4, 189-225.
Gopinath, S.P., et al. (1999). Comparison of jugular venous oxygen saturation and brain tissue Po_2 as monitors of cerebral ischemia after head injury. *Crit Care Med,* 27, 2337-45.
Gupta, A.K., et al. (1999). Measuring brain tissue oxygenation compared with jugular venous oxygen saturation for monitoring cerebral oxygenation after traumatic brain injury. *Anesthesia Analg,* 88, 549-53.

Hoffman, W.E., et al. (1998). Regional tissue $p_{bt}O_2$, pco_2, pH, and temperature measurement. *Neurologic Res,* 20(Suppl), S81-S84.

Integra NeuroSciences. (2001). *LICOX CMP Brain Oxygen Monitoring System Operations Manual.* Plainsboro, NJ: Integra Neuro Sciences, 1-32.

Keller, E., et al. (2000). Changes in cerebral blood flow and oxygen metabolism during moderate hypothermia in patients with severe middle cerebral artery infarction. *Neurosurg Focus,* 8, 1-4.

Littlejohns, L.R., and Bader, M.K. (2001). Guidelines for the management of severe head injury: Clinical application and changes in practice. *Crit Care Nurse,* 21, 48-55.

Littlejohns, L.R., Bader, M.K., and March, K. (2003). Brain tissue oxygen monitoring in severe brain injury. I: research and usefulness in critical care. *Crit Care Nurse,* 23, 17-25.

McKiney, B.A., and Parmley, C.I. (1998). Effects of injury and therapy on brain parenchyma Po_2, Pco_2, and pH and ICP following severe closed head injury. *Acta Neurochirurgica,* 71(Suppl), 177-82.

Meixensberger, J., et al. (1993). Studies of tissue Po_2 in normal and pathological human brain cortex. *Acta Neurochirugica,* 59(Suppl), 58-63.

Meixensberger, J., et al. (1997). Quality and therapeutic advances in multi-modality neuromonitoring following head injury. In Bauer, B.L., and Khun, T.J., eds. *Severe Head Injuries.* Berlin: Springer Verlag, 99-108.

Narayan, R.K., et al. (1982). Intracranial pressure: To monitor or not to monitor. *J Neurosurg,* 56, 650-9.

Smythe, P.R., and Samra, S.K. (2002). Monitors of cerebral oxygenation. *Anesthesiol Clin N Am,* 20, 293-313.

Valadka, A.B., et al. (1998). Relationship of brain tissue Po_2 to outcome after severe head injury. *Crit Care Med,* 26, 1576-81.

van den Brink, W.A., et al. (1998). Monitoring brain oxygen tension in severe head injury. The Rotterdam experience. *Acta Neurochir,* 71(Suppl), 190-4.

van den Brink, W.A., et al. (2000). Brain oxygen tension in severe head injury. *Neurosurgery,* 46, 868-78.

van Santbrink, H., et al. (1996). Continuous monitoring of partial pressure of brain tissue oxygen in patients with severe head injury. *Neurosurgery,* 38, 21-31.

van Santbrink, H., Maas, A., and Avezaat, C.J.J. (1996). Continuous monitoring of partial pressure of brain tissue oxygen in patients with severe head injury. *Neurosurgery,* 38, 21-31.

Vinas, F.C. (2001). Bedside invasive monitoring techniques in severe brain injured patients. *J Neurologic Res,* 23, 157-66.

Wilkins, S.H., and Rengachary, S.S. (1996). Cerebral blood flow. In: *Neurosurgery.* 2nd ed., Vol. II, 1997-2006.

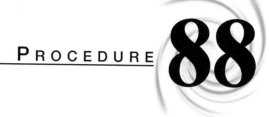
http://evolve.elsevier.com

PROCEDURE **88**

Intracranial Bolt Insertion (Assist), Monitoring, Care, Troubleshooting, and Removal

PURPOSE: Intracranial bolts are used to continuously monitor intracranial pressure (ICP) and calculate cerebral perfusion pressure (CPP) and assess cerebral compliance and autoregulation. Since intracranial bolts are not placed in the ventricular system, they cannot treat elevated ICP by draining cerebrospinal fluid (CSF).

Jacqueline Sullivan
Liza Severance-Lossin

PREREQUISITE NURSING KNOWLEDGE

- Knowledge of neuroanatomy and physiology
- Knowledge of aseptic technique
- Understanding of the setup of the neurologic drainage and pressure monitoring system (see Procedure 92).
- ICP is the fluid pressure of CSF in the intraventricular, subarachnoid, intraparenchymal (brain tissue), epidural, or subdural spaces.
- Cerebral (brain) tissue, cerebral blood, and CSF comprise three distinct volumes within the closed compartment of the skull. Any changes in one or a combination of these volumes will result in adjustments of the remaining volumes in order to keep the total volume of the intracranium constant—a compensatory mechanism also known as *intracranial compliance.*
- Despite fluctuations in systemic blood pressure, cerebral blood flow remains constant because of systemic blood pressure and intracranial pressure regulation and chemical stimuli, including changes in PCO_2, PO_2, and pyruvic acid.
- Table 88-1 lists systemic and intracranial pressure ranges necessary for intact cerebral autoregulation.
- Normal ICP ranges from 0 to 15 mm Hg (or 0 to 20 cm H_2O).[15]
- CPP is a calculated value that indirectly reflects the adequacy of cerebral blood flow; it is calculated by subtracting the ICP from the mean systemic arterial blood pressure (CPP = MAP − ICP). CPP reflects both

the systemic ability (MAP) to deliver blood to the brain and the resistance (ICP) that must be overcome in order to perfuse the brain.
- Normal CPP ranges from 60 to 160 mm Hg. Some experts recommend protecting cerebral perfusion by maintaining CPP within the minimum range of 70 to 90 mm Hg.[25]
- CPP below 50 mm Hg demonstrates inadequate cerebral perfusion.
- CPP less than 30 mm Hg results in cerebral tissue hypoxia and irreversible neuronal damage.
- Loss of cerebral autoregulation may occur when CPP remains out of the range of 50 to 150 mm Hg; that is, cerebral blood vessels no longer react to maintain CPP in response to changes in blood pressure.[1,3,7,17,24,25]
- Intracranial bolts may be placed in the subdural, subarachnoid, or intraparenchymal (brain tissue) spaces (Fig. 88-1). Only the ventricles, however, collect enough CSF to drain for therapeutic purposes, and therefore only intraventricular catheters can both treat and monitor ICP. Intracranial bolts have a lower relative risk for infection and hemorrhage because they are less invasive than

TABLE 88-1	Parameters Required for Cerebral Autoregulation Preservation
Intracranial pressure (ICP) less than or equal to 30 mm Hg	
Mean arterial pressure (MAP) within range of 60 to 160 mm Hg	
Cerebral perfusion pressure (CPP) within range of 50 to 150 mm Hg	

720

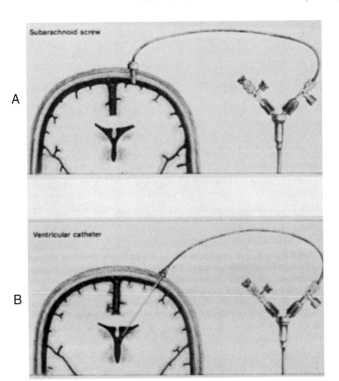

FIGURE 88-1 Anatomic placement of intracranial monitoring devices. **A,** Subarachnoid bolt. **B,** Intraventricular catheter. (*From Cardona V.D., et al. [1988]. Trauma Nursing. From Resuscitation Through Rehabilitation. Philadelphia: W.B. Saunders.*)

intraventricular catheters[5,10,11,18,21]; brain tissue can, however, herniate into the hollow bolt system, dampening the waveform, and damaging the parenchyma.[8] Intraventricular catheters can be rezeroed after insertion; intracranial bolt measurements are subject to drift since they are zeroed only prior to insertion.[12,13,18,19,21]

- A variety of intracranial bolts are currently available for monitoring ICP, including traditional fluid-coupled devices, fiberoptic systems, and microsensors. Fluid-coupled devices require the use of external strain gauge transducers; other systems do not.[16] The air-fluid interface of the external strain gauge transducer for a subdural or subarachnoid bolt should be placed at the level of the foramen of Monro, or immediately outside the cranium[14,15] (see Fig. 92-1).
- ICP waveform morphology reflects transmission of arterial and venous pressures through CSF and brain tissue. A normal ICP waveform has three distinct pressure oscillations or peaks (Fig. 88-2):
  - ❖ P1, also known as the *percussion wave,* reflects myocardial systole.

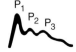

FIGURE 88-2 Components of the intracranial pressure waveform: P1, P2, and P3.

- ❖ P2, also known as the *tidal wave,* reflects myocardial diastole and ends on the dicrotic notch. P2 elevations occur with loss of cerebral compliance. P2 pressure oscillation amplitudes approach and surpass P1 pressure oscillations during periods of decompensation and loss of intracerebral compliance (Fig. 88-3).
- ❖ P3, known as the *dicrotic wave,* occurs immediately after the dicrotic notch and slopes into the diastolic baseline position. P3 oscillations correlate with venous fluctuations.[9,15,20]
- With loss of cerebral autoregulation the ICP waveform assumes a mirror-like image of the arterial waveform. If cerebral autoregulation is not intact (see Table 88-1), a rise in systemic blood pressure will cause both cerebral blood flow and the ICP to increase.[8]
- Trends over time in continuous ICP monitoring may demonstrate ICP wave patterns: *a* waves, *b* waves, and *c* waves.
- *a* waves, also known as *plateau waves,* occur in severe intracranial hypertension. *a* waves consist of sudden ICP escalations up to 50 to 100 mm Hg, which last 5 to 20 minutes and frequently accompany neurologic deterioration or cerebral herniation (Fig. 88-4).
- *b* waves are sharp rhythmic oscillations that occur every 30 seconds to 2 minutes; *b* waves may escalate up to 20 to 50 mm Hg and may precede plateau waves (Fig. 88-5).
- *c* waves demonstrate ICP elevations of up to 20 mm Hg and occur every 4 to 8 minutes; there is no evidence that they are clinically significant[20] (Fig. 88-6).
- Contraindications for intracranial bolt placement may include intracranial infection or coagulopathies.[5,6,23]
- Traditional therapeutic methods for lowering ICP include, but are not limited to, corticosteroid administration, osmotic diuresis, loop diuresis, hyperventilation, sedation, paralysis, normothermia or hypothermia, CSF drainage, and induced therapeutic barbiturate coma.[1,4,15,17,24] Use of these methods varies depending on the etiology of elevated ICP and individual patient conditions. Research-based guidelines for management of ICP for patients with traumatic brain injury have been widely disseminated and used in recent years.[3,4,14]

EQUIPMENT

- Antiseptic solution (e.g., 2% chlorhexidine-based preparation)
- Sterile gloves, surgical caps, masks, goggles or face shields, and sterile surgical gowns
- Sterile towels, half-sheets, and drapes
- Local anesthetic (lidocaine 1% or 2% without epinephrine)
- 5- or 10-ml Luer-Lok syringe with 18-G needle (for drawing up lidocaine) and 23-G needle (for administering lidocaine)
- Twist drill and bits (provided by a variety of manufacturers in both generic and custom kits)
- Sutures (2-0 nylon, 3-0 silk, 4-0 Vicryl)
- Scalpel with No. 11 blade
- Scalp retractor

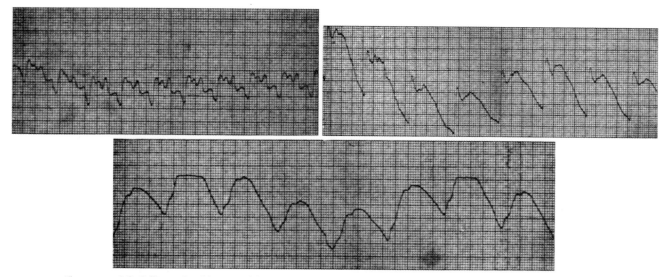

FIGURE 88-3 Example of intracranial pressure waveform with P2 elevation indicating decreased cerebral compliance.

- Forceps
- Sterile scissors
- Sterile needle holder
- Disposable cautery
- Suction and sterile suction apparatus
- Bone wax or gel-foam
- Light source
- Intracranial bolt: plastic or metal (for all systems)

- Fiberoptic or microsensor bolt catheter (if using these)
- Sterile dressing (sterile 4 × 4 gauze pads or occlusive dressing)
- Silk tape (1- and 2-inch rolls)
  Note: Many of the disposable surgical supplies listed above are available in generic and custom kits supplied by the ICP monitoring device manufacturers. Check kit labels for contents.

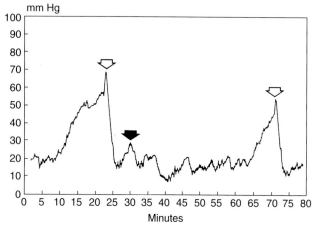

FIGURE 88-4 *a* or plateau waves. *Open arrows* indicate plateau elevations in intracranial pressure. Note that when intracranial pressure fails, it does not return to baseline preceding the first wave *(closed arrow)*. *(From Marshall S.B., et al. [1990].* Neuroscience Critical Care: Pathophysiology and Patient Management. *Philadelphia: W.B. Saunders.)*

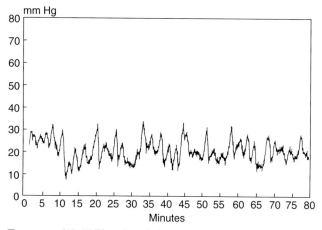

FIGURE 88-5 Elevations in intracranial pressure represent *b* waves. The intracranial pressure rise is steep and rapid, but to heights less than those observed with *a* waves and much briefer. *(From Marshall S.B., et al. [1990].* Neuroscience Critical Care: Pathophysiology and Patient Management. *Philadelphia: W.B. Saunders.)*

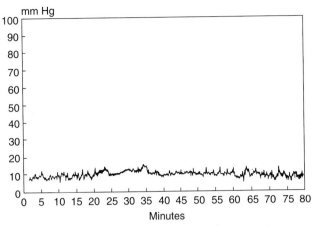

FIGURE 88-6 Lundberg or *c* waves. The intracranial pressure changes are much less impressive than those in *a* or *b* waves and reflect changes in arterial blood pressure. *(From Marshall S.B., et al. [1990]. Neuroscience Critical Care: Pathophysiology and Patient Management. Philadelphia: W.B. Saunders.)*

Additional equipment, as needed, includes the following:
- Two 4-inch gauze rolls (optional; needed if performing complete head dressing ["turban"] over insertion site dressing)
- Razor
- Fluid-coupled system: transducer cable, external strain gauge transducer, pressure tubing, three-way stopcock, 0.9% sodium chloride solution without preservative (see Procedure 92)
- Fiberoptic system: microprocessor (stand-alone monitor), preamp connector cable, monitoring cable to connect microprocessor (stand-alone monitor) to primary bedside monitoring system, fiberoptic intracranial bolt catheter with calibration screwdriver
- Sensor system: microprocessor (stand-alone monitor), microprocessor/sensor cable, monitoring cable to connect microprocessor (stand-alone monitor) to primary bedside monitoring system, intracranial bolt sensor catheter with calibration tool

PATIENT AND FAMILY EDUCATION

- Assess patient and family understanding of intracranial bolt ICP monitoring. ➥*Rationale:* Tailoring explanations to patient's and family's specific needs may alleviate stress.
- Explain the procedure for insertion of the intracranial bolt. Review the expected monitoring and patient care postinsertion. Review the family's role in maintaining an optimal ICP by limiting patient stress. ➥*Rationale:* Explanation of expected interventions may allay patient and family anxiety, encourage questions, and promote therapeutic family interaction.

- Explain the expected outcomes of intracranial bolt use. ➥*Rationale:* The patient and family may experience less stress if aware of the goals and anticipated duration of intracranial bolt monitoring use.

PATIENT ASSESSMENT AND PREPARATION

Patient Assessment

- Assess the patient's neurologic status. ➥*Rationale:* Familiarity with the patient's baseline clinical neurologic status enables the nurse to identify changes that may occur during or as a result of intracranial bolt placement.
- Observe for early signs of increased ICP, such as decreased level of consciousness, restlessness, agitation, lethargy, vomiting, motor weakness, or pupillary constriction dysfunction.[15] Observe for late signs of increased ICP such as loss of consciousness, posturing (decortication, decerebration), sluggish or absent pupillary light reflexes, respiratory pattern changes, Cushing's triad of vital sign changes (bradycardia, increased systolic blood pressure, widening pulse pressure).[15,20] ➥*Rationale:* Patients requiring placement of ICP monitoring devices are at risk for or are actually experiencing elevated ICP. Clinical neurologic assessment establishes a clinical correlate for quantitative ICP measurement data.
- Assess the patient's current laboratory profile, including complete blood count (CBC) or platelet count, international normalized ratio (INR), and partial thromboplastin time (PTT). ➥*Rationale:* Baseline coagulation studies determine the risk for bleeding during intracranial bolt insertion.[8,15]

Patient Preparation

- Ensure that the patient and family understand preprocedural teaching. Answer questions as they arise and reinforce information as needed. ➥*Rationale:* Reinforces understanding of previously taught information.
- Ensure that informed consent has been obtained. ➥*Rationale:* Protects the rights of the patient and makes an informed decision possible for the patient or family.
- Administer preprocedure analgesia or sedation, as indicated. ➥*Rationale:* Patients must remain very still during intracranial bolt insertion and may require sedation and analgesia to tolerate the procedure. In crisis situations patients may be unconscious and experiencing cerebral herniation, requiring very little sedation or analgesia for procedural tolerance.
- Assist the patient to a supine position with the head of the bed elevated 30 to 45 degrees with the neck in a midline, neutral position.[15] ➥*Rationale:* This position provides the necessary access for intracranial bolt insertion and enhances jugular venous outflow, contributing to possible reduction in intracranial pressure.

Procedure for Intracranial Bolt Insertion (Assist), Monitoring, Care, Troubleshooting, and Removal

Steps	Rationale	Special Considerations
1. Wash hands.	Reduces the transmission of microorganisms; standard precautions.	
2. Assemble the neurologic monitoring system (see Procedure 92).	Preparation of the external transducer allows immediate measurement of the ICP on insertion.	A variety of sterile, preassembled systems are available from ICP monitoring device manufacturers.
3. Flush the system, if applicable, with preservative-free 0.9% NaCl solution (see Procedure 92).	Removes air from the system.	
4. Turn on the bedside monitor and microprocessor (stand-alone monitor) if using fiberoptic or sensor devices.	Ensures that the monitoring equipment is functional and permits an immediate recording of the ICP on insertion.	
5. Prepare and check the suction.	Provides safety during the insertion process.	Suctioning may be needed during ICP Bolt placement to control bleeding or remove small fragments of bone or tissue from insertion site.[15]
6. Assist as needed with identifying the optimal area for placement of the device.	Facilitates placement.	Generally the nondominant hemisphere is the optimal location for placement of the intracranial bolt.[15,20]
7. Wash hands and don nonsterile gloves.	Reduces the transmission of microorganisms; standard precautions.	
8. Assist as needed with shaving and cleansing the insertion site with the antiseptic solution.	Reduces the microorganisms and minimizes the risk for infection.	
9. Assist as needed with draping the patient's head and upper thorax with sterile half-sheets and drapes.	Protects the insertion site from contamination.	
10. Open the sterile trays and have accessible the previously prepared neurologic monitoring system.	Facilitates the efficiency of insertion and ensures immediate ICP monitoring on insertion.	A variety of preassembled sterile trays containing disposable surgical instruments (as listed on the equipment list) are available from ICP monitoring device manufacturers. Check the list of sterile tray contents for the presence of the necessary equipment before opening the tray.
11. Level and zero the monitoring System (see Procedure 92). A. The air-fluid interface of the zeroing stopcock should be leveled at the foramen of Monro (top of the external auditory canal). Fiberoptic and sensor systems are leveled at the same location. B. Zero the system.	Ensures accuracy of the monitored data.	

Procedure	for Intracranial Bolt Insertion (Assist), Monitoring, Care, Troubleshooting, and Removal—*Continued*	
Steps	**Rationale**	**Special Considerations**
12. Perform the correlation procedure for fiberoptic systems: A. Ensure that the cable connects the microprocessor to the pressure module of the primary bedside monitoring system. B. Depress the "Cal/Step" soft key on the fiberoptic microprocessor until the number "0" appears on the microprocessor monitoring screen. Press three more times, until the "0" reappears on the screen. C. Continue to hold the "Cal/Step" soft key in the depressed position with one hand while pressing the zero option on the primary bedside monitoring system. D. When the number "0" appears on the bedside monitoring screen (it should still be appearing on the microprocessor screen also), release both soft keys on both monitors.	Ensures correlation between the fiberoptic microprocessor and the primary bedside monitoring system. Integration of the ICP data with the primary monitoring system data permits use of the centralized alarm system and trending of the ICP data with other multisystemic monitored data.	Although this procedure is called "Cal/Step," its purpose is not calibration in the traditional sense. It ensures correlation between the fiberoptic microprocessor and the primary bedside monitoring system.
13. Ensure health care providers don surgical caps, masks, goggles or face shields, and sterile gloves and gowns.	Provides an aseptic environment.	
14. Assist as needed with insertion.	Facilitates the insertion process.	
15. After the bolt is secured, cleanse around the insertion site with the antiseptic solution and apply an occlusive dressing.[2,22]	Reduces contamination by microorganisms.	Apply a complete head dressing ("turban") in addition to the insertion site dressing if desired.
16. Obtain and document the opening ICP (initial ICP reading once continuous monitoring is initiated immediately following insertion). Assess the ICP waveform morphology (e.g., P1, P2, P3). Obtain a hard-copy recording of the ICP waveform and include it in the medical record/chart.	Provides initial baseline data for the quantitative ICP measurement and qualitative assessment of the ICP waveform morphology.[10]	Waveform morphology data yield information related to the status of cerebral compliance and autoregulation.
17. Calculate and document CPP.	Provides initial indirect assessment of cerebral perfusion.[1,7,12,16,17]	
18. Discard disposable supplies, and wash hands.	Reduces the transmission of microorganisms; standard precautions.	
19. Perform a postprocedural neurologic assessment and compare it with the preprocedure baseline assessment.	Identifies any neurologic changes occurring during the procedure and the potential need for intervention.	
20. Evaluate the integrity of the intracranial bolt and functioning of the monitoring system.	Ensures accuracy and reliability of monitoring.	

Procedure continues on the following page

Procedure	**for Intracranial Bolt Insertion (Assist), Monitoring, Care, Troubleshooting, and Removal**—*Continued*

Steps	**Rationale**	**Special Considerations**
Troubleshooting		
1. Assess the integrity of the intracranial bolt device. If a dampened or aberrant ICP waveform appears on the monitor display screen:	Brain tissue or blood may occlude any of the various intracranial bolt devices, resulting in a dampened waveform. Occlusion may require manipulation or replacement.	Intracranial bolt manipulation is not a nursing responsibility in most institutions. Notify the physician or advanced practice nurse for assistance as needed.
A. Assess the tubing for air bubbles, which may dampen the waveform in the pressure monitoring system.	Fluid-coupled system may develop a leak or air bubbles, requiring a change of pressure tubing or external strain gauge transducer.[16]	Notify the physician or advanced practice nurse if the system requires changing.
B. Correct the ICP monitoring device malfunction according to the manufacturer's guidelines and institutional policy.	A fiberoptic or sensor system may be damaged, requiring replacement of the catheter. Excessively high readings (e.g., 888, 999) registered by a fiberoptic catheter usually indicate damaged fibers and the need for catheter placement.	Manufacturer's instruction and troubleshooting manuals can provide instructions for identifying and correcting common problems.
C. Using aseptic technique, change the neurologic monitoring system if needed (see Procedure 92).		
2. Assess the ICP monitor for evidence of mechanical failure (i.e., error messages on the monitor screen).	The neurologic monitoring system may need to be rezeroed. Loose cables and connecting devices may contribute to mechanical failure.	Notify the physician or advance practice nurse if unable to successfully resolve mechanical failure or zeroing issues involving the intracranial bolt. Device replacement may be necessary.
Removal of Intracranial Bolt		
1. Prepare sterile gloves, suture materials, sterile hemostat, sterile scissors, clamp, or twist drill.	Facilitates the procedure.	A sterile, palm-sized twist drill handle may facilitate removal of intracranial bolts. In fiberoptic or microsensor systems, the fiberoptic or microsensor catheter is removed first, followed by the actual intracranial bolt.
2. Ensure health care providers don masks, goggles or face shields, and sterile gloves.	Reduces the transmission of microorganisms; standard precautions.	
3. Assist the physician or advanced practice nurse as needed with removal of the intracranial bolt.	Facilitates the removal process.	
4. Apply an antiseptic solution and sterile occlusive dressing after the device is removed.	Prevents contamination by microorganisms.	
5. Dispose of used supplies and the device in the appropriate container and wash hands.	Reduces the transmission of microorganisms; standard precautions.	

Expected Outcomes

- Accurate and reliable ICP monitoring, CPP calculation, and assessment of cerebral compliance and autoregulation
- Maintenance of ICP within range of 0 to 15 mm Hg or as prescribed
- Early detection of elevated ICP trends
- Protection of cerebral perfusion (CPP within a range of 60 to 160 mm Hg) or as prescribed

Unexpected Outcomes

- CSF infection
- CSF leakage
- Dislodgment or occlusion of the intracranial bolt
- Pneumoencephalopathy (rare)
- Cerebral hemorrhage (rare)

Patient Monitoring and Care

Steps	Rationale	Reportable Conditions
		These conditions should be reported if they persist despite nursing interventions.
1. Monitor the patient's neurologic status and vital signs during the procedure.	May indicate any unexpected, although rare, multisystem consequences of intracranial bolt insertion.	• Change in neurologic status • Abnormal vital signs
2. Assess the ICP waveform trends during the insertion procedure.	The ICP waveform may show *a* or *b* waveform trends with the associated need for intervention.	• Abnormal waveform trends
3. Set the alarm limits based on the parameter goals.	Goals for ICP management are individualized for each patient based on etiology, comorbidity, and management strategies.	• Abnormal ICP • Abnormal waveforms
4. Assess the ICP hourly. The ICP should be read on the "mean" setting.	Determines the neurologic status.	• ICP elevations • ICP deviations • Sustained ICP elevations of 20 mm Hg or greater require immediate reporting/intervention
5. Perform neurologic assessments at least every hour or more frequently if indicated, including Glasgow Coma Scale (GCS), pupillary light reflex, motor assessment, and vital signs.	Neurologic assessments should be compared with the ICP, providing clinical confirmation of, and correlation with, monitored ICP data.[6,15,21]	• Changes in GCS • Changes in pupil response • Changes in vital signs • Changes in motor strength
6. Assess the ICP waveform for dampening or abnormalities.	Waveform dampening may render the ICP monitoring data inaccurate. ICP waveform assessment of P1, P2, and P3 demonstrates the status of cerebral compliance and autoregulation.[9,15,20]	• ICP waveform changes indicating loss of cerebral compliance or cerebral autoregulation should be reported immediately.
7. Assess ICP waveform trends at least hourly.	The presence of *a* or *b* ICP waveform trends reveals severity of ICP elevation and may indicate need for clinical intervention.[15,17]	• *a* waveform trends • *b* waveform trends
8. Calculate the CPP hourly (or more often, if indicated).	Adequate cerebral perfusion is indirectly assessed by CPP. Each patient may have specific CPP limits for reporting, depending on pathophysiology, individual clinical condition, and practitioner preference.	• CPP of less than 60 mm Hg should be reported to the practitioner immediately because of the imminent risk for cerebral ischemia or infarction.

Procedure continues on the following page

Patient Monitoring and Care—*Continued*

Steps	Rationale	Reportable Conditions
9. Assess the integrity of the intracranial bolt system at least hourly.	Hourly system inspection ensures accuracy and safety of monitoring and reduces contamination by microorganisms.[2,11]	
10. Zero the neurologic monitoring system during the initial setup, after insertion, if connections between the transducer and the monitoring cable become dislodged, and when the values do not fit the clinical picture.	Ensures accuracy of the monitoring process.	
11. Provide a safe environment through repeated explanation, sedation, or analgesia as needed, using mechanical restraints as a last resort.	Patient safety and prevention of unintentional removal of the intracranial bolt can be achieved through a variety of measures tailored to meet the individualized patient profile. Unintentional dislodging of the bolt must be avoided, because it can result in pneumoencephalopathy or excessive CSF drainage.	• Patient restlessness • Device dislodgment
12. Change the dressing as indicated by institutional policy or practitioner preference.	Practices regarding frequency of the dressing change and site care for ICP Monitoring devices vary considerably. Although anecdotal publications exist, currently there are no evidence-based guidelines for ICP monitoring device dressing changes. At minimum, sources recommend changing dressings that are loose or soiled.[2,11,22,23]	• Significant drainage • Signs and symptoms of infection
13. Change the ICP monitoring system as indicated in institutional policy using aseptic technique.	Limits risk for infection at insertion site or within CSF pathways. There is considerable variability regarding optimal frequency for ICP monitoring system changes. Some clinicians recommend changing system setup every 24, 48, or even 72 hours. Others prefer not to invade or change systems at arbitrary intervals. However, there is little clinical or laboratory research available to guide these decisions.[2,11]	

Documentation

Documentation should include the following:

- Patient and family education
- Time of insertion of the intracranial bolt, including any difficulties or abnormalities experienced during the insertion procedure
- Initial ICP reading
- Initial CPP calculation
- Description of CSF (clarity, color, characteristics, etc.) if observed during intracranial bolt insertion
- Patient's tolerance of the procedure

- Insertion site assessment
- Recording of ongoing hourly assessment of ICP reading, CPP calculation, ICP waveform morphology (P1, P2, P3, including assessment of cerebral compliance and autoregulation), and ICP waveform trends (including *a* or *b* waveform trends)
- Description of expected or unexpected outcomes
- Nursing interventions used to treat ICP or CPP deviations and expected or unexpected outcomes

References

1. Andrews, B.T. (1993). *Neurosurgical Intensive Care.* New York: McGraw-Hill.
2. Bader, M.K., Littlejohns, L., and Palmer, S. (1995). Ventriculostomy and intracranial pressure monitoring: In search of a 0% infection rate. *Heart & Lung: J Acute & Crit Care,* 24, 166-75.
3. Bullock, R., et al. (1996). *Guidelines for Management of Severe Head Injury.* New York: The Brain Trauma Foundation.
4. Bullock, R., et al. (1996). Guidelines for the management of severe head injury. *J Neurotrauma,* 13, 639-734.
5. Clark, W.C., et al. (1989). Complications of intracranial pressure monitoring in trauma patients. *Neurosurgery,* 25, 20-4.
6. Constantini, S., et al. (1988). Intracranial pressure monitoring after elective intracranial surgery: A retrospective study of 514 consecutive patients. *J Neurosurgery,* 69, 540-4.
7. Czosnyka, M., et al. (1997). Continuous assessment of cerebral vasomotor reactivity in head injury. *Neurosurgery,* 41, 11-4
8. Deyo, D.J., Yancy, V., and Prough, D.S. (2000). Brain function monitoring. In: Grenvik, A., ed. *Textbook of Critical Care.* 4th ed. Philadelphia: W.B. Saunders, 1816-24.
9. Germon, K. (1988). Interpretation of ICP pulse waves to determine intracerebral compliance. *J Neurosci Nurs,* 20, 344-9.
10. Germon, K. (1994). Intracranial pressure monitoring. *Crit Care Nurs Q,* 17, 21-32.
11. Hickman, K.M., Mayer, B.L., and Muwaswes, M. (1990). Intracranial pressure monitoring: Review of risk factors associated with infection. *Heart & Lung: J Acute & Crit Care,* 19, 84-90.
12. Hollingsworth-Friedlund, P., Vos, H., and Daily, E. (1988). Use of fiberoptic pressure transducer for intracranial pressure measurements: A preliminary report. *Heart & Lung,* 17, 111-20.
13. Khan, S.H., et al. (1998). Comparison of percutaneous ventriculostomies and intraparenchymal monitor: A retrospective evaluation of 156 patients. *Acta Neurochirurgica,* 71(Suppl), 50-2.
14. Lang, E.W., and Chestnut, R.M. (1994). Intracranial pressure: Monitoring and management. *Neurosurgic Crit Care,* 4, 573-604.
15. Lee, K.R., and Hoff, J.T. (1996). Intracranial pressure. In: Youmans, J.R., ed. *Neurological Surgery.* Philadelphia: W.B. Saunders, 505-7.
16. Lieberman, D.M., Maltz, P.G., and Rosegay, H. (2002). History of the strain gauge in measurement of the intracranial pressure. *J Trauma,* 52, 172-87.
17. Marshall, S.B., et al. (1990). *Neuroscience Critical Care: Pathophysiology and Patient Management.* Philadelphia: W.B. Saunders.
18. Mendelow, A.D., et al. (1983). A clinical comparison of subdural screw pressure measurements with ventricular pressure. *J Neurosurgery,* 58, 45-50.
19. Miller, J.D., Bobo, H., and Kapp, J.P. (1996). Inaccurate pressure readings for subarachnoid bolts. *Neurosurgery,* 19, 253-5.
20. North, B. (1997). Intracranial pressure monitoring. In: Reilly, P., Bullock, R., eds. *Head Injury.* London: Chapman & Hall, 210-216.
21. North, B., and Reilly, P. (1986). Comparison among three methods of intracranial pressure recording. *Neurosurgery,* 18, 730-2.
22. O'Grady, N.P., et al. (2002). Centers for Disease Control and Prevention (CDC) Hospital Infection Control Practices Advisory Committee. CDC guidelines for the prevention of intravascular catheter-related infections, 2002. *MMWR,* 1(RR10), 1-26.
23. Rebuck, J.A., et al. (2000). Infection related to intracranial pressure monitors in adults: Analysis of risk factors and antibiotic prophylaxis. *J Neurol, Neurosurg & Psychiatry,* 69, 381-4.
24. Ropper, A.H., ed. *Neurological and Neurosurgical Intensive Care.* 3rd ed. New York: Raven.
25. Rosner, M., and Daughton, S. (1990). Cerebral perfusion pressure management in head injury. *J Trauma,* 30, 933-41.

Additional Readings

Feldman, Z., et al. (1992). Effect of head elevation on intracranial pressure, cerebral perfusion pressure, and cerebral blood flow in head injured patients. *J Neurosurg,* 76, 201-11.
Schneider, G.H., et al. (1993). Influence of body position on jugular venous oxygen saturation, intracranial pressure, and cerebral perfusion pressure. *Acta Neurochir,* 59(Suppl), 107-12.
Winkelman, C. (2000). Effect of backrest position on intracranial and cerebral perfusion pressures in traumatically brain-injured adults. *Am J Crit Care,* 9, 373-80.

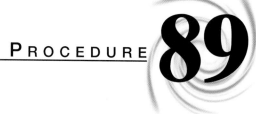
PROCEDURE **89**

Intraventricular Catheter Insertion (Assist), Monitoring, Care, Troubleshooting, and Removal

P U R P O S E : Intraventricular catheters are used to measure and continuously monitor intracranial pressure (ICP), calculate cerebral perfusion pressure (CPP), and assess cerebral compliance and autoregulation. Intraventricular catheters can also be used to treat elevated intracranial pressure by draining cerebral spinal fluid (CSF) from the lateral ventricles.

Jacqueline Sullivan
Liza Severance-Lossin

PREREQUISITE NURSING KNOWLEDGE

- Knowledge of neuroanatomy and physiology
- Knowledge of aseptic technique
- Understanding the setup of the neurologic drainage and pressure monitoring system (see Procedure 92)
- ICP represents the fluid pressure of CSF in the intraventricular, subarachnoid, intraparenchymal (brain tissue), epidural, or subdural spaces.
- Approximately 90 to 150 ml of CSF circulate within the CSF pathways in the brain and spinal subarachnoid space. Under normal circumstances a total of 20 ml of CSF is in the lateral ventricles and the cranial CSF pathways; the remainder is in the subarachnoid space surrounding the spinal cord. If cerebral edema is present, CSF may be shunted from the ventricles to the space surrounding the spinal cord.[1]
- The choroid plexus lines the lateral ventricles and secretes CSF at a rate of 0.35 ml per minute, or approximately 20 ml per hour. CSF is eventually reabsorbed into the venous circulation via subarachnoid villi. Although increased ICP does not have a substantial effect on CSF production, it may increase the rate of CSF resorption.[1]
- An intraventricular catheter is usually placed in the lateral ventricle, providing access for CSF drainage. Intraventricular catheters are the only ICP monitoring devices with capabilities for both treating and monitoring ICP (see Fig. 88-1).[6,11]

- Intraventricular catheters are the most invasive type of ICP monitoring devices and have the highest relative associated risk for infection and hemorrhage.[8,11]
- Fluid-coupled devices require use of external strain gauge transducers; other systems do not[7] (see Procedure 92). Fluid pressure is best measured in a lateral ventricle, which contains the largest accumulated volume of CSF in the normal brain. The external reference point that indicates the level of the lateral ventricles (specifically the foramen of Monro) is the top of the external auditory canal[4,6,12] (see Fig. 92-1).
- Fiberoptic and sensor ventricular catheter systems are capable of simultaneous ICP monitoring and CSF drainage; fluid-coupled systems are not. Fluid-coupled intraventricular catheters may be used in one of two ways: (1) as continuous ICP monitoring devices with intermittent CSF drainage capabilities or (2) as continuous CSF drainage devices with intermittent ICP monitoring (see Procedure 92).
- ICP waveform morphology reflects transmission of arterial and venous pressures through CSF and brain tissue. A normal ICP waveform has three distinct pressure oscillations or peaks, referred to as P1, P2, and P3 (see Fig. 88-2).
  - ❖ P1, known as the *percussion wave,* reflects myocardial systole.
  - ❖ P2, known as the *tidal wave,* reflects myocardial diastole and ends on the dicrotic notch. P2 elevations occur with loss of cerebral compliance. P2 pressure oscillation

amplitudes approach and surpass P1 pressure oscillations during periods of decompensation and loss of intracerebral compliance.

  ❖ P3, known as the *dicrotic wave,* occurs immediately after the dicrotic notch and slopes into the diastolic baseline position. P3 oscillations correlate with venous fluctuations.[6,12]

- Cerebral autoregulation is a protective mechanism which ensures adequate cerebral blood flow despite changes in systemic blood pressure. Cerebral autoregulation does not protect the brain if specific physiologic conditions are not met (see Table 88-1).[3]

- If cerebral autoregulation is not intact (see Table 88-1), a rise in systemic blood pressure will cause both cerebral blood flow and ICP to increase.[3] With loss of cerebral autoregulation the ICP waveform assumes a mirror-like image of the arterial waveform.

- Trends over time in continuous ICP monitoring may demonstrate ICP wave patterns: *a* waves, *b* waves, and *c* waves.

  ❖ *a* waves, also known as *plateau waves,* occur in severe intracranial hypertension. *a* waves consist of sudden ICP escalations up to 50 to 100 mm Hg that last 5 to 20 minutes and frequently accompany neurologic deterioration or cerebral herniation (see Fig. 88-4).

  ❖ *b* waves are sharp rhythmic oscillations that occur every 30 seconds to 2 minutes; *b* waves may escalate up to 20 to 50 mm Hg and may precede plateau waves (see Fig. 88-5).

  ❖ *c* waves demonstrate ICP elevations of up to 20 mm Hg and occur every 4 to 8 minutes; there is no evidence that they are clinically significant.[4,12] (see Fig. 88-6).

- Contraindications for intraventricular catheter placement may include intracranial infection, coagulopathies, and excessive cerebral edema with collapsed ("slit") ventricles.

- Traditional therapeutic methods for lowering ICP include, but are not limited to, corticosteroid administration, osmotic diuresis, loop diuresis, hyperventilation, sedation, paralysis, normothermia or hypothermia, CSF drainage, and induced therapeutic barbiturate coma.[5,6] Use of these methods varies depending on the etiology of the elevated ICP and individual patient conditions. Research-based guidelines for the management of ICP in patients with traumatic brain injury (TBI) have been widely disseminated and used in recent years.[2,4,6,9,12]

EQUIPMENT

- Antiseptic solution (e.g., 2% chlorhexidine-based preparation)
- Sterile gloves, surgical caps, masks, goggles or face shields, and sterile surgical gowns
- Sterile towels, half-sheets, and drapes
- Local anesthetic (lidocaine 1% or 2% without epinephrine)
- 5- or 10-ml Luer-Lok syringe with 18-G needle (for drawing up lidocaine) and 23-G needle (for administering lidocaine)

- Twist drill and bits (provided by a variety of manufacturers in both generic and custom kits)
- Sutures (2-0 nylon, 3-0 silk, 4-0 Vicryl)
- Scalpel with No. 11 blade
- Scalp retractor
- Forceps
- Sterile scissors
- Sterile needle holder
- Disposable cautery
- Suction and sterile suction apparatus
- Bone wax or gel-foam
- Light source (e.g., headlamp)
- Intraventricular catheter (silastic, fiberoptic, or microsensor)
- Sterile dressing (sterile 4 × 4 gauze pads or occlusive dressing)
- Silk tape (1- and 2-inch rolls)
  Note: Many of the disposable surgical supplies listed above are available in generic and custom kits supplied by ICP monitoring device manufacturers. Check kit labels for necessary contents.

Additional equipment, as needed, includes the following:

- Razor
- Fluid-coupled system: transducer cable, external strain gauge transducer, pressure tubing, three-way stopcock, 0.9% sodium chloride solution without preservative (may use sterile intravenous solution); sterile CSF drainage system (collection tubing, chamber, and bag) (see Procedure 92).
- Fiberoptic system: microprocessor (stand-alone monitor), preamp connector cable, monitoring cable to connect microprocessor (stand-alone monitor) to primary bedside monitoring system, fiberoptic intraventricular catheter with calibration screwdriver, sterile CSF drainage system (collection tubing, chamber, and bag).
- Sensor system: microprocessor (stand-alone monitor), microprocessor/sensor cable, monitoring cable to connect the microprocessor (stand-alone monitor) to the primary bedside monitoring system, intraventricular sensor catheter with calibration tool, sterile CSF drainage system (collection tubing, chamber, and bag).
  Note: A variety of preassembled sterile CSF drainage systems are now available in generic and custom kits from ICP monitoring device manufacturers.

PATIENT AND FAMILY EDUCATION

- Assess patient and family understanding of the intraventricular ICP monitoring and treatment. ➥*Rationale:* Tailoring explanations to the patient's and family's specific needs may alleviate stress.
- Explain the procedure for insertion of the intraventricular catheter. Review the expected monitoring and patient care postinsertion. Review the family's role in maintaining an optimal ICP by limiting patient stress. ➥*Rationale:* Explanation of expected interventions may allay patient and family anxiety, encourage questions, and promote therapeutic family interaction.

• Explain the expected outcomes of the intraventricular catheter. ➤➤*Rationale:* The patient and family may experience less stress if they are aware of the goals and expected duration of the intraventricular catheter monitoring.

PATIENT ASSESSMENT AND PREPARATION

Patient Assessment

• Assess the patient's neurologic status. ➤➤*Rationale:* Familiarity with baseline clinical neurologic status enables the nurse to identify changes that may occur during or as a result of intraventricular catheter insertion.
• Observe for early signs of increased ICP, such as decreased level of consciousness, restlessness, agitation, lethargy, vomiting, motor weakness, or pupillary constriction dysfunction. Observe for late signs of increased ICP, such as loss of consciousness, posturing (decortication, decerebration), sluggish or absent pupillary light reflexes, unequal pupils, respiratory pattern changes, and Cushing's triad of vital sign changes (bradycardia, increased systolic blood pressure, widening pulse pressure). ➤➤*Rationale:* Patients requiring placement of ICP monitoring devices are at risk for or are actually experiencing elevated ICP. Clinical neurologic assessment establishes a clinical correlate for quantitative ICP measurement data.

• Assess the patient's current laboratory profile, including complete blood count (CBC) or platelet count, international normalized ratio (INR), and partial thromboplastin time (PTT). ➤➤*Rationale:* Baseline coagulation studies determine the risk for bleeding during intraventricular catheter insertion.

Patient Preparation

• Ensure that the patient and family understand preprocedural teaching. Answer questions and reinforce information as needed. ➤➤*Rationale:* Reinforces understanding of previously taught information.
• Ensure that informed consent has been obtained. ➤➤*Rationale:* Protects the rights of the patient and makes an informed decision possible for the patient or family.
• Administer preprocedure analgesia or sedation, as indicated. ➤➤*Rationale:* Patients must remain very still during intraventricular catheter insertion and may require sedation and analgesia to tolerate the procedure. In crisis situations patients may be unconscious and experiencing cerebral herniation, requiring very little sedation or analgesia for procedural tolerance.
• Assist the patient to a supine position with the head of the bed at 30 to 45 degrees with the neck in a midline, neutral position. ➤➤*Rationale:* This position provides necessary access for intraventricular catheter insertion and enhances jugular venous outflow, contributing to possible reduction in intracranial pressure.

Procedure for Intraventricular Catheter Insertion (Assist), Monitoring, Care, Troubleshooting, and Removal		
Steps	**Rationale**	**Special Considerations**
1. Wash hands.	Reduces the transmission of microorganisms; standard precautions.	
2. Assemble and flush the fluid-coupled system with the external strain gauge transducer (see Procedure 92).	Preparation of the external transducer and CSF drainage system ensures the ability to measure the ICP immediately upon insertion.	In some institutions a single-pressure transducer system is used to obtain an external strain gauge transducer. **Depending on institution policy, either leave the system intact or remove the flush bag and tubing after the transducer is flushed and cap the end of the tubing with a sterile cap.**
3. Turn on the bedside monitor and microprocessor (stand-alone monitor) if using fiberoptic or sensor devices.	Ensures that the monitoring equipment is functional and permits the immediate recording of the ICP on insertion.	
4. Prepare and check suction.	Provides safety during the insertion process.	Suctioning or cautery may be needed during intraventricular catheter placement to control bleeding or remove small fragments of bone or tissue from the insertion site.

Procedure	for Intraventricular Catheter Insertion (Assist), Monitoring, Care, Troubleshooting, and Removal—*Continued*	
Steps	**Rationale**	**Special Considerations**
5. Assist as needed with identifying the optimal area for placement of the device.	Facilitates placement.	Generally the nondominant hemisphere is the optimal location for placement of the intraventricular catheter.[5]
6. Wash hands and don nonsterile gloves.	Reduces the transmission of microorganisms; standard precautions.	
7. Assist as needed with shaving and cleansing the insertion site with an antiseptic solution.	Reduces the microorganisms and minimizes the risk for infection.	
8. Assist as needed with covering the patient's head and upper thorax with sterile half-sheets and drapes.	Protects the insertion site from contamination.	

9. Level and zero the monitoring system (see Procedure 92).
  A. The air-fluid interface of the zeroing stopcock should be leveled at the foramen of Monro (top of the external auditory canal). Fiberoptic and sensor systems are leveled at the same location.
  B. Zero the system.
	Ensures accuracy of the monitored data.	Fiberoptic/sensor systems do not require periodic zeroing procedures during continued catheter use.[4,6]

10. Perform the correlation procedure for fiberoptic systems:
  A. Ensure that the cable connects the microprocessor to the pressure module of the primary bedside monitoring system.
  B. Depress "Cal/Step" soft key on the fiberoptic microprocessor several times, watching until the number "0" appears on the microprocessor monitoring screen.
  C. Continue to hold the "Cal/Step" soft key in the depressed position with one hand while pressing the zero option on the primary bedside monitoring system.
  D. When the number "0" appears on the bedside monitoring screen (it should still be appearing on the microprocessor screen also), release both soft keys on both monitors.
	Ensures correlation between the fiberoptic microprocessor and the primary bedside monitoring system. Integration of the ICP data with the primary monitoring system data permits use of the centralized alarm system and trending of the ICP data with other multisystemic monitored data.	Although this procedure is called "Cal/Step," it is not calibration in the traditional sense. It ensures correlation between the fiberoptic microprocessor and the primary bedside monitoring system.

11. Assemble the sterile CSF drainage system (see Procedure 92).	Prepares the equipment.	Depending on the institution, the drainage tubing may be primed after insertion with CSF.
12. Attach the sterile CSF drainage system distal to the external transducer in the fluid-coupled system and distal to the insertion end of the catheter in the fiberoptic and the sensor systems (see Procedure 92).	Prepares the equipment.	Depending on the institution, the CSF drainage system may be lowered after insertion until flow appears to ensure the correct location of the intraventricular catheter.

Procedure continues on the following page

Procedure **for Intraventricular Catheter Insertion (Assist), Monitoring, Care, Troubleshooting, and Removal**—*Continued*

Steps	Rationale	Special Considerations
13. After securing the intraventricular catheter, cleanse around the insertion site with an antiseptic solution. Apply an occlusive dressing.	Protects the site from contamination by microorganisms.	
14. Obtain the opening ICP (initial ICP reading once continuous monitoring is initiated immediately following insertion). Assess the ICP waveform morphology (e.g., P1, P2, P3). Obtain a hard-copy recording of the ICP waveform and include it in the medical record.	Provides initial baseline data for the quantitative ICP measurement and qualitative assessment of the ICP waveform morphology.[12]	Waveform morphology reflects cerebral compliance and autoregulation.
15. Calculate and document the CPP.	Provides an initial indirect assessment of cerebral perfusion.[1,3,6,11]	
16. Discard disposable supplies, and wash hands.	Reduces the transmission of microorganisms; standard precautions.	
17. Perform a postprocedural neurologic assessment and compare with the preprocedural baseline assessment.	Identifies any neurologic changes occurring during the procedure and the potential need for additional interventions.	
18. Observe the CSF drainage in the collection system.	Evaluates the CSF drainage and determines the patency of the system.	
Troubleshooting		
1. Assess the integrity of the intraventricular catheter. If a dampened or aberrant ICP waveform appears on the monitor display screen:	Brain tissue or blood may occlude any of the various intraventricular catheter devices, resulting in a dampened waveform. Occlusion may require catheter irrigation, manipulation, or replacement.	Responsibility for pressure tubing change and flushing of the intraventricular catheter system varies among institutions. Intraventricular catheter irrigation and manipulation is not a nursing responsibility in most institutions. Notify the physician or advanced practice nurse for assistance as needed. The ability to drain CSF is determined by the patient's condition.
A. Assess the tubing for air bubbles, which may dampen the pressure monitoring system and remove if possible. B. Correct the ICP monitoring device malfunction according to the manufacturer's guidelines and institutional policy. C. Using aseptic technique, change the ICP monitoring system if needed (see Procedure 92).	Some air bubbles can be displaced into the ventricular drainage chamber by opening the stopcock and allowing a few ml of CSF to drain. The manufacturer's instructions and troubleshooting manuals can provide instructions for identifying and correcting common problems.	
2. Assess the ICP monitor for evidence of mechanical failure (i.e., error messages on the monitor screen).	The neurologic monitoring system may need to be rezeroed. Loose cables and connecting devices may contribute to mechanical failure. Excessively high readings (e.g., 888, 999) registered by fiberoptic catheters usually indicate damaged fibers and the need for catheter replacement.	Notify the physician or the advanced practice nurse if unable to successfully resolve mechanical failure or zeroing issues involving intraventricular catheters. Catheter replacement may be necessary.

Procedure	for Intraventricular Catheter Insertion (Assist), Monitoring, Care, Troubleshooting, and Removal—*Continued*		
Steps	**Rationale**	**Special Considerations**	

Steps	Rationale	Special Considerations
3. Assess the patency of the CSF drainage system by ensuring the flow of CSF through the CSF drainage system. Flush the CSF drainage system and change the system using aseptic technique, if necessary (see Procedure 92).	The CSF drainage system may become occluded by cerebral tissue, blood clots, or sediment as these substances pass through the intraventricular catheter along with CSF.	Notify the physician or advanced practice nurse if a significant amount of cerebral tissue, blood, or sediment is found in the intraventricular catheter or the CSF drainage system, indicating possible occurrence of further pathologic conditions. **Responsibility for flushing the intraventricular catheter tubing varies among institutions. Intraventricular catheter irrigation and manipulation is usually not a nursing responsibility in most institutions. Notify the physician or advanced practice nurse for assistance as needed.**
Removal of an Intraventricular Catheter		
1. Prepare sterile gloves, suture materials, sterile hemostat, sterile scissors, and clamp or twist drill for assisting with the intraventricular catheter removal.	Ensures efficiency of removal procedure.	A sterile, palm-sized twist drill handle may facilitate removal of the intraventricular catheter inserted through intracranial bolts.
2. Ensure health care providers don sterile gloves or masks with face shields or goggles.	Reduces the transmission of microorganisms; standard precautions.	
3. Assist with the removal of the intraventricular catheter.	Facilitates the removal process.	Culture the tip of intraventricular catheter as prescribed.
4. Apply an antiseptic solution and sterile occlusive dressing after the device is removed.	Minimizes contamination by microorganisms.	
5. Dispose of used supplies and the device in the appropriate container and wash hands.	Reduces the transmission of microorganisms; standard precautions.	

Expected Outcomes

- Accurate and reliable ICP monitoring, CPP calculation, and assessment of cerebral compliance and autoregulation
- Maintenance of ICP within range of 0-15 mm Hg or as prescribed
- Early detection of elevated ICP trends
- Management of elevated ICP
- Protection of cerebral perfusion by maintaining CPP within a range of 60 to 160 mm Hg
- Ability to manage elevated ICP through CSF drainage

Unexpected Outcomes

- CSF infection
- CSF leakage
- Dislodging or occlusion of the intraventricular catheter
- Pneumoencephalopathy (rare)
- Cerebral hemorrhage (rare)

Patient Monitoring and Care

Steps	Rationale	Reportable Conditions
		These conditions should be reported if they persist despite nursing interventions.
1. Monitor the patient's neurologic and vital signs during the procedure.	Determines patient status during the procedure.	- Changes in neurologic status - Abnormal vital signs

Procedure continues on the following page

Patient Monitoring and Care—*Continued*

Steps	Rationale	Reportable Conditions
2. Assess the ICP hourly.[10] The ICP should be read on the "mean" setting. Adjust the pressure scale according to the patient's individualized ICP reading to capture the ICP waveform and accurate digital reading. Perform a neurologic assessment at least every hour, or more frequently if indicated, including the level of consciousness and Glasgow Coma Scale (GCS), pupillary light reflex, motor assessment, and vital signs.	The ICP, although continuously monitored, should be assessed and recorded on at least an hourly basis.[10] A neurologic assessment should also be performed and compared with the ICP to provide clinical confirmation of and correlation with the monitored ICP data.	• ICP elevations • ICP abnormalities • Sustained ICP elevations of 20 mm Hg or greater require immediate reporting and intervention • Changes in neurologic assessment • Changes in vital signs
3. Set the alarm limits based on parameter goals.	Goals for ICP management are individualized for each patient based on etiology, comorbidity, and management strategies.	• Abnormal ICP • Abnormal waveforms
4. Note the ICP waveform trends during the insertion procedure.	ICP waveform trends may show *a* or *b* waves, requiring intervention.[6-8]	• *a* or *b* waveform trends
5. Assess the ICP waveform trends at least hourly.[12]	Ensures early detection of any waveform trends requiring clinical intervention.	• *a* or *b* waveform trends
6. Calculate the CPP hourly (or more often if indicated).	Provides an indirect assessment of cerebral blood flow. Each patient may have specific CPP parameters for reporting, depending on individual clinical condition and provider preference.	• Changes in CPP • CPP less than 60 mm Hg (indicates suboptimal cerebral blood flow and imminent risk for cerebral ischemia/infarction)
7. Assess the intraventricular catheter system at least hourly.	Ensures accuracy and safety of monitoring and prevents contamination by microorganisms; may reveal new or progressing pathology.	• Frank blood or clots in the CSF drainage bag may indicate intracranial bleeding. • Absence of CSF drainage may indicate an occluded catheter, increased cerebral swelling, or overdrained ventricles. • Excessive drainage may lead to infarction and herniation.
8. Change the head and insertion site dressings and assess the insertion site as indicated by institutional policy or provider preference.	Permits assessment of device integrity and direct visualization of the insertion site. Prevents contamination of insertion site by soiled, wet, or loose dressing. Practices regarding frequency of head dressing change and site care for ICP monitoring devices vary considerably. Responsibility for insertion site dressing change and head dressing change is institutionally specific.	• Significant drainage on ICP insertion site dressing or head dressing • Signs and symptoms of infection
9. Assess comfort level of the patient.	Determines whether analgesia is needed.	• Unrelieved pain
10. Provide a safe environment, preventing unintentional dislodgment of the ICP monitoring device through repeated explanation, sedation, and analgesia as needed, using mechanical restraints only as a last resort.	Unintentional dislodgment of the catheter must be avoided because it can result in pneumoencephalopathy or excessive CSF drainage. Goals for ICP management are individualized for each patient based on etiology, comorbidity, and management strategies.	• Dislodged device • Abnormal ICP • Abnormal waveforms

Patient Monitoring and Care—*Continued*

Steps	Rationale	Reportable Conditions
11. Zero the neurologic monitoring system during the initial set up, after insertion, if connections between the transducer and the monitoring cable become dislodged, and when the values do not fit the clinical picture.	Ensures accuracy of the monitoring process.	
12. Change the ICP monitoring system and CSF drainage system, using aseptic technique as indicated by institutional policy.	Limits the risk for infection at the insertion site and within CSF pathways. There is considerable variability regarding optimal frequency for the ICP monitoring system changes. Check institutional policy.	• Signs of infection at the catheter insertion site
13. Using aseptic technique, obtain a routine CSF specimen from the intraventricular catheter using the sampling port of the CSF drainage system (see Procedure 92). Send the CSF specimen for laboratory analysis, including culture and sensitivity, Gram stain, cell count, glucose, and protein.	Provides early detection in cases where CSF infection occurs during or as a result of intraventricular catheter monitoring. Insufficient data exist to support decisions on the frequency of routine CSF sampling from intraventricular catheters. It is therefore recommended to follow institutional policy.	• Signs or symptoms of infection • Elevated white blood cell count • Elevated protein • Decreased glucose

Documentation

Documentation should include the following:

- Insertion of the intraventricular catheter, including CSF (clarity, color, other characteristics) and any difficulties of abnormalities experienced during the insertion procedure
- Opening ICP reading
- Initial CPP calculation
- Tolerance of procedure
- Insertion site assessment

- Digital and waveform hard-copy recording of the ongoing assessment of the ICP readings, CPP calculations, ICP waveform morphology (including cerebral compliance and autoregulation), and ICP waveform trends (including *a, b,* and *c* waveform trends)
- Nursing interventions used to treat ICP or CPP deviations and expected or unexpected outcomes
- Amount of CSF drainage

References

1. Barker, E., ed. (2002). *Neuroscience Nursing: A Spectrum of Care*. St. Louis: Mosby.
2. Bullock, R., et al. (1996). Guidelines for the management of severe head injury. *J Neurotrauma, 13,* 639-734.
3. Czosnyka, M., et al. (1997). Continuous assessment of the cerebral vasomotor reactivity in head injury. *Neurosurgery, 41,* 11-20.
4. Deyo, D.J., Yancy, V., and Prough, D.S. (2000). Brain function monitoring. In: Grenvik, A., ed. *Textbook of Critical Care.* 4th ed. Philadelphia: W.B. Saunders, 1816-24.
5. Greenberg, M. (2001). *Handbook of Neurosurgery.* New York: Thieme Medical Publishers, 615.
6. Lee, K.R., and Hoff, J.T. (1996). Intracranial pressure. In: Youmans, J.R., ed. *Neurological Surgery.* Philadelphia: W.B. Saunders, 505-7.
7. Lieberman, D.M., Maltz, P.G., and Rosegay, H. (2002). History of the strain gauge in measurement of the intracranial pressure. *J Trauma, 52,* 172-87.
8. Lozier, A.P., et al. (2002). Ventriculostomy-related infections: a critical review of the literature. *Neurosurgery, 51,* 170-81.
9. March, K. (2000). Intracranial pressure monitoring and assessing intracranial compliance in brain injury. *Crit Care Nurs Clin N Am, 12,* 429-36.
10. Marmarou, A., et al. (1991). NINDS Traumatic Coma Data Bank: Intracranial pressure monitoring methodology, *J Neurosurgery, 75,* S21-S27.
11. Mendelow, A.D., et al. A clinical comparison of subdural screw pressure measurements with ventricular pressure. *J Neurosurgery, 58,* 45-50.
12. North, B. (1997). Intracranial pressure monitoring. In: Reilly, P., and Bullock, R., eds. *Head Injury.* London: Chapman & Hall, 210-6.

Additional Readings

Bader, M.K. (1996). Ask the experts. What is the recommended external reference point for zeroing an intracranial monitoring system at the foramen of Monro? *Crit Care Nurse,* 19, 92-3.
Pope W. (1998). External ventriculostomy: A practical application for the acute care nurse. *J Neurosci Nurs, 30,* 185-90.

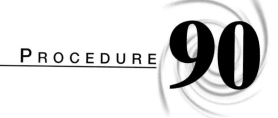

PROCEDURE **90**

Jugular Venous Oxygen Saturation Monitoring: Insertion (Assist), Care, Troubleshooting, and Removal

P U R P O S E : Jugular venous oxygen saturation (Sjvo₂) catheters are used to measure and continuously monitor the oxygen saturation of hemoglobin in the blood after cerebral perfusion. Sjvo₂ data and calculations involving this data help determine cerebral oxygen use, cerebral metabolic demand, and adequacy of cerebral oxygen delivery.

Jacqueline Sullivan
Liza Severance-Lossin

PREREQUISITE NURSING KNOWLEDGE

- Knowledge of neuroanatomy and physiology
- Knowledge of aseptic technique
- $Sjvo_2$ monitoring can help determine the balance between the brain's metabolic needs and the body's ability to meet those needs. Patients with increased intracranial pressure (ICP), potential compromise in cerebral perfusion, or alterations leading to cerebral ischemia are candidates for $Sjvo_2$ catheter monitoring.[5,8]
- Coagulopathies, local infection, cervical spine injury, local neck trauma, and impaired cerebral venous drainage generally contraindicate placing an $Sjvo_2$ catheter.
- 80% to 90% of cerebral blood drains from both hemispheres into the right internal jugular vein; the right internal jugular vein is therefore the optimal vessel for measuring and monitoring $Sjvo_2$. The $Sjvo_2$ catheter tip is positioned at the location of the jugular bulb of the internal jugular vein[1] (Fig. 90-1).
- In the presence of focal intracranial pathology, patterns of venous drainage may change, resulting in differences in right and left $Sjvo_2$ measurements. Although other modalities can monitor regional oxygenation of the brain tissue, $Sjvo_2$ gives a global picture.[2,9,12,16,20,24] Simultaneous

bilateral jugular bulb saturation measurements have been recommended in specific circumstances to capture regional variations in oxygenation; alternatively, other monitoring technology may be used in place of or in addition to $Sjvo_2$ monitoring.[11,13,17,19,25]
- The normal range for $Sjvo_2$ values is between 55% and 70%.[5,8]
- In the absence of anemia or sudden increases in the fraction of inspired oxygen, $Sjvo_2$ values over 75% suggest "luxury perfusion" globally, although areas of regional ischemia or infarction may still exist.[4,10,11,13,14,17,22]
- $Sjvo_2$ desaturation is a clinical emergency indicating potential systemic or cerebral decompensation. Table 90-1 describes potential causes of $Sjvo_2$ desaturation. Significant correlations exist between repeated $Sjvo_2$ desaturation events and poor outcomes in patients with severe traumatic brain injury and other cerebral pathologies.[3,4,5,7,8,21]
- $Sjvo_2$ values below 54% indicate relative cerebral hypoperfusion.
- $Sjvo_2$ values below 40% demonstrate global cerebral ischemia.
- Formulas and normal ranges for $Sjvo_2$ catheter data and calculations (e.g., $Sjvo_2$, $AVjDo_2$, Ceo_2) are included in Tables 90-2 and 90-3.

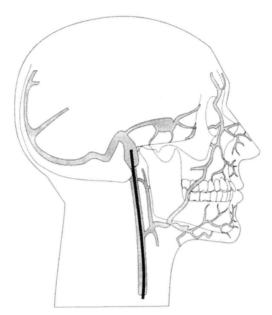

FIGURE 90-1 Placement of the jugular bulb venous catheter. *(From Kidd, K.C., and Criddle, L. [2001]. Using jugular venous catheters in patients with traumatic brain injury.* Crit Care Nurse, *21, 16-22.)*

- Arteriovenous jugular oxygen content difference ($AVjDo_2$) and cerebral extraction of oxygen (Ceo_2) are indirect clinical indicators of cerebral oxygen uptake, enabling providers to titrate clinical interventions according to cerebral oxygen uptake and cerebral metabolic demand in addition to intracranial pressure (ICP). $AVjDo_2$ calculation requires data obtained from both systemic arterial and jugular venous blood gas analysis. Ceo_2 calculation does not require data from blood gas analysis. Although $AVjDo_2$ and Ceo_2 measurements are expected to trend in the same direction, only $AVjDo_2$ calculation considers hemoglobin.
- $Sjvo_2$ values are inversely proportional to Ceo_2 and $AVjDo_2$ values:
  - If cerebral blood flow and cerebral oxygen delivery do not meet cerebral metabolic demand, $Sjvo_2$ decreases, whereas Ceo_2 and $AVjDo_2$ increase.
  - If cerebral blood flow and cerebral oxygen delivery exceed cerebral metabolic demand, $Sjvo_2$ increases, whereas Ceo_2 and $AVjDo_2$ decrease.
  - Increases in $AVjDo_2$ indicate increased oxygen uptake by cerebral cells; decreases in $AVjDo_2$ indicate decreased oxygen uptake by cerebral cells.
  - Increases in Ceo_2 indicate increased oxygen uptake by cerebral cells; decreases in Ceo_2 indicate decreased oxygen uptake by cerebral cells.
- A decision tree for clinical interventions based on $Sjvo_2$, $AVjDo_2$, and Ceo_2 data is shown in Table 90-4.
- $Sjvo_2$ catheters are available as 4-Fr fiberoptic oximetric catheters. These fiberoptic catheters require optical module cables and stand-alone oximetric monitors (processors) to provide a continuous display of $Sjvo_2$ values. Depending on equipment available, data can also be integrated into the bedside monitoring system. A pediatric central venous pressure (CVP) catheter can provide

TABLE 90-1	Etiology of Decrease in $Sjvo_2$

Anemia
Decreased cardiac output
Systemic hypotension
Arterial oxygen desaturation
Decreased cerebral blood flow
Increased cerebral metabolic demand (increased cerebral metabolic rate of oxygen)

TABLE 90-2	Formulas for Calculations Using $Sjvo_2$ Data
Calculations	**Formula**
$AVjDo_2$ (ml/dl)	Cao_2 (ml/dl) $-$ $Cjvo_2$ (ml/dl)
Cao_2 (ml/dl)	$1.34 \times Hgb \times Sao_2 + 0.0031 \times Pao_2$
$Cjvo_2$ (ml/dl)	$1.34 \times Hgb \times Sjvo_2 + 0.0031 \times Pjvo_2$
Ceo_2 (%)	Sao_2 (%) $-$ $Sjvo_2$ (%)
$CMRo_2$ (ml/100 g/min)	$\dfrac{CBF \text{ (ml/100 g/min} \times AVjDo_2 \text{ (ml/dl)}}{100}$
O_2ER (%)	$Sao_2 - Sjvo_2/Sao_2$ or Ceo_2/Sao_2
CMRL (ml/100 g/min)	$\dfrac{AVDL \text{ (ml/dl)} \times CBF \text{ (ml/100 g/min)}}{100}$
AVDL (ml/dl)	Arterial lactate (ml/dl) $-$ jugular Venous lactate (ml/dl)

AVDL, arteriovenous difference of lactate; *AVjDo₂,* arteriovenous jugular oxygen content difference; *Cao₂,* arterial oxygen content saturation; *CBF,* cerebral blood flow; *Ceo₂,* cerebral extraction of oxygen; *Cjvo₂,* jugular venous oxygen content saturation; *CMRL,* cerebral metabolic rate of lactate; *CMRo₂,* cerebral metabolic rate of oxygen; *Hgb,* hemoglobin; *O₂ER,* global cerebral oxygen extraction ratio; *Sao₂,* oxygen saturation in arterial blood; *Sjvo₂,* jugular venous oxygen saturation.

TABLE 90-3	Normal Ranges for Sjvo₂ Data and Calculations
Sjvo₂ Data	**Normal Ranges**
$Sjvo_2$	55%-70%
$AVjDo_2$	3.5-8.1 ml/dl
Ceo_2	24%-42%

Sjvo₂, jugular venous oxygen saturation; *AVjDo₂*, arteriovenous jugular oxygen content difference; *Ceo₂*, cerebral extraction of oxygen.

access for periodic blood samples from the internal jugular vein to calculate $Sjvo_2$, but cannot continuously monitor oxygen saturation.

EQUIPMENT

- Antiseptic solution (e.g., 2% chlorhexidine-based preparation)
- Surgical caps, masks, goggles, sterile gloves, and gowns
- Sterile towels, half-sheets, and drapes
- Local anesthetic (lidocaine 1% or 2% without epinephrine)
- 5- or 10-ml Luer-Lok syringe with an 18-G needle (for drawing up lidocaine) and a 23-G needle (for administering lidocaine)
- Central venous catheter insertion tray (various types available from several manufacturers)
- 5-Fr percutaneous transvenous introducer catheter
- 4-Fr fiberoptic oximetric $Sjvo_2$ catheter (available from several manufacturers)
- Optical module and connecting fiberoptic cable
- Oximetric monitor (processor)
- 500-ml bag of 0.9% sodium chloride intravenous solution (heparinized or nonheparinized, depending on physician preference or institutional standard)
- Bifurcated or dual lumen pressure tubing
- Pressure bag or device
- Sterile occlusive central venous catheter dressing
  Additional equipment as needed includes the following:
- Sterile needle driver and sutures if not provided in the central line kit
- Module and cable to connect the oximetric monitor to the bedside monitor

PATIENT AND FAMILY EDUCATION

- Assess patient and family understanding of $Sjvo_2$ catheter monitoring and its purpose. ➤*Rationale:* Clarification and repeated explanations may reinforce understanding and decrease anxiety for the patient and family.
- Explain the insertion process, patient monitoring, care and expected outcomes involved in $Sjvo_2$ catheter use. ➤*Rationale:* Knowing what to expect may reduce patient and family anxiety, as well as identify the need for clarification or additional information.

PATIENT ASSESSMENT AND PREPARATION

Patient Assessment

- Assess the patient's neurologic status. ➤*Rationale:* Baseline data provide information necessary to recognize changes during or as a result of catheter insertion.[23]
- Assess the patient for evidence of local infection or local neck trauma. ➤*Rationale:* These conditions are contraindications for $Sjvo_2$ catheter placement as they may impede venous drainage.
- Obtain current laboratory profile including complete blood count (CBC), partial thromboplastin time (PTT), and International Normalized Ratio (INR). ➤*Rationale:* Baseline coagulation studies are necessary to determine the safety of $Sjvo_2$ catheter insertion.

Patient Preparation

- Ensure that the patient understands preprocedural teaching. Answer questions as they arise, and reinforce information as needed. ➤*Rationale:* Evaluates and reinforces understanding of previously taught information.
- Administer preprocedure analgesia or sedation as indicated. ➤*Rationale:* Patients will be expected to remain still during $Sjvo_2$ catheter insertion and may require sedation or analgesia to tolerate the procedure. Alternatively, in crisis situations, patients may be unconscious and experiencing severe neurologic depression or instability, requiring little if any sedation or analgesia for procedural tolerance.

TABLE 90-4	Clinical Interventions Based on Sjvo₂ Data				
Sjvo₂	**AVjDo₂**	**Ceo₂**	**O₂ER**	**CBF Status (relative to CMRo₂)**	**Clinical Intervention**
Decreased	Increased	Increased	Increased	Decreased (cerebral hypoperfusion, ischemia, infarction)	Normalize CO_2 Hypervolemic hemodilution Induced systemic hypertension
Increased	Decreased	Decreased	Decreased	Increased ("luxury perfusion," relative cerebral hyperemia)	Hyperventilation Diuresis

Sjvo₂, jugular venous oxygen saturation; *AVjDo₂*, arteriovenous jugular oxygen content difference; *Ceo₂*, cerebral extraction of oxygen; *O₂ER*, global cerebral oxygen extraction ratio; *CBF*, cerebral blood flow; *CMRo₂*, cerebral metabolic rate of oxygen; *CO₂*, carbon dioxide.

Procedure for Assisting With SjvO$_2$ Catheter Insertion Procedure

Steps	Rationale	Special Considerations
1. Wash hands.	Reduces the transmission of microorganisms; standard precautions.	
2. Using aseptic technique, assemble and flush the double-pressure transducer system removing all air bubbles (see Procedure 75).	Prepares and eliminates air from the monitoring system. The bifurcated tubing will provide a joint flush system for both the 5-Fr percutaneous introducer catheter and the 4-Fr fiberoptic SjvO$_2$ catheter.	Although continuous SjvO$_2$ monitoring does not require invasive pressure monitoring, one of the two jugular catheter lumens (preferably the 4-Fr SjvO$_2$ catheter), if attached to a continuous invasive monitoring system, can provide a continuous recording of jugular venous pressure waves.
3. Turn on the oximetric processor (stand-alone monitor). Follow manufacturer instructions to perform in vitro calibration before catheter insertion, if required.	Ensures that the monitoring equipment is functional and prepares for in vitro calibration procedure if required by the particular SjvO$_2$ catheter and monitor manufacturer.	Unlike SvO$_2$ catheters, not all SjvO$_2$ catheters require in vitro calibration before insertion. Check the manufacturer's instructions regarding in vitro calibration before proceeding with insertion. *All* SjvO$_2$ catheters *do* require performance of the in vivo calibration procedure after insertion.
4. Ensure that the patient is supine with the neck in the neutral position and the head elevated 30 to 45 degrees.	Head elevation provides necessary accessibility for the SjvO$_2$ catheter insertion and enhances jugular venous outflow, contributing to a possible reduction in ICP.	Most candidates for SjvO$_2$ catheter monitoring are experiencing elevated ICP and require ICP monitoring.
5. Note and document the patient's baseline ICP in this position.	Provides baseline preinsertion ICP data necessary for evaluating the influence of the continuous indwelling SjvO$_2$ catheter on the ICP.	
6. Turn the patient's head away from the selected side for SjvO$_2$ catheter insertion. Note and document the patient's ICP.	The lateral head position may inhibit jugular venous outflow and cause an elevated ICP. Lateral head positioning before the insertion procedure demonstrates the patient's ability to tolerate the procedure.	Most initial SjvO$_2$ catheter insertion attempts involve use of the right internal jugular vein because 80% to 90% of the cerebral venous blood empties into the right internal jugular vein.[5]
7. Ensure that health care providers don caps, masks, goggles or face shields, sterile gloves, and gowns.	Provides aseptic environment.	
8. Prepare the selected insertion site with the antiseptic solution.	Reduces the microorganisms and minimizes the risk for infection.	
9. Drape the upper thorax and the neck with sterile half-sheets and drapes.	Protects the insertion site from contamination.	

Procedure continues on the following page

Procedure for Assisting With SjvO$_2$ Catheter Insertion Procedure—*Continued*

Steps	Rationale	Special Considerations
10. Assist as needed with opening the sterile CVP insertion tray and with setting up the sterile field using aseptic technique. Add 5-Fr percutaneous introducer catheter and 4-Fr fiberoptic SjvO$_2$ catheter using aseptic technique. Have the bifurcated or dual lumen pressure tubing or flush system available to flush catheter before insertion.	Facilitates the efficiency of insertion and avoids contamination by microorganisms.	CVP insertion trays are available from a variety of manufacturers. Check contents of the tray before opening.
11. Assist as needed with insertion.	Facilitates insertion process.	
12. Aspirate blood from each lumen and then flush each lumen.	Confirms the patency of both jugular catheter lumens before connecting to the flush system.	
13. Attach the bifurcated or dual lumen pressure tubing to the introducer and the fiberoptic catheters.	Prepares equipment.	
14. Monitor the patient throughout the insertion procedure: neurologic exam, vital signs, pain, and ICP.[23]	Ensures patient comfort, safety, and success of the insertion attempt.	Lateral head positioning during SjvO$_2$ catheter insertion may cause an elevated ICP.
15. Apply an occlusive dressing to the insertion site.	Prevents contamination of the insertion site by microorganisms.	
16. Set the alarms.	Alarms will signal changes in oxygenation.	
17. Ensure that radiology is called for skull or cervical radiographs.	Optimum placement of the SjvO$_2$ catheter tip is at the level of the jugular bulb of the internal jugular vein.[5,8] The SjvO$_2$ catheter tip position is confirmed radiographically to determine catheter position high in the jugular bulb, preferably above the upper border of the second cervical vertebra.[1,6]	Jugular bulb placement of the SjvO$_2$ catheter provides optimal sampling of jugular venous blood, reflecting oxygen saturation immediately following cerebral venous outflow and emptying. Some providers recommend anterior-posterior films.[1]
18. Obtain a jugular venous blood gas sample and perform an in vivo calibration procedure, following monitor manufacturer's instructions.	In vivo calibration ensures reliability between the continuously monitored SjvO$_2$ data and the SjvO$_2$ data obtained by laboratory analysis.	
19. Discard used supplies, and wash hands.	Reduces the transmission of microorganisms; standard precautions.	

Procedure	for Troubleshooting SjvO$_2$ Catheter		
Steps	**Rationale**	**Special Considerations**

Problem 1: Poor Light Intensity

Steps	Rationale	Special Considerations
1. Identify the low light intensity.	Fiberoptic technology provides continuous monitoring of SjvO$_2$ by analyzing reflected light signals.[6,8]	
2. Check the fiberoptic catheter for occlusion.	Low light intensity may indicate damage to the fiberoptics or catheter occlusion.[6]	
3. Cleanse the access port closest to the insertion site and attach a sterile Luer-Lok syringe.	Minimizes the risk for infection.	
4. Draw back on the syringe until blood returns freely and a normal light intensity displays.	Ensures optimal light intensity.	
5. If unable to aspirate blood or restore normal light intensity, notify the physician or advance practice nurse.	Catheter may need replacing.	

Problem 2: High Light Intensity

Steps	Rationale	Special Considerations
1. Identify the high light intensity.	High light intensity indicates vessel wall artifact. In this case SjvO$_2$ values will usually read 85% to 95%; such readings are inaccurate except in cases of brain death.	
2. Attempt to restore the normal light intensity by adjusting or slightly turning the patient's head to restore a neutral neck alignment.	Vessel wall artifact often happens during turning or positioning; repositioning corrects it.	Rarely, practitioners must reposition the catheter itself.[6,8]

Problem 3: Sampling and Calibration Errors

Steps	Rationale	Special Considerations
1. Identify sampling or calibration error.	Slow aspiration of the jugular venous sample avoids contamination of the sample with extracerebral venous blood.[15]	Some providers believe that changes in the blood flow characteristics or movement of the catheter tip during aspiration of the jugular venous sample will contribute to in vivo calibration errors. These issues require further investigation.
2. Avoid in vivo calibration errors by *slowly* aspirating (1 ml of blood over 1 minute) the jugular venous sample for in vivo calibration.	Slow aspiration of blood is needed to obtain a mixed venous oxygen sample.	

Problem 4: Coiling of the SjvO$_2$ Catheter

Steps	Rationale	Special Considerations
1. Identify rhythmic fluctuations in SjvO$_2$ trends.	Coiling of the SjvO$_2$ catheter within the internal jugular vein may cause rhythmic fluctuations in SjvO$_2$ trends that are unrelated to changes in ICP, cerebral perfusion pressure, and systemic blood pressure.[6]	
2. Consider obtaining a radiograph to assess if the catheter is coiled in the internal jugular vein.	Light intensity may remain within an acceptable range even in the presence of coiling of the SjvO$_2$ catheter.	

Procedure continues on the following page

Procedure **for Troubleshooting SjvO$_2$ Catheter**—*Continued*

Steps	Rationale	Special Considerations
3. If coiling is confirmed, consider preparing for catheter replacement.		
Problem 5: SjvO$_2$ Desaturation		
1. Identify SjvO$_2$ desaturation.	SjvO$_2$ desaturations are emergent events requiring immediate interventions for restoration or enhancement of cerebral blood flow and cerebral oxygen delivery.[3,4,5,7,8,21]	
2. Confirm the SjvO$_2$ data by obtaining a jugular venous blood gas sample for laboratory analysis.	Monitored desaturations should be confirmed by laboratory analysis to rule out monitor malfunction.[5,6,8]	
3. Perform an in vivo calibration.		

Procedure **for Removal of the SjvO$_2$ Catheter**

Steps	Rationale	Special Considerations
1. Prepare sterile gloves, suture removal equipment, sterile hemostat, and sterile scissors.	Prepares for the procedure.	
2. Wash hands and don nonsterile gloves and a face shield.	Reduces the transmission of microorganisms; standard precautions.	
3. Inactivate the alarm system.	Monitoring is no longer needed.	
4. Turn the stopcocks on the flush system to the "off" position and assist with catheter removal.	Facilitates the removal process.	
5. Apply antiseptic solution and a sterile occlusive dressing after the device is removed.	Reduces the contamination by microorganisms.	
6. Dispose of the used supplies and the device in the appropriate container; wash hands.	Reduces the transmission of microorganisms; standard precautions.	

Expected Outcomes

- Accurate and reliable SjvO$_2$ monitoring and AVjDo$_2$ and Ceo$_2$ calculations
- Optimization of the balance between cerebral perfusion, cerebral oxygenation, and cerebral metabolic demand
- Early detection and management of compromised cerebral perfusion and impaired cerebral oxygenation

Unexpected Outcomes

- Carotid artery puncture
- Excessive bleeding
- Venous infection (line sepsis)
- Impaired cerebral venous drainage or increased ICP
- Internal jugular venous thrombosis
- Pneumothorax (rare)
- Injury to stellate ganglion, phrenic nerve, or cervical ganglion (rare)

Patient Monitoring and Care

Steps	Rationale	Reportable Conditions
		These conditions should be reported if they persist despite nursing interventions.
1. Assess the patient's baseline neurologic status, vital signs, and ICP immediately after insertion.[23]	Presence of an internal jugular catheter may affect jugular venous outflow, causing an increased ICP. Some experts consider a sustained increase in ICP of more than 5 mm Hg over the baseline preinsertion value to be an indication for $SjvO_2$ catheter removal.[5,8]	• Change in neurologic status, vital signs, and ICP
2. Note and record the initial $SjvO_2$ value and calculate the baseline $AVjDO_2$, CeO_2, and O_2ER data.	Baseline $SjvO_2$ data allow the nurse to track patient trends in cerebral oxygen extraction and cerebral metabolism.	• Changes in $SjvO_2$ values and $AvjDO_2$, CeO_2, and O_2ER calculations
3. Provide a safe environment, preventing unintentional dislodging of the $SjvO_2$ catheter by providing repeated explanation and sedation or analgesia as needed. Use mechanical restraints only as a last resort.	Unintentional dislodging of the $SjvO_2$ catheter may result in excessive blood loss or jugular venous thrombosis.	• Catheter dislodgment • Any evidence of clotting
4. Continuously monitor $SjvO_2$.	$SjvO_2$ values higher than 75% suggest "luxury perfusion" globally; yet areas of regional ischemia or infarction may still be present. $SjvO_2$ values lower than 54% represent cerebral hypoperfusion. $SjvO_2$ values lower than 40% represent global cerebral ischemia. Repeated patterns of $SjvO_2$ desaturation predict a poor outcome in patients with severe head injury.[2]	• $SjvO_2$ values outside the range of 55%-70%
5. Measure ICP hourly and more frequently as indicated.	Assesses the effects of the internal jugular catheter. Sustained ICP elevations of over 20 mm Hg indicates the potential onset of intracranial hypertension.	• Changes in ICP • Sustained increases in ICP of more than 5 mm Hg over the baseline preinsertion value
6. Calculate CeO_2 and O_2ER hourly if indicated. Obtain blood gas analysis samples necessary for calculating $AVjDO_2$ as indicated. Consider calculating the cerebral metabolic rate of lactate and the cerebral metabolic rate of oxygen, as indicated.	CeO_2 and O_2ER derive from continuously monitored data (e.g., SaO_2, $SjvO_2$). $AVjDO_2$ calculation requires data from both arterial and jugular venous blood gas samples (i.e., PaO_2, $PjvO_2$). The cerebral metabolic rate of lactate is used during decreases in $SjvO_2$ as confirmatory data. The cerebral metabolic rate of oxygen calculation requires availability of cerebral blood flow measurement.[6,8,22]	• CeO_2 higher than 42% and $AvjDO_2$ higher than 8.1 ml/dl (indicate increased cerebral oxygen uptake and increased cerebral metabolic demand) • CeO_2 below 24% and $AvjDO_2$ below 3.5 ml/dl (decreased cerebral oxygen uptake and decreased cerebral metabolic demand)
7. Obtain a jugular blood gas sample and perform an in vivo calibration as recommended by manufacturer.	In vivo calibration with laboratory analysis of a jugular venous blood gas sample confirms decreases in continuously monitored $SjvO_2$ values.[5,8,15]	

Procedure continues on the following page

Patient Monitoring and Care—*Continued*

Steps	Rationale	Reportable Conditions
8. Assess the integrity of the $SjvO_2$ catheter monitoring system at least hourly.	Hourly inspection ensures accuracy and safety of the monitoring system.	
9. Change the occlusive dressing as per institutional policy for central venous lines.	No recommendation has been made by the Centers for Disease Control (CDC) for the frequency of routine central catheter dressing changes, but the CDC recommends replacing dressings when they become damp, loose, or soiled or when inspection of the site is necessary.[18]	• Signs and symptoms of infection
10. Change the intravenous flush solution and tubing for the $SjvO_2$ catheter per institutional policy.	Specific recommendations are not available for $SjvO_2$ monitoring; the CDC does state that the hemodynamic flush system for pulmonary artery catheter monitoring can be safely used for 96 hours.[18]	
11. After removal of the catheter, observe for signs of bleeding from the insertion site.	Identifies complications.	• Bleeding

Documentation

Documentation should include the following:

- Insertion of the $SjvO_2$ catheter, difficulties or abnormalities experienced during insertion
- The ICP during and after insertion
- The depth in centimeters of the catheter inserted
- Initial $SjvO_2$ recording
- Initial CeO_2 and $AVjDo_2$ calculations

- CVP dressing and insertion site assessment
- Hourly $SjvO_2$, CeO_2, and $AVjDo_2$ data, or as prescribed
- Hourly recording of ICP data
- Significant changes in $SjvO_2$, CeO_2, or $AVjDo_2$ values and interventions used to treat causes of those changes
- Expected and unexpected outcomes and interventions

References

1. Bankier, A.A., et al. (1995). Position of jugular oxygen saturation catheter in patients with head trauma: Assessment by use of plain films. *Am J Roentgenology,* 164, 437-41.
2. Chieregato, A., et al. (2002). Detection of early ischemia in severe head injury by means of arteriovenous lactate differences and jugular bulb oxygen saturation. Relationship with CPP, severity indexes and outcome. Preliminary analysis. *Acta Neurochirurgica,* 81(Suppl), 289-93.
3. Citerio, G., et al. (1998). Jugular saturation ($SjvO_2$) monitoring in subarachnoid hemorrhage (SAH). *Acta Neurochirurgica,* 71(Suppl), 316-9.
4. Cormio, M.A., Valadka, A.B., and Robertson, C.S. (1999). Elevated jugular venous oxygen saturation after severe head injury. *J Neurosurg,* 90, 9-15.
5. Cruz, J. (1998). The first decade of continuous monitoring of jugular bulb oxyhemoglobin saturation: Management strategies and clinical outcome. *Critical Care Medicine,* 26, 344-51.
6. Dearden, N.M., and Midgley, S. (1993). Technical considerations in continuous jugular venous oxygen saturation measurement. *Acta Neurochirurgica,* 59(Suppl), 91-7.
7. Fandino, J., et al. (2000). Cerebral oxygenation and systemic trauma related factors determining neurological outcome after brain injury. *J Clinical Neuroscience,* 7, 226-33.

8. Feldman, Z., and Robertson, C.S. (1997). Monitoring of cerebral hemodynamics with jugular bulb catheters. *Crit Care Clinics,* 13, 51-77.
9. Gupta, A.K., et al. (1999). Measuring brain tissue oxygenation compared with jugular venous oxygen saturation for monitoring cerebral oxygenation after traumatic brain injury. *Anesthesia and Analgesia,* 88, 549-53.
10. Imberti, R., Bellinzona, G., and Langer, M. (2002). Cerebral tissue Po2 and $SjvO_2$ changes during moderate hyperventilation in patients with severe traumatic brain injury. *J Neurosurg,* 96, 97-102.
11. Keller, E., et al. (2002). Jugular venous oxygen saturation thresholds in trauma patients may not extrapolate to ischemic stroke patients: Lessons from a preliminary study. *J Neurosurg Anesthesiology,* 14, 130-6.
12. Kiening, K.L., et al. (1996). Monitoring of cerebral oxygenation in patients with severe head injuries: Brain tissue Po2 versus jugular vein oxygen saturation. *J Neurosurg,* 85, 751-7.
13. Komiyama, M., et al. (1999). Marked regional heterogeneity in venous oxygen saturation in severe head injury studied by superselective intracranial venous sampling. *Neurosurg,* 45(6), 1469-72.
14. Lubbers, D.W., Baumgartl, H., and Zimelka, W. (1994). Heterogeneity and stability of local Po2 distribution within the brain tissue. *Adv Exp Med Biol,* 345, 567-74.

15. Matta, B.F., and Lam, A.M. (1997). The rate of blood withdrawal affects the accuracy of jugular venous bulb oxygen saturation measurements. *Anesthesiology,* 86, 806-8.

16. McLeod, A.D., et al. (2003). Measuring cerebral oxygenation during normobaric hyperoxia: A comparison of tissue microprobes, near-infrared spectroscopy, and jugular venous oximetry in head injury. *Anesthesia and Analgesia,* 97, 851-6.

17. Metz, C., et al. (1998). Monitoring of cerebral oxygen metabolism in the jugular bulb: Reliability of unilateral measurements in severe head injury. *J Cereb Blood Flow and Metab,* 18, 332-43.

18. O'Grady, N.P., et al. (2002). Guidelines for the prevention of intravascular catheter-related infections. *Am J Infect Control,* 30, 476-89.

19. Rossi, S., et al. (2001). Brain oxygen tension, oxygen supply, and consumption during arterial hyperoxia in a model of progressive cerebral ischemia. *J Neurotrauma,* 18, 163-74.

20. Schell, R.M., and Cole, D.J. (2000). Cerebral monitoring: Jugular venous oximetry. *Anesthesia and Analgesia,* 90, 559-66.

21. Sheinberg, M., et al. (1992). Continuous monitoring of jugular venous oxygen saturation in head-injured patients. *J Neurosurg,* 76, 212-7.

22. Stochetti, N., et al. (1994). Cerebral venous oxygen saturation studied with bilateral samples in internal jugular veins. *Neurosurg,* 34, 38-44.

23. Struchen, M.A., et al. (2001). The relation between acute physiological variables and outcome on the Glasgow Outcome Scale and Disability Rating Scale following severe traumatic brain injury. *J Neurotrauma,* 18, 115-25.

24. van Santbrink, H., Maas, A.I., and Avezaat, C.J. (1996). Continuous monitoring of partial pressure of brain tissue oxygen in patients with severe head injury. *Neurosurg,* 38, 21-31.

25. White, H., and Baker, A. (2002). Continuous jugular venous oximetry in the neurointensive care unit: A brief review. *Can J Anaesth,* 49, 623-9.

Additional Readings

Chatfield, D., and Rees-Pedlar, S. (2001). Jugular venous oxygen saturation: Is it relevant to the nurse? *Nursing in Critical Care,* 6, 187-91.

Gibbs, E.L., Lennox, W.G., and Nims, L.F. (1942). Arterial and cerebral venous blood. Arterial-venous differences in man. *J Biol Chem,* 144, 325-32.

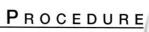
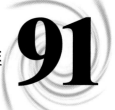

PROCEDURE **91**

Lumbar Subarachnoid Catheter Insertion (Assist) for Cerebral Spinal Fluid Pressure Monitoring and Drainage

P U R P O S E :   Patients with conditions ranging from the central nervous system to thoracoabdominal aneurysms may benefit from therapeutic levels of CSF pressure. Lumbar subarachnoid catheters are used for cerebrospinal fluid (CSF) pressure monitoring and drainage.

Liza Severance-Lossin
Patricia A. Blissitt
Jacqueline Sullivan

PREREQUISITE NURSING KNOWLEDGE

- Knowledge of the anatomy and physiology of the vertebral column, spinal meninges, and CSF circulation, including the location of the lumbar cistern
- Knowledge of aseptic technique
- Because the same meningeal layers encompass the brain and the spinal cord, normal CSF pressure in the lumbar subarachnoid space is analogous to normal intracranial pressures and ranges from 0 to 15 mm Hg.[13,24] Further research is required to ascertain therapeutic levels after surgical interventions.[1,24]
- Lumbar subarachnoid catheters (lumbar drains, intrathecal catheters) require lumbar puncture (LP) for insertion.[14,16] Lumbar subarachnoid catheters permit nurses to note any CSF pressure elevations and to maintain pressures within normal limits by draining CSF without directly accessing the intracranial compartment.
- Patients with CSF leaks may require lower CSF pressures to allow any tears in the dura mater to approximate edges and heal.[10]
- Similarly, patients with a normal pressure hydrocephalus may benefit from lumbar subarachnoid catheters during acute exacerbation episodes, when frequent lumbar punctures would be the alternative.[11,14]
- Lumbar subarachnoid drainage can be used instead of a ventriculostomy to decrease intracranial hypertension

or remove blood from the subarachnoid space.[9,21] CSF drainage has been reported to protect the spinal cord during surgical procedures requiring cross clamping of the thoracic aorta.[1,5,6] Maintaining pressure at 10 to 15 mm Hg or less via CSF drainage may correlate with fewer spinal cord deficits in patients undergoing thoracoabdominal aneurysm repair, but neurologic complications can also result.[2,6,7,12,17,22,26]

- Complications that may result from the use of a lumbar subarachnoid catheter include infection, epidural or subdural hematomas, overdrainage of CSF, pneumocephalus, and paraplegia.[3,4,7,23,26]

EQUIPMENT

- Antiseptic solution (e.g., 2% chlorhexidine-based preparation)
- Sterile gloves
- Surgical caps and masks
- Sterile surgical gowns
- Sterile towels, half-sheets, and drapes
- Local anesthetic (lidocaine 1% or 2% without epineprine)
- 5- or 10-ml Luer-Lok syringe for drawing up lidocaine and 23-G needle for administering lidocaine
- Sutures (2-0 nylon, 3-0 silk, 4-0 Vicryl)
- Forceps
- Sterile scissors
- Sterile needle holder

- Preservative-free normal saline
- Lumbar catheter
- Lumbar puncture tray with spinal needle
- Sterile occlusive dressing
- Silk tape (1- and 2-inch rolls)
- External transducer with pressure tubing
- Pressure cable
- External CSF drainage and monitoring system
  Additional supplies as needed include the following:
- Rolled towels or small pillows to support the patient during positioning
- 3-way stopcock
- Nonvented caps

PATIENT AND FAMILY EDUCATION

- Assess the patient and family understanding of the lumbar subarachnoid catheter system. ➤*Rationale:* Any necessary clarification may limit anxiety for the patient and family.
- Explain insertion, patient monitoring, and care involving the lumbar subarachnoid catheter. ➤*Rationale:* Knowing what to expect can minimize anxiety and encourage questions regarding goals, duration, and expected outcomes of the lumbar subarachnoid catheter.

PATIENT ASSESSMENT AND PREPARATION

Patient Assessment

- Assess the patient's neurologic status, including motor function in the lower extremities and bowel and bladder function. ➤*Rationale:* Provides baseline data.
- Assess the patient's current laboratory profile, including complete blood count (CBC), partial thromboplastin time (PTT), and international normalized ratio (INR). ➤*Rationale:* Baseline coagulation studies determine the risk for bleeding during and after lumbar subarachnoid catheter insertion.

Patient Preparation

- Ensure that informed consent has been obtained. ➤*Rationale:* Protects the rights of the patient and makes an informed decision possible for the patient.
- Administer preprocedure analgesia or sedation as prescribed. ➤*Rationale:* The patient will be expected to be very still during lumbar subarachnoid catheter insertion and monitoring and therefore may require sedation or analgesia to tolerate the procedure.

Procedure for Lumbar Subarachnoid Catheter Insertion (Assist)

Steps	Rationale	Special Considerations
1. Wash hands.	Reduces the transmission of microorganisms; standard precautions.	
2. Assemble a fluid-filled neurologic monitoring system (see Procedure 92).	Facilitates monitoring after catheter insertion.	The system consists of a transducer, stopcock, nonvented cap, and pressure tubing as needed based on the manufacturer's design.
3. Connect the neurologic monitoring system to the monitor (see Procedure 92).	Facilitates insertion and immediate lumbar subarachnoid CSF pressure monitoring upon insertion.	Ensure that the waveform chosen for CSF monitoring is read on the "mean setting." Set alarm limits.
4. Assemble and flush the sterile CSF drainage system compatible with the lumbar subarachnoid catheter device.	Prepares the equipment.	Some practitioners will allow CSF to flush the system after inserting the catheter.
5. Assist the patient to a side-lying position (see Fig. 97-1).	Provides access for the lumbar puncture and catheter insertion.	
6. Assist as needed with cleansing the intended insertion site with the antiseptic solution.	Minimizes the risk for infection, and protects the insertion site from recontamination.	
7. Assist as needed with draping the patient with sterile sheets and opening sterile trays.	Prepares for catheter insertion.	
8. Set the drip chamber at the level of the transducer (Figs. 91-1 and 91-2).	Ensures accurate readings on which to base therapy.	The membrane at the top of the drip chamber allows zeroing without opening the fluid-coupled system

Procedure continues on the following page

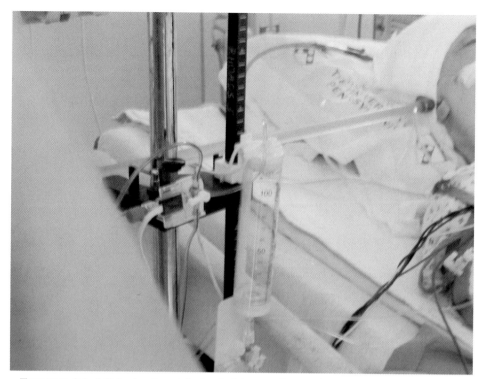

FIGURE 91-1 Drip chamber at the level of the transducer and the external auditory meatus.

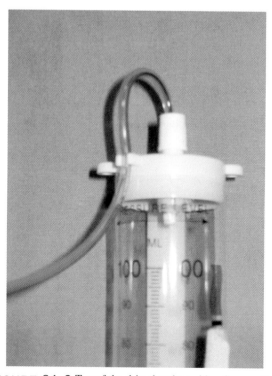

FIGURE 91-2 Top of the drip chamber with reference line.

Procedure for Lumbar Subarachnoid Catheter Insertion (Assist)—*Continued*

Steps	Rationale	Special Considerations
		to air. The membrane must remain dry in order to permit accurate readings.
9. Level the drip chamber and the transducer as prescribed or per institution standard.	Prepares the neurologic monitoring system.	For neurosurgical patients, the transducer remains at shoulder level if supine and at the external auditory meatus if sitting.[10,11,14] Thoracic surgical patients may have the transducer placed at the phlebostatic axis. Follow institution standard.
10. Turn the stopcock off to the patient and zero the monitoring system at the anatomic reference point.	Allows the monitor to use atmospheric pressure as a reference for zero.	
11. Assist as needed with the catheter insertion.	Facilitates insertion.	Surgeons may insert the catheter intraoperatively.
12. Note the initial CSF pressure.	Guides therapy.	
13. Apply an occlusive sterile dressing to the catheter insertion site.	Reduces contamination of the insertion site by microorganisms.	
14. Secure the catheter with tape, being careful not to alter the catheter position.	Reduces the potential for catheter dislodgment.	
15. Remove the fluid bag and fast flush device from the neurologic monitoring system and cap the end.	Prepares the system.	
16. Attach the fluid-filled neurologic monitoring system to the lumbar drain and drainage system.		
17. Turn the stopcock off to the patient and zero the monitoring system.	Ensures accurate data on which to base therapy.	If the drip chamber is at the level of the transducer and the membrane at the top of the drip chamber is dry, there is no need to open the fluid-filled system to air.
18. Observe the waveform morphology, obtain a strip of the waveform, and measure the CSF pressure.	Provides initial baseline data. Confirms correct placement of the catheter.	Lumbar subarachnoid CSF pressure waveform data are similar to traditional ICP waveform data.
19. Place the drip chamber at the level determined by the practitioner for maintenance of optimal lumbar subarachnoid CSF pressure.	Prevents over- or underdrainage of CSF.	Follow institution standard.
20. Turn the stopcock to monitor or to continuously drain. Follow institution standard.	Allows the system to function.	Set alarms if continuously monitoring.
21. Discard used supplies and wash hands.	Reduces the transmission of micro-organisms; standard precautions.	
Troubleshooting 1. If the CSF waveform is dampened:	Dampening of the waveform can indicate catheter occlusion or risk for catheter displacement.	Catheter occlusion may result from precipitate in the CSF.
A. Assess the integrity of the lumbar subarachnoid catheter device and correct problems if possible.	Loose connections may cause dampened waveforms as well as increase the risk for infection.	

Procedure continues on the following page

Procedure for Lumbar Subarachnoid Catheter Insertion (Assist)—*Continued*

Steps	Rationale	Special Considerations
B. Assess the monitoring system for disconnections and reconnect the system if needed.	Loose cables and connecting devices may contribute to mechanical failure.	
C. Assess the drip chamber for the correct position and readjust the position if needed (see Figs. 91-1 and 91-2).	The membrane at the top of the drip chamber allows zeroing without opening the fluid-coupled system to air. If the membrane becomes wet, it will no longer permit accurate readings and the drip chamber must be changed.	Changing the drip chamber involves changing the entire CSF drainage system. Responsibility for changing the CSF drainage system varies among institutions and is usually not a nursing responsibility in most institutions. Notify the physician or advanced practice nurse for assistance as needed.
2. Assess for the sudden absence of the pressure waveform or significant changes in pressure measurements without an apparent clinical cause. A. Ensure connections are tight. B. Ensure leveling is correct. C. Rezero the system.	Ensures accurate measurement of CSF pressure.	Notify the physician or advanced practice nurse if unable to identify a reversible cause. The CSF drainage system or the catheter may need to be replaced because of catheter dislodgment or blockage.
3. Assess the flow of CSF through the drainage system by briefly lowering the drip chamber.	Avoids increases in CSF pressure caused by equipment malfunction.	It may be necessary to flush or change the system. Follow institution standard as to who is responsible for flushing the system.

Assisting With Removal of a Lumbar Subarachnoid Catheter

Steps	Rationale	Special Considerations
1. Prepare sterile gloves, sterile suture removal materials, and a sterile hemostat for assisting with the lumbar subarachnoid catheter removal.	Facilitates the removal procedure.	
2. Wash hands and don a mask with eye shield or goggles and sterile gloves.	Reduces the transmission of microorganisms.	
3. Assist the physician or advanced practice nurse as needed with removal of the catheter.	Facilitates catheter removal.	Culture the catheter tip as prescribed. Culture of the lumbar subarachnoid catheter may reveal evidence of a CSF infection.
4. Apply a sterile occlusive dressing.	Reduces the contamination by microorganisms.	
5. Discard used supplies and wash hands.	Reduces the transmission of microorganisms; standard precautions.	

Expected Outcomes

- Accurate and reliable CSF pressure monitoring
- CSF pressure within range of 0 to 15 mm Hg
- Early detection and management of elevated CSF pressure through CSF drainage[9,14,19]
- Resolution of any CSF leak[10]
- Resolution of symptoms associated with normal pressure hydrocephalus[11]
- Prevention of spinal cord damage or reversal of late-onset symptoms associated with thoracoabdominal aneurysm repair[8,18]

Unexpected Outcomes

- CSF leak or symptoms associated with excessive drainage[8,17]
- CSF infection[4,17]
- Dislodgment or occlusion of lumbar subarachnoid catheter[15]
- Tension pneumocephalus[20]
- Motor function deficits along myotome distribution of thoracic or lumbar spinal cord[3,20,25]
- Catheter site pain
- Sensory dysfunction involving dermatome distribution of thoracic or lumbar spinal cord[3,20,25]
- Bladder or bowel dysfunction[20,26]

Patient Monitoring and Care

Steps	Rationale	Reportable Conditions
		These conditions should be reported if they persist despite nursing interventions. • Change in level of consciousness • Change in sensation of lower extremities • Change in motor function of lower extremities • Changes in bowel and bladder function • Changes in vital signs
1. Monitor the patient's neurologic status during the procedure.	Neurologic status changes may result from irritation of spinal nerves associated with subarachnoid catheter placement,[16,17] spinal cord damage related to thoracoabdominal aneurysm repair,[17,23,25,26] subdural hematoma formation, herniation, or tension pneumocranium resulting from overdrainage of CSF.[3,7,9,10,23,26]	
2. Administer sedation and analgesia as needed.	Assessment of patient for pain and procedural tolerance facilitates patient comfort, safety, and success of insertion attempt.	• Unrelieved discomfort
3. Every hour, assess and record the lumbar subarachnoid CSF pressure and the amount of CSF drainage. Assess the CSF waveform morphology hourly.[20,24]	Determines neurologic status.	• Changes in CSF pressure • Changes in CSF drainage • Changes in the CSF waveform morphology
4. Assess the integrity of the lumbar subarachnoid catheter system at least hourly.	Determines accurate functioning of the system.	• Loose connections or other openings in the catheter system
5. Zero the fluid-filled pressure monitoring system during initial set-up or before insertion, after insertion if disconnection occurs between the transducer and the monitoring cable, if disconnection occurs between the monitoring cable and the monitor, and when the values obtained do not fit the clinical picture.	Ensures accuracy of the monitored data.	
6. Assess the insertion site and change the dressing when loose or soiled. Follow institution standard for dressing changes.	Although the current CDC recommendations address dressing changes on central lines only when loose or soiled, no such evidence-based recommendations exist for lumbar subarachnoid catheters.	• Signs or symptoms of infection • Significant drainage at the catheter insertion site
7. Continue ongoing assessment of neurologic status: A. Sensation B. Motor function of lower extremities C. Bowel and bladder function D. Comfort level	Changes in neurologic status or comfort level may indicate dislodgment of the lumbar subarachnoid catheter, spinal cord damage related to thoracoabdominal aneurysm repair, or poorly managed CSF drainage.	• Change in level of consciousness • Change in sensation of lower extremities • Change in motor function of lower extremities • Changes in bowel and bladder function

Procedure continues on the following page

Patient Monitoring and Care—*Continued*

Steps	Rationale	Reportable Conditions
8. Limit patient mobility as prescribed.	Patients may be permitted to sit or ambulate with specific guidelines for placement or clamping of the drainage system.	• Inability to maintain limits on patient mobility
9. Prevent dislodgment of the lumbar subarachnoid catheter through repeated explanation, sedation/analgesia or, as a last resort, the use of mechanical restraints.	Catheter dislodgment may result in excessive drainage of CSF.	• Dislodged catheter
10. Change the CSF pressure monitoring and drainage systems according to institution standard.	Although the current CDC recommendations address changes every 96 hours on invasive lines such as pulmonary artery catheters, no such evidence-based recommendations exist for lumbar subarachnoid catheters.	
11. Obtain or assist with obtaining CSF specimens as prescribed by accessing the sampling port on the CSF drainage system using strict aseptic technique. Follow institution standard.	There currently are insufficient data to guide or support decisions on the necessary frequency of routine CSF sampling from lumbar subarachnoid catheters.[4]	• Elevated white blood cell (WBC) count • Elevated protein • Decreased glucose in CSF fluid

Documentation

Documentation should include the following:

- Insertion of the lumbar subarachnoid catheter, including opening CSF pressure, any difficulties or abnormalities, and patient tolerance
- Insertion site assessment
- CSF description (e.g., clarity, color, characteristics)
- Hourly measurement of CSF pressure and amount of drainage
- Hard copy of the waveform recording at baseline, every 8 hours, and with abnormal changes
- Description of expected or unexpected outcomes
- Nursing interventions used to treat elevated CSF pressure and expected or unexpected outcomes

References

1. Berendes, J.N., et al. (1982). Mechanism of spinal cord injury after cross clamping of the descending thoracic aorta. *Circulation*, 66, 112-5.
2. Blaisdell, F.W., and Cooley, D.A. (1962). The mechanism of paraplegia after temporary thoracic aortic occlusion and its relationship to spinal fluid pressure. *Surgery*, 51, 351-6.
3. Cina, C.S., et al. (2004). Cerebrospinal fluid drainage to prevent paraplegia during thoracic and thoracoabdominal aortic aneurysm surgery: A systematic review and meta-analysis. *J Vasc Surg*, 40, 36-44.
4. Coplin, W.M., et al. (1999). Bacterial meningitis associated with lumbar drains: A retrospective cohort study. *J Neurol Neurosurg & Psychiatry*, 67, 468-73.
5. Coselli, J.S., et al. (2002). Cerebrospinal fluid drainage reduces paraplegia after thoracoabdominal aortic aneurysm repair: Results of a randomized clinical trial. *J Vasc Surg*, 35, 631-9.
6. Crawford, E.S., et al. (1991). A prospective randomized study of cerebrospinal fluid drainage to prevent paraplegia after high-risk surgery on the thoracoabdominal aorta. *J Vasc Surg*, 13, 36-45.

7. Dardik, A., et al. (2002). Subdural hematoma after thoracoabdominal aortic aneurysm repair: An underreported complication of spinal fluid drainage? *J Vasc Surg*, 36, 47-50.
8. Fleck, T.M., et al. (2003). Cerebrospinal fluid drainage after thoracoabdominal aortic aneurysm repair. *Anesthesiology*, 99, 1019-20.
9. Fritsch, M.J., et al. (1997). Controlled external lumbar drain as treatment for therapy resistant intracranial hypertension—case report. *Zentralblatt fur Neurochirurgie*, 58, 192-5.
10. Greenberg, M.S. (2001). CSF fistula. In: *Handbook of Neurosurgery*. New York: Thieme, 167-71.
11. Greenberg, M.S. (2001). Normal pressure hydrocephalus. In: *Handbook of Neurosurgery*. New York: Thieme, 192-4.
12. Griffiths, I.R., et al. (1978). Spinal cord compression and blood flow. I: The effect of raised cerebrospinal fluid pressure on spinal cord blood flow. *Neurology*, 28, 1145-51.
13. Guyton, A.C., and Hall, J.E. (2000). Cerebral blood flow, the cerebrospinal fluid, and brain metabolism. In: Guyton, A.C., and Hall, J.E., eds. *Textbook of Medical Physiology*. 10th ed. Orlando, FL: Harcourt, 709-17.

14. Haan, J., and Thomeer, R.T. (1988). Predictive value of temporary external lumbar drainage in normal pressure hydrocephalus. *Neurosurg,* 22, 388-91.

15. Hahn, M., Murali, R., and Couldwell, W.T. (2002). Tunneled lumbar drain. *J Neurosurg,* 96, 1130-1.

16. Holroyd, K.J., and Merritt, W.T. (1995). Insertion of a lumbar drain using a pediatric central venous catheter guidewire. *Anesthesiology,* 83, 430-1.

17. Khan, S.N., and Stansby, G. (2004). Cerebrospinal fluid drainage for thoracic and thoracoabdominal aortic aneurysm surgery. *Cochrane Database of Systematic Reviews.* 4, CD003635.

18. Khong, B., et al. (2000). Reversal of paraparesis after thoracic aneurysm repair by cerebrospinal fluid drainage. *Can J Anaesth,* 49, 992-5.

19. Klimo, P., Jr., et al. (2004). Marked reduction of cerebral vasospasm with lumbar drainage of cerebrospinal fluid after subarachnoid hemorrhage. *J Neurosurgery,* 100, 215-24.

20. Marshall, S.B., et al. (1990). *Neuroscience Critical Care: Pathophysiology and Patient Management.* Philadelphia: W.B. Saunders.

21. Munch, E.C., et al. (2001). Therapy of malignant intracranial hypertension by controlled lumbar cerebrospinal fluid drainage. *Crit Care Med,* 29, 976-81.

22. Mutch, W.A. (1995). Control of outflow pressure provides spinal cord protection during resection of descending thoracic aortic aneurysms. *J Neurosurg Anesth,* 7, 133-8.

23. Roland, P.S., et al. (1992). Complication of lumbar spinal fluid drainage. *Otolaryngol Head Neck Surg,* 107, 564-9.

24. Saether, O.D., et al. (1996). Cerebral haemodynamics during thoracic and thoracoabdominal aortic aneurysm repair. *Eur J Vasc Endovasc Surg,* 12, 81-5.

25. Wada, T., et al. (2001). Prevention and detection of spinal cord injury during thoracic and thoracoabdominal aortic repairs. *Ann Thorac Surg,* 1, 80-4.

26. Weaver, K.D., et al. (2001). Complications of lumbar drainage after thoracoabdominal aortic aneurysm repair. *J Vasc Surg,* 34, 623-7.

Additional Readings

Bethel, S.A. (1999). Use of lumbar cerebrospinal fluid drainage in thoracoabdominal aortic aneurysm repairs. *J Vasc Nurs,* 17, 53-8.

Houle, P.J., et al. (2000). Pump-regulated lumbar subarachnoid drainage. *Neurosurgery,* 46, 929-32.

Overstreet, M. (2003). How do I manage a lumbar drain? *Nursing,* 33, 74-5.

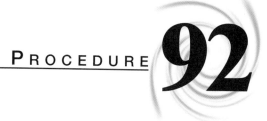
Neurologic Drainage and Pressure Monitoring System

P U R P O S E : A neurologic drainage and pressure monitoring system is used to monitor intracranial pressure (ICP) and, in the presence of pathology, to alleviate increased intracranial pressure by draining cerebral spinal fluid (CSF) from the ventricular system.

D. Nathan Preuss

PREREQUISITE NURSING KNOWLEDGE

- Knowledge of neuroanatomy and physiology
- Understanding of the assembly and maintenance of the neurologic monitoring system, care for the insertion site, and drainage techniques. All require the strictest of aseptic techniques.
- The normal range for intracranial pressure (ICP) is 0-15 mm Hg or 0-20 cm of H_2O. This measurement reflects the pressure of cerebral spinal fluid (CSF) within the intraventricular, subarachnoid, intraparenchymal, epidural, and subdural spaces.
- Cerebral perfusion pressure (CPP) is a derived mathematical calculation that indirectly reflects the adequacy of cerebral blood flow. The CPP is calculated by subtracting the ICP from the mean arterial pressure (MAP); thus CPP = MAP − ICP (see Procedures 88 and 89 for additional information related to CPP).
- Increased ICP has one common cause: namely, a disproportionate increase in one or more of the volumes of the brain (blood, CSF, or tissue) as a result of head trauma, hydrocephalus, tumor, edema, subarachnoid or intraparenchymal hemorrhage (see Procedure 89 for additional information related to the Monro-Kellie hypothesis).
- The intracranial bolt and the microsensor systems are used to monitor the ICP in the subarachnoid, subdural, and intraparenchymal spaces. When inserted and transduced at the level of the foramen of Monro (external auditory meatus), they will produce a value and a waveform that reflects the ICP. These catheters are sentinels for increased ICP but are not designed for treatment of increased ICP by CSF drainage because of the lack of

CSF in the designated spaces. The ventriculostomy and drain when transduced at the level of the foramen of Monro will produce a number and waveform reflecting the ICP and, if the ICP is increased, will allow the clinician to drain CSF (see Fig. 88-1).
- CSF is formed within the lateral ventricles of the cerebrum by the choroids plexus. From the lateral ventricles, fluid traverses the intraventricular foramina into the third ventricle. Here, presumably, the choroid plexus of the third ventricle contributes fluid, which then passes through the aqueduct of Sylvius into the fourth ventricle, where the choroid plexus in the roof of the fourth ventricle makes further additions. The fluid then enters into the subarachnoid space with the major portion of the fluid rising through the foramen of Magendie and foramen of Luschka. Some fluid passes into the subarachnoid space but the major portion rises through the tentorial notch and finds its way over the surface of the hemispheres to be absorbed finally by the arachnoid villi and arachnoid granulations where it drains into the venous system.
- CSF is a clear colorless liquid of low specific gravity that has between 2 and 3 lymphocytes/c/mm. There are approximately 90 to 150 ml of CSF circulating within the CSF pathways in the brain and spinal subarachnoid space. There is a total of 20 ml of CSF within the lateral ventricles and the cranial CSF pathways in nonpathologic conditions. The remaining circulating CSF is found within the distensible compartments of the subarachnoid space surrounding the spinal cord. CSF is secreted at the rate of 0.35 ml per minute or approximately 20 ml per hour.
- ICP waveform morphology reflects transmission of arterial and venous pressure through the CSF and brain parenchyma. A normal ICP waveform has three distinct

pressure oscillations or peaks referred to as P1, P2, and P3.[8] P1, also known as the percussion wave reflects myocardial systole. P2, also known as the tidal wave, reflects myocardial diastole and ends on the dicrotic notch. P3, the dicrotic wave, is located immediately after the dicrotic notch and slopes into the diastolic baseline position (see Fig. 88-2). P3 oscillations are correlated with venous fluctuations. P2 elevations are known to occur with the loss of cerebral compliance. P2 pressure oscillation amplitudes approach and surpass P1 pressure oscillations during periods of decompensation and loss of intracerebral compliance (see Fig. 88-3). Changes in ICP waveform morphology may also reflect loss of cerebral autoregulation. With the loss of autoregulation the ICP waveform may resemble an arterial waveform.

- Continuous ICP monitoring data trends may demonstrate three discrete ICP wave trends. These ICP trends are *a, b,* and *c* waves.[8] The *a* waves, also known as plateau waves, occur in severe intracranial hypertension, are characterized by sudden ICP escalations up to 50 to 100 mm Hg, have a duration of 5 to 20 minutes, and frequently are accompanied by neurologic deterioration or cerebral herniation (see Fig. 88-4). The *b* waves are sharp rhythmic oscillations that occur with a frequency of every 30 seconds to 2 minutes. The *b* waves may escalate up to 20 to 50 mm Hg and may precede plateau waves (see Fig. 88-5). The *c* waves demonstrate ICP elevations up to 20 mm Hg and can occur with a frequency of every 4 to 8 minutes. They are not thought to be clinically significant (see Fig. 88-6).

- Management of brain injury is focused on preventing secondary brain injury, namely, a decrease in cerebral oxygen delivery due to hypotension, hypoxemia, cerebral edema, intracranial hypertension, or abnormalities in cerebral blood flow. Early intervention in addition to intraventricular drainage in cases of increased ICP should include a decrease in environmental stimuli, elevation of the head of the bed, aligning the head and neck in a straight position to promote venous drainage, and avoidance of constrictive devices about the neck that might impede arterial flow to the brain and venous drainage from the brain. Avoid turning, excitation, straining, and hyperthermia.

- Further perfusion measures should include monitoring of pulmonary artery wedge pressures, mean arterial pressure, and cerebral perfusion pressure. Mean arterial pressure and cerebral perfusion pressure parameters will depend on the cause of the increased ICP as well as the pre- and post-treatment plans. In the case of hypertensive issues involving hemorrhagic or nonhemorrhagic stroke, the mean arterial pressure should be maintained at less than 90 mm Hg to prevent rebleeding and a cerebral perfusion pressure greater than 70 mm Hg will be required to maintain the best possible cerebral perfusion pressure. Similar parameters are required in the case of unsecured non-ruptured aneurysms. Posttreatment scenarios of secured aneurysms in the presence of a deteriorating neurologic exam and vasospasm will require MAPs greater than 90 mm Hg. Additional treatment strategies include

"triple H" therapy (hypervolemia, hypertension, and hemodilution).[4,12,13] This is achieved by means of frequent fluid challenges based on Starling curve results and the use of vasopressors.

- Patients will require daily and as-needed assessment of the complete blood count, blood chemistry, liver and renal function, as well as levels of medications such as Dilantin.

- Increased ICP requires the use of certain pharmacologic agents to include antihypertensives, antipyretics with fever, anticonvulsants (e.g., Dilantin), and corticosteroids. Extreme cases of increased ICP may require neuromuscular blocking agents (e.g., vecuronium), amnesiacs (e.g., propofol), or barbiturates (e.g., pentobarbital). In the case of barbiturate coma, continuous EEG monitoring for burst suppression is required to achieve the desired decrease in cerebral oxygen consumption and electrical stimuli.[5]

EQUIPMENT

- Pressure monitor tubing kit, including a transducer, a three-way stopcock, and nonvented caps
- External drainage system, including tubing, collection chamber, and drainage bag
- One pressure cable for the monitoring system
- 250 ml of preservative-free normal saline (may use sterile intravenous solution)
- Monitoring system (central and bedside monitor)
- Pressure monitoring cable and module
- Nonvented caps
- Three 3-ml syringes
- Antiseptic solution
- Laboratory forms and specimen labels
- Two blood specimen tubes (plain red-top tubes)
- Three sterile needles for sampling
  Additional equipment, as needed, includes the following:
- An antibiotic for the flush system if prescribed by the physician[6]
- Fiberoptic systems require a microprocessor (stand alone monitor) and a preamp connector cable to connect the microprocessor to the primary bedside monitor, in addition to the sterile CSF collection system.
- Sensor systems require a microprocessor sensor cable and a monitoring cable to connect the microprocessor (stand alone monitor) to the primary bedside monitor, in addition to the sterile CSF collection system.
- Caps, mask, sterile drapes, sterile gloves, and gowns are required for assembly of the external ventricular drainage system.

PATIENT AND FAMILY EDUCATION

- This procedure may be performed at the bedside or in an operating room. A neurologically intact patient may need to be sedated, paralyzed, and intubated. ➤*Rationale:* Patient cooperation during cranial access is of utmost importance. Following treatment and in the presence of an intact neurologic exam, the patient may be extubated. However, the patient and family should be aware that the patient may need to remain intubated to maintain a patent airway, ensure adequate oxygenation, in order to maintain a normal ICP and cerebral perfusion pressure.

- Assess the patient and the family for their understanding of cranial pressure monitoring. ➤➤*Rationale:* Knowledge is an expressed need and information helps decrease anxiety.
- Explain the waveforms on the bedside monitor and explain how this pressure will be continually monitored and, in the case of increased ICP, that the drain will be opened and CSF will be drained to alleviate the pressure. ➤➤*Rationale:* This prepares the patient and the family for what to expect.

PATIENT ASSESSMENT AND PREPARATION

Patient Assessment

- Obtain a baseline assessment to include level of consciousness, orientation, verbal abilities, motor strength, and cranial nerve integrity. ➤➤*Rationale:* This provides baseline data.
- Obtain the patient's past medical and surgical history to include use of aspirin, anticoagulants, prior craniotomies, the presence of aneurysm clips, embolic materials, permanent balloon occlusions, detachable coils, or a ventroperitoneal shunt. ➤➤*Rationale:* The information obtained determines and guides future treatment based on the neurologic exams and evidence from radiology and angiography.

Patient Preparation

- Ensure that the patient understands preprocedural teaching. Answer questions as they arise and reinforce information as needed. ➤➤*Rationale:* Evaluates and reinforces understanding of previously taught information.
- Initiate intravenous (IV) access or assess the patency of the IV. ➤➤*Rationale:* Readily available IV access is necessary if the patient needs to be sedated or paralyzed or needs other medications.

Procedure	**for Pressure Monitoring and Drainage**	
Steps	**Rationale**	**Special Considerations**
External Ventricular Drainage (EVD) System Assembly		
1. Prepare the setup: A. Wash hands. B. Open a sterile sheet to create a sterile surface for assembly. C. Open items to be assembled using sterile technique. D. Place them on the sterile surface. E. Put on cap, mask, gowns, and sterile gloves to use for assembly.	Reduces the transmission of microorganisms; standard precautions. Ensures aseptic technique.	
2. Obtain a 250-ml bag of preservative-free normal saline flush solution.	Prepares the solution needed to flush air from the system.	**At no time is this system placed under pressure.** **Never place the flush solution in a pressure bag.** **Never fast-flush the system except to prime the tubing.**
3. Spike the prepared bag with the pressure monitoring tubing.	Prepares the equipment.	
4. Connect the end of the external ventricular drainage (EVD) system tubing to the distal stopcock of the pressure monitor tubing (Fig. 92-1). Tighten all the connections.	Ensures that the system is secure and is a sterile closed system.	
5. Close the clamps between the drip chamber and the external ventricular drainage collection bag (see Fig. 92-1).	Ensures the ability to measure hourly drainage in the drip chamber.	When the drip chamber is full, the clamps are opened on the tubing between the drip chamber and the collection bag to drain the drip chamber. Then the tubing is reclamped.

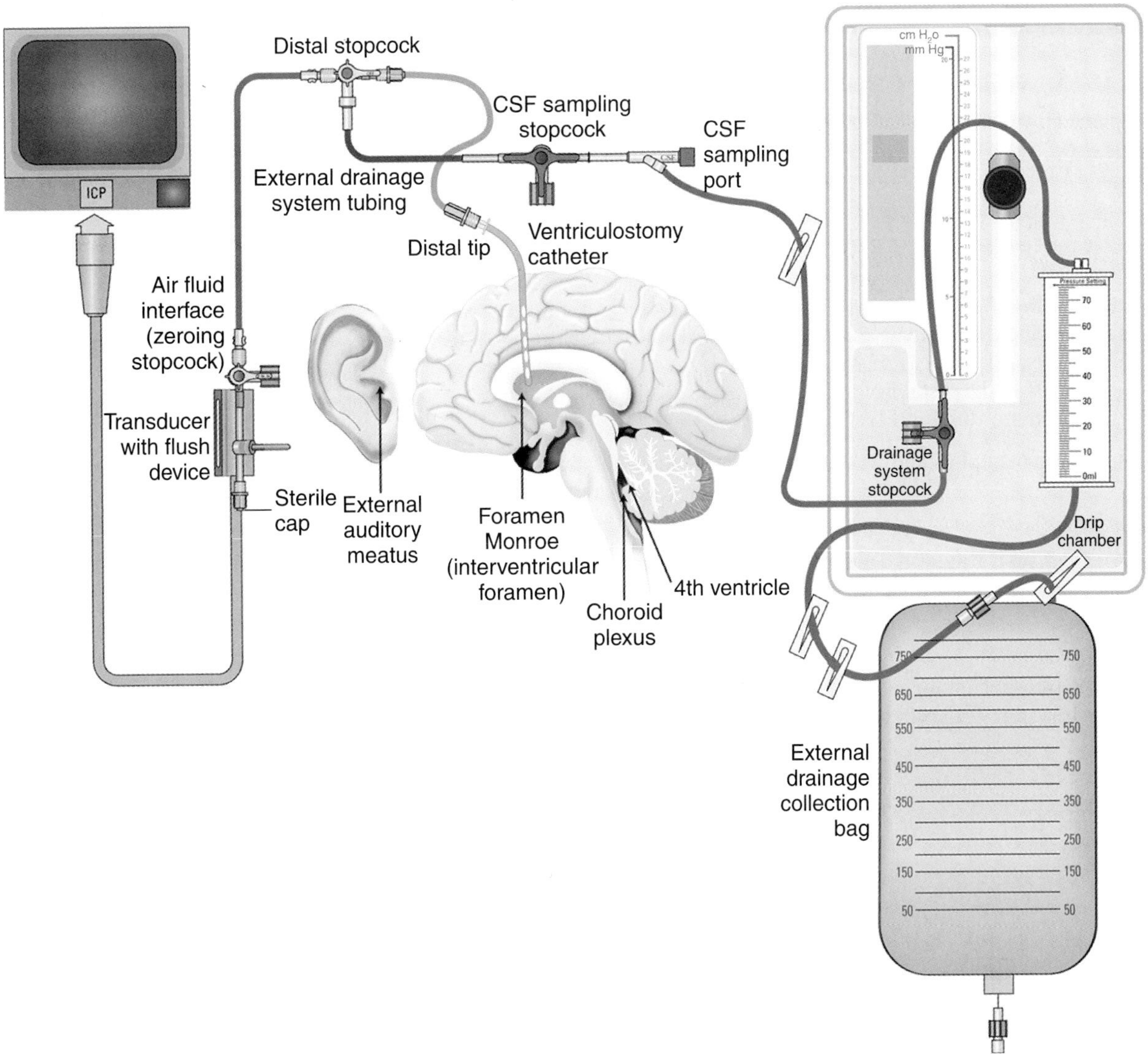

FIGURE 92-1 External ventricular drainage system. *(Drawing by Paul Schiffmacher, Thomas Jefferson University, Philadelphia, PA.)*

Procedure	for Pressure Monitoring and Drainage—*Continued*	
Steps	**Rationale**	**Special Considerations**
6. Using the flush device next to the transducer, flush the entire system, including the pressure tubing, transducer, stopcocks, and the external ventricular drainage system until the fluid enters the drip chamber (see Fig. 92-1).	Eliminates air from the system. If air is left in the tubing, it may alter the numeric value or prevent the flow of CSF.	Some systems contain a porous filter at the top of the drip chamber. If this filter becomes wet because of CSF backup or spillage, CSF will not flow. The entire system must be replaced. If for any reason there is no CSF flow, always check or replace the system and associated equipment before calling the physician to manipulate the catheter.

Procedure continues on the following page

Procedure | for Pressure Monitoring and Drainage—*Continued*

Steps	Rationale	Special Considerations
7. Replace all vented caps with nonvented caps.	Vented caps are used by the manufacturer to permit sterilization of the entire system. These caps need to be replaced with sterile nonvented caps to prevent bacteria and air from entering the system.	
8. After flushing the pressure monitor tubing and the external ventricular drainage system tubing, turn the distal stopcock off to the distal tip of the pressure monitor tubing (Fig. 92-2).	The stopcock in this position readies the entire system for connection to the ventriculostomy catheter.	Prevents the backflow of fluid into the drip chamber.
9. Discard used supplies and wash hands.	Reduces the transmission of microorganisms; standard precautions.	
Remove the Flush Bag and Tubing from the System		
1. Wash hands	Reduces the transmission of microorganisms; standard precautions.	Follow institution policy for removing the flush system.
2. Turn the transducer stopcock off to the flush system (Fig. 92-3).	Prevents air from entering the transducer.	**Extreme caution must be taken when manipulating stopcocks to prevent flushing fluid into the brain.**

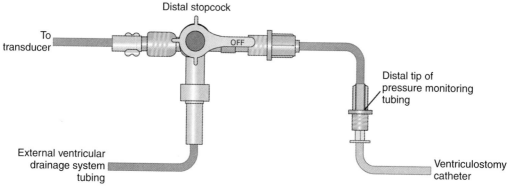

FIGURE 92-2 Distal stopcock turned off to the distal tip of the pressure monitor tubing. *(Drawing by Paul Schiffmacher, Thomas Jefferson University, Philadelphia, PA.)*

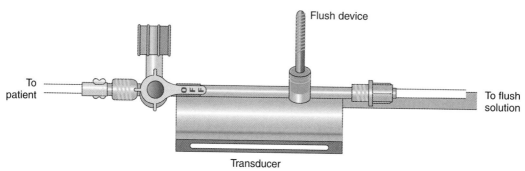

FIGURE 92-3 Transducer stopcock turned off to the flush solution. *(Drawing by Paul Schiffmacher, Thomas Jefferson University, Philadelphia, PA.)*

Procedure for Pressure Monitoring and Drainage—*Continued*

Steps	Rationale	Special Considerations
3. Remove the flush bag and tubing.	Prevents accidental flushing of fluid into the brain.	
4. Place a sterile nonvented cap on the exposed end of the transducer.	Maintains a sterile closed system.	
5. Open the stopcock to the transducer.	Allows for transmission of the pressure signal.	
6. Wash hands.	Reduces the transmission of microorganisms; standard precautions.	
Monitoring Setup		
1. Turn on the bedside monitor.	Prepares the monitor.	
2. Plug a pressure cable into the appropriate pressure module or jack in the bedside monitor (see Fig. 92-1).	The signal is transmitted to the computer so that it may be transmitted to the oscilloscope for display.	
3. Attach a transducer cable to the pressure tubing.	Prepares the equipment.	
4. Turn on the intracranial pressure (ICP) parameter.	Visualizes correct waveform.	
5. Set the appropriate scale for the measured pressure.	Necessary for visualization of the complete waveform and to obtain readings. Waveforms vary in amplitude, depending on the pressure within the system.	The scale for ICP monitoring is commonly set at 30 mm Hg. The normal ICP for an adult is within the range of 0-15 mm Hg.[3,5]
6. Set the monitor alarm limits.	Goals for ICP management are individualized for each patient based upon etiology, pathophysiology, and management strategies.	
Leveling the Transducer		
1. Wash hands.	Reduces the transmission of microorganisms; standard precautions.	
2. Position the patient in the supine position with the head of the bed elevated as prescribed by the physician.	Prepares the patient.	The head of the bed is usually placed at 20-30 degrees to aid in increasing venous return.[11]
3. Place the air-fluid interface (zeroing stopcock) at the level of the external auditory meatus (see Fig. 92-1).	The external auditory meatus approximates the level of the foramen of Monro (interventricular foramen).[1,2,9] This represents a point of communication between the third and lateral ventricle.	
4. Wash hands.	Reduces the transmission of microorganisms; standard precautions.	
Zeroing the Transducer		
1. Wash hands.	Reduces the transmission of microorganisms; standard precautions.	Follow institution standard.

Procedure continues on the following page

Procedure for Pressure Monitoring and Drainage—*Continued*

Steps	Rationale	Special Considerations
2. Turn the transducer stopcock off to the patient.	Prepares the system for the zeroing procedure.	
3. Remove the nonvented cap from the stopcock, opening the stopcock to air.	Allows the monitor to use atmospheric pressure as a reference for zero.	
4. Push and release the zeroing button on the bedside monitor. Observe the digital reading until it displays a value of zero.	The monitor will automatically adjust itself to zero. Zeroing negates the effects of atmospheric pressure.	Some monitors require that the zero be turned and adjusted manually. Some systems also may require calibration. See the manufacturer's guidelines for specific information.
5. Place a new, sterile nonvented cap on the stopcock.	Maintains sterility.	
6. Turn the stopcock so that it is open to the transducer.	Permits pressure monitoring.	
7. For insertion of an intracranial bolt or an intraventricular catheter, see Procedures 88 and 89.		
8. Wash hands.	Reduces the transmission of microorganisms; standard precautions.	
Monitoring Intracranial Pressure		
1. The ventriculostomy catheter will be connected to the distal tip of the pressure monitor tubing by the physician (see Fig. 92-2).	Connects the system.	
2. Turn the distal stopcock off to the external ventricular drainage system (Fig. 92-4).	Allows for monitoring of the ICP.	
3. Position the head of the bed as directed by the physician.	Allows for accurate and consistent monitoring of the ICP.	
4. Record the ICP value.	Provides a value for ongoing assessment.	
5. Record a waveform strip.	Identifies the ICP waveform.	The normal ICP waveform has three distinct pressure oscillations or peaks. These are referred to as P1, P2, and P3 (see Fig. 88-2).[7]

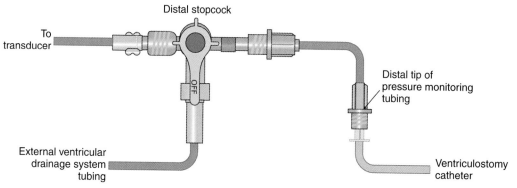

FIGURE 92-4 Distal stopcock turned off to the external drainage system tubing. (*Drawing by Paul Schiffmacher, Thomas Jefferson University, Philadelphia, PA.*)

Procedure for Pressure Monitoring and Drainage—*Continued*

Steps	Rationale	Special Considerations
6. Continuously monitor and assess the ICP waveform trends.	Assesses for changes in the ICP and waveforms.	Deviations may require immediate intervention and should be reported to the physician. If an EVD is in the monitoring position, special care must be paid to the bedside neurologic exam with regard to the potential for deterioration. The catheter may become obstructed with clot, tissue, or protein. Note any changes in flow before obstruction. Notify the physician, who may need to irrigate the catheter to re-establish patency. Other maneuvers may include turning or stimulating a cough. Some institutional policies allow the critical care nurse to irrigate the catheter with a limited amount of preservative-free saline.
Draining an EVD		
1. The physician will set the ICP parameter that initiates CSF drainage.	For example, if the physician prescribes the ICP to be maintained at less than 15 mm Hg, drainage of CSF will be initiated if the patient's ICP is greater than 15 mm Hg.	
2. Wash hands.	Reduces the transmission of microorganisms; standard precautions.	
3. To drain the CSF, turn the distal stopcock of the pressure monitoring tubing off to the transducer (Fig. 92-5).	This will allow the flow of CSF from the ventricles.	**Never leave a draining EVD unattended.** Excessive drainage may cause overdrainage and a possible collapse of the ventricles, with resulting tearing of the bridging veins of the brain causing a subdural hematoma.[11]

Procedure continues on the following page

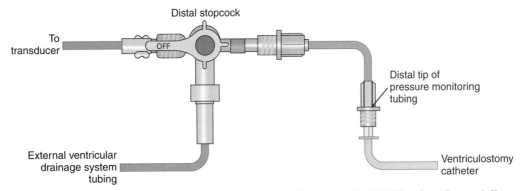

FIGURE 92-5 Distal stopcock turned off to the transducer. *(Drawing by Paul Schiffmacher, Thomas Jefferson University, Philadelphia, PA.)*

Procedure for Pressure Monitoring and Drainage—*Continued*

Steps	Rationale	Special Considerations
4. Allow 5 ml of CSF to enter the drip chamber (see Fig. 92-1).	Prevents overdrainage of CSF.	**Never leave a draining EVD unattended.**
5. Turn the distal stopcock off to the external ventricular drainage system (see Fig. 92-4) and note the ICP value.	Check the ICP value to determine whether the parameter is met.	
6. If the goal was not met, repeat steps 3 to 5 until the ICP parameter is met.	Recheck the ICP value to determine whether the parameter is met.	If the patient's CSF is being continuously drained, note and record the amount of drainage every hour. **Never leave a draining EVD unattended.**
7. Wash hands.	Reduces the transmission of microorganisms; standard precautions.	
CSF Sampling		
1. Obtain a physician prescription for a CSF sample, including the frequency.	Prepares for the test.	CSF sampling may include glucose, cell count, protein, culture, and Gram stain. If a comparison of serum glucose and CSF glucose is prescribed, a serum glucose sample should be obtained at the same time as the CSF sampling.
2. Obtain the supplies for sampling: three 3-ml syringes, two blood specimen tubes, antiseptic solution, sterile gloves, lab forms, and specimen labels.	Prepares the equipment.	
3. Wash hands and don sterile gloves.	Reduces the transmission of microorganisms and body fluids; standard precautions.	
4. Cleanse the CSF sampling port with an antiseptic solution (Fig. 92-6).	Aseptic technique.[10,14]	
5. Attach the sampling needles to the syringes.	Prepares the equipment.	
6. Cleanse the tops of the blood specimen tubes with the antiseptic solution.	Aseptic technique.	

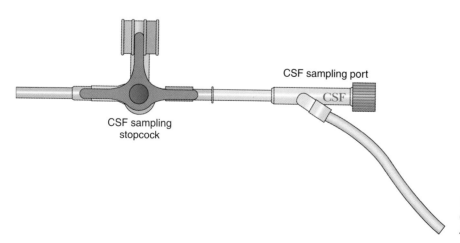

CSF sampling port

CSF

CSF sampling stopcock

FIGURE 92-6 CSF sampling port. *(Drawing by Paul Schiffmacher, Thomas Jefferson University, Philadelphia, PA.)*

Procedure for Pressure Monitoring and Drainage—*Continued*

Steps	Rationale	Special Considerations
7. Turn the distal stopcock of the pressure monitor tubing off to the transducer (see Fig. 92-5).	Allows for direct sampling of CSF from the ventriculostomy catheter.	
8. Turn the drainage system stopcock off to the drip chamber (Fig. 92-7).	Allows for direct sampling of CSF from the ventriculostomy catheter.	
9. Withdraw a 1-ml discard sample from the CSF sampling port (see Fig. 92-6).	Clears the tubing for the CSF sample.	
10. Withdraw two 1-ml samples from the CSF sampling port and inject each into a blood specimen tube.	Obtains the prescribed sample.	One sample is used for laboratory studies, and the other is used for culture and Gram stain, if prescribed by the physician.

Procedure continues on the following page

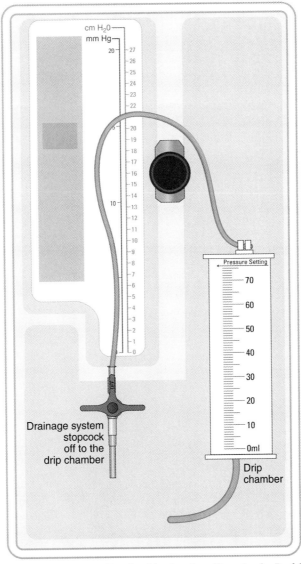

FIGURE 92-7 Drainage system stopcock off to the drip chamber. (*Drawing by Paul Schiffmacher, Thomas Jefferson University, Philadelphia, PA.*)

Procedure for Pressure Monitoring and Drainage—*Continued*

Steps	Rationale	Special Considerations
11. Turn the distal stopcock to resume monitoring and turn the drainage system stopcock open to the drip chamber.	Continues monitoring.	
12. Label the blood specimen tubes and send to the laboratory for analysis.	Prepares the specimen for analysis.	
13. Discard used supplies and wash hands.	Reduces the transmission of microorganisms and body fluids; standard precautions.	Discard sharps in appropriate biohazard container.

Expected Outcomes

- Neurologic drainage and/or pressure monitoring system is set up aseptically
- The external auditory meatus is correctly identified
- Air-fluid interface of the transducer is leveled at the external auditory meatus
- The monitoring system is zeroed
- Accurate and reliable monitoring of ICP
- Continuous flow of CSF when drainage is initiated
- Immediate management of increased ICP
- Improved neurologic functioning

Unexpected Outcomes

- Loose connections within the external ventricular drainage system
- Stopcocks left open to air without nonvented caps
- Air bubbles within the system
- CSF infection
- CSF leak
- Dislodgment or occlusion of the EVD
- Pneumocephalus
- Cerebral hemorrhage (rebleed from subarachnoid hemorrhage)
- Lack of CSF flow
- Subdural hematoma

Patient Monitoring and Care

Steps	Rationale	Reportable Conditions
		These conditions should be reported if they persist despite nursing interventions.

1. Continuously monitor the EVD:
  A. ICP
  B. CPP
  C. CSF drainage
	Assesses neurologic status.	• Any gradual or sudden increase in the ICP, with or without accompanying neurologic changes.
		• Lack of drainage in the presence of significant increased ICP requires immediate reporting to the physician. This may indicate an occlusion of the catheter.
		• Persistent large volumes of CSF totaling more than 200 ml each day may require the insertion of a VP shunt.

2. Zero the external ventricular drainage system during the initial setup or before insertion, then after insertion, again if connections between the transducer and the monitoring cable become dislodged, if connections between the monitoring cable and the monitor become dislodged, and when the values do not fit the clinical picture.	Ensures accuracy of the monitoring process.	
3. When changing the patient's position, maintain the reference level of the EVD at the external auditory meatus.	Minimizes the risk for underdrainage, overdrainage, or false values.	• Increase or decrease in CSF drainage • The inability to obtain CSF drainage • Changes in ICP
4. Check the system every hour and as needed.	Ensures that all connections are tightly secured and that there are no cracks in the system. Ensures that the	

Patient Monitoring and Care—*Continued*

Steps	Rationale	Reportable Conditions
	system is closed with nonvented caps on all stopcocks. Ensures that the system is free of air bubbles.	
5. Set the alarm parameters relative to the ICP goal established by the physician.	Provides immediate alarm for high pressures.	• Changes in ICP
6. All drainage events should be measured and recorded as part of the intake and output.	Assesses CSF drainage.	• Increase or decrease in CSF drainage
7. If the patient is being continuously drained, record the output every 1 to 2 hours. Maintain the reference point at the external auditory meatus.	Assesses CSF drainage.	• Increase or decrease in CSF drainage
8. Change the dressing at the insertion site daily or as prescribed.	Maintains sterility and provides an opportunity for site assessment.	• Signs or symptoms of infection • Loosened sutures

Documentation

Documentation should include the following:

- Initial opening ICP
- Initial CPP
- Ongoing description of CSF to include clarity and color
- Insertion site assessment
- Record a strip of the ICP waveform at the start of each shift

- Description of expected and unexpected outcomes
- Hourly to every-2-hour output or amount drained intermittently
- Hourly ICP/CCP
- Hourly neurologic assessment

References

1. Bisnaire, D., and Robinson, L. (1997). Accuracy of leveling intraventricular collection drainage systems. *J Neurosci Nurs,* 29, 261-8.
2. Cummings, R. (1992). Understanding external ventricular drainage. *J Neurosci Nurs,* 24, 84-7.
3. Czosnyka, M., and Pickard, J.D. (2004). Monitoring and interpretation of intracranial pressure. *J Neurol Neurosurg Psychiatry,* 75, 813-21.
4. Dennis, L.J., and Mayer, S.A. (2001). Diagnosis and management of increased intracranial pressure. *Neurology India,* 49(Suppl 1), S37-50.
5. Dunn, L.T. (2002). Raised intracranial pressure. *J Neurol Neurosurg Psychiatry,* 73(Suppl I), i23-7.
6. Flibotte, J.J., et al. (2004). Continuous antibiotic prophylaxis and cerebral spinal fluid infection in patients with intracranial pressure monitors. *Neurocritical Care,* 1, 61-8.
7. Kirkness, C.J., et al. (2000). Intracranial pressure waveform analysis: Clinical and research implications. *J Neurosci Nurs,* 32, 271-7.
8. March, K. (2000). Intracranial pressure monitoring and assessing intracranial compliance in brain injury. *Crit Care Nurs Clin North Am,* 12, 429-36.
9. Ng, I., Lim, J., and Wong, H.B. (2004). Effects of head posture on cerebral hemodynamics: Its influences on intracranial pressure, cerebral perfusion pressure, and cerebral oxygenation. *Neurosurg,* 54, 593-8.
10. O'Grady, N.P., et al. (2002). Guidelines for the prevention of intravascular catheter-related infections. *Am J Infect Control,* 30, 476-89.
11. Pope, W. (1998). External ventriculostomy: A practical application for the acute care nurse. *J Neurosci Nurs,* 30, 185-90.
12. Rees, G., et al. (2002). Subarachnoid hemorrhage: A clinical overview. *Nurs Stand,* 16, 47-56.
13. Vos, H.R. (1993). Making headway with intracranial hypertension. *Am J Nurs,* 93, 29-35.
14. Wisinger, D., and Mest-Beck, L. (1990). Ventriculostomy: A guide to nursing management. *J Neurosci Nurs,* 22, 365-9.

Additional Readings

American Association of Neuroscience Nurses. (1997). *Core Curriculum for Neuroscience Nurses.* Chicago: Author.
Bader, M.K. (1999). What is the recommended external reference point for zeroing an intracranial pressure monitoring system at the foramen of Monro? *Crit Care Nurse,* 19, 92-3.
Dunham, C.M., et al. (2004). Cerebral hypoxia in severely brain-injured patients is associated with admission Glasgow Coma Scale score, computed tomographic severity, cerebral perfusion pressure, and survival. *J Trauma,* 56, 482-91.
Lozier, A.P., et al. (2002). Ventriculostomy-related infections: A critical review of the literature. *Neurosurg,* 51, 170-82.
Piper, I., et al. (2001). The Camino intracranial pressure sensor: is it optimal technology? An internal audit with a review of current intracranial pressure monitoring technologies. *Neurosurg,* 49, 1158-65.
Vinas, F.C. (2001). Bedside invasive monitoring techniques in severe brain-injured patients. *Neurol Res,* 23, 157-66.

PROCEDURE **93**

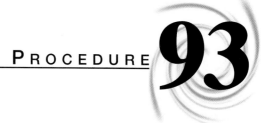

AP
Transcranial Doppler Monitoring

PURPOSE: Transcranial Doppler (TCD) measures blood flow velocities in the major branches of the circle of Willis through an intact skull. This measurement supports the grading of vasospasm severity, localization of intracranial stenoses or occlusions, detection of cerebral emboli, monitoring of hemodynamic changes with impaired intracranial perfusion, and assessment of the impact of therapeutic interventions on intracranial hemodynamics.[1-8]

Anne W. Wojner-Alexandrov
Andrei V. Alexandrov

PREREQUISITE NURSING KNOWLEDGE

- Knowledge of neuroanatomy and physiology
- Clinical and technical competence related to TCD sonography
- Noninvasive assessment of the intracranial vasculature is indicated for patients with a subarachnoid hemorrhage, ischemic stroke, cerebral emboli, impaired vasomotor reactivity, cerebral circulatory arrest, and other neurovascular disorders.
- Successful ultrasound penetration through the skull is possible through intracranial windows, which either lack bone (burr holes, flaps) or consist of thinner bone structure compared with the overall cranial bone thickness. Four windows are available for insonation: temporal, orbital, foraminal, and submandibular windows (Fig. 93-1).[1,2-4,11,15]
- The transtemporal window allows insonation of the middle cerebral artery (MCA), the anterior cerebral artery (ACA), the posterior cerebral artery (PCA), and the anterior and posterior communicating arteries (AComA and PComA).[1,2-4,11,15]
- The transorbital window allows insonation of the ophthalmic artery (OA) and the internal carotid artery (ICA) siphon.[1,2-4,11,15]

- The transforaminal window allows insonation of the vertebral arteries (VA) and the basilar artery (BA).[1,2-4,11,15]
- The submandibular window allows insonation of the ICA as it enters the skull.[1,2-4,11,15] TCD locates both the depth and direction of arterial blood flow relative to the transducer position and the ultrasonic beam direction. Flow moving toward the transducer is displayed as a waveform with a positive velocity spectrum, whereas flow moving away from the transducer is displayed as a waveform with a negative velocity spectrum.[1,2-4,11,15]
- TCD measures cerebral blood flow velocities that should not be equated to cerebral blood flow (CBF) volume. TCD is an indirect reflection of CBF.[2,11,15]
- The examination should begin with maximum power and gate settings (e.g., power 100%, gate 10 to 15 mm) to expedite identification of the temporal window and various arterial segments. Once a good temporal window is established, the power may be reduced to adhere to the FDA principles of (1) *As Low As Reasonably Achievable* (ALARA) and (2) minimization of overall time of patient exposure to ultrasound. Transorbital examination should always be performed with minimal power (e.g., 10%) to avoid potential side effects from the heating of orbital structures.[1,2-4,11,15]
- The highest-velocity signals for each arterial segment studied, as well as any abnormal or unusual waveforms, should be measured and stored in the system's computer.[3]
- Criteria for normal insonation depths, flow direction, and mean flow velocities are used to identify arteries appropriately and to diagnose abnormalities[3,11,15] (Table 93-1 and Fig. 93-2).

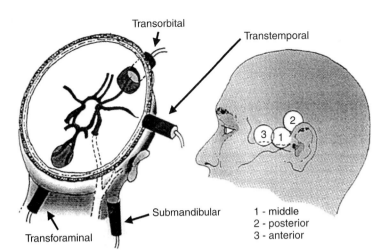

FIGURE 93-1 Four windows of transcranial Doppler insonation (left image, clockwise): orbital, temporal, submandibular, and foraminal. The temporal window has three aspects (right image): 1, middle: 2, posterior; 3, anterior. (*From Alexandrow A.V. [1998]. Transcranial Doppler Ultrasonography. Houston, Tx: University of Texas Medical School.*)

1 - middle
2 - posterior
3 - anterior

- Criteria for determination of a normal examination are listed in Table 93-2.[3]
- Criteria supporting differential diagnosis are listed in Table 93-3.[3]
- *Hemispheric index* (Lindegaard ratio) helps to differentiate vasospasm severity and hyperdynamic blood flow changes. HI = MFV ipsilateral MCA/MFV ipsilateral ICA. Normal values are less than 3.[9,10]
- *Pulsatility of flow* refers to vessel resistance and is measured by the pulsatility index (PI); normal range for PI is 0.6 to 1.1.[2,3] PI (Gosling-King) = [velocity (peak systole) − velocity (end diastole)] ÷ velocity (mean).
- Hyperventilation increases the PI and decreases mean flow velocity.[3,11,15]
- Hypercapnia decreases PI and increases mean flow velocity.[3,11,15]
- Anatomic variations in the circle of Willis are common.[2,3,11,15]

- Inability to find an artery by TCD should *not* be interpreted as arterial occlusion in the absence of other abnormal flow findings (e.g., secondary signs such as high resistance and flow diversion).[2,3]
- Clinical conditions and the effects of medications (dehydration or increased blood viscosity, hypertension or hypotension) should correlate with examination findings.[2,3,11,15]
- Although subjective, differentiation of Doppler sounds assists with identification of arterial segments and altered flow patterns.[2,3,11,15]
- Proximal extracranial, focal intracranial, and distal circulatory conditions are determinants of waveform patterns.[2,3,11] Waveform classification in patients with ischemic strokes is standardized by use of the Thrombolysis in Brain Ischemia (TIBI) Grading Scale (Table 93-4 and Fig. 93-3).[8] The TIBI grading system was prospectively validated against angiography, and it has excellent reproducibility with greater than 90% agreement in waveform interpretation among expert TCD users.[6,7] TIBI system was implemented in a multicenter randomized clinical trial of ultrasound enhanced thrombolysis for acute ischemic stroke to demonstrate superior recanalization rates when systemic tissue plasminogen activator (TPA) therapy was monitored with TCD compared with TPA given without ultrasound.[5]
- New technology using power motion Doppler (PMD or M-Mode) can be used to facilitate window and vessel identification and guide spectral Doppler sampling and may reduce the time and effort necessary to learn TCD (see Fig. 93-4).[4,12]

TABLE 93-1	Depth, Direction, and Mean Flow Velocities for Circle of Willis Arteries*		
Artery	**Depth (mm)**	**Flow Direction****	**MFV for Adults**
M1 MCA	45-65	Toward	32-82 cm/s
A1 ACA	62-75	Away	18-82 cm/s
ICA siphon	60-64	Bidirectional	20-77 cm/s
OA	50-62	Toward	Variable
PCA	60-68	Bidirectional	16-58 cm/s
BA	80-100	Away	12-66 cm/s
VA	45-80	Away	12-66 cm/s

*Depth and MFV ranges may vary slightly between reference studies.
**Toward* the probe indicates a positive (+) waveform; *away* from the probe indicates a negative (−) waveform.
M1 MCA, A1 ACA, first segments of the middle and anterior cerebral arteries; *ICA*, internal carotid artery; *OA*, ophthalmic artery; *PCA*, posterior cerebral artery; *BA*, basilar artery; *VA*, vertebral artery.
Adapted with permission from Alexandrov, A.V. (1998). Transcranial Doppler sonography: Principles, examination technique and normal values. *Vasc Ultrasound Today*, 10, 141-60.

EQUIPMENT

- A pulse-wave TCD system
- A 2-MHz probe (single or bilateral)
- Acoustic transmission gel
- Nonsterile gloves
- Tissues
- Head-phones (optional)

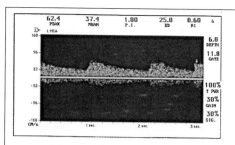

A normal waveform with sharp systolic flow acceleration, stepwise diastolic deceleration, and pulsatility index (PI) range of 0.6 – 1.1.

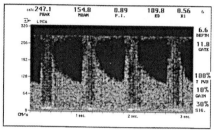

A focal significant MFV increase, with moderate vasospasm (MCA MFV range 120-200 cm/sec, MCA/ICA MFV ratio 3-6). Severe MCA spasm produces MFV greater than 200 cm/sec and ratio greater than 6.

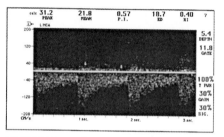

A blunted waveform indicates near occlusion with flow diversion to a branching vessel. Differential diagnosis includes the presence of a proximal ICA obstruction.

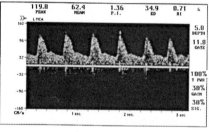

A high resistance waveform with PI greater than or equal to 1.2 can be found with systemic hypertension, increased cardiac output, distal vasospasm or increased ICP after other reasons are excluded.

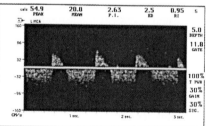

A reverberating flow waveform shows diastolic flow reversal due to ICP equal or exceeding CPP. If found in both MCA and BA, this waveform indicates cerebral circulatory arrest.

FIGURE 93-2 Typical middle cerebral artery (MCA) waveforms. Vertical scale is in cm/s; horizontal scale is in seconds. Direction of flow: (+)— toward the probe, (–)—away from the probe. Velocity and pulsatility values *(left to right):* peak systolic, mean, pulsatility index (PI), end diastolic (ED), resistance index (RI). Depth indicates depth of insonation in cm. Gate is the diameter of sample volume in mm. Power and gain setting are given in percentages.

TABLE 93-2   Criteria for Normal TCD Findings

1. Optimal windows of insonation, permitting identification of all proximal arterial segments
2. Direction of flow and depths consistent with criteria in Table 93-1
3. Side-to-side difference between flow velocities in homologous arteries is less than or equal to 30%
4. Presence of a normal velocity ratio: MCA greater than or equal to ACA greater than or equal to ICA siphon greater than or equal to PCA greater than or equal to BA greater than or equal to VA
5. Positive end-diastolic flow velocity of 20%-50% of the peak systolic velocity values
6. Low-resistance flow pattern, with PI between 0.6 and 1.1 in all intracranial arteries when $Paco_2$ between 35 and 45 mm Hg
7. High-resistance flow pattern with PI greater than or equal to 1.2 in the OA only
8. High-resistance flow patterns with PI greater than or equal to 1.2 in all arteries during hyperventilation or elevated BP

Reprinted with permission from Alexandrov, A.V. (1988). Transcranial Doppler sonography: Principles, examination technique and normal values. *Vasc Ultrasound Today,* 10, 141-60.

TABLE 93-3 Differential Diagnosis

Problem	Findings	Differential Diagnosis
Arterial stenosis	Focal MFV increase above normal values, turbulence, bruits Flow diversion to adjacent arteries Flow alteration distal to site of stenosis (deceleration, low PIs)	Primary arterial stenosis Compensatory flow increase Adjacent artery occlusion Hyperemia
Arterial near occlusion	Blunted waveform Focal decrease in MFV Slow systolic acceleration Slow flow deceleration Flow diversion to adjacent arteries	Near occlusion at the site of insonation Arterial occlusion proximal to insonation site Incorrect vessel identification
Arterial occlusion	No detectable flow Good unilateral window of insonation High-resistance flow proximal to occlusion Flow diversion to adjacent arteries	Primary arterial occlusion Incorrect vessel identification Mass effect
Arterial vasospasm*	Proximal vasospasm: Focal or diffuse elevation of MFV without parallel FV increase in feeding extracranial arteries; HI greater than 3 Distal vasospasm: Focal increase in flow pulsatility (PI greater than or equal to 1.2), indicating increased resistance distal to site of insonation Increase in MFV in the involved and adjacent arteries may not be present	Vasospasm Hyperemia Vasospasm with hyperemia Altered cerebral autoregulation Increased intracranial pressure
Increased intracranial pressure	Decreased EDV or absent end-diastolic flow Rapid flow deceleration PI greater than or equal to 1.2 Note that these findings may be present in patients with increased cardiac output or elevated blood pressure, as well as in elderly individuals	The presence of PI greater than or equal to 1.2 and positive end-diastolic flow in all arteries may be caused by the following: Hyperventilation Hypertension Increased ICP Unilateral PI greater than or equal to 1.2 may be caused by the following: Compartmental ICP increase Stenoses distal to the site of insonation PI greater than or equal to 2.0 associated with absent end-diastolic flow is caused by extreme elevations in ICP and possible cerebral circulatory arrest
Cerebral circulatory arrest	Reversed end-diastolic flow or reverberating flow pattern *or* Minimal systolic flow acceleration with no end-diastolic flow *or* Absent flow signals in all intracranial arterial systems	Possible or probable circulatory arrest; measure both MCA and BA for 30 minutes; then reassess (transient arrest may occur during transient ICP increase or low blood pressure values)

BA, basilar artery; *EDV,* end-diastolic velocity; *FV,* flow velocity; *HI,* hemispheric index; *ICP,* intracranial pressure; *MCA,* middle cerebral artery; *MFV,* mean flow velocity; *PI,* pulsatility index.
*Vasospasm criteria have been well established for the proximal MCA.[9,13,14] Fewer criteria and validation studies are available for the posterior circulation vessel and the anterior cerebral artery.[2,13,14] Institutions may set other cut-off numbers for possible vasospasm in these vessels.

Additional equipment, as needed, includes the following:
- Smaller monitoring transducer(s) with removable handles
- Head-frame for monitoring transducer(s) fixation

PATIENT AND FAMILY EDUCATION

- Explain the purpose of the diagnostic test and the procedure for testing. ➛➛***Rationale:*** Decreases patient and family anxiety.
- Explain the need for the patient to remain still and quiet during the procedure. ➛➛***Rationale:*** Elicits patient cooperation and facilitates the examination.
- Explain that the procedure will not cause any discomfort to the patient. ➛➛***Rationale:*** Decreases patient and family anxiety.

AP This procedure should be performed only by physicians, advanced practice nurses, and other health care professionals (including critical care nurses) with additional knowledge, skills, and demonstrated competence per professional licensure or institutional standard.

PATIENT ASSESSMENT AND PREPARATION

Patient Assessment

- Note pertinent patient history. ➛➛***Rationale:*** The TCD may be used to assist with the diagnosis and management of a number of intracranial arterial conditions, including vasospasm, hyperemia, stenosis, occlusion, intracranial

TABLE 93-4 TIBI Flow Grade Definitions

For credentialing purposes, interpret flow signals above the baseline. Supporting flow information may be gained from the entire image.

For interpretation, assume all images are optimized (i.e., appropriate gain, power, window, angle, sample volume, depth).

0. Absent

Absent flow signals are defined by the lack of regular pulsatile flow signals despite varying degrees of background noise.

1. Minimal

A: Systolic spikes of variable velocity and duration

B: Absent diastolic flow during all cardiac cycles based on a visual interpretation of periods of no flow during end diastole (ED). Reverberating flow is a type of minimal flow.

Caution: Despite absent ED flow by visual interpretation, TCD equipment may erroneously report end diastolic (ED) velocity figures due to noise artifacts. Do not rely on machine ED velocity measurements to determine the presence or absence of end diastolic flow.

2. Blunted

A: Flattened or delayed systolic flow acceleration of variable duration compared with control

B: Positive end diastolic (ED) velocity

C: A pulsatility index (PI) less than 1.2

Caution: Flow velocities are usually greater than 20% lower than those in the comparison side.

Caution: With low velocities, blunted versus minimal signals may be hard to differentiate. Blunted is distinguished by the visual presence of end diastolic flow.

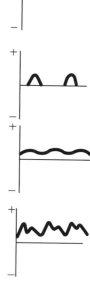

3. Dampened

A: Normal systolic flow acceleration

B: Positive end diastolic (ED) velocity

C: Decreased mean velocities by greater than or equal to 30% compared with control (calculate if close)

Caution: With subtle velocity/PI difference, look for dampened waveforms to have a more pulsatile shape.

Caution: Dampened versus blunted signals can be differentiated by dampened signals having a clear peak systolic complex (initially sharp systolic upstroke without flattening).

Caution: Dampened versus normal signals can be distinguished by dampened having a more abrupt down-slope of late systole and early diastole and other signs of obstruction, i.e., flow diversion (flow velocity ACA greater than MCA—where flow velocities below the baseline are greater than those above the baseline)

4. Stenotic

A: Mean flow velocities of greater than or equal to 80 cm/s AND velocity difference of greater than or equal to 30% compared with the control side (calculate if close); if velocity difference is less than 30%, look for additional signs of stenosis, such as turbulence, spectral narrowing

OR

B: If both affected and comparison sides have MFV less than 80 cm/s due to low end diastolic velocities, mean flow velocities greater than or equal to 30% compared with the control side (calculate if close) AND signs of turbulence.

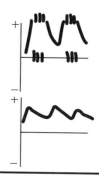

5. Normal

A: Less than 30% mean velocity difference compared with control (calculate if close)

B: Similar waveform shapes compared with control

Caution: Hypertensive individuals may have symmetric, high-resistance signals with PI greater than or equal to 1.2 and low end diastolic velocities.

Caution: Normal versus blunted signals can be differentiated by normal waveforms having initial sharp systolic upstrokes even if the rest of the waveform shows slow deceleration (note slower heart rate).

© 2000 Health Outcomes Institute, Inc.

---

hypertension, cerebral circulatory arrest, cerebral embolization, and vasomotor or autoregulation testing.

- Obtain the patient's blood pressure by arterial line or cuff. ➤*Rationale:* The arterial blood pressure may contribute to the flow velocity and waveform pattern.

- Assess preload or hydration state. ➤*Rationale:* Dehydration may decrease flow velocity because of an increase in blood viscosity and decreased preload pressures.

- Assess for hyperventilation or hypercapnia. ➤*Rationale:* The carbon dioxide level may promote vasoconstriction (hyperventilation) or vasodilation (hypercapnia).

- Assess for other factors that may affect velocity findings (e.g., age, Hct, Hgb, metabolic demand). ➤*Rationale:* Velocities decrease with age; anemia and increased metabolic demand increase velocities.

- Measure intracranial pressure (ICP) and determine cerebral perfusion pressure (CPP) and other intracranial dynamics available (e.g., SpO_2, $Sjvo_2$, brain tissue oxygenation).

➤*Rationale:* These factors may influence the pulsatility of flow and end-diastolic velocities.

- Assess the patient's neurologic status. ➤*Rationale:* Provides baseline data.

Patient Preparation

- Ensure that the patient understands preprocedural teaching. Answer questions as they arise and reinforce information as needed. ➤*Rationale:* Evaluates and reinforces understanding of previously taught information.

- Assist the patient with positioning. Supine is the best position for insonation via the transtemporal, transorbital, or submandibular windows. If the patient is alert and hemodynamically and neurologically stable, assist the patient to a sitting position for insonation through the transforaminal window; if the patient is unable to sit for transforaminal insonation, assist the patient to turn his or her head laterally; if the latter is not feasible, examine the

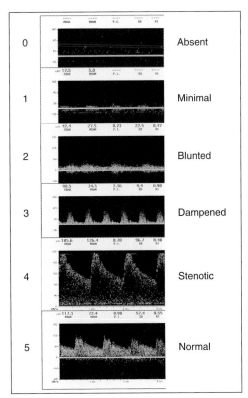

FIGURE 93-3 Thrombolysis in Brain Infarction (TIBI) Grading Scale. *(Copyright Health Outcomes Institute, The Woodlands, Texas.)*

patient supine with a smaller transducer with a removable handle or a monitoring probe. ➤*Rationale:* The transtemporal, transorbital, and submandibular windows are accessible with the patient in the supine position, whereas the transforaminal window requires a sitting position for proper probe angulation (see Fig. 93-1).

• Ask the patient to close his or her eyes for insonation

via the transorbital window. ➤*Rationale:* The probe is placed lightly, without pressure, on the eyelid and angled slightly medially to detect OA and ICA siphon flow signals.

• If necessary, ask the patient to hold his or her breath during insonation via the submandibular window. ➤*Rationale:* Breathing may produce audible and visual artifacts, obstructing assessment of the waveform.

Procedure | for Transcranial Doppler Monitoring

Steps	Rationale	Special Considerations
1. Wash hands and don nonsterile gloves.	Reduces the transmission of microorganisms and body secretions; standard precautions.	
Transtemporal Insonation 1. Set the depth at 50 to 56 mm.	Depth of 50 to 56 mm allows insonation of the M1 MCA.	
2. Set the power to maximum or 100%.	Optimizes the ability to identify the arterial waveforms.	
3. Apply gel to the probe or skin and place the probe above the zygomatic arch and aim slightly upward and anterior to the contralateral ear.	Accesses the transtemporal window (see Fig. 93-1).	No temporal window or a sub-optimal window can be found in 5% to 15% of the population.

Procedure continues on the following page

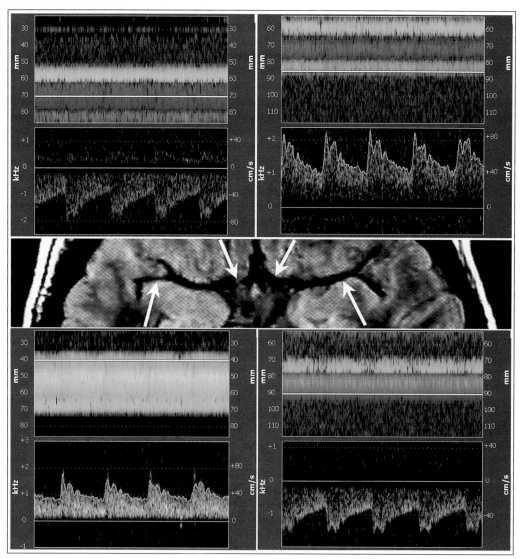

FIGURE 93-4 Power Motion Doppler (M-Mode). Top frame of each Doppler waveform identifies flow moving toward the probe *(above the baseline),* and flow moving away from the probe *(below);* depth is used to denote vessel insonated. *(Copyright Futura/Blackwell Sciences.)*

Procedure for Transcranial Doppler Monitoring—*Continued*

Steps	Rationale	Special Considerations
4. Find a flow signal directed toward the probe that meets MCA flow criteria (see Table 93-1).		
5. Follow the signal until it disappears by holding the probe in a constant position and changing the depth to shallow 40-45 mm and deeper 65-70 mm settings.	Verifies MCA identification; limits operator error.	
6. Find the ICA bifurcation at 65 mm and obtain both MCA and ACA signals.	ICA bifurcation is visualized at a depth of 65 mm; a bidirectional MCA/ACA waveform is noted.	

Procedure for Transcranial Doppler Monitoring—*Continued*

Steps	Rationale	Special Considerations
7. Follow the ACA signal to a depth of 70 to 75 mm.	ACA insonation begins at a depth of 70 to 75 mm.	The contralateral ACA may be insonated at a depth of more than 75 mm in the case of a unilateral suboptimal transtemporal window.
8. Return to the bifurcation and reset the depth to 62 mm while slowly rotating the probe posteriorly by 10 to 30 degrees to find the PCA.	The PCA is commonly detected at depths of 60 to 64 mm.	
9. Find the P1 PCA signal directed toward the probe and the P2 PCA signal directed away from the probe.		
10. Record and print findings, including at least waveforms, mean flow velocities, and PIs for all arteries insonated.		Activation of the "envelope" function may be necessary. The envelope is a continuous trace of maximum velocities during the cardiac cycle. If optimized to closely follow the maximum velocities without artifacts, the envelope provides automated calculations of MFV and flow pulsatility that are updated dependent on the display sweep speed.

Transorbital Insonation

Steps	Rationale	Special Considerations
1. Decrease the power to the minimum or 10%.	Limits eye exposure to ultrasound.	
2. Set the depth at 52 mm.	Aides in locating the ophthalmic artery (OA).	
3. Place the transducer gently over the eyelid without applying pressure, and turn the transducer slightly medially.	Aligns the ultrasound beam with the OA stem.	
4. Determine flow pulsatility and direction in the distal ophthalmic artery.	PI is equal to or greater than 1.2 because OA is an anastomosis with a high-resistance arterial system (extracranial carotid branches).	
5. Confirm findings at 55-60 mm.	Follow the OA course to the ICA siphon.	
6. Reset the depth to 60 to 64 mm and find the ICA siphon flow signals.	The ICA siphon can have bidirectional low-resistance flow signals.	
7. Record and print findings, including peak systolic, end-diastolic, and mean flow velocities, as well as PI for both the ICA and OA.	Document flow velocity and pulsatility in the ICSA siphon, and flow direction and pulsatility in the OA (results of Doppler spectral analysis for final report).	

Procedure continues on the following page

Procedure for Transcranial Doppler Monitoring—*Continued*

Steps	Rationale	Special Considerations

Transforaminal Insonation

1. Use maximum or 100% power.

2. Set the depth at 75 mm. | The VA/proximal BA junction is insonated at 75 mm. |

3. Place the probe at midline, 1 inch below the skull edge; aim toward the bridge of the nose. | Allows the ultrasound beam penetration through the foramen magnum. |

4. Identify flow directed away from the probe. | Vertebrobasilar arteries normally carry flow from the neck toward the brain (e.g., away from the probe). |

5. Increase the depth to 80 mm, then 90 mm, and 100 mm to follow the BA from proximal to distal segments. | The proximal BA is insonated at 80 mm, the mid-BA is insonated at 90 mm, and the distal BA is insonated at 95 to 100 mm or more. |

6. Confirm findings while slowly decreasing the depth of insonation. | A tortuous BA may be difficult to insonate; operator errors are common. |

7. Set the depth at 60 mm and reposition the probe laterally, aiming at the eye. | Switch from the basilar to the terminal vertebral artery. |

8. Find the VA flow directed away from the probe and follow it at 40 to 60 mm and 60 to 80 mm; repeat examination on the opposite side. | The intracranial portions of the right and left VA are insonated at depths between 40 and 80 mm. |

9. Record and print findings, including peak systolic, end-diastolic, and mean flow velocities, as well as PI for both the BA and bilateral VA. | Assess flow velocity, pulsatility and direction in the vertebrobasilar arteries. |

Submandibular Insonation

1. Set the depth at 50 to 60 mm, place the probe laterally under the jaw, and aim upward and medially. | Locate the distal ICA prior to its entrance to the skull. | Calculate the hemispheric index (HI): HI = MFV MCA/MFV ICA. Normal values are less than 3. HI is used to differentiate between M1-MCA vasospasm after subarachnoid hemorrhage and "hyperemia," or a hyperdynamic state. |

2. Find a low-resistance flow directed away from the probe that meets ICA criteria (see Table 93-1). | A high-resistance flow pattern is consistent with the external carotid artery, *not* the ICA. |

3. Repeat the examination on the opposite side. | Assess the contra-lateral ICA to complete a bilateral spectral Doppler study. |

4. Record and print findings, including at least waveforms, mean flow velocities, and PIs for both the right and left ICAs. | Assess flow velocity to calculate the hemispheric index, or the so-called Lindegaard ratio. |

5. Clean the gel from the patient's head. | Promotes comfort. |

Procedure for Transcranial Doppler Monitoring—*Continued*

Steps	Rationale	Special Considerations
6. Discard gloves, and wash hands.	Reduces the transmission of microorganisms; standard precautions.	

Expected Outcomes

- Determination of normal or pathologic flow conditions (notify physician of pathologic flow findings or inability to obtain flow velocities)
- Recommendation, as needed, for definitive angiographic examination and treatment
- Recognition of technical limitations, including operator skill

Unexpected Outcomes

- Inability to insonate via temporal window in 2% of patients after subarachnoid hemorrhage, aneurysm, or surgical obliteration, or edema and in up to 15% to 20% of other adult patients with intact skulls
- Underestimation of highest detectable velocity because of operator skill

Patient Monitoring and Care

Steps	Rationale	Reportable Conditions
		These conditions should be reported if they persist despite nursing interventions.
1. Monitor respiratory and cardiovascular status during procedure: A. $Paco_2$ B. Mean arterial pressure C. Cardiac rhythm D. Use of vasoactive medications if used during the procedure	Velocity is affected by systemic hemodynamics, as well as the vasomotor response of the resistance vessels in the brain (e.g., arterioles). TCD is not associated with the development of changes in the respiratory or cardiovascular status; instead, it is influenced by these changes, should they occur.	• Changes in respiratory status • Changes in cardiovascular status
2. When conducting the examination with a headframe, loosen the probe fixation after 1 hour and assess the skin. Minimize contact with skin incisions as much as possible.	Tight fixation by a headframe may be required to achieve better sound transmission and a constant angle of insonation.	• Skin breakdown • Unrelieved discomfort
3. When monitoring for brain embolization, note the timing of events associated with emboli detection (e.g., placement or removal of aortic cross-clamp during cardiac surgery with cardiopulmonary bypass).	Continuous monitoring with TCD has shown an association between specific operative events during cardiac surgery using cardiopulmonary bypass and the detection of brain emboli on TCD.	• Events that may affect emboli detection

Documentation

Documentation should include the following:

- Patient and family education
- Patient name, age, gender, and medical record number (should be included on every page of the written report including waveforms and interpretation)
- Clinical diagnosis (indication for testing)
- Significant, clinically detectable neurologic findings
- Arterial blood pressure, $Paco_2$, cardiac output, ICP (when feasible), and other intracranial dynamics during examination

- Preload as measured by PAWP and CVP to confirm hydration status
- Flow velocity spectra (waveforms), MFV, and PI in the arteries insonated
- Hard copies of arterial waveforms
- Presence of suboptimal windows indicated in the report
- Interpretation
- Unexpected outcomes
- Additional interventions

AP This procedure should be performed only by physicians, advanced practice nurses, and other health care professionals (including critical care nurses) with additional knowledge, skills, and demonstrated competence per professional licensure or institutional standard.

References

1. Aaslid, R., Markwalder, T.M., and Nornes, H. (1982). Noninvasive transcranial Doppler ultrasound recording of flow velocity in basal cerebral arteries. *J Neurosurg,* 57, 769-74.
2. Alexandrov, A.V. (2004). *Cerebrovascular Ultrasound in Stroke Prevention and Treatment.* Oxford: Blackwell-Futura Publishing.
3. Alexandrov, A.V. (1998). Transcranial Doppler sonography: Principles, examination technique and normal values. *Vasc Ultrasound Today,* 10, 141-60.
4. Alexandrov, A.V., Demchuk, A.M., and Burgin, W.S. (2002). Insonation method and diagnostic flow signatures for transcranial power motion (M-mode) Doppler. *J Neuroimaging,* 12, 236-44.
5. Alexandrov, A.V., et al. (2004). Ultrasound-enhanced systemic thrombolysis for acute ischemic stroke. *N Engl J Med,* 351, 2170-8.
6. Burgin, W.S., et al. (2000). TCD criteria for recanalization after thrombolysis for MCA stroke. *Stroke,* 31, 1128-32.
7. Burgin, W.S., et al. (2001). Validity and reliability of the thrombolysis in brain infarction (TIBI) flow grades. *Stroke,* 32, 324-5.
8. Demchuk, A.M., et al. (2001). Thrombolysis in brain ischemia Doppler flow grades predict clinical severity, early recovery, and mortality in patients treated with IV TPA. *Stroke,* 32, 89-93.
9. Lindegaard, K.F., et al. (1987). Cerebral vasospasm diagnosis by means of angiography and blood velocity measurements. *Acta Neurochir (Wien),* 100, 12-24.
10. Lindegaard, K.F. (1999). The role of transcranial Doppler in the management of patients with subarachnoid haemorrhage: A review. *Acta Neurochir,* 72(Suppl), 59-71.
11. McCartney, J.R., Thomas-Lukes, K.M., and Gomez, C.R. (1997). *Handbook of Transcranial Doppler.* New York: Springer.
12. Moehring, M.A., and Spencer, M.P. (2002). Power M-mode transcranial Doppler ultrasound and simultaneous single gate spectrogram. *Ultrasound Med Biol,* 28, 49-57.
13. Sloan, M.A. (1996). Transcranial Doppler monitoring of vasospasm after subarachnoid hemorrhage. In: Tegeler, C.H., Baikian, V.L., and Gomez, C.R., eds. *Neurosonology.* St. Louis: C.V. Mosby, 156-71.
14. Sloan, M.A., et al. (2004). Assessment: Transcranial Doppler ultrasonography: Report of the Therapeutics and Technology Assessment Subcommittee of the American Academy of Neurology. *Neurology,* 62, 1468-81.
15. Tegeler, C.H., Babikian, V.L., and Gomez, C.R. (1996). *Neurosonology.* St. Louis: C.V. Mosby.

Additional Readings

Newell, D.W. (1996). Trauma and brain death. In: Tegeler, C.H., Baikian, V.L., and Gomez, C.R. *Neurosonology.* St. Louis: C.V. Mosby, 189-99.
Stump, D.A., and Newman, S.P. (1996). Embolus detection during cardiopulmonary bypass. In: Tegeler, C.H., Baikian, V.L., and Gomez, C.R., *Neurosonology.* St. Louis: C.V. Mosby, 252-8.
Wojner, A.W. (2004). Integrated systemic and intracranial hemodynamics. In: Alexandrov, A.V. *Cerebrovascular Ultrasound in Stroke Prevention and Treatment.* Oxford: Blackwell-Futura Publishing, 41-61.

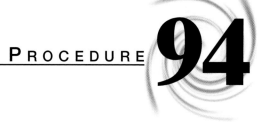

SECTION THIRTEEN

Special Neurologic
Procedures

Cerebrospinal Fluid Drainage
Assessment

P U R P O S E :   This procedure describes the collection and assessment of cerebrospinal drainage. It is important to identify cerebrospinal fluid leaks to decrease the risk for central nervous system infection and pneumocephalus.[2,3]

Phyllis Dubendorf

PREREQUISITE NURSING KNOWLEDGE

- Knowledge of neuroanatomy and physiology
- Cerebrospinal fluid (CSF) is produced primarily in the lateral ventricles and circulates in the subarachnoid space, located between the dura and the arachnoid.
- CSF leaks may occur with any breech of the dura commonly resulting from trauma or surgery. Although rare, CSF leaks can occur spontaneously.
- Most CSF leaks spontaneously resolve in 7 to 10 days; however, some may require interventions such as insertion of a lumbar drain device, blood patch, or open closure.
- CSF leaks predispose the individual to central nervous system (CNS) infection by allowing the entry of bacteria into the subarachnoid space.
- CSF leaks may predispose the individual to the development of pneumocephalus by allowing entry of air to a potential area of lower pressure.
- CSF leaks may manifest as the following (Fig. 94-1):
  ❖ Rhinorrhea (leakage of fluid from the nose)
  ❖ Otorrhea (leakage of fluid from the ear)
  ❖ Postnasal drip
- A CSF leak can sometimes be identified by a characteristic *halo* or *ring sign:* fluid absorbed by linen may create a collection of blood encircled with a larger concentric "halo" of clear or yellowish fluid. The reliability of the halo sign is controversial.[2]
- CSF can be identified by a laboratory assay of quantitative glucose (greater than 30 mg/dl is suggestive of CSF); however, false positives occur frequently. Urine glucose sticks are extremely sensitive to the presence of

glucose, and their use also yields a frequent false-positive result.
- CSF can be identified definitively by laboratory assay to detect the presence of beta-2-transferrin, a glycoprotein found in CSF but not in tears, nasal exudates, or serum.[1,2,4,5]

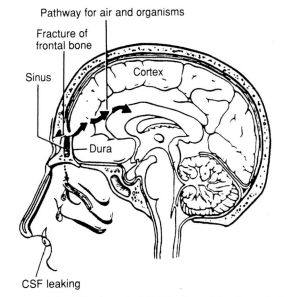

Pathway for air and organisms

Fracture of frontal bone

Sinus

Cortex

Dura

CSF leaking

FIGURE 94-1 Cerebrospinal fluid leak resulting from skull fracture. This diagram depicts a CSF leak from the nose (rhinorrhea), but CSF drainage also may be experienced from the ear (otorrhea), nasopharyngeally (described as postnasal drip), and, rarely, in tears. *CSF,* cerebrospinal fluid. *(From Shyder, M. and Jackie, M. [1981]. Neurologic Problems: A Critical Care Nursing Focus. Englewood, NJ: R.J. Brady.)*

- The presence of a CSF leak requires an increase in monitoring key neurologic indicators, such as vital signs, level of consciousness, nuchal rigidity, and photophobia.

EQUIPMENT

- Nonsterile gloves
- Small sterile container (test tube or specimen cup)
- Gauze
- Tape
- Specimen label
- Laboratory form

PATIENT AND FAMILY EDUCATION

- Explain the procedure and the reason for identification of the drainage. ➤*Rationale:* Reinforces the need for the procedure and allows the patient and family to ask questions.
- Review the signs and symptoms of meningeal irritation (e.g., stiff neck, photophobia, headache, and positive Kernig's and Brudzinski's sign) and CNS infection (e.g., fever, chills, headache, nausea, vomiting, confusion, delirium, seizures, rash). ➤*Rationale:* Recognition of meningeal signs and symptoms supports the diagnosis of a CNS infection and facilitates treatment.

PATIENT ASSESSMENT AND PREPARATION

Patient Assessment

- Obtain vital signs. ➤*Rationale:* Vital signs may be used to support the diagnosis of CNS infection.
- Perform a neurologic assessment. ➤*Rationale:* Deterioration of the neurologic assessment may be used to support the diagnosis of a CNS infection.
- Assess for the presence of meningeal signs (e.g., photophobia, headache, nuchal rigidity). ➤*Rationale:* These signs may be used to support the diagnosis of a CNS infection.

Patient Preparation

- Ensure that the patient and family understand preprocedural teaching. Answer questions as they arise and reinforce information as needed. ➤*Rationale:* Evaluates and reinforces understanding of previously taught information.
- Position the patient comfortably and in a position that facilitates fluid drainage and collection (e.g., left lateral side lying with legs and neck flexed). ➤*Rationale:* The presence and rate of CSF leakage may depend on the position of the patient's head.

Procedure | for Cerebrospinal Fluid Drainage Assessment

Steps	Rationale	Special Considerations
1. Wash hands and don nonsterile gloves.	Reduces the transmission of micro-organisms; standard precautions.	
2. If applicable, remove any sterile dressing the patient has that covers the flow of drainage.	Facilitates the collection of fluid.	
3. Collect fluid at the drainage site in a small sterile container.	Enables laboratory evaluation.	Obtain at least 1 ml of fluid for evaluation. This may be a time-consuming process if the leak is very slow.
4. Apply a new sterile dressing (if applicable).	Absorbs drainage.	
5. Discard gloves and soiled dressings, and wash hands.	Reduces the transmission of microorganisms; standard precautions.	
6. Label the sample and complete the laboratory form for detection of beta-2-transferrin.	Identifies the patient and test needed.	Beta-2-transferrin is a glycoprotein found in CSF.

Expected Outcomes

- Collection of sample for analysis
- Determination of CSF leak

Unexpected Outcomes

- Inability to obtain a sufficient amount of fluid for evaluation
- Laboratory unable to evaluate the sample
- Development of a CNS infection
- Development of a pneumocephalus

Patient Monitoring and Care

Steps	Rationale	Reportable Conditions
		These conditions should be reported if they persist despite nursing interventions.
1. Monitor the patient's neurologic status (using the Glasgow Coma Score) before and after collection of the CSF and as indicated.	Provides data for ongoing diagnosis and treatment.	• Changes in neurologic status
2. Change the sterile dressing every day and as needed.	Provides a subjective means of measuring the amount of drainage.	• Change in drainage volume or character
3. Monitor for signs and symptoms of meningitis.	Signs and symptoms of meningitis may indicate the need for further testing and evaluation.	• Change in level of consciousness • Temperature greater than 101.5°F • Photophobia • Nuchal rigidity • Seizure • Headache
4. Monitor for signs and symptoms of pneumocephalus.	Signs and symptoms of pneumocephalus may indicate the need for further testing and evaluation.	• Headache • Nuchal rigidity • Photophobia • Change in level of consciousness
5. Patients experiencing rhinorrhea should be encouraged *not* to strain or blow his or her nose.	Straining, blowing the nose or sneezing causes an increase in CSF pressure and can increase drainage.	

Documentation

Documentation should include the following:

- Patient and family education
- Patient's neurologic status
- Area from which the drainage is flowing
- Color, amount, and character of drainage

- Date, time, and amount of drainage collected for evaluation
- Unexpected outcomes
- Additional interventions

References

1. Gilroy, J. (2000). *Basic Neurology*. 3rd ed. New York: McGraw Hill.
2. Greenberg, M.S. (2001). *Handbook of Neurosurgery*. 5th ed. Lakeland, FL: Greenberg Graphics.
3. Hickey, J.V. (2003). *The Clinical Practice of Neurological and Neurosurgical Nursing*. 5th ed. Philadelphia: J.B. Lippincott.
4. Knight, J.A. (1997). Advances in the analysis of cerebrospinal fluid. *J Clin Lab Sci*, 27, 93-104.
5. Weaver, J.P., Davison, R.I., and Tabar, V. (2003). Cerebrospinal fluid aspiration. In: Irwin, et al., eds. *Procedures and Techniques in the Intensive Care Unit*. 3rd ed. Philadelphia: Lippincott Williams & Wilkins, 187-95.

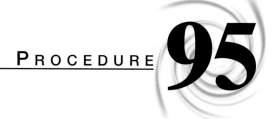

PROCEDURE **95**

External Warming/Cooling Devices

P U R P O S E :   An external warming device is applied to increase an undesirably low body temperature. An external cooling device is applied to reduce an undesirably high body temperature and to decrease cellular metabolism.

Eileen M. Kelly

PREREQUISITE NURSING KNOWLEDGE

- The *hypothalamus* is the primary thermoregulatory center for the body; it maintains normothermia through internal regulation of heat production or heat loss. Superficial or shell-zone temperature information is transmitted by thermal receptors in the skin and subcutaneous tissue to the posterior hypothalamus through the spinal cord. Thermoreceptors in the brain, heart, and other deep organs transmit the core-zone temperature. Effective temperature regulation depends on the ability of the posterior hypothalamus to receive and integrate the signals received from the core and shell zones.
- Terms associated with temperature should be known (Table 95-1).
- The hypothalamus regulates temperature in the range of approximately 36.4° to 37.3°C (97.5° to 99.4°F). By initiating physiologic responses to changes above or below this range, the hypothalamus coordinates heat loss or gain. Vasoconstriction and vasodilatation control the distribution and flow of blood to the organs, viscera, and skin surface; thus the amount of heat loss to the environment is influenced by vasomotor activity. In response to heat loss, shivering and vasoconstriction occur, the muscles tense and the extremities are drawn closer to the body, and the person seeks warmth. In response to heat gain, sweating and vasodilatation occur, muscles relax, and the person seeks coolness.
- Heat flows from a higher temperature to a lower temperature until the gradient between the two temperatures

diminishes. Conduction, convection, radiation, and evaporation transfer heat as follows:
- ❖ *Conduction* occurs when a warmer object comes in direct contact with one of a lower temperature.
- ❖ *Convection* occurs when air or liquid carries heat away from or to an object.
- ❖ *Radiation* occurs when thermal energy passes through air or space.
- ❖ *Evaporation* occurs when heat is lost to the surrounding air.
- Alteration in thermoregulation can result from a primary central nervous system injury or disease (e.g., subarachnoid hemorrhage, spinal cord injury, or neoplasm) and metabolic conditions (e.g., diabetes mellitus; toxic levels

TABLE 95-1	Terms Associated With Temperature
Term	**Definition**
Euthermia	Range of body temperature associated with health
Hypothermia	Temperature below 36.4°C
Induced hypothermia	Intentional cooling by surface means (transfer of heat from the skin to the coolant circulating through the coils of the cooling device) or central means (circulatory heat exchange in a cardiopulmonary bypass machine)
Fever	Response to a pyrogen; the hypothalamus either resets its range higher, maintaining thermoregulation, or there is a change in the sensitivity of the hypothalamus neuron activity to warmth and coldness[3]
Hyperthermia	Dysfunction of thermoregulation caused by an injury to the hypothalamus or by a person's heat loss mechanisms being overwhelmed by high environmental heat

of ethanol alcohol or other drugs, such as barbiturates and phenothiazines).

- *Body temperature* is the measurement of the presence or absence of heat. Body heat is generated, conserved, redistributed, or dissipated during all physiologic processes. Factors such as age, circadian rhythm, and hormones influence body temperature.

- Body temperature may be measured by a variety of thermometers and body sites. Electronic or digital thermometers are used to obtain rectal, oral, and axillary temperatures. Thermistors within catheters or probes measure rectal, nasopharyngeal, esophageal, bladder, brain, and pulmonary artery temperatures. Infrared thermometers measure tympanic membrane and temporal artery temperatures.

- *Core temperature* represents the temperature of internal sites ranging from the rectum to the tympanic membrane. Variations in temperatures normally occur in the body (Table 95-2).

- Site choice for temperature monitoring is based on the clinical data needed and on the patient's condition, safety, comfort, and environmental factors (e.g., room temperature), the indication for a catheter or a probe (e.g., pulmonary artery catheter), and the availability of equipment.

- A consistent temperature site must be monitored during the application of a warming or cooling device.

- Table 95-3 outlines techniques to increase heat gain.

- *Shivering* is an involuntary shaking of the body. It is caused by contraction or twitching of the muscles and is a physiologic method of heat production.

- Shivering increases the metabolic rate, carbon dioxide (CO_2) production, oxygen consumption, and myocardial work. If cardiopulmonary compensation does not occur to meet these demands, anaerobic metabolism occurs, resulting in acidosis.

- Early detection of shivering can be accomplished by palpating the mandible and feeling a "humming" vibration.[1,4] Electrocardiogram (ECG) artifact from skeletal muscle is seen on the bedside monitor. If not detected early, shivering can progress to visible twitching of the head or neck, then to visible twitching of the pectorals or trunk, and then to generalized shaking of the entire body and teeth chattering.

- At a body temperature below 35°C, the basal metabolic rate can no longer supply sufficient body heat, and an exogenous source of heat is needed.

TABLE 95-3	Techniques to Increase Heat Gain
Mechanism of Heat Transfer	**Techniques to Increase Heat Gain**
Radiation	Warming lights, warm environment, room temperature, blankets
Conduction	Warm blankets, circulating water blanket, continuous arteriovenous rewarming, cardiopulmonary bypass
Convection	Thermal fans, circulating air blanket
Evaporation	Head and body covers; warm, humidified oxygen

- *Hypothermia* may be categorized as mild (34° to 36.5°C), moderate (27.5° to 33.9°C), deep (17° to 27.4°C), or profound (less than 16.9°C).

- Hypothermia may be caused by an increase in heat loss, a decrease in heat production, an alteration in thermoregulation, and a variety of clinical conditions.

- An increase in heat loss may occur from the following:
  - ❖ Environmental exposure
  - ❖ Near drowning
  - ❖ Induced vasodilatation caused by high levels of ethanol alcohol, barbiturates, and general anesthesia
  - ❖ Dermal dysfunction (e.g., burns)
  - ❖ Iatrogenic conditions (e.g., administering cold intravenous fluids, hemodialysis, cardiopulmonary bypass)

- A decrease in heat production is associated with the following:
  - ❖ Endocrine conditions (e.g., hypothyroidism)
  - ❖ Malnutrition
  - ❖ Diabetic ketoacidosis
  - ❖ Neuromuscular insufficiency (e.g., resulting from a pharmacologic paralysis caused by a neuromuscular blocking agent or anesthetic agents)

- Clinical conditions associated with hypothermia are sepsis, hepatic coma, and systemic inflammatory response syndrome.

- The significant physiologic alterations that occur with hypothermia depend on the degree of hypothermia present and the cause of the hypothermia (Table 95-4).

- Severe hypothermia may mimic death; resuscitative efforts should be initiated despite the absence of vital signs.

- Rewarming should not occur faster than 2°C per hour. Rapid rewarming can cause a rewarming acidosis, shivering, hypovolemic shock, temperature afterdrop, and temperature overshoot.

- *Afterdrop* is a decrease in core temperature after rewarming is discontinued.

- *Overshoot* occurs when the thermoregulator mechanisms rebound or overcompensate. Terminating active external rewarming at 36° to 36.5°C may prevent temperature overshoot.

- *Rewarming acidosis* results from the increase in CO_2 production associated with the temperature increase and from the return of accumulated acids in the peripheral circulation to the heart.

TABLE 95-2	Normal Variations in Body Temperature Based on a Rectal Temperature of 37°C
Type of Temperature Measurement	**Degrees Lower Than Rectal Temperature**
Oral	0.3-0.5°C
Esophageal	0.2°C
Pulmonary artery	0.2-0.3°C
Tympanic membrane	0.05-0.25°C
Bladder	0.1-0.2°C
Axillary	0.6-0.8°C

TABLE 95-4	Physiologic Responses to Hypothermia

Central Nervous System

Decreased cerebral blood flow
Progressive paralysis of the central nervous system
Reduced cerebral metabolic demand

Cardiovascular System

Decreased heart rate, contractility, and cardiac output
Delayed depolarization in pacemaker tissue
Electrocardiogram characteristics: increased PR, QRS, and QT intervals;
   J wave (a deflection of the QRS-ST junction); ST elevation; and
   T wave inversion
Decreased transmembrane resting potential resulting in atrial fibrillation
   or ventricular fibrillation

Pulmonary System

Hypoventilation
Decreased cough reflex
Increased airway secretions
Paralysis of mucociliary mechanism

Gastrointestinal System

Hypomotility
Decreased hepatic metabolism
Decreased insulin release from the pancreas
Stress ulceration

Renal System

Impaired renal tubular transport causing decreased sodium and water
   reabsorption
Decreased antidiuretic hormone
Fluid shift from the vascular compartment to the interstitial spaces

Acid-Base Balance

Decreased systemic carbon dioxide production
Early respiratory alkalosis
Eventual metabolic acidosis in severe hypothermia

Hematologic System

Shift of oxyhemoglobin dissociation curve to the left, causing decreased
   oxygen delivery to tissues
Increased blood viscosity
Coagulopathy caused by inhibition of the enzyme reactions of the
   coagulation cascade and splenic sequestration of platelets

Immunologic System

Leukocyte sequestration in the spleen
Decreased neutrophil function
Reduced collagen deposition

- *Rewarming shock* occurs when hypothermic vasoconstriction masks hypovolemia. If the patient's circulating volume is insufficient during rewarming vasodilatation, there is a sudden decrease in blood pressure, systemic vascular resistance (SVR), and preload.
- *Hyperthermia* occurs when the thermoregulator system of the body absorbs or produces more heat than it is able to release.
- *Malignant hyperthermia* is a rare, hereditary condition of the skeletal muscle that occurs on exposure to a triggering agent or agents. The triggering agents most commonly associated with malignant hyperthermia are anesthetic agents, particularly inhalation anesthetics and succinylcholine. Malignant hyperthermia involves instability of the muscle cell membrane, which causes a sudden increase in myoplasmic calcium and skeletal muscle contractures.

- The earliest indication of malignant hyperthermia is an increase in end-tidal carbon dioxide ($ETCO_2$) of 5 mm Hg more than the patient's baseline. If the $ETCO_2$ is not being monitored, the earliest sign is tachycardia, occurring within 30 minutes of anesthesia induction. Tachycardia is followed by ventricular ectopy, which may progress to ventricular tachycardia and ventricular fibrillation. Muscle rigidity usually begins in the extremities, chest, or jaws.
- A cooling device is used to treat malignant hyperthermia after administration of the triggering agent is stopped and a muscle relaxant (e.g., dantrolene sodium) is given. The muscle relaxant blocks the release of calcium from the sarcoplasmic reticulum without affecting calcium uptake.[1]
- *Heat stroke* occurs when the outdoor temperature and humidity are excessive and heat is transferred to the body. The high humidity prevents cooling by evaporation. Other signs are hypotension, tachycardia, tachypnea, mental status changes from confusion to coma, and possibly seizures. The skin is hot and dry, and sweating may occur. The rectal temperature is greater than 104° to 106°F. Initial interventions include support of airway, breathing, and circulation. Rapid cooling of the patient is the main treatment priority with a goal of reducing the temperature to 101° to 102°F within 1 hour.
- *Fever* occurs in response to a pyrogen. During fever, the hypothalamus retains its function, and *shivering* and diaphoresis occur to gain or lose body heat. Fever may be an adaptive response and may be considered beneficial. However, a febrile state increases the heart rate and metabolic rate and may be detrimental to a critically ill patient. The decision to reduce a fever needs to be based on the patient's physical and hemodynamic stability during the fever.
- Some external warming or cooling devices transfer warmth or coolness to the patient by conduction. Warmed or cooled fluids circulate through coils in a thermal blanket or pad that is commonly placed under the patient.
- Other external devices transfer warmth to the patient by convection. A device used only for warming blows warm air through microperforations on the underside of a blanket that is placed on the patient. Warm air is directed through the blanket onto the patient's skin.
- Specific information about controls, alarms, troubleshooting, and safety features is available from each manufacturer and must be understood by the nurse before using the equipment.

EQUIPMENT

- Warming or cooling device
- Sheet or bath blanket
- Nonsterile gloves
- Temperature probe, cable, and module to monitor the patient's temperature (varies based on the type of site and thermometer selected and available)
- Cardiac monitoring (see Procedure 54)

Additional equipment to have available as needed includes the following:
- Hemodynamic monitoring (see Procedure 75)
- Distilled water

PATIENT AND FAMILY EDUCATION

- Explain the reason for the use of a warming or cooling device and standard of care, including monitoring of the temperature, expected length of therapy, comfort measures, and parameters for discontinuation of the device. ➻*Rationale:* Encourages the patient and family to ask questions and verbalize concerns about the procedure.
- Assess the patient and family understanding of the warming or cooling therapy. ➻*Rationale:* Clarification and reinforcement of information is needed during times of stress and anxiety.
- Encourage the patient to notify the nurse of any discomfort. ➻*Rationale:* Facilitates early relief and minimizes discomfort.
- If a warm air device will be used, explain the rationale for removing the patient's gown. Reassure the patient and family that privacy will be respected. ➻*Rationale:* The patient and family will know what to expect.

PATIENT ASSESSMENT AND PREPARATION

Patient Assessment

- Assess risk factors, medical history, the cause of the patient's underlying condition, and the type and the length of temperature exposure. ➻*Rationale:* Assists in anticipating, recognizing, and responding to the patient's responses and potential side effects to therapy.
- Assess the patient's medication therapy. ➻*Rationale:* Medications such as vasopressors and vasodilators may affect heat transfer, increase the potential for skin injury, and contribute to an adverse hemodynamic response.
- Obtain a core (pulmonary artery, urinary, or rectal) temperature. ➻*Rationale:* Determines baseline temperature. Determines when a warming or cooling device is needed.
- Obtain vital signs and hemodynamic values (if using pulmonary artery monitoring). ➻*Rationale:* Determines baseline cardiovascular data. Initially, cold temperatures activate the sympathetic nervous system, resulting in tachycardia, vasoconstriction, and shivering. Rewarming may result in vasodilatation and hypotension. Heart failure may occur with malignant hyperthermia and heat stroke.
- Monitor the patient's cardiac rhythm. ➻*Rationale:* Determines the baseline cardiac rhythm. Hypothermia has a negative chronotropic effect on pacemaker tissue, which may lead to bradycardia and atrioventricular heart block. Hypothermia may cause repolarization abnormalities, producing ST segment elevation and T wave inversion.

A hypothermic heart is susceptible to atrial and ventricular fibrillation. Tachycardia and ventricular dysrhythmias may occur if the patient is hyperthermic.

- Assess the patient's electrolytes, glucose, arterial blood gas, and coagulation study results. ➻*Rationale:* Alterations in temperature balance may result in acid-base imbalance, coagulopathy, electrolyte imbalance, and hypoxemia. Hypothermia inhibits insulin release from the pancreas, but glucose levels remain normal in mild hypothermia because shivering increases glucose utilization. Hyperglycemia occurs at temperatures less than 32°C because shivering ceases.
- Assess the patient's level of consciousness and neurologic function. ➻*Rationale:* Determines baseline neurologic status. A change in mental status, level of consciousness, and impaired neurologic function may occur because of an undesirable high or low temperature or from the condition causing the alteration in temperature. Fatigue, muscle incoordination, poor judgment, weakness, hallucinations, lethargy, and stupor may occur with hypothermia. Seizures may occur with hyperthermia.
- Assess the patient's ventilatory function. ➻*Rationale:* Hypoventilation, suppression of cough, and mucociliary reflexes associated with hypothermia may lead to hypoxemia, atelectasis, and pneumonia. Hypothermia shifts the oxygenation dissociation curve to the left, and less oxygen is released from oxyhemoglobin to the tissues. Because of peripheral vasoconstriction, pulse oximetry is unreliable. Hyperthermia shifts the oxygenation dissociation curve to the right, and oxygen is readily released from oxyhemoglobin.
- Assess the patient's bowel sounds, abdomen, and gastrointestinal function. ➻*Rationale:* Determines baseline status. Patients experiencing hypothermia may develop an ileus because of decreased intestinal motility. Vomiting and diarrhea may occur with hyperthermia.
- Assess the patient's skin integrity. ➻*Rationale:* Provides baseline data. An externally applied warming or cooling device can cause or exacerbate skin injury. Preexisting conditions such as diabetes and peripheral vascular disease increase the patient's risk for skin injury.

Patient Preparation

- Ensure that the patient and/or family understand preprocedural teaching. Answer questions as they arise, and reinforce information as needed. ➻*Rationale:* Evaluates and reinforces understanding of previously taught information.
- If a warm air device will be used, remove the patient's gown and top sheet. ➻*Rationale:* The warm air device works by convection and should be in direct contact with the patient's skin for optimal results.
- If the patient is hypothermic, cover the patient's head with a blanket or towel or an aluminum cap. ➻*Rationale:* Minimizes additional heat loss.

Procedure for External Warming/Cooling Devices

Steps	Rationale	Special Considerations
1. Wash hands and don nonsterile gloves.	Reduces the transmission of microorganisms; standard precautions.	
2. Obtain a method for continuously monitoring the patient's core temperature.	Continuous core temperature monitoring is necessary when using external warming or cooling devices.	Some warming or cooling devices have an adapter for connecting a temperature probe from the patient directly to the device.
3. Plug the device into a grounded outlet.	Establishes a power source.	

Use of a Warming or Cooling Fluid Device

Steps	Rationale	Special Considerations
1. Place a sheet or bath blanket between the patient and the circulating fluid blanket.	Protects the skin.	Avoid applying additional sheets or blankets because efficient heating or cooling occurs with maximal contact between the thermal pad and the patient's skin.
2. Fill the reservoir in the unit with distilled water to the indicated full level.	The reservoir must contain enough water for the machine to function properly.	

3. Attach the hoses to the circulating fluid blanket.
  A. Check that the clamps are closed before connecting the hoses from the device to the blanket.
  B. After connecting the hoses, make sure all connections are tight before unclamping.
  C. Check for kinks in the hoses.
	Allows the flow of warmed or cooled water to the blanket.	Prevents water spraying.

4. Press the start switch on.	Activates the device.	

5. Set the controls
  A. Manual control
    (1) Press the manual control switch on.
    (2) Choose the set point for the temperature of the circulating fluid. If cooling, set the temperature at 23.9°C.
 	
    (3) Turn the warming or cooling device off when the desired temperature is reached.
  B. Automatic control
    (1) Connect the temperature probe to the unit 1 minute before pressing a control mode switch.
    (2) Select the automatic mode and the set point.
	The device maintains the circulating fluid in the blanket at the temperature set point. If cooling a fluid, the temperature set at 23.9°C prevents shivering.[5]
	The temperature goal is achieved.
	
	Prevents triggering of the temperature probe alarm.
	
	In the automatic mode, the unit warms or cools the circulating fluid in the blanket based on the set point (desired temperature) for the patient. A rectal or skin probe connected to the unit monitors the patient's temperature.
		The patient's temperature must be continuously monitored by a method other than the cooling or warming device.
		
		Most warming or cooling devices sound an alarm if the probe relays a low temperature (30°C), indicative of probe dislodgment.
		The unit operates only if the patient's temperature probe is connected to the unit. Lights on the display panel indicate whether the unit is heating or cooling at any given time.

Procedure for External Warming/Cooling Devices—*Continued*

Steps	Rationale	Special Considerations
(3) Obtain the patient's temperature from the readout on the display unit.	Indicates the patient's temperature.	
(4) Take the patient's temperature with another thermometer and compare it with the readout on the device's display unit.	Ensures the warming or cooling device's temperature probe is functioning and correlates with the patient's temperature obtained by another method.	
(5) The warming or cooling device will automatically shut itself off when the desired patient temperature is reached.	The temperature goal is achieved.	Continue to monitor the patient's temperature by pressing on the monitor only switch.
(6) Wash hands.	Reduces the transmission of microorganisms; standard precautions.	
Use of a Warm Air Device		
1. Connect the air blanket to the hose attached to the device.	Prepares the equipment.	
2. Turn the device on and select the temperature of the air that will flow through the blanket.	The blanket inflates as air blows from the hose into it.	A warm air device can increase a patient's temperature 2° to 3°C per hour.
3. Remove the patient's gown, sheet, and blankets. Then place the circulating air blanket on top of the patient.	The device warms the patient by directing warm airstreams directly onto the patient's skin.	Maintain privacy.
4. Place a bath blanket or sheet over the circulating air blanket.	Prevents heat loss.	The patient's temperature must be continuously monitored.
5. Wash hands.	Reduces the transmission of microorganisms; standard precautions.	

Expected Outcomes

- External warming or cooling device applied
- Desirable core body temperature achieved

Unexpected Outcomes

- Unable to achieve desired core body temperature
- Hemodynamic instability
- Cardiac dysrhythmias
- Acid-base imbalance
- Shivering
- Skin injury

Patient Monitoring and Care

Steps	Rationale	Reportable Conditions
		These conditions should be reported if they persist despite nursing interventions.
1. Perform a physical assessment of all systems every 1 to 2 hours.	Alterations in temperature affect every system. The condition causing the change in temperature may worsen or be refractory to treatment.	- Significant changes in assessment
2. Continuously monitor the patient's core temperature.	Assesses the patient's response to warming or cooling.	- Continued hypothermia or hyperthermia

Procedure continues on the following page

Patient Monitoring and Care—*Continued*

Steps	Rationale	Reportable Conditions
3. Measure the patient's blood pressure every 15 minutes for the first hour and as frequently as indicated by the patient's condition.	Vasodilatation occurs with rewarming, and vasoconstriction may occur with cooling.	• Hypotension or hypertension
4. Palpate the patient's mandible for "humming" vibration and observe for shivering.	Aides in the early detection and prompt treatment of shivering.	• Shivering • Decreased mixed venous oxygenation saturation • Continued shivering despite prescribed medications
5. Examine the patient's skin condition hourly.	Detects signs or symptoms of skin irritation so that the temperature of the device can be adjusted or padding can be placed between the skin and the device.	• Signs or symptoms of skin irritation or injury
6. Continuous cardiac monitoring.	Detects cardiac dysrhythmias associated with warming or cooling.	• Cardiac dysrhythmias
7. Obtain arterial blood gas results as prescribed and as indicated.	Detects hypoxemia and acid-base imbalances.	• Abnormal arterial blood gas results
8. Ensure patient comfort.	Minimizes discomfort.	• Unrelieved discomfort

Documentation

Documentation should include the following:

- Patient and family education
- Patient's temperature and site of temperature assessment
- Vital signs and hemodynamic status
- Physical assessment findings
- Cardiac rhythm

- Type of warming or cooling device used
- Time external warming or cooling initiated and terminated
- Patient comfort
- Unexpected outcomes
- Additional interventions

References

1. Caruso, C.C., et al. (1992). Cooling effects and comfort of four cooling blanket temperatures in humans with fever. *Nursing Research*, 2, 68-72.
2. Henker, R., and Shaver, J. (1994). Understanding the febrile state according to an individual adaptation framework. *AACN Clin Iss Crit Care Nurs*, 2, 186-93.
3. Holtzclaw, B. (1993). Monitoring body temperature. *AACN Clin Iss Crit Care Nurs*, 1, 44-55.
4. Holtzclaw, B. (1997). Temperature problems in the postoperative period. *Crit Care Nurs Clin North Am*, 5, 368-74.
5. Miranda, A., et al. (1997). Malignant hyperthermia. *Am J Crit Care*, 5, 368-74.

Additional Readings

Aragon, D. (1999). Temperature management in trauma patients across the continuum of care: The TEMP group. *AACN Clinical Issues*, 1, 113-23.
Charkoudian, N. (2003). Skin blood flow on adult human thermoregulation: How it works, when it does not and why. *Mayo Clinic Proceedings*, 5, 603-12.
Falllis, W. (2002). Monitoring temperature in trauma patients: New research and technologies. *J Emerg Nurs*, 5, 471-2.

Grossman, S., Bautista, C., and Sullivan, L. (2002). Using evidence-based practice to develop a protocol for postoperative surgical intensive care unit patients. *DCCN-Dimensions of Critical Care Nursing*, 5, 204-14.
Henker, R., et al. (2001). Comparison of fever treatments in the critically ill: A pilot study. *Am J Crit Care*, 10, 276-80.
Holtzclaw, B.J. (2001). Circadian rhythmicity and homeostatic stability in thermoregulation. *Biologic Res Nurs*, 4, 221-35.
Keegan, M., Sharbrough, F., and Lanier, W. (1999). Shivering complicating the treatment of neurologically impaired surgical and intensive care unit patients. *Anesthesiology*, 3, 874-9.
Koschel, M. (2001). Rewarming a hypothermic patient: Raise the core temperature slowly and carefully. *Am J Nurs*, 5, 85.
Mayer, S., et al. (2001). Clinical trial of an air-circulating cooling blanket for fever control in critically ill neurologic patients. *Neurology*, 3, 292-8.
McGowan, J. (1999). Management of hypothermias in adults. *Nurs Crit Care*, 2, 59-62.
Schmitz, T., Bair, N., and Levine, C. (1995). A comparison of five methods of temperature measurement in febrile intensive patients. *Am J Crit Care*, 4, 286-92.
Sund-Levander, M., and Wahren, L. (2000). Assessment and prevention of shivering in patients with severe cerebral injury: A pilot study. *J Clin Nurs*, 1, 55-61.

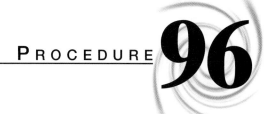

PROCEDURE **96**

Ice-Water Caloric Testing for Vestibular Function (Assist)

P U R P O S E : Caloric testing for vestibular function (oculovestibular reflex) is a diagnostic procedure that tests vestibular function in the awake patient and the functional connectivity between the medulla and the midbrain in the comatose patient.[2] Caloric testing can be used as part of brain death evaluation.

Phyllis Dubendorf

PREREQUISITE NURSING KNOWLEDGE

- Knowledge of neuroanatomy and physiology
- The oculovestibular reflex is elicited by introducing iced water or normal saline into the external auditory canal of patients with intact tympanic membranes.[2] The vestibular portion of the eighth cranial nerve (acoustic) is stimulated and transmits this impulse via the medial longitudinal fasciculus to two of the cranial nerve nuclei involving extraocular eye movements (cranial nerves III and VI). Stimulation of this reflex results in deviation of the eyes (Fig. 96-1).
- A *normal response* in the *awake* patient is nystagmus, initially a slow component toward the irrigated ear, then a faster component *away* from the irrigated ear toward the midline. If warm water is used for testing, there is a slow component of nystagmus initially *away* from the irrigated side, then a faster component *toward* the irrigated ear, hence the mnemonic COWS—Cold: Opposite; Warm: Same.[1-3]
- A *normal response* in the *comatose* patient usually results in stimulation of the slow component only and results in reflex conjugate eye movement *toward* the cold-water irrigated ear[3] (Fig. 96-2).
- An abnormal (dysconjugate) or absent response to cold water testing in the unconscious patient *may* indicate brain stem dysfunction and a poor prognosis; however, this test alone is not definitive.
- This test is *contraindicated* in patients with a perforated tympanic membrane.

- Agents or conditions that can potentially interfere with the oculovestibular reflex include the following:
  - ❖ Ototoxic medications
  - ❖ Neurosuppressant medications, such as barbiturates, phenytoin, sedatives, and tricyclic antidepressants
  - ❖ Aminoglycosides
  - ❖ Neuromuscular blockade
  - ❖ Anticholinergics
  - ❖ Preexisting vestibular disease, active labyrinth disease (Meniere's disease)
  - ❖ Preexisting cranial nerve disorders involving cranial nerves III and VI (oculomotor and abducens)
  - ❖ Facial trauma involving the auditory canal and petrous bone
- This test should be performed bilaterally, if possible, with an observation of at least 1 minute and at least 5 minutes between irrigations.
- This test may produce decorticate or decerebrate posturing in the *unconscious* patient because of the noxious nature of the stimulus. It is extremely uncomfortable and may produce nausea and vomiting in the *awake* patient.
- Additional clinical data, such as lack of spontaneous respirations, doll's eyes (oculocephalic reflex), no response to painful stimulation, nonreactive pupils, absent corneal reflexes, and abnormal diagnostic studies, are required to support the diagnosis of brain death (see Procedure 147).

EQUIPMENT

- 50- to 60-ml syringe with Luer-Lok end
- 18- or 20-G angiocatheter with needle removed

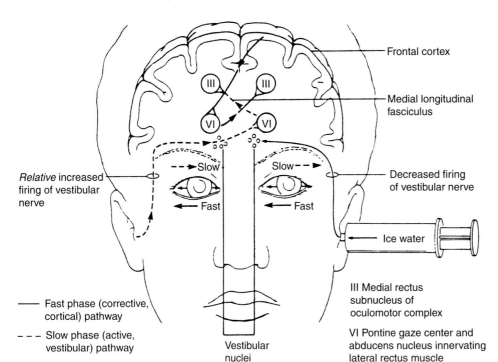

FIGURE 96-1 Physiology of the oculovestibular reflex. Cold-water irrigation of a patient will elicit this reflex if both the cerebral hemisphere and the brainstem are intact. The signal passes through the pathways from the medulla to the midbrain, resulting in a slow movement of the eyes toward the irrigated ear. Then, as the impulse travels to the intact ipsilateral hemisphere, a rapid corrective movement of the eyes (nystagmus away from the irrigated ear) can be observed. (*From* Patient Care Magazine, *Medical Economics Publishing: 1981:29.*)

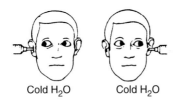

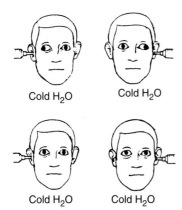

FIGURE 96-2 Cold-water caloric responses in the comatose patient. If the patient's brainstem is intact, the normal response to cold-water irrigation is slow movement toward the irrigated ear. When the brainstem is not intact, an abnormal (dysconjugated) or absent response may be observed. (*From Plum F, Posner J, [1980]. The Diagnosis of Stupor and Coma. 3rd ed. Philadelphia: F.A. Davis.*)

- Small basin
- Iced water or normal saline
- Towels and protective bedding
- Disposable nonsterile gloves
- Otoscope to assess the integrity of the tympanic membrane

PATIENT AND FAMILY EDUCATION

- Discuss the purpose of the test with the patient and family. ➡️***Rationale:*** Prepares the patient and family for what to expect.
- Discuss the unpleasant sensations that may be experienced by the awake patient, if applicable. ➡️***Rationale:*** The awake patient may experience nausea, dizziness, pain, or vomiting.

PATIENT ASSESSMENT AND PREPARATION

Patient Assessment

- Obtain vital signs. ➡️***Rationale:*** Establishes baseline values for the patient.
- Perform a neurologic assessment including the following: eye opening, verbal, and motor responses, cranial nerve function, and respiratory pattern. ➡️***Rationale:*** Establishes baseline neurologic function to support the presence or absence of voluntary or reflexive activity.
- Review the patient's current medications. ➡️***Rationale:*** Some medications may interfere with the oculovestibular response.
- Assess the patient's medical history of cranial nerve dysfunction. ➡️***Rationale:*** The occurrence of preexisting

vestibular disease may produce unreliable results related to oculovestibular testing.

- Assess the patient's current medical history. ➤➤*Rationale:* Identifies medical conditions that may affect the patient's responsiveness.
- Assist with inspection of the patient's tympanic membranes to ensure that both membranes are intact and that the auditory canals are not blocked with cerumen. ➤➤*Rationale:* Iced caloric testing is contraindicated in patients with a perforated eardrum. The presence of cerumen may impede or prevent the flow of irrigant to the semicircular apparatus.

Patient Preparation

- Ensure that the patient and family understands preprocedural teaching. Answer questions as they arise and reinforce information as needed. ➤➤*Rationale:* Evaluates and reinforces understanding of previously taught information.
- Assist the patient in positioning his or her head in a neutral position with the head of bed elevated to 30 degrees. ➤➤*Rationale:* Places the lateral semicircular canals in a vertical position, which allows maximal stimulation and optimizes venous jugular drainage. This position may be deferred if the patient experiences cardiovascular decompensation that requires alternative positioning.

Procedure for Ice-Water Caloric Testing for Vestibular Function (Assist)

Steps	Rationale	Special Considerations
1. Wash hands and don nonsterile gloves.	Reduces the transmission of microorganisms; standard precautions.	
2. Place a protective pad under the patient.	Absorbs the iced irrigant.	
3. Verify that the integrity of the tympanic membrane has been assessed.	This test is contraindicated for patients with a perforated tympanic membrane.	
4. Assist with the instillation of 50 ml of iced water or normal saline into the external auditory canal. The instillation should occur from over 30 seconds to 3 minutes, to allow adequate time for stimulation.	Stimulates oculovestibular reflex.	The physician or advanced practice nurse may elect to use up to 100 ml of iced water or normal saline. More than one examiner is needed to simultaneously inject the irrigant and ensure that the patient's eyes are open in order to assess extraocular movements.
5. Observe the patient's eyes for a response for up to 1 minute.	Determines the response to instillation.	
6. Assist with irrigation of iced water or normal saline into the opposite external auditory canal.	Both sides must be assessed for responses.	A 5-minute interval between irrigations is recommended.
7. Assess the patient's response to the procedure.	The noxious stimuli may cause posturing in the comatose patient and dizziness, nausea, pain, and vomiting in the patient who is awake.	
8. Discard supplies in appropriate receptacles; wash hands.	Reduces the transmission of microorganisms; standard precautions.	

Expected Outcomes

- Successful assessment of brainstem function in the comatose patient
- Successful assessment of vestibular function in the awake patient

Unexpected Outcomes

- Test cannot be completed.
- Ocular movement is dysconjugated.

Patient Monitoring and Care

Steps	Rationale	Reportable Conditions
		These conditions should be reported if they persist despite nursing interventions. • Hypotension or hypertension • Bradycardia or tachycardia • Ventricular or atrial dysrhythmias • Changes in breathing patterns
1. Monitor vital signs and cardiac rhythm before and after the procedure.	Patients with severe neurologic dysfunction may exhibit changes in cardiovascular and respiratory function because of involvement of the brain stem structures.	
2. Monitor neurologic status before and after the procedure.	Determines neurologic responses.	• Deterioration in neurologic responses

Documentation

Documentation should include the following:

• Patient and family education
• Date and time of testing
• Patient's baseline neurologic status and responses
• Presence of intact tympanic membrane
• Temperature and amount of irrigant

• Time between stimulus and response
• Description of extraocular movement
• Untoward responses
• Neurologic status preprocedure and postprocedure
• Additional interventions

References

1. Greenberg, M.S. (2001). *Handbook of Neurosurgery.* New York: Thieme.
2. Hickey, J. (2003). *The Clinical Practice of Neurological and Neurosurgical Nursing.* 5th ed. Philadelphia: J.B. Lippincott.
3. Serra, A., and Leigh, J. (2002). Diagnostic value of nystagmus: Spontaneous and induced ocular oscillations. *J Neurol Neurosurg & Psychiatry, 73,* 615-6.

Additional Readings

Plum, F., and Posner, J. (1983). *The Diagnosis of Stupor and Coma.* 3rd ed. Philadelphia: F.A. Davis.
Samuels, M. (1993). The evaluation of comatose patients. *Hosp Pract, 28,* 165-82.
Valli, P., et al. (2002-2003). Convection, buoyancy, or endolymph expansion: What is the actual mechanism responsible for the caloric response of semicircular canals? *J Vestibul Res, 12,* 155-65.

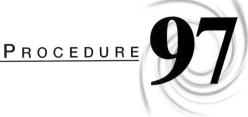

http://evolve.elsevier.com

PROCEDURE **97**

Lumbar Puncture (Perform)

PURPOSE: A lumbar puncture (LP) is performed to obtain a cerebrospinal fluid (CSF) sample, measure CSF pressure, drain CSF or to access the subarachnoid space for infusion of medications or contrast agents.[1-5]

Anne W. Wojner-Alexandrov
Marc Malkoff

PREREQUISITE NURSING KNOWLEDGE

- Knowledge of anatomy and physiology of the vertebral column, spinal meninges, and CSF circulation, including the location of the lumbar cistern
- Technical and clinical competence in performing LPs
- Knowledge of sterile technique
- The presence of meningeal irritation caused by either infectious meningitis or subarachnoid hemorrhage may promote discomfort when the patient is placed in the flexed, lateral decubitus position for the LP.
- Computed tomography (CT) or magnetic resonance imaging (MRI) supersede the routine use of LP for many diagnoses.[3,4]
- Indications for LP include the following:[1-4]
  - ❖ Suspected central nervous system infection
  - ❖ Clinical examination suggestive of subarachnoid hemorrhage accompanied by negative CT scan findings
  - ❖ Suspected Guillain-Barré syndrome
  - ❖ Suspected multiple sclerosis
  - ❖ Intrathecal administration of medications
  - ❖ Imaging procedures requiring infusion of contrast agents
  - ❖ Measurement of CSF pressure
  - ❖ CSF drainage in hydrocephalus, pseudotumor cerebri, CSF fistula

- Contraindications for LP include the following:[1-4]
  - ❖ Increased intracranial pressure with mass effect
  - ❖ Superficial skin infection localized to the site of entry
  - ❖ Bleeding diathesis (relative contraindication)
  - ❖ Platelet count less than 50,000/mm[1]
  - ❖ INR greater than 1.5
  - ❖ Patient receiving anticoagulation (e.g., heparin, warfarin)
- Normal CSF values include the following:[1-4]
  - ❖ Opening pressure 50 to 200 mm H_2O (elevated pressure, greater than 250 mm H_2O)
  - ❖ White blood cells less than 5/mm[1]
  - ❖ Glucose, 60% to 70% of serum blood glucose
  - ❖ Protein, 15 to 45 mg/dL
  - ❖ Clear, colorless appearance
  - ❖ Negative culture
- Recommended CSF tests include the following:[3,4]
  - ❖ Tube #1, Biochemistry
    - ○ Glucose
    - ○ Protein
    - ○ Protein electrophoresis (if clinically indicated)
  - ❖ Tube #2, Bacteriology
    - ○ Gram stain
    - ○ Bacterial culture
    - ○ Fungal culture (if clinically indicated); requires larger volume
    - ○ Tuberculosis culture (if clinically indicated); requires larger volume
  - ❖ Tube #3, Hematology
    - ○ Cell count
    - ○ Differential
  - ❖ Tube #4, Optional Studies as Indicated

❖ Venereal disease research laboratory (VDRL) test
❖ Oligoclonal bands
❖ Myelin protein
❖ Cytology

EQUIPMENT

• Sterile gloves, caps, masks with eye shields or goggles, and gowns
• Sterile drapes
• Sterile gauze pads
• Antiseptic solution
• Fenestrated drape
• Manometer with three-way stopcock
• Lidocaine, 1% to 2% (without epinephrine)
• 3- to 5-ml syringe
• 20-, 22-, and 25-G needles
• 20- or 22-G spinal needles
• Four numbered, capped test tubes
• Adhesive strip or sterile dressing supplies
• Specimen labels
• Laboratory forms
• Glucometer/phlebotomy equipment for serum glucose
• Many supplies are available in a lumbar tray
  Additional equipment, as needed, includes the following:
• Rolled towels or small pillows to support the patient during positioning

PATIENT AND FAMILY EDUCATION

• Explain the purpose of the LP procedure to the patient and family. ➤*Rationale:* Decreases patient and family anxiety.
• Explain the need for the patient to remain still and quiet in a lateral decubitus position with his or her head and neck flexed and knees bent up toward the chest, or sitting bent over a bed table (Fig. 97-1). ➤*Rationale:* Elicits patient cooperation during the examination; the intervertebral space widens in these positions, facilitating entry of the spinal needle into the subarachnoid space.[2,3,4]
• Explain that the procedure may produce some discomfort and that a local anesthetic agent will be injected to minimize pain. ➤*Rationale:* Prepares the patient and family for what to expect.
• Explain that the patient will need to lie flat for 1 to 4 hours after the LP. ➤*Rationale:* Minimizes postprocedural headache.[3,4]

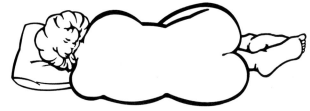

FIGURE 97-1 The lateral decubitus (fetal) position appropriate for lumbar puncture. The patient's knees are drawn up tightly to the chest, and the patient flexes the chin down to the chest. This increases the intraspinous space to facilitate needle insertion.

PATIENT ASSESSMENT AND PREPARATION

Patient Assessment

• Note pertinent patient history. ➤*Rationale:* An LP is performed to assist with the diagnosis and management of a number of neurologic disease processes (see list of indications for LP).
• Obtain a baseline neurologic assessment, including assessment for increased ICP, before performing the LP. ➤*Rationale:* Increased ICP during the LP may place the patient at risk for a downward shift in intracranial contents when the pressure is suddenly released in the lumbar subarachnoid space.[1-5]
• Assess for coagulopathies, active treatment with heparin or warfarin, local skin infections in close proximity to the site, or pertinent medication or contrast material allergies. ➤*Rationale:* Identifies potential risks for bleeding, infection, and allergic reactions.
• Assess the patient's ability to cooperate with the procedure. ➤*Rationale:* Sudden, uncontrolled movement may result in needle displacement with associated injury or need for reinsertion.
• Identify through history and clinical examination vertebral column deformities or tissue scarring that may interfere with the ability to successfully carry out the procedure. ➤*Rationale:* Scoliosis, lumbar surgery with fusion, and repeated LP procedures may interfere with successful cannulation of the subarachnoid space.[4]
• Assess for signs and symptoms of meningeal irritation, which include the following:
  ❖ Nuchal rigidity
  ❖ Photophobia
  ❖ Brudzinski's or Kernig's sign
  ❖ Fever
  ❖ Headache
  ❖ Nausea or vomiting
  ❖ Nystagmus
  ➤*Rationale:* Establishes a baseline of neurologic function before the introduction of the needle into the subarachnoid space.

Patient Preparation

• Ensure that the patient and family understand preprocedural teaching. Answer questions as they arise and reinforce information as needed. ➤*Rationale:* Evaluates and reinforces understanding of previously taught information.
• Obtain informed consent. ➤*Rationale:* Protects the rights of the patient and makes a competent decision possible for the patient; however, under emergency circumstances, time may not allow the form to be signed.
• Obtain the patient's history of allergic reactions. ➤*Rationale:* Rules out an allergy to lidocaine, the antiseptic solution, and the analgesia or sedation.
• Position the patient in the lateral decubitus position near the side of the bed, with his or her head and neck flexed and knees bent up toward the head. If difficulty is

encountered, an alternative position is to have the patient sit on the edge of the bed leaning over the bed table. Also consider performing the LP under fluoroscopy if the patient is morbidly obese or has vertebral column deformities.

➤**Rationale:** The intervertebral space widens in these positions facilitating the entry of the spinal needle into the subarachnoid space.

Procedure for Lumbar Puncture (Perform)

Steps	Rationale	Special Considerations
1. Wash hands.	Reduces the transmission of microorganisms; standard precautions.	
2. With the patient in the position for examination, identify the intervertebral spaces of L3-L4, L4-L5, and L5-S1; the L3-L4 intervertebral space is level with the iliac crests (Fig. 97-2).	The LP is performed below the level of the conus medullaris, which ends at the L1-L2. The most common site used for an LP is the L4-L5 interspace, but the L3-L4 or the L5-S1 interspace may be used when cannulation of the L4-L5 interspace is not possible.[3,4]	An imaginary line is drawn by the practitioner between the two iliac crests. Administer sedation or analgesic as needed to facilitate positioning.
3. Wash hands and don personal protective equipment.	Reduces the transmission of microorganisms; standard precautions.	
4. Set up a sterile field on the bedside stand. A. Preassemble the manometer, attaching the three-way stopcock; set to the side.	Prepares equipment for use in the procedure.	

Procedure continues on the following page

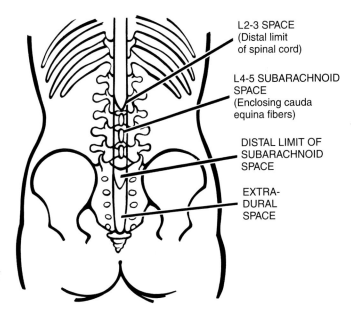

L2-3 SPACE
(Distal limit
of spinal cord)

L4-5 SUBARACHNOID
SPACE
(Enclosing cauda
equina fibers)

DISTAL LIMIT OF
SUBARACHNOID
SPACE

EXTRA-
DURAL
SPACE

FIGURE 97-2 The body of the spinal cord ends at L2-3. The region below, L4-5, encloses the cauda equina (a bundle of lumbar and sacral nerve roots) within the subarachnoid space. It is this area that is appropriate for lumbar puncture.

Procedure for Lumbar Puncture (Perform)—*Continued*		
Steps	**Rationale**	**Special Considerations**
B. Open the test tubes and place them in order of use in the tray slots.		Have the critical care nurse or assistant prepare the numbered labels for the test tubes; ensure that the tubes are labeled in the order in which they are filled to facilitate laboratory differentiation of a traumatic tap versus a subarachnoid hemorrhage.
C. Draw up approximately 3 ml of 1% lidocaine using a 20-G needle. Change to a 25-G needle for a superficial injection; change to a 22-G, 1.5-inch needle for a deeper injection.[3]		
5. Cleanse the skin over the L4-L5 puncture site, including one intervertebral space above and below the site with the antiseptic solution. Allow to air-dry; cover with a fenestrated drape.	Prepares the site for the LP; reduces incidence of infection.	
6. Administer a local anesthetic using a 25-G needle, raising a wheal in the skin. Inject a small amount into the posterior spinous region using a 22-G needle.[3]	Reduces discomfort associated with needle insertion.	
7. Insert a 22- or 20-G spinal needle through the skin into the intervertebral space of L4-L5, with the needle at an angle of 15 degrees cephalad, aiming toward the umbilicus and level with the sagittal midplane of the body.	Facilitates the passage of the needle between intervertebral spaces toward the dura mater.	If bone is encountered on needle insertion, pull back slightly, correct the angle to between 15 and 40 degrees cephalad, and reinsert. Use the interspace above (L3-L4) or below (L5-S1) the original L4-L5 insertion site, should difficulty with advancement of the needle be encountered despite correction of insertion angle.[3,4] Variations in the anatomic configuration of the vertebral column, a history of vertebral column surgery, or repeat LPs may necessitate needle insertion at a different level.
8. Once the needle has been advanced approximately 3 to 4 cm, withdraw the stylus and check the hub for CSF. If CSF is not present, replace the stylus and advance slightly. Once CSF is draining, advance the needle another 1 to 2 mm.	In most adults, a 3- to 4-cm insertion depth is sufficient to enter the subarachnoid space.	A "popping" sensation is often associated with penetration of the dura mater.
9. Attach the stopcock of the manometer to the needle. Have the patient straighten his or her legs and relax his or her position. Measure the opening pressure, and note the color of the fluid in the manometer.	Flexing the legs or straining to maintain a position may artificially elevate the CSF pressure.	Have the patient lie down on his or her side for the LP measurement.
10. Consider performing the Queckenstedt test.	The Queckenstedt test is used to assess for an obstruction of	Normal findings reflect a sharp increase in spinal subarachnoid CSF

Procedure for Lumbar Puncture (Perform)—*Continued*

Steps	Rationale	Special Considerations
A. Ask the critical care nurse to simultaneously compress the jugular veins for 10 seconds. B. Watch for a change in subarachnoid CSF pressure on the manometer.[3,4]	CSF flow in the spinal subarachnoid space; the practitioner must ensure proper placement of the spinal needle for test findings to be accurate. Test findings are often unreliable.[3]	pressure on compression of the jugular veins; on release, pressure returns to precompression levels. A lack of change in CSF pressure indicates an obstruction of CSF flow. The Queckenstedt test is contraindicated in patients with increased intracranial pressure.
11. Obtain laboratory samples: A. Position the first test tube over the stopcock port. B. Turn the stopcock and drain CSF from the manometer into the first test tube. C. Return the stopcock to the off position and discard the manometer. D. Continue filling test tubes from the hub of the spinal needle; a minimum of 1 to 2 ml CSF should be collected in the first three test tubes. The second and fourth test tubes may require up to 8 ml CSF depending on the tests ordered (e.g., fungal or tuberculosis testing).[3,4]	By draining CSF from the manometer into the test tubes, the CSF volume withdrawn is minimized.[4] Allows for progressive clearing of CSF blood in the case of a traumatic tap.[2,4,5]	In subarachnoid hemorrhage, CSF with the same consistency of blood is drained in all four test tubes. In the case of a traumatic tap, progressive clearing of bloody CSF occurs as drainage continues.
12. Cover the opening of the needle with a sterile, gloved finger. Replace the stylus and withdraw the needle.[3,4]	Prevents unnecessary CSF loss and facilitates needle withdrawal without traction on the spinal nerve roots. Reduces the contamination by microorganisms.	Minimizes postprocedural headache. If a lumbar subarachnoid catheter is inserted, refer to Procedure 91.
13. Cover the puncture site with an adhesive strip or sterile dressing.	Decreases the incidence of infection.	
14. Place the patient in a supine position immediately after the procedure.[1,2,4]	The patient's weight acts as site pressure and facilitates dural closure. Some practitioners advocate placing the patient in a prone position for 1 to 4 hours after the LP to facilitate dural closure.[3,5]	It remains unclear whether prone or supine positioning better expedites closure of the dura mater after the LP.
15. Label and send specimens to the laboratory. If there is no same-day serum glucose measurement, consider obtaining a serum glucose sample.	Obtains CSF analysis and assists with the differential. If CSF glucose is elevated, consider whether there is concomitant hyperglycemia.	
16. Discard used supplies and wash hands.	Reduces the transmission of microorganisms; standard precautions.	

Expected Outcomes

- Determination of characteristics of CSF that support establishment of diagnosis
- Recommendation for definitive treatment that promotes restoration of health or optimal functional status
- Postprocedure headache may occur in 10% to 25% of patients undergoing LP and is usually self-limiting[4]; the incidence of headache is reduced with the use of smaller-gauge spinal needles and prone positioning for 1 to 4 hours postprocedure.[3,4]
- No change in neurologic status postprocedure

Unexpected Outcomes

- In cases of supratentorial mass or severely elevated intracranial pressure, a shift in intracranial contents (brain herniation) may be promoted by the sudden decrease in pressure incurred with LP.[1-5]
- Injury of the periosteum or spinal ligaments may produce local back pain.[3,4]
- Infectious meningitis may result from improper technique that produces contamination.[1-5]
- Traumatic taps may result from inadvertently puncturing the spinal venous plexuses; usually this is a self-limiting process, but it may result in hematoma in patients with bleeding disorders.[3,4]
- Transient lower extremity pain may occur from irritation of a spinal nerve.[1-5]
- Persistent CSF leak from the puncture site is associated with nonclosure of the dura.
- Inability to obtain a CSF specimen because of practitioner skill level, patient intolerance of the procedure, pathologic blockage of CSF flow, or aberrant anatomy.

Patient Monitoring and Care

Steps	Rationale	Reportable Conditions
		These conditions should be reported if they persist despite nursing interventions. • Deterioration in neurologic status • Transient lower extremity motor or sensory changes associated with spinal nerve irritation
1. Monitor the patient's neurologic status, the patient's procedural tolerance, and the development of new onset pain or numbness in the lower extremities throughout the procedure.	Changes in neurologic status may be related to sudden intracranial decompression with brain herniation or local irritation of a spinal nerve by the needle.	
2. Monitor for postprocedural headache.	Headache occurs in 10% to 25% of patients after a LP.	• Intractable postprocedural headache
3. Monitor for drainage from the puncture site.	Persistent drainage may indicate an unresolved CSF leak.	• Drainage from the LP site • Dural tear requiring patch or closure
4. Monitor neurologic status for 24 hours after the LP.	Lower extremity motor or sensory changes may indicate a hematoma at the puncture site.	• Spinal hematoma requiring emergent surgical evacuation
5. Monitor the effectiveness of supine positioning in preventing or treating postprocedural headache.	Determines level of comfort.	• Unrelieved headache
6. Consider administration of mild analgesic agent and increasing intravenous fluid rate for the first 4 hours postprocedure or increase the patient's oral fluid intake, depending on the patient's headache severity, hydration/fluid status, existing preload indices (when available), and ability to tolerate increased intravascular volume.	Additional treatment measures may be necessary to manage postprocedural headache.	• Intractable postprocedural headache • Dural tear requiring patch or closure • Intravascular fluid volume overload or deficit

Documentation

Documentation should include the following:

- Patient and family education
- Performance of the procedure, significant findings, CSF appearance, and opening pressure
- Amount of CSF removed
- Patient tolerance of the procedure
- Change in neurologic status associated with the procedure
- CSF specimens obtained
- Unexpected outcomes
- Additional interventions

References

1. Ahyu, S.N., et al., eds. (2001). *The Washington Manual of Medical Therapeutics.* 30th ed. St. Louis: Department of Medicine, Washington University.
2. Aminoff, M.J. (2003). Nervous system. In: Tierney, L.M., McPhee, S.J., and Papadakis, M.A., eds. *Current Medical Diagnosis and Treatment.* New York: McGraw-Hill.
3. Bleck, T.P. (1999). Clinical use of neurologic diagnostic tests. In: Weiner, W.J., and Goetz, C.G., eds. *Neurology for the Non-Neurologist.* 4th ed. Philadelphia: Williams & Wilkins, 27-37.
4. Pfenninger, J.L., and Fowler, G.C. (2003). *Procedure for Primary Care Physicians.* 2nd ed. St. Louis: Mosby.
5. Pike, T.L., and Rossoll, L.W. (1995). Lumbar puncture. In: Proehl, J.A. *Emergency Nursing Procedures.* 2nd ed. Philadelphia: W.B. Saunders.

Additional Readings

Manthous, C.A., et al. (2003). Informed consent in medical procedures. *Chest,* 124, 1978-84.
Nikas, D.L. (1998). The neurologic system. In: Alspach, J.A.G., ed. *Core Curriculum for Critical Care Nursing.* 5th ed. Philadelphia: W.B. Saunders, 339-463.
Roos, K.L. (2003). Lumbar puncture. *Seminars in Neurology,* 105-14.
Scheld, W.M., Whittley, R.J., and Durach, D.T. (1997). *Infections of the Central Nervous System.* 2nd ed. New York: Raven Press.
Sudlow, C., and Warlow, C. (2003). *Epidural Blood Patching for Preventing and Treating Post-Dural Puncture Headache.* The Cochrane Library. UK: John Wiley & Sons.
Weaver, J.P., Davidson, R.I., and Tabor, U. (2003). Cerebrospinal fluid aspiration. In: Irwin, R.S., et al., eds. *Procedures and Techniques in Intensive Care Medicine.* 3rd ed. Philadelphia: Lippincott Williams & Wilkins, 187.

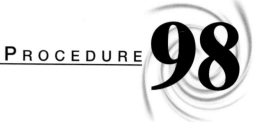

Lumbar and Cisternal Punctures (Assist)

PURPOSE: Lumbar and cisternal punctures provide access to the subarachnoid space to allow for sampling of cerebrospinal fluid, infusion of medications or contrast agents, and placement of drainage catheters.

Phyllis Dubendorf

PREREQUISITE NURSING KNOWLEDGE

- Knowledge of neuroanatomy and physiology
- A lumbar puncture (L3-L4, L4-L5) is usually performed to obtain a cerebrospinal fluid sample.
- A cisternal puncture (C1-C2) is performed if a lumbar puncture is not possible or appropriate for the patient because of positioning or anatomic restrictions.
- Indications for lumbar or cisternal puncture are as follows:
  - ❖ Cerebrospinal fluid (CSF) analysis may be indicated in the differential diagnosis of subarachnoid hemorrhage, central nervous system (CNS) infection, CNS autoimmune processes, and some CNS tumors.
  - ❖ Lumbar punctures may also be used as therapy to treat hydrocephalus due to cerebrospinal fluid fistulas and pseudotumor cerebri, to deliver medications or contrast material into the subarachnoid space, or to access the subarachnoid space for placement of a lumbar subarachnoid drain.
- Contraindications for lumbar or cisternal puncture are as follows:
  - ❖ Lumbar or cisternal punctures are contraindicated if the patient has a known or suspected intracranial mass or elevated intracranial pressure (ICP), noncommunicating hydrocephalus, infection in the region to be used for puncture, or is coagulopathic or therapeutically anticoagulated.[3] If CSF analysis is necessary, the patient may require pretreatment with fresh frozen plasma, platelets, cryoprecipitate, or the specific factor needed to correct a hematologic abnormality.[1]
  - ❖ Lumbar and cisternal punctures are *cautioned against* in patients suspected of having aneurysmal subarachnoid hemorrhage and in patients with complete spinal blocks.

In such cases, a lumbar puncture may be performed if the CT scan of the patient's head does not indicate signs of increased intracranial pressure, such as significant cerebral swelling, hematoma, intracranial tissue shifts, or herniation through dural tissues.
- The preferred positioning for a lumbar puncture is side lying with the neck flexed (see Fig. 97-1). If the lumbar puncture is not successful in this position, or if the patient cannot tolerate this position, the patient may also be positioned sitting on the side of the bed, leaning over a bedside table or stand. This procedure may also be performed under fluoroscopy for patients with marked obesity or spinal deformities. Optimal positioning is required to avoid the risk for a "dry tap," or an unsuccessful puncture attempt. Repeated attempts at puncture increase the risk for infection and patient discomfort.[6]
- The preferred positioning for a cisternal puncture is side lying with the neck flexed. Proper positioning widens the interspinous process space and facilitates the passage of the needle (Fig. 98-1).

EQUIPMENT

- Sterile gloves, caps, masks with eye shield, and gowns
- Sterile drapes
- Sterile gauze pads
- Antiseptic solution (e.g., 2% chlorhexidine-based preparation)
- Fenestrated drape
- Manometer with a three-way stopcock
- 1% to 2% lidocaine (without epinephrine)
- 3- to 5-ml syringe
- 20-, 22-, and 25-G needles
- 20- or 22-G spinal needles

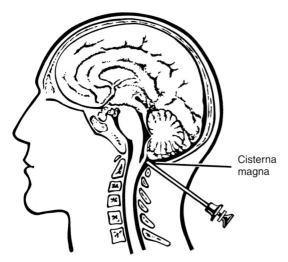

FIGURE 98-1 The cisterna magna is located at the base of the skull between the second cervical vertebra and under the posterior rim of the foramen magnum.

- Four consecutively numbered, capped test tubes
- Adhesive strip or sterile dressing supplies
- Specimen labels
- Laboratory forms
- Glucometer/phlebotomy supplies for testing concurrent serum glucose
  Additional equipment, as needed, includes the following:
- Alcohol pads or swab-sticks
- Disposable razor (for cisternal puncture)
- Two overbed tables (one for sterile field; one to position patient, if necessary)
- Rolled towels or small pillows to support the patient during positioning
- Emergency medications and resuscitative equipment (for cisternal puncture)

PATIENT AND FAMILY EDUCATION

- Explain the purpose of the procedure to the patient and family. ➤*Rationale:* Reinforces understanding of the procedure and decreases anxiety.
- Explain positioning requirements for the lumbar or cisternal puncture. ➤*Rationale:* Cooperation with positioning requirements will facilitate the procedure.
- Explain that the procedure may cause some mild discomfort; the patient will receive local anesthesia and may also receive some mild analgesia, if appropriate. ➤*Rationale:* Relieves anxiety about experiencing pain, facilitates optimal positioning, and allows the patient to verbalize concerns.
- Explain positioning restrictions required after the procedure. ➤*Rationale:* Compliance with positioning may improve patient comfort and diminish the risk for complications postprocedure.

PATIENT ASSESSMENT AND PREPARATION

Patient Assessment

- Obtain vital signs. ➤*Rationale:* Establishes baseline values for the patient.
- Perform a neurologic assessment, including mental status and motor and sensory function. ➤*Rationale:* Establishes baseline neurologic function before the insertion of a needle into the proximity of sensitive neurologic tissue.
- Assess the patient's current laboratory profile, including complete blood cell count, platelets, prothrombin time, partial thromboplastin time, bleeding time, and international normalized ratio. ➤*Rationale:* Establishes baseline values and identifies any coagulopathies that require intervention before the cisternal or lumbar puncture.
- Assess for signs and symptoms of meningeal irritation, including the following:
  - ❖ Nuchal rigidity
  - ❖ Photophobia
  - ❖ Brudzinski's sign (flexion of the knee in response to flexion of the neck)
  - ❖ Kernig's sign (pain in the hamstrings upon extension of the knee with the hip at 90-degree flexion)
  - ❖ Fever
  - ❖ Headache
  - ❖ Nausea or vomiting
  - ❖ Nystagmus
  ➤*Rationale:* Establishes baseline neurologic function before introduction of a needle into the subarachnoid space.

Patient Preparation

- Ensure that the patient and family understand preprocedural teaching. Answer questions as they arise and reinforce information as needed. ➤*Rationale:* Evaluates and reinforces understanding of previously taught information.
- Ensure that informed consent was obtained. ➤*Rationale:* Protects the rights of the patient and makes a competent decision possible for the patient; however, under emergency circumstances, time may not allow the form to be signed.
- Position patient as follows:
  - ❖ For a lumbar puncture, position the patient in a lateral decubitus position with his or her knees tightly drawn to the chest and the neck flexed or assist the patient to the edge of the bed and use the bedside table for support.[2]
  - ❖ For a cisternal puncture, position the patient comfortably in a side-lying position with the head and jaw supported or over a table with the crown of the head and jaw supported. ➤*Rationale:* Facilitates entry of the spinal needle.

Procedure for Lumbar and Cisternal Punctures (Assist)

Steps	Rationale	Special Considerations
1. Wash hands.	Reduces the transmission of microorganisms; standard precautions.	
2. Ensure that the patient is in the proper position.	Ensures spinal alignment and allows for access to the area.	The patient should be able to tolerate a side-lying position with his or her head flat. For *lumbar punctures,* to help the patient maintain this position, the nurse should place his or her arm behind the patient's head and his or her other arm around the knees. For *cisternal punctures,* to maintain this position, support the crown of the head and the jaw.
3. Administer analgesia and/or sedation as needed.	May be needed to facilitate positioning of the patient and to relieve anxiety.	
4. Wash hands and don cap, mask with eye shield, gown, and nonsterile gloves.	Reduces the transmission of microorganisms; standard precautions.	
5. Assist as needed with skin preparation using antiseptic solution (e.g., 2% chlorhexidine-based preparation).	Reduces microorganisms and helps prevent infection.	For *cisternal puncture* only, the nape of the neck must be shaved.
6. Assist in draping the area with sterile drapes.	Decreases the risk for contamination and provides a sterile field for the procedure.	Draping may be deferred during cisternal puncture so as not to obscure anatomic landmarks.
7. Assist in identifying the appropriate anatomic site for puncture.	*Lumbar punctures:* below the level of L3 to prevent damage to the spinal cord (the body of the spinal cord ends at L1-L2). *Cisternal punctures:* the skull base is used to select for puncture.	An imaginary line is drawn vertically between the iliac crests, and a second line is imagined horizontally across the spinous processes. These lines should intersect the L3-L4 area, and the puncture can be performed here or one level below at L4-L5. The second cervical vertebra is the *first* palpable spinous process. The needle is inserted slightly above this level.
8. Assist with administration of local anesthesia.	Prevents or decreases the pain from the needle insertion.	Initially, the skin is injected; then a deeper injection of anesthetic is administered to the interspinous ligament.
9. Once the needle is in place, instruct the patient to relax and breathe normally and to avoid holding his or her breath.	Increased muscle tension or intrathoracic pressure may falsely elevate CSF pressure.	Patients undergoing lumbar puncture may also straighten their legs, because leg flexion can increase intrathoracic pressure.
10. Using aseptic technique, assist in attaching the manometer to the spinal needle via a three-way stopcock.	Prepares the equipment.	
11. Obtain the CSF pressure measurement.	Readings taken at the cisternal area or with the patient in a sitting position are of little value because of altered pressure mechanics. Normal CSF pressure readings taken at the lumbar area range from 50 to 200 mm H$_2$O. The opening	The meniscus should show minimal fluctuation related to pulse and respiration.

Procedure for Lumbar and Cisternal Punctures (Assist)—*Continued*

Steps	Rationale	Special Considerations
	pressure in a traumatic tap will be within normal limits, compared with the opening pressure in patients with subarachnoid hemorrhage and meningitis.	
12. Assist in performing the Queckenstedt test, if not contraindicated, by simultaneously compressing the jugular veins for 10 seconds, while observing for a change in subarachnoid CSF pressure on the manometer.[3]	Used if an obstruction in the spinal subarachnoid space is suspected. A normal response indicates that the pathway between the skull and the lumbar needle is patent. This maneuver is **contraindicated** in patients with known or suspected elevated intracranial pressure; a sudden release of CSF pressure distally can result in herniation.	Normally there is a rapid increase in CSF pressure with resultant decrease when compression is released. If there is a complete or partial spinal block, the level will not rise, or it will rise slowly, and will remain elevated when the jugular veins are released. No increase in CSF pressure may be caused by improper needle placement.
13. Assist with the collection of CSF specimens: A. Stabilize the manometer system with one hand. B. Turn the stopcock with the other hand. C. Obtain the CSF specimen(s). D. Return the stopcock to the closed position.	Obtains needed CSF specimen(s).	Aseptic technique must be used, and care is taken to avoid rapid loss of CSF.
14. Label each tube in order of collection with the type of specimen, patient name, and the order in which the specimen was collected (e.g., "#1 of 3").	Differentiates between subarachnoid hemorrhage and traumatic tap by evaluating each numbered specimen.	Red blood cell (RBC) dissipation through consecutive samples is indicative of a traumatic tap; consistent RBC presence is indicative of a subarachnoid hemorrhage. Also, the supernatant of centrifuged CSF should be clear if the tap was traumatic and xanthrochromic if blood has been present for several hours and has undergone hemolysis.
15. Obtain a serum glucose from the patient.	Allows for comparison of the serum glucose and the CSF glucose concentration.	Hyperglycemia increases CSF glucose concentration and may interfere with the interpretation of the CSF results.
16. Apply a dressing to the puncture site once the needle is removed.	Reduces the incidence of infection.	
17. Assist the patient to a supine, flat position.	Decreases CSF pressure at the puncture site and facilitates closure of the wound.	Assist the patient to the prone position if prescribed.
18. Discard used supplies and wash hands.	Reduces the transmission of microorganisms; standard precautions.	
19. Send the specimens to the laboratory.	Ensures the specimen is sent for laboratory analysis.	

Expected Outcomes

- Lumbar or cisternal puncture completed
- CSF samples obtained
- Patient's vital signs and level of consciousness stable before, during, and after the procedure
- No headache, neck stiffness, local pain at puncture site, leg spasms, or elevated temperature related to the procedure

Unexpected Outcomes

- Significant change in vital signs, change in level of consciousness, signs of herniation (e.g., pupillary changes, bradycardia, and increased systolic blood pressure)[3]
- Inability to void spontaneously (if able to before procedure)
- CSF not obtained or unable to complete procedure
- Prolonged headache, stiff neck, and photophobia and acute increase in temperature related to the procedure
- Excessive drainage at the puncture site
- New and persistent complaints of pain, numbness, tingling, weakness, or paralysis in the lower extremities
- Cranial neuropathy[5]
- Spinal or paraspinal abscess
- Implantation of epidermal tumors
- Vasovagal syncope
- Seizure
- Pneumocephalus[4]

Patient Monitoring and Care

Steps	Rationale	Reportable Conditions
		These changes should be reported if they persist despite nursing interventions. • Respiratory depression • Motor or sensory changes • Changes in level of consciousness • Change in vital signs • Bowel or bladder dysfunction[3]
1. Monitor the patient's neurologic, respiratory, and cardiovascular status during the procedure.	Pain or abnormal sensation radiating down one or both legs may result from spinal nerve irritation, and this may necessitate a change in patient or needle position. Respiratory depression or an altered level of consciousness may result from cisternal needle proximity to the medulla.	
2. Assess vital signs and perform systematic neurologic assessments every 15 minutes for the first hour, every 30 minutes twice, then every hour for the next 4 hours, and as indicated for the following 24 hours after the procedure.	A change in vital signs or neurologic assessment could indicate acute hematoma formation, injury to a spinal nerve, infection, or herniation.	• Change in vital signs • Motor or sensory changes • Changes in level of consciousness
3. Monitor the needle puncture site.	Identifies complications at the site.	• Persistent bleeding at the site • Drainage of clear, serous fluid
4. Monitor the patient for pain or discomfort.	Identifies traumatic complications of needle placement.	• Severe, persistent back or leg pain not evident before the procedure
5. Instruct the patient to remain flat in bed for 1 to 4 hours or for the length of time prescribed. Patient may turn from side to side.	A postdural puncture headache is the most common complication after a lumbar puncture. A headache can develop within 72 hours and may last for 3-5 days.[2] Postprocedure positioning restrictions remain controversial, but a flat position is helpful in relieving the headache associated with CSF withdrawal and leakage at the puncture site.	• Headache
6. Ensure adequate oral or intravenous fluid intake.	Facilitates repletion of CSF.	• Intravascular fluid overload or deficit

Documentation

Documentation should include the following:

- Patient and family education
- Date and time of procedure
- Opening pressure
- Status of puncture site
- Specimens sent to the laboratory for analysis
- Amount and character of CSF collected
- Patient's baseline assessment and tolerance of procedure
- Any unexpected outcomes
- Additional interventions

References

1. Adams, S.C. (2000). *Neurology in Primary Care*. Philadelphia: F.A. Davis.
2. Govenar, J. (2000). Handling headache after dural puncture. *RN*, 63, 26-31.
3. Hickey, J.V. (2003*). The Clinical Practice of Neurological and Neurosurgical Nursing*. 5th ed. Philadelphia: J.B. Lippincott.
4. Kozikowski, P., and Cohen, P. (2004). Lumbar puncture associated with pneumocephalus: Report of a case. *Anesthesia & Analgesia,* 98, 524-6.
5. Nishio, I., Williams, B., and Williams, J. (2004). Diplopia: A complication of dural puncture. *Anesthesiology,* 100, 158-64.
6. Weaver, J.P., Davidson, R.I., and Tabar, V. (2003). Cerebrospinal fluid aspiration. In: Irwin, R.S., et al., eds. *Procedures and Techniques in Intensive Care Medicine*. 5th ed. Philadelphia: Lippincott Williams & Wilkins.

Additional Readings

Davis, A.E. (1998). Neurological patient assessment. In: Kinney, M.R., et al., eds. *AACN's Clinical Reference for Critical Care Nursing*. 4th ed. St. Louis: C.V. Mosby, 663-83.
Evans, R.W. (1998). Complications of lumbar puncture. *Neurol Clin,* 16, 83-105.
Roos, K. (2003). Lumbar puncture. *Seminars in Neurology,* 23, 105-14.
Safa-Tisseront, V., et al. (2001). Effectiveness of epidural blood patch in the management of post-dural puncture headache. *Anesthesiology,* 95, 334-9.
Tate, J. (2000). Eye on diagnostics. Looking at lumbar puncture in adults. *Nursing,* 30, 91.

SECTION FOURTEEN

Traction Management

External Fixation Device Insertion (Assist)

P U R P O S E :   Cervical external fixation devices or skeletal cervical traction devices (tongs) are applied to the skull to immobilize and align the cervical spine and decrease the risk of secondary spinal cord injury. Realignment and immobilization provides time for healing of fractures or supportive structures.

Joanne V. Hickey
Janis L. Namink

PREREQUISITE NURSING KNOWLEDGE

- Knowledge of neuroanatomy and physiology
- The nurse needs to be knowledgeable about the anatomy and physiology of the spine, spinal cord, and supporting ligaments and especially the special anatomy of the cervical vertebrae, the cervical spinal nerves, and innervated dermatome. In addition, the nurse must understand the pathophysiology of vertebral and spinal cord trauma, especially spinal shock, early ascending edema, and related clinical deterioration of respiratory and vasomotor tone.
- The nurse needs to be knowledgeable about the signs and symptoms of new injury or extension of spinal cord injury and the needed interventions.
- Cervical spine immobilization is instituted to stabilize the cervical vertebral column when the cervical vertebral column has become unstable as a result of vertebral fracture, vertebral dislocation, vertebral fracture-dislocation, or injury to the soft tissue ligaments that support the cervical vertebral column.[2]
- Cervical spine immobilization may be required as the definitive treatment or as part of preoperative management. An unstable cervical spinal injury may require long-term cervical traction (approximately 6 to 8 weeks) and immobility to stabilize the spine. Cervical traction may be used preoperatively to reduce a dislocation before the patient undergoes surgery. The definitive method used to treat cervical fractures depends on the injury classification, as well as physician or institutional preference.

- Tongs consist of a stainless steel body with pins attached at each end or a graphite body with titanium pins. They are used in institutions where magnetic resonance imaging (MRI) is available (Fig. 99-1).
- Cervical spine traction is provided with the use of tongs that are applied to the outer table of the skull to stabilize the cervical spine when it has become unstable as a result of cervical spinal fracture or dislocation, cervical spinal cord injury, degenerative processes of the cervical vertebrae, or spinal surgery (Fig. 99-2).
- Immobilization reduces dislocations and assists in achieving vertebral alignment. It also reduces the risk for further injury to the vertebrae, ligaments, or spinal cord in the case of an unstable vertebral column.
- There are a number of treatment options available to manage cervical injuries. The specific treatment for a particular patient depends on the type of injury, the level of injury (e.g., C2 as compared with C6), and the specific classification of the injury, as well as patient characteristics.
- Cervical tongs are available in a variety of types: Crutchfield, Gardner-Wells, and Vinke tongs and a halo ring. The shape, features, insertion site, and placement vary slightly, but the purpose, principles, and care are the same. Physician preference is an important deciding factor in choosing the specific type of cervical external fixation device to be used.
- The insertion of Crutchfield and Vinke tongs necessitates an incision to expose the skull. Two holes are made in the outer table of the skull with a twist drill, and the pins are

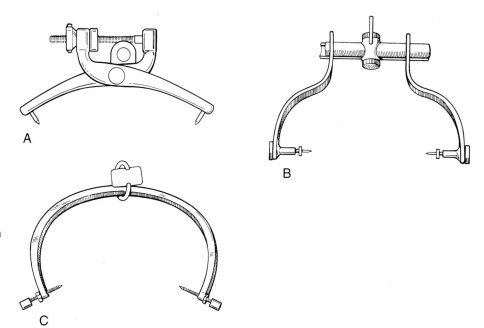

FIGURE 99-1 All three types of cervical tongs consist of a stainless steel body and a pin with a sharp tip attached to each end. **A,** Crutchfield tongs are placed about 5 inches apart in line with the long axis of the cervical spine. **B,** Vinke tongs are placed on the parietal bones, near the widest transverse diameter of the skull. **C,** Gardner-Wells tongs are inserted slightly above the patient's ears.

inserted and tightened until there is a firm fit. Gardner-Wells tongs are inserted by placing the razor-sharp pin edges to the prepared areas of the scalp and tightening the screws until the spring-loaded mechanism indicates that the correct pressure has been achieved. To decrease the possibility of tong displacement, all types of pins are well seated into the outer table of the skull and angled inward.[2]

- Cervical traction also may be applied using a halo ring device. This is a stainless steel or graphite ring that is attached to the skull by four stabilizing pins (two anterior and two posterolateral) (Fig. 99-3). The pins are threaded through holes in the ring, screwed into the outer table of the skull, and locked in place. Direct traction may be applied to the ring device with a rope and pulley system or by attaching the ring to a body vest, which allows for mobility of the patient.

EQUIPMENT

- Tongs or halo ring
- Insertion tray, including either the specific type of tongs to be used or the halo ring with insertion pins
- Local anesthetic: lidocaine 1% to 2% (with or without epinephrine, depending on the physician's preference)
- Needles (18- and 23-G)
- Sterile and nonsterile gloves
- Gowns and protective glasses
- Antiseptic solution (e.g., 2% chlorhexidine-based preparation)
- Sterile sponges
- Sterile drill and bits

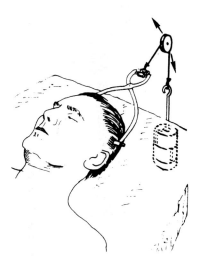

FIGURE 99-2 Continuous traction provided by weight applied to a cervical external fixation device via a rope-and-pulley system. *(From McRae, R. [1989].* Practical Fracture Treatment. *2nd ed. Edinburgh: Churchill-Livingstone.)*

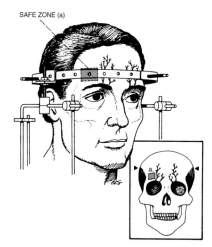

SAFE ZONE (a)

FIGURE 99-3 Placement of halo pins and ring. The anterior pins are placed anterolaterally 1 cm above the orbital ridge. This "safe zone" avoids the temporalis muscle laterally and an orbital nerve plexus and frontal sinus medially. *(From Batte, M., et al. [1989].* The halo skeletal fixator: principles of applications and maintenance. *Clin Orthop, 239, 14.)*

- Traction assembly for the bed
- Rope
- S and C hooks (to attach to the distal end of the rope for weight application)
- Weights to attach to the traction
- Torque wrench for the Halo apparatus
  Additional equipment, as needed, includes the following:
- Hair clipper or razor
- Emergency equipment

PATIENT AND FAMILY EDUCATION

- Explain the procedure and reason for cervical traction. Clarify or reinforce information as expressed by the patient or family. Discuss use of any special equipment, such as a special bed, which may be needed. ➤*Rationale:* Decreases the patient's and family's anxiety.
- Explain the patient's role in assisting with insertion of the tongs. ➤*Rationale:* Elicits patient cooperation and facilitates insertion.
- Explain that the procedure can be uncomfortable when the incisions are made but that an anesthetic will be used. ➤*Rationale:* Prepares the patient for possible discomfort and promotes cooperation.

PATIENT ASSESSMENT AND PREPARATION

Patient Assessment

- Conduct a complete neurologic assessment that includes cranial nerves, motor strength of major muscles, sensory (assess light touch and pain, noting highest dermatome level), and deep tendon (biceps, triceps, patella, and Achilles) and superficial reflexes (abdomen, anal wink). ➤*Rationale:* Provides baseline data for comparison of post-insertion assessments to determine neurologic compromise or extension of spinal cord injury.
- Assess the patient's vital signs. ➤*Rationale:* Provides baseline data for comparison of postinsertion assessments.
- Assess the patient's respiratory pattern and auscultate lung sounds. Note the use of accessory respiratory muscles and any signs or symptoms of dyspnea. ➤*Rationale:* Establishes baseline data to determine any compromise to respiratory function as a result of the procedure.
- Inspect the scalp for abrasions, lacerations, or sites of infection. ➤*Rationale:* Identifies any potential sites of infection that may contraindicate the insertion of a cervical fixation device into the infected area.
- Assess level of pain, discomfort, or anxiety. ➤*Rationale:* Establishes data for decision making regarding the need for analgesia or anxiolytics for comfort and cooperation during the insertion procedure.

Patient Preparation

- Ensure that the patient and family understand preprocedural teaching. Answer questions as they arise and reinforce information as needed. ➤*Rationale:* Evaluates and reinforces understanding of previously taught information.
- Ensure that informed consent was obtained. ➤*Rationale:* Ensures that a competent decision was made.
- Ensure that the head of the bed is flat and that the patient's head is in a neutral position by whatever approved means (e.g., hard collar, manual traction) have been instituted. ➤*Rationale:* Prevents extension of injury or spinal cord injury.

Procedure	for Assisting With Insertion of an External Fixation Device	
Steps	**Rationale**	**Special Considerations**
1. Order a bed with an orthopedic traction frame and other equipment (e.g., weights, rope, pulley system) that is attached to the bed.	Traction must be ready to reduce the potential for movement of the head and neck.	May require assistance from other departments; therefore, plan ahead to coordinate.
2. Wash hands; don nonsterile gloves, gowns, and protective glasses.	Reduces the transmission of microorganisms; standard precautions.	
3. Cleanse the potential pin sites with an antiseptic solution.	Decreases skin surface bacteria.	
4. Assist the physician with tong insertion:	Facilitates the procedure.	Because of the high risk for extension of cervical injury, this procedure usually is performed by a neurosurgeon, who can respond rapidly to extension of injury, if it occurs.
A. Assist with local anesthesia administration.	Decreases patient discomfort during pin insertion.	
B. Wash hands and don sterile gloves.	Decreases bacteria in the prepared area.	
C. Stabilize the patient's head during the procedure.	Maintains alignment of the cervical spine and provides support to the injured areas.	Cervical stabilization can be maintained with the use of a hard collar, Philadelphia collar, or other devices that prevent head rotation and neck flexion

Procedure for Assisting With Insertion of an External Fixation Device—*Continued*

Steps	Rationale	Special Considerations
		or extension. A soft collar is *not* considered a stabilizing device. Utmost care must be taken to prevent head and neck flexion or extension. Be prepared for the possibility of respiratory insufficiency, respiratory arrest, hypotension, or cardiac arrest.
5. Monitor the patient for changes in respiratory function, neurologic deterioration, and pain.	Identifies evidence of untoward effects or complications related to the procedure.	In addition to untoward effects, the patient may require additional reassurance, support, sedation, and analgesia.
6. Follow hospital policy for pin site care (e.g., apply occlusive dressings [see Procedure 101] or leave exposed to air).	Maintains asepsis.	
7. Assist with application and connection to traction as needed (see Procedure 102). A. Maintain the patient's head in a neutral position. B. Assist with application of the weights as prescribed. C. Ensure that weights are unobstructed and hanging freely.	Ensures accurate and safe use of the traction. Safeguards against extension of injury. Ensures safe use of equipment and maintains principles of traction.	
8. Discard used supplies, and wash hands.	Reduces the transmission of microorganisms; standard precautions.	

Expected Outcomes

- External fixation device inserted
- Head and neck immobilized to allow for alignment, stabilization, and healing of fractures
- Improved or stable neurologic function (motor and sensory)
- Patient discomfort minimized

Unexpected Outcomes

- Slippage of tongs, pins, or external fixation device
- Extension or deterioration of neurologic deficits or spinal cord injury
- Respiratory compromise or arrest
- Hypotensive episode
- Pain
- Bleeding at pin site

Patient Monitoring and Care

Steps	Rationale	Reportable Conditions
		These conditions should be reported if they persist despite nursing interventions.
1. Neurologic assessment every 5 minutes during the procedure, including level of consciousness, movement or intact function in arms and legs, mastication, and eyelid closure.	Facilitates early recognition of neurologic deterioration. Bitemporal tongs may interfere with these functions.	• Any deterioration or extension of baseline neurologic function (e.g., loss of more dermatomal sensation; decrease in motor strength)
2. Assessment of respiratory function (respiratory rate, pulse	Early identification of hypoxia or respiratory distress from	• Changes in respiratory function (e.g., decrease in SaO_2, increase or

Procedure continues on the following page

Patient Monitoring and Care—*Continued*

Steps	Rationale	Reportable Conditions
oximetry, lung sounds) before, during, and after the procedure.	extension of neurologic deterioration. Decrease in peripheral oxygen saturation may be an early indicator of respiratory compromise.	decrease in respiratory rate, abnormal lung sounds)
3. Provide emotional support and reassurance to the patient during the procedure.	Decreases anxiety and facilitates patient cooperation.	• Unrelieved anxiety
4. Monitor pin sites for hemostasis immediately after the procedure, every 15 minutes times four, every 30 minutes times two, and hourly, as indicated.	The scalp is vascular, and there may be continued bleeding at the pin sites that require assessment and cleansing.	• Evidence of bleeding
5. Check the security of the traction, bed frame, and bed.	The traction frame is attached to the bed and must be secure. The head of the bed may be placed on shock blocks to provide countertraction.	• Break in the integrity of the traction equipment or the bed frame
6. Maintain the patient's head flat on the bed and ensure that the bed is flat, although the head of the bed frame may be on shock blocks to provide countertraction.	The head must be flat on the bed to maintain a neutral position. Countertraction is often provided to prevent the patient from being pulled toward the top of the bed.	• Neck or head twisted or out of neutral alignment • Evidence of slippage of countertraction
7. Prepare the patient for a bedside confirmatory x-ray of the cervical spine.	An x-ray is taken to verify alignment of the cervical spine.	• Abnormal x-ray results
8. If additional weights are added or removed by the physician in an attempt to realign the cervical spine, increase the frequency of neurologic checks. Expect more frequent cervical x-rays to verify alignment.	Monitors for possible risk for secondary injury.	• Neurologic and/or respiratory deterioration

Documentation

Documentation should include the following:

- Patient and family education
- Type of cervical traction applied
- Date, time, and name of physician applying traction
- Anesthetic used
- Sedation used
- Amount of weight applied to the traction

- Ongoing comprehensive assessment data and action taken for abnormal response
- Verification of proper functioning and security of traction equipment
- Occurrence of unexpected outcomes
- Patient response to care
- Additional interventions

References

1. Berardo, L.M. (2001). Evidence-based practice for pin site care in injured children. *Orthopedic Nursing,* 20, 29-34.
2. Hickey, J.V. (2003). Vertebral and spinal cord injuries. In: Hickey, J.V., ed. *The Clinical Practice of Neurological and Neurosurgical Nursing.* 5th ed. Philadelphia: J.B. Lippincott, 430-49.

Additional Readings

Davis, A. (1998). Sensory and motor disorders. In: Kinney, M.R., et al., eds. *AACN Clinical Reference for Critical Care Nursing.* 4th ed. St. Louis: C.V. Mosby, 711.

Lee, T.T., and Green, B. (2002). Advances in the management of acute spinal cord injury. *Orththopedic Clinics of North America,* 33, 311-5.
Maher, A.B., Salmond, S.W., and Pellino, T.A. (2002). *Orthopedic Nursing.* 3rd ed. Philadelphia: W.B. Saunders, 296.
McCloskey, J.C., and Bulechek, G.M., eds. *Iowa Intervention Project: Nursing Interventions Classification (NIC).* 3rd ed. St. Louis: Mosby.
Mollabasby, A. (1997). Immobilization techniques in cervical spine injury: cervical orthoses, skeletal traction, and halo devices. *Topics Emerg Med,* 12, 3.

PROCEDURE **100**

Halo Traction Care

PURPOSE: A halo ring with or without a halo vest is designed to provide immobility to the cervical spine when the cervical spine has become unstable as a result of cervical spinal fracture or dislocation, cervical spinal cord injury, degenerative processes of the cervical vertebrae, or spinal surgery. This procedure focuses on the management of the patient who requires external cervical fixation when a halo vest and struts attached to a halo ring are used. Halo traction also decreases the risk of a secondary spinal cord injury.

Joanne V. Hickey
Joanne L. Monroig

PREREQUISITE NURSING KNOWLEDGE

- Knowledge of neuroanatomy and physiology
- The nurse needs to be knowledgeable about the anatomy and physiology of the spine, spinal cord, and supporting ligaments and especially the special anatomy of the cervical vertebrae, the cervical spinal nerves, and innervated dermatome. In addition, the nurse must understand the pathophysiology of vertebral and spinal cord trauma, especially spinal shock, early ascending edema, and related clinical deterioration of respiratory and vasomotor tone.
- The nurse needs to be knowledgeable about the signs and symptoms of new injury or extension of spinal cord injury and the needed interventions.
- There are a number of treatment options available to manage cervical injuries. The specific treatment for a particular patient depends on the type of injury, the level of injury (e.g., C2 as compared with C6), and the specific classification of the injury, as well as patient characteristics.
- Cervical spine immobility and traction are available with the aid of a number of devices. The most common types of cervical devices are Crutchfield, Gardner-Wells, and Vinke tongs and a halo ring with pins. The shape, features, insertion site, and placement vary slightly, but the purpose, principles, and care are the same. Physician preference is an important deciding factor in choosing the

specific type of cervical fixation device to be used. The halo approach is very popular because of its versatility.
- A halo ring device is a stainless steel or graphite ring that is attached to the skull by four stabilizing pins (two anterior and two posterolateral) (see Fig. 99-3). The pins are threaded through holes in the ring, screwed into the outer table of the skull, and locked in place. Direct traction may be applied to the ring device with a rope and pulley or by attaching the ring to a body vest with struts, which allows for mobility of the patient.
- After the halo ring and pins are inserted, traction can be applied by the serial addition of weights to a rope-and-pulley device attached to the ring. The physician will use serial x-rays of the cervical spine to assist in determining the optimal amount of traction (measured in pounds) needed to reduce a fracture and provide optimal alignment. Additional weight is added gradually and followed with an x-ray. Excessive traction may cause stretching of and damage to the spinal cord; **the addition of traction is managed by the physician.**
- With the halo ring and pins in place, traction can be discontinued and a halo vest and struts added for long-term immobilization of the cervical neck (Fig. 100-1). The advantage to this approach is that the patient can ambulate if he or she is neurologically intact, or his or her head can be elevated and the patient can get up to a chair.
- Patients with a halo ring, pins, and traction applied with weights are cared for similarly to patients in cervical tongs (see Procedure 99).

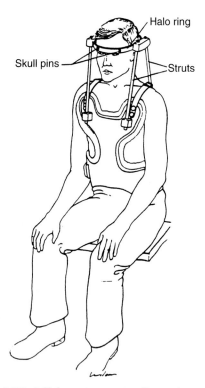

Halo ring

Skull pins

Struts

FIGURE 100-1 Halo-vest apparatus. Supportive struts and ring are attached to plastic vest, thereby applying cervical traction while allowing for patient mobility. *(From Coalbert, M.F., Kincaide, S.L. [1990]. Halo immobilization device. In: Kincaide S.L., Lohrman J., eds.* Critical Care Nursing Procedures. *Philadelphia: BC Decker, 286.)*

- The nurse must be familiar with the components of the halo-vest device, including how to access the anterior chest to administer cardiopulmonary resuscitation (CPR) in case of cardiac arrest. Refer to information from the manufacturer of the halo vest for specific information on emergency access to the chest. Some vests have "hinge" closures for quick access to the chest. If the patient is resuscitated, avoid touching the bars of the traction with the defibrillator.
- The halo-vest side panels may be opened simultaneously only when the patient is flat and supine.
- Since the halo jacket limits movement of the head, the patient must be taught to scan the environment for objects in his or her path that could lead to falls.
- The halo jacket changes the center of gravity and limits movement, thus requiring adaptations for performing ADLs.

EQUIPMENT

- Halo device (in place)
- Soap and a basin of warm water
- Wash cloth and towel
- Alcohol
- Lotion
- Nonsterile gloves
- Sheepskin liner, as needed

PATIENT AND FAMILY EDUCATION

- Explain skin care and turning and positioning procedures and the reason for cervical traction. ➤*Rationale:* Decreases the patient's and family's anxiety.
- If the patient is ambulatory, explain modifications in meeting basic needs such as bathing, toileting, eating, dressing, ambulation precautions, and safety needs. ➤*Rationale:* Develops self-care skills and awareness of special safety precautions.
- For patients who will be discharged home wearing a halo-vest device, begin a comprehensive teaching program with the patient and family. ➤*Rationale:* Prepares the patient and family for care in the home environment.
- Explain that it is unsafe to drive, ride a motorcycle, bicycle, or operate machinery while in a halo. ➤*Rationale:* Recognizes that the patient cannot turn his or her head.
- Explain that if the pins become loose, contact the physician immediately. Inform the patient and family not to adjust the pins. ➤*Rationale:* Prepares the patient and family for care in the home.

PATIENT ASSESSMENT AND PREPARATION

Patient Assessment

- Perform a complete neurologic assessment (Fig. 100-2, Fig. 100-3, Table 100-1). ➤*Rationale:* Provides baseline data.
- Obtain vital signs. ➤*Rationale:* Provides baseline data.
- Assess for difficulty with swallowing and risk for aspiration. ➤*Rationale:* Identifies a high-risk patient and the need to modify oral intake strategies.
- Assess the skin at the edges of the vest and where the vest overlaps for redness or abrasion especially over bony prominences. ➤*Rationale:* Identifies skin irritation related to the halo-vest device.
- Check the fit of the vest for tightness or looseness. ➤*Rationale:* Identifies the need for change or modification of the vest. Patient weight loss may contribute to vest looseness.
- Check the vest for loose straps, dirt, odor, or evidence of the need to repair the vest. ➤*Rationale:* The vest may need to be repaired or the liner changed.

Patient Preparation

- Ensure that the patient and family understand pre-procedural teaching. Answer questions as they arise and reinforce information as needed. ➤*Rationale:* Evaluates and reinforces understanding of previously taught information.
- Assist the patient as he or she lies supine in a neutral position with proper body alignment. ➤*Rationale:* Keeps the patient safe and accessible for inspection.
- Observe the sides and back of the vest and adjacent skin with the patient standing, if possible. ➤*Rationale:* Provides an opportunity to inspect all areas in which the skin and vest come in contact.

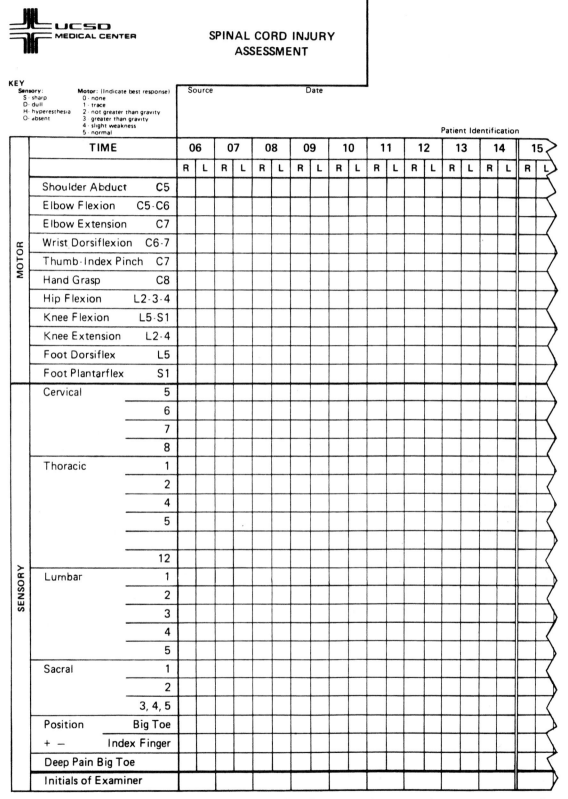

FIGURE 100-2 Sample of flow sheet documentation form for motor and sensory testing. *(From University of California-San Diego Medical Center.)*

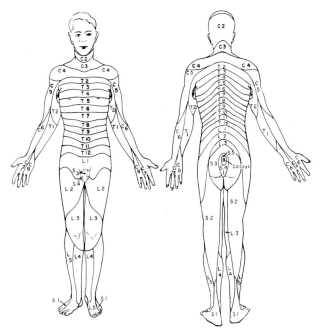

FIGURE 100-3 Sensory dermatomes: guidelines for sensory testing. *(From Barr, M.L., Kiernan, J.A. [1988].* The Human Nervous System: An Anatomical Viewpoint. *5th ed. Philadelphia: J.B. Lippincott, 81.)*

TABLE 100-1	**Assessment of Muscle Strength**
Motor Score	**Indicators**
5	Normal muscle strength; can maintain high degree of function against maximal resistance.
4	The muscle can go through its normal range of motion, but it can be overcome by increased resistance.
3	The muscle can go through its normal range of motion against gravity only; it cannot tolerate external resistance.
2	The muscle contracts weakly; it does not have sufficient strength to overcome gravity.
1	Visible or palpable muscle contractions may be seen or felt, but there is no movement in the limb.
0	Complete paralysis; no evidence of motor function.

Adapted from Hickey, J. (1997). *The Clinical Practice of Neurological and Neurosurgical Nursing.* 4th ed. Philadelphia: J.B. Lippincott.

Procedure   for Halo Traction Care

Steps	Rationale	Special Considerations
1. Wash hands.	Reduces the transmission of microorganisms; standard precautions.	
2. Maintaining alignment, position the patient on his or her side; then unbuckle one side of the halo vest while maintaining spinal alignment.	Gains access to the underlying skin.	Inadvertent rotation of the shoulders or hips may result in torsion of the spinal cord. Follow the manufacturer recommendations for unbuckling.
3. Assess the patient's skin.	Determines skin integrity.	Insensate patients may be more vulnerable to skin breakdown. The halo should fit snugly but not cause pain over pressure areas. The fit of the halo is checked daily. The sternum, ribs, scapulae, and clavicle areas are especially at high risk for skin breakdown.
4. Bathe the skin with soap and water. Alcohol may also be used.	Cleanses the skin. Alcohol does not leave a film like soap and water; it also leaves a cool clean, feeling to the skin.	Dry the skin thoroughly and avoid excessive lotion or powder, because these agents tend to mat the sheepskin liner.
5. Auscultate breath sounds.	Identifies adventitious breath sounds.	Breath sounds may be decreased at the bases in patients with poor diaphragm and intercostal muscle function.
6. Perform anterior and posterior chest physiotherapy, if indicated.	May enhance secretion maintenance and facilitate airway clearance.	There may be a slight decrease in vital capacity related to vest placement.

Procedure for Halo Traction Care—*Continued*

Steps	Rationale	Special Considerations
7. Rebuckle the vest.	Maintains cervical traction.	Ensure that the strap is secured for proper fit.
8. Turn the patient to the opposite side, keep the head of the bed flat, and repeat steps 2 through 7.	Facilitates assessment of the opposite side of the patient's body.	
9. Change the anterior sheepskin liner as needed:	Provides comfort and cleanliness and protects the skin.	Follow the hospital protocol for who changes the liner and the recommended procedure for the change. The anterior portion of the sheepskin liner may require frequent changes because of secretions or drainage from a tracheostomy or from spills while eating.
A. Don nonsterile gloves	Protects the skin from the soiled sheepskin.	
B. Place the patient supine with the head of the bed flat.	Provides support and alignment.	
C. Unbuckle both side straps of the vest.	Provides access to the sheepskin.	
D. Remove the soiled anterior sheepskin liner.		
E. Match the clean liner to the Velcro guides on the anterior vest and press it into place.	Secures the liner in place.	
F. Buckle both sides of the vest.	Maintains cervical traction.	
10. Change the posterior sheepskin liner as needed:	Promotes comfort and protects the skin.	Follow the hospital protocol as to who changes the liner and the recommended procedure for the change.
A. Don nonsterile gloves.	Protects the skin from the soiled sheepskin.	
B. Position the patient with the head of the bed flat and the patient turned to the side-lying position. Alternately, you can turn the patient prone with a pillow under the chest and a pillow under the head if patient's respiratory status tolerates this position.	Provides support and protects the skin.	
C. Unbuckle one side of the halo vest.	Provides support and alignment.	
D. Roll the soiled liner to the corresponding portion of the posterior vest and roll the remainder to the center of the vest.	Simplifies the liner change.	
E. Match half the clean liner to the corresponding portion of the posterior vest and roll the remainder to the center of the vest.	Provides comfort and protects the skin.	
F. Buckle the side strap.	Maintains cervical traction.	
G. Roll the patient to the opposite side.	Accesses the liner.	
H. Unbuckle the side strap, and remove the remainder of the soiled liner.		
I. Unroll the clean liner, and match to the corresponding Velcro strips on the vest.	Secures the liner in place.	
J. Buckle the side strap.	Maintains cervical traction.	
11. Discard supplies and wash hands.	Reduces the transmission of microorganisms; standard precautions.	

Expected Outcomes

- Cervical alignment is maintained.
- The underlying skin remains intact and free of irritation.
- The vest is functional, fits well, and is clean and odorless.
- The pin sites are clean.
- Mobility is maintained if the patient is neurologically intact.
- The patient's safety is maintained.

Unexpected Outcomes

- Slippage of the tongs, pins, or external fixation device
- Interruption of continuous traction
- Extension or deterioration of neurological deficits or spinal cord injury
- Signs and symptoms of infection (e.g., bleeding, skin breakdown, looseness of pins)
- Muscle deconditioning or orthostatic hypotension
- Skin irritation around the vest
- Respiratory distress
- Injury from fall while ambulating with a halo vest

Patient Monitoring and Care

Steps	Rationale	Reportable Conditions
		These conditions should be reported if they persist despite nursing interventions.
1. Monitor motor/sensory function every 2 to 4 hours.	Determines neurologic deterioration.	• Any deterioration or extension of baseline neurologic function (e.g., loss of more dermatomal sensation; decrease in motor strength)
2. Monitor for dyspnea, hypoxia, or decreasing tidal volumes (monitor pulse oximetry and measure tidal volumes).	Assesses for hypoxia or respiratory distress from extension of neurologic deterioration or compromised respiratory function from vest constriction. A decrease in peripheral oxygen saturation or a decrease in tidal volume may be early indicators of respiratory compromise.	• Decreased oxygen saturation • Decreased tidal volumes from baseline • Dyspnea
3. Check the fit of the vest, especially if the patient has lost or gained significant weight.	The vest may be too big if significant weight loss occurs or too small if improperly fitted originally or with weight gain.	• Inability to securely fit the vest.
4. At least once each shift, observe the skin at the edges of the vest and where the vest overlaps. Replace the vest liner if it is wet or soiled.	Promotes comfort and skin integrity.	• Skin irritation noted; the liner is wet or dirty and needs replacement. Follow the hospital protocol as to who changes the liner and the recommended procedure for the change.
5. Wash exposed skin with warm water and soap; rinse well and dry. Be careful not to wet the liner.	Maintains cleanliness of skin and protects the liner.	• If assistance is needed with liner replacement
6. Provide pin care (see Procedure 101).	Monitors pin sites and prevents infection.	• Evidence of infection
7. Check the integrity of the halo, pins, struts, and vest.	Provides for safe use of equipment and appropriate therapy.	• Any break in the integrity of the equipment
8. Move the patient and the halo vest as a unit to avoid pressure that may dislodge the pins. **Never use the struts attaching the halo to the vest for moving a patient.**	Prevents dislodgment of pins and injury.	• Evidence of dislodgment of pins or the halo

Patient Monitoring and Care—*Continued*

Steps	Rationale	Reportable Conditions
9. Support the patient with pillows when positioning the patient in the proper body alignment.	Prevents dislodgment of the halo-vest device.	• Evidence of dislodgment of the pins or halo
10. Discuss possible changes in body image related to the halo-vest device; provide emotional support.	There is a dramatic change in body image with the wearing of the halo-vest device that needs to be acknowledged.	• Maladaption to altered body image
11. Discuss safety in ambulation and fall prevention (e.g., scanning with eyes to compensate for inability to move head; walking slower).	Because of the immobilization of the head and neck, the patient is at risk for falls.	• Patients that are at high risk for falls
12. Keep the wrenches nearby in case of emergency.	Supports basic safety procedures.	• Assistance needed with use of the wrenches

Documentation

Documentation should include the following:

- Patient and family education
- Date, time, and name of the physician applying halo vest
- Skin and pin assessment
- Integrity of the vest
- Neurologic (motor/sensory assessment) and pulmonary assessment (tidal volume, pulse oximetry)

- Liner changes
- Date and time of chest physiotherapy performed
- Occurrence of unexpected outcomes
- Patient response to care
- Additional interventions

Additional Readings

Bernardo, L.M. (2001). Evidence-based practice for pin site care in injured children. *Orthopedic Nursing,* 20, 29-34.

Davis, A. (1998). Sensory and motor disorders. In: Kinney, M.R., et al., eds. *AACN Clinical Reference for Critical Care Nursing.* 4th ed. St. Louis: C.V. Mosby, 711.

Hickey, J.V. (2003). Vertebral and spinal cord injuries. In: Hickey, J.V., ed. *The Clinical Practice of Neurological and Neurosurgical Nursing.* 5th ed. Philadelphia: J.B. Lippincott, 420-34.

Maher, A.B., Salmond, S.W., and Pellino, T.A. (2002). *Orthopedic Nursing.* 3rd ed. Philadelphia: W.B. Saunders, 296.

McKenzie, L.L. (1999). In search of a standard for pin site care. *Orthopedic Nursing,* 19, 73-8.

Mollabasby, A. (1997). Immobilization techniques in cervical spine injury: Cervical orthoses, skeletal traction, and halo devices. *Topics Emerg Med,* 12, 3.

Schoen, D.H. (2000). *Adult Orthopaedic Nursing.* Philadelphia: Lippincott Williams & Wilkins, 188.

Zejdlik, C.P. (1992). Maintaining skeletal system integrity. In: Zejdlik, C.P. *Management of Spinal Cord Injury.* 2nd ed. Boston: Jones & Bartlett, 425-40.

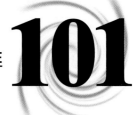

PROCEDURE 101

Tong and Halo Pin Site Care

PURPOSE: Tong and halo pin site care is provided to assess the pin insertion sites for signs and symptoms of infection, loosening, or displacement. In addition, pin care provides for removal of exudates at the pin site and for cleansing of each pin site.

Joanne V. Hickey
Jacqueline M. Davis

PREREQUISITE NURSING KNOWLEDGE

- Knowledge of neuroanatomy and physiology
- The nurse needs to be knowledgeable about the anatomy and physiology of the spine, spinal cord, and supporting ligaments and especially the special anatomy of the cervical vertebrae, the cervical spinal nerves, and innervated dermatome. In addition, the nurse must understand the pathophysiology of vertebral and spinal cord trauma, especially spinal shock, early ascending edema, and related clinical deterioration of respiratory and vasomotor tone.
- The nurse needs to be knowledgeable about the signs and symptoms of new injury or extension of spinal cord injury and the needed interventions.
- The insertion of Crutchfield and Vinke tongs necessitates an incision to expose the skull. Two holes are made in the outer table of the skull with a twist drill, and the pins are inserted and tightened until there is a firm fit. Gardener-Wells tongs are inserted by placing the razor-sharp pin edges on the prepared areas of the scalp and tightening the screws until the spring-loaded mechanism indicates that the correct pressure has been achieved. All types of pins are well seated into the outer table of the skull and angled inward to decrease the possibility of tong displacement (see Fig. 99-1).
- Cervical traction also may be applied using a halo ring device, which is a stainless steel or graphite ring attached to the skull by four stabilizing pins (two anterior and two posterolateral) (see Fig. 99-3). The pins are threaded through holes in the ring, screwed into the outer table of the skull, and locked in place.
- Once inserted, the cervical fixation device requires special care of the skin at the pin insertion site (called pin site care) to prevent infection and to monitor for it. Because the pins are inserted through the skin and into the bone, local infections can develop and proliferate and may result in cranial osteomyelitis. Tong and pin site care is essentially the same for all cervical fixation devices.
- Definitive guidelines for the specific use of solutions, use or nonuse of a dressing, and frequency of pin care have not been established and depend on institutional guidelines. A solution of hydrogen peroxide (H_2O_2) and normal saline is often used as a cleansing agent. Generally, pin sites do not require a dressing unless there is excessive drainage at the site.

EQUIPMENT

- Approximately eight cotton-tipped applicators
- Nonsterile gloves
- Approximately 60 ml cleansing solution (commonly a solution of half hydrogen peroxide and half sterile normal saline is used)
- Sterile container for cleansing solution
- Approximately 30 ml of normal saline for rinsing the pin sites after cleansing (in a sterile container)

Additional equipment, as needed, includes the following:

- Razor or hair clippers
- Dressing supplies

PATIENT AND FAMILY EDUCATION

- Explain the procedure and reason for pin care. ➻***Rationale:*** Decreases patient and family anxiety.

- Explain the patient's role in assisting with the procedure. ➤➤*Rationale:* Elicits patient cooperation and facilitates the procedure.
- Teach the family if they will be performing pin site care for the patient after discharge. ➤➤*Rationale:* Elicits family cooperation and comfort in performing the procedure.

PATIENT ASSESSMENT AND PREPARATION

Patient Assessment

- Assess the patient's scalp for signs and symptoms of skin irritation; carefully inspect the pin sites for signs and symptoms of infection (e.g., redness, edema, or drainage).

➤➤*Rationale:* Identifies skin breakdown, irritation, or pin-site infection.
- Assess the patient's level of pain, discomfort, and anxiety. ➤➤*Rationale:* Establishes comfort level and need for intervention to facilitate patient cooperation with pin care.

Patient Preparation

- Ensure that the patient and family understand preprocedural teaching. Answer questions as they arise and reinforce information as needed. ➤➤*Rationale:* Evaluates and reinforces understanding of previously taught information.
- Assist the patient to a supine position. ➤➤*Rationale:* Facilitates access to the pins for care.

Procedure for Tong and Halo Pin Site Care

Steps	Rationale	Special Considerations
1. Wash hands and don nonsterile gloves.	Reduces the transmission of microorganisms; standard precautions.	
2. Mix 1 oz of hydrogen peroxide with 1 oz of normal saline in a sterile container.	Prepares the cleansing solution for pin care.	Solutions may be kept in a covered sterile container for 24 hours. Label the date and time the solution was prepared.
3. Place 1 oz of normal saline in a second sterile container.	Prepares the solution for rinsing off the hydrogen peroxide.	
4. Cleanse the area around each pin and tong with a cotton-tipped swab and half-strength hydrogen peroxide–normal saline solution. Clean in a single sweeping motion. Gently repeat as needed with a new swab each time. Use separate swabs for each site to decrease the chance of cross-contamination.	Removes drainage, prevents excessive exudates, and cleanses the area.	Serous drainage may be present the first 2 to 3 days after insertion.
5. Rinse the site with cotton-tipped swabs and normal saline.	Removes the hydrogen peroxide and any further exudate.	Apply a dressing if excessive drainage and notify the physician.
6. Discard used supplies and wash hands.	Reduces the transmission of microorganisms; standard precautions.	

Expected Outcomes

- Pin or tong sites remain intact.
- Pin or tong sites remain free of infection.

Unexpected Outcomes

- Infection at pin or tong site that is local, extends into bone, or becomes systemic
- Loose pins
- Skin irritation or injury
- Bleeding at the pin site
- Pain at the pin site

Patient Monitoring and Care

Steps	Rationale	Reportable Conditions
		These conditions should be reported if they persist despite nursing interventions. • Evidence of infection
1. Administer pin care every 4 to 8 hours and as indicated.	Keeps pin sites clean and provides an opportunity for monitoring pin sites.	
2. Examine each pin site for evidence of bleeding, swelling, drainage, infection, or pin loosening.	Determines the presence of infection or slippage of pins.	• Evidence of bleeding, infection, or drainage; pin dislodgment
3. Obtain a sample of drainage if signs of infection are present.	Identifies presence of infectious organisms for further treatment.	• Positive culture of exudate; signs of infection
4. Monitor for pain or discomfort and treat with analgesics as prescribed.	Determines evidence of possible infection or slippage of pin.	• Unrelieved pain

Documentation

Documentation should include the following:

- Patient and family education
- Condition of skin on scalp
- Condition of skin at pin or tong sites
- Evidence of redness, drainage, or infection

- Occurrence of unexpected outcomes
- Patient response to care
- Additional interventions
- Pin site care performed

Additional Readings

Bernardo, L.M. (2001). Evidence-based practice for pin site care. *Orthopaedic Nursing, 20,* 29-34.

Davis, A. (1998). Sensory and motor disorders. In: Kinney, M.R., et al., eds. *AACN Clinical Reference for Critical Care Nursing.* 4th ed. St. Louis: C.V. Mosby, 711.

Davis, P., et al. (2001). Pin site management. Towards a consensus: part 2. *J Orthopaedic Nurs, 5,* 125-30.

Hickey, J.V. (2003). Vertebral and spinal cord injuries. In: Hickey, J.V. *The Clinical Practice of Neurological and Neurosurgical Nursing.* 5th ed. Philadelphia: J.B. Lippincott, 407-450.

Lee-Smith, J., et al. (2001). Pin site management. Towards a consensus: part 1. *J Orthopaedic Nurs, 5,* 37-42.

Maher, A.B., Salmond, S.W., and Pellino, T.A. (1998). *Orthopaedic Nursing.* 2nd ed. Philadelphia: W.B. Saunders, 296.

McKenzie, L.L. (1999). In search of a standard for pin site care. *Orthopaedic Nursing,* 73-8.

Mollabasby, A. (1997). Immobilization techniques in cervical spine injury: Cervical orthoses, skeletal traction, and halo devices. *Top Emerg Med, 12,* 3.

Schoen, D.H. (2000). *Adult Orthopaedic Nursing.* Philadelphia: Lippincott Williams & Wilkins, 188.

Zejdlick, C.P. (1992). Halo pin site care. In: *Management of Spinal Cord Injury.* New York: Jones Bartlett, 435-6.

Zejdlick, C.P. (1992). Tong site care. In: *Management of Spinal Cord Injury.* New York: Jones Bartlett, 429.

PROCEDURE **102**

Traction Maintenance

PURPOSE: Once the external cervical fixation device (tongs) is applied to the skull, the nurse cares for the patient who is immobilized on complete bed rest. Traction must be maintained on a continuous basis, often for a period of weeks, until realignment or healing is completed.

Joanne V. Hickey
Cindy Hudgens

PREREQUISITE NURSING KNOWLEDGE

- Knowledge of neuroanatomy and physiology
- The nurse needs to be knowledgeable about the anatomy and physiology of the spine, spinal cord, and supporting ligaments and especially the special anatomy of the cervical vertebrae, the cervical spinal nerves, and innervated dermatome. In addition, the nurse must understand the pathophysiology of vertebral and spinal cord trauma, especially spinal shock, early ascending edema, and related clinical deterioration of respiratory and vasomotor tone.
- The nurse needs to be knowledgeable about the signs and symptoms of new injury or extension of spinal cord injury and the needed interventions.
- After the cervical tongs are inserted, traction is applied by the serial addition of weights to a rope-and-pulley device attached to the tongs (see Fig. 99-2). The physician will use serial x-rays of the cervical spine to assist in determining the optimal amount of traction (measured in pounds) needed to reduce a fracture and provide optimal alignment. Additional weight may be added gradually, followed with an x-ray. Excessive traction may cause stretching of and damage to the spinal cord; the addition of weight to the traction is managed by the physician.[1]
- Once the cervical tongs are in place, the patient is maintained on strict bed rest. In order to facilitate turning, the patient may be placed on a special bed or turning frame (Fig. 102-1).
- The principles of traction are the foundation of managing any patient in traction. Such key points as never raising the traction weights, never disconnecting the traction, and

never allowing the traction weights to rest on the floor or other obstructing objects must be followed.

EQUIPMENT

- Cervical traction system in place (including rope, pulley system, weights)
- Pillows
Additional equipment, as needed, may include the following:
- Positioning devices
- Specialty bed (e.g., Roto-Kinetic or Stryker frame)

PATIENT AND FAMILY EDUCATION

- Explain the procedure and the reason for the traction. ➤*Rationale:* Decreases patient and family anxiety.
- Explain the patient's role in maintaining the traction. ➤*Rationale:* Elicits patient cooperation.
- Explain how the patient's basic needs will be met during the confinement to bed and the maintenance of traction. Explain any special procedures that will be instituted, such as pin care or turning. ➤*Rationale:* Reassures the patient and family that the patient will be cared for and his or her needs will be met.

PATIENT ASSESSMENT AND PREPARATION

Patient Assessment

- Conduct a complete neurologic assessment that includes cranial nerves, motor strength of the major muscles, sensory reflexes (assess light touch and pain, noting highest

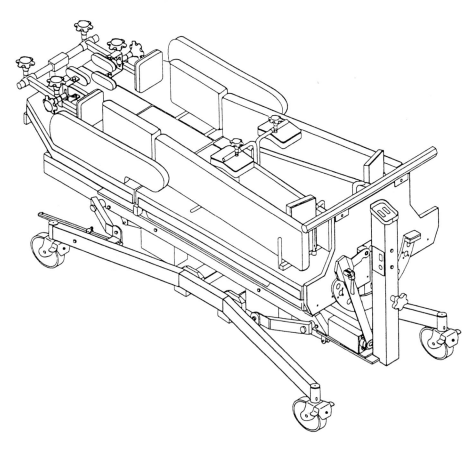

FIGURE 102-1 The Rotating Kinetic Treatment Table.® The patient is positioned and balanced on the table. The motor mechanism allows the patient to be rotated side to side, thereby displacing weight and assisting to relieve pressure areas. Cervical traction may be applied via a tension system at the head of the bed. Kinetic therapy can also facilitate pulmonary care of the patient, allowing easy access to the thoracic area for physiotherapy and coughing. (*Courtesy Kinetic Concepts Incorporated, San Antonio, Texas.*)

dermatome level), deep tendon reflexes (biceps, triceps, patellar, and Achilles), and superficial reflexes. ➤*Rationale:* Establishes database to determine any change in neurologic function.

• Assess the patient's comfort. ➤*Rationale:* Pain in the head, neck, or at the pin sites may suggest misalignment, pin site infection, or slippage of traction.

Patient Preparation

• Ensure that the patient and family understand preprocedural teaching. Answer questions as they arise and reinforce information as needed. ➤*Rationale:* Evaluates and reinforces understanding of previously taught information.

• Ensure that body alignment is maintained and that the patient is positioned in the middle of the bed. ➤*Rationale:* Facilitates comfort and even distribution of the traction.

• Check the orthopedic traction frame, knots, and pulleys for secure attachment and function. Check the ropes and weights to be sure that they are hanging freely. ➤*Rationale:* Maintains function and prevents slippage of the orthopedic equipment.

Procedure | for Traction Maintenance

Steps	Rationale	Special Considerations
1. Wash hands.	Reduces the transmission of microorganisms; standard precautions.	
2. Ensure that the orthopedic frame and traction equipment are intact.	Promotes patient safety.	
3. Maintain the weights so that they hang freely at all times.	Obstruction to free hanging of the weights will eliminate traction and could precipitate adverse neurologic responses in the patient. **Do not raise the traction at any time.**	Inform the physician immediately if there is any interruption of the traction, because a cervical radiograph may be necessary to assess cervical alignment.

Procedure for Traction Maintenance—*Continued*

Steps	Rationale	Special Considerations
4. Ensure that there are no knots in the rope that could rest on a pulley.	Could interfere with the prescriptive adequacy of the weights and traction.	
5. Maintain the patient in a straight line (centered on the bed), in a neutral position and aligned with the pulleys and ropes.	Alignment ensures optimal traction that is balanced (does not pull on one side of the body more than on the other side) and prevents traction slippage and pain.	Reposition as necessary; ensure adequate help to prevent extension of a cervical injury.
6. When turning, log-roll with at least three caregivers.	Maintains alignment.	**Begin turning only when prescribed by the physician.** Turning or moving the patient in a neutral position using a triple log-rolling technique requires coordination of turning and preplanning.
7. Use pillows and special positioning devices to maintain the patient in body alignment.	Prevents misalignment and possible extension of a cervical injury.	Do not use pillows under the patient's head; maintain the patient flat on the bed; use pillows to support alignment and maintenance of a neutral position.
8. Wash hands.	Reduces the transmission of microorganisms; standard precautions.	

Expected Outcomes

- The orthopedic traction frame and all traction equipment are secure and functional.
- Proper body alignment of the patient is maintained.
- The patient is comfortable and safe.

Unexpected Outcomes

- Slippage of tongs, pins, or external fixation device
- Interruption of continuous traction
- Extension or deterioration of neurologic deficits or spinal cord injury
- Pain

Patient Monitoring and Care

Steps	Rationale	Reportable Conditions
		These conditions should be reported if they persist despite nursing interventions.
1. Frequent neurologic assessment every 2 to 4 hours and as indicated; include cranial nerve assessment, especially mastication and eyelid closure, because bitemporal tongs may interfere with these functions.	Determines neurologic status.	- Any deterioration or extension of baseline neurologic function (e.g., loss of more dermatomal sensation; decrease in motor strength)
2. Vital signs every 2 to 4 hours and as indicated.	Determines cardiovascular stability.	- Changes in vital signs
3. Respiratory assessment (e.g., lung sounds and use of accessory muscles) every 2 to 4 hours and as indicated (Table 102-1).	Provides early identification of atelectasis, pneumonia, respiratory distress, or extension of neurologic deterioration.	- Decreased lung sounds - Increased sputum - Yellow-green sputum - Elevated temperature - Use of accessory muscles

Procedure continues on the following page

TABLE 102-1	Acute Physiologic Responses to Immobility and Spinal Cord Injury		
Body System	**Physiologic Response to Immobility**	**Physiologic Response to Spinal Cord Injury**	**Assessment Parameters**
Integumentary	Pressure → ischemia → integumentary disruption	Protective motor and sensory functions lost or impaired below the level of the lesion	Inspect bony prominences. Identify preexisting skin disruptions. Assess specific pressure areas related to traction devices and positioning.
Pulmonary	Decreased chest expansion Secretions pool CO_2 retention → respiratory acidosis	Lost or impaired neuromuscular stimulus to the diaphragm, internal and external intercostals, abdominal muscles, and accessory muscles	Observe the thorax for symmetrical chest expansion. Identify breathing patterns. Auscultate breath sounds. Respiratory parameters (NIF/FVC). Supplemental O_2 ABG/pulse oximetry Identify associated pulmonary injury.
Cardiovascular	Increased cardiac workload Thrombus formation Orthostasis	Decreased vasomotor tone Loss of sympathetic response Poor venous return Poikilothermia Spinal shock → autonomic dysreflexia	Monitor vital signs, rhythm interpretation, and hemodynamic parameters. Monitor body/skin temperature. Organ perfusion assessment: level of consciousness and urine output
Musculoskeletal	Muscle atrophy Joint immobility → contractures	Loss/impairment of voluntary motor function Flaccid → spastic paralysis	Identify level of lesion. Serial motor/sensory examinations. Assess joint mobility (flaccidity/spasticity). Identify traction and applied weights correctly.
Neurologic	Increased vasovagal/response, bradycardia, hypotension	Neurogenic shock Spinal shock	After spinal shock—assess for autonomic dysreflexia.
Gastrointestinal	Paralytic ileus	Neurogenic bowel	Monitor for absent to hypoactive bowel sounds, inability to tolerate enteral nutrition.
Genitourinary	Bladder atony	Neurogenic bladder Areflexic to eventually reflex voiding	Monitor urine output. Assess for bladder distension.

Patient Monitoring and Care—*Continued*

Steps	Rationale	Reportable Conditions
4. Cardiac assessment every 2 to 4 hours (see Table 102-1).	Provides early identification of cardiac dysrhythmias or decompensation.	• Dysrhythmias • Abnormal heart sounds • Hemodynamic instability
5. Peripheral vascular assessment every 2 to 4 hours; consider deep vein thrombosis (DVT) prophylaxis (e.g., anticoagulation and sequential compression boots).	Provides early identification of peripheral vascular insufficiency and deep vein thrombosis (DVT).	• Peripheral vascular changes • Signs of DVT
6. Gastrointestinal assessment every 4 to 8 hours; consider gastric prophylaxis.	Provides early identification of paralytic ileus and gastric distension; prevention of gastric hemorrhage.	• Abdominal distension, nausea, vomiting, decreased bowel sounds, constipation
7. Genitourinary assessment every 4 to 8 hours.	Provides early identification of urinary tract infection (UTI) and neurogenic bladder.	• Low or high output, distended bladder, signs and symptoms of UTI
8. Skin assessment every 2 to 4 hours (Tables 102-1 and 102-2).	Provides early recognition of skin breakdown.	• Evidence of skin breakdown
9. Musculoskeletal assessment every 8 hours (see Table 102-1).	Provides early recognition of musculoskeletal contractures.	• Increased spasticity or malpositioning of an extremity

TABLE 102-2 High-Risk Focus Area Skin Assessment Guide

High-Risk Skin Areas

Devices/Positions	Forehead	Occiput	Chin	Ear	Clavicle	Scapula	Shoulder	Upper Arm	Elbow	Forearm	Wrist	Thumb Webbing	Axilla	Sternum	Ribs	Iliac Crest: anterior	Iliac Crest: posterior	Sacrum	Groin	Trochanter	Thigh	Knee	Calf	Ankle	Heel	Toe	Pin Sites
Halo-vest device	✓				✓	✓	✓							✓	✓												✓
High-top sneakers																								✓	✓	✓	
Resting arm splints									✓	✓	✓	✓															
Resting foot splints																						✓	✓	✓	✓		
Rotating kinetic table		✓		✓		✓	✓		✓				✓		✓	✓	✓			✓					✓	✓	
Stryker frame: prone	✓		✓		✓	✓			✓							✓						✓				✓	
Stryker frame: supine		✓				✓			✓								✓	✓							✓		
Tenodesis splints										✓	✓	✓															
Tongs: Gardner-Wells		✓																									✓
Crutchfield		✓																									✓
Vinke		✓																									✓

Patient Monitoring and Care—*Continued*

Steps	Rationale	Reportable Conditions
10. Nutritional assessment every 8 hours.	Determines nutritional status.	• Decreased intake, poor skin turgor, intolerance of nutrition
11. Assess anxiety level, pain, and coping.	Provides early recognition of anxiety, depression, agitation, and pain.	• Anxiety, depression, agitation, pain, or other untoward responses
12. Perform pin care every 4 to 8 hours (see Procedure 101).	Monitors skin and assesses for infection.	• Evidence of infection
13. Reposition and turn, maintaining neutral body alignment every 2 hours.	Maintains skin integrity. Prevents complications of immobility.	• Impaired skin integrity
14. Respiratory management (e.g., deep breathing, suctioning, incentive spirometer, quad coughing, chest physical therapy, ventilatory management.)	Supports respiratory function and oxygenation of all body organs.	• Decreased or increased respirations • Abnormal lung sounds • Decreased oxygen saturation
15. Consider bladder and bowel programs.	Supports adequate emptying of bladder and pattern of bowel activity.	• Bladder distension • Constipation • Decrease in or absence of bowel signs
16. Perform range of motion every 2 to 4 hours and apply splints and other positioners.	Maintains intact motor function.	• Evidence of contractures, deformities, functional loss
17. Offer emotional support and other diversional therapy.	Supports patient and family through the continuum of care and keeps them actively involved.	
18. Consult support services as needed.	Support services can provide items such as prism glasses to help the patient see, read, and increase visual field.	

Documentation

Documentation should include the following:

- Patient and family education
- Ongoing comprehensive assessment data and action taken for abnormal data
- Verification of proper functioning and security of traction equipment (e.g., weights hanging freely, traction rope knot against pulley).

- Occurrence of unexpected outcomes
- Patient response to care
- Additional interventions

Reference

1. Hickey, J.V. (2003). *The Clinical Practice of Neurological and Neurosurgical Nursing.* 5th ed. Philadelphia: J.B. Lippincott, 430-33.

Additional Readings

Davis, A. (1998). Sensory and motor disorders. In: Kinney, M.R., et al., eds. *AACN Clinical Reference for Critical Care Nursing.* 4th ed. St. Louis: C.V. Mosby, 711-32.

Maher, A.B., Salmond, S.W., and Pellino, T.A. (1998). *Orthopedic Nursing.* 2nd ed. Philadelphia: W.B. Saunders, 296-350.

Mollabasby, A. (1997). Immobilization techniques in cervical spine injury: Cervical orthoses, skeletal traction, and halo devices. *Topics Emerg Med,* 12, 26-33.

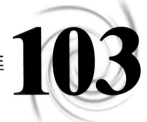
PROCEDURE

103

Epidural Catheters: Assisting With Insertion and Pain Management

P U R P O S E : An epidural catheter is used to deliver medication directly into the epidural space surrounding the spinal cord, thereby providing site-specific analgesia. Epidural pain management is used for short-term (e.g., acute, obstetric, postoperative, trauma) or long-term (e.g., chronic pain, advanced cancer pain) management.

Robyn Dealtry

PREREQUISITE NURSING KNOWLEDGE

- State boards of nursing may have detailed guidelines involving epidural analgesia. Each institution providing this therapy also has policies and guidelines pertaining to epidural therapy. The nurse should be aware of state guidelines and institution policies.
- Understanding of the principles of aseptic technique
- The epidural catheter placement and the continuing pain management of the patient should be under the supervision of an anesthesiologist, nurse anesthetist, or an acute pain service to ensure positive patient outcomes.[22,23]
- The spinal cord and brain are covered by three membranes, called *meninges:* (1) the outer layer is the dura mater; (2) the middle layer is the arachnoid, which lies just below the dura and, with the dura, forms the dural sac; (3) the inner layer, the pia mater, adheres to the surface of the spinal cord and the brain. The cerebrospinal fluid (CSF) circulates in the subarachnoid space, also called the *intrathecal space.*
- The epidural space lies between the dura mater and the bone and ligaments of the spinal canal (Fig. 103-1).
- The epidural space (potential space) contains fat, large blood vessels, connective tissue, and spinal nerve roots.
- Analgesia via an epidural catheter may be given by continuous, intermittent, or a patient-controlled epidural analgesia (PCEA) pump system.
- A variety of medication options are available, including local anesthetics, opiates, mixtures of local anesthetics and opiates, alpha$_2$-adrenergic agonists[14] and other agents

(e.g., midazolam, ketamine, and neostigmine).[15,21] All medications should be preservative-free for epidural administration.

- The pharmacology of agents given for epidural analgesia, including side effects and duration of action, should be understood.
- Knowledge of signs and symptoms of profound motor and sensory blockade or overmedication is essential. Intravenous (IV) access and immediate availability of an opioid antagonist and vasopressors are necessary.
- According to the American Pain Society,[2] the most common reason for unrelieved pain in hospitals is the failure of staff to routinely and adequately assess pain and pain relief. Many patients silently tolerate unrelieved pain if not specifically asked about it.
- The Agency for Health Care Policy and Research[1] urges health care professionals to accept the patient's self-report as "the single most reliable indicator of the existence and intensity" of pain. Behavioral observations are unreliable indicators of pain levels.
- Pain is an unpleasant sensory and emotional experience that arises from actual or potential tissue damage or is described in terms of such damage.[8] No matter how successful or how deftly conducted, surgical operations produce tissue trauma and release potent mediators of inflammation and pain.
- Pain is just one response to the trauma of surgery. In addition to the major stress of surgical trauma and pain, the substances released from injured tissue evoke "stress hormone" responses in the patient. Such responses promote breakdown of body tissue; increase metabolic rate,

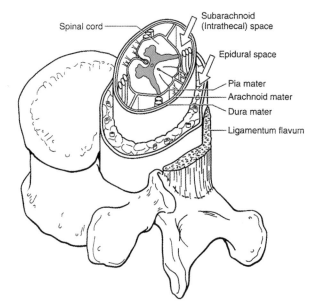

Subarachnoid (Intrathecal) space

Spinal cord

Epidural space

Pia mater
Arachnoid mater
Dura mater
Ligamentum flavum

FIGURE 103-1 Spinal anatomy. The spinal cord is a continuous structure extending from the foramen magnum to approximately the first or second lumbar vertebral interspace. *(From McCaffery, M., and Pasero, C. [1999]. Pain: Clinical Manual. St. Louis: Mosby.)*

blood clotting, and water retention; impair immune function; and trigger a "fight-or-flight" alarm reaction with autonomic features (e.g., rapid pulse) and negative emotions.[1,3,4,13]

- Pain itself may lead to shallow breathing and cough suppression in an attempt to "splint" the injured site, followed by retained pulmonary secretions and pneumonia.[11,12,13] Unrelieved pain also may delay the return of normal gastric and bowel function in the postoperative patient.[10]
- Epidural analgesia provides a number of well-documented advantages in the postoperative period with attenuation of the surgical/trauma stress response, including excellent analgesia, earlier extubation, less sedation, decreased incidence of pulmonary complications, reduction in blood loss, earlier return of bowel function, decreased deep venous thrombosis, earlier ambulation, earlier discharge from high-acuity units, and shorter hospital stays.[4,9,11,12,13,16,17,18,24]

EQUIPMENT

- One epidural catheter kit or the following supplies:
  - ◇ One 25-G × ⅝-inch (0.5 × 16 mm) injection needle
  - ◇ One 23-G × 1¼-inch (0.6 × 30 mm) injection needle
  - ◇ One 18-G × 1½-inch (1.2 × 40 mm) injection needle
  - ◇ One 5-ml Luer-Lok syringe
  - ◇ One 20-ml Luer-Lok syringe
  - ◇ One Luer-Lok loss-of-resistance syringe
  - ◇ One 18-G × 3¼-in (1.3 × 80 mm) epidural needle (pink)
  - ◇ One 0.45 × 0.85 mm epidural catheter
- One introducer stabilizing catheter guide
- One screw-cap Luer-Lok catheter
- One screw-cap Luer-Lok catheter connector

- One 0.2 μm epidural flat filter
- Topical skin antiseptic, as prescribed (e.g., 2% chlorhexidine nonalcohol-based preparation)
- Sterile towels
- Sterile forceps
- Sterile gauze 4 × 4 pads
- Sterile gloves, face masks with eye shields, sterile gowns
- 20 ml normal saline
- 5 to 10 ml local anesthetic as prescribed (e.g., 1% lidocaine) (local infiltration)
- 5 ml local anesthetic as prescribed (e.g., to establish the block)
- Test dose (e.g., 3 ml 2% lidocaine with epinephrine 1:200,000)
- Occlusive or transparent dressing to cover the epidural catheter entry site
- Tape to secure the epidural catheter to the patient's back and over the patient's shoulder
- Labels stating "Epidural only" and "Not for intravenous injection"
- Pump for administering analgesia (e.g., volumetric pump/dedicated for epidural use with rate and volume limited, which has the ability to be locked to prevent tampering and preferably is color-coded [e.g., yellow color] or a patient-controlled epidural analgesia pump)
- Dedicated epidural portless administration set
- Specific observation chart for patient monitoring of the epidural infusion
- Prescribed medication analgesics and local anesthetic medications
- Equipment for monitoring blood pressure, heart rate, and pulse oximetry

Additional equipment, as needed, includes the following:

- Ice or alcohol swabs for demonstrating block, if desired
- Emergency medications
- Respiratory equipment: oxygen mask and tubing, intubation equipment, hand-held resuscitation bag and tubing, and flow-meter

PATIENT AND FAMILY EDUCATION

- Explain the reason and purpose of the epidural catheter. If available, supply easy-to-read written information. ➤*Rationale:* Helps the patient and the family know what to expect; this may reduce anxiety.
- Explain to the patient and family that the insertion procedure can be uncomfortable but that a local anesthetic will be used to facilitate comfort. ➤*Rationale:* Promotes patient cooperation and comfort and facilitates insertion; decreases anxiety and fear.
- During therapy, instruct the patient to report side effects or changes in pain management (e.g., suboptimal analgesia, numbness of extremities, loss of motor function of extremities, acute onset of back pain, loss of bladder and bowel function, itching, and nausea and vomiting). ➤*Rationale:* Aids patient's comfort level and identifies side effects and impending serious complications.

PATIENT ASSESSMENT AND PREPARATION

Patient Assessment

- Assess the patient for local infection and generalized sepsis. ➤➤*Rationale:* Increases the risk for epidural infection (e.g., epidural abscess).[22] Septicemia and bacteremia are contraindications for epidural catheter placement.
- Assess the patient's concurrent anticoagulation therapy. ➤➤*Rationale:* Heparin (unfractionated and low-molecular-weight heparin) and heparinoids administered concurrently increase the risk for epidural hematoma and paralysis.[8,19,20] Care must be taken with insertion and removal of the epidural catheter when patients are receiving anticoagulation therapy. Anticoagulants and fibrinolytic medications may increase the risk for epidural hematoma and spinal cord damage and paralysis. If used, anticoagulants must be withheld before insertion and removal of the epidural catheter.[8,9] Removal of the epidural catheter should be directed by the physician. Nonsteroidal antiinflammatory medications (NSAIDs) do not pose an increased risk for epidural hematoma and therefore may be administered while the epidural is in progress. Assessment of sensory and motor function must be regularly performed during epidural analgesia for patients receiving anticoagulation. Special institutional guidelines must be observed.
- Obtain the patient's vital signs. ➤➤*Rationale:* Provides baseline data.
- Assess the patient's pain. ➤➤*Rationale:* Provides baseline data.

Patient Preparation

- Ensure that the patient and family understand preprocedural teaching. Answer questions as they arise and reinforce information as needed. ➤➤*Rationale:* Evaluates and reinforces understanding of previously taught information.
- Ensure that informed consent has been obtained. ➤➤*Rationale:* Protects the rights of the patient and makes a competent decision possible for the patient.
- Wash the patient's back with soap and water and open the gown in the back. ➤➤*Rationale:* Cleanses skin and allows easy access to the patient's back.

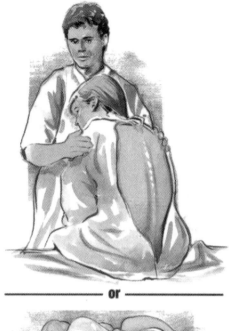
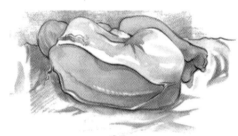

FIGURE 103-2 Patient positioning for placement of epidural catheter. *(Courtesy Astra Pharmaceuticals, London, England.)*

- Consider nothing by mouth (NPO), especially if sedation or general anesthesia are to be employed. ➤➤*Rationale:* Decreases the risk for vomiting and aspiration.
- Establish intravenous (IV) access or ensure the patency of IV lines. ➤➤*Rationale:* The need to treat hypotension or respiratory depression may occur.
- Position the patient on his or her side in the knee-chest position or have the patient sit on the edge of the bed and lean over a bedside table with a pillow for comfort (Fig. 103-2). ➤➤*Rationale:* Both positions open up the interspinous spaces, aiding in epidural catheter insertion.
- Reassure the patient. ➤➤*Rationale:* May reduce anxiety and fears.

Procedure	**for Pain Management: Epidural Catheters (Assisting With Insertion and Initiating Continuous Infusion)**	
Steps	**Rationale**	**Special Considerations**
1. Wash hands and don nonsterile gloves, gowns, and masks with eye shields.	Reduces the transmission of microorganisms and body secretions; standard precautions.	
2. Obtain the prepared epidural fluid with medication from the pharmacy as prescribed.	The medication should be prepared by aseptic technique by the pharmacy under laminar flow or prepared commercially to decrease the risk for an epidural infection.[22]	All epidural solutions are preservative-free to avoid untoward reactions.

Procedure continues on the following page

Procedure **for Pain Management: Epidural Catheters (Assisting With Insertion and Initiating Continuous Infusion)**—*Continued*

Steps	Rationale	Special Considerations
3. Connect the epidural tubing to the prepared epidural fluid with medication and prime the tubing.	Removes air from the infusion system.	
4. Ensure that the patient is in position for catheter placement (see Fig. 103-2).	Facilitates ease of insertion of the epidural catheter.	
5. Assist as needed with the antiseptic preparation of the intended insertion site.	Reduces the transmission of microorganisms into the epidural space.[22]	
6. Assist with holding the patient in position or consider sedation, if necessary.	Movement of the back may inhibit placement of the catheter.	
7. Assist the physician or advanced practice nurse as needed with the epidural catheter placement.	Facilitates catheter insertion.	
8. After the epidural catheter is inserted, assist as needed with application of an occlusive dressing.	Reduces the incidence of infection.	Use of a transparent stabilizing dressing allows for ongoing assessment of the insertion site for infection, leakage, or dislodgment.
9. Secure the epidural filter to the patient's shoulder with gauze padding.	Avoids disconnection between the epidural catheter and filter. Gauze padding prevents discomfort and skin pressure from the filter.	
10. The physician or advanced practice nurse will administer a bolus dose of medication.	Facilitates a therapeutic level of analgesia and confirms correct catheter position.	If a local anesthetic is used for the bolus, monitor the blood pressure frequently for 20 minutes, assessing for possible hypotension. Some analgesics (e.g., morphine) may take up to 1 hour to be effective.
11. Connect the prescribed medication infusion system.	Prepares the infusion system.	

12. Initiate therapy:
  A. Place the system in the epidural pump or the PCEA pump and set the rate and volume to be infused.
  B. Attach an "Epidural only" label to the epidural tubing and tape over the ports or preferably use a portless system.
 	
  C. Do not use a burette.
  D. Lock the key pad on the epidural or PCEA pump.
	No other solution or medication (e.g., antibiotic or total parenteral nutrition) should be given through the epidural catheter.
	Inadvertent intravenous administration of some epidural solutions can cause serious adverse reactions including hypotension and cardiovascular collapse.
		Responses to epidural analgesia vary individually, and epidural analgesia is tailored according to individual responses.

13. Assess the effectiveness of the analgesia. A. Determine the pain score (0-10 scale).	Excellent pain scores should be reported at rest, and very little pain should be experienced with deep breathing, coughing and movement.	

Procedure	**for Pain Management: Epidural Catheters (Assisting With Insertion and Initiating Continuous Infusion)**—*Continued*	
Steps	**Rationale**	**Special Considerations**
B. Test the level of the epidural block with ice or an alcohol swab.	The ideal epidural block should be just above and just below the surgical incision or the trauma site (see the dermatomes described in Fig. 103-3).	
14. Discard used supplies and wash hands.	Reduces the transmission of microorganisms; standard precautions.	

Procedure	**for Epidural Catheters (Bolus Dose Administration) Without a Continuous Infusion**	
Steps	**Rationale**	**Special Considerations**
1. Wash hands and don nonsterile gloves, gowns, and mask with face shield.	Reduces the transmission of microorganisms and body secretions; standard precautions.	
2. Boldly label the epidural catheter used for intermittent bolus dosing[12] (suggest color coding).[5,12]	Reduces the risk for administration of medication into intravenous lines.	

Procedure continues on the following page

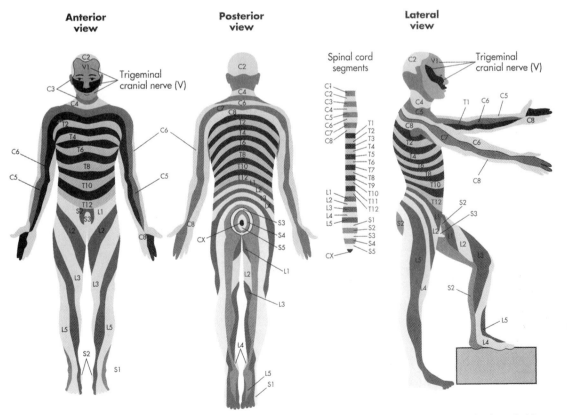

FIGURE 103-3 Dermatomes. Segmental dermatome distribution of spinal nerves to the front, back, and side of the body. *C,* cervical segments; *T,* thoracic segments; *L,* lumber segments; *S,* sacral segments; *CX,* coccygael segment. Dermatomes are specific skin surface areas innervated by a single spinal nerve or group of spinal nerves. Dermatome assessment is done to determine the level of spinal anesthesia for surgical procedures and postoperative analgesia when epidural local anesthetics are used. *(From McCaffery, M., amd Pasero, C. [1999]. Pain: Clinical Manual. St. Louis: Mosby.)*

Procedure	for Epidural Catheters (Bolus Dose Administration) Without a Continuous Infusion—*Continued*

Steps	Rationale	Special Considerations
3. Identify the correct patient and medication by utilizing the "5 rights" of medication administration.[5]	Reduces erroneous administration of medication.[5]	
4. Inform the patient of the procedure.	Prepares the patient for the quick relief of pain.	
5. Prepare the bolus dose as prescribed.	Use only preservative-free dilutant.[12]	Do not use multidose vials because this increases the risk for contamination and the risk for an epidural infection.[12]
6. Prepare and cleanse the epidural filter with an antiseptic agent.	Do not use an alcohol-based preparation. Use aqueous chlorhexidine.[12]	Preparations with alcohol are neurotoxic to the epidural space.
7. Utilize a sterile technique to administer the epidural bolus:	Administers medication.	Follow state and institution guidelines as to who is able to provide bolus doses.
A. Connect the syringe with the bolus medication to the catheter port.	Prepares for injection.	
B. Aspirate the epidural catheter. **Note:** If more than 0.5 ml of blood is aspirated, do not inject. Notify the physician.	The epidural catheter may have migrated into an epidural vessel.	
C. Administer the medication slowly. **Note:** If excessive pressure occurs, assess for kinks in the catheter and/or reposition the patient.	Some resistance will be felt because the diameter of the epidural space is small and the epidural filter will be in place.	Excessive pressure may be more pronounced if the epidural catheter is placed at the lumbar dermatome as opposed to the thoracic dermatome. If resistance continues to impair administration of a bolus dose, contact the physician.
8. Assess the effectiveness of the medication.	Pain should be relieved or decreased.	Report unrelieved or excessive pain.
9. Monitor vital signs	An epidural bolus may cause hypotension or increased sedation.	Report untoward decrease in blood pressure and sedation.
10. Discard used supplies and wash hands.	Reduces the transmission of micro-organisms; standard precautions.	

Expected Outcomes

- The epidural catheter is inserted into the epidural space.
- Pain is minimized or relieved.
- The patient experiences little or no sedation.
- The patient experiences little or no numbness and no motor loss in the limbs.

Unexpected Outcomes

- Inability to insert the epidural catheter
- Suboptimal pain relief
- Oversedation or drowsiness
- Respiratory depression or hypoxia
- Hypotension
- Motor blockade of limbs
- Sensory loss in the limbs
- Patchy block (e.g., uneven pain relief)
- Unilateral block (e.g., pain relief on one side of the body only)
- Nausea and vomiting
- Pruritus
- Urinary retention
- Accidental dural puncture into the subarachnoid space

Expected Outcomes	Unexpected Outcomes—*Continued*
	• Dural puncture headache • Epidural catheter tip migration into a vessel or adjacent structure • Redness or signs of skin breakdown at pressure area sites (e.g., sacrum, heels) • High epidural block • Total spinal blockade • Occlusion of epidural catheter • Accidental epidural catheter dislodgment • Leakage from the epidural catheter insertion site • Cracked epidural filter • Local anesthetic toxicity • Anaphylaxis • Epidural hematoma[6,7] • Epidural abscess • Nerve or spinal cord injury • Accidental connection of the epidural solution to the intravenous fluids • Cardiopulmonary arrest

Patient Monitoring and Care

Steps	Rationale	Reportable Conditions
		These conditions should be reported if they persist despite nursing interventions.
1. Assess the patient's level of sedation using a sedation scale every 1-2 hours, or more frequently if needed, during the first 12-24 hours of therapy in an opioid-naïve patient.[5,12] S = Sleeping, easily aroused; requires no action. 1 = Awake and alert; requires no action. 2 = Occasionally drowsy, easy to arouse; requires no action. 3 = Frequently drowsy, arousable, drifts off to sleep during conversation; decrease the opioid dose. 4 = Somnolent, minimal or no response to stimuli; discontinue opioid and consider use of naloxone (Narcan) (also see Fig. 105-1).	Sedation precedes opioid-related respiratory depression. A sudden change in sedation scale may indicate that the epidural catheter may have migrated into an epidural blood vessel or the intrathecal space.	• Increasing sedation and drowsiness or sudden change in sedation scale
2. Assess the patient's level of pain using a pain scale every 1-2 hours, or more frequently if needed, during the first 12-24 hours of therapy in an opioid-naïve patient.[5,12] Record the patient's subjective level of pain, using the numerical rating scale (NRS), of 0 to 10: 0 = No pain 5 = Moderate pain 10 = Worst possible pain	Describes patient response to pain therapy. A low pain score is expected both at rest and during movement. Analgesic goal is safe, steady pain control at a low level that is acceptable to the patient (e.g., less than 2/10 pain scale at rest and less than 4 during movement).	• Moderate-to-severe pain scores

Procedure continues on the following page

Patient Monitoring and Care—*Continued*

Steps	Rationale	Reportable Conditions
3. Assess respiratory rate every 1 to 2 hours and prn.	Provides data for diagnosis of respiratory depression.	• Increasing respiratory depression or sudden change in respiratory rate combined with increasing somnolence
4. Assess heart rate every 1 to 2 hours and prn.	Tachycardia may indicate a condition such as shock. Bradycardia may indicate opioid overmedication and sympathetic blockade by the local anesthetic.	• Change in heart rate • Abnormal heart rate • Abnormal cardiac rhythm

5. Assess blood pressure every 1 to 2 hours and prn. If hypotension occurs:
  A. Turn off the epidural infusion and call the physician, advanced practice nurse, or the acute pain service.
  B. Place the patient in a supine, flat position.
  C. Administer IV fluids as prescribed or according to protocol.
  D. Administer vasopressor medications as prescribed.
	Epidural solutions containing a local anesthetic may cause peripheral and venous dilation, providing a "sympathectomy." The hypotensive effect of a local anesthetic is most common when a patient's fluid status is decreased. Epidural analgesia may not be the sole cause of hypotension but may reveal hypovolemia.	• Hypotension

6. Monitor the infusion rate hourly. Ensure that the control panel is locked if using the volumetric infusor or ensure that the PCA program is locked in via key or code access.	Ensures that the medication is administered safely.	
7. Monitor oxygen saturation regularly or continuously as per institutional policy.	Assesses oxygenation.	• Oxygen saturation less than 93% or a decreasing trend in oxygenation
8. Obtain the patient's temperature every 4 hours; assess more frequently if febrile.	Increasing hyperpyrexia could signify an epidural space infection or systemic infection that is a potential risk when an epidural catheter is in place.	• Temperature greater than 101°F (38.5°C)
9. Assess the epidural catheter site every 4-8 hours and as needed.	Identifies site complications and infection. An epidural abscess is a very rare but serious complication. Patient recovery without neurologic injury depends largely on early recognition.[12]	• Redness • Tenderness or increasing diffuse back pain • Pain or paresthesia during epidural injection induration • Swelling or presence of exudate
10. Monitor urine output.	Provides data regarding urinary retention and possible early signs of epidural abscess or epidural hematoma.[12]	• Urinary incontinence • Change in bladder function • Lack of urination for greater than 6 to 8 hours
11. Monitor sensory or motor loss (e.g., leg numbness or inability to bend knees) (see Fig. 103-3).	Motor or sensory loss in the extremities may be an early warning sign of an epidural abscess or hematoma or may indicate an excessive dose of a local anesthetic. An epidural hematoma is a very rare but serious complication; if undetected, it may result in permanent paralysis.[5,12]	• Change in sensory or motor function in extremities • Sudden onset of back pain with decreasing motor weakness • Loss in bladder and bowel function (e.g., incontinence)

Patient Monitoring and Care—*Continued*

Steps	Rationale	Reportable Conditions
12. Assess for tingling around lips.	If a local anesthetic is used in the epidural solution, tingling around the lips may indicate impending local anesthetic toxicity.	• Tingling around the lips
13. Assess for tinnitus.	If a local anesthetic is used in the epidural solution, ringing in the ears can be a sign of toxicity.	• Tinnitus • Decreasing or sudden change in patient's hearing
14. Monitor and check skin integrity of sacrum and heels every 2 hours and as needed. Change patient's position as needed.	If a local anesthetic is used in the epidural solution, check for pressure points and decubitus ulceration (patient may have sensory loss in lower limbs).[5]	• Increasing redness or blistering of the skin on the sacrum or heels
15. Change the epidural catheter insertion site dressing as prescribed or if soiled, wet or loose.	Provides an opportunity to cleanse the area around the catheter and to assess for signs and symptoms of infection that may indicate early signs of an epidural abscess.	• Swelling • Site pain • Redness • Leakage of epidural solution or drainage
16. Assess for the presence of nausea or vomiting.	Antiemetics may need to be administered; the medication may need adjustment (e.g., opiates may need to be decreased or removed if nausea and vomiting is not well controlled).	• Unrelieved nausea and vomiting
17. Assess for the presence of pruritus.	Epidural opiates may cause itching. Medications such as antihistamines (may cause sedation) or other low-dose opioid antagonists may be necessary to relieve pruritus. IV ondansetron (Zofran) at the time therapy is initiated has been shown to prevent pruritus.[25]	• Itching • Redness • Rashes
18. Label the epidural pump and consider placing the epidural pump on one side of the patient's bed and all other pumps on the other side of the bed.[5]	May aid in minimizing the risk for mistaking the epidural infusion for an IV infusion system. Cardiopulmonary arrest and seizures may occur if the epidural solution is infused intravenously.	• Infusion of IV fluid into the epidural space • Infusion of epidural solution into the IV

Documentation

Documentation should include the following:

- Patient and family education
- Any difficulties in insertion
- Type of dressing used
- Confirmation of epidural catheter placement (e.g., decrease in blood pressure, demonstrable block to ice (see Fig. 103-3)
- Site assessment
- Assessment of pain, including levels of motor and sensory blockade (documented on an appropriate flow chart at regular intervals; see Fig. 103-3)
- Sedation score assessment

- Vital signs and oxygen saturation
- Epidural analgesic medication and medication concentration being infused and infusion rate per hour
- Bolus dose administration and patient response following bolus dose, including effectiveness of pain relief
- Occurrence of unexpected outcomes and/or side effects
- Nursing interventions taken
- Pump settings when programmed for PCEA
- Medication concentrations, continuous infusion rate, bolus dose, lockout interval, and 1 or 4 hour limit

References

1. Acute Pain Management Guideline Panel. (1992). *Acute Pain Management: Operative or Medical Procedures and Trauma. Clinical Practice Guidelines.* AHCPR Pub. 92-0032. Rockville, MD: Agency for Health Care Policy and Research, Public Health Service, U.S. Department of Health and Human Services.

2. American Pain Society. (1999). *Principles of Analgesic Use in the Treatment of Acute and Cancer Pain.* 4th ed. Glenview, IL: Author.

3. Barratt, S.M., et al. (2002). Multimodal analgesia and intravenous nutrition preserves total body protein following major upper gastrointestinal surgery. *Regional Anaesthesia & Pain Medicine,* 27, 15-22.

4. Beattie, W.S. (2001). Epidural analgesia reduces postoperative myocardial infarction: A meta-analysis. *Anesthesia & Analgesia,* 9, 853-8.

5. Dealtry, R. (2002). Epidural analgesia/pain management. *Hospital Based Nursing Practice Manual.* Sydney, Australia: Westmead Hospital.

6. Horlocker, T.T., and Wendel, D.J. (2000). Neurological complications of spinal and epidural anesthesia. *Regional Anesthesia & Pain Medicine,* 25, 83-9.

7. Horlocker, T.T., et al. (2003). Regional anesthesia in the anticoagulated patient: Defining the risks. *Regional Anesthesia & Pain Medicine,* May/June, 28, 172-97.

8. ISAP Subcommittee on Taxonomy. (1979). Pain terms: A list with definitions and notes on usage. *Pain,* 6, 249.

9. Jorgensen, H., et al. (2000). Epidural local anaesthetics versus opioid-based analgesic regimens on postoperative gastrointestinal paralysis, PONV, and pain after abdominal surgery. *Cochrane Database of Systemic Reviews,* (4), CD001893.

10. Kehlet, H. (1997). Multimodal approach to control postoperative pathophysiology and rehabilitation. *Brit J Anaesthesia,* 78, 606-17.

11. Kehlet, H., and Holte, K. (2001). Effect of postoperative analgesia on surgical outcome. *Brit J Anaesthesia,* 87, 62-72.

12. McCaffery, M., and Pasero, C. (1999). *Pain: Clinical Manual.* St. Louis: Mosby.

13. National Health and Medical Research Council. (1999). *Acute Pain Management: Scientific Evidence.* Canberra. Available at: www.nhmrc.health.gov.au/public/pdf/cp57.pdf.

14. Niemi, G., and Breivik, H. (2002). Epinephrine markedly improves thoracic epidural analgesia produced by a small-dose infusion of ropivacaine, fentanyl, and epinephrine after major thoracic or abdominal surgery: A randomized, double-blinded crossover study with and without epinephrine. *Anaesthesia & Analgesia,* 94, 1598-605.

15. Nishiyama, T., Yokoyama, T., and Hanaoka, K. (1998). Midazolam improves postoperative epidural analgesia with continuous infusion of local anaesthetics. *Canadian J Anaesthesia,* June, 45, 551-5.

16. Park, W.Y., Thompson, J., and Lee, K.K. (2001). Effect of epidural anesthesia and analgesia on perioperative outcome:

A randomized controlled Veterans' Administration study. *Ann Surg,* 234, 560-71.

17. Rigg, J.R.A., et al. (2002). Epidural anaesthesia and analgesia and outcome of major surgery: A randomized trial. *Lancet,* 359, 1276-82.

18. Rodgers, A., et al. (2000). Reduction of postoperative mortality and morbidity with epidural or spinal anaesthesia: Results from overview of randomised trials [Review]. *Brit Med J,* 321, 1493-7.

19. Stoll, A., and Sanchez, M. (2002). Epidural hematoma after epidural block: Implications for its use in pain management. *Surg Neurol,* April, 57, 235-40.

20. Vandermeulen, E. (1999). Is anticoagulation and central neural blockade a safe combination? *Current Opinion in Anaesthesiology,* 12, 539-42.

21. Walker, S.M., et al. (2002). Combination spinal analgesic chemotherapy: A systemic review. *Anaesthesia & Analgesia,* Sept., 95, 674-715.

22. Wang, L.P., Hauerberg, J., and Schmidt, J.F. (1999). Incidence of spinal epidural abscess after epidural analgesia. *Anaesthesiology,* 91, 1928-36.

23. Werner, M.U., et al. (2002). Does an acute pain service improve postoperative outcome? *Anesthesia & Analgesia,* 95, 1361-72.

24. Wheatley, R.G., Schug, S.A., and Watson, D. (2001). Safety and efficacy of postoperative epidural analgesia. *Brit J Anaesthesia,* 87, 47-61.

25. Yeh, H.M., et al. (2000). Prophylactic intravenous ondansetron reduces the incidence of intrathecal morphine-induced pruritus in patients undergoing cesarean delivery. *Anesthesia & Analgesia,* July, 91, 172-5.

Additional Readings

Ballanytne, J.C., and Carr, D.B. (1998). The comparative effects of postoperative analgesic therapies on pulmonary outcome: Cumulative meta-analyses of randomised, controlled trials. *Anesthesia & Analgesia,* 86, 598-612.

Ballantyne, J.C., McKenna, J.M., and Ryder, E. (2003). Epidural analgesia-experience of 5628 patients in a large teaching hospital derived through audit. *Acute Pain,* 4, 89-97.

Benedetti, J.C. (1987). Intraspinal analgesia: An historical overview. *Acta Anaesth Scand,* 31(Suppl), 85, 17-24.

Liu, S.S., et al. (1998). Patient-controlled epidural analgesia with bupivacaine and fentanyl on hospital wards: Prospective experience with 1,030 surgical patients. *Anesthesiology,* 3, 688-95.

Macintyre, P.E., and Ready, B.L. (2001). Epidural and intrathecal analgesia. In: Macintyre, P.E., and Ready, B.L., eds. *Acute Pain Management: A Practical Guide.* London: W.B. Saunders, 114-118.

McCaffery, M. (1997). Practical tips for relieving your patient's pain. *Nursing 97,* April, 42-3.

McCaffery, M., and Ferrell, B. (1997). Nurses' knowledge of pain assessment and management: How much progress have we made? *J Pain Sympt Manage,* 14, 175-88.

P R O C E D U R E **104**

Peripheral Nerve Stimulators

P U R P O S E :   Peripheral nerve stimulators are used in association with the administration of neuromuscular blocking agents to assess nerve impulse transmission at the neuromuscular junction of the skeletal muscle.

Janet G. Whetstone Foster

PREREQUISITE NURSING KNOWLEDGE

- Peripheral nerve stimulators (PNSs) are used to assess neuromuscular transmission (NMT) when neuromuscular blocking agents (NMBAs) are given to block skeletal muscle activity.
- NMBAs are given in the intensive care unit, along with sedatives and opioids, most commonly to decrease the work of breathing and facilitate mechanical ventilation in patients with severe lung injury. Neuromuscular blocking agents are also used to assist with the management of increased intracranial pressure following a head injury, severe muscle spasms associated with seizures, tetanus, and drug overdose, and for preservation of delicate reconstructive surgery.[9]
- NMBAs do not affect sensation or level of consciousness. Because NMBAs lack amnesic, sedative, and analgesic properties, sedatives and analgesics should *always* be given concurrently to minimize the patient's awareness of blocked muscle activity and discomfort; these drugs should be initiated *before* NMBAs, because neuromuscular blockade hinders the assessment of anxiety and pain.[9]
- Numerous medications such as aminoglycosides and other antibiotics, beta blockers, calcium channel blockers, diuretics, steroids, benzodiazepines, local and inhalational anesthetics, and conditions such as acidosis and various electrolyte imbalances potentiate the effects of neuromuscular blocking agents[3,14,15,16,17]; thus the level of blockade is subject to variation, necessitating vigilant monitoring with a PNS, and titration of the NMBA.
- The muscle twitch response to a small electrical stimulus delivered by the PNS corresponds to an estimated number

of nerve receptors blocked by the NMBAs and assists the clinician in the assessment and titration of the medication dosage. The level of blockade is estimated by observing the muscle twitch after stimulating the appropriate nerve with a small electrical current delivered by the PNS.
- The train-of-four (TOF) method of stimulation is most commonly used for ongoing monitoring in the critical care unit. After delivering four successive stimulating currents to a selected peripheral nerve with the PNS, in the absence of significant neuromuscular blockade, four muscle twitches follow. The four twitches signify that 75% or less of the receptors are blocked. Three twitches correspond to approximately 80% blockade, and one to two twitches in response to four stimulating currents correlate with approximately 85% to 90% blockade of the neuromuscular junction receptors.[10] One to two twitches is the recommended level of block, although the appropriate level has not yet been determined through research in the critically ill population.[9] Zero twitches may indicate that 100% of receptors are blocked, which exceeds the desired level of blockade for patients in the critical care unit (Table 104-1).
- The stimulating current is measured in milliamperes (mA). The usual range of mA required to stimulate a peripheral nerve and elicit a muscle twitch is 20 to 50 mA, although it may be necessary to increase the current to 80 mA, the highest setting on the instrument.
- Some stimulators do not indicate the mA. Instead, digital or dialed numbers ranging from 1 to 10 represent the range of mA from 20 to 80 mA. When using these instruments, the usual setting is 2 to 5, although a setting of 10 is sometimes necessary. Other stimulators (with and without digital displays) automatically adjust the voltage

TABLE 104-1 Train-of-Four Stimulation as a Correlation of Blocked Nerve Receptors

TOF (Number of Twitches)	% of Receptors Blocked (Approximately)[10]
0/4	100
1/4	90
2/4	85
3/4	80
4/4	75 or less

output relative to resistance and deliver the current accordingly.[4]

- The ulnar nerve in the wrist is recommended for testing, although the facial and the posterior tibial nerves may also be used.
- Peripheral nerve monitoring is used in conjunction with the assessment of clinical goals, and clinical decisions should never be made solely on the basis of the twitch response.
- Titration of the medication according to clinical assessment and muscle twitch response may help provide a sufficient level of blockade without overshooting the goal. Overshooting the level of blockade by using excessive doses of NMBAs is of special concern in the critically ill patient because it may predispose the patient to prolonged paralysis and muscle weakness, reported extensively in the literature.[1,9] Monitoring with a PNS during the administration of NMBAs results in the use of less medication, hastens recovery of spontaneous ventilation, and accelerates restoration of NMT,[11] which is necessary for resumption of muscle activity. Though some patients experience severe muscle weakness following neuromuscular blockade, peripheral nerve monitoring during NMBA therapy facilitates prompt recovery of NMT when therapy is terminated.[1]

EQUIPMENT

- Peripheral nerve stimulator
- Two pre-gelled electrode pads (the same as is used for electrocardiography monitoring)
- Two lead wires packaged with the peripheral nerve stimulator

Additional equipment, as needed, includes the following:

- A bipolar touch stimulator probe may be substituted for the pre-gelled electrodes and lead wires
- Scissors if needed for hair removal

PATIENT AND FAMILY EDUCATION

- Explain the purpose of peripheral nerve monitoring; for example, assessing the effect and guiding the dosage of medication. ➸***Rationale:*** May decrease anxiety.
- Describe the equipment to be used. ➸***Rationale:*** May decrease anxiety.
- Describe the experience of the stimuli as a slight prickly sensation. ➸***Rationale:*** The use of sensation descriptors is effective in reducing anxiety.
- Explain that the electrodes require periodic changing, which feels like removing a bandage. ➸***Rationale:*** May elicit decreased anxiety.

PATIENT ASSESSMENT AND PREPARATION

Patient Assessment

- Assess the patient for the best location for electrode placement. Consider criteria such as edema, hair, diaphoresis, wounds, dressings, and arterial and venous catheters. ➸***Rationale:*** Improves conduction of stimulating current through dermal tissue.
- Assess the patient for a history or the presence of hemiplegia, hemiparesis, or peripheral neuropathy. ➸***Rationale:*** Motor response to nerve stimulation of the affected limb may be diminished; receptors may be resistant to NMBAs and lead to excess doses.[4,8]
- Assess whether burns are present or whether topical ointments are being used. ➸***Rationale:*** In patients with burns or topical ointments, for whom electrode adherence is difficult, a bipolar touch probe may be more effective than the electrode pads and lead wires. Poor electrode adherence interferes with the conduction of the stimulating current.

Patient Preparation

- Ensure that the patient and family understand preprocedural teaching. Answer questions as they arise and reinforce information as needed. ➸***Rationale:*** Evaluates and reinforces understanding of previously taught information.
- Clip hair at the electrode placement sites if necessary. ➸***Rationale:*** Improves electrode contact, which facilitates current flow to the nerve.
- Whenever possible, apply the electrodes and test the TOF response to determine the adequacy of the location prior to initiating a NMBA. ➸***Rationale:*** Improves the reliability of the interpretation of the TOF response. May not be possible if the initiation of the NMBA is emergent.
- Whenever possible, determine the supramaximal stimulation (SMS) level prior to initiating NMBAs. The SMS is the level at which additional stimulating current elicits no further increase in the intensity of the four twitches. ➸***Rationale:*** Helps establish adequate stimulating current; improves reliability of testing. May not be possible if the initiation of the NMBA is emergent.

Procedure for Peripheral Nerve Stimulators

Steps	Rationale	Special Considerations
Testing the Ulnar Nerve		
1. Wash hands.	Reduces the transmission of microorganisms; standard precautions.	
2. Extend the arm, palm up, in a relaxed position (Fig. 104-1).	The ulnar nerve is superficial and easy to locate.	
3. Apply two pre-gelled electrodes over the path of the ulnar nerve (see Fig. 104-1). Place the distal electrode on the skin at the flexor crease on the ulnar surface of the wrist, as close to the nerve as possible. Place the second electrode approximately 1 to 2 cm proximal to the first, parallel to the flexor carpi ulnaris tendon. *(Level II: Theory-based, no research data to support recommendations; recommendations from expert consensus group may exist.)*	Enables stimulation of the ulnar nerve. Skin resistance causes the greatest impediment to current flow, which can be reduced through clean, dry skin and secure electrodes.[4] The electrode gel enhances conduction. Maintaining the electrodes as close as possible in alignment with the nerve minimizes artifact from direct muscle stimulation.[3]	Ensure that the patient's wrist is clean and dry.
4. Use caution in selecting the site of the electrode placement in order to avoid direct stimulation of the muscle rather than the nerve.	Direct muscle stimulation elicits a response similar to the TOF, making it difficult to evaluate blocked nerve impulse transmission.	In patients with hemiplegia, place the electrodes on the unaffected limb because resistance to NMBAs on the affected side may lead to excess doses.[4,8] In patients with limbs immobilized due to orthopedic casts, use the unaffected limb because possible resistance to some NMBAs on the affected limb may lead to excess doses.[6]

Procedure continues on the following page

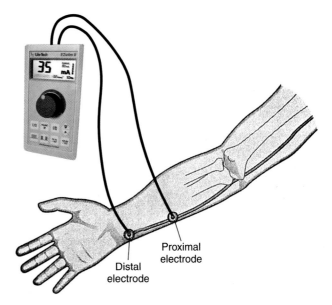

FIGURE 104-1 Placement of electrodes along the ulnar nerve.

Procedure for Peripheral Nerve Stimulators—*Continued*

Steps	Rationale	Special Considerations
5. Plug in the lead wires to the nerve stimulator, matching the negative (black) and positive (red) leads to the black and red connection sites.	Necessary for the conduction of electrical current.	
6. Attach the lead wires to the electrodes. Connect the negative (black) lead to the distal electrode over the crease in the palmer aspect of the wrist. Connect the positive (red) lead to the proximal electrode.	Prepares the equipment.	
7. Turn on the PNS and select a low mA (10 to 20 mA is typical).	Excessive current results in overstimulation and can cause repetitive nerve firing.	Patients with diabetes mellitus may require higher stimulating current than nondiabetic patients because of impaired motor nerve fibers and nerve endings.[12]
8. Depress the TOF key and through visual and tactile assessment, determine twitching of the thumb, and count the number of twitches. Do not count finger movements, only the thumb.	Finger movements result from direct muscle stimulation. The quality of the twitches may be subtle and decrease in amplitude with increasing edema; detection using both visual and tactile methods increases sensitivity and accuracy.	Placing the operator's hand over the fingers helps reduce interpretation of artifactual movement. Use the dominant hand for tactile assessment since it may more accurately detect the TOF response.[13]
9. Maintain a consistent mA current with each stimulation.	Increases reliability and validity in the quality of the twitch response.	
10. Discard used supplies and wash hands.	Reduces the transmission of microorganisms; standard precautions.	
Testing the Facial Nerve		
1. Place one electrode on the face at the outer canthus of the eye and the second electrode approximately 2 cm below, parallel with the tragus of the ear (Fig. 104-2).	Stimulates the facial nerve. Maintaining the electrodes as close as possible in alignment with the nerve minimizes artifact from direct muscle stimulation.[3]	Ensure that the patient's face is clean and dry. When wounds, edema, invasive lines, and other factors interfere with ulnar nerve testing, the facial

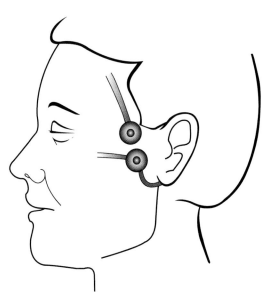

FIGURE 104-2 Placement of electrodes along the facial nerve.

Procedure for Peripheral Nerve Stimulators—*Continued*

Steps	Rationale	Special Considerations
		or posterior tibial nerves may be substituted. The risk for direct muscle stimulation is greater, however, with resulting underestimation of blockade. Also, the alternate nerves correlate less well with blockade of the diaphragm.[10,6]
2. Plug the lead wires into the nerve stimulator, matching the black and red leads to the black and red connection sites.	Necessary for conduction of the electrical current.	
3. Attach the lead wires to the electrodes. Connect the negative (black) lead to the distal electrode at the tragus of the ear. Connect the positive (red) lead to the proximal electrode at the outer canthus of the eye.	Prepares the equipment.	
4. Turn on the PNS and select a low mA (10 to 20 mA is typical).	Excessive current results in overstimulation and can cause repetitive nerve firing.	
5. Depress the TOF key and through visual and tactile assessment, determine twitching of the muscle above the eyebrow and count the number of twitches.	Determines the neuromuscular blockade at the junction between a branch of the facial nerve and orbicularis muscle.	
6. Discard used supplies and wash hands.	Reduces the transmission of microorganisms; standard precautions.	
Testing the Posterior Tibial Nerve		
1. Place one electrode approximately 2 cm posterior to the medial malleolus in the foot (Fig. 104-3).	Stimulates the posterior tibial nerve. Maintaining the electrodes as close as possible in alignment with the nerve minimizes artifact from direct muscle stimulation.[3]	Ensure that the patient's foot is clean and dry.
2. Place the second electrode approximately 2 cm above the first (see Fig. 104-3).		

Procedure continues on the following page

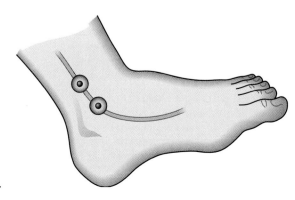

FIGURE 104-3 Placement of electrodes along the posterior tibial nerve.

Procedure for Peripheral Nerve Stimulators—*Continued*

Steps	Rationale	Special Considerations
3. Plug the lead wires into the nerve stimulator, matching the black and red leads to the black and red connection sites.	Necessary for conduction of the electrical current.	
4. Attach the lead wires to the electrodes. Connect the negative (black) lead to the distal electrode 2 cm posterior to the medial malleolus in the foot. Connect the positive (red) lead to the proximal electrode 2 cm above the medial malleolus.	Prepares the equipment.	
5. Turn on the PNS and select a low mA (10 to 20 mA is typical).	Excessive current results in overstimulation and can cause repetitive nerve firing.	
6. Depress the TOF key and observe the plantar flexion of the great toe, counting the number of twitches.	Determines the neuromuscular blockade at the junction between the posterior tibial nerve and the flexor hallucis brevis muscle.	
7. Discard used supplies and wash hands.	Reduces the transmission of microorganisms; standard precautions.	

Determine the Supramaximal Stimulation (SMS)

Steps	Rationale	Special Considerations
1. Increase the mA in increments of 10 until four twitches are observed.		
2. Note the amount of mA that corresponds to four vigorous twitches. Administer one to two more TOF stimuli.	If there is no increase in intensity of the muscle twitch when the mA is increased, the SMS is the level at which four vigorous twitches were observed.	For example, if a strong response is observed at 30 mA, raise the current to 40 mA. If there is no increase in intensity of the twitch, the SMS is 30 mA. If there is an increase, raise the mA to 50. If there is an additional increase in twitch intensity, raise it to 60. If the intensity shows no further increase, the SMS is 50 mA.

Determine the TOF Response During NMBA Infusion

Steps	Rationale	Special Considerations
1. Retest the TOF 10 to 15 minutes after a bolus dose and/or continuous infusion of NMBA is given/initiated/changed.	Evaluates the level of blockade provided.	Always assess electrode condition and placement before testing.
2. If more than one or two twitches occur and neuromuscular blockade is unsatisfactory for clinical goals, increase the infusion rate as prescribed or according to hospital protocol and retest in 10 to 15 minutes.	Signifies that less than 85% to 90% of receptors are blocked.	
3. Retest every 4 to 8 hours after clinically stable and a satisfactory level of blockade is achieved.	Evaluates the level of blockade and avoids under- and overestimation of blockade.	

Procedure for **Peripheral Nerve Stimulators**—*Continued*

Steps	Rationale	Special Considerations

Troubleshooting When There are Zero Twitches

Steps	Rationale	Special Considerations
1. Change the electrodes and ensure that the patient's skin is clean and dry.	Drying of the gel or poor contact due to moisture or soiling compromises conduction.	
2. Check the lead connections and the PNS for mechanical failure and change the battery if needed.	One of the most common causes of PNS malfunction is low battery voltage.[2]	
3. Increase the stimulating current.	The current may be inadequate to stimulate the nerve, especially for increasingly edematous patients.	
4. Retest another nerve (the other ulnar nerve or facial or posterior tibial nerves).	Avoids overestimating the level of blockade with false zero twitch responses.	
5. If there are no other explanations for a zero response, check the NMBA infusion for the rate, dose, and concentration. Reduce the infusion rate of the NMBA as prescribed or according to hospital protocol.	Excessive neuromuscular blockade produces absence of a twitch response and, if allowed to persist, may contribute to prolonged paralysis and/or severe weakness.	

Expected Outcomes

- Slight discomfort is experienced during the TOF test.
- The muscles of the thumb twitch, rather than the fingers, when the ulnar nerve is stimulated.
- The twitch response approximates the number of blocked peripheral nerve receptors; for example, four twitches before initiating the NMBA infusion and one to two twitches when a desired level of blockade is achieved.
- The NMBA dosage is titrated according to the TOF test and clinical goals.
- Resumption of four twitches occurs within 2 hours when the NMBA is discontinued.[10]

Unexpected Outcomes

- Moderate to severe discomfort from the TOF test
- Impaired skin integrity when the electrodes are removed.
- The fingers twitch when the ulnar nerve is stimulated as a result of artifact. If the thumb does not twitch, this signifies direct muscle rather than ulnar nerve stimulation.
- Resumption of four twitches does not occur within 2 hours of discontinuation of NMBA.[10]

Patient Monitoring and Care

Steps	Rationale	Reportable Conditions
		These conditions should be reported if they persist despite nursing interventions.
1. Cleanse and thoroughly dry the skin before applying electrodes.	Improves the electrode adherence.	
2. Change the electrodes whenever they are loose or when the gel becomes dry.	Optimizes conduction of the stimulating current.	
3. Select the most accessible site with the smallest degree of edema and hair and with no wounds, catheters, or dressings that would impede accurate electrode placement over the selected nerve.	Facilitates ease in testing, electrode adherence, and the conduction of current.	

Procedure continues on the following page

Patient Monitoring and Care—*Continued*

Steps	Rationale	Reportable Conditions
4. Never use the "Single Twitch," "Tetany," or "Double Burst" settings if available on the PNS.	These methods are less accurate and may cause extreme discomfort.[10]	
5. Assess the patient's oxygenation and ventilation, neurologic function, and tissue perfusion prior to increasing the rate of the NMBA infusion.	The patient may demonstrate subtle movement of the extremities with an acceptable TOF response. Clinical decisions should never be made solely on the TOF test results.	• Excessive patient movement despite acceptable TOF • Change in vital signs • Decreased oxygenation (e.g., measured via arterial blood gas or pulse oximetry) • Change in neurologic function
6. Extreme caution must be exercised to prevent the PNS lead wires from contacting an external pacing catheter or pacing lead wires.	Direct electrical current can be conducted from the PNS through the pacing wires to the heart.	• Cardiac dysrhythmias or change in patient condition
7. Perform the TOF testing every 4 to 8 hours during NMBA infusion after the patient is clinically stable and a satisfactory level of neuromuscular blockade is achieved.	Determines an effective dose of NMBA.	• Abnormal TOF results
8. Consider objective methods of sedation monitoring, such as bispectral index monitoring (see Procedure 86) or evoked potentials, during NMBA therapy.[5]	Muscle paralysis during therapy with NMBAs hinders sedation assessment with subjective instruments.	

Documentation

Documentation should include the following:

- Patient and family education
- The time, baseline SMS mA, most recent mA, TOF twitch response, and the nerve site tested
- The TOF response as 0/4, 1/4, 2/4, 3/4, or 4/4
- Dosage of NMBA

- Assessment data (e.g., neurologic, pulmonary, cardiovascular)
- Unexpected outcomes
- Troubleshooting attempts
- Additional interventions

References

1. Foster, J. (2001). *Functional Recovery Following Neuromuscular Blockade in Mechanically Ventilated Adults.* Unpublished dissertation.
2. Foster, J., Kish-Wallace, S., and Keenan, C. (2002). National practice with assessment and monitoring of neuromuscular blockade. *Crit Care Nursing Q,* 25, 27-40.
3. Gooch, J.L., et al. (1991). Prolonged paralysis after treatment with neuromuscular blocking agents. *Crit Care Med,* 19, 1125-31.
4. http://www.usyd.edu.au/su/anaes/lectures/nmj_monitoring_clt/nmj_monitoring.html. Accessed June 2003.
5. Jacobi, J., et al. (2002). Clinical practice guidelines for the sustained use of sedatives and analgesics in the critically ill adult. *Crit Care Med,* 30, 119-40.
6. Kim, K.S., et al. (2003). The duration of immobilization causes the changing pharmacodynamics of mivacurium and rocuronium in rabbits. *Anesth Analg,* 96, 438-42.
7. Larsen, P.B., et al. (2002). Acceleromyography of the orbicularis oculi muscle II: Comparing the orbicularis oculi and adductor pollicis muscles. *Acta Anaesthesiol Scand,* 46, 1131-6.

8. Muller, R., et al. (2002). Neuromuscular monitoring in a patient with hemiparesis. Resistance of the paralyzed musculature to non-depolarizing muscle relaxants. *Anaesthetist,* 51, 644-9.
9. Murray, M., et al. (2002). Clinical guidelines for sustained neuromuscular blockade in the adult critically ill patient. *Crit Care Med,* 30, 142-56.
10. Nagelhout, J.J., and Naglaniczny, K.L. (2001). *Nurse Anesthesia.* 2nd ed. Philadelphia: W.B. Saunders.
11. Rudis, M.I., et al. (1997). A prospective, randomized, controlled evaluation of peripheral nerve stimulation versus standard clinical dosing of neuromuscular blocking agents in critically ill patients. *Crit Care Med,* 25, 575-83.
12. Saitoh, Y., et al. (2003). Monitoring of neuromuscular block after administration of vecuronium in patients with diabetes mellitus. *Br J Anaesth,* 90, 480-6.
13. Saitoh, Y., et al. (1999). Tactile evaluation of fade of the train-of-four and double-burst stimulation using the anaesthetist's non-dominant hand. *Br J Anaesth,* 83, 275-8.
14. Segredo, V., et al. (1990). Pharmacokinetics of vecuronium after long-term administration (abstract). *Anesth Analg,* 70, S1-450.

15. Silverman, D.G., and Mirakhur, R.K. (1994). Effects of patient status and condition on nondepolarizing relaxants. In: Standaert, D.G. *Neuromuscular Block in Perioperative and Intensive Care.* Philadelphia: J.B. Lippincott, 11-22.
16. Torda, T. (1980). The nature of gentamicin-induced neuromuscular block. *Br J Anesth,* 52, 325-8.
17. Viby-Mogensen, J. (1985). Interaction of other drugs with muscle relaxants. *Sem in Anesth,* 4, 52-64.

Additional Readings

Arbor, R. (2003). Continuous nervous system monitoring, EEG, the bispectral index, and neuromuscular transmission. *AACN Clinical Issues,* 14, 185-207.
Johnson, K.L., et al. (1999). Therapeutic paralysis of critically ill trauma patients: Perceptions of patients and their family members. *Am J Crit Care,* 8, 490-8.

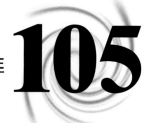
PROCEDURE **105**

Patient-Controlled Analgesia

P U R P O S E : Patient-controlled analgesia (PCA) under-scores patients' authority over their own pain. Nurses are responsible for maintaining the intravenous delivery system and, through frequent assessments and patient advocacy, for ensuring that patients are able to meet their own needs for pain management.

Liza Severance-Lossin

PREREQUISITE NURSING KNOWLEDGE

- Pain is an unpleasant sensory and emotional experience that arises from actual or potential tissue damage or is described in terms of such damage.[2]
- According to the American Pain Society, the most common reason for unrelieved pain in hospitals is the failure of staff to routinely and adequately assess pain and pain relief.[3]
- Pain can lead to shallow breathing and cough suppression, which can lead to retained pulmonary secretions, atelectasis, and pneumonia. Unrelieved pain may delay recovery and prolong hospital stays.[2,3,19]
- The Agency for Healthcare Research and Quality (AHRQ) (previously known as the Agency for Health Care Policy and Research) urges health care professionals to accept the patient's self-report as "the single most reliable indicator of the existence and intensity" of pain.[2] Behavioral observations by health care professionals and family members correlate poorly with many patient populations' self-report and frequently result in undertreatment of pain.[10,14-17,20,24,29,31,34,35,38,40,44]
- Studies and meta-analyses have shown that patient satisfaction with pain management increases with the use of PCA.[5,11,22,23,41]
- PCA has been found in many countries to be effective in the relief of pain following various surgical procedures as well as during exacerbations of chronic medical conditions and in ambulatory settings.[5,11,21,22,25,26,32,39,41-43,45]

- PCA can be an effective method of pain relief for patients of all ages.[11,13,20,21,26,28]
- Patient-controlled analgesia (PCA) may be administered by a continuous (basal) infusion along with patient-initiated boluses or solely by patient-initiated boluses.
- Patient assessments at regular intervals should include an evaluation of the patient's pain, inquiry regarding common side effects such as constipation and nausea, and a thorough assessment of both level of consciousness and respiratory effort.[2,3,6,27]
- PCA pump settings should be confirmed at regular intervals.[7,27,46] Table 105-1 lists medications that are incompatible with morphine and hydromorphone.

TABLE 105-1	Medications That are Incompatible With Commonly Used PCA Opioids
Opioid	**Incompatible With These Medications**
Hydromorphone	Amphotericin B cholesteryl sulfate complex, diazepam, minocycline, phenobarbital, phenytoin, sargramostim, sodium bicarbonate, tetracycline, thiopental
Morphine	Acyclovir, alatrofloxacin, aminophylline, amobarbital, chlorothiazide, amphotericin B cholesteryl sulfate complex, cefepime, chlorpromazine, doxorubicin liposome, floxacillin, fluorouracil, furosemide, haloperidol, heparin, meperidine, minocycline, phenobarbital, phenytoin, pentobarbital, prochlorperazine edisylate, promethazine, sargramostim, sodium bicarbonate, thiopental, TPN

From Lexi-Comp, Inc.

- Although individual patient responses vary, pain relief generally precedes sedation.[3,27] Sedation generally precedes respiratory depression.[3,27] Studies show little risk for respiratory depression in patients using PCA and no increased risk in patients using PCA versus intramuscular narcotic use.[6,22] Incidences requiring naloxone reversal of narcotic infusions have often been related to human and programming errors.[6,7,46]
- Patients need to balance the need for adequate pain management with the need to remain alert.[14] Others may fear "becoming addicted" to pain medicine. Patients who fear addiction should be informed of the extremely low likelihood of addiction resulting from the use of PCA.[3,33]
- A history of substance use is not a contraindication for PCA.[4,18] On the contrary, unrelieved and chronic pain could lead to a relapse in the recovering patient.[47] Patients in recovery may be cross-tolerant and therefore often require higher doses to achieve pain relief.[9] Patients who are on methadone maintenance and are experiencing acute pain will require analgesia in addition to their usual doses of methadone.[37] Patients in recovery, like other patients, need regular reassessment of pain, nonpharmacologic pain management options, and a nonjudgmental, supportive health care team.[1,30,36]
- Patients who may be poor candidates for PCA include the following:
  ❖ Anyone incapable of pressing a button (e.g., patients with spinal cord injury or rheumatoid arthritis)
  ❖ Anyone unable to understand and follow the directions for use (e.g., patients with a decreased level of consciousness or with developmental disabilities)

EQUIPMENT

- Patient-controlled analgesia pump
- PCA antisiphon tubing with injector
- IV pump
- IV tubing
- Prescribed medication (in syringe with plunger if not using tubing injector)
- Alcohol wipes
- Normal saline or other compatible intravenous (IV) fluid
  Additional equipment as needed includes:
- Emergency medications
- Ambu bag and oxygen

PATIENT AND FAMILY EDUCATION

- Review an appropriate pain rating scale with the patient.[8] The World Health Organization states that goals for pain management should be less than 4 on a scale of 0 to 10. ➥*Rationale:* Ensures the patient understands the pain

rating scale and enables the nurse to obtain a baseline assessment.

- Review the principles of PCA use with the patient and family members. If a basal rate has been prescribed, inform the patient that pain medication will be infusing at all times. Explain that if the pain is not relieved with this steady dose, extra medicine can be delivered (e.g., every 10 minutes); make sure the patient knows what the lockout interval is. If the patient's pain needs are not met, the dosage can and will be changed to meet those needs. ➥*Rationale:* May reduce anxiety and preconceptions about PCA use. Many patients choose to remain undermedicated, expressing concern that they will become addicted. No data show an increased risk for addiction for patients using PCA.[4] Former substance users should be counseled about the risk for relapse with unrelieved pain.[47]
- In most circumstances the patient should be the only one to deliver the demand dose. If family members want to be able to press the delivery button for the patient (e.g., if the patient is asleep), review with them the need to watch for sedation, which will generally precede a decreased respiratory drive. ➥*Rationale:* The patient should remain alert enough to administer his or her own dose.
- Instruct the patient and family members to report common side effects such as constipation, nausea or vomiting, pruritus, or oversedation. ➥*Rationale:* Identifies side effects for the patient and family.

PATIENT ASSESSMENT AND PREPARATION

Patient Assessment

- Assess the patient's level of consciousness using a sedation scale[12,27,38] (Fig. 105-1). ➥*Rationale:* Sedation will generally precede respiratory depression; a patient who is less alert should be closely monitored if PCA is prescribed.
- Review the patient's medication allergies. ➥*Rationale:* Reviewing medication allergies before administering a new medication will decrease the chances of an allergic reaction.
- Assess the patient's pain and document intensity, location, and characteristics.[2,3,27] ➥*Rationale:* A baseline assessment will permit accurate gauging of the PCA's efficacy.

Patient Preparation

- Ensure that the patient understands teaching. Answer questions as they arise and reinforce information as needed. ➥*Rationale:* Evaluates and reinforces the understanding of previously taught information.
- Obtain IV access or ensure patency of the IV. ➥*Rationale:* Analgesia is delivered intravenously.

Richmond Agitation Sedation Scale (RASS)*

Score	Term	Description	
+4	Combative	Overtly combative, violent, immediate danger to staff	
+3	Very agitated	Pulls or removes tube(s) or catheter(s); aggressive	
+2	Agitated	Frequent non-purposeful movement, fights ventilator	
+1	Restless	Anxious but movements not aggressive vigorous	
0	Alert and calm		
−1	Drowsy	Not fully alert, but has sustained awakening (eye-opening/eye contact) to *voice* **(**greater than or equal to**10 seconds)**	Verbal stimulation
−2	Light sedation	Briefly awakens with eye contact to *voice* **(**less than **10 seconds)**	Verbal stimulation
−3	Moderate sedation	Movement or eye opening to *voice* **(but no eye contact)**	Verbal stimulation
−4	Deep sedation	No response to voice, but movement or eye opening to *physical* stimulation	Physical stimulation
−5	Unarousable	No response to *voice* or *physical* stimulation	Physical stimulation

Procedure for RASS Assessment

1. Observe patient
   a. Patient is alert, restless, or agitated. **(score 0 to +4)**
2. If not alert, state patient's name and *say* to open eyes and look at speaker.
   b. Patient awakens with sustained eye opening and eye contact. **(score −1)**
   c. Patient awakens with eye opening and eye contact, but not sustained. **(score −2)**
   d. Patient has any movement in response to voice but no eye contact. **(score −3)**
3. When no response to verbal stimulation, physically stimulate patient by shaking shoulder and/or rubbing sternum.
   e. Patient has any movement to physical stimulation. **(score −4)**
   f. Patient has no response to any stimulation. **(score −5)**

* Sessler CN, et al. *The Richmond Agitation-Sedation Scale: Validity and Reliability in Adult Intensive Care Patients.* Am J Respir Crit Care Med 2002; 166:1338-1344, Ely EW, et al. *Monitoring Sedation Status Over Time in ICU Patients: The Reliability and Validity of the Richmond Agitation Sedation Scale (RASS).* JAMA 2003; 289:2983-2991.

FIGURE 105-1 Example of a sedation scale.

Procedure for Starting Patient-Controlled Analgesia

Steps	Rationale	Special Considerations
1. Review the prescription for the patient-controlled analgesia, including the medication, concentration, basal rate, bolus amount, and time lockout on the bolus.	Provides necessary information.	Check for medication allergies or sensitivities. Ensure coverage for common side effects such as pruritus, constipation, or nausea. Many institutions also require a prescription for immediate availability of naloxone.
2. Obtain a PCA pump, PCA antisiphon tubing with injector,	Prepares the necessary equipment.	Some manufacturers do not use tubing-specific injectors; in this

Procedure for Starting Patient-Controlled Analgesia—*Continued*

Steps	Rationale	Special Considerations
IV pump, IV tubing, normal saline or other compatible IV solution, and the prescribed medication.		case the injector will be the plunger of the medication syringe.
3. Wash hands.	Reduces the transmission of microorganisms; standard precautions.	
4. Remove the antisiphon tubing and the injector from the packaging; unscrew the cap of the medication syringe and attach the antisiphon tubing.	Prepares the equipment.	
5. Manually purge the tubing.	Removes air from the system.	If the injector is the syringe plunger, attach the antisiphon tubing to the syringe and manually purge. The PCA may offer the option of purging via the PCA pump.
6. Insert the syringe into the PCA pump by first placing the injector flange in the bottom of the machine at a 45-degree angle and then snapping the barrel into the syringe-holder.	Prepares the PCA system.	If using a syringe pump, snap the syringe barrel into the pump with the flange in (not above) the flange holder. Pinch the pusher block to open; then slide down to meet the plunger. Release the pusher block to hold the plunger.
7. Place the medication syringe so that the markings and labels are visible.	Ensures ready identification of the medication.	
8. Spike the intravenous infusion (e.g., normal saline or other compatible IV solution) with the IV tubing and flush the tubing.	Removes air from the system.	
9. Thread the IV tubing through the IV pump.	Prepares the infusion pump.	
10. Connect the IV tubing to the Y-site on the PCA tubing and ensure all tubing is flushed.	Prepares the system and prevents an air bolus.	
11. Cleanse the IV cap with alcohol and connect the PCA tubing to IV.	Connects the PCA to the IV.	
12. Enter the medication name and concentration, the basal rate, the bolus amount, and the time lockout for boluses.	Prepares the system.	
13. Review the pump settings with a second RN to confirm that all data have been accurately programmed.	Adverse events may be due to programming errors.	
14. Program the normal saline or other compatible IV solution at a rate to provide not less than the minimum rate for a peripheral IV per institutional policy.	Ensures the delivery of the prescribed medication. Highly concentrated medications, such as hydromorphone, may be administered in bolus doses	The medication's basal rate and normal saline combined should total the institution's minimum IV fluid rate. If the PCA is programmed for bolus dosing

Procedure continues on the following page

Procedure for Starting Patient-Controlled Analgesia—*Continued*

Steps	Rationale	Special Considerations
	of less than 1 ml, which would not reach the patient quickly through most IV tubing without a normal saline infusion.	only, set the normal saline at the minimum rate for a peripheral IV.
15. Label the PCA pump and the IV infusion pump.	Ensures quick and clear identification of IV fluids and PCA medications.	
16. Label the IV tubing and the PCA tubing.	Ensures identification of IV fluids and PCA medications infusing via each IV tubing.	
17. Secure the PCA tubing at two points of tension.	Prevents accidental removal of the IV.	
18. Discard used supplies and wash hands.	Reduces the transmission of microorganisms; standard precautions.	

Expected Outcomes

- Pain consistently reported at or less than 4 on a scale of 0 to 10
- No unmanaged side effects

Unexpected Outcomes

- Extravasation
- Oversedation or respiratory depression
- Persistent pain greater than 4 on a scale of 0 to 10

Patient Monitoring and Care

Steps	Rationale	Reportable Conditions
		These conditions should be reported if they persist despite nursing interventions. • Extravasation
1. Ensure that the medication is infusing properly through the IV.	New infusions may precipitate extravasation; an IV catheter may become dislodged through patient movement.	
2. Assess the patient's pain and level of sedation according to institutional policy.[12,27,38]	Monitors effectiveness of therapy; identifies need for adjustment. Institutional assessment policies should take into account the expected duration and peak of the medication in use.	• Pain rating greater than 4 persists despite correct PCA use • Altered level of consciousness • Change in respiratory status (e.g., respiratory rate, oxygenation via pulse oximetry)
3. Ensure patient comprehension of PCA use and analgesic goal.	Comprehension can be assessed by patient report and by reviewing the PCA history for frequency of attempts.	• Patient unable to use PCA • Inability to achieve analgesia goal
4. Assess for the presence of side effects such as nausea, pruritus, or constipation.	Many side effects from opioid use can be relieved. Side effects can often be managed if pain control is adequate.	• Nausea • Pruritus • Constipation

Documentation

Documentation should include the following:

- Medication, concentration, basal rate, bolus dose, and lockout interval (cosigned by another RN after initiation of treatment and with all changes thereafter)
- Patient's baseline and follow-up pain scores using a consistent scale
- Patient's baseline and follow-up sedation scores using a consistent scale

- Total dose of medication administered per shift and time the PCA pump was cleared, per institutional policy
- Patient teaching and any reinforcement needed
- Side effects
- Unexpected outcomes
- Additional interventions

References

1. American Academy of Family Practitioners, et al. (2002). Promoting Pain Relief and Preventing Abuse of Pain Medications: Critical Balancing Act. A Joint Statement From 21 Health Organizations and the Drug Enforcement Administration. *J Pain & Symptom Manage,* 24, 147.
2. American Pain Management Guideline Panel. (1992). *Acute Pain Management: Operative or Medical Procedures and Trauma. Clinical Practice Guidelines.* AHCPR Pub. 92-0032. Rockville, MD: Agency for Health Care Policy and Research, Public Health Service, U.S. Department of Health and Human Services.
3. American Pain Society. (1999). *Principles of Analgesic Use in the Treatment of Acute and Cancer Pain.* 4th ed. Glenview, IL: Author.
4. Anonymous. (1997). The use of opioids for the treatment of chronic pain. A consensus statement from the American Academy of Pain Medicine and the American Pain Society. *Clin J Pain,* 13, 6-8.
5. Ballantyne, J.C., et al. (1993). Postoperative patient-controlled analgesia: A meta-analysis of initial randomized controlled trials. *J Clin Anesthesia,* 5, 182-93.
6. Bennett, R., et al. (1982). Patient controlled analgesia. *Ann Surg,* 195, 700-5.
7. Brown, S.L., et al. (1997). Human error and patient-controlled analgesia pumps. *J Intraven Nurs,* 20, 311-6.
8. Chumbley, G.M., Hall, G.M., and Salmon, P. (2003). Patient-controlled analgesia: What information does the patient really want? *J Adv Nurs,* 39, 459-71.
9. Collin, E., and Cesselin, F. (1991). Neurobiological mechanisms of opioid tolerance and dependence. *Clin Neuropharmacol,* 14, 465-88.
10. Desbiens, N.A., and Mueller-Rizner, N. (2000). How well do surrogates assess the pain of seriously ill patients? *Crit Care Med,* 28, 1347-52.
11. Egbert, A.M., et al. (1990). Randomized trial of postoperative patient-controlled analgesia versus intramuscular narcotics in frail elderly men. *Arch Int Med,* 150, 1897-1903.
12. Ely, E.W., et al. (2003). Monitoring sedation status over time in ICU patients: The reliability and validity of the Richmond Agitation and Sedation Scale (RASS). *JAMA,* 289, 2983-91.
13. Gagliese, L., et al. (2000). Age is not an impediment to effective use of patient-controlled analgesia by surgical patients. *Anesthesiology,* 93, 601-10.
14. Graves, D., et al. (1983). Patient controlled analgesia. *Annals Int Med,* 99, 360-6.
15. Grossman, S.A., et al. (1991). Correlation of patient and caregiver ratings of cancer pain. *J Pain & Symptom Manage,* 6, 53-7.
16. Guru, V., and Dubinsky, I. (2000). The patient vs. caregiver perception of acute pain in the emergency department. *J Emerg Med,* 18, 7-12.
17. Hall-Lord, M.L., Larsson, G., and Steen, B. (1998). Pain and distress among elderly intensive care unit patients: Comparison of patients' experiences and nurses' assessments. *Heart & Lung: J Acute & Critical Care,* 27, 123-32.
18. Hord, A.H. (1992). Postoperative analgesia in the opioid-dependent patient. In: Sinatra, R.S., et al., eds. *Acute Pain: Mechanisms and Management.* St. Louis: Mosby Yearbook, 390-8.
19. Horn, S.D., et al. (2002). Association between patient-controlled analgesia pump use and postoperative surgical site infection in intestinal surgery patients. *Surg Infections,* 3, 109-18.
20. Iafrati, N.S. (1986). Pain on the burn unit: Patient vs nurse perceptions. *J Burn Care Rehab,* 7, 413-6.
21. Keita, H., et al. (2003). Comparison between patient-controlled analgesia and subcutaneous morphine in elderly patients after total hip replacement. *Brit J Anaesthesia,* 90, 53-7.
22. Kleiman, R., et al. (1987). PCA vs regular IM injections for severe postop pain. *Am J Nurs,* 87, 1491-2.
23. Lebovits, A.H., et al. (2001). Satisfaction with epidural and intravenous patient-controlled analgesia. *Pain Med,* 2, 280.
24. Lobchuk, M.M., et al. (1997). Perceptions of symptom distress in lung cancer patients: I. Congruence between patients and primary family caregivers. *J Pain & Symptom Manage,* 14, 136-46.
25. Macintyre, P.E. (2001). Safety and efficacy of patient-controlled analgesia. *Brit J Anaesthesia,* 87, 36-46.
26. Mann, C., et al. (2000). Comparison of intravenous or epidural patient-controlled analgesia in the elderly after major abdominal surgery. *Anesthesiology,* 92, 433-41.
27. McCaffery, M., and Beebe, A. (1999). *Pain: Clinical Manual for Nursing Practice.* St. Louis: Mosby.
28. Monitto, C.L., et al. (2000). The safety and efficacy of parent-/nurse-controlled analgesia in patients less than six years of age. *Anesthesia & Analgesia,* 91, 573-9.
29. Nekolaichuk, C.L., et al. (1999). Assessing the reliability of patient, nurse, and family caregiver symptom ratings in hospitalized advanced cancer patients. *J Clin Oncol,* 17, 3621-30.
30. Pasero, C.L., and Compton, P. (1997). Pain management in addicted patients. *Am J Nurs,* 4, 17-9.
31. Pasero, C., and McCaffery, M. (2001). The undertreatment of pain. *Am J Nurs* 101, 62-5.
32. Pettersson, P.H., Lindskog, E.A., and Owall, A. (2000). Patient-controlled versus nurse-controlled pain treatment after coronary artery bypass surgery. *Acta Anaesthesiologica Scandinavica,* 44, 43-7.
33. Porter, J., and Jick, H. (1980). Addiction rare in patients treated with narcotics. *N Engl J Med,* 302, 123.
34. Puntillo, K.A., et al. (1997). Relationship between behavioral and physiological indicators of pain, critical care patients' self-reports of pain, and opioid administration. *Crit Care Med,* 25, 1159-66.
35. Redinbaugh, E.M., et al. (2002). Factors associated with the accuracy of family caregiver estimates of patient pain. *J Pain & Symptom Manage,* 23, 31-8.

36. Savage, S.R. (1998). Principles of pain treatment in the addicted patient. In: Graham, A.W., Schultz, T.K., and Wilford, B.B., eds. *Principles of Addiction Medicine.* 2nd ed. Chevy Chase, MD: American Society of Addiction Medicine, 919-43.

37. Schulz, J.E. (1997). The integration of medical management with recovery. *J Psychoactive Drugs,* 29, 233-7.

38. Sessler, C.N., et al. (2002). The Richmond Agitation Sedation Scale: Validity and reliability in intensive care patients. *Am J Resp & Crit Care Med,* 166, 1338-44.

39. Shapiro, B.S., Cohen, D.E., and Howe, C.J. (1993). Patient-controlled analgesia for sickle-cell-related pain. *J Pain & Symptom Manage,* 8, 22-8.

40. Sheiner, E.K., et al. (1999). Ethnic differences influence caregivers' estimates of pain during labour. *Pain,* 81, 299-305.

41. Snell, C.C., Fothergill-Bourbonnais, F., and Durocher-Hendriks, S. (1997). Patient-controlled analgesia and intramuscular injections: A comparison of patient pain experiences and postoperative outcomes. *J Adv Nurs,* 25, 681-90.

42. Swanson, G., et al. (1989). Patient-controlled analgesia for chronic cancer pain in the ambulatory setting: A report of 117 patients. *J Clin Oncol,* 7, 1903-8.

43. Tanskanen, P., Kytta, J., and Randell, T. (1999). Patient-controlled analgesia with oxycodone in treatment of postcraniotomy pain. *Acta Anaesthesiologica Scandinavica,* 43, 42-5.

44. Teyske, K., Daut, R.L., and Cleeland, C.S. (1983). Relationships between nurses' observations and patients' self-reports of pain. *Pain,* 16, 289-96.

45. Thurlow, J.A., et al. (2002). Remifentanil by patient-controlled analgesia compared with intramuscular meperidine for pain relief in labour. *Brit J Anaesthesia,* 88, 374-8.

46. Vicente, K.J., et al. (2003). Programming errors contribute to death from patient-controlled analgesia: A case report and estimate of probability. *Can J Anaesthesia,* 50, 328-32.

47. Wesson, D.R., et al. (1993). Prescription of opioids for treatment of pain in patients with addictive disease. *J Pain & Symptom Manage,* 8, 289-96.

Additional Readings

Koh, P., and Thomas, V.J. (1994). Patient-controlled analgesia (PCA): Does time saved by PCA improve patient satisfaction with nursing care? *J Adv Nurs,* 20, 61-70.

Reiff, P.A., and Miziolek, M.M. (2001). Troubleshooting tips for PCA. *RN,* 4, 33-7.

PROCEDURE **106**

Peripheral Nerve Blocks (Assist)

P U R P O S E :   Peripheral nerve blocks are administered via a catheter that is placed within a specific anatomic area to provide site-specific (e.g., femoral, brachial plexus, axillary, intrapleural, extrapleural, paravertebral, tibial, sciatic, and lumbar plexus) prolonged anesthesia and/or analgesia for postoperative and trauma pain management.

Robyn Dealtry

PREREQUISITE NURSING KNOWLEDGE

- State boards of nursing may have detailed guidelines involving peripheral nerve blockade. Each institution providing this therapy also has policies and guidelines pertaining to peripheral nerve blockade. The nurse should be aware of state and institution guidelines and policies.
- The use of peripheral nerve blocks requires skilled and knowledgeable clinicians.[13]
- The catheter placement and the continuing management of the patient should be under the direct supervision of an anesthesiologist, nurse anesthetist, or an acute pain service.[11,24]
- Understanding of the principles of aseptic technique
- Peripheral nerve blocks are used as part of a preemptive and multimodal analgesic technique to provide safe and effective postoperative pain management with minimal side effects.[13,25]
- The basis for the efficacy and utility of peripheral nerve blockade in patients with acute pain is by the interruption of nociceptive input at its source or by blocking nociceptive transmissions in the peripheral nerve.[6,18] In addition to blocking nociceptors in the incision, a continuous infusion may wash away pain-mediating substances, such as histamine, bradykinin, and prostaglandins.[22]
- There are a number of ways in which peripheral nerve blocks with local anesthetics can be used to treat acute pain regionally. These vary from wound infiltration to continuous peripheral nerve blockade using catheters that will provide many hours or days of optimal analgesia following surgery or trauma.[10,11,15]

- In the outpatient setting, peripheral nerve blocks have facilitated early ambulation and discharge by decreasing side effects, such as drowsiness, nausea, and vomiting.[1] In addition, peripheral nerve blocks allow patients to remain conscious and preserve their protective reflexes (e.g., gag reflex) while avoiding the need for airway manipulation and intubation. This reduces the potential side effects and complications of general anesthesia.[13]
- Catheters may be placed by the surgeon under direct vision either adjacent to, or into a nerve sheath (e.g., sciatic or tibial during surgery for lower limb amputation).[11] Catheters may also be placed after surgery (e.g., intercostal, intrapleural, axillary, brachial plexus, femoral, and paravertebral).
- Continuous peripheral nerve blockade improves postoperative analgesia, patient satisfaction, and rehabilitation compared with intravenous opioids for upper and lower extremity procedures.[3,4,18,20,21]
- A "three-in-one" peripheral nerve block can be used for analgesia after proximal lower limb orthopedic surgery. A "three-in-one" peripheral nerve block provides analgesia to block three nerves, including the lateral femoral cutaneous, femoral, and obturator nerves. This block is as effective as epidural analgesia, with fewer side effects (e.g., urinary retention, nausea, and risk for spinal subarachnoid hemorrhage in anticoagulated patients).[3,11,23]
- Some forms of plexus analgesia (e.g., brachial plexus analgesia) in the postoperative setting may serve two purposes: (a) pain relief and (b) sympathetic blockade, which increases blood flow and may improve outcome in some cases (i.e., digit reimplantation).[11,20]
- The anatomic position of the specific catheter placement is clearly defined and documented after insertion

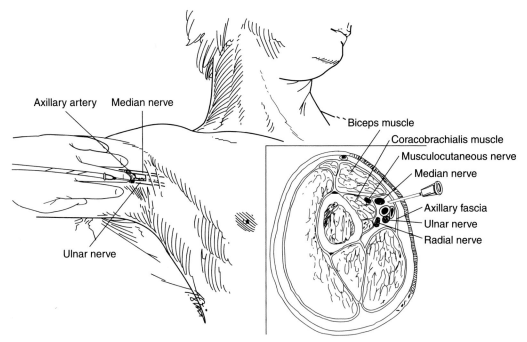

FIGURE 106-1 Location for needle insertion for an axillary block. *(From Sinatra, R.S. [1992].* Acute Pain: Mechanisms & Management. *St. Louis: Mosby.)*

(e.g., femoral, brachial plexus, axillary, intrapleural, extrapleural, paravertebral, tibial, sciatic, and lumbar plexus).[3,5] This is illustrated in Figs. 106-1, 106-2, and 106-3.

- Radiologic confirmation[3] of the catheter position may be required to avoid suboptimal outcomes (e.g., pneumothorax).
- The peripheral nerve block may be performed with or without a nerve stimulator device, depending on the physician's preference.[17-20]

- Analgesia via a catheter may be administered as a continuous infusion utilizing a volumetric pump system or by a patient controlled regional infusion system.[11,17,22,23]
- Medication administered is usually a local anesthetic. Other agents have been utilized as an adjunct on a one-time-only basis (e.g., opioids, clonidine and neostigmine).[14]
- The pharmacokinetics and pharmacodynamics of local anesthetics and other agents utilized, including side effects and duration of action, should be clearly understood.

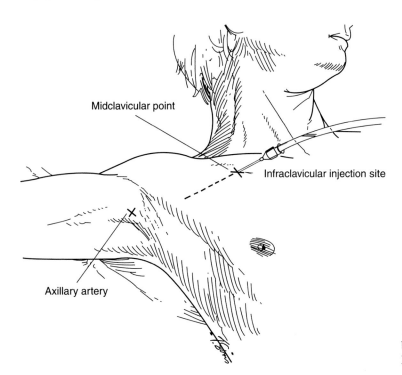

FIGURE 106-2 Needle insertion for an axillary block. *(From Sinatra, R.S. [1992].* Acute Pain: Mechanisms & Management. *St. Louis: Mosby.)*

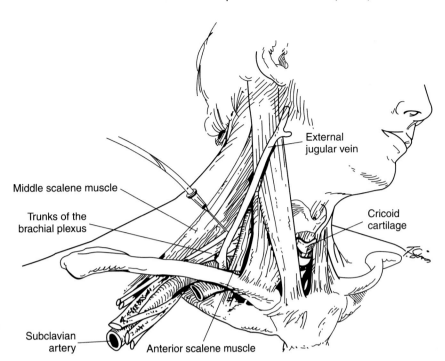

FIGURE 106-3 Landmarks for inter scalene brachial plexus block. *(From Sinatra, R.S. [1992]. Acute Pain: Mechanisms & Management. St. Louis: Mosby.)*

Labels in figure: External jugular vein; Middle scalene muscle; Trunks of the brachial plexus; Cricoid cartilage; Subclavian artery; Anterior scalene muscle

- Local anesthetic medications used for peripheral nerve blocks provide surgical analgesia (i.e., loss of pain sensation) and anesthesia (i.e., loss of all sensation). The duration of action for each anesthetic medication depends on several factors, including the volume injected, concentration of the medication, site of injection, and absorption. The addition of a vasoconstrictor, such as epinephrine, constricts blood vessels and reduces vascular uptake, which further prolongs the duration of action of the local anesthetic.[13]
- Epinephrine should not be used in peripheral nerve blocks in areas where there are end arteries, such as ear lobes, the nose, digits, and the penis. Vasoconstrictor medications may cause spasm of blood vessels, resulting in necrosis.[16]
- Knowledge of signs and symptoms of profound motor and sensory blockade or overmedication is essential. Note: Sensory and motor blockade may be acceptable or desirable depending on the physician's goals and preference.
- According to the American Pain Society,[2] the most common reason for unrelieved pain in hospitals is failure of the staff to routinely and adequately assess pain and pain relief. Many patients silently tolerate unrelieved pain if not specifically asked about it.
- The Agency for Health Care Policy and Research[1] urges health care professionals to accept the patient's self-report as "the single most reliable indicator of the existence and intensity" of pain. Behavioral observations are unreliable indicators of pain levels.
- Pain is an unpleasant sensory and emotional experience that arises from actual or potential tissue damage or is described in terms of such damage.[8] No matter how successful or how deftly conducted, surgical operations produce tissue trauma and release potent mediators of inflammation and pain.[1,9]

- Pain is just one response to the trauma of surgery. In addition to the major stress of surgical trauma and pain, the substances released from injured tissue evoke "stress hormone" responses in the patient. Such responses promote breakdown of body tissue; increase metabolic rate, blood clotting, and water retention; impair immune function; and trigger a "fight-or-flight" alarm reaction with autonomic features (e.g., rapid pulse) and negative emotions.[1,2,4,9,15]
- Pain itself may lead to shallow breathing and cough suppression in an attempt to "splint" the injured site, followed by retained pulmonary secretions and pneumonia.[1,2,9,15] Unrelieved pain also may delay the return of normal gastric and bowel function in the postoperative patient.[2,4]
- Peripheral nerve blockade is contraindicated in patients with a history of coagulopathy, preexisting neuropathies, anatomic or pathologic deviations at the injection site, and systemic disease or infection.[13]

EQUIPMENT

- One epidural catheter kit
- Set for continuous plexus anesthesia with/without an adaptor for a nerve stimulator
- Topical skin antiseptic, as prescribed (e.g., 2% chlorhexidine-based preparation)
- Sterile towels
- Sterile forceps
- Sterile gauze 4 × 4 pads
- Sterile gloves, face masks with eye shields, sterile gowns
- 20 ml normal saline
- 5 to 10 ml local anesthetic as prescribed (1% lidocaine) for local infiltration
- Local anesthetic as prescribed (to establish the block)
- Occlusive dressing supplies to cover the catheter entry site

- Gauze and tape to secure the catheter to the patient's body
- Labels stating "Local anesthetic only" and "Not for intravenous injection"
- Pump for administering analgesia (e.g., volumetric pump/dedicated for peripheral nerve block infusion with rate and volume limited, and preferably a different color from epidural and intravenous infusion pumps, or patient-controlled analgesic pump [PCA])
- Specific observation chart for patient monitoring of the peripheral nerve block infusion
- Prescribed analgesics and local anesthetics
- Equipment for monitoring BP, heart rate, and SpO_2
  Additional equipment, as needed, includes the following:
- Ice or alcohol swabs for demonstrating sensory block
- Emergency medications
- Respiratory equipment: oxygen mask and tubing, intubation equipment, hand-held resuscitation bag and tubing, and flow meter
- Nerve stimulator

PATIENT AND FAMILY EDUCATION

- Explain the reason and purpose of the catheter. If available, supply easy-to-read patient information. ➥*Rationale:* The patient and the family know what to expect; may reduce anxiety.
- Explain to the patient and family that the procedure can be uncomfortable but that a local anesthetic will be used to facilitate comfort. ➥*Rationale:* Elicits patient's cooperation and comfort and facilitates insertion; decreases anxiety and fear.
- During therapy, instruct the patient to report side effects or changes in pain management (e.g., suboptimal analgesia, profound numbness of extremities [beyond the goal of therapy], lightheadedness, metallic taste, circumoral numbness, dizziness, blurred vision, tinnitus, loss of hearing and seizures).[13] ➥*Rationale:* Aids patient's comfort level and identifies side effects.
- Teach the patient to protect the affected extremity. ➥*Rationale:* Increases patient safety and protects the limb from injury and trauma (e.g., burns).[13]
- If a PCA pump is used, educate the patient and family on its use (see Procedure 105). ➥*Rationale:* Provides education and adequate analgesia.

PATIENT ASSESSMENT AND PREPARATION

Patient Assessment

- Observe the patient for local infection or generalized sepsis. ➥*Rationale:* Increases the risk for infection at the site of catheter insertion. Septicemia and bacteremia are contraindications for peripheral nerve block catheter placement and/or continuation of therapy.
- Assess the patient's concurrent anticoagulant and fibrinolytic therapy. ➥*Rationale:* Heparin (unfractionated and low-molecular-weight heparin) and heparinoids and fibrinolytic agents administered concurrently increase the risk for vessel trauma (e.g., hematoma). Care must be taken with insertion and removal of the peripheral nerve block catheter when patients are on anticoagulant and fibrinolytic therapy.[7] Special institutional guidelines must be observed.
- Obtain the patient's vital signs. ➥*Rationale:* Provides baseline data.
- Assess the patient's pain. ➥*Rationale:* Provides baseline data.

Patient Preparation

- Ensure that the patient and family understand preprocedural teaching. Answer questions as they arise, and reinforce information as needed. ➥*Rationale:* Evaluates and reinforces understanding of previously taught information.
- Ensure that informed consent has been obtained. ➥*Rationale:* Protects the rights of the patient and makes a competent decision possible for the patient.
- Wash the specific anatomic area of the patient's body with soap and water and open the gown to expose the site for injection while maintaining the patient's privacy and dignity. ➥*Rationale:* Cleanses the skin and allows easy access to the specific anatomic area of the patient's body.
- Consider nothing by mouth (NPO), especially if sedation or general anesthesia is to be employed. ➥*Rationale:* Decreases the risk for vomiting and aspiration.
- Establish intravenous (IV) access or ensure the patency of IV lines. ➥*Rationale:* The need to treat convulsions, cardiovascular depression, respiratory arrest, and coma may occur.
- Position the patient as appropriate, according to which anatomic area of the body is to be blocked. ➥*Rationale:* Aids in correct positioning of the catheter.
- Reassure the patient. ➥*Rationale:* May reduce anxiety and fears.

Procedure | for Peripheral Nerve Blocks

Steps	Rationale	Special Considerations
1. Wash hands and don gloves, gowns, and masks with eye shields.	Reduces the transmission of microorganisms and body secretions; standard precautions.	
2. Obtain the prescribed peripheral nerve block medication.	The medication should be prepared by aseptic technique by the pharmacy under laminar flow or prepared commercially to decrease the risk for infection.	All peripheral nerve block solutions are preservative-free to avoid untoward reactions.[5]

Procedure for Peripheral Nerve Blocks—*Continued*		
Steps	**Rationale**	**Special Considerations**
3. Connect the correct tubing to the prepared infusion and prime the tubing.	Removes air from the infusion system.	
4. Ensure that the patient is in position for catheter placement.	Facilitates ease of insertion of the peripheral nerve block catheter.	
5. Assist as needed with the antiseptic preparation of the intended insertion site.	Reduces the transmission of microorganisms into the nerve sheath or plexus space.	
6. Assist with holding the patient in position or consider sedation, if necessary.	Movement of the body may inhibit placement of the catheter.	
7. Assist the physician as needed with the catheter placement.	Facilitates catheter insertion.	
8. After the peripheral nerve catheter is inserted, assist as needed with the application of an occlusive dressing.	Reduces the incidence of infection.	
9. Secure the filter to the patient's body with a gauze padding and tape.	Avoids disconnection between the peripheral nerve catheter and the filter. Gauze padding prevents discomfort and skin pressure from the filter.	
10. The physician will administer a bolus dose of medication.	Facilitates a therapeutic level of analgesia and ensures correct catheter placement.	Monitor vital signs, including pain score. Emergency medications and equipment must be available.
11. Connect the prescribed medication infusion system.	Prepares the infusion system.	
12. Initiate therapy: A. Place the system in a volumetric pump and set the rate and volume to be infused.	Do not give any other solution or medication via this catheter. Inadvertent administration of some IV medications into the peripheral nerve block catheter may cause nerve or tissue damage.	Responses to peripheral nerve block analgesia vary individually, and analgesia is tailored according to individual responses.
B. Attach a "Local anesthetic only—Not for intravenous injection" label to the tubing and tape over the ports or use a portless system.[5] C. Do not use a burette.[5] D. Lock the key pad on the volumetric or PCA pump.	Inadvertent administration of local anesthetic intravenously can cause hypotension and cardiovascular collapse/arrest.	
13. Assess the quality of the analgesia. A. Determine the pain score based on a scale of 0 to 10.	Excellent pain scores should be reported at rest, and very little pain should be experienced with deep breathing, coughing and movement.	
B. Test the level of the epidural block with ice or an alcohol swab.	The ideal peripheral nerve block should be just above and just below the surgical incision or the trauma site (see the dermatomes described in Fig. 103-3).	
14. Discard used supplies, and wash hands.	Reduces the transmission of micro-organisms; standard precautions.	

Expected Outcomes

- Regional analgesic catheter inserted; accurate placement confirmed by radiologic means when appropriate[3]
- Pain minimized or relieved[5,11]
- No patient sedation or respiratory depression[11,15]
- Reduced need for parenteral opioids, thereby also reducing opioid side effects[14,20]
- Reduction in neuropathic pain states, especially following limb amputation[10]

Unexpected Outcomes

- Inability to insert the catheter
- Untimely or erroneous medication administration[5]
- Suboptimal analgesia
- Adverse medication reactions not recognized
- Altered skin integrity due to decreased sensory and motor loss[5,13]
- Accidental dislodgment of the catheter delivery system
- Leakage from the catheter insertion site
- Cracked filter on the delivery system
- Inadvertent injection into a blood vessel
- Ipsilateral Horner's syndrome and hoarseness[5,13]
- Nerve or vessel trauma[5,13]
- Hemorrhage/hematoma[5,13]
- Sepsis[5]
- Anaphylaxis
- Permanent neurologic injuries and damage[5,13]
- Local anesthetic toxicity (e.g., tachycardia, hypertension, metallic taste, dizziness, blurred vision, circumoral numbness, tinnitus, decreased hearing, seizures)[13]

Patient Monitoring and Care

Steps	Rationale	Reportable Conditions
		These conditions should be reported if they persist despite nursing interventions.
1. Assess the patient's level of sedation using a sedation scale every 1 hour for the first 6 hours, then every 2 hours or more frequently if needed. S = Sleeping, easily aroused; requires no action 1 = Awake and alert; requires no action. 2 = Occasionally drowsy, easy to arouse; requires no action. 3 = Frequently drowsy, arousable, drifts off to sleep during conversation; decrease the opioid dose. 4 = Somnolent; minimal or no response to stimuli; discontinue opioid and consider use of naloxone (Narcan) (see Fig. 105-1).	Sedation precedes opioid related respiratory depression.	• Increasing sedation and drowsiness or change in sedation score. • Report and provide ventilatory and circulatory support

2. Assess the patient's level of pain using a pain scale every 1 hour for the first 6 hours, then every 2 hours or more frequently if needed. Record the patient's subjective level of pain, using the numeric rating scale (0 to 10).[12]
  0 = No pain
  5 = Moderate pain
  10 = Worst possible pain
	Describes patient response to pain therapy. A low pain score is expected. Rating pain in this objective manner helps determine appropriate treatment measures.[13]	• Moderate to severe pain scores

3. Assess the levels of motor and sensory blockade (see Fig. 103-3).	Ensures effectiveness of analgesia and maintenance of the block at the correct level.	• Signs and symptoms of overmedication
4. Monitor the infusion rate hourly. Ensure that the control panel is locked if using a volumetric infusor or ensure that the PCA program is locked via a key or code access.	Ensures that medication is administered safely and securely.	

Patient Monitoring and Care—*Continued*

Steps	Rationale	Reportable Conditions
5. Monitor oxygen saturation continuously if parenteral opioids are administered (e.g., via IV PCA).	Assesses oxygenation.	• Oxygen saturation less than 93% or decreasing trend in oxygenation
6. Obtain temperature every 4-8 hours; assess more frequently if febrile.	Increasing hyperpyrexia could signify infection.	• Temperature greater than 101°F (38.5°C)
7. Assess the catheter site every 4-8 hours and as needed.	Identifies site complications.	• A change in the integrity of the peripheral nerve block insertion site (e.g., redness, tenderness, or swelling or the presence of exudate on the dressing)
8. Observe for signs and symptoms of peripheral nerve migration into a blood vessel.	The catheter is no longer in the correct position.	• Unexpected change in sedation scale • Drowsiness • Dizziness • Blurred vision • Slurred speech • Poor balance • Circumoral numbness
9. Monitor sensory or motor loss according to the defined goal of therapy.	Motor or sensory loss may result from the local anesthetic infusion. *Note*: With peripheral nerve blockade sensory loss is usually acceptable and often desirable. Motor loss is not desirable, but often acceptable.	• Unexpected change in sensory or motor function beyond defined goal of therapy (i.e., interference with respiration or excessive spread of local anesthetic beyond defined area of recommendation)
10. Assess for circumoral numbness.[13]	Local anesthetic is used in the solution and circumoral numbness may indicate local anesthetic toxicity.	• Tingling around the lips
11. Assess for tinnitus and loss of hearing.[13]	If a local anesthetic is used in the peripheral nerve block solution, ringing in the ears can be a sign of local anesthetic toxicity.	• Decreasing or sudden change in the patient's hearing
12. Monitor and check the skin integrity of the pressure points relating to the location of the peripheral nerve block (e.g., elbow, sacrum and heels). Change patient's position as needed.[5,13]	If a local anesthetic is used in the solution, check for decubitus ulceration (patient may have sensory loss in areas adjacent to the area of the peripheral nerve block).	• Increasing redness or blistering of the skin on pressure points
13. Change the peripheral nerve block catheter insertion site dressing as prescribed or if soiled, wet, or loose. *Note:* Usually the dressing is left intact for the duration of therapy unless wet or loose.[5]	Provides an opportunity to cleanse the area around the catheter and to assess for signs and symptoms of infection.	• Signs of site infection (e.g., swelling, pain, redness, or presence of drainage) • Leakage of the peripheral nerve block solution
14. Label the peripheral nerve block pump and consider placing the pump on one side of the patient's bed and all other pumps on the other side of the bed.[5]	Aids in minimizing the risk for mistaking the local anesthetic infusion for an IV infusion system.[5]	

Documentation

Documentation should include the following:

- Patient and family education
- Patient tolerance of procedure
- Catheter location
- Type of dressing used
- Confirmation of peripheral nerve block catheter placement (e.g., radiologic confirmation)
- Site assessment
- Assessment of pain and levels of motor and sensory blockade documented on an appropriate flow chart (see Fig. 103-3).

- If PCA is used, document medication concentration, PCA bolus dose, continuous infusion, lockout interval, hourly limits, and total dosage.
- Regional analgesic medication and medication concentration being infused and infusion rate
- Bolus dose administration (if appropriate) and patient response following a bolus dose, including quality of pain relief
- Occurrence of unexpected outcomes
- Nursing interventions taken
- Date and time of discontinuation of treatment

References

1. Acute Pain Management Guideline Panel. (1992). *Acute Pain Management: Operative or Medical Procedures and Trauma. Clinical Practice Guidelines*. AHCPR Pub. 92-0032. Rockville, MD: Agency for Health Care Policy and Research, Public Health Service, U.S. Department of Health and Human Services.
2. American Pain Society. (1999). *Principles of Analgesic Use in the Treatment of Acute and Cancer Pain*. 4th ed. Glenview, IL: Author.
3. Capdevila, X., et al. (2002). Continuous three-in-one block for postoperative pain after lower limb orthopedic surgery: Where do the catheters go? *Anaesthesia & Analgesia,* 94, 1001-6.
4. Capdevila, X., et al. (1999). Effects of perioperative analgesic technique on the surgical outcome and duration of rehabilitation after major knee surgery. *Anesthesiology,* 91, 8-15.
5. Dealtry, R. (2002). Regional analgesia/pain management. *Nursing Practice Manual*. Sydney, Australia: Westmead Hospital.
6. Enneking, F.K., and Wedel, D.J. (2000). The art and science of peripheral nerve blocks. *Anesthesia & Analgesia,* 90, 1-2.
7. Horlocker, T.T., et al. (2003). Regional anesthesia in the anticoagulated patient: Defining the risks. *Region Anesthesia & Pain Medicine,* May/June, 28, 172-97.
8. ISAP Subcommittee on Taxonomy. (1979). Pain terms: A list with definitions and notes on usage. *Pain,* 6, 249.
9. Kehlet, H., and Holte, K. (2001). Effect of postoperative analgesia on surgical outcome. *Brit J Anaesthesia,* 87, 62-72.
10. Kiefer, R.T., et al. (2002). Continuous brachial plexus analgesia and NMDA-receptor blockade in early phantom limb pain: A report of two cases. *Pain Med,* 3, 156-60.
11. Macintyre, P.E., and Ready, B.L. (2001). Other techniques in acute pain management. In: Macintyre, P.E., and Ready, B.L., eds. *Acute Pain Management: A Practical Guide*. London: W.B. Saunders.
12. McCaffery, M., and Pasero, C. (1999). Assessment. In: McCaffery, M., and Pasero, C., eds. *Pain: Clinical Manual*. St. Louis: Mosby.
13. Murauski, J.D., and Gonzalez, K.R. (2002). Peripheral nerve blocks for postoperative analgesia. *AORN J,* 75, January, 134-54.
14. Murphy, D.B., McCartney, C.J., and Chan, V.W. (2000). Novel analgesic adjuncts for brachial plexus block: A systemic review. *Anesthesia & Analgesia,* 90, 1122-8.
15. National Health and Medical Research Council. (1999). *Acute Pain Management: Scientific Evidence*. Canberra. Available at: www.nhmrc.health.gov.au/public/pdf/cp57.pdf.
16. Park, G., and Fulton, B. (1991). Local anesthetic techniques—Practical procedures. In: Park, G., and Fulton, B., eds. *The Management of Acute Pain*. Oxford: Oxford University Press.
17. Pham-Dang, C., et al. (2003). Continuous peripheral nerve blocks with stimulating catheters. *Region Anesthesia & Pain Medicine,* March/April, 28, 83-8.
18. Poon, L. (2003). The use of naropin (ropivacaine HCL) for interscalene blocks using a catheter for post-operative pain relief. *Block of the Month,* Sept., AstraZeneca NSW, Australia.
19. Salinas, F.V. (2003). Location, location, location: Continuous peripheral nerve blocks and stimulating catheters. *Region Anesthesia & Pain Medicine,* March/April, 28, 79-82.
20. Sevarino, F.B., and Preble, L.M. (1992). Other modalities for acute pain management. In: Sevarino, F.B., and Preble, L.M., eds. *A Manual for Acute Postoperative Pain Management*. New York: Raven Press.
21. Singelyn, F., et al. (1998). Effects of intravenous patient-controlled analgesia with morphine, continuous epidural analgesia, and continuous three-in-one block on postoperative pain and knee rehabilitation after unilateral total knee arthroplasty. *Anesthesia & Analgesia,* 87, 88-92.
22. Singelyn, F.J., et al. (2001). Extended femoral nerve sheath block after total hip arthroplasty: Continuous versus patient-controlled techniques. *Anesthesia & Analgesia,* 92, 455-9.
23. Weissman, S.L., and Scott III, J.F. (1992). Peripheral nerve blocks for use in acute pain. In: Sinatra, R.S., et al., eds. *Acute Pain: Mechanisms & Management*. St. Louis: Mosby Yearbook.
24. Werner, M.U., et al. (2002). Does an acute pain service improve postoperative outcome? *Anesthesia & Analgesia,* 95, 1361-72.
25. Woolf, C.J., and Chong, M.S. (1993). Preemptive analgesia: Treating postoperative pain by preventing the establishment of central sensitization. *Anesthesia & Analgesia,* 77, 362-79.

Additional Readings

Cousins, M.J., and Bridenbaugh, P.O. (1998). *Neural Blockade in Clinical Anesthesia and Management of Pain*. Philadelphia: J.B. Lippincott.

Morphet, S. (2000). Nerve blocks for anaesthesia and analgesia of the lower limb—A practical guide: femoral, lumbar plexus, sciatic. *Practical Procedures*. Available at: www.nda.ox.ac.uk/wfsa/htm/ull/u1112_01.htm). Accessed Sept. 26, 2003.

Meier, G., and Buttner, J. (2003). Pocket compendium of peripheral nerve blocks. *Regional Anaesthesia*. Munich: Arcus Publishing Company. Available at: www.anaesthesia-az.com.

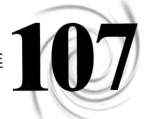
UNIT IV
Gastrointestinal System

SECTION SIXTEEN

Special Gastrointestinal Procedures

PROCEDURE **107**

Esophagogastric Tamponade Tube

PURPOSE: Esophagogastric tamponade therapy is used to provide temporary control of bleeding from gastric or esophageal varices.

Michael W. Day

PREREQUISITE NURSING KNOWLEDGE

- Tamponade therapy exerts direct pressure against the varices with the use of a gastric or esophageal balloon and may be used for cases unresponsive to medical therapy or those too hemodynamically unstable to undergo endoscopy and/or sclerotherapy.[1,2,3]
- Esophagogastric tamponade tubes are used to control bleeding from either gastric or esophageal varices. The suction lumens allow the evacuation of accumulated blood from the stomach or esophagus. The suction lumens also allow for the intermittent instillation of saline to assist in the evacuation of blood or clots.
- There are three types of tubes available for esophagogastric tamponade therapy. The two most common are the Sengstaken-Blakemore and the Minnesota tubes. The three-lumen Sengstaken-Blakemore tube (Fig. 107-1) has a gastric and esophageal balloon and a gastric suction lumen. The four-lumen Minnesota tube (Fig. 107-2) has gastric and esophageal balloons and separate gastric and esophageal suction lumens. The third, the Linton or Linton-Nachlas tube, has a gastric balloon and separate gastric and esophageal suction lumens and is used only for treatment of bleeding gastric varices. The Minnesota tube is considered the standard for esophagogastric tamponade therapy because it allows for suction above and below the balloons.[2,4]
- Esophagogastric tamponade tubes may be introduced by either the nasogastric or orogastric routes. The tubes are then advanced through the oropharynx and esophagus and into the stomach.

- Contraindications include esophageal strictures or recent esophageal surgery.[3]
- Because of the risk for aspiration, the patient may require endotracheal intubation (see Procedure 2) prior to placement of the tube.[1,2,3,5]
- Sedation should be considered[1] but should be minimal considering the possibility of liver damage and alterations in the metabolism of medications.[3]

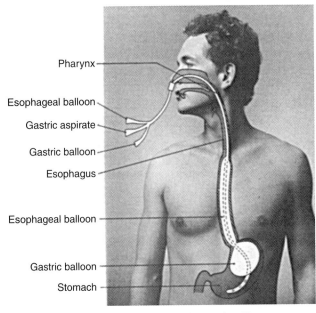

Pharynx

Esophageal balloon

Gastric aspirate

Gastric balloon

Esophagus

Esophageal balloon

Gastric balloon

Stomach

FIGURE 107-1 Sengstaken-Blakemore tube. *(From Swearingen, P.L. [1991]. Photo Atlas of Nursing Procedures. Reading, MA: Addison-Wesley.)*

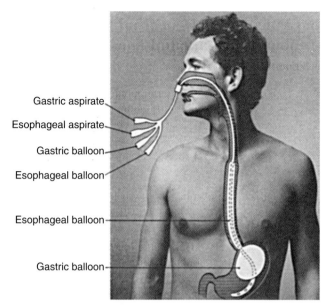

Gastric aspirate

Esophageal aspirate

Gastric balloon

Esophageal balloon

Esophageal balloon

Gastric balloon

FIGURE 107-2 Minnesota four-lumen tube. *(From Swearingen, P.L. [1991]. Photo Atlas of Nursing Procedures. Reading, MA: Addison-Wesley.)*

EQUIPMENT

- Tamponade tube (Sengstaken-Blakemore, Minnesota, or Linton-Nachlas)
- Irrigation kit (or catheter-tipped, 60-ml syringe and basin)
- Nasogastric (NG) tube(s)—one for Minnesota or Linton-Nachlas tube; two for Sengstaken-Blakemore tube
- Normal saline (NS) for irrigation
- Water-soluble lubricant
- Topical anesthetic agent
- Bite block or oral airway
- pH testing paper
- Sphygmomanometer or pressure gauge
- Four rubber-shod clamps
- Adhesive tape
- Two suction setups and tubing
- Endotracheal suction equipment
- Cardiac monitor
- Atropine or transcutaneous pacemaker
- Scissors to be kept at bedside
  Additional equipment (to have available based on patient need) includes the following:
- Rubber cube sponge (used for nasal intubation)
- Balanced suspension traction apparatus with 1 to 3 pounds of weights, or football helmet with face mask or guard
- Suture material to secure NG tube to the Sengstaken-Blakemore tube

PATIENT AND FAMILY EDUCATION

- Explain the reason and procedure for the tube insertion. ➵*Rationale:* Decreases patient anxiety.
- Explain the patient's role in assisting with the passage of the tube and maintenance of tamponade traction. ➵*Rationale:* Elicits patient cooperation during the insertion and tamponade therapy.

- Explain that the procedure can be uncomfortable, because the gag reflex may be stimulated, causing the patient to be nauseated or to vomit. ➵*Rationale:* Elicits patient cooperation during the insertion.

PATIENT ASSESSMENT AND PREPARATION

Patient Assessment

- Signs and symptoms of major blood loss
  - ❖ Tachycardia
  - ❖ Hypotension
  - ❖ Decreased urine output
  - ❖ Decreased filling pressures (PAP, PCWP, CVP)
  - ❖ Decreased platelets
  - ❖ Decreased hematocrit and hemoglobin
  ➵*Rationale:* Esophageal or gastric varices can cause significant blood loss.
- Baseline cardiac rhythm. ➵*Rationale:* Passage of a large-bore tube down the esophagus may cause vagal stimulation and bradycardia.
- Baseline respiratory status (i.e., rate, depth, pattern, and characteristics of secretions). ➵*Rationale:* Use of topical anesthetic agents in the nares or oropharynx may alter the gag or cough reflex, increasing the risk for aspiration. Passage of a large-bore tube may impair the airway. Large amounts of blood in the stomach predispose a patient to vomiting and potential aspiration.
- If anticipating nasal intubation:
  - ❖ Absolute contraindication: history of transphenoidal hypophysectomy. ➵*Rationale:* This type of surgical procedure may predispose placement of the tube into the cranial vault.
  - ❖ Assess for past medical history of nasal deformity, surgery, trauma, epistaxis, or coagulopathy. ➵*Rationale:* Increases the risk for complications and bleeding with nasal insertion.
  - ❖ Evaluate patency of nares. Occlude one naris at a time and ask the patient to breathe through the nose. Select the naris with the best air flow. ➵*Rationale:* Choosing the most patent naris will ease insertion and may improve patient tolerance of the tube.
  - ❖ Nausea or vomiting. ➵*Rationale:* Nausea or vomiting increases the risk for aspiration during insertion of the tube.
  - ❖ Mental status. ➵*Rationale:* Patients with altered mental status should be intubated prophylactically to prevent airway complications.

Patient Preparation

- Ensure that patient understands preprocedural teaching. Answer questions as they arise and reinforce information as needed. ➵*Rationale:* Evaluates and reinforces understanding of previously taught information.
- Measure the tube from the bridge of the nose to the earlobe to the tip of the xiphoid process (see Fig. 111-3). Mark the length of tube to be inserted. ➵*Rationale:* Estimating the

length of tube to be inserted will help place the distal tip in the stomach.

• If patient is alert, place him or her in high-Fowler or semi-Fowler position. If the patient is unconscious or obtunded, place patient head-down in the left lateral position. Cover the patient's chest with a towel. ➼*Rationale:* Facilitates the passage of the tube into the stomach and reduces the risk for aspiration.

Procedure for Inserting Esophagogastric Tamponade Tube

Steps	Rationale	Special Considerations
1. Wash hands and don personal protective equipment.	Reduces risk for transmission of microorganisms and body secretions; standard precautions.	
2. Attach the gastric balloon port to the sphygmomanometer or pressure gauge (Fig. 107-3).	Measuring the pressure of the gastric balloon as it is inflated immediately upon insertion may prevent its inflation in the esophagus, causing esophageal rupture.	
3. Test the tamponade tube balloon integrity:	Ensures integrity of esophageal balloon.[3,6,8,9]	
A. If applicable, inflate the esophageal balloon with the volume indicated in the package insert. *(Level I: Manufacturer's recommendation only.)*		
B. Inflate the gastric balloon with 100, 200, 300, 400, and 500 ml of air, noting the pressure reading at each stage of inflation. *(Level I: Manufacturer's recommendation only.)*	Knowing the pressure required at each stage of inflation may prevent inadvertent perforation of the esophagus after insertion.[6,8,9]	
C. Hold the air-filled balloon(s) under water to test for air leaks. *(Level I: Manufacturer's recommendation only.)*	Ensures integrity of balloon(s).[6,8,9]	
D. Actively and completely deflate the balloon(s) and clamp. *(Level I: Manufacturer's recommendation only.)*	Deflated balloon will ease insertion.	

Procedure continues on the following page

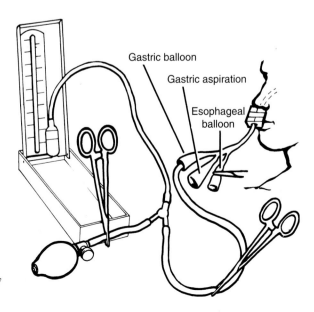

FIGURE 1O7-3 Inflation of esophageal balloon. *(Courtesy Davol, Inc.)*

Procedure for Inserting Esophagogastric Tamponade Tube

Steps	Rationale	Special Considerations
4. Insert a nasogastric tube (see Procedure 111), lavage the stomach, and remove tube. *(Level II: Theory-based, no research data to support recommendations; recommendations from expert consensus group may exist.)*	Emptying the stomach of blood will decrease the risk for aspiration and blocking the tube with blood clots.[3,4]	
5. Lubricate balloons and distal 15 cm of tube with water-soluble lubricant.	Minimizes mucosal injury and irritation during insertion; facilitates insertion.	Use only water-soluble lubricant. Oil-based lubricants, such as petroleum jelly, may cause respiratory complications if inadvertently aspirated.
6. Apply the topical anesthetic agent to the posterior oropharynx (and nostril if nasally inserted). *(Level IV: Limited clinical studies to support recommendations.)*	Decreases discomfort caused by insertion.[6,8,9]	Caution: gag and cough reflexes may be compromised by topical anesthetic, increasing the risk for aspiration. Keep emergency intubation equipment easily available.
7. Insert oral airway (see Procedure 9) or bite block. *(Level II: Theory-based, no research data to support recommendations; recommendations from expert consensus group may exist.)*	Prevents patient from biting on tube or inserter's fingers.	Remove dentures, if present.
8. Insert tube into mouth or selected nostril and advance into stomach to at least the 50 cm mark on the tube or 10 cm beyond the estimated length needed to reach the stomach. *(Level I: Manufacturer's recommendation only.)*	Ensures placement of entire gastric balloon in stomach.[6,8,9]	Heart rate may decrease as a result of vagal stimulation. Administer atropine or initiate transcutaneous pacing for symptomatic bradycardia. Nasal route is not recommended in patients with coagulopathy.[3]
9. Lavage stomach via gastric suction port with NS until clear of large blood clots. *(Level I: Manufacturer's recommendation only.)*	Ensures patency and prevents clots from blocking the tube.[6,8,9]	
10. Connect gastric suction port to intermittent suction at 60 to 120 mm Hg. *(Level II: Theory-based, no research data to support recommendations; recommendations from expert consensus group may exist.)*	Provides for evacuation of gastric contents and for assessment of continued bleeding.[3]	
11. Connect esophageal suction port to intermittent suction at 120 to 200 mm Hg (Minnesota tube only). *(Level II: Theory-based, no research data to support recommendations; recommendations from expert consensus may exist.)*	Provides for evacuation of secretions and for assessment of continued bleeding.	
12. Confirm tube placement: A. Aspirate drainage from gastric suction port. *(Level I: Manufacturer's recommendation only.)*	Prevents gastric balloon from being inflated in the esophagus, causing rupture. With pH testing, gastric placement will show a pH less than 5.5. Intestinal placement will show a pH greater than 6.0. Pulmonary secretions have an alkaline pH.[7]	The ability to simply aspirate fluid from the tube is often interpreted as confirmation of gastric intubation. Several reports[7,8] have shown that fluid can also be aspirated after endotracheal intubation. Common practice for many years has been to evaluate tube placement by placing a stethoscope over the stomach

Procedure for Inserting Esophagogastric Tamponade Tube—*Continued*		
Steps	**Rationale**	**Special Considerations**

		and instilling 20 to 50 ml of air via syringe. There are numerous reports in the literature of false-positive results using this method (see Procedure 111).
B. *Slowly* inflate the gastric balloon with increments of 100 ml of air, up to a total 500 ml, observing the pressure on the sphygmomanometer or pressure gauge at each increment. (If the pressure exceeds preinflation pressure for a particular volume by more than 15 mm Hg, withdraw all of the air and advance tube an additional 10 cm.) *(Level II: Theory-based, no research data to support recommendations; recommendations from expert consensus group may exist.)*	A pressure difference of more than 15 mm Hg indicates that the gastric balloon is in the esophagus.[4,6,8,9]	
C. Upon full inflation of the gastric balloon, clamp the gastric balloon lumen with a rubber-shod clamp. Obtain abdominal x-ray. *(Level II: Theory-based, no research data to support recommendations; recommendations from expert consensus group may exist.)*	Outline of gastric balloon can be visualized on x-ray. Ensures placement of entire gastric balloon with the stomach.[2-3,8-9]	
13. Upon x-ray confirmation of placement, withdraw the tube until slight resistance is met and double-clamp with rubber-shod clamp. *(Level I: Manufacturer's recommendation only.)*	Inflated balloon fills stomach and creates tamponade effect.[4,5] Positions gastric balloon at gastroesophageal junction.[4,5] Clamps prevent air leak from gastric balloon.[3,6,8,9]	
14. Place tape marker around tube as it exits the mouth or nose. *(Level III: Laboratory data, no clinical data to support recommendations.)*	Reference point to assess movement of tube.	
15. Inflate esophageal balloon if bleeding is not controlled by gastric tamponade.	Produces direct pressure on esophageal vessels.	Maintain esophageal balloon pressures as prescribed.
A. Clamp the tube and disconnect the sphygmomanometer or pressure gauge from the gastric balloon port and attach it to the esophageal balloon port. *(Level I: Manufacturer's recommendation only.)*		
B. Gradually inflate the esophageal balloon to 25 to 45 mm Hg. *(Level I: Manufacturer's recommendation only.)*	Higher pressures may cause esophageal necrosis.[4,6,8]	Patient may experience chest pain with inflation.
C. Double-clamp esophageal balloon port with rubber-shod clamps. *(Level I: Manufacturer's recommendation only.)*	Prevents air leaks from esophageal balloon.	
16. If bleeding has not stopped, apply gentle traction on the tube. *(Level II: Theory-based, no research data to support recommendations; recommendations from consensus group may exist.)*	Fixes position of gastric balloon and exerts pressure on varices.[3,6,8,9]	

Procedure continues on the following page

Procedure for Inserting Esophagogastric Tamponade Tube—*Continued*

Steps	Rationale	Special Considerations
A. Apply gentle traction with 1 to 3 pounds of weight attached to tube using balance suspension traction (Fig. 107-4). B. Tape tube to sponge cube at naris, if tube is passed nasally. Or C. Apply football helmet to patient and tape tube to chin or faceguard (Fig. 107-5).		Pad the inside of helmet to ensure a snug fit and to prevent pressure ulcer formation on back of head.[3]
17. Place the head of the bed at 30 to 45 degrees. *(Level IV: Limited clinical data support recommendations.)*	Promotes comfort and prevents aspiration.[8,9]	
18. Insert an NG tube (see Procedure 111) to just above esophageal balloon. (Sengstaken-Blakemore tube only). *(Level II: Theory-based, no research data to support recommendations; recommendations from expert consensus group may exist.)* A. Secure the NG tube to the tamponade tube with a suture where it exits the mouth. B. Connect to intermittent suction 120 to 200 mm Hg.	Removes secretions and accumulated blood.[3,6]	
Discontinuing Tamponade Therapy		
19. Discontinue tamponade therapy in stages. *(Level I: Manufacturer's recommendation only.)*	Provides for gradual reduction in tamponade in order to assess cessation of bleeding.[4]	Never deflate gastric balloon while esophageal balloon remains inflated. A deflated gastric balloon may allow an inflated esophageal

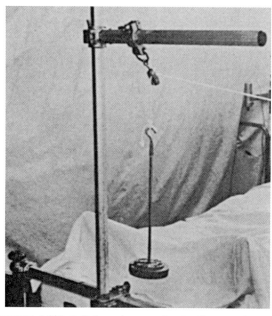

FIGURE 107-4 Balanced suspension traction securing tamponade tube and placement. *(From DeGroot, K.D., & Damato, M. [1987].* Critical Care Skills. *Norwalk, CT: Appleton & Lange.)*

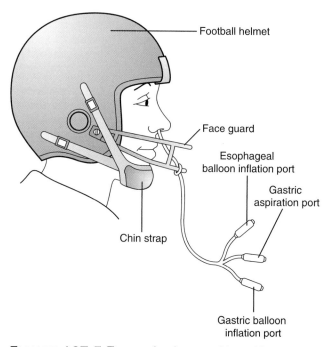

FIGURE 107-5 Tamponade tube secured in position with helmet.

Procedure **for Inserting Esophagogastric Tamponade Tube**—*Continued*

Steps	Rationale	Special Considerations
		balloon to migrate in the airway. *If the airway becomes obstructed, immediately cut both balloon ports to deflate the balloons and remove the tube immediately.*
A. Deflate esophageal balloon by unclamping the esophageal balloon port and aspirating with an irrigation syringe to actively deflate the balloon.		
B. Observe for the recurrence of bleeding over 24 hours. If bleeding recurs, reinflate the esophageal balloon.	Bleeding may recur with the release of pressure.[8]	
C. If no further bleeding is noted, deflate the gastric balloon by unclamping the gastric balloon port and aspirating with an irrigation syringe to actively deflate the balloon.		
D. Observe for the recurrence of bleeding over 24 hours. If bleeding recurs, reinflate the gastric balloon.	Bleeding may recur with the release of pressure on the gastric varices.[9]	
20. If bleeding has not recurred in 24 hours, cut the balloon lumens with scissors and remove tube slowly. *(Level II: Theory-based, no research data to support recommendations; recommendations from expert consensus group may exist.)*	Ensures complete balloon deflation before removal.[9]	

Expected Outcomes	Unexpected Outcomes
• Cessation of variceal bleeding • Gastric decompression and evacuation	• Inappropriate placement of tamponade tube • Gastric or esophageal necrosis • Esophageal rupture • Airway obstruction • Cardiac dysrhythmias (during insertion or removal) • Aspiration of gastric or oropharyngeal contents • Erosion of mucosa around nares

Patient Monitoring and Care

Steps	Rationale	Reportable Conditions
		These conditions should be reported if they persist despite nursing interventions. • Continued bleeding
1. Maintain tamponade therapy as needed: maximum of 24 to 36 hours for esophageal balloon; 48 to 72 hours for gastric balloon. *(Level II: Theory-based, no research data to support recommendations; recommendations from expert consensus group may exist.)*	Longer inflation time may cause necrosis or ulceration.[6,8]	

Procedure continues on the following page

Patient Monitoring and Care—*Continued*

Steps	Rationale	Reportable Conditions
2. Provide nares care every 2 hours when tube is inserted nasally. A. Remove dried blood or secretions from nasal orifice and proximal nares. B. Apply lubricating ointment or gel to keep mucosa moist.	Prevents drying and ulcerations of mucosa.	• Breakdown of tissue around nares
3. Provide oral care every 2 hours. Swab mouth with cleansing agents and mechanical debriders.	Prevents drying and ulcerations of mucosa.	• Mouth, tongue, or lip ulcerations
4. Provide frequent oral suctioning. *(Level II: Theory-based, no research data to support recommendations; recommendations from expert consensus group may exist.)*	Esophageal balloon prevents swallowing of secretions and saliva.[6]	• Bloody oral secretions
5. Monitor esophageal balloon pressure hourly. Maintain esophageal balloon pressures at 25 to 45 mm Hg (pressures will vary with respirations and may intermittently reach 70 mm Hg). *(Level II: Theory-based, no research data to support recommendations; recommendations from expert consensus group may exist.)*	Prevents excessive pressure on esophageal tissues.[6] Sudden loss of pressure may indicate rupture of balloon or esophagus.	• Continued esophageal bleeding • Sudden loss of balloon pressure
6. Decrease esophageal balloon pressure by 5 mm Hg every 3 hours until pressure is 25 mm Hg, without evidence of bleeding. *(Level II: Theory-based, no research data to support recommendations; recommendations from expert consensus group may exist.)*	Using the lowest possible pressure to create tamponade effect will reduce the possibility of necrosis.[8]	• Continued esophageal bleeding
7. Completely deflate the esophageal balloon for 30 minutes every 8 hours. *(Level II: Theory-based, no research data to support recommendations; recommendations from expert consensus group may exist.)*	Intermittent relief of the pressure may prevent necrosis of esophageal tissue.[3]	• Continued esophageal bleeding
8. Evaluate for recurrence of variceal bleeding. *(Level II: Theory-based, no research data to support recommendations; recommendations from expert consensus group may exist.)*	Bleeding may occur despite tamponade therapy.	• Continued bleeding
9. Monitor for airway patency and respiratory status. *(Level II: Theory-based, no research data to support recommendations; recommendations from expert consensus group may exist.)*	Presence or movement of a large-bore tube may impair the upper airway.	• Tachypnea • Stridor • Cough
10. Keep scissors at the bedside to immediately deflate the balloons. *(Level II: Theory-based, no research data to support recommendations; recommendations from expert consensus group may exist.)*	Inadvertent deflation of the gastric balloon may allow blockage of the airway by the esophageal balloon.[3,4]	

Patient Monitoring and Care—*Continued*

Steps	Rationale	Reportable Conditions
11. Obtain a abdominal x-ray every 24 hours or sooner if there is any indication of displacement of the tube.[3] *(Level II: Theory-based, no research data to support recommendations; recommendations from expert consensus group may exist.)*	Inadvertent deflation of the gastric balloon may allow blockage of the airway by the esophageal balloon.[3,4]	
12. Monitor gastric output. Irrigate gastric suction port with 50 ml of NS every 30 minutes, or as needed, to keep lumen patent. *(Level I: Manufacturer's recommendation only.)*	Blood clots may occlude the gastric lumen.[6]	• Continued gastric bleeding • Change in characteristics of output (color, quantity)
13. Monitor esophageal output. Irrigate esophageal suction port (or NG with Sengstaken-Blakemore) with 5 to 10 ml of NS every 2 to 4 hours, or as needed, to keep patent. *(Level I: Manufacturer's recommendation only.)*	Blood clots may occlude the esophageal suction lumen (or NG tube).[6]	• Continued esophageal bleeding • Change in characteristics of drainage (color, quantity)

Documentation

Documentation should include the following:

- Patient and family education
- Date and time of insertion
- Name of provider inserting tube, if other than nurse documenting
- Tube type
- Any difficulties with insertion
- Patient tolerance of insertion, including pressures with specific balloon volumes
- Confirmation of placement by pH testing paper and abdominal x-ray
- Type and maintenance of traction device
- Amount and type of suction applied to various lumens

- Esophageal or gastric balloon pressures
- Periodic deflation of esophageal balloon
- Appearance and volume of gastric and esophageal drainage, if present
- Nasal or oral care
- Maintenance of traction
- Tube site assessments (nasal or oral)
- Unexpected outcomes
- Nursing interventions
- Deflation sequence of tubes

References

1. Bass, N.M., and Yao, F.Y. (2003). Portal hypertension and variceal bleeding. In: Feldman, M., Friedman, L.S., and Sleisenger, M.H., eds. *Sleisenger and Fordtran's Gastrointestinal and Liver Disease: Pathophysiology/Diagnosis/Management.* 7th ed. Philadelphia: W.B. Saunders, 1487-1575.
2. Barefield, L.B. (October 7, 1998). Personal communication.
3. Chung, R.T., and Podolsky, D.K. (2001). Cirrhosis and its complications. In: Brunwald, E., et al., eds. *Harrison's Principles of Internal Medicine.* 15th ed. New York: McGraw-Hill, 1754-66.
4. Davol, Inc. (1985). *Blakemore Esophageal-Nasogastric Tube: Instructions for Passing the Esophageal Balloon for the Control of Bleeding for Esophageal Varices.* Cranston, RI: Author.
5. Davol, Inc. (1985). *Minnesota Four Lumen Esophagogastric Tamponade Tube for Control of Bleeding from Esophageal Varices.* Cranston, RI: Author.

6. Gow, J.P., and Chapman, R.W. (2001). Modern management of oesophageal varices. *Postgrad Med J,* 77, 75-81.
7. Metheny, N., et al. (1993). Effectiveness of pH measurements in predicting feeding tube placement: An update. *Nurs Res,* 43, 324-31.
8. Pavini, M.T., and Puyana, J.C. (2003). Management of acute esophageal variceal hemorrhage with gastroesophageal balloon tamponade. In: Irwin, R.S., and Rippe, J.M., eds. *Irwin and Rippe's Intensive Care Medicine.* 5th ed. Philadelphia: Lippincott Williams & Wilkins, 171-6.
9. Stacy, K.M. (2002). Gastrointestinal disorders and therapeutic management. In: Urban, L.D., Stacy, K.M., and Lough, M.E., eds. *Thelan's Critical Care Nursing: Diagnosis and Management.* 4th ed. St. Louis: Mosby, 807-27.

Additional Reading

Harry, R., and Wendon, J. (2002). Management of variceal bleeding. *Curr Opin Crit Care,* 8, 164-70.

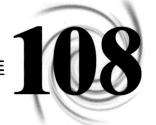
PROCEDURE **108**

Gastric Lavage in Hemorrhage and Overdose

PURPOSE: In hemorrhage, gastric lavage is used to localize the site and severity of upper gastrointestinal (GI) bleeding, monitor for continued bleeding, cleanse the stomach of blood and clots in preparation for endoscopy or endoscopic treatments (such as scleral therapy), decrease or prevent absorption of a high nitrogen load, and prevent aspiration of blood. In overdose, gastric lavage is used to evacuate drugs or toxins and therefore prevent or minimize both the serious consequences of systemic absorption of drugs or toxins and damage to the GI tissue.

JoAnne K. Phillips

PREREQUISITE NURSING KNOWLEDGE

- The potential benefit of gastric lavage is noted in two different patient populations: the patient experiencing gastrointestinal (GI) hemorrhage and the patient who has ingested a potentially life threatening amount of poison.
  - ❖ GI hemorrhage: The patient who has experienced a major GI hemorrhage may present with signs and symptoms of volume loss, as well as a decrease in oxygen-carrying capacity. These symptoms include tachycardia, hypotension, decreased hemodynamic filling pressures, pallor, cold and clammy skin, and decreased urine output. The benefit of lavage in GI hemorrhage is to empty the stomach of blood and clots to facilitate evaluation of the source of bleeding. Gastric lavage is accomplished by instilling large amounts of neutral fluid (normal saline or tap water) and draining the gastric contents and lavage fluid out. Patients with esophageal varices or a recent history of GI surgery should be carefully evaluated for the risk/benefit ratio before gastric lavage is performed.[6]
  - ❖ Overdose: The second indication for gastric lavage is in the patient who is suspected of ingesting a life-threatening amount of drug or toxin. The American Academy of Clinical Toxicology does not recommend the use of gastric lavage in the management of poison unless the procedure can be done within 60 minutes of ingestion and the patient has taken a potentially

life-threatening amount of poison.[1,2,8,12,13] Indications for performing gastric lavage after 60 minutes include the ingestion of enteric-coated, sustained-release, or long-acting medication or in patients with decreased GI motility.[3] Gastric lavage is contraindicated if the patient has consumed strong corrosives or hydrocarbons (e.g., gasoline). Several methods may be used to remove drugs or toxins from the GI tract. In addition to gastric lavage, induced vomiting, the administration of activated charcoal, and whole bowel irrigation may play a role. The administration of activated charcoal in addition to gastric lavage must be approached cautiously, because it may result in an increase risk for aspiration, increased rate of intubation, and increase in admissions to the intensive care unit.[4]

- Gastric lavage following overdose or toxin ingestion has variable efficacy. The amount of toxin or drug recovered depends on variables such as time from ingestion, whether liquid or pills were ingested, specific agent ingested, and size of lavage tube used. Even if lavage is performed close to the time of ingestion, not all the ingested toxin will be recovered.

- As with GI hemorrhage, ravaging or cleansing of the stomach is accomplished by instilling large amounts of neutral fluid (normal saline or tap water) into the stomach and then draining the gastric contents and lavage fluid out of the stomach.

- Nonintubated patients who require gastric lavage must be alert and have adequate pharyngeal and laryngeal reflexes.

If the patient is not able to protect his or her airway, he or she should be intubated before gastric lavage is performed.[12] All patients undergoing gastric lavage should be positioned in the left lateral or semi-Fowler position to prevent aspiration. If the gag reflex is not intact, the patient should be endotracheally intubated before gastric lavage is attempted.[12]

- Passage of the lavage tube may cause vagal stimulation and precipitate bradydysrhythmias.

EQUIPMENT

- Lavage tube
  - ❖ Number 32- to 40-Fr gastric tube (e.g., Ewald)[15] *or*
  - ❖ Number 16- to 18-Fr gastric tube or sump tube
- Irrigating kit with 50- to 60-ml irrigating syringe
- Water-soluble lubricant
- Lavage fluid (NS or tap water)
- Disposable basin for aspirate
- Suction source and connecting tubing
- Rigid pharyngeal suction-tip (Yankauer) catheter
- Topical anesthetic agent
- Bite block or oral airway
- Stethoscope
- Emergency intubation equipment
- Endotracheal suction equipment
- Cardiac monitor
- Pulse oximeter
- Automatic blood pressure cuff
- Nonsterile gloves
- Eye and face protection
- Barrier gowns

  Additional equipment (to have available based on patient need) includes the following:
- Specimen container for aspirate (for overdose)
- Absorptive agent for instillation (for overdose, if prescribed)
- Emergency medications

PATIENT AND FAMILY EDUCATION

- Explain the indications and procedure for gastric lavage. ➤*Rationale:* Decreases patient and family anxiety.
- Explain the patient's role in assisting with passage of the tube and lavage of the stomach. ➤*Rationale:* Elicits patient's cooperation during the procedure.
- Explain the purpose of the cardiac monitor, automatic blood pressure cuff, and pulse oximeter. ➤*Rationale:* Decreases patient and family anxiety.
- Evaluate patient and family need for information on prevention of accidental ingestion of drugs or toxic agents. ➤*Rationale:* Patient and family may be unaware or uninformed that the agent or drug is (potentially) toxic.
- Evaluate patient and family need for information on emergency treatment for accidental ingestion of drug or toxic agents. ➤*Rationale:* Emergency first aid measures

may be helpful with some ingestions to decrease potential toxicity or systemic absorption.

PATIENT ASSESSMENT AND PREPARATION

Patient Assessment

- Baseline respiratory, cardiovascular, and neurologic assessments; hemodynamic status; cardiac rhythm; and vital signs. ➤*Rationale:* Passage of the lavage tube may cause vagal stimulation and precipitate bradydysrhythmias. In the overdose patient, toxic levels of certain classes of drugs (e.g., tricyclic antidepressants) can cause electrocardiogram (ECG) changes. Gastric lavage has been shown to cause ECG changes.[3,18]
- Baseline pulse oximetry. ➤*Rationale:* Gastric lavage has been shown to cause changes in oxygen saturation.
- Signs and symptoms of major blood loss, are as follows:
  - ❖ Tachycardia
  - ❖ Hypotension
  - ❖ Decreased hemodynamic filling pressures
  - ❖ Pallor, cold and clammy skin
  - ❖ Decreased urine output.
  ➤*Rationale:* Esophageal or gastric varices can cause significant blood loss.
- History of esophageal varices, recent esophageal or gastric surgery. ➤*Rationale:* Varices or recent surgery may predispose the patient to complications during tube insertion.
- Baseline coagulation studies, hematocrit and hemoglobin, and liver function tests (GI hemorrhage patient and overdose cases where toxin ingested is liver toxic). ➤*Rationale:* Provides for baseline information so that patient progress can be more accurately monitored.
- Adequacy of gag reflex. ➤*Rationale:* For the overdose patient, induced vomiting may be the treatment of choice if the patient is alert and awake with an adequate gag reflex, making lavage unnecessary. Lack of an adequate gag reflex will indicate the need for endotracheal intubation prior to beginning lavage.
- Type of drugs or toxic substances ingested, as well as quantity ingested (for the overdose patient). ➤*Rationale:* Certain substances may require neutralization before attempting tube evacuation. A poison control center should be contacted if the practitioner is unsure that lavage is indicated. Side effects can be anticipated if the drugs or toxins that were swallowed and the quantity are known.
- Careful skin assessment (overdose patient). ➤*Rationale:* May give evidence regarding route (needle tracks) and name of drug or toxin ingested. Various drugs can cause cutaneous changes. Changes to look for include diaphoresis, bullae, acneiform rash, flushed appearance, and cyanosis.
- Odors present (overdose patient). ➤*Rationale:* Some toxins have a distinctive odor, aiding in identification of substance ingested.
- 12-lead ECG. ➤*Rationale:* For the overdose victim, the drug or toxin ingested may be cardiotoxic. For the patient

with a GI hemorrhage, co-morbid disease states may increase risk for tissue hypoxia and ischemia.

- Serum toxicology screen, urinalysis and urine toxicology screen, and anion gap (overdose victim). ➤*Rationale:* Provides baseline information for diagnosis so that intervention can be made appropriately and patient progress can be more accurately monitored.
- Arterial blood gas (ABG). ➤*Rationale:* Overdose victims with hypoventilation and GI hemorrhage patients with significant blood loss or comorbid disease are at risk for hypoxia, hypercapnea, and/or acid-base disorders.

Patient Preparation

- Ensure that patient understands preprocedural teaching. Answer questions as they arise and reinforce information as needed. ➤*Rationale:* Evaluates and reinforces understanding of previously taught information.

- Place the patient on a cardiac monitor, automatic blood pressure cuff, and pulse oximeter. Set up oropharyngeal suction. ➤*Rationale:* Allows for close cardiovascular and respiratory monitoring during the procedure and makes suction available for procedure.
- Establish and maintain intravenous (IV) access. For the GI hemorrhage patient, two large-bore (18-G or larger) IVs are essential. ➤*Rationale:* IV access is necessary for emergency IV medication administration and volume resuscitation in the case of GI hemorrhage.
- Position patient in left lateral or semi-Fowler position. ➤*Rationale:* Facilitates passage of the tube into the stomach. The left lateral position is the position of choice to prevent aspiration if the patient should vomit.
- Apply oxygen by nasal prongs or mask (GI hemorrhage patient or overdose patient as indicated). ➤*Rationale:* Supplemental oxygen will optimize the patient's oxygen saturation.

Procedure for Gastric Lavage in Hemorrhage and Overdose

Steps	Rationale	Special Considerations
1. Wash hands and don nonsterile gloves, eye and face protection, and a barrier gown.	Reduces transmission of microorganisms; standard precautions.	
2. Coat 6 to 10 cm of the distal end of the lavage tube with water-soluble lubricant.	Minimizes mucosal injury and irritation during insertion of the tube.	
3. Place the bed in a semi-Fowler's position with the head of the bed up 10-20 degrees, a slight reverse Trendelenburg. Place the patient in the left lateral decubitus position.	The left lateral decubitus position maximizes access to the stomach and minimizes pyloric emptying.[15,18] The slight reverse Trendelenburg position will also decrease movement of stomach contents into the duodenum.	Ensure adequate ventilation and oxygenation while the patient is positioned for gastric lavage.
4. Insert a large orogastric tube (see Procedure 111).	A large-bore Ewald tube (number 32 to 40 Fr) is preferred for the evacuation of blood, clots, undigested pills, or pill fragments. A smaller-bore tube may become occluded with solid material. A smaller-bore tube may be used with liquid poisons.[7]	Do not pass nasally, because severe nasal trauma may occur. If the patient does not have an intact gag reflex, endotracheal intubation should be done first.[3,12]
A. Measure distance from patient's bridge of nose to ear and then from earlobe to tip of xiphoid process (see Fig. 111-3). Mark this distance on the tube.		
B. Anesthetize posterior oropharynx with topical anesthetic agent, as ordered.	Decreases discomfort caused by passing tube.	The gag reflex may be compromised by topical anesthesia, increasing the risk for aspiration. Have emergency intubation equipment available.
C. Insert oral airway (see Procedure 9) or bite block.	Prevents patients from biting on tube or inserter's fingers.	Remove patient dentures.
D. Position tube toward posterior pharynx over tongue.		Heart rate may decrease as a result of vagal stimulation,

Procedure for Gastric Lavage in Hemorrhage and Overdose—*Continued*

Steps	Rationale	Special Considerations
		especially if the patient has ingested toxic amounts of digoxin. Have atropine (or transcutaneous pacer) ready and use as necessary. Have oropharyngeal suction available.
E. Pass tube slowly into stomach (approximately 20 in). Encourage patient to attempt to swallow while passing tube.	Rapid passage of tube may stimulate vomiting and increase risk of aspiration.	
Or		
5. Insert (number 16 to 18 Fr) gastric tube or sump (see Procedure 111).	The larger lumen (18 Fr) helps prevent the drainage ports from becoming occluded with clots or pill fragments. In overdose, a smaller lumen may be used with ingestion of liquid agents or liquefied tablets or capsules.	
6. Aspirate with syringe for return of stomach contents. The aspirate can be tested with pH paper to confirm gastric placement (acid pH).[11] *(Level V: Clinical studies in more than one patient population and situation.)*	The position of the lavage tube must be confirmed to be in the stomach because of the risk for endotracheal placement of the lavage tube and subsequent pulmonary complications. X-ray confirmation of lavage tube placement has been suggested in the literature.[14] With pH testing, gastric placement will often show a pH less than 5.5. Intestinal placement will usually show a pH greater than 6.0. Pulmonary secretions have an alkaline pH.[11] A pH test strip with multiple comparative color columns increases the probability of obtaining accurate pH estimation. A test strip with a wide range (such as 1 to 10) is preferred.	
7. After placement is confirmed, aspirate gastric contents through lavage tube using irrigating syringe.	Manual aspiration will withdraw gastric contents and toxic agents or blood and clots out of the stomach.	In cases of overdose, save specimen in specimen container and send to laboratory for analysis.
8. Perform intermittent lavage (using either room-temperature saline or tap water). *(Level III: Laboratory data, no clinical data to support recommendations.)*	In overdose, lavage aids in diluting toxic agents and removing them from the stomach before absorption. In GI hemorrhage, lavage aids in breaking up clots and rinsing the stomach of blood. Removing blood clots by lavage may be helpful in allowing the stomach to contract and tamponade bleeding vessels.[9] Room-temperature solutions have been shown to be effective in clearing the stomach of clots and promoting hemostasis.[4,5]	No benefit has been shown in using iced saline over room temperature tap water or saline for lavage with GI bleeding.[16,17] However, use of NS may lead to hypernatremia in patients with renal failure.[7]
A. Instill lavage fluid into lavage tube using irrigating syringe (for adults, use 100 to 150 ml of fluid[7]).		For the elderly patient, the lavage fluid should be slightly warmed to prevent hypothermia. (Bottles of NS may be submerged in warm water before use as an irrigant.)

Procedure continues on the following page

Procedure for Gastric Lavage in Hemorrhage and Overdose—*Continued*

Steps	Rationale	Special Considerations
B. Aspirate gastric contents through lavage tube using irrigating syringe. *Or*	Evacuates stomach contents and clots or ingested toxic agents.	The amount returned should equal the amount instilled.
C. Connect lavage tube to less than 80 mm Hg suction (GI hemorrhage patient).	Low levels of suction should be used to prevent suction-induced mucosal damage.	
D. For GI hemorrhage patients, continue intermittent lavage until returns are clear and free of clots.	In GI hemorrhage lavage, it aids in breaking up clots and rinsing the stomach of blood. Room-temperature solutions have been shown to be effective in clearing the stomach of clots and promoting hemostasis.[5] No benefit has been shown in using iced saline over room-temperature tap water or saline for lavage with GI bleeding.[12,17]	The lavage fluid should be slightly warmed in the elderly patient to prevent hypothermia. (A fluid or blood warmer may be used to warm the irrigant as it infuses.) The use of NS may lead to hypernatremia in patients with renal failure.[7]
E. In the overdose patient, once returns are clear, continue lavage using an additional 1 to 2 L of fluid. *(Level IV: Limited clinical studies to support recommendations.)*	In overdose patients, performing gastric lavage with an additional 1 to 2 L after the aspirate is clear has been shown to allow recovery of more of the ingested materials as compared with lavage only until the aspirate is clear.[19] In overdose, lavage also aids in diluting toxic agents and removing them from the stomach before absorption.	
9. Remove orogastric tube, if indicated. If the lavage tube is not able to be removed easily, the patient may be experiencing esophageal spasm and the tube may be impacted. *(Level IV: Limited clinical studies to support recommendations.)*	Glucagon, given either via the subcutaneous or intramuscular route, can decrease esophageal spasm and allow removal of impacted lavage tubes. Contraindications to the use of glucagon include a history of pheochromocytoma, insulinoma, or Zollinger-Ellison syndrome.[17]	
A. Clamp lavage tube with rubber-shod clamp.	Prevents leakage of contents remaining within lumen and possible aspiration of contents during removal.	
B. Pull tube out slowly and steadily.	Minimizes risk for vomiting.	
10. Insert nasogastric (NG) tube, if needed (see Procedure 111). For the overdose patient, instill medications as ordered. The NG tube should be clamped after medication instillation.	For the overdose victim, an NG tube provides access to the stomach for administration of activated charcoal. Activated charcoal is used for absorption of the residual substance ingested (unable to be removed by lavage). If the patient is alert and has an intact gag reflex, activated charcoal can be swallowed.	NG tube should be inserted in all patients with upper GI bleeding to decompress the stomach. The data do not suggest that insertion of an NG tube will initiate or potentiate bleeding in patients with esophageal varices.[10]
For the GI hemorrhage patient, the tube may be connected to suction.	For the GI hemorrhage patient, the NG tube may also allow for close assessment of further bleeding. However, the presence of an NG tube can cause further mucosal damage during insertion or if connected to suction.	

Procedure for Gastric Lavage in Hemorrhage and Overdose—*Continued*

Steps	Rationale	Special Considerations
11. Dispose of equipment in appropriate receptacle.	Standard precautions.	
12. Remove barrier gown, face and eye protection, and gloves. Wash hands.	Reduces transmission of microorganisms.	
13. Document procedure in patient record.		

Expected Outcomes

- Evacuation of blood and clots from the stomach
- Prevention of blood aspiration
- Prevention of absorption of high nitrogen load
- Prevention or minimization of systemic complications secondary to the absorption of drugs or toxic agents
- Minimization of mucosal damage by toxic agents

Unexpected Outcomes

- Endotracheal intubation rather than gastric intubation with lavage tube
- Esophageal perforation
- Trauma to the nose, throat, or esophagus
- Epistaxis if NG route is used for lavage
- Hypothermia in the elderly patient
- Bradydysrhythmias
- Pulmonary aspiration of gastric contents
- Movement of gastric contents into the duodenum, potentially increasing the amount of toxin absorbed
- Fluid and electrolyte imbalance
- Laryngospasm
- Hypoxia/hypercapnia
- Combative behavior[1,2]

Patient Monitoring and Care

Steps	Rationale	Reportable Conditions
		These conditions should be reported if they persist despite nursing interventions.
1. Monitor vital signs every 15 minutes throughout the procedure and every hour following lavage for at least 4 hours or longer, depending on patient condition.	Continued blood loss or side effects of drugs or toxins ingested may cause changes in vital signs. Cold lavage fluid may cause hypothermia in the elderly patient.	• Increase in heart rate 10 to 20 beats above baseline • Decrease in blood pressure 20 to 30 mm Hg below baseline • Respiratory rate lower than 8 or higher than 24 breaths per minute • Temperature lower than 97.5°F (36.5°C) or higher than 101°F (38°C)
2. Monitor neurologic status continuously throughout procedure and after lavage.	Side effects from toxic agents ingested or significant blood loss may lead to decrease in level of consciousness.	• Decreasing level of consciousness • Loss of gag reflex
3. Monitor respiratory status continuously throughout procedure and after lavage: A. Pulse oximetry B. Respiratory rate C. Work of breathing	Aspiration is a potential complication because of change in level of consciousness, loss of gag reflex, or vomiting. Pulse oximetry values have been shown to decrease during gastric lavage, especially in older smokers.[3]	• Decrease in oximetry below baseline, or 92% • Increase in respiratory rate above baseline • Complaints of shortness of breath
4. Monitor cardiac status continuously throughout procedure and after lavage: A. Heart rate	Bradydysrhythmias may be caused by passage of the lavage tube. Toxic effect of drugs ingested may also cause ECG changes,	• Heart rate less than 60 beats per minute with or without a decrease in blood pressure below baseline

Procedure continues on the following page

Patient Monitoring and Care—*Continued*

Steps	Rationale	Reportable Conditions
B. Heart rhythm C. ECG intervals D. Signs and symptoms of decreased cardiac output	including prolongation of the PR, QRS, and QT intervals. ECG changes have been shown during gastric lavage, especially in older smokers.[3]	• Chest pain, diaphoresis, change in level of consciousness, and shortness of breath • Change in ECG rhythm or length of PR, QRS, and QT intervals from baseline
5. Assess for normal pharyngeal function. After lavage, keep patient in left lateral position with slight head elevation until normal gag reflex returns.	Topical anesthesia will decrease the gag reflex and increase the risk for aspiration. The left lateral position is the position of choice to prevent aspiration should the patient not be able to control secretions or emesis.	• Prolonged absence of gag reflex
6. For the GI hemorrhage patient A. Measure blood volume loss.	Aids in assessment of fluid balance and fluid resuscitation requirements.	• Bright red emesis or bleeding from the lavage tube or NG tube
B. Monitor for recurrence of bleeding, color, and consistency of gastric drainage, serial hemoglobin and hematocrit, postural vital signs, urine output, and change in level of consciousness.	Bleeding may recur. Be aware that a decrease in hemoglobin value may be delayed after an acute bleed.	• Decrease in hemoglobin or hematocrit below baseline. • Decrease in blood pressure 20 to 30 mm Hg below baseline • Increase in pulse 10 to 20 beats per minute above baseline • Urine output less than 30 ml/hr • Increasing confusion or decreasing level of consciousness
C. Administer NS or lactated Ringer's injection at 150 to 200 ml/hr. Switch to administration of packed cells when available for volume replacement.	Replaces volume and prevents hemorrhagic shock. If blood is not readily available, resuscitate with NS; 300 ml of NS for every 100 ml of estimated blood lost.	• Continued bleeding
D. Administer antacids, histamine$_2$ (H$_2$) blockers, sucralfate, or proton pump inhibitors (PPI) as ordered by physician or advanced practice nurse.	Antacids neutralize gastric acid. H$_2$ blockers decrease gastric acid secretion. Sucralfate reacts with gastric acid, forming a paste, which adheres to ulcer sites. PPI's inhibits the proton pump in the parietal cells of the stomach, suppressing gastric acid secretion.	
E. If clinically indicated, evaluate blood ammonia levels in patients with liver failure.	The ammonia level provides an estimate of the nitrogen load that has been absorbed and helps determine the need for agents (e.g., Lactulose) to prevent the absorption of ammonia from the bowel.	• Rising serum ammonia level • Increasing confusion or decreasing level of consciousness
7. For the overdose victim A. Evaluate the patient's need for follow-up psychiatric support for suicide ideation. B. Institute suicide precautions until patient has been cleared by psychiatric services. This includes removal of objects from patient's room that could be used by patient to harm self.	The drug or toxin ingestion may be a result of suicidal ideations.	• Patient reporting intent to harm self • Patient reporting that ingestion was a suicide attempt

Patient Monitoring and Care—*Continued*

Steps	Rationale	Reportable Conditions
C. In the hours and days following ingestion, repeat laboratory tests, including electrolytes, glucose, blood urea nitrogen and creatinine, liver function, and drug or toxin levels.	Laboratory tests ordered will depend on the drug or toxins ingested. Lavage may cause electrolyte abnormalities. Liver function tests may be necessary if the drug is toxic to the liver. Drug or toxin level tests will validate the clearance of the drug or toxin from the patient's system.	• Deviation of test results outside normal limits

Documentation

Documentation should include the following:

- Patient and family education
- History of ingestion of drug or toxin *or* upper GI bleeding
- Date, time, and reason for lavage
- Type and size of lavage tube inserted
- Patient tolerance of tube placement and lavage procedure
- Verification of lavage tube placement (method used)
- Type and amount of lavage fluid used
- Unexpected outcomes

- Nursing interventions
- Amount and characteristics of aspirate
- Assessment of gastric drainage after lavage
- Name and dose of medications given after the lavage
- Aspirated specimen sent to laboratory for analysis
- Size of NG tube inserted after lavage
- Patient tolerance of NG tube insertion
- Referral to psychiatry if suicide is suspected

References

1. American Academy of Toxicology. *Position Statement: Gastric Lavage.* Available at: www.clintox.org. Accessed July 14, 2003.
2. American Academy of Toxicology. *Position Statement: Single Dose Activated Charcoal.* Available at: www.clintox.org. Accessed July 14, 2003.
3. Blazys, D. (2000). Use of lavage in treating overdose. *J Emerg Nurs,* 26, 343.
4. Bond, G.R. (2002). The role of activated charcoal and gastric emptying in gastrointestinal decontamination. *Ann Emerg Med,* 39, 273.
5. Bryant, L.R., et al. (1972). Comparison of ice water with iced saline solution for gastric lavage in gastroduodenal hemorrhage. *Am J Surg,* 124, 570-2.
6. Conrad, S. (2002). Acute upper gastrointestinal bleeding in critically ill patients: Causes and treatment modalities. *Crit Care Med,* 30, S365.
7. Grierson, R., et al. (2000). Gastric lavage for liquid poisons. *Ann Emerg Med,* 35, 435.
8. Jones, A.L., and Volans, G. (1999). Management of self-poisoning. *BMJ,* 319, 1414.
9. Krumberger, J.M., and Hammer, B. (1998). GI disorders. In: McKinney, M.R., et al., eds. *AACN Clinical Reference for Critical Care.* 4th ed. Philadelphia: Mosby.
10. Marik, P.E. (2001). Management of GI bleed. In: *Handbook of Evidence-Based Medicine.* New York: Springer.
11. Metheny, N., et al. (1993). Effectiveness of pH measurements in predicting feeding tube placement: An update. *Nurs Res,* 43, 324-31.
12. Mokhlesi, B., et al. (2003). Adult toxicology in critical care: Part I: General approaches to the intoxicated patient. *Chest,* 123, 577.

13. Riordan, M., Rylance, G., and Berry, K. (2002). Poisoning in children 1: General management. *Arch Dis Child,* 87, 392.
14. Sabga, E., et al. (1997). Direct administration of charcoal into the lung and pleural cavity. *Ann Emerg Med,* 30, 695-7.
15. Shannon, M. (2000). Primary care: Ingestion of toxic substances by children. *N Engl J Med,* 342, 186.
16. Stotland, B.R., and Ginsberg, G.G. (2001). Upper GI bleeding. In: Lanken, P.N., ed. *The ICU Manual.* Philadelphia: W.B. Saunders.
17. Thoma, M.A., and Glauser, J.M. (1995). Use of glucagon for removal of an orogastric lavage tube. *Am J Emerg Med,* 13, 219-22.
18. Tucker, J.R. (2000). Indications for, techniques of, complications of, and efficacy of gastric lavage in the treatment of the poisoned child. *Curr Opin Peds,* 12, 163.
19. Weinman, S.A. (1993). Emergency management of drug overdose. *Crit Care Nurse,* 13, 45-51.

Additional Readings

Bitterman, R.A. (1989). Upper gastrointestinal hemorrhage. *Emerg Med,* 21, 77-8, 83-4, 86.
Erickson, T.B. (1996). Dealing with the unknown overdose. *Emerg Med,* 28, 74, 79-83, 84, 86-8.
Harris, C.R., and Kingston, R. (1992). Gastrointestinal decontamination: Which method is best? *Postgrad Med,* 92, 116, 118-22, 125, 128.
Hoffman, R. (1992). Choices in gastric decontamination. *Emerg Med,* 24, 212, 214, 217, 221-4.
Mokhlesi, B., et al. (2003). Adult toxicology in critical care: Part II: Specific poisonings. *Chest,* 123, 897.

PROCEDURE **109**

Monitoring Gastrointestinal Perfusion With a Gastric Tonometer

PURPOSE: The gastric tonometer measures gastric intramucosal carbon dioxide (CO_2), which reflects intramucosal blood flow and perfusion. Increases in gastric intramucosal CO_2 may suggest that a patient is experiencing covert shock and can be useful in guiding resuscitation.

Andrea Marshall

PREREQUISITE NURSING KNOWLEDGE

- Normal gastrointestinal anatomy and physiology should be understood.
- Understanding the physiologic concepts related to oxygen delivery, oxygen consumption and oxygen utilization is necessary.
- The physiologic consequences of shock should be understood.
- Knowledge of changes that occur in the gut during critical illness and the links to the development of multiple organ failure[1] is essential.
- Knowledge of nasogastric tube insertion, care, and removal (see Procedure 111).
- A gastric tonometer (Fig. 109-1) is identical to a Salem Sump with the addition of a silicone balloon near the tip of the catheter.
- The silicone balloon is permeable to carbon dioxide (CO_2). Based on the principle of diffusion CO_2 from the gastric mucosa will move into the lumen of the stomach and then into the tonometer balloon where CO_2 levels can be measured (Fig. 109-2).[19,20]
- Physiologically, the basis for the use of gastric tonometry is related to the concepts of covert shock and the intense vasoconstriction that occurs first in the splanchnic region during shock. Splanchnic vasoconstriction can occur in the absence of overt signs of shock such as tachycardia and hypotension. Vasoconstriction results in a decreased

splanchnic blood flow and an increase in regional CO_2 levels, because of slower removal of CO_2 from the area and/or the development of anaerobic metabolism. Gastric tonometry measures increases in gastric intramucosal CO_2, thus providing an early warning for the development of shock.[6,8]

- Increases in gastric intramucosal CO_2 can occur in response to gastric hypoperfusion,[22,24] anaerobic metabolism,[23] systemic increases in CO_2, such as in chronic obstructive pulmonary disease[33] or buffering of hydrogen ions with bicarbonate.[15]
- Gastric tonometry allows for the measurement of gastric intramucosal CO_2 levels. Many abbreviations for gastric intramucosal CO_2 exist and include the partial pressure of gastric (Pg_{CO_2}), partial pressure of tonometer CO_2 (Pt_{CO_2}), partial pressure of regional CO_2 (Pr_{CO_2}), or the partial pressure of intramucosal CO_2 (Pi_{CO_2}). Pg_{CO_2} will be used throughout this procedure.
- Normal levels of Pg_{CO_2} range from 35-50 mm Hg but need to be evaluated within the clinical context of the patient.
- From the measurement of Pg_{CO_2}, additional calculated values are obtained. The $P(g-a)_{CO_2}$ gap (also referred to as the CO_2 gap) calculates the difference between gastric intramucosal and arterial CO_2, thus taking into account any systemic increases in carbon dioxide values.[33]
- Pg_{CO_2} and arterial bicarbonate values are used, within a modified Henderson-Hasselbalch equation, to calculate gastric intramucosal pH (pHi). Although this calculation is reported in the literature, its reliability in the clinical

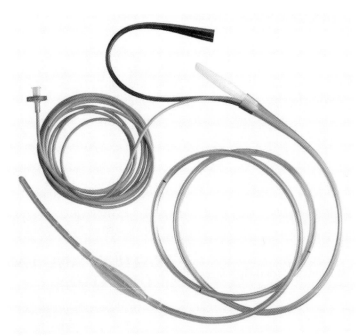

FIGURE 109-1 The Tonometry Catheter. *(Reproduced with permission, Datex-Ohmeda, Helsinki, Finland.)*

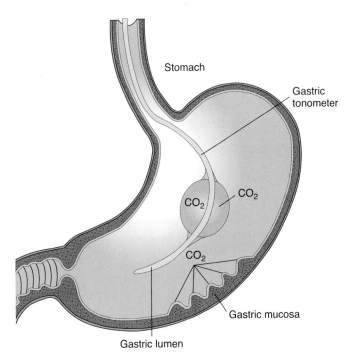

FIGURE 109-2 Principles of gastric tonometry.

setting is questioned because it is based on the assumption that the arterial bicarbonate is the same as the bicarbonate in the mucosa. This assumption has not yet been validated.[3,6,31]

- The measurement of $PgCO_2$ using a gastric tonometer can also be influenced by the following factors:
  - ❖ Position of tonometer[11,36]
  - ❖ Use of histamine$_2$ receptor antagonists[15,21,34]
  - ❖ Enteral feeding[17,18,19,27]
  - ❖ Systemic hypercarbia[33,35]
  - ❖ Systemic acidosis
  - ❖ Procedural error[9]
  - ❖ Use of saline as the tonometric medium[25,32]

EQUIPMENT

- ❖ Gastric tonometer (available in the following sizes: 8 Fr, 14 Fr, 16 Fr, and 18 Fr)
- ❖ Water-soluble lubricant
- ❖ Nonsterile gloves
- ❖ 20- to 50-ml syringe with catheter tip or adapter
- ❖ Normal saline (NS) for irrigation
- ❖ Two emesis basins
- ❖ Ice
- ❖ Ice chips or cup of tap water with straw
- ❖ Suction source with connecting tubing
- ❖ Rubber band
- ❖ Safety pin
- ❖ Pink tape or tube attachment device (Plastic Adhesive Tape; Hy-tape Surgical Products Corporation, Yonkers, NY) or tube attachment device
- ❖ pH test paper
- ❖ Tongue blade

Additional equipment, (to have available based on patient need) includes the following:

- Tincture of benzoin
- Guaiac test materials
- Tonocap™ TC-200 (Datex-Ohmeda, Helsinki, Finland) (Fig. 109-3)
  or
- M-TONO (Datex-Ohmeda, Helsinki, Finland) (Fig. 109-4)
- 5-ml syringe
- Arterial blood gas syringe
- Saline tonometry
- NS or phosphate buffered solution
- 5-ml syringe
- Two arterial blood gas syringes

PATIENT AND FAMILY EDUCATION

- Explain reason for tonometer insertion. ➤➤*Rationale:* To decrease patient anxiety.
- Explain patient's role in assisting with tube insertion. ➤➤*Rationale:* Elicits patient cooperation and facilitates insertion.
- Explain that the procedure can be uncomfortable because the gag reflex may be stimulated, causing the patient to feel nauseated or to vomit. ➤➤*Rationale:* Elicits patient cooperation and facilitates insertion.
- Explain that tonometer is similar to a conventional nasogastric tube with the additional capability of measuring gastric mucosal CO_2, which can be used to guide patient treatment. ➤➤*Rationale:* To decrease anxiety and confusion with equipment changes that may be perceived as unnecessary.

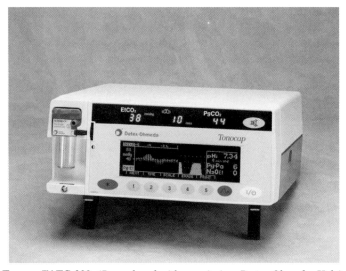

FIGURE 109-3 Tonocap™ TC-200. *(Reproduced with permission, Datex-Ohmeda, Helsinki, Finland.)*

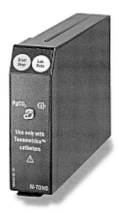

FIGURE 109-4 The Tonometry Module, M-TONO.
(Reproduced with permission, Datex-Ohmeda, Helsinki, Finland.)

PATIENT ASSESSMENT AND PREPARATION

Patient Assessment

- Obtain past medical history of nasal deformity, epistaxis, surgery, trauma, varices, or recent esophageal or gastric surgery. ➤*Rationale:* These conditions increase the risk for complications from tube placement.
- Ensure patency of nares, if nasogastric (NG) intubation is planned. This can be done by occluding one nostril at a time, asking the patient to breathe, and selecting the nostril with the best airflow. ➤*Rationale:* Choosing the most patent nostril will ease insertion and may improve patient tolerance of tube.
- Obtain immediate history of ingestion of drugs or toxins. ➤*Rationale:* Allows preparation for immediate evacuation or neutralization of gastric contents to prevent absorption and tissue damage.
- Obtain immediate history of facial or head injury, sinusitis, transphenoidal pituitary resection, and after basilar skull fracture.[8,13] ➤*Rationale:* To decrease risk for inadvertent tube placement into the brain, orogastric tube placement should be used.
- Signs of gastric distention include the following:
  ❖ Nausea
  ❖ Vomiting
  ❖ Absence of or hypoactive bowel tones
  ➤*Rationale:* Accumulation of secretions or air in the stomach increases the risk for vomiting and aspiration and provides baseline for later comparison.
- Determine need for analysis of gastric contents (e.g., pH, guaiac, drug screen). ➤*Rationale:* Knowing whether samples are needed before the procedure is initiated will allow the practitioner to have necessary supplies available and to obtain samples in a timely manner.
- Determine whether patient is intubated. ➤*Rationale:* Intubation may make nasogastric tube insertion more difficult and assistance may be needed to perform the procedure.
- Determine whether arterial access is present. ➤*Rationale:* If saline tonometry is used, an arterial blood gas will be needed to be taken to determine arterial bicarbonate and CO_2, which are used to calculate the pHi and $PgCO_2$ gap, respectively.

Patient Preparation

- Ensure that patient understands preprocedural teaching. Answer questions as they arise, and reinforce information as needed. ➤*Rationale:* Evaluates and reinforces understanding of previously taught information.
- If patient is alert, place patient in high Fowler or semi-Fowler's position. If patient is obtunded or unconscious, place patient head down in the left lateral position. Cover the chest with a towel. ➤*Rationale:* Facilitates passage of tube into the stomach and minimizes risk for aspiration. Inserting an NG tube into an obtunded patient may require the assistance of an additional person. Placing the obtunded or unconscious patient head down provides safety against aspiration should the patient vomit during the procedure.
- Measure the tube from the bridge of the nose to the earlobe to the tip of the xiphoid process (see Fig. 111-3). Mark the length of tube to be passed (a small piece of tape works well and can be easily removed). ➤*Rationale:* Estimates the length of the tube to be passed to ensure placement into the stomach.

Procedure for Monitoring Gastrointestinal Perfusion With a Gastric Tonometer

Steps	Rationale	Special Considerations
Tonometer Insertion		
1. Determine whether saline or air tonometry is to be used.	If using saline tonometry, equipment for arterial blood gas sampling will need to be acquired. If air tonometry is used, the appropriate equipment (either the Tonocop or M-Tono) will need to be obtained and placed at the bedside.	
2. Select appropriate gastric tonometer.	Gastric tonometers are available in 8 Fr, 14 Fr, 16 Fr and 18 Fr sizes.	Some tonometers are for use only with Datex-Ohmeda Tonometry Monitors (8 Fr, 14 Fr, 16 Fr, and 18 Fr). A 16 Fr tonometer is available for use with saline tonometry or the Tonocap.
3. Insert Gastric tonometer tube (see Procedure 111).	The gastric tonometer is inserted as per conventional nasogastric tube insertion.	
4. Determine position of gastric tonometer on chest x-ray. *(Level IV: Limited clinical studies to support recommendations.)*	Measured $Pgco_2$ can differ depending on the position of the tonometer balloon within the gastrointestinal tract.[11]	Currently, gastric tonometry is used more commonly than small bowel tonometry in the clinical setting. Although it is argued that small bowel tonometry is more accurate than gastric tonometry,[36] further studies are needed. If the catheter is placed too close to the duodenum, pyloric reflux may increase $Pgco_2$.[13]
Measurements With Saline (or Phosphate-Buffered Solution) Tonometry		
1. Flush the side lumen of the stopcock, attached to the gastric tonometer, with NS or phosphate-buffered solution.	Flushing the side lumen of the stopcock with NS ensures that a strictly anaerobic sampling environment is maintained.	The presence of air within the sampling system will contribute to measurement error and sample dilution because of the lack of stability of CO_2 in NS. This would result in measurement bias and lower measured $Pgco_2$.[13]
2. Inject 2.5 ml of NS into the balloon. *(Level IV: Limited clinical studies to support recommendations.)*	NS is the medium in which CO_2 becomes dissolved and can thus be measured in an arterial blood gas machine. Phosphate buffered solutions can also be used as the tonometric medium in the place of NS.[16]	Measurement of $Pgco_2$ with NS is problematic for several reasons. CO_2 is very unstable in NS.[2,25,26,29,32] Additionally, blood gas machines are calibrated for the determination of $Pgco_2$ in blood. Some blood gas machines have a minimal amount of bias, whereas the bias in others can be large.[4,26,31] The use of phosphate-buffered solutions has demonstrated an improvement in measurement of $Pgco_2$.[16]

Procedure	for Monitoring Gastrointestinal Perfusion With a Gastric Tonometer—*Continued*	
Steps	**Rationale**	**Special Considerations**
3. Turn the tonometer lumen to off.	Ensures NS stays within the tonometer balloon and is not contaminated by air.	NS must not come into contact with air because this could result in movement of CO_2 from the NS into the air, resulting in loss of CO_2 and lower $PgCO_2$ measurements.[14]
4. Note the time NS was injected into the balloon.	Time of NS injection is necessary to determine equilibration period.	Equilibration periods are needed to determine the steady state $PgCO_2$ from a time-dependent correction factor (Table 109-1).
5. Let NS equilibrate in the balloon for 30 to 90 minutes. *(Level I: Manufacturer's recommendations only.)*	Equilibration allows for CO_2 to move from the gastric mucosa to the gastric lumen and into the tonometer balloon.[30]	Equilibration times for $PgCO_2$ vary within the gastrointestinal tract. Full equilibration within the stomach is thought to occur after 90 minutes.[23] Others[12] suggest that 90 minutes may be an insufficient period for equilibration.
6. Aspirate 1 ml of NS and discard through the side lumen of the stopcock. *(Level IV: Limited clinical studies to support recommendations.)*	Allows for removal of NS from sampling line so that only tonometer balloon NS is sampled. Failure to remove dead space from the sampling line may result in dilution of the sample, lowering $PgCO_2$ measurement. Catheter dead space has been identified as a possible source of error during tonometry. It is suggested that rinsing the sampling line to remove NS containing carbon dioxide may result in improved accuracy of measurements,[28] particularly when short dwell times are used.	

Procedure continues on the following page

TABLE 109-1	Equilibration Periods and Corresponding TRIP NGS Catheter Correction Factors at 37°C

Equilibration Period = Sampling Time − Infusion Time

Equilibration Period (min)	**Correction Factor***
10	1.62
20	1.36
30	1.24
45	1.17
60	1.13
>90	1.12

*These factors have been determined in vitro.
Reprinted with permission from Datex-Ohmeda.

Procedure	**for Monitoring Gastrointestinal Perfusion With a Gastric Tonometer**—*Continued*	

Steps	Rationale	Special Considerations
7. Slowly aspirate fluid until resistance is met.	Slow aspiration reduces the risk for pulling air into the system. All saline must be aspirated from the balloon until increased resistance is felt.	
8. Record the sampling time. (*Level I: Manufacturer's recommendations only.*)	Time of NS evacuation is necessary to determine equilibration period.	Equilibration periods are needed to determine the steady state $PgCO_2$ from a time-dependent correction factor (see Table 109-1).
9. Obtain an arterial blood sample (see Procedure 60 or 79) and determine arterial HCO_3^- and $PaCO_2$ in the arterial blood gas machine. (*Level I: Manufacturer's recommendations only.*)	Arterial blood gas sample is necessary to obtain $PaCO_2$ (used to determine $P[g-a]CO_2$ gap) and arterial bicarbonate (used to determine gastric mucosal pH—pHi).	Traditionally, gastric pHi has been calculated using the arterial bicarbonate and $PgCO_2$ in the Henderson-Hasselbalch equation (Table 109-2). This approach is problematic because arterial bicarbonate may not necessarily reflect mucosal bicarbonate. Regional bicarbonate may be lower because of local ischemic lactic acidosis; thus the pHi may be overestimated.[12] Likewise, increases in $PgCO_2$ that correspond with arterial CO_2 may result in a decrease in pHi. Calculation of the $P(g-a)CO_2$ gap allows for the correction of systemic hypercarbia. For example, a patient with respiratory dysfunction who has CO_2 retention will have an elevated $PgCO_2$ reading not associated with hypoperfusion or hypoxia.[33,35]

TABLE 109-2	**The Modified Henderson-Hasselbalch Equation for Calculating pHi**

$$pHi = 6.1 + log_{10}\left[\frac{HCO_3^-}{PiCO_{2(ss)} \times 0.03}\right]$$

$PiCO_{2(ss)}$	Steady-state adjusted $PiCO_2$ of tonometer (Table 109-1)
6.1	pK for the HCO_3^-/CO_2 system in plasma at 37°C
HCO_3^-	Actual bicarbonate concentration in mmol/L of arterial blood sample
0.03	Solubility of CO_2 in plasma at 37°C

Procedure **for Monitoring Gastrointestinal Perfusion With a Gastric Tonometer**—*Continued*

Steps	Rationale	Special Considerations
10. Keeping the sample at room temperature, immediately analyze saline from gastric tonometer in arterial blood gas machine. (*Level IV: Limited clinical studies to support recommendations.*)	Length of time to analysis of saline from the gastric tonometer allows more time for diffusion of CO_2 out of the NS.[12] It has been suggested that the tonometer saline sample be treated in the same manner as an arterial blood gas sample. Some have recommended placing the sample on ice.[23] It is now known that temperature influences the solubility of CO_2 in solution. Current recommendations are for the sample be kept at room temperature.[7]	CO_2 is unstable in NS, and diffusion out of solution can lead to underestimation of the $PgCO_2$.[2] Measurement error inherent in the analysis of CO_2 in saline[29] using an arterial blood gas machine also creates difficulty with the accuracy of $PgCO_2$ measurement using the saline method.
11. Convert $PgCO_2$ to steady state. (*Level 1: Manufacturer's recommendation only.*)	A time-dependent correction factor, based on the equilibration period, is applied to the $PgCO_2$ to determine the steady-state $PgCO_2$ (see Table 109-1).	Time-dependent correction factors were determined in vivo.
12. Calculate gastric intramucosal pH (pHi) if necessary.	A modified Henderson-Hasselbalch equation (see Table 109-2) is used to calculate pHi.	Arterial bicarbonate values are used within the Henderson-Hasselbalch (see Table 109-2) equation to calculate the pHi. This practice is questionable since the assumption that arterial bicarbonate closely approximates tissue bicarbonate has not been validated.[3,6,31]
13. Calculate difference between gastric and arterial CO_2 (P[g-a]CO_2) if necessary.	Calculation of the Pa(g-a)CO_2 gap is done by subtracting the $PaCO_2$ from the $PgCO_2$ allowing for correction of systemic acid-base disturbances.	Most published data on tonometry is based on the assessment of pHi. The advantage of using the P(g-a)CO_2 gap is that this simple equation does not use systemic acid-base data. The advantages as a prognostic marker and target or therapeutic interventions will become better established as research reporting the P(g-a)CO_2 gap develops.[30]
14. Document in patient record.		

Measurements With Air Tonometry (Tonocap)

1. Ensure tonometer inserted is able to be used with the Tonocap monitor.	Tonometer specifications differ, and not all tonometers can be used with the Tonocap monitor.	
2. Before connecting the patient, attach a clean airway sampling line to the connector on the D-fend water trap. The D-fend water trap container must be empty and clean.	The Tonocap allows for monitoring of end-tidal CO_2 ($ETCO_2$). Use of the D-fend water trap allows for moisture in the exhaled gases to be collected, thus keeping the airway sampling line clear.	End-tidal CO_2 monitoring can be assessed against the $PaCO_2$. If both values are similar, the $ETCO_2$ can be used to determine the CO_2 gap, negating the need for repeated arterial blood gas samples.[33]
3. Turn the Tonocap monitor on; allow to warm up for 5 minutes.	As soon as the patient is connected to the monitor, the $ETCO_2$ will be measured and values displayed.	

Procedure continues on the following page

Procedure	for Monitoring Gastrointestinal Perfusion With a Gastric Tonometer—*Continued*	
Steps	**Rationale**	**Special Considerations**
4. Attach tonometer sampling line with bacterial filter to the connector on the monitor below the water trap.	Once connected, the Tonocap will test the presence of the catheter (initialization) and fill the tonometer balloon with 4 ml of room air.	
5. Following initialization, the Tonocap will test the presence of the catheter every 5 minutes. The cycling time will be set for every 15 minutes.	The recommended cycle time is 15 minutes. Cycling time can be changed by selecting the $PgCO_2$ row in the SETUP menu. Choose from manual, 10, 15, 30, 60 minutes. If manual measurements are chosen, $PgCO_2$ is measured by pressing the $*$ key. Manual measurements can be done only if 5 minutes have elapsed since the last measurements.	
6. If calculation of pHi is required, obtain an arterial blood gas sample (see Procedure 60 or 79). Note the time arterial blood gas sample is taken. (*Level IV: Limited clinical studies to support recommendations.*)	Arterial blood gas sample is necessary to obtain the arterial bicarbonate (used to determine gastric mucosal pH, or pHi). Arterial PCO_2 can be used to determine the $P(g-a)CO_2$ gap. Alternatively, if $ETCO_2$ and $PaCO_2$ values are similar, $P(g-a)CO_2$ gap can be estimated by subtracting the $ETCO_2$ from the $PgCO_2$. Calculation of the $P(g-a)CO_2$ gap allows for the correction of systemic hypercarbia. For example, a patient with respiratory dysfunction who has CO_2 retention will have an elevated $PgCO_2$ reading that is not associated with hypoperfusion or hypoxia.[33,35]	Traditionally, gastric pHi has been calculated using the arterial bicarbonate and tonometer CO_2 in the Henderson-Hasselbalch equation (see Table 109-2). This approach is problematic because arterial bicarbonate may not reflect mucosal bicarbonate. Regional bicarbonate may be lower because of local ischemic lactic acidosis; thus the pHi may be overestimated.[12] Likewise, increases in tonometer CO_2 that correspond with arterial CO_2 may result in a decrease in pHi.
7. Once arterial blood gases are obtained, enter the $PaCO_2$ and HCO_3^- values into the Tonocap.	SETUP brings up the $PaCO_2$ value. Enter value with key arrows. Press NEXT to highlight pHa. Enter value. Move highlight to DELAY and with arrow keys set the amount of minutes since analysis sample was taken. Press NEXT to highlight STORE. Press an arrow key. The monitor will calculate the pHi value using the $PaCO_2$/pHa entered and the latest $PgCO_2$ value and will display the new pHi value.	Note that $PaCO_2$ can be entered as mm Hg or kPa.
8. Document in patient record.		

Procedure	for Monitoring Gastrointestinal Perfusion With a Gastric Tonometer—*Continued*	
Steps	**Rationale**	**Special Considerations**

Measurements With Air Tonometry (M-Tono)—For Use With Datex-Ohmeda Monitors Only

1. Attach integrated sampling line to M-Tono module; press START.	The monitor will automatically inject 4 ml of room air into the balloon. After 10 minutes, air is automatically withdrawn from the tonometer balloon and CO_2 is measured in the M-Tono by an infrared sensor. To compensate for incomplete equilibration, a correction factor is applied. The sample is then returned to the balloon to allow quicker equilibrium times. The cycle is then repeated in 10-minute intervals. The steady state of the $PgCO_2$ measurement takes place after the second or third measurement cycle (approximately 30 minutes).	The first one or two CO_2 samples are contaminated by air carry-over from the sampling line, thereby diluting the CO_2 sample drawn from the balloon.
2. Obtain an arterial blood gas (see Procedure 60 or 79) if pHi or $P(g-a)CO_2$ gap needs to be calculated. (*Level IV: Limited clinical studies to support recommendations.*)	Arterial blood gas sample is necessary to obtain the arterial bicarbonate (used to determine gastric mucosal pH, or pHi). $PaCO_2$ can be used to determine $P(g-a)CO_2$ gap. Alternatively, if $ETCO_2$ and $PaCO_2$ values are similar, $P(g-a)CO_2$ gap can be estimated by subtracting the $ETCO_2$ from the $PgCO_2$. Calculation of the $P(g-a)CO_2$ gap allows for the correction of systemic hypercarbia. For example, a patient with respiratory dysfunction who has CO_2 retention will have an elevated $PgCO_2$ reading that is not associated with hypoperfusion or hypoxia.[33,35]	Traditionally, gastric pHi has been calculated using the arterial bicarbonate and $PgCO_2$ in the Henderson-Hasselbalch equation (see Table 109-2). This approach is problematic because arterial bicarbonate may not necessarily reflect mucosal bicarbonate. Regional bicarbonate may be lower because of local ischemic lactic acidosis; thus the pHi may be overestimated.[12] Likewise, increases in $PgCO_2$ that correspond with $PaCO_2$ may result in a decrease in pHi.
3. Enter arterial blood gas values by pressing the LAB DATA key on the M-Tono module.	The monitor will calculate $P(g-a)CO_2$ gap and pHi and will display values as well as trends.	
4. Repeat measurements as required.		
5. Disconnect the catheter system from the monitor whenever it is switched off or turned to standby.		
6. Document in patient record.		

Expected Outcomes

- Measurement of $PgCO_2$ and evaluation of measurements to guide therapeutic interventions
- Decompression of stomach
- Gastric emptying

Unexpected Outcomes

- Tube placement in the trachea or lungs
- Tube placement in the esophagus or duodenum
- Nasal bleeding from Tonometer insertion or from removal with Tonometer balloon inflated
- Skin ulceration, sinusitis, esophageal-tracheal fistula, gastric ulceration, or oral infections
- Vagal response during insertion or from gag reflex stimulation

Patient Monitoring and Care

Steps	Rationale	Reportable Conditions
		These conditions should be reported if they persist despite nursing interventions.
1. Maintain and check tube patency every 4 hours and as needed.	Prevents gastric distention and associated patient discomfort.	• Inability to establish patency
2. Monitor output (color, amount, type, pH, guaiac) every 4 hours and as needed.	Provides data for diagnosis and fluid balance.	• Increasing output or sudden change in output (increase or decrease) • Frank blood or "coffee-ground," black, or brown returns • Positive guaiac • Abnormal pH
3. Calculate output into patient's overall intake and output record.	Volume loss from gastric secretions can cause patients to become hypovolemic; large volumes may need to be replaced with appropriate intravenous fluids.	• Increasing output or sudden change in output (increase or decrease)
4. Assess oral cavity and perform oral care every 2 hours and as needed.	Patients with orogastric or NG tubes in place tend to mouth-breathe, drying their mouths and increasing the risk for mucosal breakdown and ulceration. Tube presence may also predispose a patient to sinusitis or oral infections.	• Ulceration, drainage, foul odor
5. Monitor insertion site of tube for redness, swelling, drainage, bleeding, or skin breakdown. Use only water-soluble lubricants at site.	Many critically ill patients have fragile skin and have associated conditions that predispose them to skin breakdown. Frequent monitoring and subsequent repositioning of the tube can prevent serious damage.	• Redness • Swelling • Drainage • Bleeding • Skin breakdown at insertion site
6. Irrigate the tube, using air or NS, per institutional standards and as needed.	Assists in maintaining patency of tube and facilitates drainage.	• Inability to irrigate tube
7. Maintain tube to suction as ordered.	Low (20 to 80 mm Hg) intermittent suction is recommended to minimize gastric mucosal irritation yet provide for adequate drainage.	
8. Monitor vital signs per unit standards. Perform respiratory and gastrointestinal assessment every 2 hours.	Change in vital signs or respiratory or gastrointestinal assessments may be early warning signs of the development of complications.	• Sudden change in vital signs • Unexplained respiratory distress • Increased abdominal distention, change in bowel tones
9. Reposition and retape tube every 24 hours or when tape is soiled.	Decreases risk for tissue damage to mouth or nares.	
10. Monitor Pg_{CO_2} as indicated by patients clinical condition.	Increased Pg_{CO_2} may indicate deterioration in the patient's clinical condition. Conversely, a decrease in Pg_{CO_2} from previously high levels may be an indicator of clinical improvement. A $P(g\text{-}a)_{CO_2}$ gap between 10-20 mm Hg may indicate deterioration in the patient's condition. A $P(g\text{-}a)_{CO_2}$ gap greater than 20 mm Hg is considered a sign of significant gastrointestinal mucosal hypoperfusion.	• Increased Pg_{CO_2} above normal levels identified by the institution or an increase in Pg_{CO_2} from the patient's norm

Patient Monitoring and Care—*Continued*

Steps	Rationale	Reportable Conditions
	A rapid drop in P_{gCO_2} without any physiologic cause may indicate a kink in the tubing.[30] If P_{gCO_2} is lower than Pa_{CO_2} check for leaks in the tonometer catheter. Aspirate stomach if it is suspected that stomach has been inflated with oxygen following hand bagging of the patient with O_2.[30]	
11. Identify confounding variables that may contribute to incorrect P_{gCO_2} readings. *(Level VI: Clinical studies in a variety of patient populations and situations to support recommendations.)*	Check position of tonometer by x-ray. Migration of the tonometer into the small bowel or esophagus will influence evaluation of measurements since regional CO_2 in these areas differs from P_{gCO_2}. Enteral feeding may generate CO_2 and cause an increase in the P_{gCO_2} unrelated to mucosal perfusion.[17,18] The suggested interval between feeding and tonometric measurements is 60 minutes, although this has not been well researched. Data showing an increase in P_{gCO_2} related to feeding was collected in the initial period following initiation of enteral feeding[17,18,19]; however, one study demonstrates stabilization in P_{gCO_2} at 24 and 48 hours after feeding was initiated.[19] Further research is required in this area. Administration of H_2 antagonists is suggested to prevent the buffering of gastric acid with bicarbonate, which causes an increase in the P_{gCO_2} of normal subjects in which inadequate perfusion is unlikely.[15] Further data have not supported this finding in the critically ill,[5,21] whose ability to produce gastric acid appears to be impaired.[10]	• Incorrect position of tonometer
12. Fully deflate tonometer balloon and adjust stopcock so that the balloon is open to air before removal.	An inflated balloon will increase the diameter of the tonometer and cause injury to the nasal passage during removal.	
13. Air tonometry: disconnect tonometer from Tonocap or M-Tono when not in use.	Allows tonometer balloon to empty, reducing stress on the balloon and ensuring the balloon is empty should the tonometer be removed.	
14. Check tonometer for evidence of blockage or leaking. The Tonocap and M-Tono will display the message "CHECK CATHETER."	This may occur when P_{gCO_2} is very low or less than ET_{CO_2}. Check the sampling line and Leur-Lok connections. If failure persists and if tonometer used does not have an integrated sampling line, replace sampling line. If failure persists, change tonometer.	

Documentation

Documentation should include the following:

- Patient and family education
- Insertion of orogastric or NG tube
- Tube type and size
- Any difficulties in insertion
- Patient toleration
- Tonometer position; how placement was confirmed
- Appearance and volume of gastric secretions, if present

- $Pgco_2$, pHi and $P(g-a)co_2$ gap
- Amount and type of irrigation fluid (if appropriate)
- Oral care
- Tube site assessments
- Unexpected outcomes
- Nursing interventions
- Management of enteral feeding during tonometer measurements

---

References

1. Ackland, G., Grocott, M.P., and Mythen, M.G. (2000). Understanding gastrointestinal perfusion in critical care: So near, and yet so far. *Crit Care,* 4, 269-81.
2. Barry, B., et al. (1998). Comparison of air tonometry with gastric tonometry using saline and other equilibrating fluids: An in vivo and in vitro study. *Intensive Care Med,* 24, 777-84.
3. Benjamin, E., et al. (1992). Sodium bicarbonate administration affects the diagnostic accuracy of gastrointestinal tonometry in acute mesenteric ischaemia. *Crit Care Med,* 2, 1181-3.
4. Boyd, O., et al. (1993). Comparison of clinical information gained from routine blood-gas analysis and from gastric tonometry for intramural pH. *Lancet,* 341, 142-5.
5. Calvet, X., et al. (1995). Effect of ranitidine in gastric intramucosal pH determinations in critically ill patients. *Am J Resp Crit Care Med,* 151, A334.
6. Cerny, V., and Cvachoveck, K. (2000). Gastric tonometry and intramucosal pH—Theoretical principles and clinical application. *Physiol Res,* 49, 289-97.
7. Chapman, M.V., et al. (1999). Temperature dependent errors using gastrointestinal goniometry: An in vivo study. *Br J Anapest,* S1, A580.
8. Dabrowski, G.P., et al. (2000). A critical assessment of endpoints of shock resuscitation. *Surg Clin North Am,* 80, 825-44.
9. Ferguson, A.P. (1996). Gastric tonometry: Evaluating tissue oxygenation. *Crit Care Nurse,* 16, 48-55.
10. Groeneveld, A.B.J. (1996). Gastrointestinal exocrine failure in critical illness. In: Rombeau, J.L., and Takala, J., eds. *Gut Dysfunction in Critical Illness.* Berlin: Springer.
11. Guzman, J.A., Lacoma, F.J., and Kruse, J.A. (1998). Gastric and esophageal intramucosal Pco_2 ($Pico_2$) during endotoxemia. *Chest,* 113, 1078-83.
12. Hameed, S.M., and Cohn, S.M. (2003). Gastric tonometry— the role of mucosal pH measurement in the management of trauma. *Chest,* 123, 475S-81S.
13. Hamilton, M.A., and Mythen, M.G. (2000). *Intragastric Luminal Tonometry in Intensive Care. Clinical Window.* Datex-Ohmeda. Available at: www.datex-ohmeda.com/ clinical/cw_prev_02_article1.htm. Accessed August 13, 2003.
14. Heard, S.O. (2003). Gastric tonometry. *Chest,* 123, 469S-74S.
15. Heard, S.O. (1998). Suppression of gastric acid secretion: Preventing excess gas. *Intensive Care Med,* 24, 1123-25.
16. Knichwitz, G., et al. (1996). Gastric tonometry: Precision and reliability are improved by a phosphate buffered solution. *Crit Care Med,* 24, 512-6.
17. Levy, B., et al. (1998). Gastric versus duodenal feeding and gastric tonometric measurements. *Crit Care Med,* 26, 1991-4.
18. Marik, P.E., and Lorenzana, A. (1996). The effect of tube feeding on the measurement of gastric intramucosal pH. *Crit Care Med,* 24, 1498-1500.
19. Marshall, A., and West, S. (2003). Gastric tonometry and enteral nutrition: A possible conflict in critical care nursing practice. *Am J Crit Care,* 12, 349-56.
20. Marshall, A.P., and West, S.H. (2004). Gastric tonometry and monitoring gastrointestinal perfusion: Using research to support nursing practice. *Nurs Crit Care,* 9, 3, 123-33.
21. Maynard, N., et al. (1994). Influence of intravenous ranitidine on gastric intramucosal pH in critically ill patients. *Crit Care Med,* 22, A79.
22. Meisner, F.G., et al. (2001). Changes in $P(i)co_2$ reflect splanchnic mucosal ischaemia more reliably than changes in pHi during haemorrhagic shock. *Langenbecks Arch Surg,* 386, 333-8.
23. Mythen, M., and Faehnrich, J. (1996). Monitoring gut perfusion. In: Rombeau, J.L., and Takala, J., eds. *Gut Dysfunction in Critical Illness.* Berlin: Springer.
24. Naguib, K., et al. (2000). Is regional tonometry a reliable index of tissue oxygenation? A comparative study with conventional global monitoring. *Middle East J Anesth,* 15, 515-28.
25. Oud, L., Sobek, S.B., and Kruse, J.A. (1996). Poor in vivo reproducibility of gastric intramucosal Pco_2 measurement by saline-balloon tonometry. *Crit Care Med,* 24 Suppl, A47.
26. Riddington, D., et al. (1994). Measuring carbon dioxide tension in saline and alternative solutions: Quantification of bias and precision in two blood gas analyzers. *Crit Care Med,* 22, 96-100.
27. Roykyta, R., et al. (2001). Impact of enteral feeding on gastric tonometry in healthy volunteers and critically ill patients. *Acta Anaesthesiol Scand,* 45, 564-9.
28. Steverink, P.J.G.M., et al. (1998). Catheter deadspace: A source of error during tonometry. *Br J Anaesth,* 80, 337-41.
29. Takala, J., et al. (1994). Saline Pco_2 is an important source of error in the assessment of gastric intramucosal pH. *Crit Care Med,* 22, 1877-9.
30. Takala, J. (2002). *Gastrointestinal Tonometry.* Finland: Datex-Ohmeda.
31. Tang, W., et al. (1994). Gastric intramucosal Pco_2 as monitor of perfusion failure during hemorrhagic and anaphylactic shock. *J App Physiol,* 76, 572-7.
32. Tzelepis, G., et al. (1996). Comparison of gastric air tonometry with standard saline tonometry. *Intensive Care Med,* 22, 1239-43.
33. Uusaro, A., et al. (2000). Gastric mucosal end-tidal Pco_2 difference as a continuous indicator of splanchnic perfusion. *Br J Anaesth,* 85, 563-9.
34. Vaisanen, O., et al. (2000). Ranitidine or dobutamine alone or combined has no effect on gastric intramucosal-arterial Pco_2 difference after cardiac surgery. *Intensive Care Med,* 26, 45-51.
35. Vincent, J.L., and Creteur, J. (1998). Gastric mucosal pH is definitely obsolete—please tell us more about gastric mucosal Pco_2. *Crit Care Med,* 26, 1479-81.
36. Walley, K.R., et al. (1998). Small bowel tonometry is more accurate than gastric tonometry in detecting gut ischaemia. *J App Physiol,* 85, 1770-7.

Additional Readings

Boswell, S.A., and Scalea, T.M. (2003). Sublingual capnometry. *AACN Clin Issues,* 14, 176-84.

Brown, S.D., and Gutierrez, G. (1997). Does gastric tonometry work? Yes. *Crit Care Clinics,* 12, 569-85.

Fiddian-Green, R.G. (1992). Tonometry: Theory and applications. *Intensive Care World,* 9, 60-5.

Fiddian-Green, R.G. (1992). Tonometry: Part 2: Clinical use and cost implications. *Intensive Care World,* 9, 130-5.

Gomersall, C.D., et al. (1997). Gastric tonometry and prediction of outcome in the critically ill: Arterial to intramucosal pH gradient and carbon dioxide gradient. *Anaesthesia,* 52, 619-23.

Hamilton, M.A., and Mythen, M.G. (2001). Gastric tonometry: Where do we stand? *Current Opin Crit Care,* 7, 122-7.

Kolkman, J.J., Otte, J.A., and Groeneveld, A.B.J. (2000). Gastrointestinal luminal P_{CO_2} tonometry: An update on physiology, methodology and clinical applications. *Br J Anaesth,* 84, 74-86.

Ruffolo, D.C., and Headley, J.M. (2003). Regional carbon dioxide monitoring. *AACN Clinical Issues,* 14, 168-75.

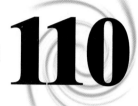

http://evolve.elsevier.com

P R O C E D U R E **110**

Intraabdominal Pressure Monitoring

P U R P O S E : Intraabdominal pressure (IAP) measurement is indicated in patients who are at risk for the development of intraabdominal hypertension (IAH) or abdominal compartment syndrome (ACS). IAH and ACS result when the abdominal contents expand in excess of the capacity of the abdominal cavity.[1,2,4-6,9-13]

John J. Gallagher

PREREQUISITE NURSING KNOWLEDGE

- Understanding of gastrointestinal anatomy and physiology is required.
- Knowledge of aseptic technique is essential.
- Possible causes of IAH and ACS include the following:
  - ❖ Intraperitoneal blood
  - ❖ Third space resuscitation fluid
  - ❖ Peritonitis
  - ❖ Ascites
  - ❖ Gaseous bowel distention
- Additionally, the presence of intraabdominal packing, use of pneumatic antishock garments, insufflation of the peritoneum during laparoscopic procedures, and full closure of the abdominal wall in the presence of visceral edema have been implicated in the development of IAH and ACS (Table 110-1).
- Elevated intraabdominal compartment pressures may result in decreased blood flow to organs in the abdominal cavity and can adversely affect the functioning of multiple organ systems[1,2,5-13] (Table 110-2).
- IAP measurements should be correlated with associated organ system pathology to determine the presence of IAH/ACS and the need for surgical intervention.
- Several methods are described in the literature to measure IAP.[3,10,11,14] These include direct intraperitoneal measurement using a peritoneal dialysis catheter, the intragastric method via a nasogastric (NG) tube, the rectal route, and through a urinary catheter in the bladder.
- Measurement of bladder pressures via an indwelling urinary catheter is the most widely accepted method for clinical use and may be performed with equipment readily available in the critical care environment.

- Compartment syndrome can result in any confined anatomic space where there is an increase in pressure.
- The elevation of pressure within the compartment can cause compression or occlusion of arterial blood flow, resulting in ischemia, tissue necrosis, and irreversible organ failure if blood flow is not restored.
- The bladder acts as a passive reservoir and will accurately reflect intraabdominal pressure (IAP) when the intravesicular volume is 100 ml or less.[8]
- Bladder pressures may be measured using a standard pressure transducer monitoring set connected to the patient's urinary drainage system (see Procedure 75).
- Bladder pressures reflective of the IAP are measured in millimeters of mercury (mm Hg) and may be classified

TABLE 110-1	Patients at Risk for Development of Intraabdominal Hypertension and Abdominal Compartment Syndrome[1,2,7,9-12]

1. Trauma/abdominal surgery[1]
   - Blunt or penetrating abdominal trauma/intraperitoneal hematoma
   - Pelvic fractures/retroperitoneal hematoma
   - Damage-control abdominal surgery/abdominal packing/primary closure
   - Visceral tissue edema secondary to ischemia and fluid resuscitation
   - Pneumoperitoneum during laparoscopic procedures
   - Liver transplant
2. Pneumatic antishock garments
3. Ruptured abdominal aortic aneurysm
4. Cirrhosis/ascites
5. Small bowel obstruction
6. Hemorrhagic pancreatitis
7. Neoplasm
8. Obstetrical conditions
   - Preeclampsia
   - Pregnancy-related disseminated intravascular coagulation/hemorrhage

892

TABLE 110-2	Physiologic Changes Associated With Intraabdominal Hypertension and Abdominal Compartment Syndrome[2,7,9-13]
Organ System (IAP Range of Initial Organ System Impact)	**Rationale**
Cardiovascular (IAP low-to-moderate range) ↑ CVP, PAP, PCWP, SVR ↓ CO (more pronounced with hypovolemia) ↓ Venous return from lower extremities (risk for DVT)	Increased abdominal pressure prevents venous return (preload reduction) and impedes arterial outflow (increase in afterload). Transmitted backpressure from the abdominal cavity falsely elevates CVP, PAP, PCWP, PVR, and SVR.
Renal (IAPs low to moderate) ↓ Renal blood flow → ↓ GFR → ↓ urine output	Increased intraabdominal pressure compresses the renal parenchyma, reducing blood flow and urine output.
Pulmonary (IAP moderate-to-severe range) ↑ Intrathoracic pressures ↑ Peak inspiratory pressures ↓ Tidal volume → hypercarbia + ↓ PaO_2 ↓ Compliance	Increased intraabdominal pressure causes an increase in intrathoracic pressure and limits diaphragm excursion, resulting in hypoventilation and hypoxia.
Neurologic (IAP low-to-moderate range) ↑ ICP ↓ CPP	Increased intraabdominal pressure impedes venous outflow from the brain, increasing cerebral venous congestion.
Gastrointestinal/hepatic effect (IAP low-to-moderate range) ↓ Celiac and portal blood flow ↓ Lactate clearance ↓ Mucosal blood flow → ↓ intramucosal pH (pHi)	Increased intraabdominal pressure reduces perfusion to the abdominal organs.

CPP, cerebral perfusion pressure; *CVP*, central venous pressure; *DVT*, deep vein thrombosis; *GFR*, glomerular filtration rate; *IAP*, intraabdominal pressure; *ICP*, intracranial pressure; *PAP*, pulmonary artery pressure; *PCWP*, pulmonary capillary wedge pressure; *PVR*, pulmonary vascular resistance; *SVR*, systemic vascular resistance.

as normal (0 mm Hg to subatmospheric), mildly elevated (10 to 20 mm Hg), moderately elevated (greater than 20 to 40 mm Hg) and severely elevated (greater than 40 mm Hg).[6,11]

- Pressures between 0 and 15 mm Hg normally are seen after abdominal surgery; however, measurements in the upper portion of this range also may indicate early IAH. Bladder pressures of greater than 15 mm Hg indicate onset of IAH and generally are associated with early organ system pathology.[2,10] Pressures in the moderate to severe range are associated with marked alterations in cardiovascular function, anuria or oliguria, and impaired respiratory function[2,6,10-13] (see Table 110-2). It is accepted surgical practice to perform surgical decompression of the abdomen in patients with IAPs of 20 to 25 mm Hg, associated with clinical assessment findings that indicate IAH/ACS.[2,8]

EQUIPMENT

- Nonsterile gloves
- Cardiac monitor and pressure cable for interface with the monitor
- 500- or 1000-ml IV bag of normal saline (NS) solution with appropriate-size pressure bag
- Pressure transducer system, including pressure tubing with flush device, transducer, and two stopcocks
- 60-ml Luer-Lok syringe
- Clamp
- Povidone-iodine pads or swab-sticks
- 18-G needle or angiocatheter

PATIENT AND FAMILY EDUCATION

- Explain the procedure of bladder pressure measurement and its purpose to the patient and family. ➤➤*Rationale:* Decreases patient and family anxiety. Understanding of

how the procedure is done will assist in the patient's ability to cooperate.

- Inform the patient that he or she will feel "fullness" in the bladder when saline is injected into the bladder during the procedure. ➤➤*Rationale:* Decreases patient anxiety. Prepares patient for what to expect.

PATIENT ASSESSMENT AND PREPARATION

Patient Assessment

- Obtain a patient health history to uncover risk factors predisposing the patient to IAH or ACS. These conditions are outlined in Table 110-1. ➤➤*Rationale:* Patients with these conditions may experience an increase in abdominal cavity fluid collection or tissue edema, placing them at risk for IAH and ACS.
- Assess the patient for signs of IAH or ACS, including decreased cardiac output and blood pressure, oliguria and anuria, increased peak inspiratory pressures (PIPs), hypercarbia and hypoxia, increased intracranial pressure (ICP), increase in abdominal girth, and abdominal wall rigidity (see Table 110-2). ➤➤*Rationale:* These physical findings indicate pathophysiologic organ system changes associated with the onset and presence of IAH and ACS.

Patient Preparation

- Ensure that the patient and family understand preprocedural teaching. Answer questions as they arise and reinforce information as needed. ➤➤*Rationale:* Evaluates and reinforces understanding of previously taught information.
- Ensure the presence of a conventional (single-lumen) urinary catheter connected to a closed drainage system. ➤➤*Rationale:* A urinary catheter with a closed drainage system is required to obtain bladder pressure measurements.

Multilumen irrigation urinary catheters also may be used, but are not required.

- Place the patient in the supine, flat position (if this can be tolerated) in preparation for bladder pressure measurement. ➤**Rationale:** The supine, flat position reduces the effect of downward pressure from the abdominal organs on the bladder, reducing the chance that IAP will be falsely elevated. Patients who cannot tolerate the supine position (head injury, respiratory compromise) may have measurements taken with the head of the bed elevated; however, the same position should be used for all subsequent measurements to obtain comparable readings.

Procedure | for Intraabdominal Pressure Monitoring

Steps	Rationale	Special Considerations
1. Wash hands and don gloves.	Reduces the transmission of microorganisms; standard precautions.	
2. Assemble the entire pressure transducer system as shown (Fig. 110-1), flush the system with NS, and pressurize the system to 300 mm Hg, using the pressure bag.	Ensure all air is out of the system. Pressurizing the system will allow for easier filling of the syringe.	To minimize air bubbles in the system, do not pressurize the system before flushing the tubing with fluid.

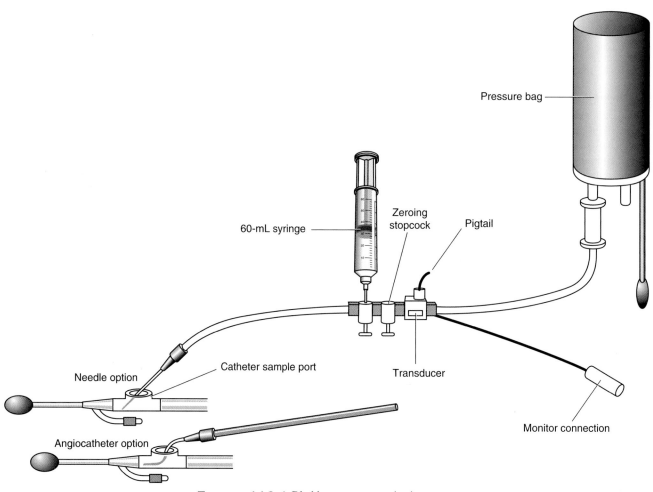

FIGURE 110-1 Bladder pressure monitoring setup.

Procedure **for Intraabdominal Pressure Monitoring**—*Continued*

Steps	Rationale	Special Considerations
3. Attach the 60-ml syringe to the distal stopcock and attach the needle to the end of the tubing (see Fig. 110-1).	The syringe is used to fill the bladder with saline from the IV bag.	If an angiocatheter is used, do not attach it to the end of the tubing until after step 7, when it has been threaded into the urinary drainage system sampling port.
4. Connect the pressurized system to the pressure module of the monitoring system with the transducer cable. Select a 30- or 60-mm Hg scale.	Connects the system for monitoring. The 30- or 60-mm Hg scale will be sufficient to measure the majority of IAP ranges.	
5. Level the fluid interface (zeroing stopcock) to the symphysis pubis.	The symphysis pubis approximates the level of the bladder and should be used as the reference point.	Marking the position ensures consistent use of the same reference point. The transducer may be secured to an IV pole beside the patient and leveled in the standard fashion, or it may be placed on the patient at the level of the symphysis pubis.
6. Zero the intraabdominal pressure monitoring system (see Procedure 75).	Negates the effect of atmospheric pressure. Ensures accuracy of the system with the established reference point.	
7. Clamp the bladder drainage system just distal to the catheter and drainage bag connection on the drainage bag tubing.	Prevents drainage of saline out of the bladder during bladder filling.	
8. Cleanse the sampling port on the urinary drainage system with povidone and aseptically insert the needle or angiocatheter into the sampling port. *If using the angiocatheter, insert the angiocatheter and thread the catheter into the port; remove the needle and connect the catheter to the pressure tubing.*	Cleansing the sampling port reduces the incidence of nosocomial urinary tract infection (UTI) from system contamination.	Either a needle for intermittent connection of the pressure transducer to the catheter system or an angiocatheter threaded through the sampling port that remains in place continuously can be used. The angiocatheter method prevents the need for repeated punctures of the sampling port and may reduce the chance of needle stick injury.[1] It has also been hypothesized that this technique may reduce the incidence of UTI.
9. Turn the stopcock attached to the syringe off to the patient and open to the pressure bag and syringe. Activate the fast-flush mechanism (pigtail) while pulling back on the syringe plunger to fill the syringe to 50 ml.		
10. Turn the stopcock off to the pressure bag and open to the syringe and patient. Inject the 50 ml of saline into the bladder.	The fluid-filled bladder will accurately reflect IAP. Using a volume of 50 ml will prevent overdistention of the bladder and false elevation of the bladder pressure.	

Procedure continues on the following page

Procedure **for Intraabdominal Pressure Monitoring**—*Continued*

Steps	Rationale	Special Considerations
11. Expel any air seen between the clamp and the urinary catheter by opening the clamp and allowing the saline to flow back past the clamp; then reclamp.	Air in the system may dampen the pressure reading.	
12. Run a strip of the waveform.	Intraabdominal pressure should be determined from the graphic strip, because the effect of ventilation can be identified.	Use of the numeric IAP pressure displayed on the monitor should not be used. This numeric reading is a "mean" pressure value, reflecting the average of both inspiratory and expiratory IAP, rather than just the expiratory IAP.
13. Measure the intraabdominal pressure at end expiration (Fig. 110-2).	Measurement is most accurate as the effects of pulmonary pressures are minimized.	
14. Once a reading has been obtained, remove the needle from the sampling port and unclamp the drainage system. If an angiocatheter has been used, it should be left in the sampling port with the entire transducer system left connected. *The urinary drainage system should be left unclamped between readings.*	Removing the needle and unclamping the drainage system will discontinue pressure measurement and resume the normal urinary drainage function of the catheter system.	Although the angiocatheter/transducer system remains attached, bladder pressures cannot be continuously measured. Monitoring requires clamping the drainage system and filling the bladder to obtain a reading. Continuous connection of the system simply prevents repeated punctures of the sampling port.
15. Record the bladder pressure on the patient flow sheet and remember to subtract the 50 ml of instilled saline from the hourly urine output.	The volume of instilled normal saline will falsely elevate hourly urine output if it is not subtracted.	
16. Report IAP readings as per protocol, if they are trending upward, or if they are associated with other assessment findings indicating the development of IAH and ACS.	Early detection and surgical intervention to relieve high IAPs is essential to reduce the morbidity and mortality associated with IAH and ACS.	
17. Discard used supplies and wash hands.	Reduces transmission of microorganisms; standard precautions.	

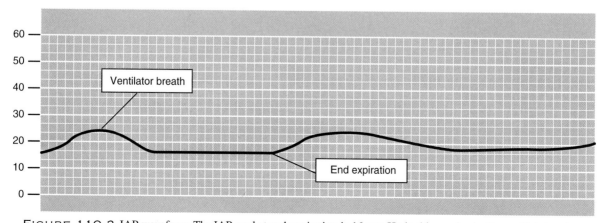

FIGURE 110-2 IAP waveform. The IAP read at end-expiration is 16 mm Hg in this mechanically ventilated patient.

Expected Outcomes

- Intraabdominal pressure monitoring achieved
- Compartment pressure within normal limits
- Elevated compartment pressure detected and therapeutic intervention initiated

Unexpected Outcomes

- Inability to monitor intraabdominal pressure
- Inaccurate pressure readings obtained
- Development of a nosocomial UTI secondary to urinary drainage system manipulation
- Patient discomfort

Patient Monitoring and Care

Steps	Rationale	Reportable Conditions
		These conditions should be reported if they persist despite nursing interventions.
1. Assess the patient for signs of increasing intraabdominal pressure, including: A. Decrease in blood pressure and cardiac output B. Oliguria or anuria C. Increase in peak inspiratory pressures D. Hypoxia and hypercarbia E. Elevated intracranial pressure (ICP) F. Increase in abdominal girth G. Increase in the tenseness of the abdomen wall	Patients may develop symptoms slowly over time. The symptoms may mimic other clinical conditions such as acute respiratory distress syndrome (ARDS), acute renal failure, congestive heart failure, and intracranial hypertension.	• Decrease in blood pressure and cardiac output • Oliguria or anuria • Increase in peak inspiratory pressures • Hypoxia and hypercarbia • Elevated ICP • Increase in abdominal girth • Increase in the tenseness of the abdomen wall
2. Monitor intraabdominal pressures every 2 to 4 hours or more frequently, depending on clinical need.	Serial measurements will detect a trended increase in IAPs, reflecting development of ACS.	• IAPs greater than 15 mm Hg • IAPs less than 15 mm Hg if associated with other clinical findings suggestive of IAH/ACS
3. Monitor for signs and symptoms of UTI.	Frequent breaks in the integrity of the urinary drainage system may contribute to the development of UTI.	• Temperature elevation • Elevated white blood cell count • Increased sediment or cloudiness of urine

Documentation

Documentation should include the following:

- Patient and family education
- Assessment findings before obtaining intraabdominal pressures
- Intraabdominal pressure value
- Postprocedure assessment
- Changes in the patient's assessment indicating onset of IAH/ACS

- The amount of fluid instilled into the bladder to be subtracted from the hourly urine output
- Unexpected outcomes
- Additional interventions
- Reportable conditions

References

1. Balogh, Z., et al. (2002). Secondary abdominal compartment syndrome is an elusive early complication of traumatic shock resuscitation. *Am J Surg,* 184, 538-43.
2. Cheatham, M.L. (1999). Intraabdominal hypertension. *New Horiz,* 7, 96-115.
3. Cheatham, M.L., and Safcak, K. (1998). Intraabdominal pressure: A revised method for measurement. *J Am Coll Surg,* 186, 594-5.
4. Chen, R.J., Fang, J.F., and Chen, M.F. (2001). Intra-abdominal pressure monitoring as a guideline in the nonoperative management of blunt hepatic trauma. *J Trauma-Injury, Infection & Crit Care,* 51, 44-50.
5. Citerio, G., et al. (2001). Intra-abdominal pressure monitoring increases intracranial pressure in neurotrauma patients: A prospective study. *Crit Care Med,* 29, 1466-71.
6. Cullen, D., et al. (1989). Cardiovascular, pulmonary, and renal effects of massively increased intraabdominal pressure in critically ill patients. *Crit Care Med,* 17, 118-22.
7. Gracias, V.H., et al. (2002). Abdominal compartment syndrome in the open abdomen. *Arch Surg,* 137, 1298-1300.
8. Kron, I., Harman, K., and Nolan, S.P. (1984). The measurement of intraabdominal pressure as a criterion for abdominal re-exploration. *Ann Surg,* 199, 28-30.
9. Losanoff, J.E. (1999). Abdominal compartment syndrome: Prompt recognition and treatment. *Am Surg,* 65, 93-4.
10. Lozen, Y. (1999). Intraabdominal hypertension and abdominal compartment syndrome in trauma: Pathophysiology and interventions. *AACN Clin Iss,* 10, 104-12.
11. MacDonnell, S.P. (1996). Comments on the abdominal compartment syndrome: The physiological and clinical

consequences of elevated intraabdominal pressure. *J Am Coll Surg,* 183, 419-20.

12. McNelis, J., et al. (2002). Abdominal compartment syndrome in the surgical intensive care unit. *Am Surg,* 68, 18-23.

13. Ridings, P., et al. (1995). Cardiopulmonary effects of raised intraabdominal pressure before and after intravascular volume. *J Trauma,* 39, 1071-5.

14. Sanchez, N.C., et al. (2001). What is normal intra-abdominal pressure? *Am Surg,* 67, 243-8.

Additional Reading

Gallagher, J.J. (2000). Ask the expert: Describe the procedure for monitoring intra-abdominal pressure via an indwelling urinary catheter. *Crit Care Nurs,* 20, 87-91.

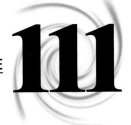
PROCEDURE **111**

Nasogastric Tube Insertion, Care, and Removal

P U R P O S E : Orogastric or nasogastric (NG) tube insertion is performed to decompress the stomach; to remove blood, secretions, ingested drugs or toxins; or to instill medications, feedings, lavage fluids, or warmed lavage fluids to correct hypothermia.

Karen K. Carlson

PREREQUISITE NURSING KNOWLEDGE

- Knowledge of anatomy of the upper gastrointestinal tract is needed.
- Orogastric or NG tubes are used for both diagnostic and therapeutic purposes. They are frequently indicated for stomach decompression and gastric contents evacuation when a patient has overdosed or hemorrhaged or has an ileus. Gastric content samples may be obtained for laboratory analysis, and medications, fluids, or feedings can be instilled.
- Orogastric or NG intubation is performed by passing a tube through either a nostril (NG) or the oral cavity (orogastric), advancing it through the oropharynx and esophagus and into the stomach.
- Orogastric intubation is specifically recommended for patients with anterior fossa skull fracture or maxillofacial injury. These patients have increased potential for inadvertent tube placement into the brain via the cribriform plate or ethmoid bone, if the tube is inserted nasally. Additionally, patients needing extra-large caliber tubes (30 to 36 Fr) for gastric emptying in drug overdoses should be orally intubated.
- A variety of tubes are available for gastric intubation. Tubes have single or double lumens, are weighted or nonweighted, and are vented or nonvented. The Levine tube is a nonvented, single-lumen tube (Fig. 111-1). This tube, used primarily for decompression, lavage, or feeding, should not be connected to suction because it may cause the tube to adhere to the mucosal surface, causing irritation. The Salem sump (Fig. 111-2), a vented, nonweighted double-lumen tube, is more commonly used when suction

is desired. The second lumen of the sump tube is the air vent, allowing air to continually irrigate the distal tip of the tube. This continual air irrigation decreases the likelihood of tube adherence to the gastric mucosa and resultant irritation.
- Small-bore, weighted, single-lumen tubes are preferred for enteral feedings (see Procedure 145).

EQUIPMENT

- Orogastric or NG tube (size range is 12 to 18 Fr for adults)
- Water-soluble lubricant
- Nonsterile gloves
- 20- to 50-ml syringe with catheter tip or adapter
- Normal saline (NS) for irrigation
- Two emesis basins
- Ice
- Ice chips or cup of tap water with straw
- Suction source with connecting tubing
- Rubber band

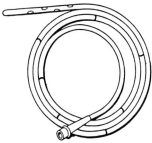

FIGURE 111-1 Nonvented single lumen (Levin) tube. *(From Norton, B.A., and Miller, A.M. [1986].* Skills for Professional Nursing Practice. *Norwalk, CT: Appleton-Century-Crofts.)*

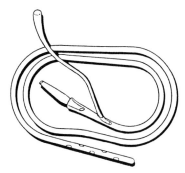

FIGURE 111-2 Vented double-lumen (Salem sump) tube. *(From Norton, B.A., and Miller, A.M. [1986]. Skills for Professional Nursing Practice.* Norwalk, CT: Appleton-Century-Crofts.)

- Safety pin
- Pink tape (Hy-tape Surgical Products Corporation, Yonkers, NY) or tube attachment device
- pH test paper
- Tongue blade
  Additional equipment (to have available depending on patient need) includes the following:
- Tincture of benzoin
- Guaiac test materials

PATIENT AND FAMILY EDUCATION

- Explain the procedure and the reason for tube insertion. ➤*Rationale:* Decreases patient anxiety.
- Explain the patient's role in assisting with passage of the tube. ➤*Rationale:* Elicits patient cooperation and facilitates insertion.
- Explain that the procedure can be uncomfortable because the gag reflex may be stimulated, causing the patient to feel nauseated or to vomit. ➤*Rationale:* Elicits patient cooperation and facilitates insertion.

PATIENT ASSESSMENT AND PREPARATION

Patient Assessment

- Obtain past medical history of nasal deformity, epistaxis, surgery, trauma, varices, or recent esophageal or gastric surgery. ➤*Rationale:* Increases the risk for complications from tube placement.
- Ensure patency of nares, if NG intubation is planned. This can be done by occluding one nostril at a time, asking the patient to breathe, and selecting the nostril with the best airflow. ➤*Rationale:* Choosing the most patent nostril will ease insertion and may improve patient tolerance of tube.
- Obtain immediate history of ingestion of drugs or toxins. ➤*Rationale:* Allows preparation for immediate evacuation or neutralization of gastric contents to prevent absorption and tissue damage.
- Obtain immediate history of facial or head injury, sinusitis, transphenoidal pituitary resection, and after basilar skull fracture[8,13] ➤*Rationale:* To decrease risk for inadvertent tube placement into the brain, orogastric tube placement should be used.

- Signs of gastric distention include the following:
  - ❖ Nausea
  - ❖ Vomiting
  - ❖ Absence of or hypoactive bowel tones
  ➤*Rationale:* Accumulation of secretions or air in the stomach increases the risk for vomiting and aspiration and provides baseline for later comparison.
- Determine need for analysis of gastric contents (e.g., pH, guaiac, drug screen). ➤*Rationale:* Knowing before the procedure is initiated if samples are needed will allow the practitioner to have necessary supplies available and to obtain samples in a timely manner.

Patient Preparation

- Ensure that patient understands preprocedural teaching. Answer questions as they arise, and reinforce information as needed. ➤*Rationale:* Evaluates and reinforces understanding of previously taught information.
- If patient is alert, place patient in high Fowler's or semi-Fowler's position. If patient is obtunded or unconscious, place him or her head-down in the left lateral position. Cover the chest with a towel. ➤*Rationale:* Facilitates passage of tube into the stomach and minimizes risk for aspiration. Inserting an NG tube into an obtunded patient may require the assistance of an additional person. Placing the obtunded or unconscious patient head-down provides safety against aspiration should the patient vomit during the procedure.
- Measure the tube from the bridge of the nose to the earlobe to the tip of the xiphoid process (Fig. 111-3). Mark the length of tube to be passed (a small piece of tape works well and can be easily removed). ➤*Rationale:* Estimates the length of the tube to be passed to ensure placement into the stomach.

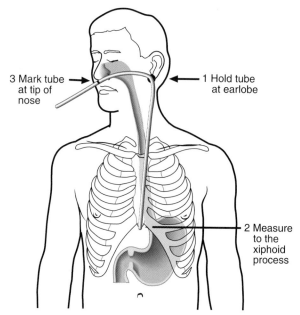

3 Mark tube at tip of nose

1 Hold tube at earlobe

2 Measure to the xiphoid process

FIGURE 111-3 Measuring nasogastric tube. *(From Luckmann, J. [1997]. Saunders Manual of Nursing Care. Philadelphia: W.B. Saunders.)*

Procedure for Nasogastric Tube Insertion, Care, and Removal

Steps	Rationale	Special Considerations
1. If tape will be used to secure the tube, prepare the tape by tearing a piece 1.5 to 2 inches long. Split the last 1 inch of the tape. Set aside.	Once the tube is in place, it will be easier to secure immediately if the tape is ready to apply.	
2. Wash hands and don personal protective equipment.	Reduces transmission of microorganisms and body secretions; standard precautions.	Immersing a rubber tube in iced water for several minutes before insertion has been recommended as a means to stiffen the tube and facilitate placement, but it may make placement more uncomfortable for the patient. Immersing a plastic tube in warm water will make the tube more flexible, facilitating placement.
3. Lubricate 6 to 10 cm of distal end of tube, using water-soluble lubricant. *(Level III: Laboratory data, no clinical data to support recommendations.)*	Minimizes mucosal injury and irritation during insertion; facilitates insertion.	It is important that only water-soluble lubricants be used in tube placement. Oil-soluble lubricants, such as petroleum jelly, cannot be absorbed by the pulmonary mucosa should the tube be inadvertently placed in the lungs. The lubricant could then cause respiratory complications.
4. For orogastric intubation: Implement direct and indirect comforting strategies throughout the procedure. *(Level IV: Limited clinical studies to support recommendations.)*	Comfort strategies have been shown to facilitate tube placement, including remaining attentive to the overall patient experience (pain, simultaneous procedures, team interaction) and using comforting talk (speech that is patterned, repetitive, and at a comfortable volume, pacing the procedure).[15,17]	
5. Position curved edge of the tube downward, inserting the tube into the oral cavity over the tongue. Aim the tube back and down toward the pharynx. When the tube hits the pharynx, have the patient flex the head forward. If patient is unable to flex his or her head, help flex it forward. If appropriate, ask the patient to take sips of water through a straw while tube is being advanced. Proceed to step 6. *(Level II: Theory based, no research data to support recommendations: recommendations from expert consensus group may exist.)*	Flexing the head of an unconscious patient will also facilitate tube placement. Having the patent take sips of water or mimic a swallowing motion causes the epiglottis to close the trachea and directs the tube toward the esophagus.	If patient is uncooperative, place an oral airway (see Procedure 9) or bite block in the mouth before attempting to place the tube to prevent the patient from biting on the tube. Having the patient flex his or her head may be especially helpful in intubated patients. If unsure whether or not cervical spine injury is present, do not flex patient's head.
6. For NG intubation: Using the more patent nare, insert the tube through the nose, aiming down and back. When the tube hits the pharynx, if patient is able, have him or her flex the	If the patient gags, coughs, or begins choking, withdraw slightly and stop insertion, allowing the patient to rest.	If resistance is met, do not force insertion, because this could damage the nasal turbinates and mucosa and cause bleeding. Having the patient flex her or his head may be especially helpful in intubated

Procedure continues on the following page

Procedure for Nasogastric Tube Insertion, Care, and Removal—*Continued*

Steps	Rationale	Special Considerations
head forward and swallow. Advance tube as patient swallows. *(Level III: Laboratory data, no clinical data to support recommendations.)*		patients. If uncertain whether or not cervical spine injury is present, do not flex patient's head.
7. If resistance is met, rotating the tube may facilitate placement.	If unable to advance tube after several attempts, notify physician or advanced practice nurse.	
8. Continue to advance the tube until the marked position on the tube is reached.	Advances tube into stomach.	
9. Confirm tube placement in stomach. A. Aspirate fluid and evaluate the pH. *(Level V: Clinical studies in more than one patient population and situation.)*	With pH testing, gastric placement will often show a pH less than 5.5. Intestinal placement will usually show a pH greater than 6.0. Pulmonary secretions have an alkaline pH.[9,11,14] A pH test strip with multiple comparative color columns increases the probability of obtaining accurate pH estimation. A test strip with a wide range (such as 1 to 10) is preferred.	Common practice for many years has been to evaluate tube placement by placing a stethoscope over the stomach and instilling 20 to 50 ml of air via syringe. There are numerous reports in the literature of false-positive results using this method, including reports of serious pulmonary complications because of tracheal tube placement.[9,5-7,19] The ability to simply aspirate fluid from the tube is often interpreted as confirmation of gastric intubation. Several reports[16,19] have shown that fluid can also be aspirated after endotracheal intubation. Also, some authors have suggested that placement can be confirmed by placing the tip of the NG tube under water and observing for bubbles. Bubbles would indicate endotracheal intubation. Although logical, this method is also unreliable.[3,9] If a tube were lodged in the mucosal wall of either the esophagus or the lung, no bubbles would result, but placement would be incorrect.
B. Aspirate fluid and evaluate its appearance. *(Level V: Clinical studies in more than one patient population and situation.)*	Gastric juice is usually clear and colorless. When pigment is present, gastric aspirate may appear off-white, tan, or grassy green (because of refluxed bile that has been exposed to gastric acid).[4,10] Small intestine aspirates are usually golden (bile-stained) and have a translucent appearance. When formula is being administered continuously, appearance of GI aspirates is less helpful in distinguishing between gastric and small bowel placement. An aspirate from the stomach, obtained during continuous feedings, may have the appearance of formula that has been mixed	

Procedure for Nasogastric Tube Insertion, Care, and Removal—*Continued*		
Steps	**Rationale**	**Special Considerations**
	with gastric juice (perhaps curdled by the presence of gastric acid). An aspirate from the small bowel during continuous feedings may be bile-stained: often it appears as unaltered formula.[12,13]	
C. Attach a pressure gauge (negative inspiratory force spring-gauge manometer) to distal tip of tube. *(Level IV: Limited clinical studies to support recommendations.)*	Tubes placed in the gastrointestinal tract will yield positive pressures (0 or greater), whereas tubes placed in the pulmonary tract will yield negative pressures (less than 0).[18]	In theory, this procedure has merit. However, in practice, there are potential problems. It is unclear how well the gauge works when used in small-bore tubes or whether occlusion of the tube's ports against the mucosa might interfere with the pressure reading. False readings are possible.
D. Attach an end-tidal carbon dioxide detector to the proximal end of the tube. Observe for color change. *(Level IV: Limited clinical studies to support recommendations.)*	If carbon dioxide is detected, the tube has been placed in the airway.[1]	Lack of color change is not completely indicative of gastric placement. False readings might occur if the tube's ports were occluded by mucosa or mucus.
10. Secure tube in position, using pink tape (Fig. 111-4), clear or adhesive dressing, or a commercially available tube holder. *(Level IV: Limited clinical studies to support recommendations.)*	Maintains tube in correct position and prevents inadvertent dislodgment. Use of pink tape (Hy-tape Surgical Products Corporation, Yonkers, NY) was found to be superior to two other methods.[2]	A variety of methods are used to secure the tube in place, including use of different types of tape, clear adhesive dressings, and commercially available tube holders. Whatever means employed, the goal is to avoid exerting pressure against the rim of the nare, because ulceration could occur.

Procedure continues on the following page

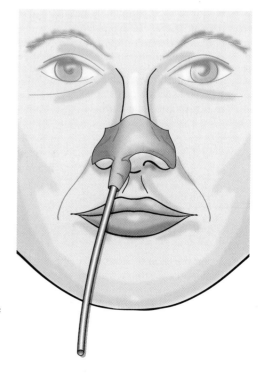

FIGURE 111-4 Pink tape method. One half of a 1.5-inch strip was applied to the nose, and the lower portion was split up to the tip of the nose. Each half of the tape was then wrapped around the tube and the strip of white water-proof tape. *(Adapted from Burns, S.M., et al. [1995]. Comparison of nasogastric tube securing methods and tube types in medical intensive care patients. Am J Crit Care, 4[3]:201.)*

Procedure for Nasogastric Tube Insertion, Care, and Removal—*Continued*

Steps	Rationale	Special Considerations
11. Attach primary lumen to suction or gravity drainage, as ordered.	Initiates therapy.	
12. Secure tube to patient's gown 10 to 12 in from nose. Loop rubber band around tube and pin rubber band to gown.	Prevents tube from pulling and putting pressure against the rim of the nose; provides additional protection against tube dislodgment.	
13. Reassess position of tube per institutional standards and patient condition and before instillation of any medication, irrigant, or feeding.	Incorrect position of tube increases risk for aspiration.	
14. Irrigate tube per institutional standards and patient condition and as needed with 20 to 30 ml NS.	Ensure tube patency.	Some institutions use air to irrigate the tube. However, there is no evidence that air is sufficient to keep a tube patent after feedings or medications have been administered via the tube.
15. Document in patient record.		
Tube Removal		
1. Wash hands and don personal protective equipment.	Reduces transmission of microorganisms and body secretions; standard precautions.	
2. Cover patient's chest with a towel.	Drainage from the tube may be present on the tube as it is removed. Covering the chest with a towel prevents soiling of patient gown and covers.	
3. Remove tape or tube holder. If tube is pinned to gown, remove pin.	Allows for easy removal of tube.	
4. Using smooth, constant motion, withdraw tube completely out of patient. *(Level III: Laboratory data, no clinical data to support recommendations.)*		
5. Wrap tube in towel and discard tube and suction canister according to institutional standard.	Provides a means for collecting any drainage on tube and moving it to a correct disposal receptacle.	
6. Provide oral or nasal care as needed.	Cleanse area where tube was in place; increases patient comfort.	
7. Document in patient record.		

Expected Outcomes

- Decompression of stomach
- Evacuation of stomach and proximal small intestine contents
- Instillation of fluid, medications, or feedings

Unexpected Outcomes

- Tube placement into trachea, bronchus, or esophagus
- Bleeding from nose, mouth, esophagus, or stomach
- Vagal response during insertion or from gag reflex stimulation
- Skin ulceration, sinusitis, esophageal-tracheal fistula, gastric ulceration, or oral infections
- Vomiting or aspiration

Patient Monitoring and Care

Steps	Rationale	Reportable Conditions
		These conditions should be reported if they persist despite nursing interventions.
1. Maintain and check tube patency every 4 hours and as needed.	Prevents gastric distention and associated patient discomfort.	• Inability to establish patency
2. Monitor output (color, amount, type, pH, guaiac) every 4 hours and as needed.	Provides data for diagnosis and fluid balance.	• Increasing output or sudden change in output (increase or decrease) • Frank blood or brown, black, or "coffee-ground" returns • Positive guaiac • Abnormal pH
3. Calculate output into patient's overall intake and output record.	Volume loss from gastric secretions can cause patients to become hypovolemic; large volumes may need to be replaced with appropriate intravenous fluids.	• Increasing output or sudden change in output (increase or decrease)
4. Assess oral cavity and perform oral care every 2 hours and as needed.	Patients with orogastric or NG tubes in place tend to mouth-breathe, drying their mouths and increasing the risk for mucosal breakdown and ulceration. Tube presence may also predispose a patient to sinusitis or oral infections.	• Ulceration, drainage, foul odor
5. Monitor insertion site of tube for redness, swelling, drainage, bleeding, or skin breakdown. Use only water-soluble lubricants at site.	Many critically ill patients have fragile skin and have associated conditions that predispose them to skin breakdown. Frequent monitoring and subsequent repositioning of the tube can prevent serious damage.	• Redness • Swelling • Drainage • Bleeding • Skin breakdown at insertion site
6. Irrigate the tube, using air or NS, per institutional standards and as needed.	Assists in maintaining patency of tube and facilitates drainage.	• Inability to irrigate tube
7. If using a sump tube, position pigtail above the level of the patient's stomach. Irrigate pigtail with 5 to 10 ml of air per institutional standards.	Prevents backflow of gastric secretions; antireflux valves are available.[20]	• Backflow of gastric contents
8. Maintain tube to suction as ordered.	Low (20 to 80 mm Hg), intermittent suction is recommended to minimize gastric mucosal irritation yet provide for adequate drainage.	
9. Monitor vital signs per unit standards. Perform respiratory and gastrointestinal assessment every 2 hours.	Change in vital signs or respiratory or gastrointestinal assessments may be early warning signs of the development of complications.	• Sudden change in vital signs • Unexplained respiratory distress • Increased abdominal distention, change in bowel tones
10. Reposition and retape tube every 24 hours or when tape is soiled.	Decreases risk of tissue damage to mouth or nares.	

Documentation

Documentation should include the following:

- Patient and family education
- Insertion of orogastric or NG tube
- Tube type and size
- Any difficulties in insertion
- Patient toleration
- How placement was confirmed

- Appearance and volume of gastric secretions, if present
- Amount and type of irrigation fluid (if appropriate)
- Oral care
- Tube site assessments
- Unexpected outcomes
- Nursing interventions

References

1. Araujo-Persa, C.E., et al. (2002). Use of capnometry to verify feeding tube placement. *Crit Care Med, 30*, 2255-9.
2. Burns, S.M., et al. (1995). Comparison of nasogastric tube securing methods and tube types in medical intensive care patients. *Am J Crit Care, 4*, 198-203.
3. Chang, J., et al. (1982). Inadvertent endobronchial intubation with nasogastric tube. *Arch Otolaryngol, 108*, 528-9.
4. Gharpure, V., et al. (2000). Indicators of post-pyloric feeding tube placement. *Crit Care Med, 28*, 2962-6.
5. Hand, W., et al. (1984). Inadvertent transbronchial insertion of narrow bore feeding tubes into the pleural space. *JAMA, 251*, 2396-7.
6. Lipman, T.O., Kessler, T., and Arabian, A. (1995). Nasopulmonary intubation with feeding tubes: Case reports and review of the literature. *J Parenter Enteral Nutr, 5*, 618-20.
7. Metheny, N. (1988). Measures to test placement of nasogastric and nasoenteric feeding tubes: A review. *Nurs Res, 37*, 324-9.
8. Metheny, N. (2002). Inadvertent intracranial placement of a nasogastric tube following transnasal transsphenoidal surgery: A case report. *AJN, 102*, 25-7.
9. Metheny, N., et al. (1990). Effectiveness of the auscultatory method in predicting feeding tube location. *Nurs Res, 5*, 262-7.
10. Metheny, N., et al. (1994). Visual characteristics of aspirates from feeding tubes as a method for predicting tube location. *Nurs Res, 43*, 282-7.
11. Metheny, N., et al. (1993). Effectiveness of pH measurements in predicting feeding tube placement: An update. *Nurs Res, 43*, 324-31.
12. Metheny, N., and Stewart, B. (2002). Testing feeding tube placement during continuous tube feedings. *Applied Nurs Res, 15*, 254-8.
13. Metheny, N., and Titler, M. (2001). Assessing placement of feeding tubes. *AJN, 101*, 36-42.
14. Metheny, N., et al. (1989). Effectiveness of pH measurements in predicting feeding tube placement. *Nurs Res, 38*, 280-5.
15. Morse, J.M., et al. (2000). Evaluating the efficiency of effectiveness of approaches to nasogastric tube insertion during trauma care. *Am J Crit Care, 9*, 325-33.
16. Nakao, M.A., Killam, D., and Wilson, R. (1983). Pneumothorax secondary to inadvertent nasotracheal placement of a nasoenteric tube past a cuffed endotracheal tube. *Crit Care Med, 11*, 210-1.
17. Penrod, J., Morse, J.M., and Wilson, S. (1999). Comforting strategies used during nasogastric tube insertion. *J Clin Nurs, 8*, 31-3.
18. Swiech, K., Lancaster, D.R., and Sheehan, R. (1994). Use of a pressure gauge to differentiate gastric from pulmonary placement of nasoenteral feeding tubes. *Appl Nurs Res, 4*, 183-9.
19. Theodore, A.C., et al. (1984). Errant placement of nasoenteric tubes: A hazard in obtunded patients. *Chest, 86*, 931-3.
20. Tucker, K., Kaiser, S., and Ahrens, T. (1991). Clinical effectiveness of a GI antireflux valve. *Heart Lung, 20*, 304.

Additional Reading

Metheny, N., et al. (1998). pH, color, and feeding tubes. *RN, 61*, 25-7.

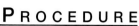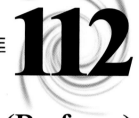

PROCEDURE **112**

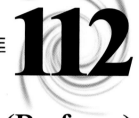

Paracentesis (Perform)

PURPOSE: Abdominal paracentesis is performed to remove fluid from the peritoneal cavity for diagnostic or therapeutic purposes.

Peggy Kirkwood

PREREQUISITE NURSING KNOWLEDGE

- Knowledge of anatomy and physiology of the abdomen is important in order to avoid unexpected outcomes.
- Intestines and bladder lie immediately beneath the abdominal surface.
- Large volumes of ascitic fluid will tend to float the air-filled bowel toward the midline, where it may be easily perforated during the procedure.
- The cecum is relatively fixed and is much less mobile than the sigmoid colon. Therefore bowel perforations are more frequent in the right lower quadrant than in the left.
- Peritoneal fluid is normally straw-colored, serous fluid secreted by the cells of the peritoneum. Grossly bloody fluid in the abdomen is abnormal.
- The peritoneal fluid collected is used to evaluate and diagnose the cause of ascites, acute abdominal conditions such as peritonitis or pancreatitis, and blunt or penetrating trauma to the abdomen.
- Therapeutic paracentesis is used to reduce intraabdominal and diaphragmatic pressures in order to relieve dyspnea and respiratory compromise and prevent peritoneal rupture.
- Ascitic fluid is produced as a result of a variety of conditions. These may include interference in venous return because of heart failure, constrictive pericarditis, or tricuspid valve insufficiency; obstruction of flow in the vena cava or portal vein; disturbance in electrolyte balance such as sodium retention; depletion of plasma proteins, because of nephrotic syndrome or starvation; lymphoma, leukemia, or neoplasms involving the liver or mediastinum; ovarian malignancy; chronic pancreatitis; or cirrhosis of the liver.
- Paracentesis is contraindicated in patients with an acute abdomen, who require immediate surgery. Coagulopathies and thrombocytopenia are considered relative contraindications. Coagulopathy should preclude paracentesis only when there is clinically evident fibrinolysis or clinically evident disseminated intravascular coagulation.
- Caution should be used when paracentesis is performed in patients with severe bowel distention, previous abdominal surgery (especially pelvic surgery), pregnancy (use open technique after first trimester), distended bladder that cannot be emptied with a Foley catheter, or obvious infection at intended site of insertion (cellulitis or abscess).
- Insertion site should be midline one third the distance from the umbilicus to the symphysis, or 2 to 3 cm below the umbilicus (Fig. 112-1). Alternate position is a point one third the distance from the umbilicus to the anterior iliac crest (left side preferred).[1]
- Ultrasound can be used prior to paracentesis to locate fluid and during the procedure to guide insertion of catheter.[10]
- A semipermanent catheter or a shunt may be an option for patients with rapidly reaccumulating ascites.[3,5,7-8]

EQUIPMENT

- Commercially prepared kit or the following:
  - ❖ Sterile gloves and mask
  - ❖ Skin-cleansing solution (povidone-iodine)
  - ❖ Sterile marking pen
  - ❖ Sterile towels or sterile drape

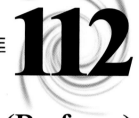

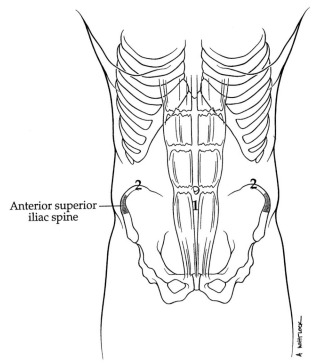

FIGURE 112-1 Preferred sites for paracentesis: **1,** Primary site is infraumbilical in midline through linea alba. **2,** Preferred alternate (lateral rectus) site is in either lower quadrant, approximately 4 to 5 cm cephalad and medical to the anterior superior iliac spine. *(From Roberts, J.R., and Hedges, J.R. [2004]. Clinical Procedures in Emergency Medicine. 4th ed. Philadelphia: W.B. Saunders.)*

- Local anesthetic for injection: 1% or 2% lidocaine with epinephrine
- 5- or 10-ml syringe with 21- or 25-G needle for anesthetic
- Trocar with stylet, needle (16-, 18-, or 20-G), or angio-catheter, depending on abdominal wall thickness
- 25- or 27-G 1½-in needle
- 20- or 22-G spinal needles
- 20-ml syringe for diagnostic tap
- 50-ml syringe if using stopcock technique
- Four sterile tubes for specimens
- Scalpel and No. 11 knife blade
- Three-way stopcock
- Sterile 1-L collection bottles with connecting tubing
- Nylon skin suture material on cutting needle (4-0 or 5-0) and needle holder
- Mayo scissors and straight scissors
- Four to six sterile 4 × 4 gauze pads
- Sterile gauze dressing with tape or adhesive strip
- Stoma bag
- Soft wrist restraints

PATIENT AND FAMILY EDUCATION

- Explain the indications, procedure, and risks to the patient and family. ➤*Rationale:* Decreases patient anxiety

and encourages patient and family cooperation and understanding of the procedure.
- Explain the patient's role in assisting with the procedure and postprocedure care. ➤*Rationale:* Elicits patient cooperation during and after the procedure.
- Explain the signs and symptoms to report, such as fever, abdominal pain, decreased urine output, bleeding, and leakage of fluid from surgical wound site. ➤*Rationale:* Unexpected outcomes may not manifest themselves for a period of time following the procedure.

PATIENT ASSESSMENT AND PREPARATION

Patient Assessment

- Past medical history and review of systems for abdominal injury, major gastrointestinal pathology, liver disease, and portal hypertension. ➤*Rationale:* Certain conditions of the gastrointestinal tract may be diagnosed and treated with paracentesis. Contraindications to paracentesis may be identified.
- Respiratory status (i.e., rate, depth, excursion, gas exchange, and use of accessory muscles). ➤*Rationale:* Paracentesis may be indicated to decrease work of breathing.
- Baseline heart rate, blood pressure, and pulse oximetry. ➤*Rationale:* Hypotension and dysrhythmias may occur with rapid changes in intraabdominal pressure.
- Baseline fluid and electrolyte status. ➤*Rationale:* Removal of peritoneal fluid may cause compartment shifting of intravascular volume, electrolytes, and proteins, leading to a decreased circulating volume.
- Bowel or bladder distention. ➤*Rationale:* Distension increases the risk for bowel or bladder perforation during the procedure.
- Abdominal girth. ➤*Rationale:* Provides information on changes in fluid accumulation within the peritoneal cavity.
- Coagulation studies (i.e., prothrombin time [PT], partial thromboplastin time [PTT], and platelets). ➤*Rationale:* Abnormal clotting studies may increase the risk for bleeding during and after the procedure. Therapy may be necessary to correct clotting abnormalities before the procedure.

Patient Preparation

- Ensure that patient understands preprocedural teaching. Answer questions as they arise and reinforce information as needed. ➤*Rationale:* Evaluates and reinforces understanding of previously taught information.
- Obtain a written informed consent form. ➤*Rationale:* Paracentesis is an invasive procedure, requiring a signed informed consent form.
- Decompress the bladder either by having the patient void or by inserting a Foley catheter. ➤*Rationale:* A distended bladder increases the risk for bladder perforation during the procedure.
- Obtain plain and upright x-rays of the abdomen before performing the procedure. ➤*Rationale:* Air is introduced during the procedure and may confuse the diagnosis later.

- Place the patient in the supine position (may tilt to side of collection slightly for improved fluid positioning). ➥*Rationale:* Fluid accumulates in the dependent areas.
- Examine abdomen for areas of shifting dullness. Find landmarks and mark appropriately. ➥*Rationale:* Shifting dullness indicates fluid.

- If the patient has altered mental status, soft wrist restraints may be needed. ➥*Rationale:* It is imperative that the patient not move his or her hands into the sterile field once it has been established.

Procedure for Performing Paracentesis

Steps	Rationale	Special Considerations
1. Wash hands and put on mask.	Reduces the transmission of microorganisms and body secretions; standard precautions.	
2. Prepare equipment and sterile field.	Facilitates easy access to needed equipment.	Maintain aseptic technique.
3. Cleanse insertion site with povidone-iodine solution.	Reduces risk for infection.	Use sterile technique.
4. Determine the site for trochar insertion.	Site should be midline one third the distance from the umbilicus to the symphysis (2 to 3 cm below the umbilicus; see Fig. 112-1). Alternate position is a point one third the distance from the umbilicus to the anterior iliac crest (left side preferred).	Avoid the rectus muscle because of increased risk for hemorrhage from epigastric vessels; surgical scars because of increased risk for perforation caused by adhesion of bowel to the wall of the peritoneum; and upper quadrants because of the possibility of undetected hepatomegaly.[1]
5. Apply sterile gloves.	Reduces transmission of microorganisms and body secretions.	
6. Apply sterile drapes to outline the area to be tapped.	Provide sterile field to decrease risk for infection.	
7. Inject area with local anesthetic (lidocaine with epinephrine preferred). Initially infiltrate skin and subcutaneous tissues; then direct needle perpendicular to the skin and infiltrate the peritoneum.	Local anesthesia minimizes pain and discomfort. Epinephrine helps eliminate unwanted abdominal wall bleeding and false-positive results.	Maximum dose of lidocaine is 30 ml of 1% or 15 ml of 2%. Assess for anesthesia of area. Resistance will be felt as the needle perforates the peritoneum.
8. Using the No. 11 blade and scalpel holder, create a skin incision large enough to allow threading a 3- to 5-mm catheter.	Allows ease of entry for the catheter.	If necessary to lavage, the opening will be large enough to thread the lavage catheter.
9. Insert an 18-gauge needle attached to a 20-ml or 50-ml syringe through the anesthetized tract into the peritoneum. Apply slight suction to the syringe as it is advanced. Grasp the needle close to the skin as it is advanced.	Provides access to peritoneal fluid for evacuation. Slight suction is applied to indicate when the peritoneum is entered and if a blood vessel is entered. Grasping the needle as it is advanced prevents accidental thrusting into the abdomen and possible viscous perforation.	Inserted through small stab wound at midline below umbilicus. A small pop is felt as needle advances through anterior and posterior muscle fascia and enters peritoneum.

Procedure continues on the following page

Procedure | **for Performing Paracentesis**—*Continued*

Steps	Rationale	Special Considerations
10. Once in the cavity, direct the needle at a 60-degree angle toward the center of the pelvic hollow. When fluid returns, fill the syringe (Fig. 112-2).	Collection of fluid for laboratory studies to provide information about the patient's status.	Usually, diagnostic tests are ordered dependent on patient's status and reason for paracentesis.[4] They may include the following: tube 1—lactate dehydrogenase (LDH), glucose, albumin; tube 2—protein, specific gravity; tube 3—cell count and differential; tube 4—save until further notice. If indicated, Gram stain, acid-fast bacillus (AFB) stain, bacterial and fungal cultures, amylase and triglycerides.[1]
11. Attach syringes or stopcock and tubing and gently aspirate or siphon fluid by gravity or vacuum into collection device. Drains may be left in and allowed to drain for 6 to 12 hours.[10] *(Level IV: Limited clinical studies to support recommendations.)*	Initiates therapy.	Monitor amount of fluid removed. Removal of large amount of fluid (greater than 5 L) may cause hypotension.[6,9,11] If large amounts are removed or hypotension is seen, consider IV albumin to maintain intravascular volume.[2,3] *There is no evidence that leaving the drain in for 24-48 hours or more is safer or more effective.[6]*
12. After the fluid is removed, gently remove the catheter and apply pressure to the wound. If the wound is still leaking fluid after 5 minutes of direct pressure, suture the puncture site using a mattress suture (see Procedure 134) and apply a pressure dressing. If there is significant leakage, apply a stoma bag over the site until drainage becomes minimal.	Keeps insertion site clean. Reduces risk for infection.	Inspect catheter to ensure it is intact.

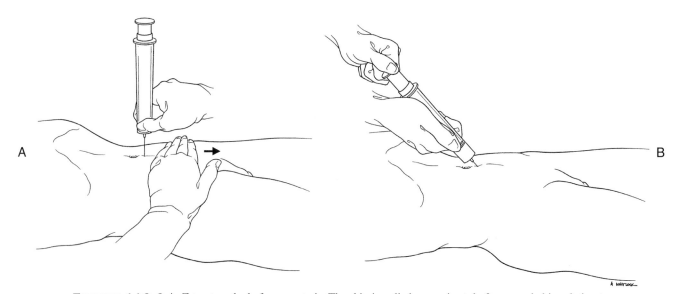

FIGURE 112-2 **A,** Z-tract method of paracentesis. The skin is pulled approximately 2 cm caudad in relation to the deep abdominal wall by the non-needle-bearing hand while the paracentesis needle is slowly being inserted directly perpendicular to the skin. **B,** After penetrating the peritoneum and obtaining fluid return, the skin is released. Note that the needle is angulated caudally. *(From Roberts, J.R., and Hedges, J.R. [2004]. Clinical Procedures in Emergency Medicine. 4th ed. Philadelphia: W.B. Saunders.)*

Procedure for Performing Paracentesis—*Continued*

Steps	Rationale	Special Considerations
13. Apply sterile dressing to wound site.	Provides a barrier to infection and collects fluid that may leak from wound site.	
14. Dispose of equipment and soiled material in appropriate receptacle.	Standard precautions.	
15. Wash hands.	Reduces transmission of microorganisms.	
16. Document in patient record.		

Expected Outcomes

- Evacuation of peritoneal fluid for laboratory analysis
- Decompression of peritoneal cavity
- Relief of respiratory compromise
- Relief of abdominal discomfort

Unexpected Outcomes

- Perforation of bowel, bladder, or stomach
- Lacerations of major vessels (mesenteric, iliac, aorta)
- Abdominal wall hematomas
- Laceration of catheter and loss in peritoneal cavity
- Incisional hernias
- Local or systemic infection
- Hypovolemia, hypotension, shock
- Bleeding from insertion site
- Ascitic fluid leak from insertion site
- Peritonitis

Patient Monitoring and Care

Steps	Rationale	Reportable Conditions
		These conditions should be reported if they persist despite nursing interventions.
1. Evaluate changes in abdominal girth.	Provides evidence of fluid reaccumulation.	• Increasing abdominal girth
2. Monitor for changes in respiratory status.	Removal of ascitic fluid should relieve pressure on the diaphragm and the resulting respiratory distress.	• Respiratory rate greater than 24 breaths per minute or significant increase from baseline • Increased depth of breathing • Irregular breathing pattern • Pulse oximetry less than 92%, or significant decrease from baseline
3. Monitor for potential complications, including bowel or bladder perforation, bleeding, and intravascular volume loss.	Paracentesis interrupts the integrity of the skin and underlying peritoneum.	• Hematuria • Hypotension • Tachycardia
4. Monitor vital signs, temperature, insertion site for drainage, or evidence of infection.	Rapid changes in intraabdominal pressure may affect heart rate and blood pressure. Infection is a complication of paracentesis.	• Hypotension • Dysrhythmias • Increased temperature • Purulent drainage from insertion site • Redness, swelling at insertion site • Abnormal laboratory results (e.g., increased white blood cells [WBCs])
5. Monitor intake and output.	Provides data for evaluation of fluid balance status.	• Inappropriate fluid balance or changes from baseline fluid status

Procedure continues on the following page

Patient Monitoring and Care—*Continued*

Steps	Rationale	Reportable Conditions
6. Monitor abdominal pain and level of weakness.	Patients often feel weak and experience abdominal discomfort for a few hours after the procedure.	• Continued pain after several hours
7. Evaluate laboratory data when returned.	Provides for evaluation of condition and aids in diagnosis.	• Red blood cells (RBCs) greater than 100,000/mm^3 • Amylase greater than 2.5 times normal • Alkaline phosphatase greater than 5.5 mg/dl • WBCs greater than 100/mm^3 • Positive culture results

Documentation

Documentation should include the following:

- Patient and family education
- Date and time of procedure
- Patient tolerance of procedure
- Assessment of insertion site after procedure
- Amount and characteristics of fluid removed

- Specimens sent for laboratory analysis
- Postprocedure vital signs, respiratory status, and abdominal girth
- Unexpected outcomes
- Nursing interventions

References

1. Ferri, F.F. (2004). Paracentesis. In: Ferri, F., ed. *Practical Guide to the Care of the Medical Patient.* 6th ed. St. Louis: Mosby, 810-12.
2. Gines, A., et al. (1996). Randomized trial comparing albumin, dextran 70, and polygeline in cirrhotic patients with ascites treated by paracentesis. *Gastroenterology,* 111, 1002-10.
3. Iyengar, T.D., and Herzog, T.J. (2002). Management of symptomatic ascites in recurrent ovarian cancer patients using an intra-abdominal semi-permanent catheter. *Am J Hosp Palliat Care,* 9, 35-8.
4. Jeffries, M.A., et al. (1999). Unsuspected infection is infrequent in asymptomatic outpatients with refractory ascites undergoing therapeutic paracentesis. *Am J Gastroenterol,* 94, 2972-6.
5. O'Neill, M.J., et al. (2001). Tunneled peritoneal catheter placement under sonographic and fluoroscopic guidance in the palliative treatment of malignant ascites. *Am J Roentgenol,* 177, 615-8.
6. Peltekian, K.M., et al. (1997). Cardiovascular, renal and neurohumoral responses to single large-volume paracentesis in cirrhotic patients with diuretic-resistant ascites. *Am J Gastroenterol,* 92, 394-9.
7. Richard, H.M., III, et al. (2001). Pleurx tunneled catheter in the management of malignant ascites. *J Vasc Interv Radiol,* 12, 373-5.
8. Rossle, M., et al. (2000). A comparison of paracentesis and transjugular intrahepatic portosystemic shunting in patients with ascites. *N Engl J Med,* 342, 1701-7.
9. Runyon, B.A. (1997). Patient selection is important in studying the impact of large-volume paracentesis on intravascular volume. *Am J Gastroentero,* 92, 371-3.
10. Stephenson, J., and Gilbert, J. (2002). The development of clinical guidelines on paracentesis for ascites related to malignancy. *Palliat Med,* 16, 213-8.
11. Vila, M.C., et al. (1998). Hemodynamic changes in patients developing effective hypovolemia after total paracentesis. *J Hepatol,* 28, 639-45.

Additional Readings

Blendis, L., and Wong, F. (2003). The natural history and management of hepatorenal disorders: From pre-ascites to hepatorenal syndrome. *Clin Med,* 3, 154-9.
Lee, C.W., Bociek, G., and Faught, W. (1998). A survey of practice in management of malignant ascites. *J Pain Symptom Manage,* 16, 96-101.
Marx, J.A. (2004). Peritoneal procedures. In: Roberts, J.R., and Hedges, J.R., eds. *Clinical Procedures in Emergency Medicine.* 4th ed. Philadelphia: W.B. Saunders, 733-49.
McNamara, P. (2000). Paracentesis—An effective method of symptom control in the palliative care setting? *Palliat Med,* 14, 62-4.
Moorson, D. (2001). Paracentesis in a home care setting. *Palliat Med,* 15, 169-70.
Tamsma, J.T., Keizer, H.J., and Meinders, A.E. (2001). Pathogenesis of malignant ascites: Starling's law of capillary hemodynamics revisited. *Ann Oncol,* 12, 1353-7.
Vila, M.C., et al. (1998). Hemodynamic changes in patients developing effective hypovolemia after total paracentesis. *J Hepatology,* 28, 639-45.

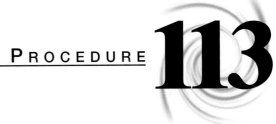

PROCEDURE **113**

Paracentesis (Assist)

PURPOSE: Abdominal paracentesis is performed to remove fluid from the peritoneal cavity for diagnostic or therapeutic purposes.

Peggy Kirkwood
Karen K. Carlson

PREREQUISITE NURSING KNOWLEDGE

- Knowledge of anatomy and physiology of the abdomen is important in order to avoid unexpected outcomes.
- Intestines and bladder lie immediately beneath the abdominal surface.
- Large volumes of ascitic fluid will tend to float the air-filled bowel toward the midline, where it may be easily perforated during the procedure.
- The cecum is relatively fixed and is much less mobile than the sigmoid colon. Therefore bowel perforations are more frequent in the right lower quadrant than in the left.
- Peritoneal fluid is normally straw-colored, serous fluid secreted by the cells of the peritoneum. Grossly bloody fluid in the abdomen is abnormal.
- The peritoneal fluid collected is used to evaluate and diagnose the cause of ascites, acute abdominal conditions such as peritonitis or pancreatitis, and blunt or penetrating trauma to the abdomen.
- Therapeutic paracentesis is used to reduce intraabdominal and diaphragmatic pressures in order to relieve dyspnea and respiratory compromise and prevent peritoneal rupture.
- Ascitic fluid is produced as a result of a variety of conditions. These may include interference in venous return because of heart failure, constrictive pericarditis, or tricuspid valve insufficiency; obstruction of flow in the vena cava or portal vein; disturbance in electrolyte balance such as sodium retention; depletion of plasma proteins, because of nephrotic syndrome or starvation; lymphoma, leukemia, or neoplasms involving the liver or mediastinum; ovarian malignancy; chronic pancreatitis; or cirrhosis of the liver.
- Paracentesis is contraindicated in patients with an acute abdomen, who require immediate surgery. Coagulopathies

and thrombocytopenia are considered relative contraindications. Coagulopathy should preclude paracentesis only when there is clinically evident fibrinolysis or clinically evident disseminated intravascular coagulation.
- Caution should be used when paracentesis is performed in patients with severe bowel distention, previous abdominal surgery (especially pelvic surgery), pregnancy (use open technique after first trimester), distended bladder that cannot be emptied with a Foley catheter, or obvious infection at intended site of insertion (cellulitis or abscess).
- Insertion site should be midline one third the distance from the umbilicus to the symphysis (2 to 3 cm below the umbilicus; see Fig. 112-1). Alternate position is a point one third the distance from the umbilicus to the anterior iliac crest (left side preferred).[1]
- Ultrasound can be used prior to paracentesis to locate fluid and during the procedure to guide insertion of catheter.[10]
- A semipermanent catheter or a shunt may be an option for patients with rapidly reaccumulating ascites.[3,5,7-8]

EQUIPMENT

- Commercially prepared kit or the following:
  - ❖ Sterile gloves and mask
  - ❖ Skin-cleansing solution (povidone-iodine)
  - ❖ Sterile marking pen
  - ❖ Sterile towels or sterile drape
  - ❖ Local anesthetic for injection: 1% or 2% lidocaine with epinephrine
  - ❖ 5- or 10-ml syringe with 21- or 25-G needle for anesthetic
  - ❖ Trocar with stylet, needle (16-, 18-, or 20-G), or angiocatheter, depending on abdominal wall thickness

❖ 25- or 27-G 11/2 -in needle
❖ 20- or 22-G spinal needles
❖ 20-ml syringe for diagnostic tap
❖ 50-ml syringe if using stopcock technique
❖ Four sterile tubes for specimens
❖ Scalpel and No. 11 knife blade
❖ Three-way stopcock
❖ Sterile 1-L collection bottles with connecting tubing
❖ Nylon skin suture material on cutting needle (4-0 or 5-0) and needle holder
❖ Mayo scissors and straight scissors
❖ Four to six sterile 4 × 4 gauze pads
❖ Sterile gauze dressing with tape or adhesive strip
❖ Stoma bag
❖ Soft wrist restraints

PATIENT AND FAMILY EDUCATION

- Explain the indications, procedure, and risks to the patient and family. ➻*Rationale:* Decreases patient anxiety and encourages patient and family cooperation and understanding of the procedure.
- Explain the patient's role in assisting with the procedure and postprocedure care. ➻*Rationale:* Elicits patient cooperation during and after the procedure.
- Explain the signs and symptoms to report, such as fever, abdominal pain, decreased urine output, bleeding, and leakage of fluid from surgical wound site. ➻*Rationale:* Unexpected outcomes may not manifest themselves for a period of time following the procedure.

PATIENT ASSESSMENT AND PREPARATION

Patient Assessment

- Past medical history and review of systems for abdominal injury, major gastrointestinal pathology, liver disease, and portal hypertension. ➻*Rationale:* Certain conditions of the gastrointestinal tract may be diagnosed and treated with paracentesis. Contraindications to paracentesis may be identified.
- Respiratory status (i.e., rate, depth, excursion, gas exchange, and use of accessory muscles). ➻*Rationale:* Paracentesis may be indicated to decrease work of breathing.

- Baseline heart rate, blood pressure, and pulse oximetry. ➻*Rationale:* Hypotension and dysrhythmias may occur with rapid changes in intra-abdominal pressure.
- Baseline fluid and electrolyte status. ➻*Rationale:* Removal of peritoneal fluid may cause compartment shifting of intravascular volume, electrolytes, and proteins, leading to a decreased circulating volume.
- Bowel or bladder distention. ➻*Rationale:* Distension increases the risk for bowel or bladder perforation during the procedure.
- Abdominal girth. ➻*Rationale:* Provides information on changes in fluid accumulation within the peritoneal cavity.
- Coagulation studies (i.e., prothrombin time [PT], partial thromboplastin time [PTT], and platelets). ➻*Rationale:* Abnormal clotting studies may increase the risk for bleeding during and after the procedure. Therapy may be necessary to correct clotting abnormalities before the procedure.

Patient Preparation

- Ensure that patient understands preprocedural teaching. Answer questions as they arise and reinforce information as needed. ➻*Rationale:* Evaluates and reinforces understanding of previously taught information.
- Obtain a written informed consent form. ➻*Rationale:* Paracentesis is an invasive procedure, requiring a signed informed consent form.
- Decompress the bladder either by having the patient void or by inserting a Foley catheter. ➻*Rationale:* A distended bladder increases the risk for bladder perforation during the procedure.
- Obtain plain and upright x-rays of the abdomen before performing the procedure. ➻*Rationale:* Air is introduced during the procedure and may confuse the diagnosis later.
- Place the patient in the supine position (may tilt to side of collection slightly for improved fluid positioning). ➻*Rationale:* Fluid accumulates in the dependent areas.
- Examine abdomen for areas of shifting dullness. Find landmarks and mark appropriately. ➻*Rationale:* Shifting dullness indicates fluid.
- If the patient has altered mental status, soft wrist restraints may be needed. ➻*Rationale:* It is imperative that the patient not move his or her hands into the sterile field once it has been established.

Procedure **for Assisting With Paracentesis**		
Steps	Rationale	Special Considerations
1. Wash hands and don mask.	Reduces transmission of microorganisms and body secretions; standard precautions.	
2. Assist in preparing equipment and sterile field.	Facilitates easy access to needed equipment.	Maintain aseptic technique.

Procedure **for Assisting With Paracentesis**—*Continued*

Steps	Rationale	Special Considerations
3. Assist physician or nurse practitioner to cleanse insertion site with povidone-iodine solution.	Reduces risk for infection.	Use sterile technique.
4. Apply sterile drapes to outline the area to be tapped.	Provide sterile field to decrease risk for infection.	
5. Assist physician or nurse practitioner to draw up local anesthetic (lidocaine with epinephrine preferred).	Local anesthesia minimizes pain and discomfort. Epinephrine helps eliminate unwanted abdominal wall bleeding and false-positive results.	Maximum dose of lidocaine is 30 ml of 1% or 15 ml of 2%. Assess for anesthesia of area. Resistance will be felt as the needle perforates the peritoneum.
6. Assist in collection of peritoneal fluid for laboratory analysis.	Collection of fluid for laboratory studies to provide information about the patient's status.	Usually diagnostic tests are ordered, depending on patient's status and reason for paracentesis.[4] These may include the following: tube 1—lactate dehydrogenase (LDH), glucose, albumin; tube 2—protein, specific gravity; tube 3—cell count and differential; tube 4—save until further notice. If indicated, Gram stain, acid-fast bacillus (AFB) stain, bacterial and fungal cultures, amylase and triglycerides.[1]
7. Assist to attach syringes or stopcock and tubing and gently aspirate or siphon fluid by gravity or vacuum into collection device. Drains may be left in and allowed to drain for 6 to 12 hours.[10] *(Level IV: Limited clinical studies to support recommendations.)*	Initiates therapy.	Monitor amount of fluid removed. Removal of large amount of fluid (greater than 5 L) may cause hypotension.[6,9,11] If large amounts are removed or hypotension seen, consider IV albumin to maintain intravascular volume.[2,3] *There is no evidence that leaving the drain in for 24-48 hours or more is safer or more effective.[6]*
8. After the fluid and catheter are removed, apply pressure to the wound. If the wound is still leaking fluid after 5 minutes of direct pressure, have the puncture site sutured (see Procedure 134) and apply a pressure dressing. If there is significant leakage, apply a stoma bag over the site until drainage becomes minimal.	Keeps insertion site clean. Reduces risk for infection.	Inspect catheter to ensure it is intact.
9. Apply sterile dressing to wound site.	Provides a barrier to infection and collects fluid that may leak from wound site.	
10. Dispose of equipment and soiled material in appropriate receptacle.	Standard precautions.	
11. Wash hands.	Reduces transmission of microorganisms.	
12. Document in patient record.		

Expected Outcomes

- Evacuation of peritoneal fluid for laboratory analysis
- Decompression of peritoneal cavity
- Relief of respiratory compromise
- Relief of abdominal discomfort

Unexpected Outcomes

- Perforation of bowel, bladder, or stomach
- Lacerations of major vessels (mesenteric, iliac, aorta)
- Abdominal wall hematomas
- Laceration of catheter and loss in peritoneal cavity
- Incisional hernias
- Local or systemic infection
- Hypovolemia, hypotension, shock
- Bleeding from insertion site
- Ascitic fluid leak from insertion site
- Peritonitis

Patient Monitoring and Care

Steps	Rationale	Reportable Conditions
		These conditions should be reported if they persist despite nursing interventions.
1. Evaluate changes in abdominal girth.	Provides evidence of fluid reaccumulation.	- Increasing abdominal girth
2. Monitor for changes in respiratory status.	Removal of ascitic fluid should relieve pressure on the diaphragm and the resulting respiratory distress.	- Respiratory rate greater than 24 breaths per minute or significant increase from baseline - Increased depth of breathing - Irregular breathing pattern - Pulse oximetry less than 92%, or significant decrease from baseline
3. Monitor for potential complications, including bowel or bladder perforation, bleeding, and intravascular volume loss.	Paracentesis interrupts the integrity of the skin and underlying peritoneum.	- Hematuria - Hypotension - Tachycardia
4. Monitor vital signs, temperature, insertion site for drainage, or evidence of infection.	Rapid changes in intraabdominal pressure may affect heart rate and blood pressure. Infection is a complication of paracentesis.	- Hypotension - Dysrhythmias - Increased temperature - Purulent drainage from insertion site - Redness, swelling at insertion site - Abnormal laboratory results (increased white blood cells [WBCs])
5. Monitor intake and output.	Provides data for evaluation of fluid balance status.	- Inappropriate fluid balance or changes from baseline fluid status
6. Monitor abdominal pain and level of weakness.	Patients often feel weak and experience abdominal discomfort for a few hours after the procedure.	- Continued pain after several hours
7. Evaluate laboratory data when returned.	Provides for evaluation of condition and aids in diagnosis.	- Red blood cells (RBCs) greater than 100,000/mm^3 - Amylase greater than 2.5 times normal - Alkaline phosphatase greater than 5.5 mg/dl - WBCs greater than 100/mm^3 - Positive culture results

Documentation

Documentation should include the following:

- Patient and family education
- Date and time of procedure
- Patient tolerance of procedure
- Assessment of insertion site after procedure
- Amount and characteristics of fluid removed

- Specimens sent for laboratory analysis
- Postprocedure vital signs, respiratory status, and abdominal girth
- Unexpected outcomes
- Nursing interventions

References

1. Ferri, F.F. (2004). Paracentesis. In: Ferri, F., ed. *Practical Guide to the Care of the Medical Patient.* 6th ed. St. Louis: Mosby, 810-12.
2. Gines, A., et al. (1996). Randomized trial comparing albumin, dextran 70, and polygeline in cirrhotic patients with ascites treated by paracentesis. *Gastroenterology,* 111, 1002-10.
3. Iyengar, T.D., and Herzog, T.J. (2002). Management of symptomatic ascites in recurrent ovarian cancer patients using an intra-abdominal semi-permanent catheter. *Am J Hosp Palliat Care,* 9, 35-8.
4. Jeffries, M.A., et al. (1999). Unsuspected infection is infrequent in asymptomatic outpatients with refractory ascites undergoing therapeutic paracentesis. *Am J Gastroenterol,* 94, 2972-6.
5. O'Neill, M.J., et al. (2001). Tunneled peritoneal catheter placement under sonographic and fluoroscopic guidance in the palliative treatment of malignant ascites. *Am J Roentgenol,* 177, 615-8.
6. Peltekian, K.M., et al. (1997). Cardiovascular, renal and neurohumoral responses to single large-volume paracentesis in cirrhotic patients with diuretic-resistant ascites. *Am J Gastroenterol,* 92, 394-9.
7. Richard, H.M., III, et al. (2001). Pleurx tunneled catheter in the management of malignant ascites. *J Vasc Interv Radiol,* 12, 373-5.
8. Rossle, M., et al. (2000). A comparison of paracentesis and transjugular intrahepatic portosystemic shunting in patients with ascites. *N Engl J Med,* 342, 1701-7.
9. Runyon, B.A. (1997). Patient selection is important in studying the impact of large-volume paracentesis on intravascular volume. *Am J Gastroenterol,* 92, 371-3.
10. Stephenson, J., and Gilbert, J. (2002). The development of clinical guidelines on paracentesis for ascites related to malignancy. *Palliat Med,* 16, 213-8.
11. Vila, M.C., et al. (1998). Hemodynamic changes in patients developing effective hypovolemia after total paracentesis. *J Hepatol,* 28, 639-45.

Additional Readings

Blendis, L., and Wong, F. (2003). The natural history and management of hepatorenal disorders: From pre-ascites to hepatorenal syndrome. *Clin Med,* 3, 154-9.

Lee, C.W., Bociek, G., and Faught, W. (1998). A survey of practice in management of malignant ascites. *J Pain Symptom Manage,* 16, 96-101.

Marx, J.A. (2004). Peritoneal procedures. In: Roberts, J.R., and Hedges, J.R., eds. *Clinical Procedures in Emergency Medicine.* 4th ed. Philadelphia: W.B. Saunders, 733-49.

McNamara, P. (2000). Paracentesis-an effective method of symptom control in the palliative care setting? *Palliat Med,* 14, 62-4.

Moorson, D. (2001). Paracentesis in a home care setting. *Palliat Med,* 15, 169-70.

Tamsma, J.T., Keizer, H.J., and Meinders, A.E. (2001). Pathogenesis of malignant ascites: Starling's law of capillary hemodynamics revisited. *Ann Oncol,* 12, 1353-7.

Vila, M.C., et al. (1998). Hemodynamic changes in patients developing effective hypovolemia after total paracentesis. *J Hepatology,* 28, 639-45.

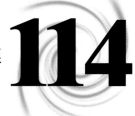
PROCEDURE **114**

Peritoneal Lavage (Perform)

P U R P O S E :   Percutaneous peritoneal lavage is performed for both therapeutic and diagnostic purposes.

Peggy Kirkwood

PREREQUISITE NURSING KNOWLEDGE

- Knowledge of anatomy and physiology of the abdomen is important to avoid unexpected outcomes.
- Intestines and bladder lie immediately beneath the abdominal surface. In children, the bladder is an abdominal organ. In adults, a full bladder is raised out of the pelvis.
- The cecum is relatively fixed and is much less mobile than the sigmoid colon. Therefore bowel perforations are more frequent in the right lower quadrant than in the left.
- A distended stomach can extend to the anterior abdominal wall.
- Peritoneal fluid is normally straw-colored, serous fluid secreted by the cells of the peritoneum. Grossly bloody fluid, a red blood cell (RBC) count of greater than 100,000/mm^3, or the presence of bacteria or bile in the return fluid in the abdomen is abnormal.
- Diagnostic lavage is used after blunt abdominal trauma, or in trauma patients with head injuries, those who are unconscious, or those with preexisting paraplegia to determine the presence of the following:
  - ❖ Hemoperitoneum (blood in lavage returns)
  - ❖ Organ injury (intestinal enzymes or microorganisms in lavage returns).
- Therapeutic lavage is used to:
  - ❖ Irrigate and cleanse purulent exudate in patients with peritonitis or intraabdominal abscess

- ❖ Warm the abdominal cavity in hypothermic patients
- ❖ Remove unwanted or toxic chemicals through peritoneal dialysis
- ❖ Obtain cytology specimens in patients with cancer
- Computed tomography (CT) frequently is used in hemodynamically stable trauma patients as the diagnostic procedure of choice.[9,14] Also, abdominal sonography and focused abdominal sonography for trauma (FAST) has been increasingly used to screen blunt abdominal trauma patients for hemoperitoneum.[3,8,13]
- In hemodynamically unstable patients, diagnostic peritoneal lavage (DPL) may be preferred by some practitioners because of its high sensitivity.[2,4,5] DPL is quick, inexpensive, safe, and highly sensitive to the presence of blood in the peritoneal cavity.[12] Hemodynamically unstable patients may also go directly to the OR for laparotomy.
- Complementary CT and DPL decreases nontherapeutic laparotomy rates and allows nonoperative management of those patients with solid-organ injury.[8]
- Peritoneal lavage is absolutely contraindicated in an acute abdomen that requires immediate surgery as indicated by free air on x-ray or penetrating abdominal trauma.
- Relative contraindications for DPL include the following[10-11]:
  - ❖ Thrombocytopenia
  - ❖ Coagulopathy
  - ❖ Severe bowel distension
  - ❖ Previous abdominal surgery, especially pelvic surgery
  - ❖ Distended bladder that cannot be emptied with a Foley catheter
  - ❖ Obvious infection at intended site of insertion (cellulitis or abscess)

- Use caution when performing DPL in patients with suspected pelvic fractures (may use a supraumbilical site) or pregnancy (use open technique with supraumbilical approach after first trimester).
- Insertion site should be midline one third the distance from the umbilicus to the symphysis, or 2 to 3 cm below the umbilicus (see Fig. 112-1). Alternate position is a point one third the distance from the umbilicus to the anterior iliac crest (left side preferred).[4]
- Ultrasound can be used prior to peritoneal lavage to locate fluid and during the procedure to guide insertion of catheter.[1,7]

EQUIPMENT

- Commercially prepared kit or the following:
  - ❖ Sterile gloves and mask or face shield
  - ❖ Skin cleansing solution (povidone-iodine)
  - ❖ Sterile marking pen
  - ❖ Sterile towels or sterile drape
  - ❖ Razor to shave area, if necessary
  - ❖ Local anesthetic for injection: 1% or 2% lidocaine with epinephrine
  - ❖ 5- or 10-ml syringe with 25- or 27-G needle for anesthetic
  - ❖ Scalpel and No. 11 knife blade
  - ❖ Trocar with stylet, or needle (16-, 18-, or 20-G), or angiocatheter, depending on abdominal wall thickness, guide wire with floppy tip, and 9- to 18-Fr peritoneal lavage catheter
  - ❖ 20-ml syringe for diagnostic tap
  - ❖ Sterile intravenous (IV) tubing (without valves) with appropriate sterile connectors for lavage catheter and IV bags
  - ❖ Sterile tubes for specimens
  - ❖ Warmed Ringer's lactate (RL), normal saline (NS), or antibiotic solution for infusion into abdomen
  - ❖ Three-way stopcock for therapeutic lavage
  - ❖ Nylon skin suture material on cutting needle (4-0 or 5-0) and needle holder
  - ❖ Four to six sterile 4 × 4 gauze pads
  - ❖ Sterile gauze dressing with tape or adhesive strip
  - ❖ Soft wrist restraints
  - ❖ Pressure bag

PATIENT AND FAMILY EDUCATION

- Explain the indications, the procedure, and the risks to the patient and family. ➥*Rationale:* Decreases patient anxiety and encourages patient and family cooperation and understanding of procedure.

- Explain the patient's role in assisting with the procedure and postprocedure care. ➥*Rationale:* Elicits patient cooperation during and after the procedure.
- Explain the signs and symptoms to report, such as fever, abdominal pain, decreased urine output, bleeding, and leakage of fluid from wound site. ➥*Rationale:* Unexpected outcomes may not manifest themselves for a period of time following the procedure.

PATIENT ASSESSMENT AND PREPARATION

Patient Assessment

- Past medical history and review of systems for abdominal injury, peritonitis, intraabdominal abscess, or pregnancy. ➥*Rationale:* Certain conditions of the gastrointestinal tract may be diagnosed and treated with peritoneal lavage. Contraindications to peritoneal lavage may be identified.
- Bowel or bladder distension. ➥*Rationale:* Distension increases the risk for bowel or bladder perforation during the procedure.
- Coagulation studies (i.e., prothrombin time [PT], partial thromboplastin time [PTT], and platelets). ➥*Rationale:* Abnormal clotting studies may increase the risk for bleeding during and after the procedure. Therapy may be necessary to correct clotting abnormalities before performing the procedure.
- Plain and upright x-rays of the abdomen (before the procedure). ➥*Rationale:* Air is introduced during the procedure and may confound the diagnosis later.

Patient Preparation

- Ensure that patient understands preprocedural teaching. Answer questions as they arise and reinforce information as needed. ➥*Rationale:* Evaluates and reinforces understanding of previously taught information.
- Obtain a written informed consent form, if possible. In a trauma situation or unresponsive patient, this may be implied consent. ➥*Rationale:* Peritoneal lavage is an invasive procedure, requiring a signed consent form.
- Have patient void or insert a Foley catheter. ➥*Rationale:* A distended bladder increases the risk for bladder perforation during the procedure.
- Insert a nasogastric tube (see Procedure 111) and attach to low intermittent suction. ➥*Rationale:* A distended stomach increases the risk for perforation during the procedure.
- Place the patient in the supine position (may tilt to side of collection slightly for improved fluid positioning). ➥*Rationale:* Fluid accumulates in the dependent areas.
- Examine abdomen for landmarks and mark appropriately. Shave area, if necessary. ➥*Rationale:* Correct placement of catheter for peritoneal lavage will minimize complications.
- If the patient has altered mental status, soft wrist restraints may be needed. ➥*Rationale:* It is imperative that the patient not move his or her hands into the sterile field once it has been established.

Procedure for Performing Peritoneal Lavage

Steps	Rationale	Special Considerations
1. Wash hands and don mask.	Reduces transmission of microorganisms and body secretions; standard precautions.	
2. Prepare equipment and sterile field and apply sterile gloves.	Facilitates easy access to needed equipment.	Maintain aseptic technique.
3. Set up lavage equipment. A. Attach IV tubing to lavage fluid and clear tubing of air. B. Attach IV tubing to one port of three-way stopcock and attach drainage collector to second port of three-way stopcock. *Or* C. Use IV tubing with a roller clamp and use the lavage fluid bag as the drainage bag.	Provides closed system for instillation and drainage of lavage fluid.	
4. Prepare insertion site with povidone-iodine solution.	Reduces risk for infection.	Use sterile technique.
5. Apply sterile drapes to outline the insertion site. Site should be in the midline about one third the distance from the umbilicus to the symphysis (usually 2 to 3 cm below the umbilicus; see Fig. 112-1). Alternate position is a point about one third the distance from the umbilicus to the anterior iliac crest (left side preferred).		Avoid rectus muscle because of increased risk for hemorrhage from epigastric vessels; avoid surgical scars because of increased risk for perforation caused by adhesion of bowel to the wall of the peritoneum; avoid upper quadrants because of possibility of undetected hepatomegaly.[6]
6. Inject area with local anesthetic (lidocaine with epinephrine preferred). Initially direct needle perpendicular to the skin and infiltrate the peritoneum with anesthetic.	Local anesthesia minimizes pain and discomfort. Epinephrine helps eliminate unwanted abdominal wall bleeding and false-positive results.	Maximum dose of lidocaine is 30 ml of 1% or 15 ml of 2%. Assess for anesthesia of area. Resistance will be felt as the needle perforates the peritoneum.
7. Using the No. 11 blade scalpel, create a vertical skin incision large enough to allow threading of a 3- to 5-mm lavage catheter. Spread the subcutaneous tissue and incise the fascia to expose the peritoneum. Nick the peritoneal membrane to pass the catheter.	To create an opening large enough to thread the lavage catheter.	When the subcutaneous tissue is nicked with the scalpel, a tough, gritty sensation will be felt.
8. Insert an 18-G needle attached to a 20-ml or 50-ml syringe perpendicular through the anesthetized tract into the peritoneum. Apply slight suction to the syringe as it is advanced. Grasp the needle close to the skin as it is advanced (see Fig. 112-2).	Provides access to peritoneal space. Slight suction is applied to indicate when the peritoneum is entered or if a blood vessel is entered. Grasping the needle as it is advanced prevents accidental thrusting into the abdomen and possible viscous perforation.	Inserted through small incision at midline below umbilicus. A small pop is felt as needle advances through anterior and posterior muscle fascia and enters peritoneum.
9. Once in the cavity, direct the needle at a 60-degree angle toward the center of the pelvic hollow. If fluid returns, fill the syringe.	Collection of fluid for laboratory studies.	A free return of 10 ml of blood is a strong positive finding for a hemoperitoneum. If blood is returned, remove the needle and prepare for immediate surgical intervention.

Procedure for Performing Peritoneal Lavage—*Continued*

Steps	Rationale	Special Considerations
10. If the tap is dry, perform the lavage technique.	Accurately assesses for hemoperitoneum.	
11. Introduce guide wire through the 18-G needle.	Provides access for insertion of the peritoneal lavage catheter.	The wire should insert easily. If there is any resistance, advance or redirect the needle until the wire feeds easily. Difficulty in advancing the catheter may indicate the stylet is not in the peritoneal cavity or that there may be adhesions.
12. Insert about half of the wire into the pelvis and remove the needle. Hold on to the guide wire continuously.	Letting go of the guide wire could allow the wire to inadvertently migrate into peritoneum.	
13. Slide the peritoneal lavage catheter over the wire, using gently twisting motions (Fig. 114-1).	Twisting motion minimizes visceral perforation and displaces abdominal contents.	Always keep a firm hold on the wire to prevent it from slipping into the peritoneal cavity.
14. Remove the wire after the catheter is in the peritoneal cavity.		Aspiration may be attempted. If it is dry, proceed to lavage.
15. Attach lavage catheter to remaining port of stopcock and tubing to withdraw peritoneal fluid.	Fluid may be gently aspirated, siphoned by gravity, or collected into a vacuum device.	Retain first 100 ml of fluid for laboratory analysis. Refer to step 23 below for specific lab tests.
16. Instill lavage fluid: A. If drainage collector is used, turn stopcock off to drainage collector. B. Open clamp on IV tubing. C. Instill 700 to 1000 ml of warmed RL, NS, or antibacterial fluid.	Directs lavage fluid into peritoneal space.	Infuse over 10 to 15 minutes. This may be done with a pressure bag to decrease time.

Procedure continues on the following page

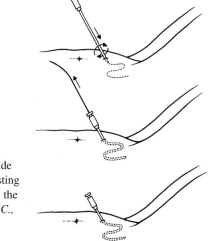

FIGURE 114-1 The plastic catheter is placed over the guide wire and inserted into the peritoneal cavity by means of a twisting motion at the skin level. After the catheter has been advanced, the guide wire is removed. (*From Pfenninger, J.L., and Fowler, G.C., eds. [2003]. Pfenninger and Fowler's Procedures for Primary Care. 2nd ed. St. Louis: Mosby.*)

Procedure for Performing Peritoneal Lavage—*Continued*

Steps	Rationale	Special Considerations
17. Rotate patient side to side (if not contraindicated).	Facilitates sampling of fluid that may accumulate in pockets on either side. Mixes solution with any free material in abdominal cavity.	
18. Drain lavage fluid: A. If drainage collector is used, turn stopcock off to IV tubing. B. If drainage collector is not used, lower IV bag to a level below the patient. C. Allow fluid to drain into drainage collector or lowered IV bag.	Directs lavage fluid from peritoneal space to drainage collector.	In therapeutic lavage, consider dwell time of fluid prior to drainage (usually 5 to 10 minutes). When draining fluid, be careful that there is not tension on the tubing.
19. Rotate patient side to side (if not contraindicated).	Facilitates drainage of fluid that may accumulate in pockets on either side.	Lavage fluid may be absorbed into intravascular space, creating a potential fluid volume excess. Twisting catheter may free the catheter from adhering to peritoneum and facilitate drainage of fluid.
20. Repeat steps 16 through 19 as needed.	Continued lavage may be needed to cleanse peritoneal space.	
21. If lavage is positive for blood, prepare patient for immediate surgery. Leave incision open and cover with sterile, NS-soaked dressing.	Immediate repair of bleeding site is needed.	
22. After the fluid is removed, gently remove the catheter and apply pressure to the wound. Suture the puncture site using a mattress suture with 4-0 nylon (see Procedure 134) and apply a dressing.	Keeps insertion site clean. Reduces risk for infection. Provides a barrier to infection and collects fluid that may leak from wound site.	Inspect catheter to ensure it is intact.
23. Prepare and send fluid specimens for laboratory analysis.	Provides information about patient status.	Have the first 100 ml of fluid analyzed for RBCs, WBCs, bilirubin, amylase, lipase, alkaline phosphate, and culture and sensitivity.
24. Dispose of equipment and soiled material in appropriate receptacle.	Standard precautions.	
25. Wash hands.	Reduces transmission of microorganisms.	
26. Document in patient record.		

Expected Outcomes

- Lavage fluid returns obtained for diagnostic evaluation
- Peritoneum cleansed of purulent exudate and microorganisms

Unexpected Outcomes

- Perforation of bowel, bladder, or stomach
- Lacerations of major vessels (mesenteric, iliac, aorta)
- Laceration of catheter or guide wire with loss in peritoneal cavity
- Local or systemic infection
- Hypovolemia, hypotension
- Bleeding from insertion site
- Inadequate drainage of lavage fluid
- Respiratory compromise

Patient Monitoring and Care

Steps	Rationale	Reportable Conditions
		These conditions should be reported if they persist despite nursing interventions.
1. Monitor for changes in respiratory status (i.e., rate, depth, and pattern).	Retained lavage fluid puts pressure on diaphragm and intraabdominal organs, causing difficulty breathing.	• Respiratory rate greater than 24 breaths per minute • Increased depth of breathing • Irregular breathing pattern • Pulse oximetry less than 92%, or significant decrease from baseline
2. Monitor for potential complications, including bowel or bladder perforation, bleeding, and intravascular volume loss.	Peritoneal lavage interrupts the integrity of the skin and underlying peritoneum.	• Acute abdominal pain, distention, rigidity, and guarding • Decreased bowel sounds • Fever, chills • Blood in urine • Hypotension • Tachycardia
3. Monitor vital signs and insertion site for drainage or evidence of infection.	Infection is a complication of peritoneal lavage.	• Increased temperature • Purulent drainage from insertion site • Redness, swelling at insertion site • Labile blood pressure
4. Monitor intake and output.	Provides data for evaluation of fluid balance status.	• Inappropriate fluid balance
5. Evaluate laboratory data when returned.	Provides for evaluation of condition and aids in diagnosis.	• RBCs greater than 100,000/mm³ • Amylase greater than 2.5 times normal • Alkaline phosphate greater than 5.5 mg/dl • Positive bilirubin • Vegetable matter present • WBCs greater than 100/mm³ • Positive culture results

Documentation

Documentation should include the following:

- Patient and family education
- Date and time of procedure
- Patient tolerance of procedure
- Assessment of insertion site after procedure
- Type and amount of fluid instilled and dwell time
- True drainage (total drainage minus lavage fluid input)

- Amount and characteristics of fluid removed
- Specimens sent for laboratory analysis
- Postprocedure vital signs, respiratory status
- Unexpected outcomes
- Nursing interventions

References

1. Bode, P.J., and van Vugt, A.B. (1996). Ultrasound in the diagnosis of injury. *Injury,* 27, 379-83.
2. Brakenridge, S.C., et al. (2003). Detection of intra-abdominal injury using diagnostic peritoneal lavage after shotgun wound to the abdomen. *J Trauma,* 54, 329-31.
3. Brown, M.A., et al. (2001). Blunt abdominal trauma: Screening US in 2,693 patients. *Radiology,* 218, 352-8.
4. Coleridge, S.T. (1998). Peritoneal lavage. In: Howell, J.M., ed. *Emergency Medicine.* Philadelphia: W.B. Saunders, 73-8.
5. Colucciello, S.A., and Marx, J.S. (2001). Blunt abdominal trauma. In: Harwood-Nuss, A.L., ed. *The Clinical Practice of Emergency Medicine.* 3rd ed. Philadelphia: Lippincott Williams & Wilkins, 460-64.

6. Ferri, F.F. (2004). Paracentesis. In: Ferri, E., ed. *Practical Guide to the Care of the Medical Patient.* 6th ed. St. Louis: Mosby, 810-2.
7. Goletti, O., et al. (1994). The role of ultrasonography in blunt abdominal trauma: Results in 250 consecutive cases. *J Trauma,* 36, 178-81.
8. Gonzalez, R.P., Ickler, J., and Gachassin, P. (2001). Complementary roles of diagnostic peritoneal lavage and computed tomography in the evaluation of blunt abdominal trauma. *J Trauma,* 51, 1128-34.
9. Jacobs, D.G., Sarafin, J.L., and Marx, J.A. (2000). Abdominal CT scanning for trauma: How low can we go? *Injury,* 31, 337-43.

10. Lindsay, M.C. (1998). Abdominal trauma. In: Aghababian, R.V., ed. *Emergency Medicine: The Core Curriculum.* Philadelphia: Lippincott-Raven, 1239-45.
11. Marx, J.A. (2004). Peritoneal procedures. In: Roberts, J.R., and Hedges, J.R., eds. *Clinical Procedures in Emergency Medicine.* 4th ed. Philadelphia: W.B. Saunders, 733-49.
12. Marx, J.A., et al. (1985). Limitations of computed tomography in the evaluation of acute abdominal trauma: A prospective comparison with diagnostic peritoneal lavage. *J Trauma,* 25, 933-937.
13. McKenney, M.G., McKenney, K.L., and Hong, J.J. (2001). Evaluating blunt abdominal trauma with sonography: A cost analysis. *AM Surg,* 67, 930-4.
14. Pal, J.D., and Victorino, G.P. (2002). Defining the role of computed tomography in blunt abdominal trauma: Use in the hemodynamically stable patient with a depressed level of consciousness. *Arch Surg,* 137, 1029-32.

Additional Readings

Biffl, W.L., et al. (2001). Evolution of a multidisciplinary clinical pathway for the management of unstable patients with pelvic fractures. *Ann Surg,* 233, 843-50.
Liu, A., Kaufmann, C., and Ritchie, R. (2001). A computer-based simulator for diagnostic peritoneal lavage. *Stud Health Technol Inform,* 81, 278-85.
Maxwell-Armstrong, C., et al. (2002). Diagnostic peritoneal lavage analysis: Should trauma guidelines be revised? *Emerg Med J,* 19, 524-5.

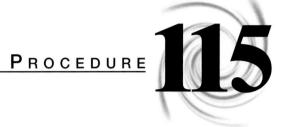

PROCEDURE **115**

Peritoneal Lavage (Assist)

PURPOSE: Percutaneous peritoneal lavage is performed for both therapeutic and diagnostic purposes.

Peggy Kirkwood
Karen K. Carlson

PREREQUISITE NURSING KNOWLEDGE

- Knowledge of anatomy and physiology of the abdomen is important in order to avoid unexpected outcomes.
- Intestines and bladder lie immediately beneath the abdominal surface. In children, the bladder is an abdominal organ. In adults, a full bladder is raised out of the pelvis.
- The cecum is relatively fixed and is much less mobile than the sigmoid colon. Therefore bowel perforations are more frequent in the right lower quadrant than in the left.
- A distended stomach can extend to the anterior abdominal wall.
- Peritoneal fluid is normally straw-colored, serous fluid secreted by the cells of the peritoneum. Grossly bloody fluid, a red blood cell (RBC) count of greater than 100,000/mm^3, or the presence of bacteria or bile in the return fluid in the abdomen is abnormal.
- Diagnostic lavage is used after blunt abdominal trauma, or in trauma patients with head injuries, those who are unconscious, or those with preexisting paraplegia to determine the presence of the following:
  - ❖ Hemoperitoneum (blood in lavage returns)
  - ❖ Organ injury (intestinal enzymes or microorganisms in lavage returns)
- Therapeutic lavage is used to:
  - ❖ Irrigate and cleanse purulent exudate in patients with peritonitis or intraabdominal abscess
  - ❖ Warm the abdominal cavity in hypothermic patients.
  - ❖ Remove unwanted or toxic chemicals through peritoneal dialysis
  - ❖ Obtain cytology specimens in patients with cancer

- Computed tomography (CT) frequently is used in hemodynamically stable trauma patients as the diagnostic procedure of choice.[9,14] Also, abdominal sonography and focused abdominal sonography for trauma (FAST) has been increasingly used to screen blunt abdominal trauma patients for hemoperitoneum.[3,8,13]
- In hemodynamically unstable patients, diagnostic peritoneal lavage (DPL) may be preferred by some practitioners because of its high sensitivity.[2,4,5] DPL is quick, inexpensive, safe, and highly sensitive to the presence of blood in the peritoneal cavity.[12] Hemodynamically unstable patients may also go directly to the OR for laparotomy.
- Complementary CT and DPL decreases nontherapeutic laparotomy rates and allows nonoperative management of those patients with solid-organ injury.[8]
- Peritoneal lavage is absolutely contraindicated in an acute abdomen that requires immediate surgery as indicated by free air on x-ray or penetrating abdominal trauma.
- Relative contraindications for DPL include the following[10-11]:
  - ❖ Thrombocytopenia
  - ❖ Coagulopathy
  - ❖ Severe bowel distension
  - ❖ Previous abdominal surgery, especially pelvic surgery
  - ❖ Distended bladder that cannot be emptied with a Foley catheter
  - ❖ Obvious infection at intended site of insertion (cellulitis or abscess).
- Use caution when performing DPL in patients with suspected pelvic fractures (may use a supraumbilical site) or pregnancy (use open technique with supraumbilical approach after first trimester).

- Insertion site should be midline one third the distance from the umbilicus to the symphysis, or 2 to 3 cm below the umbilicus (see Fig. 112-1). Alternate position is a point one third the distance from the umbilicus to the anterior iliac crest (left side preferred).[4]
- Ultrasound can be used prior to peritoneal lavage to locate fluid and during the procedure to guide insertion of catheter.[1,7]

EQUIPMENT

- Commercially prepared kit or the following:
  - ❖ Sterile gloves and mask or face shield
  - ❖ Skin cleansing solution (povidone-iodine)
  - ❖ Sterile marking pen
  - ❖ Sterile towels or sterile drape
  - ❖ Razor to shave area, if necessary
  - ❖ Local anesthetic for injection: 1% or 2% lidocaine with epinephrine
  - ❖ 5- or 10-ml syringe with 25- or 27-G needle for anesthetic
  - ❖ Scalpel and No. 11 knife blade
  - ❖ Trocar with stylet, or needle (16-, 18-, or 20-G), or angiocatheter, depending on abdominal wall thickness, guide wire with floppy tip, and 9- to 18-Fr peritoneal lavage catheter
  - ❖ 20-ml syringe for diagnostic tap
  - ❖ Sterile intravenous (IV) tubing (without valves) with appropriate sterile connectors for lavage catheter and IV bags
  - ❖ Sterile tubes for specimens
  - ❖ Warmed Ringer's lactate (RL), normal saline (NS), or antibiotic solution for infusion into abdomen
  - ❖ Three-way stopcock for therapeutic lavage
  - ❖ Nylon skin suture material on cutting needle (4-0 or 5-0) and needle holder
  - ❖ Four to six sterile 4 × 4 gauze pads
  - ❖ Sterile gauze dressing with tape or adhesive strip
  - ❖ Soft wrist restraints
  - ❖ Pressure bag

PATIENT AND FAMILY EDUCATION

- Explain the indications, the procedure, and the risks to the patient and family. ➤➤*Rationale:* Decreases patient anxiety and encourages patient and family cooperation and understanding of procedure.
- Explain the patient's role in assisting with the procedure and postprocedure care. ➤➤*Rationale:* Elicits patient cooperation during and after the procedure.
- Explain the signs and symptoms to report, such as fever, abdominal pain, decreased urine output, bleeding, and

leakage of fluid from wound site. ➤➤*Rationale:* Unexpected outcomes may not manifest themselves for a period of time following the procedure.

PATIENT ASSESSMENT AND PREPARATION

Patient Assessment

- Past medical history and review of systems for abdominal injury, peritonitis, intraabdominal abscess, or pregnancy. ➤➤*Rationale:* Certain conditions of the gastrointestinal tract may be diagnosed and treated with peritoneal lavage. Contraindications to peritoneal lavage may be identified.
- Bowel or bladder distension. ➤➤*Rationale:* Distension increases the risk for bowel or bladder perforation during the procedure.
- Coagulation studies (i.e., prothrombin time [PT], partial thromboplastin time [PTT], and platelets). ➤➤*Rationale:* Abnormal clotting studies may increase the risk for bleeding during and after the procedure. Therapy may be necessary to correct clotting abnormalities before performing the procedure.
- Plain and upright x-rays of the abdomen (before the procedure). ➤➤*Rationale:* Air is introduced during the procedure and may confound the diagnosis later.

Patient Preparation

- Ensure that patient understands preprocedural teaching. Answer questions as they arise and reinforce information as needed. ➤➤*Rationale:* Evaluates and reinforces understanding of previously taught information.
- Obtain a written informed consent form, if possible. In a trauma situation or unresponsive patient, this may be implied consent. ➤➤*Rationale:* Peritoneal lavage is an invasive procedure, requiring a signed consent form.
- Have patient void or insert a Foley catheter. ➤➤*Rationale:* A distended bladder increases the risk for bladder perforation during the procedure.
- Insert a nasogastric tube (see Procedure 111) and attach to low intermittent suction. ➤➤*Rationale:* A distended stomach increases the risk for perforation during the procedure.
- Place the patient in the supine position (may tilt to side of collection slightly for improved fluid positioning). ➤➤*Rationale:* Fluid accumulates in the dependent areas.
- Examine abdomen for landmarks and mark appropriately. Shave area, if necessary. ➤➤*Rationale:* Correct placement of catheter for peritoneal lavage will minimize complications.
- If the patient has altered mental status, soft wrist restraints may be needed. ➤➤*Rationale:* It is imperative that the patient not move his or her hands into the sterile field once it has been established.

Procedure for Assisting With Peritoneal Lavage

Steps	Rationale	Special Considerations
1. Wash hands and don mask.	Reduces transmission of microorganisms and body secretions; standard precautions.	
2. Assist in preparing equipment and sterile field.	Facilitates easy access to needed equipment.	Maintain aseptic technique.
3. Set up lavage equipment. A. Attach IV tubing to lavage fluid and clear tubing of air. B. Attach IV tubing to one port of three-way stopcock and attach drainage collector to second port of three-way stopcock. *Or* C. Use IV tubing with a roller clamp and use the lavage fluid bag as the drainage bag.	Provides closed system for instillation and drainage of lavage fluid.	
4. Assist in preparing insertion site with povidone-iodine solution.	Reduces risk for infection.	Use sterile technique.
5. Apply sterile drapes to outline the insertion site. Site should be in the midline about one third the distance from the umbilicus to the symphysis (usually 2 to 3 cm below the umbilicus; see Fig. 112-1). Alternate position is a point about one third the distance from the umbilicus to the anterior iliac crest (left side preferred).		Avoid rectus muscle because of increased risk for hemorrhage from epigastric vessels; avoid surgical scars because of increased risk for perforation caused by adhesion of bowel to the wall of the peritoneum; avoid upper quadrants because of possibility of undetected hepatomegaly.[6]
6. Assist in drawing up local anesthetic (lidocaine with epinephrine preferred).	Local anesthesia minimizes pain and discomfort. Epinephrine helps eliminate unwanted abdominal wall bleeding and false positive results.	Maximum dose of lidocaine is 30 ml of 1% or 15 ml of 2%. Assess for anesthesia of area. Resistance will be felt as the needle perforates the peritoneum.
7. If fluid returns, fill syringe and send specimen to laboratory as ordered.	Collection of fluid for laboratory studies.	A free return of 10 ml of blood is a strong positive finding for a hemoperitoneum. If blood is returned, remove the needle and prepare for immediate surgical intervention.
8. If the tap is dry, perform the lavage technique.	Accurately assesses for hemoperitoneum.	
9. Attach lavage catheter to remaining port of stopcock and tubing to withdraw peritoneal fluid.	Fluid may be gently aspirated, siphoned by gravity, or collected into a vacuum device.	Retain first 100 ml of fluid for laboratory analysis and have it analyzed for RBCs, WBCs, bilirubin, amylase, lipase, alkaline phosphate, and culture and sensitivity.
10. Instill lavage fluid: A. If drainage collector is used, turn stopcock off to drainage collector. B. Open clamp on IV tubing.	Directs lavage fluid into peritoneal space.	Infuse over 10 to 15 minutes. This may be done with a pressure bag to decrease time.

Procedure continues on the following page

Procedure for Assisting With Peritoneal Lavage—*Continued*

Steps	Rationale	Special Considerations
C. Instill 700 to 1000 ml of warmed RL, NS, or antibacterial fluid.		
11. Rotate patient side to side (if not contraindicated).	Facilitates sampling of fluid that may accumulate in pockets on either side. Mixes solution with any free material in abdominal cavity.	
12. Drain lavage fluid: A. If drainage collector is used, turn stopcock off to IV tubing. B. If drainage collector is not used, lower IV bag to a level below the patient. C. Allow fluid to drain into drainage collector or lowered IV bag.	Directs lavage fluid from peritoneal space to drainage collector.	In therapeutic lavage, consider dwell time of fluid prior to drainage (usually 5 to 10 minutes). When draining fluid, be careful that there is not tension on the tubing.
13. Rotate patient side to side (if not contraindicated).	Facilitates drainage of fluid that may accumulate in pockets on either side.	Lavage fluid may be absorbed into intravascular space, creating a potential fluid volume excess. Twisting catheter may free the catheter from adhering to peritoneum and facilitate drainage of fluid.
14. Repeat steps 11 through 13 as needed.	Continued lavage may be needed to cleanse peritoneal space.	
15. If lavage is positive for blood, prepare patient for immediate surgery. Leave incision open and cover with sterile, NS-soaked dressing.	Immediate repair of bleeding site is needed.	
16. After the fluid is removed, gently remove the catheter and apply pressure to the wound. Assist with suturing (see Procedure 134) and apply a dressing.	Keeps insertion site clean. Reduces risk for infection. Provides a barrier to infection and collects fluid that may leak from wound site.	Inspect catheter to ensure it is intact.
17. Prepare and send fluid specimens for laboratory analysis.	Provides information about patient status.	Have the first 100 ml of fluid analyzed for RBCs, WBCs, bilirubin, amylase, lipase, alkaline phosphate, and culture and sensitivity.
18. Dispose of equipment and soiled material in appropriate receptacle.	Standard precautions.	
19. Wash hands.	Reduces transmission of microorganisms.	

Expected Outcomes

- Lavage fluid returns obtained for diagnostic evaluation
- Peritoneum cleansed of purulent exudate and microorganisms

Unexpected Outcomes

- Perforation of bowel, bladder, or stomach
- Lacerations of major vessels (mesenteric, iliac, aorta)
- Laceration of catheter or guide wire with loss in peritoneal cavity
- Local or systemic infection
- Hypovolemia, hypotension
- Bleeding from insertion site
- Inadequate drainage of lavage fluid
- Respiratory compromise

Patient Monitoring and Care

Steps	Rationale	Reportable Conditions
		These conditions should be reported if they persist despite nursing interventions.
1. Monitor for changes in respiratory status (i.e., rate, depth, and pattern).	Retained lavage fluid puts pressure on diaphragm and intraabdominal organs, causing difficulty breathing.	• Respiratory rate greater than 24 breaths per minute • Increased depth of breathing • Irregular breathing pattern • Pulse oximetry less than 92%, or significant decrease from baseline
2. Monitor for potential complications, including bowel or bladder perforation, bleeding, and intravascular volume loss.	Peritoneal lavage interrupts the integrity of the skin and underlying peritoneum.	• Acute abdominal pain, distention, rigidity, and guarding • Decreased bowel sounds • Fever, chills • Blood in urine • Hypotension • Tachycardia
3. Monitor vital signs and insertion site for drainage or evidence of infection.	Infection is a complication of peritoneal lavage.	• Increased temperature • Purulent drainage from insertion site • Redness, swelling at insertion site • Labile blood pressure
4. Monitor intake and output.	Provides data for evaluation of fluid balance status.	• Inappropriate fluid balance
5. Evaluate laboratory data when returned.	Provides for evaluation of condition and aids in diagnosis.	• RBCs greater than 100,000/mm^3 • Amylase greater than 2.5 times normal • Alkaline phosphate greater than 5.5 mg/dl • Positive bilirubin • Vegetable matter present • WBCs greater than 100/mm^3 • Positive culture results

Documentation

Documentation should include the following:

- Patient and family education
- Date and time of procedure
- Patient tolerance of procedure
- Assessment of insertion site after procedure
- Type and amount of fluid instilled and dwell time
- True drainage (total drainage minus lavage fluid input)

- Amount and characteristics of fluid removed
- Specimens sent for laboratory analysis
- Postprocedure vital signs, respiratory status
- Unexpected outcomes
- Nursing interventions

References

1. Bode, P.J., and van Vugt, A.B. (1996). Ultrasound in the diagnosis of injury. *Injury,* 27, 379-83.
2. Brakenridge, S.C., et al. (2003). Detection of intra-abdominal injury using diagnostic peritoneal lavage after shotgun wound to the abdomen. *J Trauma,* 54, 329-31.
3. Brown, M.A., et al. (2001). Blunt abdominal trauma: Screening US in 2,693 patients. *Radiology,* 218, 352-8.
4. Coleridge, S.T. (1998). Peritoneal lavage. In: Howell, J.M., ed. *Emergency Medicine.* Philadelphia: W.B. Saunders, 73-8.
5. Colucciello, S.A., and Marx, J.S. (2001). Blunt abdominal trauma. In: Harwood-Nuss, A.L., ed. *The Clinical Practice of*

Emergency Medicine. 3rd ed. Philadelphia: Lippincott Williams & Wilkins, 460-4.
6. Ferri, F.F. (2004). Paracentesis. In: Ferri, E., ed. *Practical Guide to the Care of the Medical Patient.* 6th ed. St. Louis: Mosby, 810-2.
7. Goletti, O., et al. (1994). The role of ultrasonography in blunt abdominal trauma: Results in 250 consecutive cases. *J Trauma,* 36, 178-81.
8. Gonzalez, R.P., Ickler, J., and Gachassin, P. (2001). Complementary roles of diagnostic peritoneal lavage and computed tomography in the evaluation of blunt abdominal trauma. *J Trauma,* 51, 1128-34.
9. Jacobs, D.G., Sarafin, J.L., and Marx, J.A. (2000). Abdominal CT scanning for trauma: How low can we go? *Injury,* 31, 337-43.

10. Lindsay, M.C. (1998). Abdominal trauma. In: Aghababian, R.V., ed. *Emergency Medicine: The Core Curriculum.* Philadelphia: Lippincott-Raven, 1239-45.

11. Marx, J.A. (2004). Peritoneal procedures. In: Roberts, J.R., and Hedges, J.R., eds. *Clinical Procedures in Emergency Medicine.* 4th ed. Philadelphia: W.B. Saunders, 733-49.

12. Marx, J.A., et al. (1985). Limitations of computed tomography in the evaluation of acute abdominal trauma: A prospective comparison with diagnostic peritoneal lavage. *J Trauma,* 25, 933-937.

13. McKenney, M.G., McKenney, K.L., and Hong, J.J. (2001). Evaluating blunt abdominal trauma with sonography: a cost analysis. *Am Surg,* 67, 930-4.

14. Pal, J.D., and Victorino, G.P. (2002). Defining the role of computed tomography in blunt abdominal trauma: Use in the hemodynamically stable patient with a depressed level of consciousness. *Arch Surg,* 137, 1029-32.

Additional Readings

Biffl, W.L., et al. (2001). Evolution of a multidisciplinary clinical pathway for the management of unstable patients with pelvic fractures. *Ann Surg,* 233, 843-50.

Liu, A., Kaufmann, C., and Ritchie, R. (2001). A computer-based simulator for diagnostic peritoneal lavage. *Stud Health Technol Inform,* 81, 278-85.

Maxwell-Armstrong, C., et al. (2002). Diagnostic peritoneal lavage analysis: should trauma guidelines be revised? *Emerg Med J,* 19, 524-5.

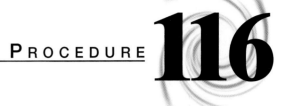
PROCEDURE **116**

Scleral Endoscopic Therapy

PURPOSE: Scleral endoscopic therapy is performed to control or prevent bleeding from esophageal varices, gastric or duodenal ulcer sites, or other selected causes of upper gastrointestinal (GI) bleeding.

Karen K. Carlson

PREREQUISITE NURSING KNOWLEDGE

- Endoscopic injection sclerotherapy (EIS) is the first choice of treatment for esophageal variceal bleeding. Rebleeding was shown to be well controlled in long-term follow-up with endoscopy and additional EIS.[5]
- A fiberoptic endoscope is passed through the esophagus and into the stomach and duodenum. Once the site of bleeding is found, a sclerosing agent can be injected through an injector needle, inserted through a port in the endoscope. The sclerosing agent is injected into the bleeding vessel, esophageal varix, or the tissue surrounding the vessel or varix.
- There are several proposed mechanisms of action of the various sclerosing agents, including esophageal or vascular smooth muscle spasm, compression of the bleeding vessel by submucosal edema or by the volume of sclerosing agent used, arterial constriction, and actual coagulation of the vessel. Ultimately, vessel thrombosis occurs.
- Scleral therapy can be combined with a number of other endoscopic therapies to promote hemostasis, including esophageal band ligation, laser therapy, thermal coagulation, and transjugular intrahepatic portosystemic shunt (TIPS).[3]
- A variety of sclerosing agents are available (Table 116-1). The physician performing the endoscopy will order the agents to be used.
- Passage of the large-bore therapeutic endoscope may stimulate the vagal response in the patient and precipitate bradydysrhythmias.
- As a result of the sedation and topical anesthetic used, the patient's gag reflex may be diminished or absent, putting the patient at risk for aspiration.

- Sedation can put the patient at risk for respiratory depression. It is recommended that a conscious sedation protocol be used to guide monitoring of the patient.

EQUIPMENT

- Endoscope (rigid or flexible; however, the flexible scope is the usual type used for upper endoscopy)
- Endoscopic injector needle (23- to 26-G, 2- to 5-mm needle; as ordered by physician)
- Three 10-ml syringes filled with sclerosing agent, as ordered by physician
- Suction setup with connecting tubing
- Rigid pharyngeal suction-tip (Yankauer) catheter
- Safety goggles for each assistant and the patient
- Nonsterile gloves
- Barrier gowns
- Nonsterile 4-inch gauze or washcloth
- Water-soluble lubricant
- Topical anesthesia
- Premedications (as ordered by physician)
- Two 30- to 60-ml syringes
- Normal saline (NS) or tap water for irrigation
- Oral airway or bite block
- Cardiac monitor
- Pulse oximeter
- Automatic blood pressure cuff
- Emergency intubation equipment
  Additional equipment, depending on patient need, includes the following:
- Nasogastric (NG) tube, Minnesota tube, or Sengstaken-Blakemore tube for esophagogastric tamponade (see Procedure 107)

TABLE 116-1	Sclerosing Agents	
Sclerosants Used for Bleeding Varices[3,4]	**Sclerosants Used for Other Causes of Upper Gastrointestinal Bleeding[3,4]**	
Sodium morrhuate (5%)	Epinephrine (1:10,000-1:20,000)	
Ethanolamine oleate (5%)	Ethyl alcohol (volumes greater than 1-2 ml can lead to tissue damage)	
Ethanolamine acetate	Thrombin	
Polidocanol (0.5%-1%)	Hypertonic saline	
Ethanol (can cause ulceration)	Polidocanol	
	Other variceal sclerosants	

PATIENT AND FAMILY EDUCATION

- Explain the procedure and indication for scleral therapy, as well as the patient's role in the procedure. ➼*Rationale:* Assists in decreasing patient and family anxiety.
- Explain that the patient will be sedated for comfort and for ease in passing the endoscope. ➼*Rationale:* Assists in decreasing patient and family anxiety.
- Explain that the patient will be monitored closely during and after the procedure. ➼*Rationale:* Assists in decreasing patient and family anxiety.

PATIENT ASSESSMENT AND PREPARATION

Patient Assessment

- Past history of upper GI bleeding and source of bleeding; baseline hematocrit and hemoglobin. ➼*Rationale:* Used as a basis for assessing bleeding or continued bleeding following scleral therapy.
- Baseline cardiac rhythm. ➼*Rationale:* Passage of a large-bore tube may cause vagal stimulation and bradydysrhythmias.
- Baseline coagulation studies (i.e., prothrombin time [PT], partial thromboplastin time [PTT], platelet count). ➼*Rationale:* Abnormal coagulation values increase the potential for bleeding after scleral therapy.
- Respiratory, hemodynamic, and neurologic assessment before the administration of any sedative agent(s). ➼*Rationale:* Baseline assessment data provide information to use as a comparison for further assessment once medications have been administered.
- Baseline vital signs and pulse oximeter reading. ➼*Rationale:* Close monitoring of vital signs and pulse oximetry during the procedure and comparison to baseline are essential to assess patient's tolerance of the procedure.
- Sedation score (Aldrete score, Ramsay scale, or the Conscious Sedation Scale are commonly used) based on blood pressure, pulse, oxygen saturation, level of consciousness, and respiratory status. ➼*Rationale:* Using a scoring system standardizes assessment of the patient's tolerance of conscious sedation.

Patient Preparation

- Ensure that patient understands preprocedural teaching. Answer questions as they arise and reinforce information as needed. ➼*Rationale:* Evaluates and reinforces understanding of previously taught information.
- Ensure that informed consent has been obtained. ➼*Rationale:* Informed consent is necessary prior to invasive procedures and before the administration of conscious sedation.
- Place the patient on a cardiac monitor and apply a pulse oximeter and automatic blood pressure cuff. ➼*Rationale:* Allows for close cardiovascular and respiratory monitoring during the procedure.
- Ensure venous access is in place. ➼*Rationale:* Venous access is needed for premedications and emergency medications.
- Ensure that the patient has been NPO for at least 4 hours before procedure. ➼*Rationale:* Undigested material in the stomach increases the risk for aspiration and decreases visualization of the GI tract.
- Have sedatives (common sedatives used include midazolam, diazepam, meperidine, and fentanyl) available (as ordered) and administer when requested. Naloxone and Romazicon should be available for narcotic or sedative reversal. ➼*Rationale:* Sedation decreases patient anxiety and allows cooperation during the procedure.
- Set up suction with connecting tubing and rigid pharyngeal suction tip attached and a catheter ready. ➼*Rationale:* Necessary for suctioning the patient's oral secretions during the procedure.
- Have atropine available at the bedside. ➼*Rationale:* Necessary if a vagal reaction occurs with the insertion and passage of the endoscope.
- Remove patient dentures. ➼*Rationale:* Dentures interfere with safe passage of the endoscope.
- Protect patient's eyes with goggles or a waterproof covering. ➼*Rationale:* Provides protection against accidental exposure to blood or the sclerosing agents. Sclerosing agents are eye irritants.

Procedure for Assisting With Scleral Endoscopic Therapy

Steps	Rationale	Special Considerations
1. Wash hands and don barrier gown and nonsterile gloves.	Reduces transmission of microorganisms; standard precautions.	
2. Don protective goggles.	Provides protection against accidental spraying with blood or sclerosing agent.	
3. Position patient in the left lateral position. *(Level II: Theory-based, no research data to support recommendations; recommendations from expert consensus group may exist.)*	The left lateral position allows predictable views of the stomach as the scope is advanced. This position allows secretions to collect in the dependent areas of the mouth for ease of suctioning and is the position of choice to prevent aspiration should the patient vomit.	
4. Perform or assist the physician with gastric lavage (see Procedure 108).	Large amounts of blood or clots in the stomach or esophagus can impair visualization of varices and increase the risk for aspiration during the procedure.	
5. Administer premedications as ordered.	Allows patient cooperation during the endoscopy and facilitates passage of the endoscope.	
6. Assist physician or nurse practitioner with insertion of the endoscope.		
A. Anesthetize the posterior pharynx with topical agent as requested.	Decreases discomfort caused by passage of endoscope.	
B. Insert oral airway (see Procedure 9) or bite block.	Prevents patient from biting the endoscope or inserter's fingers.	
C. Lubricate 20 to 30 cm of distal end of endoscope with water-soluble lubricant. (Many physicians or nurse practitioners prefer to lubricate the scope themselves.)	Minimizes mucosal injury and irritation and facilitates ease of passage of the endoscope.	
D. Encourage patient to simulate swallowing while tube is being passed.	Swallowing maneuver causes epiglottis to close trachea and directs endoscope into esophagus.	
E. Suction oral pharynx as needed.	Because of the diminished gag reflex and the presence of the endoscope in the patient's pharynx, oral secretions may not be able to be swallowed. Blood from the GI tract may be vomited and could be aspirated due to the diminished gag reflex.	Gag and cough reflexes may be compromised by topical anesthetics, and the patient may vomit as the endoscope is passed, increasing the risk for aspiration. Have emergency intubation equipment available. Monitor heart rate, rhythm, and respiratory status during endoscopy.
7. Inject irrigant via endoscope as requested.	Cleanses area to increase visualization of the tissue.	
8. Manipulate sclerosing needle as requested (Fig. 116-1).	Ensures that the sclerosing needle is in proper position for injection and does not injure tissue during movement of endoscope.	Needle must be retracted prior to manipulation of endoscope.
9. Inject sclerosing agent as requested.		The volume of sclerosant used varies, depending on the agent used and condition being treated.

Procedure continues on the following page

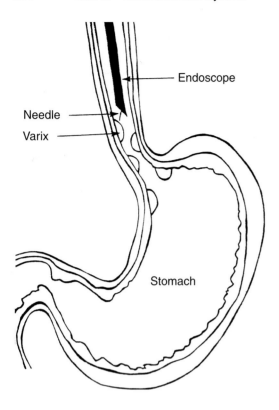

FIGURE 116-1 Injection of sclerosing agent into engorged varix. *(From Pierce, J.D., Wilkerson, E., and Griffiths, S.A. [1990]. Acute esophageal bleeding and endoscopic injection therapy. Crit Care Nurse, 10:67-72.)*

Procedure for Assisting With Scleral Endoscopic Therapy—*Continued*

Steps	Rationale	Special Considerations
10. Insert NG tube (see Procedure 111) or esophagogastric tamponade tube (see Procedure 107) after removal of endoscope, as requested.	NG tube provides assessment of continued or recurrent bleeding. Esophagogastric tamponade tube may be used to apply pressure to oozing varices.	Suction applied to a NG tube can cause mucosal damage and/or disrupt fragile varices and initiate bleeding. A chest x-ray may be performed to rule out aspiration or esophageal perforation.
11. Dispose of equipment in appropriate receptacles. The endoscope should be returned to the GI laboratory for proper disinfection.	Standard precautions.	
12. Wash hands.	Reduces transmission of microorganisms.	
13. Document in patient record.		

Expected Outcomes

- Hemostasis at site of GI bleeding without recurrent bleeding or prevention of bleeding from esophageal varices
- Stabilization of hematocrit and hemoglobin

Unexpected Outcomes

- Continued or recurrent bleeding from injected varices or ulcer site
- Esophageal sloughing or ulceration
- Esophageal perforation
- Substernal chest pain
- Fever
- Temporary dysphagia
- Allergic response to sclerosing agent
- Aspiration pneumonia
- Pleural effusion
- Atelectasis
- Bacteremia/sepsis

Patient Monitoring and Care

Steps	Rationale	Reportable Conditions
		These conditions should be reported if they persist despite nursing interventions.
1. Monitor cardiovascular, respiratory, and neurologic status every 15 min during and after endoscopy until patient returns to preprocedure status, then every 30 min to 1 hour for 2 to 4 hours. Includes: A. Level of consciousness B. Vital signs C. Oximetry D. Electrocardiogram	Changes in vital signs, heart rhythm, and oximetry may indicate complications related to the procedure.	• Altered level of consciousness from baseline • Oximetry reading below baseline • Pulse above or below baseline • Fever greater than 101°F • Decrease in blood pressure 20 to 30 mm Hg below baseline
2. Assess pain status.	May indicate continued bleeding or reaction to sclerosant.	• Same pain as experienced before procedure • New onset of chest pain
3. Monitor output from NG tube or any vomitus.	Signs of continued or recurrent bleeding.	• Bright red vomitus or NG drainage
4. Monitor serial hematocrit and hemoglobin results.	Continued fall in the hematocrit and hemoglobin indicates continued or recurrent bleeding.	• Decreasing hematocrit and hemoglobin below baseline
5. Monitor postural vital signs once the patient is able to be out of bed.	Postural changes indicate volume loss.	• Decrease in blood pressure 20 to 30 mm Hg below baseline • Increase in pulse 10 to 20 beats per minute above baseline
6. Assess for return of normal pharyngeal function. Keep patient on left side with slight head elevation until gag, swallow, and cough reflexes are intact.	Scleral therapy can cause transient dysphagia. Topical anesthesia decreases the gag reflex and increases the risk for aspiration. The left lateral position is the position of choice to prevent aspiration should the patient not be able to control secretions or vomit.	• Prolonged absence of gag, swallow, or cough reflex
7. Provide clear liquids when ordered after return of pharyngeal function. Diet should be progressed slowly to solid food.	Food may act as an irritant to sclerosed ulcer or variceal sites	• Nausea • Vomiting of bright red blood
8. Administer antacids, histamine (H₂) blockers, sulcralfate, omeprazole, somatostatin, or octreotide as ordered. *(Level V: Clinical studies in more than one patient population and situation.)*	Antacids neutralize gastric acid. Histamine blockers decrease gastric acid secretion. Sulcralfate reacts with gastric acid, forming a paste that adheres to ulcer sites. Omeprazole inhibits the proton pump in the parietal cells of the stomach, suppressing gastric acid secretion. Somatostatin and octreotide (synthetic somatostatin) lower portal pressure by splanchnic vasoconstriction.[1-4]	
9. Continue patient and family education.	Unexpected outcomes can occur within hours or may be delayed days or weeks after scleral therapy.	

Procedure continues on the following page

Patient Monitoring and Care—*Continued*

Steps	Rationale	Reportable Conditions
A. Explain signs and symptoms to report (fever, chest pain, difficulty swallowing, vomiting bright red blood, difficulty breathing).		
B. Explain diet progression.	Improves patient compliance and decreases risk for aspiration of liquid or food before patient is ready for swallowing.	
C. Explain medication therapy.	Improves patient compliance.	

Documentation

Documentation should include the following:

- Patient and family education
- Date and time of procedure
- Initial patient assessment
- Pre- and postprocedure patient and family education
- Baseline vital signs
- Baseline pulse oximetry
- Premedications administered
- Gastric lavage (if performed) and patient's tolerance
- Vital signs and pulse oximetry during scleral therapy
- Sclerosing agents administered and amount

- Time of insertion of NG or tamponade tube (if inserted) and patient's tolerance, characteristics of any drainage from NG tube, x-ray documentation of placement of tamponade tube, and initial pressure applied
- Postscleral therapy vital signs and pulse oximetry
- Position of patient after procedure
- Assessment of gag, swallow, and cough reflexes
- Postprocedure medications administered
- Unexpected outcomes
- Nursing interventions

References

1. D'amico, G., et al. (2003). Emergency sclerotherapy versus vasoactive drugs for variceal bleeding in cirrhosis: A Cochrane meta-analysis. *Gastroenterology,* 124, 1277-91.
2. Kovacs, T.O.G., and Jensen, D.M. (2002). Recent advances in the endoscopic diagnosis and therapy of upper gastrointestinal, small intestinal, and colonic bleeding. *Med Clin North Am,* 86, 1319-56.
3. Nagell, W., et al. (2002). Primary prophylactic therapy of esophageal varices—a literature review. *Hepato-Gastoenterology,* 49, 423-7.
4. Russo, M. (2002). Variceal bleeding. *Current Treatment Options in Gastroenterology,* 5, 471-7.
5. Tomikawa, M., et al. (2002). Endoscopic injection sclerotherapy in the management of 2105 patients with esophageal varices. *Surgery,* 131(1Suppl), S171-5.

Additional Readings

Jenkins, S.A., et al. (1997). Randomised trial of octreotide for long-term management of cirrhosis after variceal haemorrhage. *BMJ,* 315, 1338-41.
Singh, P., et al. (2002). Combined ligation and sclerotherapy versus ligation alone for secondary prophylaxis of esophageal variceal bleeding: A meta-analysis. *Am J Gastroenterol,* 97, 623-9.

UNIT V
Renal System

SECTION SEVENTEEN

Renal Replacement

PROCEDURE

117

Continuous Renal Replacement Therapies

P U R P O S E : Continuous renal replacement therapies (CRRT) are used in the in-patient setting for volume regulation, acid-base control, electrolyte regulation, management of azotemia, and in some cases, immune modulation. These methods are most often used in critically ill patients whose hemodynamic status will not tolerate the rapid fluid and electrolyte shifts associated with hemodialysis or in those who require continuous removal or regulation of solutes and intravascular volume.

Rhonda K. Martin

PREREQUISITE NURSING KNOWLEDGE

- Continuous renal replacement therapy (CRRT) is an extracorporeal blood purification therapy intended to substitute for impaired renal function over an extended period of time and applied for, or aimed at being applied for, 24 hours per day.
- CRRT can be accomplished through a variety of methods, as listed below (details outlined in Table 117-1):
  - Arteriovenous slow continuous ultrafiltration (AVSCUF)
  - Venovenous slow continuous ultrafiltration (VVSCUF)
  - Continuous arteriovenous hemofiltration (CAVH)
  - Continuous arteriovenous hemodialysis (CAVHD)
  - Continuous arteriovenous hemodiafiltration (CAVHDF)
  - Continuous venovenous hemofiltration (CVVH)
  - Continuous venovenous hemodialysis (CVVHD)
  - Continuous venovenous hemodiafiltration (CVVHDF)[1,4]
- Basic knowledge of the principles of diffusion, ultrafiltration (UF), osmosis, oncotic pressure, and hydrostatic pressure—and how they pertain to fluid and solute management during dialysis—is required:
  - Diffusion: The passive movement of solutes through a semipermeable membrane from an area of higher to lower concentration until equilibrium is reached.
  - Convective transport: The rapid movement of fluid across a semipermeable membrane from an area of high pressure to an area of low pressure with transport of solutes. When water moves across a membrane along

a pressure gradient, some solutes are carried along with the water and do not require a solute concentration gradient (also called *solute drag*). Convective transport is most effective for the removal of middle- and large-molecular-weight solutes.

- Ultrafiltration (UF): The bulk movement of solute and solvent through a semipermeable membrane using a pressure movement. This is usually achieved by positive pressure in the blood compartment in the hemofilter and negative pressure in the dialysate compartment. Blood and dialysate run countercurrent. The size of the solute molecules as compared with the size of molecules that can move through the semipermeable membrane determines the degree of UF.
- Osmosis: The passive movement of solvent through a semipermeable membrane from an area of higher to lower concentration.
- Oncotic pressure: The pressure exerted by plasma proteins favoring intravascular fluid retention, as well as movement of fluid from the extravascular to the intravascular space.
- Hydrostatic pressure: The force exerted by arterial blood pressure that favors the movement of fluid from the intravascular to the extravascular space.
- Absorption: The process by which drug molecules pass through membranes and fluid barriers and into body fluids.
- Adsorption: The adhesion of molecules (solutes) to the surface of the hemofilter, charcoal, or resin.

TABLE 117-1	**Continuous Renal Replacement Therapies**					
Mode	**Principles Involved**	**Access**	**Pump Assisted**	**Indications**	**Advantages**	**Complications/Disadvantages***
Ultrafiltration Therapies						
SCUF (slow, continuous ultrafiltration)	Ultrafiltration Convection	Arteriovenous Venovenous	No Yes	Diuretic-resistant, volume-overloaded, hemodynamically unstable patient who cannot tolerate rapid fluid shifts	Continuous, gradual treatment (fewer high and low extremes)	**Anticoagulation, bleeding** **Hypotension** **Hypothermia** **Access complications (bleeding, clotting, infection)** **Requires strict monitoring of fluid and electrolyte replacement to avoid deficits or overload** **Air embolism** **ICU setting only** **Requires 1:1 nurse/patient ratio** Prolonged, large-bore arterial cannulation required Ideally need MAP of 60 mm Hg to drive extracorporeal circuit Poor control of azotemia, may need dialysis Minimal solute clearance Poor emergent treatment of hyperkalemia/acidosis Loss of limb (distal arterial ischemia)
CAVH (continuous arteriovenous hemofiltration)	Ultrafiltration Convection	Arteriovenous	No	Diuretic-resistant, volume-overloaded, hemodynamically unstable patient who cannot tolerate rapid fluid shifts Parenteral or enteral alimentation in volume overloaded patient	Continuous, gradual treatment (fewer high and low extremes) High rate of fluid removal/ replacement allows flexibility in fluid balance	**Anticoagulation, bleeding** **Hypotension** **Hypothermia** **Access complications (bleeding, clotting, infection)** **Requires strict monitoring of fluid and electrolyte replacement to avoid deficits or overload** **Air embolism** **ICU setting only** **Requires 1:1 nurse/patient ratio** Prolonged, large-bore arterial cannulation required Ideally need MAP of 60 mm Hg to drive extracorporeal circuit Poor control of azotemia, may need dialysis Poor emergent treatment of hyperkalemia/acidosis Loss of limb (distal arterial ischemia)
CVVH (continuous venovenous hemofiltration)	Ultrafiltration Diffusion Solute removal	Venovenous	Yes	Diuretic-resistant, hemodynamically unstable, volume-overloaded patient who cannot tolerate rapid fluid shifts Parenteral or enteral alimentation in volume-overloaded patient	Precise fluid control Can be done in patient with low MAP Ease of initiation Large volume of parenteral nutrition may be administered No arterial cannulation Better solute clearance than CAVH	**Anticoagulation, bleeding** **Hypotension** **Hypothermia** **Access complications (bleeding, clotting, infection)** **Requires strict monitoring of fluid and electrolyte replacement to avoid deficits or overload** **Air embolism** **ICU setting only** **Requires 1:1 nurse/patient ratio** Waste product removal not as efficient as CVVHDF Requires special pump to augment blood flow through extracorporeal circuit Requires training of ICU nurses in use of pump

Dialysis Therapies

				Indications	Advantages	Complications/Disadvantages
CAVHD (continuous arteriovenous hemodialysis)	Ultrafiltration Diffusion Solute removal Convection	Arteriovenous	No	Volume-overloaded hemodynamically unstable patient with azotemia or uremia Catabolic acute renal failure Electrolyte imbalances and acidosis Parenteral and enteral alimentation in volume overloaded, catabolic patient	Precise fluid control Ease of initiation Large volume of parenteral nutrition may be administered	**Same as CAVH** **Hyperglycemia** Hypernatremia Hypophosphatemia
CAVHDF (continuous arteriovenous hemodiafiltration)						
CVVHD (continuous venovenous hemodialysis)	Ultrafiltration Diffusion Solute removal	Venovenous	Yes	Volume-overloaded hemodynamically unstable patient with azotemia or uremia Catabolic acute renal failure Electrolyte imbalances and metabolic acidosis Parenteral and enteral alimentation in volume overloaded, catabolic patient	No arterial cannulation Precise fluid control Ease of initiation Large volume of parenteral nutrition may be administered Better solute clearance than CAVHDF Can be done in patient with low MAP	**Same as CVVH** **Hyperglycemia** Hypernatremia Hypophosphatemia
CVVHDF (continuous venovenous hemodiafiltration)						

*Complications/disadvantages appearing in boldface are common to CAVH/CAVHD/CVVH/CVVHDF.

ICU, intensive care unit; *MAP,* mean arterial pressure.

Adapted from Giuliano, K., and Pysznik, E. (1998). Renal replacement therapy in critical care: implementation of a unit-based CVVH program. *Crit Care Nurse,* 18, 40-5.

- CRRT uses an artificial kidney (i.e., hemofilter, dialyzer) with a semipermeable membrane to create two separate compartments: the blood compartment and the dialysis solution compartment. The semipermeable membrane allows the movement of small molecules (e.g., electrolytes) and middle-size molecules (creatinine, vasoactive substances) from the patient's blood into the dialysis solution but is impermeable to larger molecules (RBCs, plasma proteins).

- Each dialyzer has four ports: two end ports for blood (in one end and out the other) and two side ports for dialysis solution ultrafiltrate (in one end and out the other). In most cases, the blood and dialysate are run through the dialyzer in opposite or countercurrent directions.

- With hollow-fiber dialyzers, the blood flows through the center of hollow fibers and the dialysis solution (dialysate) flows around the outside of the hollow fibers. The advantages of hollow-fiber filters include a low priming volume, low resistance to flow, and high amount of surface area. The major disadvantage is the potential for clotting secondary to the small fiber size.

- Parallel-plate dialyzers are designed as sheets of membrane over supporting structures. Blood and dialysis solutions pass through alternate spaces of the dialyzer. The major disadvantages of this type of filter are the increase in allergic dialyzer reactions and less filter surface area.

- All dialyzers have ultrafiltration (UF) coefficients; thus the dialyzer selected will vary in different clinical situations. The higher the UF coefficient, the more rapid the fluid removal. UF coefficients are determined by in vivo measurements done by each dialyzer manufacturer.

- *Clearance* refers to the ability of the dialyzer to remove metabolic waste products or drugs from the patient's blood. The blood flow rate, the dialysate flow rate, and the solute concentration affect clearance. Clearance occurs by the processes of diffusion, convection, and UF.

- The dialysate (when used during CRRT) is composed of water, a buffer (i.e., lactate or bicarbonate), and various electrolytes. Most solutions also contain glucose. The buffer helps neutralize acids that are generated as a result of normal cellular metabolism and that usually are excreted by the kidney. The concentration of electrolytes is usually the normal plasma concentration, helping to create a concentration gradient for removal of excess electrolytes. The glucose aids in increasing the oncotic pressure in the dialysate (thus aiding in fluid removal) and in caloric replacement; although glucose comes in various concentrations, it is usually used in normal plasma concentrations to prevent hyperglycemia.

- Heparin or citrate is often used during CRRT to prevent clotting of the circuit during treatment. Saline flushes can be used alone or with other anticoagulants to maintain circuit patency.[6,7,11]

- Heparin or 4% citrate can be used to maintain vascular access patency when CRRT is not in use.[7]

- If the patient is taking ACE (angiotensin-converting enzyme) inhibitors, contact with certain filters or membranes in the CRRT system can cause an anaphylactic reaction and severe hypotension. This is due to increased levels of bradykinin, a potent vasodilator. It is recommended that ACE inhibitors be withheld for a 48-72 hour before treatment, if possible.

- Continuous renal replacement therapy can be done by either a pumped or nonpumped system. In a nonpumped system, the patient's arterial pressure provides the gradient that propels the blood through the circuit. In pumped systems, a mechanical roller pump propels the blood through the circuit. Because of the complication associated with non-pumped systems, such as variability in blood pressure, blood flow, and system performance, and the complications associated with an arterial access, pump systems are preferred. The patient's volume status and serum electrolytes are changed gradually so that patients experience fewer problems than they do with hemodialysis. Specifics of all of these therapies are outlined in Table 117-1.[2,4,8]

- SCUF (Fig. 117-1), CAVH (Fig. 117-2), CAVHD (Fig. 117-3), and CAVHDF (Fig. 117-4) are all performed using nonpumped systems. For all of these therapies, the force generated by arterial pressure drives the system; a mean arterial pressure (MAP) of 60 mm Hg is generally required for adequate UF. Both arterial and venous access catheters are required. Short, large-bore catheters are placed in the femoral artery for arterial access and in the femoral, internal jugular, or subclavian veins for venous access.

- CVVH (Fig. 117-5), CVVHD (Fig. 117-6), and CVVHDF (Fig. 117-7) use pumped systems. These therapies are used to remove both plasma water and solutes and are generally more effective than nonpumped systems. These therapies require venous access, most commonly provided by a double-lumen vascular access catheter. Because of the risk for vascular complications and decreased efficiency in non-pumped systems, pumped methods are preferred for CRRT.[1] External arteriovenous (AV) hemodialysis shunts or surgically created A-V hemodialysis anastomoses have been used in the past for CRRT;

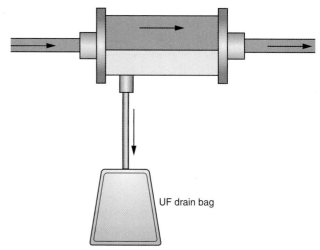

FIGURE 117-1 Slow continuous ultrafiltration (SCUF©). Fluid removal, no fluid replacement. *(Copyright Rhonda K. Martin. All rights reserved. Used with permission.)*

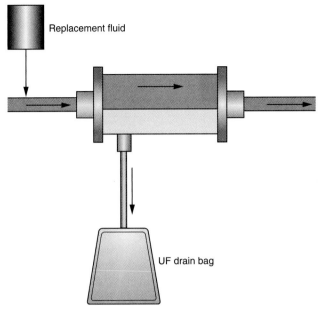

FIGURE 117-2 Continuous arteriovenous hemofiltration (CAVH©). Fluid removal and fluid replacement. *(Copyright Rhonda K. Martin. All rights reserved. Used with permission.)*

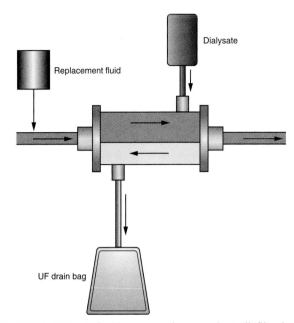

FIGURE 117-4 Continuous arteriovenous hemodiafiltration (CAVHDF©). Fluid replacement with dialysate. *(Copyright Rhonda K. Martin. All rights reserved. Used with permission.)*

because of increased incident of vascular injury, bleeding, and infection, they are NOT recommended for access for CRRT.[1] Common sites for the double-lumen vascular catheter, in order of preference, are the internal jugular vein, femoral vein, and subclavian vein.[1]

- A blood pump provides the pressure driving the system; the blood circuit consists of blood lines, a blood pump, and various monitoring devices. The blood lines carry the blood to and from the patient. The blood pump controls the speed of the blood through the circuit. The monitoring devices include arterial and venous pressure monitors, as well as an air detection monitor to prevent air that may have entered the circuit from being returned to the

patient. Anticoagulant, dialysate, and replacement fluids can also be added to the system.

- ❖ Integrated pump systems (Prisma®, Diapact®, Accura®, Aquarius®) have separate pumps for blood, dialysate, ultrafiltrate/effluent, and replacement fluids (Fig. 117-8). The pumps are controlled by a computerized control module. Blood flow rate, dialysate flow rate, anticoagulation rate, and fluid removal rates are entered by the nurse per medical orders. Dialysate, ultrafiltrate/effluent, and/or replacement fluids are

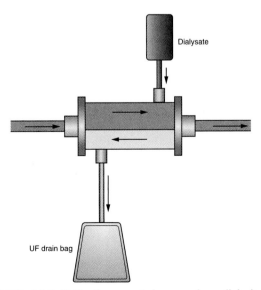

FIGURE 117-3 Continuous arteriovenous hemodialysis (CAVHD©). Fluid and solute removal with dialysate. *(Copyright Rhonda K. Martin. All rights reserved. Used with permission.)*

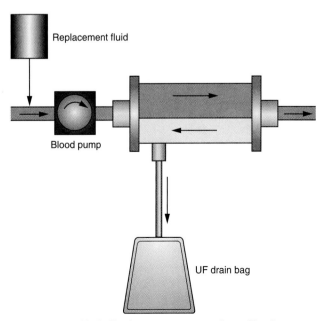

FIGURE 117-5 Continuous venovenous hemofiltration (CVVH©). Fluid removal and fluid replacement. *(Copyright Rhonda K. Martin. All rights reserved. Used with permission.)*

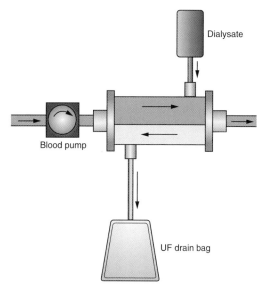

FIGURE 117-6 Continuous venovenous hemodialysis (CVVHD©). Fluid and solute removal with dialysate. *(Copyright Rhonda K. Martin. All rights reserved. Used with permission.)*

measured by weight scales on the unit. The module calculates and adjusts pump speeds to achieve the selected fluid goal. The module also records and displays treatment data.

- SCUF is used primarily to remove plasma water in small amounts (150 to 300 ml/hr). A hemofilter with a large surface area, high sieving coefficient, and low resistance is used to facilitate slow, continuous fluid removal. Replacement fluid is generally not used.
- CAVH (see Fig. 117-2) and CVVH (see Fig. 117-5) remove fluids and solutes primarily by convection. Intravenous (IV) or blood circuit replacement fluid is used

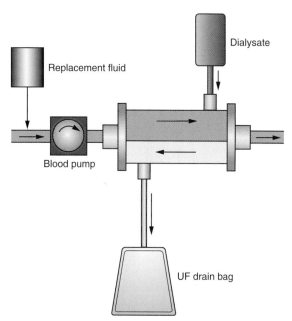

FIGURE 117-7 Continuous venovenous hemodiafiltration (CVVHDF©). Fluid replacement with dialysate. *(Copyright Rhonda K. Martin. All rights reserved. Used with permission.)*

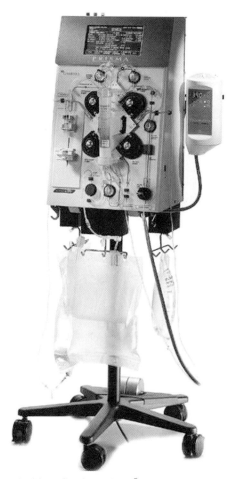

FIGURE 117-8 Gambro Prisma® CRRT Machine. *(Courtesy Gambro USA, Lakewood, Colorado.)*

continuously based on the amount of UF removed each hour and the net fluid goals for the patient.

- Continuous high-volume hemofiltration is a variant of CVVH, which requires high surface area hemofilters and uses high hourly ultrafiltration volumes, usually greater than 35 ml/hr/kg.[1]
- CAVHD (see Fig. 117-3) and CVVHD (see Fig. 117-6) are used to remove solutes primarily by diffusion. Dialysate solution is part of the setup; flow of the dialysate is countercurrent to the blood flow. Replacement fluid is not used.
- CAVHDF (see Fig. 117-4) and CVVHDF (see Fig. 117-7) remove fluids and solutes by diffusion and convection. Dialysate runs countercurrent to the blood flow. Intravenous or blood circuit replacement fluid is used continuously based on the amount of UF removed each hour and net fluid goals for the patient.
- Other extended renal replacement therapy techniques or "hybrid" techniques (sustained low efficiency dialysis [SLED], extended daily dialysis [EDD]) generally use standard hemodialysis equipment with reduced blood flow and dialysate rates to gradually remove plasma water and solutes. They are used from 4 to 12 hours a day. These procedures are described in Procedure 118.

EQUIPMENT

- Masks, goggles
- Sharps container
- Two 10-ml syringes and two 3-ml syringes
- Sterile normal saline (NS), 3 L
- Dressing supplies (sterile barrier, gauze pads, transparent dressing, tape)
- Povidone-iodine solution/swabs or chlorhexidine bactericidal solution
- Heparin (1000 units/ml) (both for priming and infusion, as ordered)
- Sterile bowl
- Two 19-G needles
- Antiseptic soap
- Hemostats
- Hemofilter system/setup
- Infusion pumps, blood pump, and/or integrated pump system
- 4 × 4 gauze pads, tape, sterile barrier
- Replacement fluid, as ordered
- Fluid warmer
- Dialysate fluid, as ordered
- Sterile gloves, clean gloves
- Alcohol wipes
- Sterile towels
- Drainage bag

Equipment for termination includes the following:

- Hemostats
- Gauze pads, tape, povidone-iodine, sterile barrier, sterile gloves
- NS, 1000 ml
- Clean gloves, goggles, mask
- Heparin (1000 units/ml *or* 5000 units/ml, depending on institution protocol) *or* 4% citrate, heparin lock caps, syringes (if using vascular catheters), labels for vascular access catheter (VAC).
- Two 10-ml syringes filled with NS

PATIENT AND FAMILY EDUCATION

- Explain the purpose of CRRT, specifically why the treatment is being performed, and the expected clinical outcomes. ➳***Rationale:*** The patient and family should understand that CRRT is necessary to perform the physiologic functions of the kidneys when fluid overload or renal failure is present (or other specific purpose for the therapy).
- Explain the procedure, including risks, anticipated length of treatment, patient positioning, and review any questions the patient may have. ➳***Rationale:*** Provides information and decreases patient anxiety.
- Explain the need for careful sterile technique for the duration of treatment. ➳***Rationale:*** It is important for the patient and family to know the importance of sterile technique to decrease the likelihood of systemic infection.
- Explain the need for careful monitoring of the patient during the treatment particularly for fluid and electrolyte imbalance. ➳***Rationale:*** The patient and family should understand that careful monitoring is a routine part of CRRT.
- Explain the signs and symptoms of possible complications during CRRT. ➳***Rationale:*** Patients and family should be fully prepared in case one of the complications occurs (e.g., hypotension, hemorrhage, manifestations of fluid/electrolyte/acid-base imbalance).
- Explain the CRRT circuit setup to the patient and family. ➳***Rationale:*** It is important for the patient and family to know that blood will be removed from the patient's body and will be visible during the CRRT treatment.

PATIENT ASSESSMENT AND PREPARATION

Patient Assessment

- Baseline vital signs/hemodynamic parameters/weight, laboratory values (blood urea nitrogen [BUN]/creatinine/electrolytes/hemoglobin/hematocrit), neurologic status. ➳***Rationale:*** Patients in renal failure often have altered baseline assessments, both in physical assessment and in the laboratory values. Having this information before treatments are started is helpful so that interventions, including the net fluid balance and dialysate fluid, can be individualized. Alterations during treatment are common because of the rapid removal of fluid and solutes.
- Catheter insertion site/vascular access site for signs and symptoms of infection. ➳***Rationale:*** Catheter insertion sites provide a portal of entry for infection, which may result in septicemia if unrecognized or untreated. If the catheter insertion site appears to be infected, further interventions (e.g., site change, culture, antibiotic treatment) may be necessary.
- Patency and the ability to easily aspirate blood from both ports. ➳***Rationale:*** Adequate blood flow is necessary during a treatment in order to facilitate optimal fluid and solute removal. Patent catheter lumens are necessary for adequate blood flow.
- Check site for presence of bruit and quality of blood flow (if using an AV fistula). ➳***Rationale:*** Physical assessment of the fistula can indicate patency of the graft, as well as the possible presence of infection.
- Adequate circulation to the distal parts of the access limb. ➳***Rationale:*** The placement of a vascular access may compromise circulation.
- Maintenance of the CRRT circuit (arterial and venous pressures, clotting, blood leaks, or breaks in the closed system). ➳***Rationale:*** CRRT treatments pose a risk to the patient if the circuit is not carefully monitored for technical problems in the system and untoward patient responses.

Patient Preparation

- Ensure that patient understands preprocedural teaching. Answer questions as they arise and reinforce information as needed. ➳***Rationale:*** Evaluates and reinforces understanding of previously taught information.
- Verify that the informed consent for treatment has been signed. ➳***Rationale:*** A signed informed consent is

necessary before implementing extracorporeal procedures such as CRRT.

- Position the patient in a comfortable position (that will also facilitate optimal blood flow through the vascular access). →*Rationale:* It is important for the patient and family to understand that movement during the procedure may affect the blood flow through the system and that

getting into a comfortable position before the initiation of therapy is important. They should also understand that different catheter sites may require different patient positions to facilitate optimal blood flow. Choose a position that will allow for setup of the sterile field. The nurse who is setting up the sterile field and initiating therapy must be able to easily reach all the necessary supplies.

Procedure for Initiating and Terminating Continuous Renal Replacement Therapy

Steps	Rationale	Special Considerations
Nonpumped Systems (SCUF, CAVH, CAVHD, CAVHDF)		
Initiation		
1. Wash hands.	Reduces transmission of microorganisms; standard precaution.	
2. Verify orders, which should include the following: (*Level II: Theory based, no research data to support recommendations: recommendations from expert consensus group may exist.*) A. Modality B. Vascular access C. Type of hemofilter/dialyzer D. Anticoagulant type, concentration, infusion rate, monitoring parameters E. Replacement fluid (if used) F. Hourly ultrafiltration rate G. Hourly net fluid goal H. Dialysate solution and rate (if used) I. Blood pressure/vital sign parameters J. Laboratory testing	Familiarizes nurse with the individualized patient treatment, reduces the possibility of error, and maintains the patency of the circuit.[10]	Ensure patient weight and laboratory values are recorded before initiation of therapy.
3. Remove hemofilter and lines from package and check that protective caps are properly placed at the end of the arterial and venous blood lines, and the hemofilter/dialyzer. *Note: Read and follow any manufacturer's recommendations for priming.*	The closed system remains intact to maintain sterility.	Inspect the hemofilter and observe the minimal distance between the priming solution and the hemofilter and the collection/measuring device. By raising the priming solution higher than the rest of the system, the amount of time required to prime the system is decreased.
4. Attach the hemofilter/dialyzer to the blood lines if not preattached, using strict aseptic technique. (*Level I: Manufacturer's recommendation only.*)	Forms the blood circuit for priming.	Follow the manufacturer's recommendations for circuit priming.
5. Check that blood line connections to hemofilter are secure.	Avoids accidental leaks or disconnections.	
6. Place the hemofilter with arterial end down (blood inlet) in the holder; lock the holder.	Positions hemofilter for priming procedure.	

Procedure for Initiating and Terminating Continuous Renal Replacement Therapy—*Continued*		
Steps	**Rationale**	**Special Considerations**
7. Hang the heparinized NS at least 48 inches above the level of the hemofilter.	Facilitates priming of the hemofilter by gravity.	Heparin dose may vary. Check the institutional protocol or order.
8. Spike the first bag, flush the tubing, and then close the clamp.	Prepares for priming.	
9. Connect the heparinized NS tubing to the end of the arterial line (blood outlet).	Used as a flushing solution to flush sterilant from filter.	
10. Attach a collection bag to the end of the venous line (blood outlet).	Used to collect the sterilant and flush.	These bags are usually provided by the manufacturer. An empty sterile IV bag can also be used.
11. Uncap the UF port on the hemofilter (across from arterial inlet port) and attach one end of the UF line.	Provides a closed, countercurrent system for collection of ultrafiltrate.	Maintains aseptic technique.
12. Connect the other end of the UF line to the closed collection/measuring device.	Completes assembly of system and facilitates measurement of the priming solution.	
13. Hang the collection system approximately 20 inches (no less than 16 inches) below the level of the hemofilter.	Priming position enhances movement of the priming solution across the membrane of the hemofilter.	Clamp the drain tube on the collection bag.
14. Check that the dialysate port on the hemofilter (across from the venous outlet port) is capped and/or clamped.	Prevents introduction of air and/or leakage.	
15. Check that all lines are securely connected.	Prevents leaks or disconnections.	
16. Close clamp on arterial blood line and venous line. For hollow fiber hemofilters/dialyzers, clamp the UF line; for parallel plate hemofilters, keep the UF line open.	Removes air and sterilant, wets the membranes, and primes the system.	"Bulldog" clamps (nonserrated cannulated clamps that prevent cutting of tubing) can be used if roller clamps are not available.
17. Wash hands.	Reduces transmission of microorganisms; standard precautions.	
18. Unclamp the arterial line and the roller clamp on the priming solution tubing; flush all connecting lines with heparinized NS.	Initiates priming of the system.	For parallel plate dialyzers: ensure that whenever there is fluid (either priming solution or blood) moving through the blood compartment of the hemofilter, the UF line remains unclamped. If the UF line is clamped during the priming procedure, there may be inadequate removal of air or collapse of some or all of the layers of the hemofilter, rendering it nonfunctional. For other filters, keep the UF line clamped.
19. Intermittently clamp and unclamp the venous line for 3 to 5 seconds. Tap the filter as needed to dislodge air.	Enhances removal of air from the blood compartment.	Make sure the other tubings and outlet ports on the blood lines (e.g., anticoagulant infusion line) are primed and free of air.

Procedure continues on the following page

Procedure **for Initiating and Terminating Continuous Renal Replacement Therapy**—*Continued*

Steps	Rationale	Special Considerations
20. When nearly all of the 1000 ml of priming solution has flowed into the system, clamp the priming line and venous line, and rotate the hemofilter/dialyzer so that the arterial line is up.	Continues priming of the ultrafiltrate compartment.	Hemofilter/dialyzer must be rinsed to remove glycerin coating, ethylene oxide (from sterilization), and all air bubbles.
21. Hang another 1000 ml of heparinized NS on the priming tubing.	For priming ultrafiltrate compartment.	
22. Open the UF line clamp, if not open. Continue priming with heparinized NS until 400 ml has collected in the UF collection/measuring device.	Ensures that ultrafiltrate compartment is thoroughly primed.	Clamping the venous line increases the pressure in the blood compartment, forcing the priming solution through the membrane, and priming the dialysate compartment.
23. Rotate the hemofilter so that the arterial line end is down.	Completes priming of the hemofilter and dialysate compartment.	
24. Unclamp the venous line and continue priming with heparinized NS.	Allows drainage of fluid from the hemofilter.	
25. Infuse 500 ml through the venous blood site, and intermittently clamp and unclamp the venous line.	Promotes purging of air bubbles from the hemofilter.	
26. When 100 ml of the heparinized NS remains in the IV bag, clamp the IV priming line and the arterial line.	Prevents introduction of air into the system.	*Caution:* Air accumulated in the blood compartment can create an air lock, which can cause a decreased UF rate, clotting, and rupture of the filter membranes. Check for air in the hemofilter/dialyzer. If air bubbles persist, continue flushing the system with heparinized NS.
27. Clamp the venous and UF lines.	Prevents loss of priming solution from system and potential for air accumulation.	
28. Flush the infusion line for the anticoagulant and attach to the infusion port on the arterial blood line (or as directed per protocol).		
29. Drain and discard the NS in UF collection device. The system is now ready for patient use.	Excludes NS priming solution from ultrafiltrate volume.	Label hemofilter/tubing with time and date.
30. Wash hands.	Reduces transmission of microorganisms.	
31. Inspect vascular access.	Provides route for hemofiltration.	Subclavian, femoral, and venipuncture access may be initiated, depending on established protocols. Ensure that patient has both an arterial access and a venous access for nonpumped systems. Inspect for signs and symptoms of exit-site infection: drainage, crusting,

Procedure for Initiating and Terminating Continuous Renal Replacement Therapy—*Continued*

Steps	Rationale	Special Considerations
		swelling, redness, exudate, or complaints of pain at the site.
32. Position hemofilter parallel and close to the patient's access, at heart level, and secure.	Positioning the hemofilter near the access decreases the resistance to pressure to propel blood through the circuit.	The arterial line is normally much shorter than the venous line to maintain the driving pressure within the system and prevent clotting.
33. Don mask and goggles and wash hands.	Reduces transmission of microorganisms; standard precautions.	
34. Prepare sterile field with sterile barrier under the vascular catheters. Place 2 × 2 pads and 4 × 4 pads onto the sterile field.	Prepares material and maintains aseptic technique.	
35. Open sterile needles and syringes. Place on sterile field.	Readies equipment and maintains aseptic technique to prevent transmission of microorganisms.	
36. Add bactericidal solution to sterile basin.	Prepares solution used to cleanse catheter. Povidone-iodine and chlorhexidine are the recommended bactericidal agents.[5,12,13]	
37. Don sterile gloves	Prevents infection.	
38. Attach 19-G needles to 10-ml syringes; fill with NS flush or flush solution according to institutional standard. (*Level I: Manufacturer's recommendations only.*)	Prepares syringe for catheter flushing.	Check the manufacturer's recommendations for flushing volumes.[3]
39. Saturate four of the 4 × 4 pads in bactericidal solution and perform a 1-minute scrub of the arterial catheter port.	Prevent introduction of infection.	Make sure to remove any crust or drainage.
40. Wrap second bactericidal-soaked 4 × 4 pad around arterial catheter port and leave in place for 3 to 5 minutes. Repeat steps 39 and 40 for the venous port.	Reduces transmission of microorganisms.[9,12,13]	
41. After 3 to 5 minutes, remove the bactericidal-soaked 4 × 4 pad and discard in appropriate receptacle.	Standard precautions.	
42. Make sure catheter clamps are closed on the arterial and venous catheters; then remove cap from arterial catheter and discard appropriately.	Provides access to arterial side of catheter. Standard precautions.	Be sure catheter clamp is closed before removing arterial limb catheter cap.
43. Attach an empty 3-ml syringe to the arterial catheter port, open the clamp, and gently	Verifies patency of arterial catheter. Note any resistance, which could mean a clotted or kinked catheter.	Never forward-flush an indwelling catheter until first aspirating. This prevents dislodgement/embolism

Procedure continues on the following page

Procedure | **for Initiating and Terminating Continuous Renal Replacement Therapy**—*Continued*

Steps	Rationale	Special Considerations
aspirate 3 ml of blood and anticoagulant. Close the clamp, remove syringe, and discard in appropriate receptacle.	Prevents bolus of anticoagulant to the patient and decreases transmission of microorganisms.	of catheter clots, and prevents an intravenous bolus of anticoagulant in the catheter from entering the patient.
44. Repeat steps 42 and 43 on the venous catheter.	Verifies patency of venous catheter. Note any resistance, which could mean a clotted or kinked catheter. Prevents bolus of anticoagulant to the patient and decreases transmission of microorganisms.	Observe for clots. A clotted or kinked catheter decreases blood flow, which reduces efficacy of the treatment.
45. Attach 10-ml syringe with NS or other flush solution to arterial port. Open clamp and flush; then close clamp.	Prevents clotting of blood until dialysis is initiated. Positive pressure prevents backup of blood into the catheter after flushing.	Syringe should be left attached to catheter limb until replaced with dialyzer tubing connector.
46. Repeat step 45 on venous port.		
47. If ordered, administer or have an assistant administer initial heparin dose via appropriate intravenous access.	Prevents clotting of the system.	
48. Remove flush syringe from arterial catheter. Attach arterial line from CRRT circuit securely to the arterial catheter port.	Connects to hemofilter.	
49. Repeat step 48 for the venous line.		
50. Open arterial and venous access clamps and arterial and venous blood line clamps.	Establishes blood flow through the system	Carefully note any air bubbles in the system. If air is noted, clamp the venous blood line and aspirate air with a 10-ml syringe. Open the venous clamp when air is removed.
51. Make sure the clamp is open on the UF tubing and position the collection bag below the level of the patient.	Promotes flow of ultrafiltrate by gravity and siphoning pressure.	The UF tubing is usually longer than blood tubing. Lowering the collection bag creates a negative, or siphoning, pressure in the tubing. The level of the UF bag helps to determine the rate of ultrafiltration. Raising the collection bag decreases the negative pressure and rate of ultrafiltration; lowering it increases the negative pressure and the rate of ultrafiltration. During initiation, the collection bag is usually raised to prevent sudden hypovolemia.
52. Observe blood flow and UF flow through the circuit.	Validates performance of the system.	Separation of blood and plasma in the circuit indicates the system is clotting.
53. Start infusion of dialysate, replacement fluids, and anticoagulants, as ordered.		

Procedure	for Initiating and Terminating Continuous Renal Replacement Therapy—*Continued*	
Steps	**Rationale**	**Special Considerations**
54. Securely tape all circuit connections and secure hemofilter and lines. Keep the hemofilter and lines visible at all times.	Prevents leaks or disconnections; ensures any leaks will be noted immediately.	Exsanguination can occur from a system leak.
55. Observe the color and volume of UF in the collection bag.	Detects rupture of the hemofilter.	Pink or blood-tinged UF may mean the membranes of the hemofilter have ruptured; exsanguination can occur. Discontinue the system immediately.
56. Measure the amount during the first 5 minutes and multiply by 12. Adjust UF collection bag level to achieve desired UF rate.	Calculating the initial volume of UF helps to determine whether fluid replacement is necessary and the amount of adjustment of the UF collection bag to increase or decrease the UF rate.	
57. Dispose of soiled materials in the appropriate containers.	Prevents infection.	
58. Wash hands	Prevents transmission of microorganisms.	
59. Prepare a fluid balance flow sheet and calculate the net fluid gain/loss prescribed each hour.	Accurate calculations of hourly fluid balance prevent hyper- and hypovolemia and ensure that clinical goals are being met.	Hourly fluid balance is usually calculated by subtracting the total output (including UF) from the total intake.
Termination		
1. Wash hands	Reduces the transmission of organisms.	
2. Stop infusions of anticoagulants, replacement fluids, dialysate, or any other system infusions; clamp lines.	Prevent infusion during and after discontinuing system.	
3. Don clean gloves.	Standard precautions.	
4. Connect a 1000-ml normal saline bag to IV tubing, and prime tubing.	Prevents air from entering system.	
5. Attach the flush tubing to the infusion port on the arterial line.	Prepares for blood return.	
6. Clamp the arterial port of the vascular access and arterial line above the infusion port.	Stops blood flow into the circuit and prevents backflow of flush into the patient.	
7. Open the clamp on the infusion port of the blood line and the NS flush. Flush the circuit until blood is returned to the patient; then clamp NS flush line.		
8. Clamp the venous blood line and venous port of the vascular access.		
9. Record the amount of NS infused and ultrafiltrate in the collection bag.	Helps to ensure accurate fluid balance.[10]	The flush solution is fluid given to the patient and must be recorded as intake. Record the UF volume before disposing of the system.

Procedure continues on the following page

	Procedure for Initiating and Terminating Continuous Renal Replacement Therapy—*Continued*		

Steps	Rationale	Special Considerations
10. Remove the tape from the vascular access connections.		
11. Prepare sterile field with sterile barrier under the vascular catheters. Place 2 × 2 pads and 4 × 4 pads onto the sterile field.	Prepares material and maintains aseptic technique.	
12. Open sterile needles and syringes. Place on sterile field.	Readies equipment and maintains aseptic technique to prevent transmission of microorganisms.	
13. Add bactericidal solution to sterile basin.	Prepares solution used to cleanse catheter. Povidone-iodine and chlorhexidine are bacteriocidal agents.[5,12,13]	
14. Don mask, goggles, and sterile gloves.	Prevent infection and contamination.	
15. Attach 19-G needles to 10-ml syringes; fill with normal saline flush or flush solution according to institutional standard.	Prepares syringe for catheter flushing.	
16. Saturate four of the 4 × 4 pads in bactericidal solution and perform a 1-minute scrub of the arterial limb of the catheter.	Prevent introduction of infection. Povidone-iodine or chlorhexidine solutions are bactericidal solutions to be used.	Make sure to remove any crust or drainage.
17. Wrap second bactericidal-soaked 4 × 4 pad around arterial limb and leave in place for 3 to 5 minutes.	Reduces transmission of microorganisms.	
18. After 3 to 5 minutes, remove the bactericidal-soaked 4 × 4 pad and discard in appropriate receptacle.	Standard precautions.	
19. Make sure catheter clamps are closed on the arterial and venous lines of the catheter; disconnect the arterial blood line from the arterial vascular access.	Opens system under sterile conditions for system termination.	Be sure catheter clamp is closed before removing arterial line.
20. Repeat step 19 on the venous system line.		
21. Attach 10 ml-syringe with NS or other flush solution to arterial port. Open clamp and flush; then close clamp.	Prevents clotting of blood until anticoagulant is instilled.	
22. Repeat step 21 on venous port.		
23. Instill heparin or 4% citrate into each access port according to institutional protocol. Use only the volume listed on the vascular access.	Maintains patency of accesses.[11,13]	Use only the amount listed on the access to avoid instilling anticoagulant into the patient. Label each catheter with date/time/anticoagulant used/nurse's initials.
24. Clamp and cap the arterial and venous catheters with sterile caps; tape securely.		

Procedure	for Initiating and Terminating Continuous Renal Replacement Therapy—*Continued*	
Steps	**Rationale**	**Special Considerations**
25. Change vascular access dressings according to institutional protocol.	Prevent infection.	
26. Dispose of soiled materials in the appropriate containers	Prevent infection.	
27. Wash hands	Prevent transmission of microorganisms.	

Pumped Systems (CVVH, CVVHD, CVVHDF)
Initiation

1. Wash hands.	Prevents transmission of microorganisms; standard precaution.	
2. Verify orders, which should include the following: *(Level II: Theory based, no research data to support recommendations;recommendations from expert consensus group may exist.)* A. Modality B. Vascular access C. Type of hemofilter/dialyzer D. Anticoagulant type, concentration, infusion rate, monitoring parameters E. Replacement fluid (if used) F. Hourly ultrafiltration rate G. Hourly net fluid goal H. Dialysate solution and rate (if used) I. Blood pressure/vital sign parameters J. Laboratory testing	Familiarizes nurse with the individualized patient treatment and reduces the possibility of error.[10]	Ensure patient weight and laboratory values are recorded before initiation of therapy.
3. Turn the system on. Set up system according to manufacturer's instructions, attach any prescribed solutions, and prepare heparin/citrate infusion (if ordered), replacement fluid, dialysate, and flush infusion (if ordered). *(Level V: Clinical studies in more than one patient population and situation)*	Correct system setup is imperative for safety and optimal functioning. Use of anticoagulants prolongs the function of the hemofilter.[1,7]	Pump must be plugged into a generator outlet as some pumps do not have battery power. Heparin, if ordered, is usually administered on a prefilter port; citrate is usually administered at the arterial port of the vascular access catheter (VAC). Replacement solutions are administered through the arterial or venous infusion port as ordered (usually arterial) using blood tubing. Connect 1 liter NS to arterial infusion port (for flushing system). Dialysate solution (if using CVVHD/DF) is connected to the outlet port of the hemofilter near the venous end using blood tubing.
A. For integrated pump units (Prisma®, Diapact®, Accura®, Aquarius®), follow the manufacturer's instructions and prompts from the control module. (1) Automated setup instructions will include: • Select therapy/modality • Calibration	Ensure correct system setup.	Each integrated pump is loaded and primed by various methods, ranging from assembly and priming of all components, to "one touch" circuit loading and priming.

Procedure continues on the following page

Procedure	**for Initiating and Terminating Continuous Renal Replacement Therapy**—*Continued*	

Steps	Rationale	Special Considerations

• Load set
• Priming
• Anticoagulant/
  dialysate/replacement
  fluid setup
• Blood flow rate/fluid
  removal rate
  (2) After priming per
      manufacturer's
      instructions, go to step 4.
  B. For nonintegrated or blood
     pump–only systems:
  (1) Turn on pump and
      ensure air detector is
      activated before
      beginning treatment.
  (2) Follow manufacturer's
      instructions for setup.
  (3) Place the hemofilter in a
      vertical position, with
      the venous side up.
      Place the UF drain bag
      below the level of the
      patient's heart after
      priming is complete.
	Prevents an air embolus.
	  Lowering the UF bag increases
	  UF rate.
		Some unit's air detectors are activated
		  after the machine is primed.

4. With the protective caps on,
   place the arterial and venous
   blood lines on the patient's
   bed near the vascular access
   catheter (VAC).
	Leave the priming bag, collection
	  bag, and the protective caps in place
	  to preserve sterility of the system
	  until the blood lines are attached
	  to the vascular access catheter.
		Some systems have a collection bag
		  for the priming solution, which
		  stays attached to the venous blood
		  line until it is attached to the VAC.

5. Don mask and goggles and
   wash hands.
	Reduces transmission of
	  microorganisms; standard
	  precautions.	

6. Prepare sterile field with sterile
   barrier under the vascular access
   catheter. Place 2 × 2 pads and
   4 × 4 pads onto the sterile field.
	Prepares material and maintains
	  aseptic technique.	

7. Open sterile needles and
   syringes. Place on sterile field.
	Readies equipment and maintains
	  aseptic technique to prevent
	  transmission of microorganisms.	

8. Add bactericidal solution to
   sterile basin.
	Prepares solution used to cleanse
	  catheter. Povidone-iodine and
	  chlorhexidine are the acceptable
	  bactericidal agents.[5,12,13]	

9. Don sterile gloves	Prevents infection.	

10. Attach 19-G needles to 10-ml
    syringes; fill with normal saline
    flush or flush solution according
    to institutional standard.
	Prepares syringe for catheter
	  flushing.
		Quinton catheters recommend 20 to
		  30 ml per lumen flushes for
		  hemocaths and permacaths.[3]

11. Saturate four of the 4 × 4 pads
    in bactericidal solution and
    perform a 1-minute scrub of the
    arterial and venous ports of
    the catheter.
	Prevent introduction of infection.	Make sure to remove any crust or
		  drainage.

Procedure	for Initiating and Terminating Continuous Renal Replacement Therapy—*Continued*	

Steps	Rationale	Special Considerations
12. Wrap second bactericidal-soaked 4 × 4 pad around arterial and venous ports and leave in place for 3 to 5 minutes.	Reduces transmission of microorganisms.	
13. After 3 to 5 minutes, remove the bactericidal-soaked 4 × 4 pad and discard in appropriate receptacle.	Standard precautions.	
14. Make sure catheter clamps are closed on the arterial and venous ports of the catheter; then remove cap from arterial limb of catheter and discard appropriately.	Provides access to arterial side of catheter. Standard precautions.	Be sure catheter clamp is closed before removing arterial limb catheter cap.
15. Attach an empty 5-ml syringe to the arterial limb, open the clamp, and gently aspirate 5-ml of blood and anticoagulant. Close the clamp, remove syringe, and discard in appropriate receptacle.	Verifies patency of arterial limb. Note any resistance, which could mean a clotted or kinked catheter. Prevents bolus of anticoagulant to the patient and decreases transmission of microorganisms.[13]	Never forward-flush an indwelling catheter until first aspirating. This prevents dislodgement/embolism of catheter clots and prevents a bolus of anticoagulant to the patient.
16. Repeat steps 14 and 15 on the venous limb.	Verifies patency of venous limb. Note any resistance, which could mean a clotted or kinked catheter. Prevents bolus of anticoagulant to the patient and decreases transmission of microorganisms.	Observe for clots. A clotted or kinked catheter decreases blood flow and reduces efficacy of the treatment.
17. Attach 10-ml syringe with NS or other flush solution to arterial port. Open clamp and flush; then close clamp.	Prevents clotting of blood until dialysis is initiated.	Note any resistance on flushing.
18. Repeat step 17 on venous port.		
19. Disconnect protective cap or priming bag from arterial blood line, attach to arterial port of the VAC, and secure the connection.	Loose connections will introduce air into the circuit.	Since the venous line is not attached to the patient, the priming solution can be discarded.
20. Open the clamps on the arterial and venous blood lines; open the arterial port of the VAC.	Opens the circuit in preparation of starting the blood pump.	
21. Turn on the blood pump at a reduced blood flow (50 ml/min).[3]	Allows for troubleshooting of the system as needed.	
22. As the blood moves through the arterial tubing, administer prefilter heparin bolus, if ordered, and start heparin or citrate infusions as ordered.	Anticoagulates the extracorporeal system.	Anticoagulant must be administered before blood reaches the hemofilter to prevent fibrin buildup, clotting, and decreased efficacy of the hemofilter.
23. Turn the blood pump off as blood approaches the end of the venous blood line; clamp the venous blood line.	Prevents blood loss.	

Procedure continues on the following page

Procedure **for Initiating and Terminating Continuous Renal Replacement Therapy**—*Continued*

Steps	Rationale	Special Considerations
24. Don a new pair of sterile gloves.	Maintains sterile technique.	
25. Disconnect the protective cap or priming bag from the venous blood tubing, attach to the venous port of the VAC, and secure the connection.	Loose connections will introduce air into the circuit.	
26. Open the clamps on the venous port of the VAC and the venous blood line.	Prepares for starting the blood pump circuit.	Do final check for air in the blood circuit.
27. Turn the blood pump on and gradually turn the blood flow rate to the ordered rate.	Prevents hypotension from rapid blood and fluid shifts.	Observe for blood leaks, air in the system, and pressure alarms.
28. Start the ordered replacement fluid solution, if ordered.	Fluid loss without replacement may cause hypotension.	Fluids should be warmed to prevent hypothermia.
29. Start dialysate infusion, if ordered.	Starts hemodialysis/hemodiafiltration.	
30. Check that all alarms are on and parameters are set.	Ensures safe delivery of therapy.	
31. Note blood pump flow rate, arterial and venous monitor pressures, amount and color of UF, and vital signs on initiation and hourly or per institutional standard.		Increased arterial monitor pressure indicates problems with the vascular access or blood inflow. Increased venous monitor pressure indicates clotting of the hemofilter or system.
32. Dispose of soiled materials in the appropriate containers.	Prevents infection.	
33. Wash hands.	Prevents transmission of microorganisms.	
34. Prepare a fluid balance flow sheet and calculate the net fluid gain/loss prescribed each hour.	Accurate calculations of hourly fluid balance prevent hyper- and hypovolemia and ensure that clinical goals are being met.	Hourly fluid balance is usually calculated by subtracting the total output (including UF) from the total intake.

Flushing

1. Wash hands.	Prevents infection.	
2. Connect NS with flushed tubing to the arterial replacement port.		
3. Clamp the arterial side of the circuit (proximal to the arterial infusion port).	Prevents any more blood from entering the circuit via the arterial port during flushing.	*Note:* Make sure that NS flush is running freely to prevent rupture or back-filtration. Hemostasis and clot formation in the arterial limb of the tubing is also a possibility if the flushing procedure is prolonged.
4. Open the NS flush while the pump continues to run. Note the amount infused.	Flushing allows the nurse to assess the patency of the system.	Flushing contributes to the patient's IV intake; the volume of fluid should be documented. When the circuit is flushed of blood, clots may be observed. Flushing will not dissolve existing clots.

Procedure	for Initiating and Terminating Continuous Renal Replacement Therapy—*Continued*	
Steps	**Rationale**	**Special Considerations**
5. If no clots are observed, turn the saline off and unclamp the arterial circuit to allow hemofiltration to continue.		If numerous clots are observed, the hemofilter may need to be replaced.
Termination		
1. Turn off all infusions into the circuit.		
2. Open NS flush solution attached to arterial infusion port. Clamp the UF line.		
3. Continue terminating, depending on type of pump:	Follow instructions on the unit for termination.	
A. For integrated pump systems, press the "End Treatment" option and follow instructions. Continue to step 4.		
B. For nonintegrated pumps: with the blood pump still running, clamp off the arterial line near the patient, open the NS flush solution, place the hemofilter with arterial end up, and return the patient's blood. Continue to step 4.	The blood should be flushed through the circuit to prevent unnecessary blood loss.	If clots are identified beyond the venous bubble trap, *stop* the pump; do *not* return blood to patient. Blood from the arterial limb of the catheter is not returned to the patient because of the possibility of clot formation, and the machine will not detect clots in that location.
4. Once hemofilter and venous line is flushed, stop the pump.		
5. When the entire circuit is clear of blood, turn off the pump and clamp off both the arterial and venous access ports and the arterial and venous circuit lines.		
6. If the line is to be discontinued, remove it now per institutional policy.		If the line is not being discontinued, flush both ports with heparin or citrate as described below.
7. Record the amount of NS infused and UF in the collection bag.	Ensures accurate fluid balance.	The flush solution is fluid given to the patient and must be recorded as intake. Record the UF volume before disposing of the system.
8. Remove the tape from the vascular access connections.		
9. Prepare sterile field with sterile barrier under the vascular catheters. Place 2 × 2 pads and 4 × 4 pads onto the sterile field.	Prepares material and maintains aseptic technique.	
10. Open sterile needles and syringes. Place on sterile field.	Readies equipment and maintains aseptic technique to prevent transmission of microorganisms.	

Procedure continues on the following page

Procedure for Initiating and Terminating Continuous Renal Replacement Therapy—*Continued*

Steps	Rationale	Special Considerations
11. Add bactericidal solution to sterile basin.	Prepares solution used to cleanse catheter. Povidone-iodine and chlorhexidine are bactericidal agents to be used.[5,12,13]	
12. Don mask, goggles, and sterile gloves.	Prevents infection and contamination.	
13. Attach 19-G needles to 10-ml syringes; fill with normal saline flush or flush solution according to institutional standard.	Prepares syringe for catheter flushing.	
14. Saturate four of the 4 × 4 pads in bactericidal solution and perform a 1-minute scrub of the arterial limb of the catheter.	Prevents introduction of infection.	Make sure to remove any crust or drainage.
15. Wrap second bactericidal-soaked 4 × 4 pad around arterial limb and leave in place for 3 to 5 minutes.	Reduces transmission of microorganisms.[9,12]	
16. After 3 to 5 minutes, remove the bactericidal-soaked 4 × 4 pad and discard in appropriate receptacle.	Standard precautions.	
17. Make sure catheter clamps are closed on the arterial and venous lines of the catheter; then disconnect the arterial blood line from the arterial vascular access.	Opens system under sterile conditions for system termination.	Be sure catheter clamp is closed before removing arterial line.
18. Repeat step 17 on the venous system line.		
19. Attach 10-ml syringe with NS or other flush solution to arterial port. Open clamp and flush; then close clamp.	Prevents clotting of blood until anticoagulant is instilled.	
20. Repeat step 19 on venous port.		
21. Instill heparin or 4% citrate into each access port according to institutional protocol. Use only the volume listed on the vascular access.	Maintains patency of accesses.	Use only the amount listed on the access to avoid instilling anticoagulant into the patient. Label each catheter with date/time/anticoagulant used/ nurse's initials.
22. Clamp and cap the arterial and venous catheters with sterile caps; tape securely.		
23. Change vascular access dressings according to institutional protocol.	Prevents infection.	
24. Dispose of soiled materials in the appropriate containers.	Prevents infection.	
25. Wash hands.	Prevents transmission of microorganisms.	

Procedure	for Initiating and Terminating Continuous Renal Replacement Therapy—*Continued*	
Steps	**Rationale**	**Special Considerations**
Emergency Termination		
1. Clamp arterial and venous vascular access ports and circuit lines.		Emergency termination is used to emergently move the patient, or for serious complications, including blood leak, hemofilter rupture, clotting, circuit disconnection, or dialyzer/circuit reaction.
2. Don mask and sterile gloves.	Prevents infection.	
3. Disconnect circuit bloodlines from the vascular access catheters.		
4. Flush VAC with NS and instill with heparin or citrate per institutional protocol.	Maintains VAC patency.	
5. Stop all infusions related to CRRT treatment.	Prevents fluid and electrolyte imbalances.	
6. Dispose of soiled material in the appropriate containers.	Prevents transmission of microorganisms.	Blood in the circuit is lost during emergency termination.
7. Wash hands	Prevents infection.	

Expected Outcomes

- VAC accessed without any complications
- Blood easily aspirated from the access site
- Accumulated fluid and waste products removed
- Acid-base balance restored
- BUN and creatinine restored to baseline levels
- Electrolytes within baseline values
- Hemodynamic stability and maintenance of optimal intravascular volume
- Nutritional status maintained

Unexpected Outcomes

- Clotting/decreased patency of the catheter lumens
- Crack in the catheter or end caps
- Bleeding from insertion site or access site
- Signs and symptoms of infection at the insertion or access site
- Dislodgment of the catheter
- Decreased circulation in the extremity with the vascular access
- Hematoma formation at the access site
- Physiologic complications (dysrhythmias, chest pain, fluid or electrolyte imbalance, complications related to anticoagulation, air embolism, hypotension, seizures, nausea and vomiting, headaches, muscle cramping, dyspnea)
- Introduction of pathogens into the circuit
- Technical problems with the blood pump during (blood leak, air leak, clotting, disconnection of circuit, hemolysis, hemofilter rupture)
- Hypothermia
- Malnutrition

Patient Monitoring and Care

Steps	Rationale	Reportable Conditions
		These conditions should be reported if they persist despite nursing interventions.
1. Perform and record a predialysis and daily weights. *(Level V: Clinical studies in more than one patient population and situation.)*	Predialysis weight is an important factor in deciding how much UF is needed during treatment. It also helps to guide ongoing treatment.[2,3]	- Abnormal increase or decrease in weight

Procedure continues on the following page

Patient Monitoring and Care—*Continued*

Steps	Rationale	Reportable Conditions
2. Perform a baseline and ongoing assessments, including the following: A. Vital signs B. Jugular vein distention C. Presence of edema D. Intake and output E. Neurologic assessment F. Pulmonary assessment *(Level V: Clinical studies in more than one patient population and situation.)*	Important to establish a baseline before initiation of treatment.[2,3,10] Monitors for complications.	• Hypotension • Hypertension • Tachycardia/bradycardia • Tachypnea/bradypnea • Fever • Hypothermia • Jugular vein distention • Crackles • Edema • Change in level of consciousness, dizziness • Change in cardiac rhythm
3. Monitor the circulation to the extremity where the VAC is located. *(Level V: Clinical studies in more than one patient population and situation.)*	To assess for any decrease in perfusion distal to the VAC site.[2-3]	• Diminished capillary refill • Diminished or absent peripheral pulses • Pale, mottled, or cyanotic • Cool to touch • Diminished or absent movement • Pain
4. Monitor electrolytes, glucose, and albumin during treatment as per institutional standard.	Must be monitored because of continued fluid and electrolyte shifts during treatment. Amino acids are also lost through the hemofilter.	• Hyper- or hypokalemia • Hyper- or hyponatremia • Hyper- or hypocalcemia • Hyper- or hypoglycemia • Hyper- or hypomagnesemia • Hyper- or hypophosphatemia • Hypoalbuminemia
5. Administer medications to correct electrolyte abnormalities as ordered during treatment. *(Level V: Clinical studies in more than one patient population and situation.)*	Patients with renal failure are predisposed to many electrolyte abnormalities. During CRRT, several medications/electrolyte replacements may be given as ordered for individual patients.[2-3] Renal diet with adjusted protein, potassium, phosphorous, carbohydrate, and fluid intake that takes into account the patient's current catabolic state, residual renal function, adequacy of dialysis, and removal of amino acids by dialysis is required.[2,3,10]	• Hyper- or hypokalemia • Hyper- or hyponatremia • Hyper- or hypocalcemia • Hyper- or hypoglycemia • Hyper- or hypomagnesemia • Hyper- or hypophosphatemia • Hypoalbuminemia • Unexpected change in weight (loss or gain)
6. Monitor the CRRT circuit (e.g., occlusions; kinks in UF, blood, or vascular access lines; position of hemofilter). *(Level V: Clinical studies in more than one patient population and situation.)*	Disconnections or introduction of air into the circuit are always possible during treatment. Bleeding or exsanguination can also occur.[4-5] Level of collection device should be approximately 16 to 20 inches below the level of the filter to allow for best gravity drainage. Clotting of the circuit is a potential complication. If hemofilter becomes excessively clotted, the extracorporeal blood volume should be returned to the patient quickly. Blood leaks from the dialyzer into the dialysate may occur and necessitate termination of treatment.	• Disconnections, cracks, or leaks • Excessive clotting • Blood leaks/hemofilter rupture • Malfunction of dialyzer or access

Patient Monitoring and Care—*Continued*

Steps	Rationale	Reportable Conditions
	In the event of a filter leak, do NOT return the circuit blood to the patient. Venous or arterial pressures that are out of range may indicate dialyzer or access malfunction.	
7. Monitor UF for rate, clarity, and air bubbles. *(Level V: Clinical studies in more than one patient population and situation.)*	A decrease in UF production can occur due to clotting of the dialyzer.[1,2,3,10] Pink or blood-tinged UF is indicative of filter leak or rupture.	• Decrease in UF production • Change in color or characteristics of UF • Air in UF
8. Administer heparin or citrate as ordered. *(Level V: Clinical studies in more than one patient population and situation.)*	Heparin or citrate is often used to prevent clotting of the circuit.[1,7] Heparin/citrate dose varies according to patient condition and laboratory values.	• Suspicion of clotting in the circuit
9. Monitor anticoagulation as per institutional standard.	Because heparin or citrate commonly are used to prevent system clotting, coagulation studies should be routinely monitored.	• Abnormal coagulation studies
10. Monitor the vascular access. *(Level V: Clinical studies in more than one patient population and situation.)*	Bleeding can occur from either the venous or arterial catheter. Clotting of the access can occur.[2,3,10]	• Decrease in access function or patency
11. Monitor condition of access site. *(Level V: Clinical studies in more than one patient population and situation.)*	Bleeding or infection can be access site complications.[2,3]	• Bleeding • Site redness/edema • Warmth • Purulent drainage • Pain or tenderness • Fever
12. Initiate and monitor rate of replacement fluids.	Prevents hypotensive episodes. Replacement fluids are dependent on patient's baseline assessment. Ringer's lactate commonly is used and infused as follows: Amount of previous hour's UF plus previous hour's total output (TO) minus previous hour's IV fluids (IV) plus desired net hourly fluid loss (FL) equals amount of replacement fluid (RF) (UF + TO) − (IV + FL) = RF.	
13. Monitor the patient for complications associated with CRRT treatment. *(Level V: Clinical studies in more than one patient population and situation.)*	Several complications are possible with CRRT.[4-5]	• Muscle cramps • Dialysis disequilibrium (headache, nausea and vomiting, hypertension, decreased sensorium, convulsions, coma) • Air embolism • Dialyzer reaction (hypotension, pruritis, back pain, angioedema, anaphylaxis) • Hypoxemia

Procedure continues on the following page

Patient Monitoring and Care—*Continued*

Steps	Rationale	Reportable Conditions
14. Monitor the blood pump for proper functioning.	Any type of equipment is subject to malfunctioning. It is important for the nurse operating the blood pump to be competent with its operation, understand troubleshooting methods, and know when to take the pump out of service to be checked by the biomedical department.	• Problems with the blood pump

Documentation

Documentation should include the following:

- Patient and family education
- Date and time of treatment initiation/filter change
- Condition of vascular access catheter regarding patency, quality of blood flow, ease of access procedure
- Date and time of VAC insertion and dressing change
- Condition of insertion site and any signs or symptoms of infection
- For pumped systems, blood flow rate and arterial and venous monitoring pressures

- Vital signs/hemodynamic parameters
- Hourly fluid balance calculation
- Patient's response to CRRT and daily progress toward treatment goals
- Unexpected outcomes
- Nursing interventions
- Daily weight
- Laboratory assessment data

References

1. *Acute Dialysis Quality Initiative Guidelines for Practice.* (2003). Available at: www.adqi.net.
2. American Nephrology Nurses Association. (1999). *ANNA Standards of Clinical Practice for Nephrology Nurses.* 3rd ed. Pitman, NJ: Author, 61-70.
3. American Nephrology Nurses Association. (1999). *Core Curriculum for Nephrology Nursing.* Pitman, NJ: Author, 323-45.
4. Bellomo, R., Ronco, C., and Mehta, R. (1996). Nomenclature for continuous renal replacement therapies. *A J Kid Dis,* 28, S2-7.
5. Centers for Disease Control, Hospital Infection Control Advisory Council. (1996). Guideline for the prevention of intravascular device-related infections. Part 1: Intravascular device-related infections: An overview. *Am J Infect Control,* 24, 262-76.
6. Davenport, A. (1997). The coagulation system in the critically ill patient with acute renal failure and the effect of an extracorporeal circuit. *Am J Kid Dis,* 30, S20-7.
7. Davenport, A., and Mehta, S. (2002). The acute dialysis quality initiative-part VI: Access and anticoagulation in CRRT. *Adv Renal Replacement Therapy,* 9, 273-81.
8. Giuliano, K., and Pysznik, E. (1998). Renal replacement therapy in critical care: Implementation of a unit-based CVVH program. *Crit Care Nurse,* 18, 40-51.

9. Goldstein, M.B. (1992). Prevention of sepsis from central venous dialysis catheters. *Semin Dialysis,* 5, 106-7.
10. Martin, R., and Jurschak, J. (1996). Nursing management of continuous renal replacement therapy. *Seminars in Dialysis,* 9, 192-9.
11. Mehta, R.L. (1996). Anticoagulation strategies for continuous renal replacement therapies: What works? *Am J Kid Dis,* 30, S8-14.
12. National Guideline Clearinghouse. (2003). *Guidelines for the Prevention of Intravascular Catheter-Related Infections.* Available at: www.guideline.gov.
13. NKF/DOQI. (2001). Clinical Practice Guidelines for Vascular Access: Update 2000. *Am J Kidney Dis,* 37, S137-81.

Additional Readings

Mehta, R., and Martin, R. (1996). Initiating and implementing a continuous renal replacement therapy program: Requirements and guidelines. *Seminars in Dialysis,* 9, 80-7.
Parker, J. (1998). *Contemporary Nephrology Nursing.* Pitman, NJ: American Nephrology Nurses Association, 577-88.
Ronco, C., and Bellomo, R. (1998). *Critical Care Nephrology.* Dordrecht, Germany: Klewa Academic Publishers.

PROCEDURE **118**

Hemodialysis

P U R P O S E : Hemodialysis is performed for volume regulation, acid-base control, electrolyte regulation, and management of azotemia.

Rhonda K. Martin

PREREQUISITE NURSING KNOWLEDGE

- Hemodialysis (Fig. 118-1) may be needed for the onset of acute renal failure, as well as for maintenance therapy for patients with chronic renal failure.
- Basic knowledge is necessary of the principles of diffusion, ultrafiltration (UF), osmosis, oncotic pressure, and hydrostatic pressure as they pertain to fluid and solute management during dialysis[1,2,10]:
  - ❖ Diffusion is the passive movement of solutes through a semipermeable membrane from an area of higher to lower concentration until equilibrium is reached.
  - ❖ Ultrafiltration is the bulk movement of solute and solvent through a semipermeable membrane using a pressure movement. This is usually achieved by positive pressure in the blood compartment of the hemofilter, and negative pressure in the dialysate compartment. Blood and dialysate run countercurrent to each other (in opposite directions). The size of the solute molecules as compared with the size of molecules that can move through the semipermeable membrane determines the degree of UF.
  - ❖ Osmosis is the passive movement of solvent through a semipermeable membrane from an area of higher to lower concentration.
  - ❖ Oncotic pressure is the pressure exerted by plasma proteins, which favors intravascular fluid retention and movement of fluid from the extravascular to the intravascular space.
  - ❖ Hydrostatic pressure is the force exerted by arterial blood pressure, which favors the movement of fluid from the intravascular to the extravascular space.

- Adsorption is the adhesion of molecules (solutes) to the surface to the hemofilter, charcoal, or resin.
- Vascular access is needed to perform hemodialysis and can be provided by a double-lumen catheter, an external arteriovenous (AV) shunt, or a surgically created AV anastomosis (e.g., fistula or graft). Common sites for the double-lumen catheter include the internal jugular, the subclavian, or the femoral vein. Common sites for the external shunt include the forearm (radial artery to cephalic vein) or the leg (posterior tibial artery to long saphenous vein). The AV fistula or graft is used for long-term dialysis management.
- Hemodialysis uses an artificial kidney (hemofilter, dialyzer) with a semipermeable membrane to create two separate compartments: the blood compartment and the dialysis solution (dialysate) compartment. The semipermeable membrane allows the movement of small molecules (e.g., electrolytes, urea, drugs) and middle-weight molecules (creatinine) from the patient's blood into the dialysate but is impermeable to larger molecules (blood cells, plasma proteins).
- Each dialyzer has four ports: two end ports for blood (in one end and out the other) and two side ports for dialysis solution (also in one end and out the other). In most cases, the blood and dialysate are run through the dialyzer in opposite or countercurrent directions.
- The hollow-fiber dialyzer is the most commonly used dialyzer. Using this dialyzer, the blood flows through the center of hollow fibers and the dialysate flows around the outside of the hollow fibers. The advantages of hollow-fiber filters include a low priming volume, low resistance to flow, and high amount of surface area. The major disadvantage is the potential for clotting secondary to the small fiber size.

961

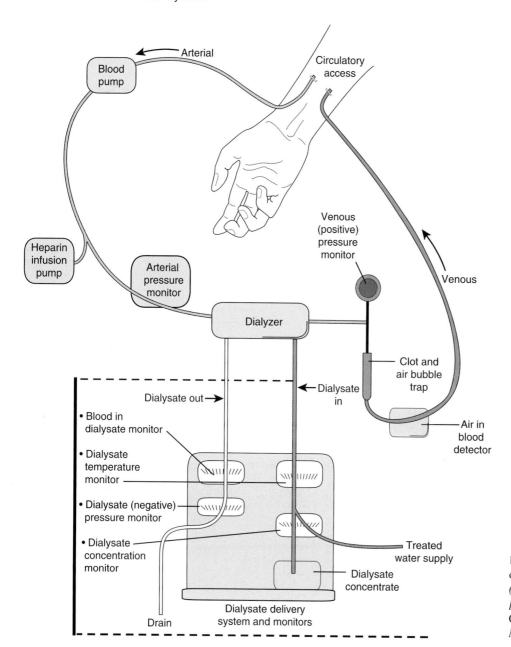

Arterial

Circulatory
access

Blood
pump

Heparin
infusion
pump

Arterial
pressure
monitor

Venous
(positive)
pressure
monitor

Venous

Dialyzer

Clot and
air bubble
trap

Dialysate
in

Dialysate out

• Blood in
dialysate monitor

• Dialysate
temperature
monitor

• Dialysate (negative)
pressure monitor

• Dialysate
concentration
monitor

Air in
blood
detector

Treated
water supply

Dialysate
concentrate

Drain

Dialysate delivery
system and monitors

FIGURE 118-1 Components of a typical hemodialysis system. *(From Thompson J.M., et al., eds. [1989].* Mosby's Manual of Clinical Nursing. *St. Louis: CV Mosby.)*

- Parallel-plate dialyzers are designed as sheets of membrane over supporting structures. Blood and dialysate pass through alternate spaces of the dialyzer. The major disadvantages of this type of filter are the increase in allergic dialyzer reactions, and lower filter surface area.
- All dialyzers have UF coefficients; thus the dialyzer selected will vary in different clinical situations. The higher the UF coefficient, the more rapid the fluid removal. UF coefficients are determined by in vivo measurements done by each dialyzer manufacturer.
- Clearance refers to the ability of the dialyzer to remove metabolic waste products from the patient's blood. The blood flow rate, the dialysate flow rate, and the solute concentration affect clearance. Clearance occurs by the processes of diffusion, convection, and UF.[2]
- The blood circuit consists of blood lines, a blood pump, and various monitoring devices. The blood lines carry the

blood to and from the patient. The blood pump controls the speed of the blood through the circuit. The monitoring devices include arterial and venous pressure monitors, as well as an air detection monitor, to prevent air entering the circuit from being returned to the patient.
- The dialysate is composed of water, a buffer (e.g., acetate or bicarbonate), and various electrolytes. Most solutions also contain glucose. The buffer helps neutralize acids that are generated as a result of normal cellular metabolism and usually are excreted by the kidney. The concentration of electrolytes is usual normal plasma concentrations, helping to create a concentration gradient for removal of excess electrolytes. The glucose, available in various concentrations, promotes the removal of plasma water.[2]
- Heparin is usually used during dialysis to prevent clotting of the circuit. In patients with coagulopathies, normal saline flushes can be used to keep the blood circuit patent.[5]

- Because large volumes of water are used during treatments to generate the dialysate, the water must be purified prior to patient use, preventing patient exposure to potentially harmful substances present in the water supply (e.g., calcium carbonate, sodium chloride, and iron).
- Other extended renal replacement therapy techniques or "hybrid" techniques (sustained low efficiency dialysis [SLED], extended daily dialysis [EDD]) generally use standard hemodialysis equipment and techniques with reduced blood flow and dialysate rates to gradually remove plasma water and solutes in the critically ill patient. They are used from 4 to 12 hours a day.[6]
- The adequacy of dialysis and assessment of the patient's residual renal function should be evaluated on a periodic basis. Adequacy of dialysis can be measured using urea kinetic modeling (Kt/V) or urea clearance. Residual renal functioning can be monitored using urine creatinine clearance. Collaboration with the nephrology team is necessary to monitor these parameters.[2,10]

EQUIPMENT

- Masks, goggles
- Sharps container
- Two 10-ml syringes and two 3-ml syringes
- Sterile normal saline (NS), 3 L
- Dressing supplies (sterile barrier, gauze pads, transparent dressing, tape)
- Povidone-iodine solution/swabs or chlorhexidine bactericidal solution
- Heparin (1000 unit/ml) (both for priming and infusion, as ordered)
- Sterile bowl
- Two 19-G needles
- Antiseptic soap
- Hemostats
- 4 × 4 gauze pads, tape, sterile barrier
- Replacement fluid, as ordered
- Dialysate fluid, as ordered
- Sterile gloves, clean gloves
- Alcohol wipes

Additional equipment for graft cannulation includes the following:
- Two 10-ml syringes
- Two 19-G needles
- NS for injection
- Two fistula needles
- Povidone-iodine swabs
- 1% lidocaine and two tuberculin syringes
- Two hemostats

Additional equipment for initiation of hemodialysis includes the following:
- Dialysis machine, tubing, dialyzer, and dialysate solution/water treatment setup
- Two hemostats
- One 30-ml syringe
- One 18-G needle

Additional equipment, to have available depending on patient need, includes the following:
- One tourniquet (AV fistula only)
- Loading dose of heparin (if ordered)

Equipment for termination of hemodialysis includes the following:
- Four hemostats
- 2 × 2 gauze pads
- NS, 1000 ml
- Nonsterile gloves
- Goggles
- Four bandages, tape
- Sharps container

PATIENT AND FAMILY EDUCATION

- Explain the procedure and review any questions the patient may have. ➤*Rationale:* Provides information and decreases patient anxiety.
- Explain the need for careful sterile technique for the duration of treatment. ➤*Rationale:* Decreases the chance of systemic infection, because pathogens can be transported throughout the entire body via the circulation.
- Explain the purpose of hemodialysis. ➤*Rationale:* Hemodialysis is necessary to perform the physiologic functions of the kidneys when renal failure is present.
- Explain the need for careful monitoring of the patient during the treatment for fluid and electrolyte imbalance. ➤*Rationale:* Dialysis treatment puts the patient at risk for imbalance because of the rapid movement of fluid and electrolytes from the patient during treatment.
- Explain the importance of input from the patient on how he or she is feeling during the treatment. ➤*Rationale:* Hypotension is a common occurrence during treatment; the patient may experience lightheadedness or dizziness if hypotension is present. Letting the patient know to expect this as a possibility should help decrease patient anxiety.
- Explain the hemodialysis circuit setup to the patient. ➤*Rationale:* It is important for the patient and family to be aware that blood will be removed from the patient's body and will be visible during the hemodialysis treatment.

PATIENT ASSESSMENT AND PREPARATION

Patient Assessment

- Baseline vital signs, weight, neurologic status, physical assessment of all body systems, fluid and electrolyte status. ➤*Rationale:* Patients in renal failure often have altered baseline assessments, both in physical assessment and in the laboratory values. Having this information before treatments are started is helpful so that interventions, including the dialysate, can be individualized. Alterations during treatment are common because of the rapid removal of fluid and solutes.

- Graft, fistula, or catheter insertion site for signs or symptoms of infection. ➤*Rationale:* Because dialysis access sites are used frequently, infection is always a potential risk. Dialysis access sites should only be used for dialysis, and not for other intravenous access needs, except in an emergency situation. Catheter insertion sites provide a portal of entry for infection, which may result in septicemia if unrecognized or untreated. If the catheter insertion site appears to be infected, further interventions (e.g., site change, culture, and antibiotic treatment) may be necessary.
- Catheter patency and the ability to easily aspirate blood from both ports. ➤*Rationale:* Adequate blood flow is necessary during a treatment in order to facilitate optimal fluid and solute removal. Patent catheter lumens are necessary for adequate blood flow.
- If using an AV fistula, assess the site for presence of bruit, erythema, swelling, and quality of blood flow. ➤*Rationale:* Physical assessment of the fistula can indicate patency of the graft, as well as the possible presence of infection.
- Adequate circulation to the distal parts of the access limb. ➤*Rationale:* The placement of a vascular access may compromise circulation.

Patient Preparation

- Ensure that patient understands preprocedural teaching. Answer questions as they arise and reinforce information as needed. ➤*Rationale:* Evaluates and reinforces understanding of previously taught information.
- Position the patient in a comfortable position (that will also facilitate optimal blood flow through the catheter and allow for the setup of a sterile field). ➤*Rationale:* Facilitating patient comfort will help to minimize the amount of patient movement during treatment, which can change the amount of blood flow through the catheter. Different catheter sites may require different patient positions to facilitate optimal blood flow.
- If using an AV fistula, ask the patient whether he or she wants lidocaine used on the access site before accessing the fistula. ➤*Rationale:* Promotes patient comfort and reduces anxiety.

Procedure for Hemodialysis

Steps	Rationale	Special Considerations
Cannulation of AV Fistula or Graft		
1. Wash hands.	Reduces transmission of microorganisms; standard precautions.	
2. Wash access site for 1 full minute with antiseptic soap using a 4 × 4 gauze pad; rinse off with water.	Reduces the transmission of microorganisms.	
3. Place arm on sterile barrier.	Maintains aseptic technique.	
4. Starting at the site for insertion, moving out in concentric circles for 2 to 3 inches, wash access area with bactericidal swabs or soaked 2 × 2 gauze pad for 1 full minute. *(Level V: Clinical studies in more than one patient population and situation.)*	Povidone-iodine solution serves as a bactericidal agent.[3,4,9]	Skin asepsis is crucial; however, the most effective method for skin cleansing has not yet been established.
5. Repeat step 4 with a new swab or 2 × 2 gauze pad.		
6. Using two 10-mL syringes and two 19-G needles, draw up prescribed flush solution in each syringe.	Prepares syringes for flushing fistula/graft.	Use an amount of heparinized saline that is consistent with institutional policy. In some cases, only saline will be used. Activated clotting times (ACTs) will provide information regarding the patient's anticoagulation status.
7. Attach flush to fistula needle tubing, and prime fistula needles.	Prevents clotting of blood in fistula needles.	

Procedure for Hemodialysis—*Continued*

Steps	Rationale	Special Considerations
8. Clamp catheter/tubing.	Prevents loss of heparinized solution and backflow of blood.	
9. Apply tourniquet to upper portion of access limb (AV fistula cannulation).	Facilitates site determination for cannulation.[1,2,9]	
10. Don nonsterile gloves and goggles.	Standard precautions.	
11. Select site to be used.	Decreases recirculation of dialyzed blood.	Arterial site should be at least 3 inches from arterial anastomosis. Venous needle must be in the direction of venous flow and, if possible, 3 inches or more from the arterial needle.
12. Grasp butterfly wings or hub of fistula needle between thumb and index finger of dominant hand with needle tip bevel-up.	Provides secure grasp of needle upon cannulation.	*Optional:* Before insertion of fistula needle, lidocaine may be injected intradermally to make a small wheal, per patient preference.
13. Remove needle guard.	Exposes fistula needle.	
14. Hold skin taut with nondominant hand.	Prevents rolling of vessel.	Prevents contamination of area to be punctured.
15. With dominant hand, insert needle at a 45-degree angle to the skin (if lidocaine was used, use same puncture site for needle).		
A. *AV fistula:* Advance bevel up to hub of the needle.	Accesses arterial vascular system.	Prevents shearing of graft material.
B. *AV graft:* As soon as tip is through the graft, rotate needle 180 degrees and advance needle to hub, with bevel down.	Accesses arterial vascular system. Bevel-down position prevents shearing of graft.	
16. Remove tourniquet before infusing NS or heparin (AV fistula).	Prevents clotting.	
17. Unclamp needle/tubing clamp and aspirate blood.	Verifies correct placement and patency of access.	
18. Infuse flush solution; reclamp catheter.	Prevents clotting and backflow of blood.	
19. Secure needle with adhesive tape over insertion site.	Maintains angle of needle so that it floats freely in the vessel/graft.	
20. Repeat steps 12 through 18 for insertion of second needle.	Cannulation of venous site.	Hemodialysis can now be initiated.
21. Discard soiled material in appropriate receptacle.	Standard precautions.	
22. Wash hands.	Reduces transmission of microorganisms.	
Accessing a Vascular Catheter		
1. Don mask and goggles and wash hands.	Reduces transmission of microorganisms; standard precautions.	
2. Prepare sterile field with sterile barriers, 2 × 2 pads, 4 × 4 pads, and transparent dressing.	Prepares material and maintains aseptic technique.	

Procedure continues on the following page

Procedure for Hemodialysis—*Continued*

Steps	Rationale	Special Considerations
3. Open sterile needles and syringes. Place on sterile field.	Readies equipment and maintains aseptic technique to prevent transmission of microorganisms.	
4. Attach 19-G needles to 10-mL syringes; prepare flush solution according to institutional standard. *(Level I: Manufacturer's recommendation only.)*	Prepares syringe for catheter flushing.	Refer to manufacturer's recommendations for amount of flush to be used
5. Add bactericidal solution to sterile basin.	Prepares solution used to cleanse catheter.	
6. Remove dressing from exit site, taking care not to contaminate or dislodge cannula.	Allows access to exit site.	Inspect for signs and symptoms of exit-site infection: drainage, crusting, swelling, redness, exudate, or complaints of pain at the site.
7. Discard soiled dressing in appropriate container.	Standard precautions.	
8. Wash hands.	Reduces transmission of microorganisms.	
9. Don sterile gloves.	Maintains aseptic technique.	
10. Place sterile barrier beneath catheter.	Sets up sterile field.	Do not touch catheter with gloves. Should gloves accidentally touch the catheter, a glove change is necessary to maintain aseptic technique.
11. Saturate four of the 4 × 4 pads in bactericidal solution and perform a 1-minute scrub of the arterial limb of the catheter.	Povidone-iodine and chlorhexidine are the only currently approved bactericidal agents.[3,4,8]	Make sure to remove any crust or drainage.
12. Wrap second bactericidal-soaked 4 × 4 pad around arterial limb and leave in place for approximately 3 to 5 minutes.	Reduces transmission of microorganisms.	
13. After 3 to 5 minutes, remove soaked 4 × 4 pad and discard in appropriate receptacle.	Standard precautions.	
14. Remove cap from arterial limb of catheter and discard appropriately.	Provides access to arterial side of catheter. Standard precautions.	Be sure slide clamp is closed before removing arterial limb catheter cap.
15. Attach an empty 3-ml syringe to the arterial limb, open the slide clamp, and gently aspirate 3-ml of blood. Close the slide clamp, remove syringe, and discard in appropriate receptacle.	Remove indwelling heparin from the catheter, and assess patency.	If you have difficulty aspirating blood, notify physician or advanced practice nurse. If serum laboratory work is required, attach another empty syringe to the arterial limb and aspirate required amount of blood.
16. Repeat steps 11 through 15 on the venous limb.	Verifies patency of venous limb; decreases transmission of microorganisms.	Observe for clots.
17. Attach flush syringe to arterial limb, open slide clamp, and gently aspirate 2 to 3 ml of blood; slowly flush catheter; then close slide clamp.	Positive pressure prevents backup of blood into the catheter after flushing.	Syringe should be left attached to catheter limb until replaced with dialyzer tubing connector.

Procedure for Hemodialysis—*Continued*

Steps	Rationale	Special Considerations
18. Repeat step 17 on venous limb.	Prevents clotting of blood until dialysis is initiated.	Syringe should be left attached to catheter limb until replaced with dialyzer tubing connector.
19. Soak two 2 × 2 pads in bactericidal solution and cleanse connection site.	Reduces infection.	
20. Remove flush syringe from arterial limb. Attach arterial line from dialysis machine securely to the arterial limb. Place the venous line from the dialysis machine in the container for priming fluid discard. Leave the recirculating adaptor in on the end.	Connects the patient to the dialysis machine.	
21. Tape connections securely.	Prevents accidental separation of lines.	
22. Open the clamps on the arterial limb of the catheter and dialysis tubing, and turn on blood pump at a slow rate (50-100 ml/min).	Primes the blood lines with blood.	
23. When the venous drip chamber located on the hemodialysis machine is pink, turn off the blood pump; clamp the venous line. Remove flush syringe from the venous limb; securely attach to the venous tubing.	Indicates blood has circulated through dialyzer to the venous line.	The venous limb should be left in clamped position.
24. Secure connections.	Prevents accidental separation of lines.	
25. Remove gloves and discard soiled material in appropriate receptacle.	Standard precautions.	
26. Wash hands. Proceed to initiation of hemodialysis.	Reduces transmission of microorganisms.	
Disconnecting From Catheter		
1. Don mask and cap and wash hands.	Reduces transmission of microorganisms; standard precautions.	
2. Open syringes, caps, needles, and 2 × 2 gauze pads; place on sterile field.	Maintains aseptic technique.	
3. Fill two syringes with desired amount of heparin, depending on type of catheter used. Fill two 10-ml syringes with NS. *(Level I: Manufacturer's recommendations only.)*	Heparin is used to maintain patency of access.[9]	
4. Place sterile barrier under catheter limbs.	Sets up a sterile field.	
5. Wrap both catheter limbs with bactericidal soaked 2 × 2 pads and scrub for 1 minute.	Povidone-iodine and chlorhexidine act as a bactericidal agents.[3,4,8]	
6. Don sterile gloves.	Maintains aseptic technique.	
7. Clamp arterial and venous limbs.	Prevents blood loss from catheters.	

Procedure continues on the following page

Procedure for Hemodialysis—*Continued*

Steps	Rationale	Special Considerations
8. Using the same povidone-iodine–soaked 2 × 2 pad to handle the dialysis tubing, disconnect arterial line from the limb and attach the NS-filled syringe.	Prevents blood from entering the tip of the catheter.	
9. Attach a 3- or 5-ml syringe with heparin, unclamp slide clamp; inject prescribed amount of heparin.	Maintains catheter patency by preventing clotting of blood.	Heparin dosage will vary depending on type of catheter used and unit policy. In some cases, catheter may be flushed with NS only. Use only the amount listed on the access to avoid instilling anticoagulant into the patient. Label each catheter with date/time/anticoagulant used/nurse's initials.[9]
10. Clamp, disconnect syringe, and cap the arterial limb.	Prevents loss of blood.	
11. Repeat steps 8 through 10 on venous limb.	Maintains patency by preventing clotting of blood.	
12. Apply povidone-iodine ointment to the catheter insertion site at each dressing change. *(Level IV: Limited clinical studies to support recommendations.)*	Lowers incidence of catheter-related infections.[9,11]	
13. Apply dressing to catheter site at each hemodialysis treatment or when the dressing become damp, loosened, or soiled. *(Level IV: Limited clinical studies to support recommendations.)*	Prevents contamination of catheter exit site.[3,4,8]	Dressing should be maintained and changed at least weekly.
14. Discard soiled material in appropriate receptacle.	Standard precautions.	
15. Wash hands.	Reduces transmission of microorganisms.	

Initiation and Termination of Hemodialysis[1,11]

Steps	Rationale	Special Considerations
1. Verify orders, which should include: A. Vascular access B. Hours of treatment C. Type of hemofilter/dialyzer D. Blood flow rate E. Anticoagulant-type, concentration, infusion rate, monitoring parameters F. Ultrafiltration goal G. Dialysate solution and rate (if used) H. Blood pressure/vital sign parameters I. Laboratory testing. *(Level IV: Limited clinical studies to support recommendations)*	Familiarizes nurse with the individualized patient treatment and reduces the possibility of error.	Ensure patient weight and laboratory values are recorded before initiation of therapy.
2. Set up dialysis machine according to manufacturer's instructions.	Ensures safe and proper assembly and allows for testing of all patient alarms and the proper functioning of the machine prior to accessing the catheter/fistula.	
3. Don gloves and goggles and wash hands.	Reduces transmission of microorganisms; standard precautions.	

Procedure for Hemodialysis—*Continued*

Steps	Rationale	Special Considerations
4. Access catheter, graft, or fistula.		
5. Wash access arm for 1 full minute with antiseptic soap and a sterile 4 × 4 gauze pad. Place arm on sterile barrier.	Reduces transmission of microorganisms and establishes a sterile field.	
6. Connect arterial access to arterial blood line.	Provides a circuit between the patient and the dialyzer.	
7. Place the venous dialyzer tubing line into the retaining clamps of the fluid receptacle on the side of the dialysis machine.	Prevents contamination of venous tubing.	Be careful not to immerse the end of the venous line below the fluid level.
8. Tape arterial cannula connections securely.	Prevents accidental disconnection.	
9. Remove clamp from arterial line.	Permits flow of blood.	
10. Adjust blood pump to 100 ml/min until blood reaches the venous drip chamber.	Slow rate prevents symptoms of rapid blood loss and allows for assessment of blood flow from the arterial limb.	Heparin loading dose, if ordered, may be given via bolus in arterial line.
11. Turn off blood pump.	Prevents blood loss from dialyzer and cannula.	
12. Clamp the end of the venous tubing below the drip chamber with a bulldog clamp.	Prevents introduction of air.	
13. Remove venous line tubing from fluid container, remove the recirculation adaptor, and connect to the venous access cannula.	Completes pathway circuit for return of blood from the dialyzer to the patient.	
14. Tape venous connections securely.	Prevents accidental separation.	
15. Remove clamp from venous tubing.	Permits flow of blood.	
16. Turn on blood pump and adjust blood flow rate.	Initiates flow of blood from patient to the dialyzer.	
17. Immediately turn on foam detector switch from bypass to alarm position.	Sets the foam detector alarm monitor to on.	The air/foam monitor detects minute air leaks.
18. Adjust the blood level in the arterial and venous drip chambers to three-quarters full.	Prevents accumulation of air in tubing and dialyzer.	
19. Turn dialyzer over so that arterial (red) port is at the top.	Establishes countercurrent flow.	
20. If patient is receiving systemic heparinization, set parameters on heparin infusion pump as prescribed.	Provides anticoagulation.	
21. Secure cannula connections and blood.	Additional precaution against accidental disconnection.	
22. Slowly increase blood pump speed to prescribed rate while continuing to assess patient (level of consciousness, complaints of chest pain, dysrhythmias, and changes in hemodynamic variables).	Prevents complications of rapid removal of blood.	If there is any question as to how well the patient will tolerate hemodialysis, the pump speed should be started at 100 ml/min and gradually increased to goal.

Procedure continues on the following page

Procedure for Hemodialysis—*Continued*

Steps	Rationale	Special Considerations
23. Set arterial and venous alarm parameters.	Sets the safety alarm system.	
24. Observe the patient's transmembrane pressure (TMP) display.	Removes desired UF.	To calculate TMP, the following formula may be used: Weight to be removed × 500 ml− KUF = TMP. (KUF is the coefficient of ultrafiltration of the dialyzer. Each type/size of dialyzer has a different KUF, which can be obtained from the package insert.)
25. Set TMP or negative pressure and alarms.	Allows for UF.	Most machines will automatically adjust based on treatment time and volume removal goal.
26. Wash hands.	Reduces transmission of microorganisms.	
27. Continuously monitor patient status and machine function throughout treatment.	Prevents complications and minimizes effects of fluid and electrolyte shifts.	Patient assessment should include vital signs and symptoms related to fluid and electrolyte shifts (e.g., cramping, hypotension, nausea, vomiting). Monitor the machine for blood flow rate, arterial and venous pressure readings, dialysate pressure, TMP, and blood circuit for clotting or air.
Termination		
1. Don nonsterile gloves and goggles and wash hands.	Reduces transmission of microorganisms; standard precautions.	
2. Move the arterial, venous, and dialysate pressure alarms to the maximum low/high limits.	Prevents machine from alarming when terminating dialysis as pressures drop.	
3. Turn TMP or negative pressure off.	Removes negative pressure, thereby stopping UF.	
4. Turn off the heparin infusion pump.	Discontinues heparinization prior to the end of dialysis, thus allowing clotting times to return to normal shortly after treatment.	May be done 30 minutes to 1 hour prior to termination of treatment, depending on institutional standard.
5. Decrease the blood pump flow rate.	Reduces blood flow.	
6. Check amount of NS; hang a new bag if necessary.	Minimizes the danger of air embolism on return of blood to patient.	NS (100-300 ml) is used to return blood to patient.
7. Maintain the blood level in the arterial and venous drip chambers at three-quarters full.	Prevents air in tubing and dialyzer.	
8. Turn off the blood pump.	Stops blood flow.	
9. Unclamp the NS flush line on the arterial side of the blood circuit. Allow flush to infuse until lines are pink-tinged.		

Procedure for Hemodialysis—*Continued*

Steps	Rationale	Special Considerations
10. Clamp the arterial tubing between patient and blood pump, and on the vascular access.	Prevents loss of blood if the tubing becomes separated.	
11. Place a sterile 4 × 4 under a VAC. Disconnect the arterial dialysis tubing from the arterial vascular access.	Prevent contamination.	
12. Turn on blood pump; simultaneously unclamp the patient end connector of the arterial tubing.	Promotes slow return of blood in tubing back to patient.	
13. Clear the blood tubing and dialyzer with saline until rinse-back is achieved.	Promotes rinse-back of blood to patient.	Satisfactory rinse-back is achieved when venous chamber has pink-tinged fluid.
14. Turn off blood pump.	Terminates flow of blood.	
15. Clamp venous access.	Prevents backflow of blood.	
16. If using a central venous catheter, flush the catheter with heparin or citrate (see Procedures 65 and 117).	Discontinues vascular access.	
17. AV fistula/AV graft: when fistula needles are used, remove both cannulas from patient's access site, one at a time. Using a sterile 2 × 2 gauze pad, apply moderate pressure to access site until bleeding has stopped.	Discontinues vascular access.	
18. Dress access site(s) with remaining sterile 2 × 2 gauze pad and bandages.	Provides protective barrier.	
19. Dispose of soiled material and equipment in appropriate disposal receptacle.	Standard precautions.	
20. Sanitize single-patient machine according to established procedure. *(Level I: Manufacturer's recommendation only.)*	Reduces transmission of microorganisms and readies it for future use.	
21. Wash hands.	Reduces transmission of microorganisms.	
22. Document in patient record.		

Expected Outcomes

- Catheter/fistula/graft accessed without any complications
- Blood easily aspirated from the access site
- Pulsating blood flow in the dialysis tubing set
- Accumulated waste products removed
- Acid-base balance restored
- Blood urea nitrogen (BUN) and creatinine restored to baseline levels
- Electrolytes restored to baseline levels
- Accumulated fluid removed; dry weight restored.
- Nutritional status maintained

Unexpected Outcomes

- Clotting or decreased patency of the AV fistula or the catheter lumens
- Poor blood flow
- Bleeding from the insertion site or access site
- Signs or symptoms of infection at the insertion or access site
- Dislodgment of the catheter
- Decreased circulation in the vascular access limb
- Hematoma formation at the access site
- Physiologic complications (dysrhythmias, chest pain, fluid-electrolyte imbalance, hypotension, seizures, nausea and vomiting, headaches, muscle cramping, dyspnea)
- Technical problems with the dialysis machine

Patient Monitoring and Care

Steps	Rationale	Reportable Conditions
		These conditions should be reported if they persist despite nursing interventions.
1. Perform and record a predialysis weight and daily weights. *(Level V: Clinical studies in more than one patient population and situation.)*	Predialysis weight is an important factor in deciding how much UF is needed during treatment. It also helps to guide ongoing treatment.[1,2]	• Abnormal increase or decrease in weight
2. Perform a baseline and ongoing assessments, including the following: *(Level V: Clinical studies in more than one patient population and situation.)* A. Vital signs B. Jugular vein distension C. Presence of edema D. Intake and output E. Neurologic assessment F. Pulmonary assessment	It is important to establish a baseline before initiation of treatment.[1,2] Monitors for complications.	• Hypotension • Hypertension • Tachycardia/bradycardia • Tachypnea/bradypnea • Fever • Hypothermia • Jugular vein distension • Crackles • Edema • Change in level of consciousness, dizziness • Change in cardiac rhythm
3. Monitor the circulation to the extremity where the graft/fistula is located. *(Level V: Clinical studies in more than one patient population and situation.)* A. Capillary refill B. Pulses distal to access C. Color/temperature of extremity D. Sensation	To assess for any decrease in perfusion distal to the graft site.[1,2]	• Diminished capillary refill • Diminished or absent peripheral pulses • Pale, mottled, or cyanotic extremity • Cool to touch • Diminished or absent movement • Pain
4. Monitor electrolytes and glucose during treatment as per institutional standard.	Must be monitored because of continued fluid and electrolyte shifts during treatment.	• Hyper- or hypokalemia • Hyper- or hyponatremia • Hyper- or hypocalcemia • Hyper- or hypoglycemia • Hyperphosphatemia
5. Administer medications to correct electrolyte abnormalities as ordered during treatment. *(Level V: Clinical studies in more than one patient population and situation.)*	Patients with renal failure are predisposed to many electrolyte abnormalities. During dialysis, several medications/electrolyte replacements may be given, as ordered for individual patients.[1,10]	
6. Monitor the dialysis circuit (e.g., occlusions, kinks, or leaks; blood or clots in vascular access lines). *(Level V: Clinical studies in more than one patient population and situation.)*	Disconnections or introduction of air into the circuit are always possible during treatment. Bleeding or exsanguination also can occur.[1,2] Clotting of the circuit is a potential complication. If hemofilter becomes excessively clotted, the extracorporeal blood volume should be returned to the patient quickly. Blood leaks from dialyzer into the dialysate may occur and would necessitate termination of treatment. Venous or arterial pressures, which are out of range, may indicate dialyzer or access malfunction.	• Disconnections, cracks, or leaks • Bleeding • Excessive clotting • Blood leaks/hemofilter rupture • Malfunction of dialyzer or access

Patient Monitoring and Care—*Continued*

Steps	Rationale	Reportable Conditions
7. Monitor UF for rate, clarity, and air bubbles. *(Level V: Clinical studies in more than one patient population and situation.)*	A decrease in UF production can occur due to clotting of the dialyzer.[1,2,10] Pink or blood-tinged UF is indicative of filter leak or rupture.	• Decrease in UF production • Change in color or characteristic of UF • Air in UF
8. Administer heparin as ordered. *(Level V: Clinical studies in more than one patient population and situation.)*	Heparin is often used to prevent clotting of the circuit.[2,5] Heparin dose varies according to patient condition and laboratory values.	• Suspicion of clotting in the circuit
9. Monitor anticoagulation as per institutional standard.	Because heparin is commonly used to prevent system clotting, coagulation studies should be routinely monitored.	• Abnormal coagulation studies

10. Monitor the patency of vascular access.
  A. Gently palpate along entire length of graft or over access for a thrill (feeling of vibration or purring under fingers).
  B. Auscultate for the presence of bruit (sounds like rushing water). *(Level V: Clinical studies in more than one patient population and situation.)*
	Bleeding can occur from either the venous or arterial catheter or AV fistula. Clotting of the access can occur.[1,11]
	
	Absence of a bruit does not confirm occlusion. Use Doppler if unable to hear a bruit with a stethoscope.
		• Decrease in access function or patency
		• Absence of bruit or thrill

11. Monitor the patient for complications associated with dialysis treatment. *(Level V: Clinical studies in more than one patient population and situation.)*	Several complications are possible with dialysis.[1,2]	• Muscle cramps • Dialysis disequilibrium (headache, nausea/vomiting, hypertension, decreased sensorium, convulsions, coma) • Air embolism • Dialyzer reaction (hypotension, pruritus, back pain, angioedema, anaphylaxis) • Hypoxemia

12. Administer medications to correct metabolic abnormalities as ordered. *(Level V: Clinical studies in more than one patient population and situation.)*	Patients with renal failure are predisposed to many metabolic abnormalities. Common medications administered to patients with renal failure include the following[1,2,7,11]:
	  A. Vitamin D and calcium carbonate to increase the serum calcium level and prevent or treat bone disease
	  B. Erythropoietin and iron to treat anemia
	  C. Deferoxamine mesylate to remove excessive iron
	  D. Phosphate binders to treat hyperphosphatemia
	Renal diet may also be prescribed, with adjusted protein, potassium, phosphorous, carbohydrate, and fluid intake that takes into account the	

Procedure continues on the following page

Patient Monitoring and Care—*Continued*

Steps	Rationale	Reportable Conditions
	patient's current catabolic state, residual renal function, adequacy of dialysis, and removal of amino acids by dialysis.[2,7,10]	
13. Place a sign above patient's bed indicating which limb has the vascular access (AV graft or fistula).	Blood pressures and blood draws should not be done on the access arm.	

Documentation

Documentation should include the following:

- Patient and family education
- Date and time of treatment initiation
- Condition of catheter or AV fistula regarding patency, quality of blood flow, ease of access procedure
- Condition of insertion site and any signs or symptoms of infection
- Presence of bruit if using an AV fistula
- Needle gauge size used for cannulation
- Type of machine used for dialysis

- Arterial and venous pressures during treatment
- Pump speed
- Length of dialysis treatment
- Vital signs throughout the treatments
- Unexpected outcomes
- Any medications/IV fluids given during treatment
- Nursing interventions
- Pre- and postdialysis weight
- Laboratory assessment data

References

1. American Nephrology Nurses Association. (1999). *ANNA Standards of Clinical Practice for Nephrology Nurses.* 3rd ed. Pitman, NJ: Author, 17-29.
2. American Nephrology Nurses Association. (1999). *Core Curriculum for Nephrology Nursing.* Pitman, NJ: Author, 123-88.
3. Centers for Disease Control, Hospital Infection Control Advisory Council. (1996). Guideline for the prevention of intravascular device-related infections. Part 1: Intravascular device-related infections: An overview. *Am J Infec Control,* 24, 262-76.
4. Centers for Disease Control, Hospital Infection Control Advisory Council. (1996). Guideline for the prevention of intravascular device-related infections. Part 2: Recommendations for the prevention of nosocomial intravascular device-related infections. *Am J Infec Control,* 24, 277-93.
5. Kellum, J.A., Mehta, R.L., and Ronco, C. (2001). Acute dialysis quality initiative. *Contrib Nephrol,* 132, 258-65.
6. Klemer, S. (2001). Sustained low-efficiency dialysis for critically ill patients requiring renal replacement therapy. *Kidney Int,* Aug., 60, 777-85.
7. Kopple, J. (1996). The nutritional management of acute renal failure in the intensive care unit. *JPEN,* 20, 3-12.
8. National Guideline Clearinghouse. (2003). *Guidelines for the Prevention of Intravascular Catheter-Related Infections.* Available at: www.guideline.gov.
9. NKF/DOQI. (2001). Clinical Practice Guidelines for Vascular Access: Update 2000. *Am J Kidney Dis,* 37, S137-81.
10. Parker, J. (1998). *Contemporary Nephrology Nursing.* Pitman, NJ: American Nephrology Nurses Association, 525-576.
11. Thomas-Hawkins, C. (1996). Nursing interventions related to vascular access infections (review). *Adv Renal Replace Ther,* 3, 218-21.

Additional Readings

Brunier, G. (1996). Care of the hemodialysis patient with a new permanent vascular access: Review of assessment and teaching. *ANNA J,* 23, 547-58.
Carbone, V. (1995). Heparin and dialyzer membranes during hemodialysis: A literature review. *ANNA J,* 22, 452-5.
Dinwiddle, L.C., et al. (1996). Comparison of measure for prospective identification of venous stenosis. *ANNA J,* 23, 593-600.
Dubose, T.D., et al. (1997). Acute renal failure in the 21st century: Recommendations for management and outcomes assessment. *Am J Kid Dis,* 29, 793-9.
Gomez, N. (2003). Practice issues in nephrology nursing: Focus on issues from ANNA's special interest groups. National Symposium Special Interest Group presentations. *Nephrology Nursing Journal: Journal of the American Nephrology Nurses' Association.* June, 30, 333, 341.
Handley, J. (1994). Rebound hypertension during hemodialysis. *ANNA J,* 21, 279.
Hartigan, M.F. (1994). Vascular access and nephrology nursing practice: Existing views and rationale for change. *Adv Renal Replace Ther,* 1, 155-62.
Himmelfarb, J., and Hakim, R.M. (1997). The use of biocompatible dialysis membranes in acute renal failure. *Adv Renal Replace Ther,* 4(2 Suppl 1), 72-80.
Kirby, S., and Davenport, A. (1996). Haemofiltration/dialysis treatment in patients with acute renal failure. *Care Critically Ill,* 12, 54-8.
Sherman, R.A., et al. (1994). Recirculation assessed: The impact of blood flow rate and low-flow method reevaluated. *Am J Kid Dis,* 23, 846-8.
Sherman, R.A. (2002). Intradialytic hypotension: An overview of recent, unresolved and overlooked issues. *Semin Dial,* 15, 141-3.
Wiseman, K.C. (1996). Clinical consult: Appropriate nursing care for hemodialysis patients with uncomplicated hypotensive events. *ANNA J,* 23, 404-5.

PROCEDURE **119**

Peritoneal Dialysis

P U R P O S E : Peritoneal dialysis (PD) is used for the removal of fluid and toxins, the regulation of electrolytes, and the management of azotemia.

Rhonda K. Martin

PREREQUISITE NURSING KNOWLEDGE

- Basic knowledge of the principles of diffusion and osmosis is necessary.
  - ❖ *Diffusion* is the passive movement of solutes through a semipermeable membrane from an area of higher concentration to one of lower concentration.
  - ❖ *Osmosis* is the passive movement of solvent through a semipermeable membrane from an area of lower concentration to one of higher concentration.
- PD uses the peritoneal membrane as the semipermeable membrane for both fluid solutes.
- Sterile dialysis fluid (dialysate) is infused into the peritoneal cavity through a flexible abdominal catheter (Fig. 119-1).

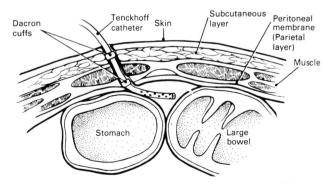

FIGURE 119-1 Tenckhoff catheter used in peritoneal dialysis. *(From Lewis, S.M., and Collier, I.C. [1987]. Medical-Surgical Nursing Assessment and Management of Clinical Problems. 2nd ed. New York: McGraw-Hill.)*

- A small-framed adult can usually tolerate 2 L to 2.5 L dialysate, whereas a large-framed adult may be able to tolerate up to 3 L in the abdominal cavity. The larger the volume of dialysate, the more effective the removal of blood urea nitrogen (BUN) and creatinine. The most limiting factor is compromise of respiratory excursion by direct pressure on the diaphragm.
- The PD dialysate contains higher concentrations of glucose than normal serum levels. This aids in the removal of water by osmosis and small-to-middle weight molecules (urea, creatinine) by diffusion. Icodextrin can also be used for this purpose.[5]
- PD involves repeated fluid exchanges or cycles; each cycle has three phases: instillation, dwell, and drain.
  - ❖ During the *instillation phase,* the dialysate is infused by gravity into the patient's abdominal cavity through an abdominal catheter.
  - ❖ During the *dwell phase,* the dialysate remains in the patient's abdominal cavity allowing osmosis and diffusion to occur. Dwell time varies based on the patient's clinical need. Using dialysate with a high concentration of glucose enhances fluid removal.
  - ❖ During the *drain phase,* the dialysate and excess extracellular fluid, wastes, and electrolytes are drained by gravity from the abdominal cavity via the abdominal catheter.
- PD can be performed either manually by using a single tubing and bag setup or by using a cycler machine (Fig. 119-2). When using a cycler machine, multiple exchanges are programmed into the machine and run automatically. Cycler machines are frequently found in the hospital setting and are often used by outpatients for their evening and night exchanges.

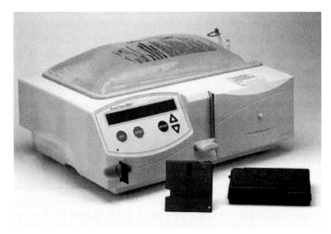

FIGURE 119-2 Baxter HomeChoice Pro PD Cycler. *(Courtesy Baxter International, Inc., Deerfield, IL.)*

- PD catheters can become clogged by the buildup of fibrin. Heparin is sometimes added to the dialysate or used as a separate flush to prevent occlusion.
- PD dialysate should be warmed to the appropriate temperature in a commercial warmer. NEVER warm the solution in a standard microwave oven, which heats unevenly and does not regulate the fluid temperature.
- The adequacy of dialysis and assessment of the patient's residual renal function should be evaluated on a periodic basis. Adequacy of dialysis can be measured using urea kinetic modeling (Kt/V) or urea clearance. Residual renal functioning can be monitored using urine creatinine clearance. Collaboration with the nephrology team is necessary to monitor these parameters.

EQUIPMENT

- Masks
- Goggles
- Sterile gloves
- Sterile gauze
- Sterile container
- Hydrogen peroxide
- Povidone-iodine solution
- Tape
- Sterile barriers
- Hemostats

  Additional equipment, to have available depending on patient need, includes the following:
- Equipment for culture (if ordered)
- Equipment for cell count/hematocrit (if ordered)

  Additional equipment for initiation of PD includes the following:
- PD tubing with drainage bag
- Warmed dialysate solution
- Cycler with tubing (if being used)

  Additional equipment for termination of PD includes the following:
- Catheter caps
- Labels for catheter

PATIENT AND FAMILY EDUCATION

- Explain the purpose of PD. ➙*Rationale:* PD is necessary to perform the physiologic functions of the kidneys when renal failure is present.
- Explain the procedure and review any questions. ➙*Rationale:* Provides information and decreases patient anxiety.
- Explain the need for careful sterile technique when accessing the abdominal catheter. ➙*Rationale:* Sterile technique is used to decrease the chance of peritoneal infection because pathogens can be introduced into the abdominal cavity via the catheter.
- Explain the three phases of PD. ➙*Rationale:* Because each phase is different, it is important for the patient to be informed of all three phases, the purpose, interventions, and possible complications of each.
- Explain the potential for feelings of fullness and possibly shortness of breath during the dwell phase. ➙*Rationale:* The pressure of the dialysate fluid on the diaphragm may cause the patient to have these feelings, which are normal for the dwell phase.

PATIENT ASSESSMENT AND PREPARATION

Patient Assessment

- Baseline vital signs, respiratory status, abdominal assessment, blood glucose level, pertinent laboratory results (potassium, sodium, calcium, phosphorus, magnesium, renal function tests, complete blood count). ➙*Rationale:* Patients in renal failure often have altered baseline assessments, according to both physical assessment and laboratory values. Having this information before treatments are started is helpful so that interventions, including the type and amount of dialysate fluid, can be individualized.
- Volume status, as indicated by the following:
  - ❖ Skin turgor
  - ❖ Mucous membranes
  - ❖ Edema
  - ❖ Breath sounds
  - ❖ Weight
  - ❖ Intake and output

  ➙*Rationale:* PD is often initiated for the control of hypervolemia. Knowing a patient's pretreatment volume status is essential to allow for the individualization of treatment goals and interventions.
- PD catheter and abdominal exit site for signs and symptoms of infection, leakage or drainage, or signs and symptoms of peritonitis:
  - ❖ Cloudy or bloody dialysate solution
  - ❖ Leakage at the catheter site
  - ❖ Subcutaneous fluid in abdomen, groin, or upper thighs
  - ❖ Abdominal pain
  - ❖ Fever

❖ Chills

❖ Rebound tenderness

➤*Rationale:* Catheter insertion site provides a portal of entry for infection resulting in septicemia or peritonitis. If the insertion site or effluent appears to be infected, further interventions (e.g., site change, culture, antibiotics) may be necessary.

• Peritoneal catheter and tubing for kinking, puncture sites, and loose connections. ➤*Rationale:* Adequate flow is essential for optimal treatment. A dysfunctional catheter can alter outcomes.

Patient Preparation

• Ensure that patient understands preprocedural teaching. Answer questions as they arise and reinforce information as needed. ➤*Rationale:* Evaluates and reinforces understanding of previously taught information.

• Assist the patient in applying his/her mask. ➤*Rationale:* Decreases the risk for airborne and nasal pathogens.

• Reposition patient to a comfortable position. ➤*Rationale:* Proper positioning is important to ensure patient comfort, optimize respiratory status, and facilitate optimal flow through the abdominal catheter.

Procedure for Peritoneal Dialysis		
Steps	**Rationale**	**Special Considerations**
PD Initiation and Discontinuation		
1. Verify PD orders, which should include: 　A. Manual or automated delivery system 　B. Dialysis solution type, volume, dextrose/isodextrin and calcium concentrations, and additional medications 　C. Fill volume/time, dwell time, drain volume/time 　D. Vital sign parameters 　E. Laboratory testing	Familiarizes nurse with the individualized patient treatment and reduces the possibility of error.	Ensure that patient weight and laboratory values are recorded before initiation of therapy and that the patient is wearing a mask and is properly positioned.
2. Don personal protective equipment; wash hands.	Reduces transmission of microorganisms; reduces contamination from airborne pathogens; standard precautions.	
3. Remove dialysate bag from protective pouch; check for expiration date, clarity, and leaks.	Assess for contamination of dialysate.	Consider obtaining and recording bag weight to accurately assess intake and output.
4. Connect and prime tubing with dialysate; clamp tubing.	Fills tubing with dialysate; decreases chance of introducing air into the abdominal cavity.	Signs of air instillation into the peritoneum include referred shoulder and back pain.
5. Wash hands and don gloves.	Reduces transmission of organisms; standard precautions.	
6. Prepare sterile field.		
7. Pour povidone-iodine into a sterile container or onto sterile 4 × 4 gauze pads.	Maintains aseptic technique.	
8. Remove catheter connector site dressing and discard.		Note odor or drainage on the old dressing.
9. Don sterile gloves.	Maintains aseptic technique.	
10. Saturate four of the 4 × 4 gauze pads in povidone-iodine solution and perform a 1-minute scrub of the catheter-cap connection.	Povidone-iodine serves as a bactericidal agent.	Make sure to remove any crust or drainage.
11. Wrap second povidone-iodine–soaked 4 × 4 gauze pad around catheter-cap connection; leave in place for approximately 3 to 5 minutes.	Reduces transmission of microorganisms.	

Procedure continues on the following page

Procedure for Peritoneal Dialysis—*Continued*

Steps	Rationale	Special Considerations
12. After 3 to 5 minutes, remove povidone-iodine–soaked 4 × 4 gauze pad; discard in appropriate receptacle.	Standard precautions.	
13. Using the nondominant hand, pick up the PD catheter with a sterile 4 × 4 gauze pad; remove cap.		
14. Connect catheter to dialysate tubing.	Ensures a tight connection.	
Instillation Cycle		
15. Unclamp and remove any clamps present on the catheter or tubing.	Provides open access between catheter and PD tubing, allowing inflow of dialysate.	
16. Set flow rate as prescribed.		Time for inflow depends on the height of the dialysate bag, position of patient, and the patency of the catheter.
17. When inflow is complete, clamp the dialysate tubing.	Helps prevent backflow.	
Dwell Cycle		
18. Begin dwell cycle.	Allow for exchange across the peritoneal membrane of fluid, toxins, and electrolytes.	Dwell time is determined by the number of cycles needed in a 24-hour period. If using a cycler, the cycles will be preprogrammed. Drainage is often routed directly into a toilet or appropriate container.
19. Discard dialysate bag.	Standard precautions.	
Drain Cycle		
20. Wash hands.	Standard precautions.	
21. Place drainage bag below midabdominal area.	Enhances gravity outflow.	If using a cycler, follow manufacturer's instructions for system setup.
22. Unclamp to permit drainage from peritoneal cavity.		Allow 15 to 20 minutes for outflow; observe and record characteristics (cloudy, bloody, clear, yellow) and amount of outflow. Reposition patient if flow stops or is sluggish. Notify physician or advanced practice nurse if drainage is cloudy or bloody.
23. Monitor vital signs as prescribed during outflow.	Assess for hypotension, tachycardia related to hypovolemia, and sudden release of intraabdominal pressure.	
24. Clamp when effluent is completely drained.	Decreases leakage and contamination.	Consider obtaining and recording bag weight to accurately assess intake and output.
25. Repeat steps 14 to 24 as ordered.		
Discontinuation of PD		
26. Don mask and goggles; wash hands.	Reduces the transmission of microorganisms; standard precautions.	

Steps	Rationale	Special Considerations
Procedure for Peritoneal Dialysis—*Continued*		
27. Observe outflow of last PD cycle.	Turning the patient from side to side ensures that patient's abdomen is empty of dialysate.	
28. Don clean gloves.		
29. Clamp both the catheter and the PD tubing.	Prevents leakage and contamination.	
30. Prepare sterile field.		
31. Pour povidone-iodine into a sterile container with sterile catheter cap.	Acts as a bactericidal agent for cap; some institutions do not use a povidone soak for new caps but instead simply attach a new sterile cap.	
32. Don sterile gloves.	Standard precautions.	
33. Remove catheter cap and place on sterile field.		
34. Using sterile 4 × 4 gauze pads, disconnect the catheter from the PD tubing.		
35. Carefully connect catheter cap to catheter.	Maintains aseptic technique	
36. Securely tape catheter to abdomen.	Prevents accidental dislodgment.	
37. Apply dressing.		Dressing should be changed on a routine basis.
38. Discard soiled materials in an appropriate receptacle.	Standard precautions.	
39. Wash hands.	Reduces transmission of microorganisms.	
Catheter Exit Site Care		
1. Don personal protective equipment and wash hands.	Reduces transmission of microorganisms; standard precautions.	
2. Prepare sterile field.	Prevents contamination of sterile supplies.	
3. Open 4 × 4 gauze pads onto sterile field.	Maintains aseptic technique.	
4. Pour hydrogen peroxide and povidone-iodine into sterile containers.	Reduces transmission of microorganisms.	
5. Remove and discard old dressing into appropriate receptacle.		Be careful not to tug or dislodge the catheter. Note any odor or drainage on old dressing.
6. Inspect catheter exit site and surrounding area for leakage, infection, or trauma.	Provides assessment for complications.	Note any pain, warmth, crusting, bleeding, tenderness, redness, or swelling that may indicate infection.
7. Gently palpate subcutaneous catheter segments and cuff.	Check for pain, erythema, edema, or accumulated drainage.	Obtain culture if drainage is present and notify physician or advanced practice nurse if the listed signs or symptoms are present.
8. Don sterile gloves.		

Procedure continues on the following page

Procedure   for Peritoneal Dialysis—*Continued*

Steps	Rationale	Special Considerations
9. Use a sterile 4 × 4 gauze pad to hold the catheter off the skin.	Helps prevent contamination of catheter by skin flora.	
10. Use a hydrogen peroxide–soaked 4 × 4 gauze pad to cleanse the catheter and surrounding skin.	Hydrogen peroxide is helpful in removing old secretions.	When cleansing skin, begin at exit site and move outward in concentric circles. Keep cleansing solutions out of the catheter sinus track.[4]
11. Use povidone-iodine–soaked 4 × 4 gauze pads to cleanse catheter *and* exit site; allow them to air dry.	Acts as a bactericidal agent.	
12. Apply a new catheter site dressing using sterile gauze or a transparent occlusive dressing.	Gauze wicks drainage away from the site.	Transparent, occlusive dressings are not recommended in the first 2 weeks after catheter placement because they allow pooling of secretions in the sinus track.[4]
13. Discard soiled supplies in an appropriate receptacle.	Standard precautions.	
14. Wash hands.	Reduces transmission of organisms.	
15. Document in patient record.		

Expected Outcomes

- Catheter and exit site maintained without any complications
- Instillation and drainage of dialysate without problems
- Respiratory status not compromised during treatment
- BUN and creatinine restored to baseline levels
- Electrolytes restored to baseline levels
- Glucose control maintained
- Accumulated fluid removed
- Nutritional status maintained
- Peritoneum and abdomen intact

Unexpected Outcomes

- Drainage/leakage from the exit site
- Poor dialysate flow during instillation or drainage
- Signs and symptoms of peritonitis
- Inability to drain the total amount of instilled dialysate
- Signs or symptoms of infection at the insertion or access site
- Dislodgment of the abdominal catheter
- Tubing disconnection
- Physiologic complications during treatment
- Introduction of pathogens into the abdominal catheter
- Diaphragmatic impingement
- Viscous perforation by PD catheter
- Malnutrition
- Protein and/or blood loss from peritonitis

Patient Monitoring and Care

Steps	Rationale	Reportable Conditions
		These conditions should be reported if they persist despite nursing interventions.
1. Perform and record a predialysis and daily weight. *(Level V: Clinical studies in more than one patient population and situation.)*	Predialysis weight is an important factor in deciding how much PD is needed during treatment. It also helps to guide ongoing treatment and nutritional status.[1-4]	• Abnormal increase or decrease in weight
2. Perform baseline and ongoing assessments, including the following: *(Level V: Clinical studies in more than one patient population and situation.)*	Important to establish a baseline before initiation of treatment.[1-4] Monitors for complications.	• Hypotension • Hypertension • Fever • Hypothermia

Patient Monitoring and Care—*Continued*

Steps	Rationale	Reportable Conditions
A. Vital signs B. Jugular vein distention C. Central venous and pulmonary artery wedge pressures, as appropriate D. Presence or absence of edema E. Skin turgor F. Mucus membranes G. Intake and output H. Pulmonary assessment, including expiratory tidal volume and peak inspiratory pressures on the ventilated patient I. Abdominal assessment		• Jugular vein distention • Elevated or decreased CVP or PAWP • Dry mucous membranes • Shortness of breath • Crackles • Edema • Abdominal distention or tenderness • Rebound tenderness • Decreased tidal volume • Increased peak inspiratory pressures
3. Monitor blood urea nitrogen (BUN), creatinine, and electrolytes during treatment at a frequency determined by your institutional standard. *(Level V: Clinical studies in more than one patient population and situation.)*	Fluids and electrolytes shift during treatment.[1-4]	• Hyperglycemia • BUN or creatinine levels abnormal for patient • Hyper- or hypokalemia • Hyper- or hyponatremia • Hyper- or hypocalcemia
4. Administer medications to correct metabolic abnormalities as ordered. *(Level V: Clinical studies in more than one patient population and situation.)*	Patients with renal failure are predisposed to many metabolic abnormalities. Common medications administered to patients with renal failure include the following[1-4]: • Vitamin D and calcium carbonate to increase the serum calcium level and prevent or treat bone disease • Erythropoietin and iron to treat anemia • Deferoxamine mesylate to remove excessive iron • Stool softeners, because constipation can impair drainage of PD fluid • Phosphate binders to treat hyperphosphatemia Renal diet may also be prescribed, with adjusted protein, phosphorous, carbohydrate, and fluid intake that takes into account the patient's current catabolic state, residual renal function, adequacy of dialysis, and removal of amino acids by dialysis.[1,6,7]	• Hyper- or hypocalcemia • Abnormal hemoglobin or hematocrit • Hyper- or hypophosphatemia • Decreased albumin or prealbumin
5. Monitor serum glucose at the beginning of the treatment and at frequencies throughout the treatment according to institutional standard. *(Level V: Clinical studies in more than one patient population and situation.)*	The glucose in the dialysate solution predisposes patients to hyperglycemia, especially diabetic patients.[1,6] Administer insulin as ordered to maintain glucose control.	• Hyper- or hypoglycemia
6. Monitor the integrity of the PD setup. *(Level V: Clinical studies in more than one patient population and situation.)*	Disconnections in the setup provide a portal of entry for pathogen that can lead to peritonitis.[1,6]	• Fever • Tachycardia • Cloudy or bloody dialysate

Procedure continues on the following page

Patient Monitoring and Care—*Continued*

Steps	Rationale	Reportable Conditions
7. Monitor for signs and symptoms of infection at catheter exit site.		• Site redness or edema • Warmth • Bleeding • Purulent drainage • Pain or tenderness • Fever
8. Monitor the ease with which the dialysate is both instilled and drained through the abdominal catheter.	Patients may need repositioning to facilitate flow through the abdominal catheter. Catheters may also become kinked or occluded. Fibrin clots can obstruct outflow; heparin may be added to the dialysate solution. If clotting is suspected, urokinase may also be used to clear the catheter. Rapid infusion can cause abdominal pain.	• Inability to instill or drain fluid through the abdominal catheter.

Documentation

Documentation should include the following:

- Patient and family education
- Date and time of treatment initiation
- Treatment/exchange number
- Condition of abdominal catheter and exit site at time of treatment
- Date and time of dressing application
- Patient weight before and after treatment

- Intake and output
- Length and parameters of treatment
- Dialysate solution used
- Vital signs/hemodynamic parameters throughout the treatment
- Unexpected outcomes
- Nursing interventions
- Laboratory assessment data

References

1. American Nephrology Nurses Association. (1999). *Core Curriculum for Nephrology Nursing.* Pitman, NJ: Author, 281-322.
2. American Nephrology Nurses Association. (1999). Peritoneal dialysis. In: *ANNA Standards of Clinical Practice for Nephrology Nurses.* 3rd ed. Pitman, NJ: Author, 71-84.
3. Bernardini, J. (1998). Nursing application: Established protocols of patient care based on published research. *Perit Dial Int,* 18, 11-33.
4. Gokal, R., et al. (1998). Peritoneal catheters and exit-site practices toward optimum peritoneal access: 1998 update. *Perit Dial Int,* 18, 11-33.
5. Kopple, J. (1996). The nutritional management of acute renal failure in the intensive care unit. *JPEN,* 20, 3-12.
6. Moberly, J., et al. (2002). Pharmacokinetics of icodextrin-based peritoneal dialysis solutions. *Kidney International,* 62(S81), 23.
7. Parker, J. (1998). *Contemporary Nephrology Nursing.* Pitman, NJ: American Nephrology Nurses Association, 603-60.

Additional Readings

Albee, B. (1995). CAPD catheter exit site healing and clean dressing techniques. *ANNA J,* 22, 482-3.
ANNA Peritoneal Dialysis Special Interest Group. (2003). Peritoneal dialysis resource guide. *Nephrol Nurs J,* 30, 535-64.
Martis, L., Chen, C., and Moberly, J.B. (1998). Peritoneal dialysis solutions for the 21st century. *Artif Organs,* 22, 13-6.
Pastan, S., and Bailey, J. (1998). Dialysis therapy. *N Engl J Med,* 338, 1428-37.

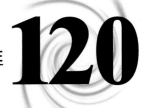
SECTION EIGHTEEN

Special Renal
Procedures

Apheresis, Plasmapheresis, and Plasma Exchange (Assist)

P U R P O S E : Apheresis techniques are used to remove cells, plasma, and other substances from blood. Plasmapheresis is used to remove plasma from the blood. These are used as adjunctive treatments in many diseases, especially in antibody-mediated conditions that produce autoantibodies.

Rhonda K. Martin

PREREQUISITE NURSING KNOWLEDGE

- Therapeutic apheresis (i.e., hemapheresis) is a technique for selective removal of cells, plasma, and substances from the patient's circulation to promote clinical improvement. There are different apheresis techniques; their names vary according to the component of the blood removed and/or replaced or substance removed:
  - ❖ Plasmapheresis is the process of removing plasma and/or proteins from the blood. Other components are returned to the patient.
  - ❖ Plasma exchange is the process of replacing the plasma removed with an equal amount of either plasma or another fluid.
  - ❖ Cytapheresis is the selective removal of the cellular components of blood. Blood is withdrawn from the patient and a specific cellular component is retained (i.e., white blood cell), the remainder of other cells and plasma is returned to the donor/patient.
  - ❖ Leukocytapheresis is the removal of white blood cells from the blood. It has been used in the treatment of autoimmune disorders (e.g., rheumatoid arthritis and systemic lupus erythematosus).
  - ❖ Erythrocytapheresis is the removal and replacement of red blood cells.
  - ❖ Plateletpheresis is the selective removal of platelets.
  - ❖ Plasma adsorption/perfusion is the removal of plasma by a hollow fiber filter. Blood is returned to the patient,

and the plasma is pumped over an adsorptive column that removes certain proteins or pathogens. The treated plasma is then returned to the patient.
  - ❖ Immunoadsorption is the removal of an antigen in the blood by a specific antibody lining the surface of a filter or cartridge.
  - ❖ Photopheresis uses pheresis techniques to remove and return blood to the patient. Photosensitizing drugs are given to the patient and while the blood is removed during pheresis, it is exposed to an ultraviolet light which will destroy certain cells (e.g., T cells in cutaneous T cell lymphoma and in solid organ transplant rejection).
- Apheresis techniques are also used for the procurement of peripheral stem cells for bone marrow transplantation.
- The plasma removed must be replaced; the most common replacement fluids are fresh-frozen plasma (FFP), thawed plasma (derived from thawed FFP and maintained at low temperatures for use within 1-5 days), albumin, and electrolyte solutions (normal saline, Plasmalyte®); other solutions include plasma expanders (solvent detergent-treated plasma). Because clotting factors are transiently reduced by plasmapheresis, fresh-frozen plasma (FFP) can also be used as a fluid replacement in patients when bleeding is an issue.
- Plasma volume is an estimate of the patient's total volume based on age, gender, height, weight, build, and hematocrit. Exchange volume is the ratio of the patient's plasma volume to be removed and replaced; this is

usually 1:1 or 1.5:1 of the patient's estimated plasma volume.

- In plasma exchange, an average of 3-5 liters of plasma is removed and replaced.[6]
- Treatments can be done with two different machines[8]:
  ❖ A centrifugal apheresis machine separates plasma and other blood components by use of a centrifuge (Fig. 120-1).
  ❖ Filtration—A hollow-fiber cell separator, permeable to plasma proteins, is used to remove the patient's plasma via an apheresis machine or continuous renal replacement machines adapted for pheresis (Fig. 120-2).
- Treatment length and frequency varies according to the disease being treated, rate of production of the substance being removed, and the patient's response to treatment. Acute conditions, such as thrombotic thrombocytopenia purpura or graft-versus-host disease, usually require daily treatments for 5-7 days. Other conditions usually require plasma exchanges two or three times weekly for up to 6 weeks. The total amount of plasma to be exchanged is used as a guide for treatment. A single treatment, referred to as a plasma exchange, usually takes 2 to 3 hours with a centrifugal machine; 2 to 6 hours with filtration methods.[6]

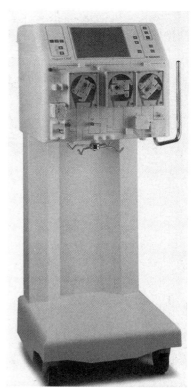

FIGURE 120-2 The B. Braun Diapact CRRT system can also be used for therapeutic plasma exchange and plasma adsorption/perfusion. *(Photo courtesy B. Braun Medical, Inc.)*

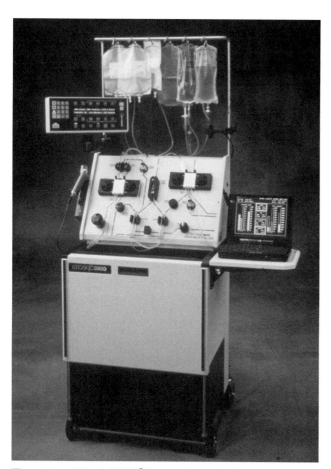

FIGURE 120-1 COBE® Spectra Apheresis System. *(Copyright COBE Laboratories Inc. Photo courtesy COBE® BCT™ Inc.)*

- Apheresis/plasmapheresis, although commonly performed in critical care units, is most often performed by health care professionals with special knowledge and skills in the apheresis/plasmapheresis process, such as local blood bank or dialysis personnel.
- The most commonly used apheresis/plasmapheresis systems uses either two large-bore peripheral venous catheters or a double-lumen central venous catheter to access the vascular system. Peripherally inserted central venous catheters or implantable venous access ports do not provide for adequate blood flow and are not acceptable for use.[8]
- The system should be primed with an anticoagulant (e.g., heparin or citrate) to prevent clotting. If citrate is used, the patient must be monitored closely for hypocalcemia. Citrate works as an anticoagulant by binding calcium (Ca^{++}), therefore decreasing the amount of Ca^{++} available for normal clotting.
- Plasmapheresis is used to treat antibody-mediated disorders, because the pathogenic antibodies are contained in the plasma. Removal of these antibodies through plasmapheresis reduces the number of circulating antibodies, temporarily decreasing the patient's symptoms.
- Conditions treated by apheresis/plasmapheresis may include the following:[11]
  ❖ Myasthenia gravis
  ❖ Guillain-Barré syndrome

* Various hematologic disorders
* Nephrologic disorders
* Rhematologic disorders
* Poisoning
* Drug overdose/drug toxicity
* Acute liver failure
* In solid organ transplantation for ABO-incompatibility and rejection
* In cytokine-mediated injury, such as sepsis, burns, and multisystem organ dysfunction syndrome (MODS); experimental use[10]

* Current indication categories for therapeutic apheresis, as endorsed by the American Association of Blood Banks and the American Society for Apheresis, are listed in Table 120-1.
* If the patient is taking ACE (angiotensin-converting enzyme) inhibitors, contact with certain filters or membranes in the apheresis/plasmapheresis system can cause an anaphylactic reaction and severe hypotension. This is due to increased levels of bradykinin, a potent vasodilator. It is recommended that ACE inhibitors be withheld for 48-72 hours prior to treatment.

TABLE 120-1   **Indication Categories for Therapeutic Apheresis-Selected Acute Conditions**

Disease	Procedure	Indication Category*
Renal and Metabolic Diseases		
Antiglomerular basement membrane antibody disease	Plasma exchange	I
Rapidly progressive glomerulonephritis	Plasma exchange	II
Hemolytic uremic syndrome	Plasma exchange	III
Renal transplantation		
Rejection	Plasma exchange	IV
Sensitization	Plasma exchange	III
Heart transplant rejection	Plasma exchange	III
	Photopheresis	III
Acute hepatic failure	Plasma exchange	III
Overdose or poisoning	Plasma exchange	III
Autoimmune and Rheumatic Diseases		
Cryoglobulinemia	Plasma exchange	II
Idiopathic thrombocytopenic purpura	Immunoadsorption	II
Raynaud's phenomenon	Plasma exchange	III
Vasculitis	Plasma exchange	III
Autoimmune hemolytic anemia	Plasma exchange	III
Rheumatoid arthritis	Immunoadsorption	II
	Lymphoplasmapheresis	II
	Plasma exchange	IV
Systemic lupus erythematosus	Plasma exchange	III
Hematologic Diseases		
ABO-mismatched marrow transplant	RBC removal (marrow)	I
	Plasma exchange (recipient)	II
Erythrocytosis or polycythemia vera	Phlebotomy	I
	Erythrocytapheresis	II
Leukocytosis and thrombocytosis	Cytapheresis	I
Thrombotic thrombocytopenia purpura	Plasma exchange	I
Posttransfusion purpura	Plasma exchange	I
Sickle cell diseases	RBC exchange	I
Myeloma, paraproteins, or hyperviscosity	Plasma exchange	II
Myeloma or acute renal failure	Plasma exchange	II
Coagulation factor inhibitors	Plasma exchange	II
Hemolytic uremic syndrome	Plasma exchange	III
Aplastic anemia or pure RBC aplasia	Plasma exchange	III
Cutaneous T cell lymphoma	Photopheresis	I
	Leukapheresis	III
Neurologic Disorders		
Acute inflammatory demyelinating polyradiculoneuropathy	Plasma exchange	I
Lambert-Eaton myasthenia syndrome	Plasma exchange	II
Multiple sclerosis		
Relapsing	Plasma exchange	III
Progressive	Plasma exchange	III
	Lymphocytapheresis	III
Myasthenia gravis	Plasma exchange	I
Acute central nervous system inflammatory demyelinating disease	Plasma exchange	II
Paraneoplastic neurologic syndromes	Plasma exchange	III
	Immunoadsorption	III
Demyelinating polyneuropathy with IgG and IgA	Plasma exchange	I
	Immunoadsorption	III

Continued

TABLE 120-1	Indication Categories for Therapeutic Apheresis–Selected Acute Conditions—*Continued*	
Disease	**Procedure**	**Indication Category***
Polyneuropathy with IgM (with or without Waldenstrom's)	Plasma exchange	II
	Immunoadsorption	III
Cryoglobulinemia with polyneuropathy	Plasma exchange	II
Multiple myeloma with polyneuropathy	Plasma exchange	III
POEMS syndrome†	Plasma exchange	III
Systemic (AL) amyloidosis	Plasma exchange	IV
Polymyositis or dermatomyositis	Plasma exchange	III
	Leukapheresis	IV
Inclusion-body myositis	Plasma exchange	III
	Leukapheresis	IV
Rasmussen's encephalitis	Plasma exchange	III
Stiff-man syndrome	Plasma exchange	III
PANDAS‡	Plasma exchange	II

*Indication categories as established by the American Medical Association: *I,* Standard therapy, acceptable but not mandatory. *II,* Available evidence tends to favor efficacy; conventional therapy usually tried first. *III,* Inadequately tested at this time. *IV,* No demonstrated value in controlled trials.
†*POEMS syndrome* = Polyneuropathy, organomegaly, endocrinopathy, monoclonal gammopathy, and skin lesions.
‡*PANDAS* = Pediatric autoimmune neuropsychiatric disorders.
From Smith, J.W., Weinstein, R., and Hillyer, K.L. (2004). Therapeutic apheresis: a summary of current indication categories endorsed by the AABB and the American Society for Apheresis. *Transfusion* 43(6), 820-22. Used with permission.

- Invasive procedures should be delayed until after the treatment, unless fresh-frozen plasma is used as a replacement fluid.
- Potential complications of pheresis techniques include the following:
  - ❖ Bleeding
  - ❖ Thrombocytopenia
  - ❖ Red blood cell (RBC) lysis/hemolysis
  - ❖ Air embolism
  - ❖ Blood leak
  - ❖ Circuit clotting
  - ❖ Hypovolemia
  - ❖ Hypotension
  - ❖ Hypothermia
  - ❖ Vascular access complications
  - ❖ Fever/chills
  - ❖ Shock
  - ❖ Anaphylaxis
  - ❖ Allergic reactions
  - ❖ Transfusion reactions
  - ❖ Electrolyte imbalances
  - ❖ Arrhythmias
  - ❖ Citrate toxicity
  - ❖ Infection

EQUIPMENT

- Blood cell separator machine
- Blood cell separator tubing set
- Replacement fluids
- Hemostats
- Appropriate laboratory specimen tubes
- Vascular access dressings and flushes

PATIENT AND FAMILY EDUCATION

- Explain the procedure, including risks, length of treatment, patient positioning, and review any questions the patient may have. ➥*Rationale:* Provides information and decreases patient anxiety.
- Explain the purpose of apheresis/plasmapheresis, specifically why this treatment is being performed, and the expected clinical outcomes. ➥*Rationale:* Plasmapheresis is used to treat antibody-mediated disorders.
- Explain the need for careful sterile technique for the duration of treatment. ➥*Rationale:* Sterile technique is important in order to decrease the chance of systemic infection, because pathogens can be transported throughout the entire body via the circulation.
- Explain the need for careful monitoring of the patient during the treatment for complications. ➥*Rationale:* Hypocalcemia, hypotension, bleeding, and hypothermia are all potential complications of plasmapheresis.
- Explain the importance of the patient letting the nurse know how he or she is feeling during the treatment. ➥*Rationale:* Patient symptoms can be important signs of complications related to the procedure. Examples include lightheadedness as a sign of hypotension and numbness and tingling as a sign of hypocalcemia.
- Explain the importance of preventing bleeding complications: pressure dressings at vascular sites, avoiding shaving, care of vascular catheter. ➥*Rationale:* Alterations in blood composition and anticoagulation can put the patient at risk for bleeding.
- Explain the plasmapheresis circuit setup to the patient and family. ➥*Rationale:* Blood will be removed from the patient's body and will be visible during the plasmapheresis treatment.

PATIENT ASSESSMENT AND PREPARATION

Patient Assessment

- Baseline vital signs, body system assessment, hemodynamic parameters (if appropriate), weight, and pretreatment fluid balance. ➤➤*Rationale:* Total body assessment should be based specifically on the patient's diagnosis and reason for treatment. Pretreatment assessment provides a baseline for comparison once the treatment is started, allowing for appropriate modification of intervention as needed. Changes in weight during and after treatment are an indicator of fluid balance.

- Pretreatment laboratory values. ➤➤*Rationale:* It is important to have baseline values of the complete blood count (CBC) with differential, platelet count, and electrolytes before these are altered by treatment. Coagulation parameters are particularly important; fibrinogen, prothrombin time (PT), activated clotting time (ACT) and partial thromboplastin time (PTT), if using heparin; ACT and ionized Ca^{++}, if using citrate. Serum sodium and serum bicarbonate levels/pH also should be evaluated in patients when citrate will be used as the anticoagulant.

Disease-specific tests should also be obtained pretreatment as needed.

- Vascular access. ➤➤*Rationale:* A properly functioning vascular access is necessary in order to perform plasmapheresis.

Patient Preparation

- Ensure that patient understands preprocedural teaching. Answer questions as they arise and reinforce information as needed. ➤➤*Rationale:* Evaluates and reinforces understanding of previously taught information.
- Assist the patient to a position of comfort that also facilitates optimal blood flow through the vascular access. ➤➤*Rationale:* Facilitating patient comfort helps to minimize the amount of patient movement during treatment. Movement can change the blood flow through the catheter. Different catheter sites may require different patient positions to facilitate optimal blood flow.

Procedure	for Assisting With Apheresis/Plasmapheresis		
Steps	**Rationale**	**Special Considerations**	
1. Verify apheresis/plasmapheresis orders and consent.	Familiarizes nurse with the individualized patient treatment and reduces the possibility of error.		

2. Review the following with the pheresis nurse:
A. Exchange volume
B. Anticoagulant
C. Replacement fluids
D. Baseline patient assessment, including
  (1) Vital signs
  (2) Jugular vein distention
  (3) Presence of edema
  (4) Intake and output
  (5) Neurologic assessment
  (6) Pulmonary assessment
  (7) Renal assessment
  (8) Parameters/treatment for heart rate and blood pressure
  (9) Laboratory monitoring
  (10) Procedure for Code Blue
	Sets joint goals and actions to provide for patient safety and optimize the patient's outcome.[9]		

3. Gather supplies for vascular access.		The process of vascular access depends on whether the site is central or peripheral.	
4. Assist in gathering the supplies for plasmapheresis.		Obtaining and sending laboratory specimens may be part of the plasmapheresis setup as the vascular system is accessed.	
5. Ensure that appropriate replacement fluid is available. Warm replacement fluids. *(Level V: Clinical studies in more than one patient population and situation.)*	Avoids chilling patient.[1-5]	Replacement fluids should be slightly warmed before infusion. Never use a microwave to warm fluids. Some patients also may require an increase in the ambient room temperature or	

Procedure continues on the following page

Procedure for Assisting With Apheresis/Plasmapheresis—*Continued*

Steps	Rationale	Special Considerations
		ventilator cascade and warming blankets to avoid hypothermia.
6. Infuse fluid boluses as needed prior to initiation.		
7. Assist with setup and priming of the plasmapheresis circuit as needed.	Ensures safe and proper assembly and complete removal of air from the circuit.	
8. Tape and secure all connections.	Prevents inadvertent disconnection of the system.	

Expected Outcomes

- Therapeutic goals achieved
- Properly functioning access site

Unexpected Outcomes

- Complications related to the treatment (e.g., hypotension, hypocalcemia, hypothermia, hypokalemia, hypernatremia, metabolic alkalosis, air embolism, blood leak, bleeding, and infection)
- Poor blood flow through the vascular access
- Bleeding from the access site
- Dislodgment of the catheter
- Hematoma formation at the access site
- Technical problems with apheresis/plasmapheresis circuit
- Hemolysis

Patient Monitoring and Care

Steps	Rationale	Reportable Conditions

1. Monitor the patient throughout and after the course of the plasmapheresis treatment.
  A. Vital signs
  B. Hemodynamic parameters
  C. Jugular vein distention
  D. Presence of edema
  E. Intake and output
  F. Neurologic assessment
  G. Pulmonary assessment
  H. Renal assessment (*Level V: Clinical studies in more than one patient population and situations.*)
  I. Plasmapheresis circuit
  J. Laboratory values as ordered (if plasma is removed, include prothrombin time/INR, fibrinogen, platelet count) (*Level V: Clinical studies in more than one patient population and situation.*)
	Patients can experience complications such as hypotension, hypothermia, blood leak, air embolism, transfusion reactions, hypocalcemia, RBC hemolysis, thrombocytopenia, citrate toxicity, and bleeding that may require intervention.[1-5,7]	*These conditions should be reported if they persist despite nursing interventions.*
		• Hypotension
		• Hypertension
		• Tachycardia/bradycardia
		• Tachypnea/bradypnea
		• Fever
		• Hypothermia
		• Jugular vein distension
		• Crackles
		• Edema
		• Change in level of consciousness
		• Dizziness
		• Change in cardiac rhythm
		• Blood leak
		• Hemolysis
		• Thrombocytopenia
		• Arrhythmias
		• Coagulopathies
		• Allergic reaction
		• Transfusion reaction

2. Monitor serum ionized Ca^{++}, magnesium, serum sodium, and	Citrate binds with Ca^{++} and can cause hypocalcemia. It also	• Hypocalcemia • Hypernatremia

Patient Monitoring and Care—*Continued*

Steps	Rationale	Reportable Conditions
serum bicarbonate levels/pH (if citrate is used as an anticoagulant).	metabolizes to sodium and bicarbonate, which may cause hypernatremia, metabolic alkalosis, and citrate toxicity.	• Metabolic alkalosis • Increased anion gap
3. Monitor ACT/PTT (if heparin is used as an anticoagulant).	These values primarily reflect the activity of the intrinsic clotting pathway.	• Prolonged ACT/PTT
4. Administer replacement fluid as needed.	Replacement fluids are important during the treatment to maintain adequate intravascular volume.	• Hypotension • Tachycardia • Decreased central venous and pulmonary artery pressures • Decreased urine output
5. Hold medication administration. *(Level V: Clinical studies in more than one patient population and situation.)*	Many medications are withheld during treatment, including vasopressors and pain medications, especially those that are protein-bound.[1-5] Some medications, such as antihypertensive agents, anticholinergic agents, Ca^{++} supplements, analgesics, and antipyretics, may be indicated during a treatment.[7]	
6. Monitor the access and dressing sites after the termination of apheresis/plasmapheresis.	Bleeding or signs or symptoms of infection can be complications of the vascular access.	• Bleeding • Redness, tenderness, pain, or warmth at the catheter insertion site • Generalized bleeding or fever
7. Appropriately label vascular access catheters containing indwelling anticoagulant.	Prevents the infusion of anticoagulant into the patient.	• Bleeding • Bruising • Oozing • Arrhythmias
8. Receive report from the pheresis nurse, including: A. Amount and type of fluids removed B. Amount and type of fluids given C. Exchange volume D. Medications given during treatment	For proper patient evaluation and documentation.	

Documentation

Documentation should include the following:

- Patient and family education
- Date and time of treatment initiation
- Condition of vascular access
- Intake/output/fluid balance
- Vital signs throughout the apheresis/plasmapheresis treatment
- Daily weight

- Patient's response to apheresis/plasmapheresis and daily progress toward treatment goals
- Unexpected outcomes
- Nursing interventions
- Laboratory assessment data

References

1. American Nephrology Nurses Association. (1999). *Core Curriculum for Nephrology Nursing.* Pitman, NJ: Author, 347-65.
2. American Nephrology Nurses Association. (1999). Therapeutic plasma exchange. In: *ANNA Standards and Guidelines of Clinical Practice for Nephrology Nurses.* 3rd ed. Pitman, NJ: Author, 97-107.
3. Busund, R., and Koukline, V. (2002). Plasmapheresis in severe sepsis and septic shock: a prospective, randomized control trial. *Intens Care Med,* 28, 1434-9.
4. Gloor, J., et al. (2003). ABO incompatible kidney transplants using both A2 and non-A2 living donors. *Transplantation,* 75, 971-7.
5. Malchesky, P., Koo, A., and Rybiccki, L. (2001). Apheresis technologies and clinical applications: The 2000 International Apheresis Registry. *Therapeutic Apheresis,* 5, 193-206.
6. McLeod, B., Price, T., and Drew, M. (1997). *Apheresis: Principles and Practice.* AABB Press.
7. Mokrzycki, M., and Kaplan, A. (1994). Therapeutic plasma exchange: Complications and management. *Am J Kid Dis,* 23, 817-27.
8. Price, C., and McCarley, P. (1993). Technical considerations of therapeutic plasma exchange as a nephrology nursing procedure. *ANNA J,* 20, 41-6.
9. Price, C., and McCarley, P. (1994). Physical assessment for patients receiving therapeutic plasma exchange. *ANNA J,* 21, 149-54, 201.
10. Reeves, J. (2002). A review of plasma exchange in sepsis. *Blood Purification,* 20, 282-8.
11. Smith, J., Weinstein, R., and Hillyer, K. (2003). Therapeutic apheresis: A summary of current indication categories endorsed by the AABB and the American Society for Apheresis. *Transfusion,* 43, 820-2.

Additional Readings

Myers, L. (2003). Thrombotic thrombocytopenia purpura-hemolytic uremic syndrome: Pathophysiology and management. *Nephrol Nurs J,* 29, 171-80.
Parker, J. (1997). *Contemporary Nephrology Nursing.* Pitman, NJ: American Nephrology Nurses Association.

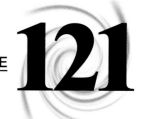
<table>
<tr><td>

UNIT VI
Hematologic System

SECTION NINETEEN

Fluid Management

</td></tr>
</table>

P R O C E D U R E **121**

Blood and Blood Component Administration

P U R P O S E :   Blood components are administered based on an individual patient's clinical need.

Maribeth Wooldridge-King

PREREQUISITE NURSING KNOWLEDGE

- The standard practice in transfusion therapy is to prescribe specific blood components (Table 121-1) based on criteria, the patient's clinical picture, and underlying pathophysiology. Although individual institutions establish criteria for blood component administration, the American Association of Blood Banks (AABB), America's Blood Centers, and the American Red Cross have developed accepted criteria in which transfusion of blood components would be considered reasonable although not mandatory.[1]
- The Joint Commission on Accreditation of Healthcare Organizations (JCAHO) requires all hospitals to have policies and procedures that address the prescription, distribution, handling, dispensing and administration of blood components, as well as monitoring the effects of blood component administration on patients.
- All blood and blood components pose a risk to the patient for the transmission of infectious agents (Table 121-2). Meticulous donor selection and laboratory testing are able to significantly reduce, but not eliminate, the risk for disease transmission. Nucleic acid amplification testing (NAT) technology detects the genetic material of viruses, thus reducing the window during which the infectious agent is undetectable and further improving blood safety. NAT, currently used to detect HIV-1 (most prevalent in the United States) and HCV, is under investigation for the detection of other infectious disease agents.
- When feasible, health care providers should consider autologous transfusion techniques (see Procedure 17), preoperative donation and perioperative collection, as recognized alternatives to allogeneic transfusions to

decrease the risks for disease transmission and immune reactions.

- All donors (1) are assessed for high-risk behavior associated with hepatitis and acquired immunodeficiency syndrome (AIDS); (2) are questioned regarding practices and circumstances that preclude them for donating; (3) have completed a health assessment, which includes questions on past and present illnesses; (4) meet certain physiologic criteria; and (5) have had the opportunity to confidentially exclude their donation from transfusion. The honesty and integrity of the donor is imperative to appropriately exclude a donor whose blood may transmit disease to recipients.
- Donor blood for allogeneic use is tested using U.S. Food and Drug Administration (FDA) licensed tests (Table 121-3). All donor units have also tested negative or the results have been deemed clinically insignificant for unexpected antibodies against red blood cell (RBC) antigens unless otherwise indicated on the label. Units intended for *autologous* use that test positive for one of the above antibodies/antigens are acceptable to transfuse with physician authorization and are labeled with a biohazard label that indicates the specific reactivity.
- The label on the blood/blood product contains the following information:
  - ❖ Product name
  - ❖ Method by which the product was prepared
  - ❖ Temperature range recommended for storage
  - ❖ Preservatives and anticoagulant if used in the preparation
  - ❖ Standard volume (assumed unless otherwise indicated on the label)
  - ❖ Number of units in a pooled component and any sedimenting agent used during cytapheresis

TABLE 121-1 | **Introduction to Transfusion: Blood Components**

Component	Major Indications	Action	Not Indicated for...	Special Precautions	Hazards	Rate of Infusion per Unit
Whole Blood	Symptomatic anemia with large volume deficit	Restoration of • Oxygen-carrying capacity • Blood volume	Condition responsive to specific component	• Must be ABO-identical • Labile coagulation factors deteriorate within 24 hours after collection	• Infectious diseases • Septic/toxic, allergic, febrile reactions • Circulatory overload • GVHD	For massive loss, fast as patient can tolerate *Usual:* 1½ to 4 hours
Red Blood Cells	Symptomatic anemia	Restoration of oxygen-carrying capacity	• Pharmacologically treatable anemia • Coagulation deficiency	Must be ABO-compatible	• Infectious diseases • Septic/toxic, allergic, febrile reactions • GVHD	As patient can tolerate but less than 4 hours *Usual:* 1½ to 4 hours
Red Blood Cells, Leukocytes Removed	• Symptomatic anemia • Febrile reactions from leukocyte antibodies and cellular products released during storage (cytokines)	Restoration of oxygen-carrying capacity	• Pharmacologically treatable anemia • Coagulation deficiency	Must be ABO-compatible	• Infectious diseases • Septic/toxic, allergic, febrile reactions (unless plasma also removed, e.g., by washing) • GVHD	As patient can tolerate but less than 4 hours *Usual:* 1½ to 4 hours
Fresh Frozen Plasma	Deficit of labile and stable plasma coagulation factors and thrombotic thrombocytopenia purpura (TTP)	Source of labile and non-labile plasma factors	Condition responsive to volume replacement	Should be ABO-compatible	• Infectious diseases • Allergic reactions • Circulatory overload	Less than 4 hours *Usual:* 30 to 80 min
Liquid Plasma and Plasma	Deficit of stable coagulation factors	Source of non-labile factors	Deficit of labile coagulation factors or volume replacement	Should be ABO-compatible	• Infectious diseases • Allergic reactions	Less than 4 hours *Usual:* 30 to 60 min
Cryoprecipitated AHF	• Hemophilia A • von Willebrand disease • Hypofibrinogenemia • Factor XIII deficiency	Provides Factor VIII, fibrinogen, vWF, Factor XIII	Conditions not deficient in contained factors	Frequent repeat doses may be necessary	• Infectious diseases • Allergic reactions	Less than 4 hours *Usual:* 15 to 30 min
• Platelets • Platelets, Pheresis	Bleeding from thrombocytopenia or platelet function abnormality	Improves hemostasis	Plasma coagulation defects and some conditions with rapid platelet destruction, e.g., idiopathic thrombocytopenic purpura (ITP) or TTP	Should not use some microaggregate filters (check manufacturer's instructions)	• Infectious diseases • Septic/toxic, allergic, febrile reactions • GVHD	Less than 4 hours *Usual:* 15 to 30 min
Granulocytes, Pheresis	Neutropenia with infection	Provides granulocytes	Infection responsive to antibiotics	• Must be ABO-compatible • Do not use depth-type microaggregate filters • Do not administer within 4 to 6 hours before or after giving amphotericin, an anti-fungal and anti-parasitic agent, to minimize the possibility of reported pulmonary side effects	• Infectious diseases • Allergic, febrile reactions • GVHD	• One unit over a 2- to 4-hour period • Closely observe for reactions

From American Association of Blood Banks. (2002). *Primer of Blood Administration.* Bethesda, MD: Author.

TABLE 121-2	Current Estimated Risks of Transfusion-Transmitted Disease in the United States[1,2]
Disease	**Level of Risk per Unit of Blood**
HIV	1:2,000,000[3]
Hepatitis B	1:150,000[3]
Hepatitis C	1:1.6,000,000[3]
HTLV-I/II	1:641,000[4]
Malaria	<1:1,000,000[3]
Chagas' disease	<1:1,000,000[3]
Babesiosis	<1:1,000,000[3]
Yersinia	<1:1,000,000[5(p638)]
Cytomegalovirus (CMV)	<1:100 of the components from CMV-seropositive donors (approximately 50% of donors) can transmit this infection, but generally it is significant only in immunoincompetent recipients[5(p633)]
Febrile nonhemolytic reaction	1:200[6]
Delayed hemolytic reaction	1:2,500 (red cell transfusions)[6]
Circulatory overload	1:10,000[6]
Acute hemolytic transfusion reaction	1:25,000 (red cell transfusions)[5]

1. There may be some geographic variation in rates for some infectious diseases, and rates change as new research data are published.
2. Risks of transfusion-transmitted bacterial septicemia currently are being assessed.
3. Bianco, C. *Infectious Risks of Blood Transfusion (Audioconference Presentation)*. Bethesda, MD: American Association of Blood Banks.
4. Schreiber, G., et al. (1996). The risk of transfusion-transmitted viral infections. The Retrovirus Epidemiology Donor Study. *N Engl J Med* 334:1685-90.
5. Brecher, M.E., ed. (2002). *Technical Manual*, 14th edition. Bethesda, MD: American Association of Blood Banks.
6. Walker, R.H. (1987). Special report: Transfusion risks. *Am J Clin Pathol* 88:374-8.
From American Association of Blood Banks. (2002). *Primer of Blood Administration*. Bethesda, MD: Author.

❖ Name, address, registration number and U.S. license number (if applicable) of the collection and processing center; expiration date and, if applicable, time (if the time is not indicated, the product expires at midnight of the date indicated)
❖ Donation (unit or pool) identification number
❖ Donor category; ABO group and Rh type

TABLE 121-3	Tests Performed on Donor Blood
Test	**Infectious Viral Agent and/or Disease**
HBsAg (hepatitis B surface antigen)	Hepatitis B virus
Antibodies to HBc (hepatitis B core antigen)	Hepatitis B virus
Antibodies to HCV[1]	Hepatitis C virus[1]
Antibodies to HIV-1/2[1]	HIV infection including AIDS[1]
HIV-1-Ag[1]	HIV infection including AIDS[1]
STS (serologic test for syphilis)	Syphilis
Antibodies to HTLV-I/II	Human T-cell lymphotropic virus
Antibodies to CMV[2]	Cytomegalovirus[2]
Alanine aminotransferase (ALT)	Liver abnormality

1. Nucleic acid amplification testing (NAT) will be performed routinely in the near future to detect these infectious viral agents and/or diseases. NAT may supplement or replace existing tests.
2. CMV testing usually is performed for any cellular blood component intended for an immunocompromised recipient, (e.g., a CMV-seronegative low birthweight neonate or a patient receiving immunosuppressive therapy.)
From American Association of Blood Banks. (2002). *Primer of Blood Administration*. Bethesda, MD: Author.

❖ Special handling information, if indicated
❖ Statements regarding recipient identification, infectious disease risk, prescription requirement, and mention of the *Circular of Information for the Use of Human Blood and Blood Components*[2]

- All blood and blood components must be maintained in a controlled environment under appropriate conditions as defined by the AABB Standards for Blood Banks and Transfusion Services.
- Identification of the recipient and blood container must be properly completed before the transfusion is initiated.
- All blood components must be administered through a filter (usually 170-260 microns) to remove clots and aggregates.
- The hematocrit is a less sensitive indicator of oxygen-carrying capacity than hemoglobin as it fluctuates with fluid status. RBCs should not be administered in the treatment of anemias that can be corrected by specific medications such as iron, vitamin B_{12}, folic acid, and erythropoietin.
- Fresh-frozen plasma (FFP) is indicated in the management of preoperative or bleeding patients who require replacement of multiple plasma coagulation factors as in those with liver disease; in patients undergoing massive transfusion therapy who have clinically significant coagulation deficiencies; in patients on warfarin who are bleeding or need to undergo an invasive procedure before vitamin K can reverse the warfarin effect; for transfusion or plasma exchange in patients with thrombotic thrombocytopenic purpura (TTP); in patients with selected congenital or acquired coagulation factor deficiencies when no specific coagulation concentrates are available; and in those patients with rare specific plasma protein deficiencies. FFP should not be administered when a coagulopathy can be corrected more effectively with specific therapy—for example, vitamin K (for patient on warfarin), cryoprecipitate AHF, or factor VIII concentrates. FFP should not be used as a volume expander when other IV solutions can be used safely and adequately. Each ml of undiluted plasma contains 1 international unit (IU) of each coagulation factor.
- Platelet transfusion may be indicated in selected cases of postoperative bleeding in which the platelet count is less than 50,000/microliter. In the setting of normal platelet function, platelets should not be transfused if the platelet count is greater than 100,000/microliter.
- Patients with a history of a febrile reaction may have their symptoms reduced by premedicating with antipyretics; mild reactions are premedicated with antihistamines; severe allergic reactions are premedicated with antipyretics, antihistamines, and hydrocortisone. Oral medications should be given 30 minutes prior to starting the transfusion to ensure effectiveness. IV medications may be given immediately prior to initiating the transfusion. Some institutions have protocols for the treatment of allergic reactions with sequential dosing of premedications that begins several hours prior to transfusion.

- No medications or IV solutions may be added to or infused through the tubing with blood or blood components, with the exception of 0.9% normal saline (NS) injections. Dextrose-containing solutions should never be used because glucose induces red cell aggregation. Medications or other solutions added to or infused with the blood or blood components must have been approved for such use by the FDA or have documentation that demonstrates that the addition to the component is safe and does not adversely affect the blood or component. Lactated Ringer's (LR) and other solutions containing calcium should never be added to or infused with components containing citrate.
- All blood and blood components should be inspected for the presence of excessive hemolysis, a color change in the blood bag when compared with the tubing segments, floccular material, cloudy appearance, or other problems; if any of these situations exist, the unit must be returned to the blood bank for further evaluation.
- Once the integrity of the unit is violated (i.e., spiked with administration set), the component expires in 4 hours, if the unit is maintained at room temperature (20° to 24°C), or in 24 hours, if the unit is refrigerated (1° to 6°C).
- Blood components may be warmed for exchange as with massive transfusions or in those patients with cold-reactive antibodies. In these situations, only an FDA-approved warming device is used to prevent hemolysis. White cell–reduced components, cytomegalovirus (CMV)–negative products, irradiated blood components, washed red cells and platelets, frozen-thawed-deglycerolized red cells, and human leukocyte antigen (HLA)–matched platelets are specially processed components. While these are expensive and time-consuming to prepare, certain situations exist in which these products are indicated.
- In nonemergent situations, informed consent is required prior to the transfusion of all blood components and plasma products. This process is documented in the medical record. Institutional policies vary as to whether a patient's signature is required to complete the informed consent process.
- In situations in which there may not be time to discuss transfusion with the patient or other decision-making individual, the health care provider ordering the transfusion must make a reasonable judgment that the patient would accept a transfusion or that an implied consent for treatment including transfusion exists. Transfusions should not be delayed in life-threatening situations if it is likely that the patient would consent to a transfusion.

EQUIPMENT

- Blood component as prescribed
- Appropriate administration set for the blood component to be transfused
- NS solution for IV administration
- One alcohol pad
- Needleless connecting device
- Nonsterile gloves
- Thermometer

Additional equipment as needed includes the following:
- Blood pump
- FDA-approved blood warmer

PATIENT AND FAMILY EDUCATION

- Explain the procedure and reason for administration of the blood component. ➤*Rationale:* Decreases anxiety and provides an opportunity to ask questions and seek clarification.
- Explain the signs and symptoms of a transfusion reaction and the need to notify the nurse if detected. ➤*Rationale:* The patient may be the first to sense the signs and symptoms of a transfusion reaction. Prompt notification of the nurse facilitates immediate intervention, decreasing the likelihood of serious sequelae.
- Evaluate the patient's need for long-term blood or blood component therapy. ➤*Rationale:* The patient may need to carry a record of transfusion, history/severity of transfusion reactions, and the requirement for premedication(s) or irradiated blood or blood components to reduce the risk for a transfusion reaction (see Procedure 125).

PATIENT ASSESSMENT AND PREPARATION

Patient Assessment

- Assess for evidence of hemorrhage with respect to recent surgery or trauma. ➤*Rationale:* Signs and symptoms of hypovolemic shock with significant blood loss (i.e., hemoglobin less than 8 g/dl) requires replacement, usually with packed RBCs. In patient's with normal hemoglobin, whole blood and RBC components should not be used as volume expanders or to increase the oncotic pressure of circulating blood.
- Assess for evidence of deficit in oxygen-carrying capacity: hemoglobin less than 8 g/dl in the presence of a compromised respiratory status and arterial blood gases. ➤*Rationale:* Significant improvement may be seen in the respiratory status, arterial blood gases, and performance of activities of daily living (ADLs) with the administration of RBCs when the hemoglobin is increased to 10 g/dl or greater.
- Assess for evidence of coagulopathies. ➤*Rationale:* FFP provides plasma proteins in those patients who are either deficient in or have defective plasma proteins.
- Assess for evidence of bleeding due to decreased circulating platelets, functionally abnormal platelets, or low platelet counts of less than 10,000/microliter secondary to cancer, marrow aplasia, or chemotherapy. ➤*Rationale:* Platelets are necessary for normal hemostasis.
- Evaluate transfusion history, the presence and severity of transfusion reactions, and/or the necessity of premedications. ➤*Rationale:* A direct relationship exists between the number of transfusions a patient has had and the number of circulating antibodies and thus the likelihood of a transfusion reaction.

- Assess the patient for the signs and symptoms consistent with those of a transfusion reaction: the presence of chills, itching, rash, hematuria, muscle aches, and/or difficulty breathing. ➥*Rationale:* These symptoms may later be mistaken for a transfusion reaction.
- Assess pretransfusion vital signs, including temperature, blood pressure, heart rate, respiratory rate, breath sounds and, if applicable, filling pressures (i.e., central venous pressure [CVP], pulmonary artery pressure [PAP], pulmonary capillary wedge pressure [PCWP]). ➥*Rationale:* Establishes baseline values when monitoring for transfusion reaction or fluid overload. Having a fever may delay the initiation of a transfusion as the symptom of a transfusion reaction may be masked and the efficacy of a platelet transfusion may be compromised.

Patient Preparation

- Ensure that the patient and family understand preprocedural teaching. Answer questions as they arise and reinforce information as needed. ➥*Rationale:* Evaluates and reinforces understanding of previously taught information.
- Ensure that informed consent has been obtained and is documented in the medical record. ➥*Rationale:* Protects the rights of the patient and ensures that a competent decision has been made by the patient.
- Verify the written prescription for transfusion. ➥*Rationale:* Required before the initiation of transfusion, the prescription should include the name of the blood component, the amount to be transfused, duration of the infusion, and if appropriate, pretransfusion medications.

- Validate that a current type (ABO and Rh) and screen (all other antibodies) is available in the blood bank. If a type and screen is not available or outdated, obtain a blood specimen for type and screen and send to blood bank. ➥*Rationale:* Type and screen specimens usually are valid for 24 to 72 hours. Check your institution's policy for the number of days the type and screen is valid. Determine whether the patient, family, or friends have donated blood for transfusion. If so, alert the blood bank that a "directed unit" should be available.
- Establish or ensure the patency of a peripheral IV line (18- to 20-G catheter is recommended; however, RBCs can safely be administered through 22- to 25-G catheters) or central venous access catheter. No harmful effects have been reported when blood components have been administered through multilumen catheters, since the solutions and blood component are rapidly diluted in large blood vessels.[3] Blood components may be administered through the proximal port of the pulmonary artery catheter. ➥*Rationale:* Larger-gauge catheter encourages flow of blood or blood components.
- Assess the vascular access line for the possibility of incompatible IV fluids. If necessary, flush the line with normal saline before and after the transfusion. ➥*Rationale:* Only NS may be infused through the same tubing as blood components.
- If indicated, administer pretransfusion medications. ➥*Rationale:* Patients who have a history of a transfusion reaction(s) may require premedications.

Procedure for Blood and Blood Component Administration

Steps	Rationale	Special Considerations
1. Obtain blood component from the blood bank.	Blood components must be returned to the blood bank within 30 minutes of their release if they not going to be transfused.	
2. With another qualified health care provider, check the blood component record against the patient's identification band, verifying the following information:	Verifying this information reduces the risk for an identification error that could result in the administration of an incompatible blood component.	If any errors or inconsistencies are noted, *do not puncture the unit or administer the blood component. Notify the blood bank immediately.* Review your institution's policies and procedures for checking blood or blood components. State laws may specify who is qualified to check patient identifiers prior to transfusion.
A. Exact spelling of the patient's first name, middle initial, and last name		If possible, have the patient state their name and spell it—first name, middle initial, and last name.
B. The patient's medical record number		

Procedure continues on the following page

Procedure for Blood and Blood Component Administration—*Continued*

Steps	Rationale	Special Considerations
C. Type of blood component D. Compatibility of patient's blood group and Rh type with the donor's blood group and Rh type (Table 121-4) E. Whether the unit of blood components has undergone any special processing F. Unit number G. Expiration date of component H. Any abnormal color or appearance of the blood component		Some patients may require special processing of blood components to reduce the risk for transfusion reaction.
3. Ensure that the registered nurses and qualified health care provider sign the transfusion record.	Validates that proper validation/identification procedures were completed.	
4. Wash hands and don nonsterile gloves.	Reduces transmission of microorganisms; standard precautions.	

TABLE 121-4	**Red Blood Cell Transfusion Selection (for RBCs Only—Not Whole Blood)**							
	Patient							
Donor	**O+**	**A+**	**B+**	**AB+**	**O Neg**	**A–**	**B–**	**AB–**
O+	+	+	+	+				
A+	–	+	–	+				
B+	–	–	+	+				
AB+	–	–	–	+				
O–	+	+	+	+	+	+	+	+
A–	–	+	–	+	–	+	–	+
B–	–	–	+	+	–	–	+	+
AB–	–	–	–	+	–	–	–	+

+ = compatible transfusion
– = not compatible (incompatible)
From American Association of Blood Banks (2002). *Primer of Blood Administration.* Bethesda, MD: Author.

Procedure for Blood and Blood Component Administration—*Continued*

Steps	Rationale	Special Considerations

5. Prepare the administration set:
    A. For Y-type administration set:
 	
        (1) Close both roller clamps.
        (2) Spike a 250-ml bag of 0.9% normal saline and prime tubing. Close roller clamp.
        (3) Attach a needle or needleless connector to the distal end of the tubing.
        (4) Spike the unit of blood or blood components.
    B. For single-tubing administration set:
        (1) Close roller clamp.
        (2) Spike the unit of blood components.
        (3) Open the roller clamp between the unit and drip chamber; prime the drip chamber, making sure the filter is covered.
        (4) Prime the remaining length of the tubing.
        (5) Close the roller clamp.
        (6) Attach a needle or needleless connector to the distal end of the tubing.
	Y-tubing is used for transfusing whole blood or red blood cells.
	Prevents spillage.
	Reduces risk for air emboli.
	
	For insertion/connection to primary administration set.
	
	Accesses unit for administration.
	
	Prevents spillage.
	Accesses the unit.
	
	Primes drip chamber to prevent damage to constituents in the blood or blood components.
	
	Reduces the risk for air emboli.
	
	Prevents spillage.
	For connection to the primary administration set.
		Blood administration sets usually have a 170-260 micron filter to trap fibrin and other debris that accumulates during blood storage. Sets usually have a maximum capacity (check with manufacturer's instructions). Y-type tubing simplifies the process of adding normal saline to the infusion and provides an immediate saline flush should a reaction occur.
		This type of administration set is commonly used for the administration of FFP. Platelets, cryoprecipitate, albumin, and granulocytes have product-specific administration sets that are supplied by either the blood bank or pharmacy.

6. Cleanse Y-port injection site proximal to the insertion site with an alcohol wipe.	Reduces transmission of microorganisms.	The IV piggyback port most proximal to the IV insertion site reduces the risk for precipitation or hemolysis in the primary tubing. FFP and platelets should be administered directly into the IV catheter; *do not piggyback.*
7. Insert the needle into the proximal port or attach the blood tubing to the needleless connector of the primary tubing. Clamp off the primary infusion.	Decreases potential for hemolysis or precipitation in primary administration.	Primary infusion set may need to be flushed with normal saline before initiating the transfusion to prevent hemolysis or precipitation in the primary administration set.
8. Release the roller clamp between the unit and the filter.	Allows the transfusion to proceed.	
9. Adjust the rate to infuse 10 to 15 drops per minute for the first 15 minutes.	Ensures patient receives only a small amount of blood components, should a transfusion reaction occur.	A major ABO incompatibility or a severe allergic reaction will usually manifest with the first 50 ml of transfused component.
10. Adjust the rate to infuse as prescribed. Transfusion should be completed within maximum of 4 hours of initiating the infusion.	Likelihood of bacterial contamination markedly increases after 4 hours of hang time.	Troubleshooting if the transfusion is infusing slowly: Ascertain that the IV access is patent and has not infiltrated; may need new IV access. Raise the height of the blood component unit to increase the rate of flow. Gently massage the unit container to resuspend the red blood cells.

Procedure continues on the following page

Procedure for Blood and Blood Component Administration—*Continued*

Steps	Rationale	Special Considerations
		Check to see whether the filter has become clogged with debris; may need to change the administration set.
11. At the completion of the transfusion, flush the administration set with NS.	Allows for the infusion of the blood in the tubing.	
12. Clamp off the blood administration set and adjust the flow of the primary infusion to the prescribed rate.	Continues primary infusion.	
13. Discard supplies and wash hands.	Reduces transmission of microorganisms; standard precautions.	Blood container and administration set should be handled as hazardous waste according to your institution's policies and procedures.
14. Assess posttransfusion vital signs.		
15. Calculate the amount of NS, blood components infused. Document on the intake and output record. Complete the transfusion record.	Maintains accuracy of intake for evaluation of fluid balance.	

Expected Outcomes

- Complete infusion of blood or blood components
- Restoration of normovolemic status
- Improved oxygen-carrying capacity
- Correction of coagulopathies
- Restoration of hemostasis

Unexpected Outcomes

- Immediate reactions: hemolytic reactions, bacterial sepsis, febrile reactions, transfusion-related acute lung injury (TRALI), allergic reactions, circulatory overload, air emboli, hypothermia, electrolyte disturbances, "citrate" intoxication (hypocalcemia) (see Procedure 125)
- Delayed reactions: delayed hemolytic reaction, transmission of infectious agents, graft-versus-host disease, alloimmunization
- Inability to infuse blood component within prescribed time or 4-hour time

Patient Monitoring and Care

Steps	Rationale	Reportable Conditions
		These conditions should be reported if they persist despite nursing interventions.
1. Monitor the vital signs during the first 15 minutes of the transfusion.	Acute transfusion reactions usually occur within the first 15 minutes of the infusion.	- If signs and symptoms of a transfusion reaction occur, ***stop the transfusion***. See Procedure 125 for more details
2. Monitor the vital signs at the completion of the transfusion as well as 1 hour after the completion of the transfusion.[3]	Detects changes that suggest a transfusion reaction.	- Mild transfusion reaction—temperature rise less than 1°C above baseline; minimal itching or localized urticaria; chills
		- Moderate transfusion reaction—temperature rise greater than 1° to 2.5°C above baseline; itching unresolved with antihistamines; urticaria unresolved with antihistamines; chills with fever unresolved with antipyretics

Patient Monitoring and Care—*Continued*

Steps	Rationale	Reportable Conditions
		• Severe transfusion reaction—temperature rise greater than 2.5°C above baseline; progressive or extensive urticaria; shock; hypotension; cyanosis; hemoglobinuria; dyspnea; back (flank) pain
3. Obtain posttransfusion laboratory values.	Determines efficacy of transfusion. One unit of PRBC should raise the nonbleeding adult's hemoglobin by 1 g/dl and the hematocrit by 3%. For FFP: monitor the prothrombin time (PT), partial thromboplastin time (PTT) or specific factor assays as prescribed. For platelets: Evaluate platelet count at 1 hour and 24 hours after transfusion to assess patient's response.[4]	• Abnormal laboratory values

Documentation

Documentation should include the following:

- Patient and family education
- Pretransfusion assessment
- Validation of informed consent
- Date and time transfusion was initiated and terminated
- Baseline and serial vital sign measurements
- Transfusion record validated by registered nurse and another qualified health care provider

- Type and amount of blood or component administered
- Appropriate laboratory values pre- and posttransfusion
- Patient's tolerance of transfusion
- Occurrence of unexpected outcomes and interventions taken

References

1. American Association of Blood Banks, America's Blood Centers, and the American Red Cross. (2002). *Circular of Information for the Use of Human Blood and Blood Components, Summary Chart of Blood Components,* July, 38-9.
2. American Association of Blood Banks, America's Blood Centers, and the American Red Cross. (2002). *Circular of Information for the Use of Human Blood and Blood Components,* July, 4.
3. American Association of Blood Banks. (2002). *Primer of Blood Administration,* Bethesda, MD: The Association, Revised 12/02, Chapter 5, 3.
4. American Association of Blood Banks, America's Blood Centers, and the American Red Cross. (2002). *Circular of Information for the Use of Human Blood and Blood Components,* July 7, 26.

Additional Readings

American Association of Blood Banks, America's Blood Centers, and the American Red Cross. (2002). *Circular of Information for the Use of Human Blood and Blood Components,* July.
American Society of Anesthesiologists Task Force on Blood Component Therapy. (1996). Practice guidelines for blood component therapy. *Anesthesiology,* 84, 732-47.
Anderson, K.C., and Ness, P.M. (1999). *Scientific Basis of Transfusion Medicine: Implications for Clinical Practice.* 2nd ed. Philadelphia: W.B. Saunders.

Davenport, R. *Informed Consent for Blood Transfusion.* Bethesda, MD: American Association of Blood Banks.
De la Roche, M.R.P., and Gautheir, L. (1993). Rapid transfusion of packed red blood cells: Effects of dilution, pressure, and catheter size. *Annals of Emergency Medicine,* Oct 22, 1551-5.
Gorlin, J., ed. (2002). *Standards for Blood Banks and Transfusion Services.* 21st ed. Bethesda, MD: American Association of Blood Banks.
Hollinger, F.B., and Kleinman, S. (2003). Transfusion transmission of West Nile virus: A merging of historical and contemporary perspectives. *Transfusion,* 43, 992-7.
Miller, R.L.S. (2002). Blood component therapy. *Urologic Nursing,* Oct, 22, 331-8.
Silliman, C.C. (1999). Transfusion-related acute lung injury. *Transfusion Medicine Review,* 13, 177-86.
Simon, T.L., Dzik, W.H., and Snyder, E.L., eds. (2002). *Principles of Transfusion Medicine.* 3rd ed. Baltimore: Williams & Wilkins.
Truilzi, D., ed. (2002). *Blood Transfusion Therapy: A Physician's Handbook.* 7th ed. Bethesda, MD: American Association of Blood Banks.
U.S. Department of Health and Human Services Food and Drug Administration, Center for Biologics Evaluation and Research. (2002). *Revised Preventive Measures to Reduce the Possible Risk of Transmission of Creutzfeldt-Jakob Disease (CJD) and Variant Creutzfeldt-Jakob Disease (vCJD) by Blood and Blood Products,* Jan. Available at: www.fda.gov/cber/gdlns/cjdvcjd.htm.

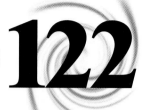

PROCEDURE **122**

Blood Pump Use

P U R P O S E : An external pressure infusion cuff is used to administer a large amount of blood or plasma to a patient with massive, life-threatening hemorrhage or to infuse viscous packed red blood cells (RBCs) within a prescribed period of time.

Maribeth Wooldridge-King

PREREQUISITE NURSING KNOWLEDGE

- Only external pressure cuffs specifically designed for blood or blood component infusions should be used. A standard sphygmomanometer cuff should never be used to administer large-volume transfusions or infusions because it does not exert uniform pressure on all parts of the component container.
- External pressure cuffs should only be used with central line catheters or large-bore (18 gauge or larger) peripheral intravenous (IV) catheters. Caution must be exercised when applying a pressurized cuff to a peripheral IV catheter in order to avoid damaging the vein.
- The applied pressure should not exceed 300 torr when pressure-transfusing components that contain red blood cells. A rapid infusion (1 unit every 5 minutes) of cold blood (1° to 6°C) may lower the temperature of the sinoatrial node to less than 30°C, at which point ventricular fibrillation can occur.[1] Warming of blood components must always be done using an FDA-approved warming device to avoid hemolysis (see Procedure 123).

EQUIPMENT

- Blood administration set
- External pressure infusion cuff
- Blood component for transfusion
- 0.9% normal saline (NS) for infusion
- Cardiac monitor
- Nonsterile gloves

PATIENT AND FAMILY EDUCATION

- Explain the rationale for using an external pressure infusion cuff. ➤➤*Rationale:* Informs patient and family regarding the purpose of the device.
- Explain that the patient may feel discomfort in his or her extremity or IV insertion site if the external pressure infusion cuff is used with a peripheral IV catheter. ➤➤*Rationale:* Pressure applied to a peripheral vein may be uncomfortable to the patient.
- Instruct patient to report any signs or symptoms of a transfusion reaction to the nurse (see Procedure 125). ➤➤*Rationale:* Facilitates prompt and immediate intervention by the nurse.

PATIENT ASSESSMENT AND PREPARATION

Patient Assessment

- If using a peripheral IV catheter, assess the IV site for redness, swelling, or pain. ➤➤*Rationale:* Signs and symptoms of an infiltration that necessitate the insertion of a new peripheral IV catheter.
- For peripheral pressurized administration, ascertain that the venous catheter is 18 gauge or larger. ➤➤*Rationale:* External pressure cuffs should not be used on peripheral venous catheters smaller than 18 G.

Patient Preparation

- Ensure that the patient and family understand preprocedural teaching. Answer questions as they arise and reinforce information as needed. ➤*Rationale:* Evaluates and reinforces understanding of previously taught information.

- Take pretransfusion vital signs, including temperature, pulse, respiration, and blood pressure. Note filling pressures, (central venous pressure [CVP], pulmonary artery pressure [PAP], and pulmonary capillary wedge pressure [PCWP]) if available. ➤*Rationale:* Documents baseline data.

- Place patient on cardiac monitor. ➤*Rationale:* Provides for rapid assessment of cardiac dysrhythmias that may occur with rapid administration of blood.

Procedure for Blood Pump Use

Steps	Rationale	Special Considerations
1. Wash hands and don nonsterile gloves.	Reduces transmission of microorganisms; standard precautions.	
2. Obtain and set up blood component for administration (see Procedure 121).	Blood component should be assembled before inserting the unit into the pump.	
3. Prime the tubing and piggyback or directly connect into the primary IV line.	Allows transfusion to proceed.	
4. Open the roller clamp on the administration set.	Rate of infusion is dependent on the amount of pressure applied to the unit, not the position of the roller clamp.	
5. Deflate the external pressure infusion cuff.	Allows for easy placement of unit of blood or blood components into the cuff.	
6. Guide the unit of blood component through the mesh or plastic covering of the cuff so that the entire unit remains within the mesh or plastic panel.	Allows pressure to be evenly applied to blood components bag.	Do not allow the top of the unit to appear above the mesh or plastic covering, because this will interfere with flow.
7. Secure the unit of blood component in place with fabric strap or Velcro closure and hang the cuff from the IV pole.	Prevents unit from slipping out of the cuff when hung from the IV pole.	
8. Inflate the external pressure infusion cuff to achieve the desired rate of flow.	Pressure of blood pump is used to adjust flow, not the position of the roller clamp.	The pressure should not exceed 300 mm Hg to avoid damaging the red blood cells, rupturing the blood bag, dislodging the IV catheter or injuring the vein. The patient may complain of discomfort in his or her extremity if a peripheral catheter is used; if appropriate, decrease the pressure to maintain patient comfort.
9. When the transfusion is complete, deflate the external pressure cuff, close the roller clamp to the blood bag, and open the roller clamp to the 0.9% NS.	Pressure is usually not needed to infuse the normal saline.	

Procedure continues on the following page

Procedure for Blood Pump Use—*Continued*

Steps	Rationale	Special Considerations
10. Flush the primary infusion tubing with 0.9% NS.	Allows the patient to receive blood sequestered in the tubing.	
11. Transfuse additional units of blood components, if prescribed.	Multiple transfusions may be necessary for life-threatening hemorrhage.	
12. When all of the transfusions are completed, don nonsterile gloves, deflate the cuff, and remove the unit of blood component.	Standard precautions.	
13. Regulate the primary IV infusion at the prescribed rate.	Continues fluid resuscitation.	Administration of crystalloid and colloids can be used in conjunction with blood replacement therapy to provide cardiovascular support.
14. Discard used supplies and wash hands.	Reduces the transmission of microorganisms; standard precautions.	Blood container and administration set should be handled as hazardous waste.
15. Document in patient record.		

Expected Outcomes

- Improved or rapid flow of blood component
- Infusion completed within prescribed time limit

Unexpected Outcomes

- Dislodgment of IV catheter
- Rupture of blood component bag
- Patient discomfort

Patient Monitoring and Care

Steps	Rationale	Reportable Conditions
		These conditions should be reported if they persist despite nursing interventions. • Redness • Swelling • Pain
1. Assess the peripheral IV site for redness, swelling, and pain during the transfusion. If signs and symptoms of infiltration occur, stop the transfusion immediately, remove the catheter, and initiate another IV catheter infusion site.	Pressurized infusion can cause catheter dislodgment.	
2. Monitor the patient's blood pressure (BP), filling pressures (CVP, PAP, and PCWP) if possible, cardiac rate and rhythm, urine output, and respiratory rate during the first 15 minutes of the transfusion, then hourly until 1 hour after completion of the transfusion.	Monitors patient response to rapid blood administration. Stored blood may be rich in potassium, leading to cardiac dysrhythmias.	• Significant change in BP, CVP, PAP, or PCWP
3. Monitor the patient for signs and symptoms of a transfusion reaction. If a transfusion reaction is suspected, **stop the transfusion!** (See Procedure 125.)	Blood component replacement therapy constitutes the infusion of a foreign substance into the recipient.	• Signs and symptoms of a transfusion reaction (see Procedure 125)

Documentation

Documentation should include the following:

- Patient and family education
- Pretransfusion assessment
- Date and time infusion is initiated and completed
- Transfusion record validated by the registered nurse and another qualified health care provider.
- Baseline and serial vital sign measurements
- Use of an external pressure cuff or blood pump
- The type and amount of the blood or blood components infused under pressure
- Appropriate laboratory value(s) pre- and posttransfusion
- Patient's tolerance of the transfusion
- Unexpected outcomes and interventions taken

Reference

1. Boyan, C.P., and Howland, W.S. (1961). Blood temperature: A critical factor in massive transfusion. *Anesthesiology, 22,* 559.

Additional Reading

American Association of Blood Banks. (2002). *Primer of Blood Administration.* Revised 12/02, Bethesda, MD: The Association.

PROCEDURE **123**

Continuous Arteriovenous Rewarming

P U R P O S E :   Continuous arteriovenous rewarming (CAVR) is used to rapidly rewarm severely hypothermic patients, reverse hypothermia-induced coagulopathy, prevent or treat adverse physiologic effects of severe hypothermia, and assist with massive fluid resuscitation in hypovolemic patients who are hypothermic.[2] The patient populations CAVR is most frequently used for are critically injured trauma patients, near-drowning patients, patients with massive gastrointestinal (GI) hemorrhage, patients with abdominal aortic aneurysm, and environmentally exposed patients.

Christine S. Schulman

PREREQUISITE NURSING KNOWLEDGE

- Knowledge of aseptic technique is essential.
- Severe hypothermia poses a number of adverse physiologic consequences in critically ill or injured patients. Cardiovascular, neurologic, GI, metabolic, and pulmonary disturbances that occur as a result of hypothermia predispose patients to numerous complications and may interfere with the patient's ability to respond to illness or trauma.
- Hypothermia-induced coagulopathies are especially life-threatening to patients with ongoing hemorrhage and are an all-too-frequent complication of aggressive fluid resuscitation with inadequately warmed fluids and blood products. Hypothermia-induced coagulopathies begin to appear when the patient's body temperature falls below 34.5°C and worsen any preexisting hemorrhage the patient may have.[4]
- Progressive hypothermia causes a left shift of the oxygen-hemoglobin dissociation curve as the patient cools. In the presence of hypothermia, hemoglobin increases its affinity for oxygen and will not release oxygen to the tissues. The resulting cellular hypoxia places additional demands on cells that are already under great physiologic stress from critical illness or injury.[1,4]
- CAVR is an arteriovenous circuit in which blood is diverted from the patient's femoral artery into special heparin-coated tubing through a rewarming chamber

and filter; it is then returned to the patient via either the subclavian, femoral, or internal jugular vein (Fig. 123-1). The system is driven by the patient's blood pressure. Patients can be rewarmed from 32° to 36°C in as little as 45 minutes. By being rapidly rewarmed, coagulopathies are reversed, the use of blood products and IV fluids is decreased, and patient mortality is improved.[3]
- The physician or advanced practice nurse inserts the arterial and venous catheters, but it is the nurse's responsibility to maintain patency of the circuit and troubleshoot the system. Only the 9-French catheters included in the CAVR vascular access kit are used; pulmonary artery (PA) catheter and angiography introducers are not large enough for the system to function properly. No stopcocks, reflux valves, or additional connection tubing can be used because they will slow blood flow and potentiate clotting of the system. Hemodynamic and laboratory monitoring, fluid and blood product resuscitation, and all other aspects of patient care can occur concurrent to CAVR.[2,5]
- Contraindications to CAVR include patients with a systolic blood pressure of less than 80 mm Hg, patients weighing less than 90 pounds, and patients with known vascular occlusive disease or compartment syndrome of the lower extremities. Systolic blood pressure usually can be supported to stay above 80 mm Hg by infusion of additional IV fluids, blood products, and vasopressors.[2]
- As patients warm, vasodilation occurs and additional IV fluids often are necessary to reverse hypovolemia.

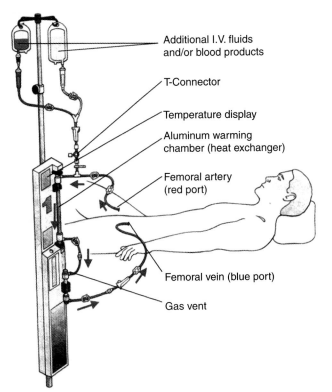

FIGURE 123-1 Continuous arteriovenous rewarming. *(Courtesy Level 1, Inc., Rockland, MA.)*

Cold, hyperkalemic, and acidotic blood returns from the previously hypoperfused lower extremities to the core circulation and can cause "reperfusion injury." This is manifested by cardiac dysrhythmias, hypotension, and acidosis and can result in adult respiratory distress syndrome, acute tubular necrosis, and multisystem organ failure.[1] This is more common with peripheral warming methods, such as warmed cotton blankets and warm air blankets, rather than with central warming methods, such as warmed peritoneal lavage, CAVR, and cardiac bypass.

EQUIPMENT

- Pulmonary artery catheter, tympanic thermometer, or bladder temperature probe to effectively monitor the patient's core temperature
- Level 1 fluid warmer (Model H-500 or H-250) or Level 1 fluid management system H-1025 (Sims Level 1 Technologies, Rockland, MA)
- Vascular access insertion tray for CAVR via Gentilello technique (Sims Level 1 Technologies, Rockland, MA)
- Nonsterile gloves
- Disposable tubing for CAVR
- Replacement filter with gas vent
- Replacement IV infusion set
- Two central line dressing kits
- Sterile or distilled water for water chamber
- Normal saline or lactated Ringer's IV solution

Additional equipment, as needed, includes the following:
- Doppler
- Additional massive fluid infusers as indicated by the patient's volume depletion

PATIENT AND FAMILY EDUCATION

- Explain the reason for CAVR. ➡️*Rationale:* Helps the patient and family understand the consequences of hypothermia as well as the plan of care.
- Explain the procedure and explain the equipment. ➡️*Rationale:* Decreases patient and family anxiety about the procedure and unfamiliar equipment at the bedside.

PATIENT ASSESSMENT AND PREPARATION

Patient Assessment

- Obtain the patient's medical history, including the length of exposure to cold, surgical procedure, or types of injuries. ➡️*Rationale:* Assists in anticipating severity of hypothermia, coagulopathy, and potential multisystem complications.
- Assess core temperature using a tympanic thermometer, bladder probe, or pulmonary artery catheter. ➡️*Rationale:* Assesses severity of hypothermia and efficacy of therapy.
- Obtain vital signs. ➡️*Rationale:* Provides baseline data.
- Obtain hemodynamic parameters, including cardiac output (CO) and index (CI), central venous pressure (CVP), pulmonary artery pressure (PAP), pulmonary capillary wedge pressure (PCWP), and systemic vascular resistance (SVR). If monitoring system is available, also measure the right ventricular ejection fraction, oxygen delivery, and oxygen consumption. ➡️*Rationale:* Identifies baseline oxygen transport and tissue perfusion.
- Assess arterial blood gas, hemoglobin, hematocrit, electrolytes, and coagulation studies. ➡️*Rationale:* Measures oxygenation, presence of metabolic acidosis, severity of hemorrhage, and severity of coagulopathy so that effectiveness of interventions can be assessed and additional interventions initiated.
- Assess patency of current IV large-bore sites. ➡️*Rationale:* Infusion of IV fluids in addition to those infused through the CAVR circuit most likely will be necessary. Multiple IV sites will be needed for infusion for supplementary blood products and resuscitation fluids.
- Assess distal pulses, color, and temperature of extremities. ➡️*Rationale:* Provides baseline data.

Patient Preparation

- Ensure that the patient and family understand preprocedural teaching. Answer questions as they arise and reinforce information as needed. ➡️*Rationale:* Evaluates and reinforces understanding of previously taught information.
- Place additional IV sites. ➡️*Rationale:* Aggressive fluid resuscitation will require more access than what is provided

The labels in the figure read:
- Additional I.V. fluids and/or blood products
- T-Connector
- Temperature display
- Aluminum warming chamber (heat exchanger)
- Femoral artery (red port)
- Femoral vein (blue port)
- Gas vent

by the CAVR circuit. Hypothermia-induced coagulopathy increases the patient's tendency to bleed, necessitating replacement of fluids and blood components.

- If central venous access or a pulmonary artery catheter is not already in place, assist the physician or advanced practice nurse with placement. ➤*Rationale:* Allows for assessment of volume status in response to fluids, assessment of core temperature with PA catheter, and central venous access in the event that vasoactive medications are needed.

- Remove any fluids from the patient's skin and change bedding frequently to keep dry linens next to the patient. Cover the patient with warm blankets or a warm air blanket; cover the patient's head with a warmed blanket, towel, or aluminum cap. ➤*Rationale:* Minimizes additional heat loss via radiation and convection.

Procedure for Continuous Arteriovenous Rewarming

Steps	Rationale	Special Considerations
1. Wash hands and don gloves.	Reduces transmission of microorganisms; standard precautions.	
2. Verify the physician's order for CAVR and infusion of additional IV fluids or blood products.	Prevents unnecessary or incorrect blood product or IV fluid administration.	Physician's order should include additional IV fluids and blood products, laboratory studies, and temperature at which therapy should be discontinued.
3. Assist the physician or advanced practice nurse with placing arterial and venous access sites.	Establishes arterial and venous access.	Access sites must be large to accommodate the 9-Fr catheters in the CAVR vascular access kit. Angiography and PA catheter introducers are too small for adequate blood flow through the circuit and should not be used. No stopcocks or extension tubing should be added to the system, because they also restrict flow.[1]
4. Push the bottom end of the heat exchanger rod *firmly* into the bottom socket and snap the heat exchanger into the guide (Fig. 123-2).	The bottom of the heat exchanger must be firmly placed; otherwise, it will not fit into the top socket.	Being too gentle will result in improper placement of the tubing, and the warmer will not run.
5. Slide the top socket up and place the top end of the exchanger into the placement tract.	Prepares the system.	
6. Slide the top heat exchanger socket down over the heat exchanger tube until the pole latch clicks into place.	Locks the warming chamber into place at both the top and bottom sockets.	
7. Snap the gas vent filter into the holder on the lower portion of the pole assembly with the orange end up.	Filters air and blood clots from the tubing.	It will only fit one way; the tubing is not long enough if placed incorrectly.
8. Plug the device into the outlet and turn it on.	Activates warmer.	Disposable tubing must be in place for the machine to turn on without alarming. If the "Check Disposable" alarm sounds despite tubing being in place, make sure that all pieces fit firmly into their holders.

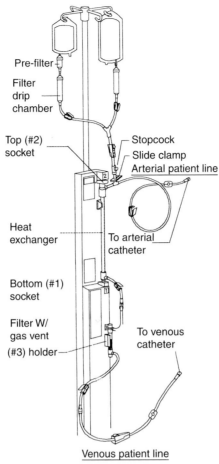

FIGURE 123-2 Insertion of CAVR tubing into Level 1 Rapid Infuser. *(Courtesy Level 1, Inc., Rockland, MA.)*

Procedure for Continuous Arteriovenous Rewarming—*Continued*

Steps	Rationale	Special Considerations
9. Perform all function and alarm checks as per manufacturer's instructions.	Safety precaution. Validates proper equipment function.	
10. Wait for temperature readout to reach operating temperature of 41°C.	Prevents cooling of the patient's blood by directing it through the warming chamber before it reaches operational temperature.	
11. Close all tubing clamps.	Prevents flow through the circuit before everything is warmed and ready.	
12. Spike one of the sides of the Y-connector with normal saline and open the clamp.	Prepares the tubing system.	This can be done while the infuser is warming to 41°C.
13. Open the clamps along the main tubing line to prime with IV fluid. Keep arterial and venous tubing clamps closed.	Prevents air embolus and facilitates blood flow through the system when the CAVR circuit is first opened.	Priming the tubing is optional; the tubing can also be primed with the patient's blood when the arterial catheter clamp is opened.

Procedure continues on the following page

Procedure **for Continuous Arteriovenous Rewarming**—*Continued*

Steps	Rationale	Special Considerations
14. Prime saline to the end of the line.	Removes air from the tubing.	
15. Close all clamps.		
16. Connect the arterial patient line to the arterial catheter. Connect the venous patient line to the venous catheter.	Blood will start to fill the tubing, driven by the patient's blood pressure.	CAVR should be withheld in patients with a systolic blood pressure (BP) less than 80 mm Hg. However, additional IV fluids, blood products, and vasopressors usually can maintain the BP above 80 mm Hg.[2]
17. Open both arterial and venous clamps. Open all clamps between arterial and venous lines.	At this point, patient rewarming is occurring.	All clamps must be wide open for CAVR to function properly. Priming the system outside of the patient allows for assessment of equipment function and arterial flow before the system is connected to the patient.
18. Infuse additional fluids and blood products into the T-connector.	Supports patient's BP and hematocrit. Helps keep system patent by ensuring good flow of fluid.	Additional IV fluids and blood products may be necessary to speed up blood flow through the circuit to keep it open, as well as to support the patient's blood pressure. May need to use pressure chambers to facilitate forward flow of the piggybacked fluids and to prevent back flow into the arterial catheter. To support blood pressure with additional fluids, use of a second rapid infuser is recommended.
19. Tape the disposable tubing to the patient's leg.	Prevents the catheters from kinking and being pulled out.	
20. Apply dry, occlusive dressings to the sites.	Prevents infection.	
21. Discard used supplies, and wash hands.	Reduces transmission of microorganisms; standard precautions.	
22. Document in patient record.		
Patient Transportation		
1. Turn the rewarmer/rapid infuser machine off.	The machine will not operate when the clamps are closed.	Fluid from the water chamber will spill out of the chamber and the aluminum heat exchanger if the machine is on when the tubing is removed from the holders.
2. Clamp the CAVR circuit distal to the arterial patient line. Using saline hanging in the pressure chamber, flush into the arterial line. Clamp both the arterial patient line and arterial catheter once the line is clear of blood.	The Level 1 infuser does not have a battery, and rewarming cannot continue when the machine is not plugged in.	It is essential that the unwarmed CAVR fluid does not cool the patient again, so CAVR must be briefly interrupted during actual transport and resumed when the patient arrives at his or her destination.
3. Open the distal clamp, and flush the remainder of the tubing clear of the patient's blood through the venous side. Clamp the venous patient line and the venous catheter.	Returns blood back to the patient. Clears blood from the circuit so that it does not clot while the system is off.	

Procedure for Continuous Arteriovenous Rewarming—*Continued*

Steps	Rationale	Special Considerations
4. Remove the heat exchanger and gas vent filter from the warming device and lay it in the bed alongside the patient.	Keeps the tubing set close to the patient and prevents it from being pulled out.	The Level 1 infuser can now be transported separately from the patient, simplifying transport.
5. Replace the heat exchanger and gas vent filter into the infuser on reaching destination.	Readies the circuit for resumption of blood flow.	
6. Plug in the machine and let it warm to 41°C.	Lets the machine reach appropriate temperature before circuit is reopened.	
7. Open all clamps, starting at arterial side of the patient, moving towards the venous side.	Opens the circuit to blood flow, allowing rewarming to resume.	
8. Assess blood flow through the circuit.	Ensures that catheters or tubing did not clot off during transport.	Patency of the circuit is dependent on brisk blood flow and effective flushing of catheters when not in use.
9. Discard supplies and wash hands.	Reduces transmission of microorganisms; standard precautions.	
Troubleshooting CAVR 1. Check arterial and venous catheter insertion sites for kinking.	Kinking will obstruct flow.	May need to support catheters with folded gauze dressings to keep them straight.
2. Check the filter for clotting.	Continuous flow of patient blood or banked blood can put the system at risk for clotting.	Change whenever flow becomes sluggish and clots are noted in the filter.
A. Change the filter by briefly clamping both arterial and venous clamps on either side of the filter and removing the filter from its holder.	Clamps tubing so that blood will not spill when the tubing is taken apart.	CAVR blood flow will be interrupted.
B. Attach the arterial end of the new filter to the tubing, invert the filter, and slowly release the arterial clamp to prime the filter with the patient's blood. Return the filter to the upright position (orange end up) and place in the holder.	Less air will be trapped in the filter if it is filled in the inverted position.	
C. Unclamp the venous clamp; allow flow through to the end of the filter. Connect the venous end of the filter to the venous tubing. Release the clamp, allowing blood to flow into the patient. Make sure all clamps are open and that the circuit is flowing briskly.	Allows circuit to be reestablished.	Keep additional CAVR filters close at hand if the patient is being massively transfused. CAVR filters are *not* compatible with regular Level 1 infusion tubing.

Procedure continues on the following page

Procedure for Continuous Arteriovenous Rewarming—*Continued*

Steps	Rationale	Special Considerations
3. If alarm sounds and "Check Disposable" light is illuminated, check to make sure the disposable tubing is properly placed in all of the holders.	The system will not run if the disposable tubing is not completely set into the machine.	Set can become easily dislodged.
4. If the alarm sounds and "Water Level" light is illuminated, check water level in chamber and replace as needed with sterile or distilled water.	System will not operate if water level is too low.	
5. If the alarm sounds and the "Overtemp" light is illuminated, then turn the machine off and use a different rapid infuser.		
6. Maintain the patient's systolic BP above 80 mm Hg with warmed crystalloids, blood products, and vasopressors as prescribed.	Systolic blood flow drives the CAVR circuit; hypotension causes the circuit to clot.	If the patient is persistently hypotensive despite fluids, blood, and vasopressors, the CAVR circuit may need to be back-flushed and discontinued. Fluids can be directly infused into the T-connector through the warmer and into the patient. A second fluid warmer to deliver fluids via another access site often is used in addition to CAVR for patients requiring massive fluid resuscitation.
Discontinuing CAVR	CAVR is discontinued when the patient's temperature reaches 36.5°C and stabilizes there for at least 2 hours.	Once the patient's temperature has reached 36.5°C, his or her temperature is considered back to normal and hypothermia-induced coagulopathies have resolved. Patients can cool down again, however, after CAVR is stopped when cool blood from the distal circulation beds returns to the core circulation. Thus it is important to not discontinue the catheters until the core temperature has been stable for at least 2 hours.[1] Catheters should not remain in place for more than 12 hours after CAVR has stopped to minimize thrombosis development.
1. Wash hands and don gloves.	Reduces transmission of microorganisms, standard precautions.	
2. Clamp the CAVR circuit distal to the arterial patient line.	Turns off the circuit flow.	
3. Using the saline hanging in pressure chamber, flush into the arterial line. Clamp both the arterial patient line and arterial catheter once the line is clear of blood. Disconnect the patient line from the arterial catheter. Cover the arterial catheter with a sterile cap.	Prevents clotting of the arterial catheter in case it needs to be used again before it is discontinued.	

Procedure for Continuous Arteriovenous Rewarming—*Continued*

Steps	Rationale	Special Considerations
4. Flush the remaining patient blood through the system into the patient using crystalloids from the T-connector until the tubing is clear.	Returns blood in the tubing back into the patient.	
5. Clamp the venous catheter clamp. Disconnect the patient line from the venous catheter. Cover the venous catheter with a sterile cap.	Closes off the CAVR circuit to the patient.	
6. Assist as needed with application of direct pressure to the catheter sites for 15 min after the catheters have been removed by the physician.	Minimizes hematoma development.	Catheters should not be removed until coagulation values have normalized. Direct pressure may be needed to stop bleeding from the site once the catheters are removed.
7. Apply occlusive dressings to sites.	Reduces incidence of infection.	
8. Discard supplies, and wash hands.	Reduces transmission of microorganisms; standard precautions.	
9. Document in patient record.		

Expected Outcomes

- Return of patient's core temperature to 36.5°C within 3 hours[4]
- Systolic BP remains above 80 mm Hg
- Restoration of intravascular volume as patient rewarms and coagulopathy reverses[4]
- Vital signs stable throughout CAVR

Unexpected Outcomes

- Patient not rewarming to 36.5°C within 3 hours
- Systolic BP remains below 80 mm Hg despite fluid resuscitation and rewarming
- Inability to restore intravascular volume despite return to normothermia
- Coagulopathies unchanged despite rewarming
- Systolic blood pressure remaining below 80 mm Hg, so that the CAVR system does not run and clots off
- Kinking arterial or venous catheters, occluding blood flow and predisposing the tubing to developing clots
- Clotting of the filter because of administration of additional blood products, leading to no flow through the CAVR circuit
- Hematoma development at the catheter insertion sites
- Loss of pulses in distal extremities in which the CAVR catheters have been placed

Patient Monitoring and Care

Steps	Rationale	Reportable Conditions
		These conditions should be reported if they persist despite nursing interventions.
1. Assess the patient's core temperature using a consistent route every 15 to 30 min.	Use of a consistent route is essential in correctly trending temperature changes, monitoring efficacy of therapy, and helping to determine when to stop CAVR.	- Unchanging temperature
2. Monitor vital signs, cardiac rhythm, and hemodynamic parameters at least every 15 min.	Cardiac dysrhythmias ranging from bradycardia to premature ventricular contractions (PVCs) and ventricular	- Changes in vital signs, cardiac rhythm, and hemodynamic parameters

Procedure continues on the following page

Patient Monitoring and Care—*Continued*

Steps	Rationale	Reportable Conditions
	fibrillation may occur with rapid rewarming. Hypotension also can occur as warming vessels dilate in the face of inadequate intravascular volume. Vital signs guide additional infusions of fluids, blood products, and vasopressors to support systolic BP above 80 mm Hg.	
3. Assess blood flow through the CAVR circuit every 15 min. Briefly slow the infusion of crystalloid infusing into the T-connector by barely closing the roller clamp. This allows the patient's blood to flow by the T-connector and show a pulsatile backflash of blood backward into the crystalloid line. Open the clamp back up to infuse crystalloids as needed to support the patient's BP and maintain a brisk flow through the circuit. If no flash is seen, the blood flow coming from the patient is sluggish or has stopped.	Ensures that system has not clotted off. Immediate troubleshooting for the cause of sluggish or stopped flow is critical to prevent clotting of the circuit.	• Unsuccessful troubleshooting attempts
4. Monitor hemoglobin, hematocrit, PT, PTT, and International Normalized Ratio (INR) at least every hour.	Guides resuscitation of blood and clotting factors to reverse hypothermia-induced coagulopathy. Helps determine presence of continued coagulopathy. Helps assess whether coagulopathy is improving as the patient's temperature rises.	• Abnormal hemoglobin, hematocrit, or coagulation values
5. Monitor urine output hourly.	Establishes perfusion status of major viscera that may be diminished during hypothermia and shock. As the patient warms and intravascular volume is restored, urine output should increase.	• Urine output less than 0.5 ml/kg/h
6. Assess catheter insertion sites a minimum of every 30 min.	Evaluates for presence of catheter kinking or hematoma development that can compromise flow through the circuit to the extremities.	• Bleeding or hematoma development
7. Assess distal pulses at least every 15 min.	Ensures that distal circulation to and from the extremities is patent around the catheters. All patients will have a femoral artery catheter. Venous sites can be jugular, subclavian, or femoral.	• Distal pulses that cannot be palpated or obtained with a Doppler; pallor in the distal extremity; pain in the extremity; decreased ability to sense or move the extremity

<table>
<tr><td colspan="2">

Documentation

Documentation should include the following:

- Patient and family education
- Time CAVR started and ended
- Temperature throughout duration of CAVR and every hour for at least 4 hours after CAVR has been stopped
- Vital signs, hemodynamic parameters, laboratory values, and urine output throughout CAVR
- Any difficulties with insertion of catheters
- Any difficulties in keeping adequate blood flow through the CAVR circuit that are not resolved with troubleshooting

- Presence of distal pulses in extremities
- Appearance of arterial and venous catheter insertion sites throughout CAVR and on removal of catheters
- Amount of IV fluids and blood products infused during CAVR
- Patient's hemodynamic and temperature response after CAVR is discontinued
- Unexpected outcomes
- Additional interventions

</td></tr>
</table>

References

1. Fritsch, D.E. (1995). Hypothermia in the trauma patient. *AACN Clin Issues Adv Pract Acute Crit Care,* 6, 196.
2. Gentilello, L.M. (1994). Practical approaches to hypothermia. *Adv Trauma Crit Care,* 9, 39.
3. Gentilello, L.M., et al. (1997). Is hypothermia in the victim of major trauma protective or harmful? *Ann Surg,* 226, 439.
4. Gubler, K.D., et al. (1994). The effect of hypothermia on dilutional coagulopathy. *J Trauma,* 36, 847.
5. Schulman, C.S., and Pierce, B. (1999). Continuous arteriovenous rewarming: A bedside technique. *Crit Care Nurse,* 19, 54.

Additional Readings

Rohrer, M.J., and Natale, A.M. (1992). Effect of hypothermia on the coagulation cascade. *Crit Care Med,* 20, 1402.
Stevens, T. (1993). Managing post-op hypothermia, rewarming, and its complications. *Crit Care Nurs Q,* 16, 60.

PROCEDURE **124**

Massive Infusion Devices

PURPOSE: Rapid infusers are used to warm and quickly infuse multiple units of blood and large amounts of intravenous (IV) fluids into patients who are hemodynamically unstable. Patients with trauma, severe gastrointestinal hemorrhage, postoperative hemorrhage, and severe intravascular losses, such as occurring from septic shock and burns, may require rapid administration of IV fluids to maintain homeostasis.

Christine S. Schulman

PREREQUISITE NURSING KNOWLEDGE

- Knowledge of aseptic technique and principles of fluid resuscitation and blood transfusions are essential.
- Use of a rapid infusion device, such as the one described in this procedure (Fig. 124-1), can warm and infuse fluids at rates from 75 to 30,000 ml/hr (Level 1, Inc., Rockland, MA). The tubing is made of soft plastic that expands to allow rapid infusion of fluids under pressure. Some rapid infusers include automated pressure chambers to compress IV bags. They allow for fast and easy bag changes and can accommodate both 1-L IV bags and 500-ml blood product bags. Pressure is maintained at a constant 300 mm Hg and is turned on and off via a simple toggle switch at the top of each pressure chamber. Older infusers simply have an IV pole from which to hang fluids, and separate inflatable pressure bags must be used.
- IV catheters for aggressive fluid resuscitation should have a large bore and short diameter to facilitate the rapid infusion of large volumes of IV fluids and blood products. Usually multiple IVs are used, including peripheral and central sites. Venous access may also be obtained surgically via a venous cutdown of the basilic or saphenous veins when peripheral access cannot be obtained.[6]
- Both crystalloid and colloid IV solutions are used for resuscitating hypovolemic, hemodynamically unstable patients. Whereas crystalloids directly increase the intravascular volume, colloids expand plasma volume by pulling interstitial fluid back into the vascular space via osmosis. Numerous crystalloid and colloid preparations are available in isotonic, hypotonic, and hypertonic preparations.
- Crystalloids and colloids must be replaced along with blood and blood products in the patient with ongoing hemorrhage. Preference for using either crystalloids or colloids varies among physicians and geographic regions around the United States.[6]
- Crystalloids most commonly used in aggressive fluid resuscitation for trauma and other severe hemorrhage are 0.9% normal saline and Ringer's lactated solution. Although both of these solutions are isotonic and suitable for restoring intravascular volume, the latter contains multiple electrolytes, similar in concentration to that of plasma, so that the patient's electrolytes remain closer to normal.
- The use of colloids such as albumin, dextran, and hetastarch will allow the effective restoration of intravascular volume with smaller amounts of fluid; however, these colloids coat red blood cells (RBCs) and platelets, which may result in type and crossmatch difficulties, as well as clotting problems. Even slight overresuscitation with colloids increases the risk for fluid overload and pulmonary edema.[6,7]
- Blood and blood products are natural colloids used to replace lost blood and restore coagulation factors. In the patient with significant ongoing hemorrhage, infusing blood and clotting factors is critical to restoring intravascular volume.

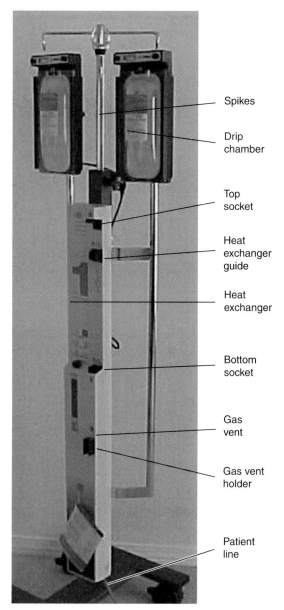

Spikes

Drip chamber

Top socket

Heat exchanger guide

Heat exchanger

Bottom socket

Gas vent

Gas vent holder

Patient line

FIGURE 124-1 Level 1 rapid infuser. *(Courtesy Level 1, Inc., Rockland, MA.)*

Type O-negative blood is the universal donor for all patients and can be given in extreme emergencies before the completion of typing and crossmatching. Packed RBCs and whole blood are used to replace oxygen-carrying components; fresh-frozen plasma, platelets, and cryoprecipitate are used to replace essential clotting factors (see Procedure 121).[6]

- When large volumes of IV fluids are being infused into patients, the fluids must be warmed to prevent hypothermia. (Although institutions vary in what constitutes large volumes, a good rule of thumb is to institute fluid rewarming measures when more than 2 L of fluid are required in less than 1 hour.)

- Hypothermia is a common consequence of aggressive fluid resuscitation and has serious physiologic consequences. Infusion of cold fluids can rapidly cool the

patient's body temperature to the point at which cardiovascular, neurologic, gastrointestinal, metabolic, and pulmonary disturbances result. Hypothermia-induced coagulopathies will exacerbate any ongoing hemorrhage and contribute to intravascular volume loss. Also, a left shift of the oxygen-hemoglobin dissociation curve occurs in hypothermic patients and in patients who receive large amounts of banked blood; thus hemoglobin increases its affinity for oxygen and will not release it to the tissues, potentially resulting in cellular hypoxia. Continuous arteriovenous rewarming (CAVR) and other interventions to minimize or reverse heat loss may be necessary if the patient's core temperature drops below 34.5°C[3-5] (see Procedures 95 and 123).

- Patients who have received multiple transfusions and aggressive fluid resuscitation are at risk for multiple complications as a result of being in shock, as well as from the fluids and blood products themselves. These sequelae may include fluid overload, adult respiratory distress syndrome, acute tubular necrosis, hypothermia, hypokalemia, hypocalcemia, hemolytic and allergic reactions, and air embolism.[7]

- Using systolic BP as a parameter to guide resuscitation may result in a patient who is underresuscitated. Catecholamine-induced vasoconstriction seen with shock, pain, anxiety, and hypothermia causes an increase in vascular tone that may not reflect true volume states. Multiple parameters must be evaluated to correctly determine a patient's resuscitation status.[1,8,9]

- Some recent literature suggests that there is no difference in mortality when controlled fluid resuscitation is used compared with aggressive fluid therapy. There is new evidence suggesting that forcing a systolic BP over 90 mm Hg with aggressive fluid resuscitation does not necessarily improve regional perfusion. Some researchers also believe that higher blood pressures may flush away newly formed clots from bleeding sites, promoting continued hemorrhage.[2,10]

EQUIPMENT

- Rapid infuser (see Fig. 124-1)
- Disposable fluid administration sets (Fig. 124-2)
- Replaceable filter with gas vent (Fig. 124-3)
- IV fluids or blood products as prescribed
- Sterile or distilled water for warmer
- Nonsterile gloves

PATIENT AND FAMILY EDUCATION

- Explain the need for rapid infusion of fluids, the purpose of warming fluids, and how the equipment operates.
  ➤*Rationale:* Decreases patient and family anxiety about unfamiliar equipment at the bedside.

- Explain that preventing hypothermia is among the top priorities in the resuscitation of the patient.
  ➤*Rationale:* Helps the patient and family understand the plan of care.

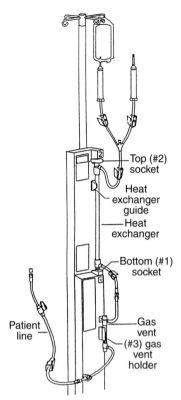

FIGURE 124-2 Placement of tubing in Level 1 rapid infuser. *(Courtesy Level 1, Inc., Rockland, MA.)*

PATIENT ASSESSMENT AND PREPARATION

Patient Assessment

- Assess blood pressure, heart rate, respiratory rate, peripheral pulses, and level of consciousness. ➤➤*Rationale:* Necessary to determine the severity of the patient's volume depletion and shock.
- Assess temperature using a tympanic thermometer, bladder probe, or pulmonary artery catheter. ➤➤*Rationale:* Necessary to assess for the development of hypothermia while large volumes of fluids are infused. Core temperatures most accurately reflect true body temperature.
- Assess patient history, including precipitating events, surgical and medical interventions thus far, and history of cardiac problems. ➤➤*Rationale:* Identifies potential or actual need for massive fluid resuscitation and risk for fluid overload.
- Assess hemodynamic parameters, including baseline central venous pressure (CVP) and, if available, pulmonary artery pressure (PAP), pulmonary capillary wedge pressure (PCWP), cardiac output (CO) and cardiac index (CI), systemic vascular resistance (SVR), and mixed venous oxygen saturation (Svo_2). Assessment of right ventricular ejection fraction, oxygen delivery and consumption, and oxygen extraction ratio should also be included if the technology is available. ➤➤*Rationale:* Provides baseline information about patient's preload, afterload, and cardiac contractility.

- Assess laboratory values to include arterial blood gases, serum electrolytes, serum lactate, base deficit, hemoglobin, hematocrit, and coagulation studies. ➤➤*Rationale:* Measures baseline oxygenation, presence of metabolic acidosis, severity of ongoing hemorrhage, and severity of coagulopathy so that the need for intervention and the effectiveness of interventions can be determined.
- Assess patency of multiple large-bore IV sites. ➤➤*Rationale:* Multiple sites are often necessary to infuse enough fluids and blood products to support the patient's vital signs. Extra sites in addition to those used for rapid infusion should be kept patent in case one of the other sites becomes nonfunctional or is accidentally pulled out.

Patient Preparation

- Ensure that the patient and family understand the need and purpose for rapid infusion. Answer questions as they arise and reinforce information as needed. ➤➤*Rationale:* Evaluates and reinforces understanding of previously taught information.
- Place additional peripheral IV sites. ➤➤*Rationale:* Aggressive fluid resuscitation requires additional IV access besides the one site being used with the rapid infuser. Backup IV sites can be used if other sites infiltrate or become pulled out; extra sites may also be used to infuse medications, such as vasopressors, that should be kept separate from rapid infusion lines. Ideal sites for large IV catheter access are the antecubital fossae, saphenous veins, and the veins of the forearm and upper arm.
- Assist the physician or advanced practice nurse with placement of central venous access or pulmonary artery catheter or both. ➤➤*Rationale:* Allows for the assessment of volume status before and after infusing fluids and blood products. Allows for assessment of core temperature with pulmonary artery catheter thermistor. Provides central venous access in the event vasoactive medications are needed.
- Place an automatic blood pressure monitor on the patient's arm that is not being infused with the rapid infusion device. Set it to check blood pressure every 5 minutes. ➤➤*Rationale:* Provides assessment of patient's hemodynamics and response to fluid replacement. This is used temporarily until an arterial line can be placed by the physician or advanced practice nurse.
- Assist the physician or advanced practice nurse with placement of an arterial line. ➤➤*Rationale:* Allows for continuous assessment of the blood pressure during resuscitation and provides convenient access for blood sampling.
- Obtain a blood sample for type and crossmatch. Two tubes should be sent if a large volume of blood is expected to be transfused. ➤➤*Rationale:* Prepares blood for transfusion.
- Obtain baseline hematocrit, chemistry panel, and coagulation studies. Repeat, as ordered, every 15-60 minutes until hemorrhage is controlled. ➤➤*Rationale:* Guides proper replacement of blood, blood products, and essential electrolytes.

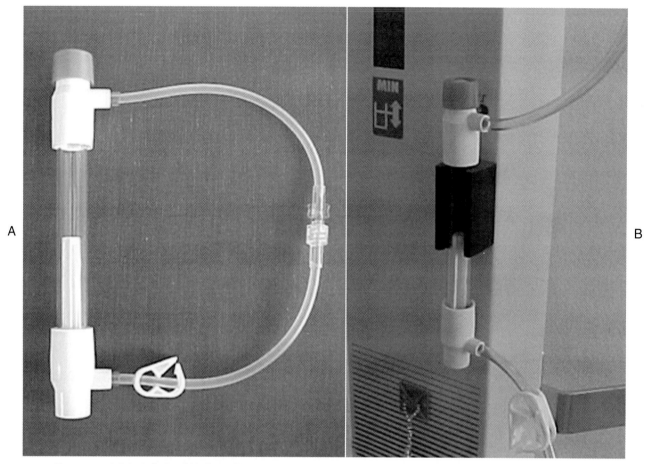

FIGURE 124-3 **A,** Rapid infuser filter showing male/female connecting ends on the right. **B,** Insertion of the filter in the Level 1 rapid infuser with the clamp open. *(Courtesy Level 1, Inc., Rockland, MA.)*

- Place a Foley catheter. ➥*Rationale:* Patients who require aggressive fluid resuscitation should have a Foley catheter placed to determine volume status and end-organ perfusion.

- Cover the patient with warm cotton blankets or a warm-air blanket. Cover the patient's head with a warmed blanket, a towel, or an aluminum cap. ➥*Rationale:* Minimizes additional heat loss.

Procedure for Massive Infusion Devices

Steps	Rationale	Special Considerations
1. Wash hands and don gloves.	Reduces transmission of microorganisms; standard precautions.	
2. Verify order for infusion of IV fluids and blood products and use of a fluid warmer.	Prevents unnecessary blood product or IV fluid administration.	The order from the physician or advanced practice nurse should include volume and type of additional IV fluids and blood products, laboratory work, and rationale for using a fluid warmer or rapid infuser.

Procedure continues on the following page

Procedure for Massive Infusion Devices—*Continued*

Steps	Rationale	Special Considerations
3. Turn on device.	Allows system to warm before moving fluid through the warming chamber.	
4. Open Y-set fluid administration package provided by the manufacturer. Close all clamps.	Prevents accidental spillage of blood or fluid. Prevents flow of fluid through circuit before machine is warmed.	
5. Spike fluid or blood with both sides of the Y-set.	Allows for smooth transition from an empty bag to the next bag.	
6. Hang fluid bags on small hooks inside the rapid infuser pressure chambers, leaving the chamber doors open (see Fig. 124-1) or place fluid bags in separate pressure bags.	It is easier to clear the tubing of air if the tubing is primed while the bags are still unpressurized.	Autotransfusion bags will not fit into the pressure chambers.
7. Push the bottom end of the heat exchanger rod *firmly* into the bottom socket, and snap the heat exchanger into the guide (see Fig. 124-2).	The bottom of the heat exchanger must be firmly placed or it will not fit into the top socket.	Being too gentle will result in improper placement of the tubing, and the warmer will not run.
8. Slide the top socket up and place the top end of the exchanger into the placement tract.	Locks the warming chamber into place at both the top and bottom sockets.	
9. Slide the top heat exchanger socket down over the heat exchanger tube until the pole latch clicks into place.		
10. Snap the gas vent filter into the holder on the lower portion of the pole assembly with the orange end up (see Fig. 124-3).	Filters air and blood clots from tubing.	Will only fit into the machine one way because the tubing is not long enough to be placed incorrectly.
11. Squeeze drip chambers so that they are half full.	Minimizes entrapment of bubbles in the tubing. Allows visualization of the drip chamber so that drip rate can be assessed.	
12. Open the clamp on one side of the Y-set.	Make sure that only one side of the Y tubing is open during priming; otherwise, fluid will be pumped from one bag to the other and not through the tubing.	
13. Remove the male Luer-Lok cap at the end of the IV tubing; open the clamps.	Will not prime unless the end cap has been removed.	
14. Remove the filter from its holder and invert it. Prime the tubing; close the roller clamp. Turn the filter back over and replace it in its holder.	Prevents entrapment of large amounts of air.	
15. Tap the filter or air eliminator against the cabinet several times. Monitor fluid line for bubbles during use.	Releases any residual trapped air.	Never administer fluids if there are air bubbles between the filter chamber and the patient connection. Run IV fluid into the trash container to rid tubing of any residual air. When no more bubbles are observed leaving the gas vent filter, all the air has been vented from the filter or air eliminator.

Procedure **for Massive Infusion Devices**—*Continued*

Steps	Rationale	Special Considerations
16. Open the roller clamp partially and slowly infuse fluid.	Infusing slowly will allow for assessment of any air bubbles. The air filter will eliminate bubbles in the tubing.	If unable to clear line of air and there is more than ¼ inch of air at the top of the filter, replace the filter.
17. Replace male Luer-Lok cap at the end of the tubing; close the clamps.		
18. Close the pressure chamber doors and latch.	Positions fluid bags for pressurization when the machines are turned on and the pressure switch is activated.	Be certain that the latch is secure before the chamber is pressurized.
19. Perform all function and alarm checks as per manufacturer's instructions.	Validates proper equipment function.	
20. Wait for the temperature readout to reach the operating temperature of 41°C.	Prevents hypothermia by making sure the chamber is warm before fluids are run through it and into the patient.	
21. Flip the toggle switch at the top of the pressure chamber to ON/+ or inflate the separate pressure bags.	Pressurizes the chambers.	The pressure automatically inflates to 300 mm Hg. Fluids will infuse via gravity flow without being pressurized; however, high flow rates cannot be achieved unless the pressure bags are inflated.
22. Connect the distal end of the tubing to the patient IV.	Prepares for infusion.	
23. Open the roller clamp to infuse the fluid.	Fluids or blood products will now infuse under pressure.	It is best to infuse one side at a time, especially when blood products are infusing, to prevent mixing of fluids and blood products. The pressure system is designed to leave a small volume remaining to prevent air emboli.
24. Set the rate by gradually opening the clamp.	Fluids given via rapid infusers are administered as boluses over short periods; roller clamps are usually left wide open until the bolus is complete.	If a slower bolus is desired, adjust the roller clamp to decrease the flow of fluid.

Changing the Bags

1. Close the top clamp on the side of the Y-connector with the empty fluid bag.		
2. Open the clamp on the side of the Y-connector with the full fluid bag; infuse the fluid.	Keeping one side of the Y-connector spiked with fluid ready to infuse is helpful when patients are severely unstable and need immediate boluses of fluid.	
3. Turn the ON/+ switch above the pressure chamber to the OFF position and remove the empty bag.	Releases pressure from the pressure chamber.	
4. Replace the empty fluid bag with a full one.	It is important to have the next bag of IV fluid ready to infuse to avoid delays in infusion in case the patient's blood pressure falls precipitously.	

Procedure continues on the following page

Procedure for Massive Infusion Devices—*Continued*

Steps	Rationale	Special Considerations
5. Close the pressure chamber door and latch; flip the control switch above the pressure chamber to ON/+.	Repressurizes chamber.	

Replacing the Filter or Air Eliminator

Steps	Rationale	Special Considerations
1. Close the clamps on the disposable fluid administration set just proximal to the filter and between the filter and the patient connection.	The filter should be replaced after 3 hours of use, after 4 units of blood, or if fluid rate slows secondary to clotting.	
2. Remove the old filter or air eliminator from the holder and place the new filter or air eliminator in the holder.	Keep the old filter or air eliminator connected to the disposable fluid administration set until ready to change to new one to minimize potential for contaminating exposed tubing ends.	
3. Disconnect the old filter or air eliminator at the upper Luer-Lok and connect the tubing to the new filter.		
4. Disconnect the patient line Luer-Lok from the old filter or air eliminator and connect to the new one.		
5. Open the clamp just proximal to the filter or air eliminator to restart fluid. Invert the filter until completely filled with fluid; then turn back to proper position and replace in holder. Open the clamp between the filter and the patient connection.	Infusion of fluid will resume.	
6. Remove the filter or air eliminator from the holder and tap until all bubbles are eliminated and reinsert. Check patient line for bubbles before opening the roller clamp.	Facilitates removal of bubbles.	If air bubbles are present, disconnect the tubing from the patient and infuse into the trash container until the line is clear of air. Reconnect to the patient and resume the infusion. If alarm sounds after setup, check to make sure filter is properly snapped into place.

Troubleshooting Alarms

Steps	Rationale	Special Considerations
1. If the alarm sounds and the disposable light is illuminated, check to make sure the disposable tubing set is properly placed in the machine.	The system will not run if the disposable tubing is not completely set into the machine.	The tubing set can become inadvertently dislodged.
2. If the alarm sounds and the water level light is illuminated, check the water level in the chamber and replace as needed with sterile or distilled water.	The system will not run if the water level is too low.	
3. If the system alarms "overtemp," turn the machine off and use a different rapid infuser.	Fluids inadequately warmed will cause hypothermia. Fluids overly warmed will cause hemolysis of red blood cells.	Notify biomedical engineering of the problem.

Transporting a Patient With a Rapid Infuser

Steps	Rationale	Special Considerations
1. Turn the rapid infuser off.	If the infuser is still on when the administration set is removed from its holder, water will spurt out of the warming chamber and aluminium tube.	

Procedure for Massive Infusion Devices—*Continued*

Steps	Rationale	Special Considerations
2. Remove the disposable administration set from its holder on the infuser and place it in the bed alongside the patient or hang it on the transport IV pole.	The rapid infusers described here do not operate on a battery. Fluids will infuse via gravity, or separate pressure bags can be used.	Fluids will run briskly via gravity drainage. If pressure is still necessary to infuse fluids, separate pressure bags will need to be used as long as the machine is not plugged in. Interventions to minimize heat loss must be in place while the infuser is not plugged in: aluminum head covering, warmed cotton blankets, and warm-air blankets will help prevent heat loss. Removing the administration set from the machine and transporting the patient separately from the infuser is less awkward and will minimize the risk for pulling out the IV lines during transport.
3. Plug the infuser into an electric outlet once you reach the intended destination.	Establishes power source.	
4. Return administration set into the infuser. Turn the machine on. Return fluid bags to pressure chambers.	The infuser is now ready to repressurize the chambers and warm the fluid. Any bubbles will be eliminated by the filter.	If bubbles are not removed and more than ¼ inch of air is at the top of the filter, the filter must be replaced.

Expected Outcomes

- Patient's blood pressure and heart rate return to baseline.
- Patient's core temperature remains above 36.0°C.
- CVP, PAP, PCWP, CO, CI, and SVR reflect return of normovolemia and hemodynamic stability.
- IV sites remain patent and infuse fluids easily.
- Urine output at least 0.5 ml/kg/hr.

Unexpected Outcomes

- Blood pressure remains below baseline despite multiple liters of fluid and blood products.
- Core temperature falls below 36.0°C so that more aggressive rewarming interventions become necessary.
- Hypothermia-induced coagulopathy develops as temperature falls below 34.5°C.
- Inability to restore normal intravascular status occurs, as seen by CVP less than 6, PCWP less than 6, CO less than 4 L/min, CI less than 2 L/min/m², or SVR greater than 1500 dynes/sec.
- Infiltration of IV sites occurs. Clotting of filter occurs.
- Anuria or oliguria with urinary output less than 0.5 ml/kg/hr occurs.

Patient Monitoring and Care

Steps	Rationale	Reportable Conditions
		These conditions should be reported if they persist despite nursing interventions.
1. Monitor the patient's vital signs every 5 to 15 minutes as indicated. As the patient becomes more stable, assessment of vital signs may be done less frequently (every 15 to 30 minutes until the blood pressure remains stable for more than 2 hours).	Determines severity of shock, responsiveness to fluids and blood products, and the need for additional fluids.	• Systolic blood pressure below 90 mm Hg despite fluid administration • Abnormal vital signs
2. Assess the patient's core temperature every 15 to 30 minutes.	Patients who are in severe shock have impaired thermogenesis.	• Worsening hypothermia or unrelieved hypothermia

Procedure continues on the following page

Patient Monitoring and Care—*Continued*

Steps	Rationale	Reportable Conditions
	This, in combination with the infusion of inadequately warmed fluids, will lead to hypothermia. Hypothermia-induced coagulopathies begin at a core temperature of 34.5°C and will exacerbate any hemorrhage already occurring. Also, severe physiologic complications from hypothermia, such as cardiovascular instability, electrolyte changes, urine concentration problems, and shifts in the oxygen-hemoglobin dissociation curve, will affect the patient's ability to respond to physiologic stress. Prevention of hypothermia is a critical goal for patients undergoing massive fluid resuscitation.[2,5]	
3. Assess the integrity of IV sites every 15 minutes.	IV sites under pressure are at higher risk for infiltration. Also, lines can be inadvertently pulled out during x-ray filming, turning, and other aspects of patient care during a massive resuscitation. It is recommended that multiple IV sites be available at all times in the event an IV infiltrates or is pulled out.	
4. Assess hemodynamic parameters every 15 to 30 minutes.	Determines intravascular volume status and responsiveness to interventions. New research suggests that patients may still be inadequately resuscitated even though vital signs, urine output, and hemodynamic parameters have returned to normal. Recent studies suggest that a complete clinical picture (including laboratory tests in conjunction with vital signs, urine output, and hemodynamic parameters) is the best way to determine whether a patient has been adequately resuscitated.[6]	• Abnormal trends in hemodynamic monitoring
5. Assess urine output every 30 to 60 minutes.	Urine output is an assessment of end-organ perfusion. If there is little or no urine being produced, it is assumed that the kidneys are not being perfused and, therefore, other major viscera are also probably not being adequately perfused. Trauma to the urinary tract	• Urine output less than 0.5 ml/kg/hr

Patient Monitoring and Care—*Continued*

Steps	Rationale	Reportable Conditions
	may interfere with accurate assessment of urine output because clots may block urine drainage and laceration to ureters may result in extravasation of urine into the peritoneum.	
6. Draw hemoglobin, hematocrit, and coagulation studies as prescribed. These are usually measured every 30 to 60 minutes or after transfusion of blood and blood components.	Determines presence of ongoing blood loss and coagulopathy.[2-5]	• Abnormal hemoglobin, hematocrit, and coagulation results
7. Draw arterial blood gases and lactic acid as prescribed and indicated.	Determines persistence of metabolic acidosis and identifies need for additional interventions to improve perfusion to major organs.[6]	• Abnormal laboratory results
8. Draw electrolytes as prescribed.	Patients undergoing large-volume resuscitation are at risk for hypokalemia, hypomagnesemia, hypocalcemia, and hypophosphatemia.[2]	• Abnormal laboratory results

Documentation

Documentation should include the following:

- Patient and family education
- Rationale for using the rapid infuser
- Blood pressure, heart rate, respiratory rate, lung sounds, and peripheral pulses throughout the resuscitation
- The patient's core temperature while the rapid infusers are used
- Hemodynamic parameters, including CVP, PAP, PCWP, CO, CI, and SVR
- Urine output, estimated blood loss, other measured output

- Laboratory results, including arterial blood gases, hematocrit, hemoglobin, electrolytes, and lactic acid
- Appearance of IV sites
- IV insertions
- Total IV fluids and blood products in intake and output record
- Unexpected outcomes
- Additional interventions

References

1. Abou-Khalil, B., et al. (1994). Hemodynamic responses to shock in young trauma patients: Need for invasive monitoring. *Crit Care Med, 22,* 633.
2. Buris, D., et al. (1999). Controlled resuscitation of uncontrolled hemorrhagic shock. *J Trauma, 46,* 216.
3. Fritsch, D.E. (1995). Hypothermia in the trauma patient. *AACN Clin Issues Adv Pract Acute Crit Care, 6,* 196-211.
4. Gentilello, L.M. (1994). Practical approaches to hypothermia. *Adv Trauma Crit Care, 9,* 39.
5. Gubler, K.D., et al. (1994). The effect of hypothermia on dilutional coagulopathy. *J Trauma, 36,* 847.
6. Koran, Z., and Newberry, L. (2003). Vascular access and fluid replacement. In: Emergency Nurses Association and Newberry, L., eds. *Sheehy's Emergency Nursing.* 5th ed. St. Louis: Mosby, 147.
7. McQuillan, K.A. (2002). Initial management of traumatic shock. In: McQuillan, K.A., et al. *Trauma Nursing: From Resuscitation Through Rehabilitation.* 3rd ed. Philadelphia: W.B. Saunders, 151.
8. Porter, J.M., and Ivatury, R.R. (1998). In search of the optimal end points of resuscitation in trauma patients: A review. *J Trauma, 44,* 908.
9. Scalea, T.M., et al. (1994). Resuscitation of multiple trauma and head injury: Role of crystalloid fluids and inotropes. *Crit Care Med, 20,* 1610.
10. Smail, N., et al. (1998). Resuscitation after uncontrolled venous hemorrhage: Does increased resuscitation volume improve regional perfusion? *J Trauma, 44,* 701.

Additional Readings

Schulman, C.S. (2002). End points of resuscitation: Choosing the right parameters to monitor. *Dimens Crit Care Nurs, 21,* 2.
Stevens, T. (1993). Managing post-op hypothermia, rewarming, and its complications. *Crit Care Nurs Q, 16,* 60.

PROCEDURE **125**

Transfusion Reaction Management

PURPOSE: Prompt recognition and treatment of a transfusion reaction may minimize the development of life-threatening sequelae.

Maribeth Wooldridge-King

PREREQUISITE NURSING KNOWLEDGE

- A *transfusion reaction* is defined as "any unfavorable event occurring in a patient during or following transfusion of blood or blood components that can be related to that transfusion. Any adverse change in a patient's condition should be considered a possible symptom of a transfusion reaction and evaluated."[1] Transfusion reactions are classified as immediate or delayed. Immediate transfusion reactions occur during the transfusion or within several hours after the transfusion has been completed.

- Immediate transfusion reactions include acute hemolytic reactions, immune-mediated platelet alloimmunization, bacterial contamination, febrile nonhemolytic reactions, transfusion-related acute lung injury (TRALI), allergic reactions, circulatory overload, hypothermia, metabolic complications, and "citrate" intoxication (hypocalcemia).

- An acute hemolytic transfusion reaction is the destruction of transfused red blood cells, usually caused by an incompatibility of antigen on the donor's cells with antibody in the recipient's circulation. Acute hemolytic transfusion reactions are most commonly caused by the administration of ABO-incompatible blood due to an error in the identification process. Serologic incompatibility that is not detected during pretransfusion testing is a much less common cause of acute hemolysis. Identifiers of the patient and blood component and the accompanying forms and labels should be reviewed immediately to detect possible errors in the identification process.

- In immune-mediated platelet alloimmunization HLA antibodies are produced in the recipient to HLA or platelet-specific antigens on transfused platelets. The survival time of the transfused platelets is markedly shortened. Nonimmune factors that may also contribute to shortened platelet survival include splenomegaly, sepsis,

fever, idiopathic thrombocytopenia purpura (ITP) and disseminated intravascular coagulation (DIC). By evaluating platelet recovery 10-60 minutes after platelet transfusion, it is possible to distinguish immune versus nonimmune refractoriness. In immune refractory states, there is poor platelet incremental change in the early posttransfusion period. In nonimmune refractory states, platelet recovery within 1 hour of infusion may be adequate, but long-term survival (24 hours) is reduced. Serologic testing can identify the presence of alloimmunization. HLA-matched platelets may be requested for patients with immune-mediated platelet destruction. HLA-matched platelets are not more effective and thus not indicated when the refractoriness is caused by nonimmune events.

- Bacterial contamination occurs rarely but can result in acute, severe, life-threatening effects, including severe chills, hypotension, and circulatory collapse. A temperature elevation of greater than 2°C (or greater than 3°F) during or immediately following a transfusion is suggestive of bacterial contamination and/or endotoxin reaction. Platelets stored at room temperature, frozen components thawed by water bath immersion, and red cell components stored at 1-6°C for several weeks have been associated with bacterial contamination. Both gram-positive and gram-negative organisms have been implicated in the septic reactions.

- Febrile nonhemolytic reactions, occurring in about 1% of transfusions, manifest with a temperature increase of more than 1°C (or 2°F) during or shortly following a transfusion when no other pyretic stimulus is identified. This reaction is thought to represent the action of antibodies against white cells or the actions of cytokines either present in the transfused component or generated by the recipient to the transfused component. These reactions occur more frequently in patients who have become alloimmunized by either transfusion or pregnancy. There are no pre- or posttransfusion tests to predict or prevent febrile reactions. Patients with severe, repeated febrile reactions may need to have leukocyte-reduced components.

- In transfusion-related acute lung injury (TRALI), a massive leakage of fluid and protein into the alveolar spaces and interstitium occurs as a result of the increased permeability of the pulmonary microcirculation, usually within 6 hours of the transfusion. Many cases of TRALI are associated with the presence of granulocyte antibodies in the donor or recipient. The exact mechanism of this reaction is not clear. Treatment consists of aggressive respiratory support.

- Allergic reactions usually consist of urticaria but may occasionally include wheezing and angioedematous reactions. Allergic reactions usually respond to antihistamines but may occasionally require corticosteroids and epinephrine in more severe cases. No laboratory tests are available to predict or prevent allergic reactions. Anaphylactic reactions are rare and most have been reported in those patients with IgA-deficiencies who have IgA antibodies of the IgE class. These patients may not have been previously transfused and become symptomatic after the infusion of a very small amount of IgA-containing plasma in any blood component. Anaphylactic reactions are life-threatening and require immediate treatment with corticosteroids and epinephrine with progression to code management.

- Circulatory overload leading to pulmonary edema is associated with the rapid infusion or the transfusion of an excessive volume of blood components. The elderly and those with chronic severe anemia (low red cell count associated with a high plasma volume) are at a particular risk. The acute expansion of the intravascular volume may exceed the ability of the cardiovascular system to compensate. Signs and symptoms include the onset of a sudden severe headache, dyspnea, tachycardia, tachypnea, crackles, and increased filling pressures, that is, central venous pressure (CVP), pulmonary artery pressure (PAP), and pulmonary capillary wedge pressure (PCWP). Patients should be given diuretics to decrease intravascular volume and in some cases the transfusion may need to be stopped. For patients at risk for or with a history of fluid overload, the blood bank may be asked to divide the unit into smaller aliquots so that the entire unit of blood can then be administered over a longer period of time.

- Hypothermia can result in cardiac arrhythmias or cardiac arrest. The rapid infusion of large volumes of refrigerated blood lowers internal body temperature and may be compounded in patients experiencing shock or undergoing surgical or anesthetic procedures that lower body temperature or disrupt thermoregulation. Warming of blood components should be considered when rapid infusion of blood components is necessary and must always be done using an FDA-approved warming device to avoid hemolysis (see Procedure 123). Hot tap water and microwaves should never be used to warm blood.

- While rare, citrate "toxicity" (hypocalcemia) occurs when there is decreased ionized calcium as a result of large quantities of circulating citrate anticoagulant. Citrate is a component of the preservative used in blood storage that chelates calcium and interferes with the coagulation cascade. The citrate is rapidly metabolized by the liver, and thus this complication is usually mild and self-limiting. However, if prolonged Q-T intervals or signs of tetany are observed, ionized calcium levels should be evaluated and calcium replacement initiated as indicated. Calcium should never be added to a unit of blood. Patients with severe liver disease or those with inadequate hepatic blood flow receiving rapid, large volume transfusions are at particular risk for citrate toxicity.

- Delayed transfusion reactions include delayed hemolytic reactions, transmission of infection (hepatitis, AIDS, malaria, syphilis, bacteria or viruses), posttransfusion purpura (PTP) and graft-versus-host disease.

- Delayed hemolytic reactions generally present 2 to 14 days following transfusion; they are usually benign and require no treatment. These reactions reflect the production of antibodies by red cell alloimmunized patients to antigens on transfused red cells. The antibodies reach a significant circulating level while the transfused cells are still in the patient's circulation. Signs and symptoms may include an unexplained fever, development of a positive DAT (direct antiglobulin test), unexplained decrease in hemoglobin/hematocrit, and an elevated LDH (lactic dehydrogenase) or bilirubin. Hemoglobinemia and hemoglobinuria, though uncommon, may also occur.

- Transmission of infectious agents may occur because the product is made from human blood. Procedures to screen donors and test the blood reduce but do not totally eliminate the risk for transmitting known and unknown infectious agents. Every effort is made to screen out potential donors with an increased risk for infection with HIV, HTLV, hepatitis, syphilis, and other agents to minimize risk to the blood supply. Cytomegalovirus (CMV) may be present in white cell–containing components from donors infected with this virus, which can persist for a lifetime despite serum antibodies. The administration of CMV-seronegative components or leukocyte-reduced components is advised for low-birth-weight (less than 1200 g) premature infants born to CMV-seronegative mothers and in certain CMV-seronegative immunocompromised patients.

- Posttransfusion purpura (PTP) is a rare complication occurring 7-10 days following blood transfusion in which there is a dramatic and sudden but self-limiting thrombocytopenia in a patient with a history of sensitization by either pregnancy or transfusion. Both autologous and allogeneic platelets are destroyed. High-dose immune globulin intravenous (IGIV) may promptly correct the thrombocytopenia.

- Graft-versus-host disease (GVHD) is a rare but extremely serious condition in which viable T lymphocytes in the transfused component engraft and react against tissue antigens in the recipient. It can occur following the transfusion of any blood component that contains even minute amounts of viable T lymphocytes. Even those components that have been leukocyte-reduced contain sufficient residual T lymphocytes to generate a reaction. Severely immunocompromised patients are at greatest risk (fetuses receiving intrauterine transfusions, recipients of transplanted marrow or peripheral blood progenitor cells, and those with severe immunodeficiency conditions). Irradiating blood components is the only known method of inactivating T lymphocytes and is the only approved means to prevent GVHD.

- Nonimmunologic hemolysis is a rare event. This complication can occur as the result of red blood cells that are subjected to excessive heat from a non-FDA approved warming device or method, the administration of hypotonic intravenous fluid concurrent with the red cell transfusion, or the transfusion of red cells under high pressure through a small-gauge or defective catheter. Other causes include effects of drugs coadministered with the transfusion, the effects of bacterial toxins, thermal damage (freezing or overheating) to blood components, or metabolic damage to transfused cells secondary to hemoglobinopathies or enzyme deficiencies.

- Metabolic complications can occur with large-volume transfusion, particularly in those with liver or kidney disease or those with preexisting circulatory or metabolic problems. These derangements include acidosis or alkalosis, reflecting the changing concentrations of citric acid and its conversion to pyruvate and bicarbonate. Hyper- or hypokalemia may also occur.

- Any fatality resulting from a complication of blood component transfusion is required to be reported to the FDA within 24 hours.

EQUIPMENT

- Intravenous solution (0.9% normal saline [NS])
- Intravenous administration set (macrodrip tubing)
- Stethoscope
- Blood pressure cuff or arterial line
- Cardiac monitor
- Pulse oximeter
- Urine specimen container
- Vacutainer holder and needle
- Blood specimen tubes
- Thermometer
- Nonsterile gloves
- Specimen labels
- Laboratory requisitions
  Additional equipment, as needed, includes the following:
- Flowmeter for oxygen
- Nasal cannula or Venturi mask
- Emergency drug box
- Emergency cart

PATIENT AND FAMILY EDUCATION

- Explain that the patient may be experiencing a transfusion reaction. ➥*Rationale:* Promotes patient and family understanding of transfusion reaction.

- Once the patient is stabilized, instruct the patient and family to include the occurrence of a transfusion reaction on the patient's medical history. ➥*Rationale:* Alerts health care providers to the potential need for premedication, the need for specially prepared component therapy, or the increased risk for transfusion reactions with future transfusions.

- Evaluate the patient's need for long-term blood or blood component administration. ➥*Rationale:* Patient may need to carry a record of transfusions containing the history of severity of transfusion reactions, the requirement for specially processed blood or blood components and/or premedications to prevent or minimize a transfusion reaction.

PATIENT ASSESSMENT AND PREPARATION

Patient Assessment

- Note the severity of previous transfusion history/ reactions, whether the patient has ever been pregnant, and the treatment to which patient responded. ➥*Rationale:* Allows the nurse to anticipate what treatment modalities may be required to interrupt this reaction.

- Assess for signs and symptoms of a transfusion reaction, particularly during the first 15 minutes of transfusion administration (Table 125-1). ➥*Rationale:* The first 10 to 15 minutes of any transfusion are most critical in regard to stopping the transfusion and limiting the exposure to the offending antigen or infectious agent.

- Assess oxygenation (SaO_2) via pulse oximeter or arterial blood gas (ABG). ➥*Rationale:* Catecholamine release as a response to the antigen-antibody reaction produces vasoconstriction in the lungs; the resulting ventilation perfusion abnormality may require oxygen administration or intubation and mechanical ventilation.

- Assess vital signs, including temperature, blood pressure, heart rate, respiratory rate, breath sounds, and if applicable, filling pressures (i.e., central venous pressure [CVP], pulmonary artery pressure [PAP], pulmonary capillary wedge pressure [PCWP]). ➥*Rationale:* Transfusion reactions will cause deviations from baseline (pretransfusion) vital signs (see Table 125-1).

Patient Preparation

- Ensure that the patient and family understand preprocedural teaching. Answer questions as they arise and reinforce information as needed. ➥*Rationale:* Evaluates and reinforces understanding of previously taught information.

- Ensure or reestablish patency of the peripheral intravenous line or central venous access device. ➥*Rationale:* Allows for infusion of crystalloid solution to support the patient's cardiovascular system and increases renal blood flow to prevent the development of acute tubular necrosis.

TABLE 125-1	Summary of Acute Transfusion Reactions				
Transfusion Reaction	**Frequency of Reaction**	**Potential Causes**	**Symptoms**	**Prevention**	**Treatment**
Febrile nonhemolytic transfusion reaction	1:5 platelets 1:10 RBCs	Recipient antibodies to donor leukocytes Bacterial contamination Inflammatory cytokine release	Increase in temperature 1°C (1.8°F) or greater within 2 hr after transfusion Chills	Premedicate with antipyretics	Antipyretics Antihistamines
Bacterial contamination	1:350 platelets 1:2,500,000 RBCs	Contamination of blood product during procurement, storage, preparation, or administration of product	Fever Chills Sepsis	Use aseptic technique when collecting blood product Properly store product Change blood tubing or filter every 4 hr Ensure transfusion takes no longer than 4 hr	Antibiotics Antipyretics
Transfusion-related acute lung injury	1:10,000 RBCs also with cryoprecipitate	Activation of complement and histamine release, resulting in increased pulmonary capillary permeability	Respiratory distress, which may be accompanied by: Fever Chills Cyanosis Hypotension	No known prevention; antihistamines and steroids may be helpful	Standard treatment of acute respiratory distress syndrome: Antipyretics Antihistamines Oxygen Fluid resuscitation Mechanical ventilation Vasopressors
Acute hemolytic reaction	1:25,000 RBCs	Administration of incompatible blood Preexisting antibodies against transfused RBCs, resulting in massive hemolysis Improper hemolysis administration (i.e., with dextrose solution)	Fever Chills Nausea Dyspnea Low back pain Hemoglobinurea Pain at infusion site Tachycardia Hypotension Cardiovascular collapse Renal failure Disseminated intravascular coagulopathy	Strictly adhere to institutional policy regarding collection of patients samples and administration of blood products Initiate transfusion of blood product slowly for the first 15 min Administer only with normal saline	Antipyretics Antihistamines Steroids Fluid resuscitation If progression to shock consider: Oxygen Epinephrine Diuretics Vasopressors
Urticarial reaction	1:1000 blood products	Recipient responds to donor proteins	Flushing Hives Itching	Transfuse plasma-free blood products Premedicate with antipyretics or antihistamines or both	Antipyretics Antihistamines
Anaphylaxis	1:1,150,000 blood products	Severe immune response to a foreign substance	Generalized flushing Dyspnea Stridor Chest pain Hypotension Nausea Abdominal cramps Loss of consciousness	Transfuse plasma-free blood products	Epinephrine Code management

RBC, red blood cell.
Adapted from Labovich, T.M. (1997). Transfusion therapy: Nursing implications. *Clin J Oncol Nurs, 3,* 63-4.

Procedure for Transfusion Reaction Management

Steps	Rationale	Special Considerations
1. **Stop the transfusion!** Notify the physician or advanced practice nurse.	Prevents additional exposure to offending antigen or infectious agent.	
2. Wash hands and don nonsterile gloves.	Reduces transmission of microorganisms; standard precautions.	
3. Disconnect the blood administration set from the primary intravenous line and cap with a sterile cap.	The remaining contents of the unit of blood are sent back to the blood bank with the administration set attached.	Institution policies and procedures regarding the disposition of the remaining unit contents may vary.
4. Replace primary intravenous tubing with a new macrodrip intravenous administration set.	Prevents the patient from receiving additional blood component that may still be in the primary tubing.	Macrodrip tubing is used for rapid volume replacement if needed.
5. Infuse crystalloid intravenous solution, usually 0.9% NS, to maintain a urine output of 100 ml/h for 24 hours or as prescribed.	Increases renal blood flow to prevent the development of acute tubular necrosis.	
6. Recheck identifiers, including the blood component label, transfusion slip, and patient's identification band to detect possible error.	The majority of acute hemolytic reactions are caused by the administration of incompatible blood due to an identification error.	
7. Obtain blood specimen(s) as per your institution's policy. Blood should be drawn from a site other than the transfusion site. If bacterial contamination is suspected, obtain a blood specimen for culture and sensitivity testing.	One sample is crossmatched with the pretransfusion sample to determine whether the correct blood was administered. The second sample is examined for hemolysis. If bacterial contamination is suspected, return blood component bag to the blood bank for culture.	Usually, blood specimens are sent to the blood bank with the suspect unit of blood or blood component. Indicate "Possible Transfusion Reaction" on the laboratory requisition.
8. Obtain urine specimen.	Determines presence of red blood cells or free hemoglobin.	
9. Complete the specific forms for a transfusion reaction.	Documents possibility of a transfusion reaction and the actions taken.	
10. Return the blood component to blood bank.	Allows the blood bank to confirm the presence or absence of a transfusion reaction.	Patients receiving multiple transfusions over time (e.g., patients with cancer or AIDS) may demonstrate signs and symptoms of a transfusion reaction; however, laboratory analysis may not verify that a reaction has occurred. You may be instructed to rehang the blood component and monitor the patient closely.
11. Discard used supplies and wash hands.	Reduces transmission of microorganisms; standard precautions.	
12. Document in patient record.		

Expected Outcomes

- Vital signs stable and within patient's baseline values
- Laboratory values within normal limits
- Renal function normal

Unexpected Outcomes

- Hemodynamic instability
- Abnormal laboratory values
- Impaired renal function
- Cardiopulmonary arrest

Patient Monitoring and Care

Steps	Rationale	Reportable Conditions
		These conditions should be reported if they persist despite nursing interventions.
1. Monitor the patient's vital signs and oxygenation as needed until stable.	Detects further compromise in cardiovascular status.	• Vital sign and Sao$_2$ abnormalities
2. Monitor and record the urinary output every hour for the next 6-12 hours.	Detects diminished renal blood flow or renal vasoconstriction, which may result in acute tubular necrosis.	• Decreasing urine output • Change in color of urine
3. Monitor blood urea nitrogen (BUN) and creatinine levels.		• Increasing BUN and creatinine
4. Monitor International Normalized Ratio (INR), prothrombin time (PT), partial thromboplastin time (PTT), and fibrinogen levels.	Extensive destruction of RBCs may result in DIC.	• Abnormal PT • Abnormal PTT • Abnormal INR • Abnormal fibrinogen levels
5. Monitor levels of lactate dehydrogenase (LDH).	LDH levels may rise markedly with lysis of red blood cells.	• Elevated LDH
6. If the patient develops signs or symptoms of shock or cardiovascular collapse, perform the following: A. Insert another large-bore IV catheter.	Allows for the rapid infusion of intravenous fluids and medications.	• Signs and symptoms of shock and cardiovascular collapse
B. Prepare and administer emergency medications as prescribed.	Supports cardiopulmonary systems.	
C. If bacterial contamination is suspected, obtain a blood specimen for culture and sensitivity testing. Return blood component bag to the blood bank for culture. Administer broad-spectrum antibiotics intravenously as prescribed.	An infusion of a contaminated unit of blood components will result in immediate signs and symptoms of shock.	• Continued fever
D. Administer oxygen therapy as prescribed. Initiate advanced cardiac life support (ACLS) protocol in the event of respiratory or cardiac arrest.	Corrects hypoxemia. Life-preserving intervention.	• Continued hypoxemia

Documentation

Documentation should include the following:

- Patient and family education
- Date and exact time of the signs and symptoms of a transfusion reaction
- Date and time infusion was discontinued
- Assessment findings
- Name of the physician or advanced practice nurse notified
- Unexpected outcomes
- Interventions taken
- Patient's response to the interventions

Reference

1. American Association of Blood Banks. (2002). *Primer of Blood Administration*. Bethesda, MD: The Association.

Additional Readings

American Association of Blood Banks. (2002). *Primer of Blood Administration*. Bethesda, MD, Dec. Available at: www.aabb.org.

American Association of Blood Banks, America's Blood Centers, and the American Red Cross. (2002). *Circular of Information for the Use of Human Blood and Blood Components*. Bethesda, MD: Author, July. Available at: www.aabb.org.

Brand, A. (2000). Immunologic aspects of blood transfusions. *Blood Review*, 14, 130-44. Available at: http://www.idealibrary.com.

Hollinger, F.B., and Kleinman, S. (2003). Transfusion transmission of West Nile virus: A merging of historical and contemporary perspectives. *Transfusion*, Aug, (43)8, 992-7.

National Institutes of Health (NIH) Clearing Center Nursing Department. (2000). *Procedure: Blood Product Administration*. Available at: www.cc.nih.gov/nursing.

U.S. Department of Health and Human Services: Food and Drug Administration Center for Biologics and Research (CBER). (2002). *Revised Preventive Measures to Reduce the Possible Risk of Transmission of Creutzfeldt-Jakob (CJD) and Variant Creutzfeldt-Jakob Disease (vCJD) by Blood and Blood Products*. Rockville, MD, Jan. Available at: http://www.fda.gov.cyber/guidelines.htm.

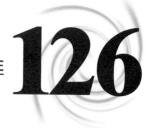

SECTION TWENTY

Special Hematologic
Procedures

PROCEDURE **126**

**Bone Marrow Biopsy and
Aspiration (Perform)**

P U R P O S E :   Bone marrow aspiration and biopsy are used to diagnose and classify various hematopoietic diseases, identify metastatic disease, monitor clinical response to treatment, and assess engraftment after stem cell transplant.

M.J. Heffernan

PREREQUISITE NURSING KNOWLEDGE

- Anatomy of the posterior and anterior iliac crest should be understood.
- Clinical and technical competence in performing a bone marrow aspirate and biopsy is necessary.
- Knowledge of sterile technique is essential.
- Institutional policies and procedures for administration of intravenous (IV) pharmacologic agents including conscious sedation (if indicated).
- Procedural care of the patient receiving conscious sedation (if indicated).
- Bone marrow aspirate is used to identify normal and abnormal hematopoietic elements. The aspirate is also used to identify malignant clones by flow cytometry, to identify chromosomal abnormalities that occur in hematologic malignancies, molecular diagnostic studies of gene re-arrangements and translocations, and to perform chimerism studies in patients after allogenic transplant.
- A bone marrow biopsy is used for morphologic analysis of hematopoietic cells and for assessing the architecture of the bone marrow that may be abnormal in certain disease states.

- Indications for bone marrow aspiration and biopsy include the following:
  - To diagnose a hematologic abnormality
  - To monitor a hematologic disease state after therapy
  - To rule out bone marrow metastasis before stem cell collection and for staging of various malignant states
  - In all patients after bone marrow transplant, to assess the status of engraftment
  - In patients after allogenic transplant, to assess for chimerism and immune reconstitution
  - To evaluate immunodeficiency syndromes or to confirm an infectious disease process in the marrow
- Contraindications to bone marrow biopsy and aspirate include *severe* bleeding dyscrasias such as hemophilia. The use of anticoagulant medications such as warfarin or Lovenox may pose serious bleeding risk; therefore coagulation studies should be obtained in these patients. Thrombocytopenia alone is not a contraindication to bone marrow examination.

EQUIPMENT

- Bone marrow aspiration and biopsy kit, which includes the following:
  - Povidone-iodine or chlorhexidine-alcohol antiseptic preparation
  - Sterile fenestrated drape
  - 1 vial lidocaine (1% or 2%)
  - 5 ml syringe for drawing up lidocaine

- ❖ Needles of appropriate lengths to anesthetize both skin and periosteum
- ❖ Sterile 4 × 4 gauze pads
- ❖ Small scalpel blade
- ❖ Bone marrow aspirate needle
- ❖ Jamshidi bone biopsy needle
- ❖ 20-ml syringe for bone marrow aspirate
- ❖ Two 10-ml syringes with needles
- ❖ Adhesive bandage
- Sterile gloves
- Required tubes for specimen processing: two EDTA (lavender top) and two sodium heparin (green top) tubes
- Glass slides
- 2½- to 3½-inch spinal needle (may be required for anesthetizing periosteum in the obese patient)
- Container for bone biopsy specimen, including appropriate fixative (10% formalin)
- 1 vial of 1000 unit/ml heparin
- 1 additional vial of lidocaine (1% or 2%)

Additional equipment for patients receiving conscious sedation:

- Pulse oximeter
- Automated blood pressure monitor
- Oxygen
- Suction
- Ambu bag
- IV pharmacologic agents for sedation (i.e., midazolam 2-4 mg, fentanyl 25-50 mcg, lorazepam 1-2 mg)
- IV opiate and benzodiazepine antagonist agents (i.e., naloxone and flumazenil)

PATIENT AND FAMILY EDUCATION

- Assess patient and family understanding of the bone marrow aspiration and biopsy procedure and the reason for it. ➼*Rationale:* Clarification of the procedure and reinforcement of information are expressed patient and family needs in times of stress and anxiety.
- Inform the patient and family that the results will be shared with them as soon as they are available. ➼*Rationale:* The patient and family are usually anxious about the results.
- Explain the actual procedure to the patient and family. ➼*Rationale:* Prepares the patient and family for what to expect and may decrease anxiety.
- Review safety requirements for patients who will receive pharmacologic agents for sedation (i.e., must have transportation and escort home and may not drive until the following day). ➼*Rationale:* Ensures patient safety and health care provider's accountability for patients receiving sedation.
- Encourage the patient to verbalize any pain experienced during the procedure. ➼*Rationale:* Additional lidocaine, pain medication, or sedation medication can be administered.
- Instruct patient and family to keep pressure dressing clean, dry, and in place for 24 hours after the procedure. ➼*Rationale:* Reduces chance syf bleeding, minimizes chance of infection at the site.

PATIENT ASSESSMENT AND PREPARATION

Patient Assessment

- Assess the need for antianxiety, analgesic medication or conscious sedation. ➼*Rationale:* If the patient is very anxious before the procedure or has experienced severe pain with previous bone marrow procedures, small doses of analgesia or sedation will promote patient comfort.
- Assess coagulation studies in patients who are taking anticoagulant medications. ➼*Rationale:* Identifies patients at risk for bleeding complications.
- Assess the ability of the patient to lie on his or her stomach or side, with the head of the bed at no greater than a 25-degree elevation. ➼*Rationale:* Access to, and control of, the posterior iliac crest is best obtained with the patient lying flat, or with the head of the bed only slightly raised, in a side-lying or prone position.
- Assess vital signs and oxygenation status. ➼*Rationale:* Provides baseline data. Ensures that the blood pressure and oxygenation status can be maintained if the patient is placed on his or her side or prone.
- Assess the posterior iliac crest by palpation. In select cases, the anterior iliac crest may be utilized as a result of positioning limitations or excessive tissue surrounding the posterior iliac crest. The sternum is used for aspiration only in very select cases because of potential fatal complications with this procedure; therefore it should be performed only by physicians. ➼*Rationale:* Identifies the most suitable area for obtaining optimal samples with a minimum of risk or discomfort for the patient.
- Assess for recent bone marrow aspiration and biopsy sites. ➼*Rationale:* It may be painful for the patient if an additional biopsy is performed at a site that has not yet healed from a previous procedure.

Patient Preparation

- Ensure that the patient and family understand preprocedural teaching and discharge instructions. Answer questions as they arise and reinforce information as needed. ➼*Rationale:* Evaluates and reinforces understanding of previously taught information. Ensures that patient and family understand postprocedure care.
- Obtain informed consent for bone marrow aspiration and biopsy and, if indicated, conscious sedation. ➼*Rationale:* Protects the rights of the patient.
- Prescribe analgesia or sedation, if needed. ➼*Rationale:* Patient may need analgesia or sedation to ensure adequate cooperation and minimize discomfort during the procedure.
- Per individual institutional policy, prepare necessary equipment and personnel for care of the patient receiving conscious sedation. ➼*Rationale:* Ensures appropriate emergency equipment and medical staff are available.
- Obtain IV access for patients receiving conscious sedation. ➼*Rationale:* A secure patent IV is necessary for administration of IV pharmacologic agents and, if necessary, emergency antagonist agents.

- Obtain a complete blood count and differential. ➛***Rationale:*** Many pathologists prefer to review a peripheral blood sample in conjunction with the marrow in order to make a complete and accurate diagnostic evaluation.
- Confirm availability of personnel who will assist with the procedure. ➛***Rationale:*** Slide preparation, specimen processing, and obtaining additional supplies require an appropriately trained assistant for the procedure.
- Assist the patient to a side-lying or prone position depending on the patient's comfort and the practitioner's preference. ➛***Rationale:*** Ensures good visualization and control of the posterior iliac crest.

Procedure for Performing Bone Marrow Biopsy and Aspiration

Steps	Rationale	Special Considerations
1. Wash hands; don protective clothing and eye goggles.	Reduces transmission of microorganisms; standard precautions.	
2. Open the bone marrow procedure tray; add any additional supplies in a manner that preserves sterility. Don sterile gloves.	Maintains sterility of the procedure.	
3. Prepare all necessary syringes, including lidocaine syringe and those requiring anticoagulant.	Ensures adequate preparation for the procedure and reduces distraction once the procedure is started.	
4. Prepare the intended site with the antiseptic swabs and place sterile drape.	Minimizes risk for infection.	
5. Using a 25-30-g needle, inject the skin with lidocaine.	A small-gauge needle lessens the discomfort associated with administering local anesthesia.	
6. Using a 21-g 1½ needle (or spinal needle if necessary) infiltrate the periosteum with lidocaine in a "peppering" fashion. It is helpful to stabilize the site of aspiration by stretching the skin with the thumb and forefinger of the opposite hand.	If the periosteum is not numb, the patient will experience extreme discomfort. Also, it is often difficult to assess the area of the posterior iliac crest in an obese patient. Use of the spinal needle will help the practitioner locate an appropriate site.	If additional lidocaine is needed, ask the assistant to invert the extra vial. If the 1½-in needle does not reach the bone, use the 3½-in spinal needle to reach it. The spinal needle can also be used to assess the geography of the posterior iliac crest and will allow the practitioner to assess the depth of the bone.
7. Advance the aspirate needle (while continuing to stretch the skin) to the periosteum with firm pressure and slight rotation; penetrate the cortex. A slight sensation of "giving" is often noticed as the marrow cavity or medulla is reached.	Slight rotation of the needle allows for smooth entry into the marrow cavity.	If the patient experiences excessive pain, it is recommended that the needle be placed in another section of bone and/or additional lidocaine be applied to the outer surface of the bone.
8. Remove the stylet, attach the 20-ml syringe and aspirate 2- to 3-ml of marrow. Immediately hand this syringe to the assistant and verify presence of spicules in the sample.	The first aspirate sample is used to make the slides and to place in the purple-top EDTA tubes for clot sections or polymerase chain reaction (PCR) studies.	

Procedure continues on the following page

AP This procedure should be performed only by physicians, advanced practice nurses, and other health care professionals (including critical care nurses) with additional knowledge, skills, and demonstrated competence per professional licensure or institutional standard.

Procedure for Performing Bone Marrow Biopsy and Aspiration—*Continued*

Steps	Rationale	Special Considerations
9. If aspirate is not obtained or is aparticulate, replace the stylet, reposition the needle, and attempt to aspirate again. With each pull, rotate the needle slightly.		At times it is difficult to obtain a bone marrow aspirate. Difficulty can occur if a patient is aplastic or if the marrow space is packed by disease. In these cases, the practitioner should try to obtain a good core biopsy specimen for pathology analysis. The touch preparation in this case becomes a crucial step in providing the pathologist with material suitable for morphologic examination.
10. Obtain additional samples as needed in the 10-ml syringe containing heparin. Place in the green-top sodium heparin tubes with the help of the assistant.	Heparinized aspirate is used for flow cytometry, chromosome analysis, and chimerism studies.	
11. Have the assistant invert all of the tubes several times.	Aspirate samples can clot quickly if not thoroughly mixed with anticoagulant.	
12. Remove the aspiration needle from the site and apply firm pressure with sterile gauze. If obtaining a bone biopsy, proceed to step 1 (next section).	Ensures adequate hemostasis and reduces chance of infection.	
13. Hold pressure for 5 minutes or until bleeding has stopped. Pressure dressing should then be applied.	Ensures adequate hemostasis and reduces chance of infection.	
Bone Marrow Biopsy		
1. Make a 5-mm skin incision, pass the Jamshidi needle through the incision, and advance the needle until the periosteum is reached.	Allows smooth entry of the marrow needle into the skin.	Some sections of bone are extremely hard, making placement of the Jamshidi needle difficult. If hard bone is encountered, another section of bone should be used. If a section of bone is extremely soft, it is often difficult to obtain an adequate biopsy, and another section of bone should be chosen.
2. Rotate the needle slightly until it is firmly seated in the bone.		
3. Remove the stylet and advance the needle approximately 1-2 cm using a slight rotating motion.		
4. Verify the length of the biopsy, using the stylet as a guide.		Optimal length of biopsy sample should be between 1.5 and 2.0 cm.
5. Before removal, the Jamshidi needle should be rotated 360 degrees in each direction 2 to 3 times. Place the thumb over the hub and gently back the needle out of the bone and skin.	Giving the Jamshidi needle a few 360-degree turns and creating a vacuum by placing a finger over the top of the needle during removal increases the likelihood that the bone core will be retained within the needle.	

Procedure for Performing Bone Marrow Biopsy and Aspiration—*Continued*

Steps	Rationale	Special Considerations
6. Apply firm pressure to the site for 5 minutes or until bleeding has stopped; apply the adhesive pressure dressing. Assist patient to supine position and place small rolled towel directly under site to apply additional direct pressure.	Reduces chance of bleeding at the site. Prevents infection.	
7. If available, attach a guide to the distal end of the biopsy needle. Using the blunt obturator supplied, remove the core sample by passing the obturator through the guide and pushing the sample out through the needle hub.	Removing the core sample this way prevents damage to the bone by not forcing it through the narrower "drill" end of the needle.	
8. With the help of the assistant, place the bone core sample on a glass slide. Using an additional glass slide, gently touch the slide against the length of the biopsy sample in order to make 3 to 4 imprints. Place core sample in specimen container with appropriate solution for processing (i.e., 10% formalin).	A touch prep can be very useful for a complete pathology analysis.	
9. Discard supplies and wash hands.	Reduces transmission of microorganisms; standard precautions.	
10. Document in patient record.		

Expected Outcomes

- Adequate bone marrow aspirate and core biopsy specimens obtained
- Spicules in the aspirate (unless the patient is aplastic); aspirate not clotted
- Minimal bleeding and discomfort (patient may feel a dull ache for a few days after the procedure)

Unexpected Outcomes

- Difficulty obtaining a bone marrow aspirate
- Excessive pain

Patient Monitoring and Care

Steps	Rationale	Reportable Conditions
		These conditions should be reported if they persist despite nursing interventions.
1. Prescribe analgesia or sedatives as needed before and during the procedure.	Promotes patient comfort.	- Unrelieved discomfort

Procedure continues on the following page

AP This procedure should be performed only by physicians, advanced practice nurses, and other health care professionals (including critical care nurses) with additional knowledge, skills, and demonstrated competence per professional licensure or institutional standard.

Patient Monitoring and Care—*Continued*

Steps	Rationale	Reportable Conditions
2. Assess vital signs, oxygenation, level of consciousness, and electrocardiogram rhythm during the procedure and until complete recovery from sedation medications.	Monitors patient response to positioning, the procedure, and medications.	• Changes in vital signs, decreases in SaO_2, changes in cardiac rhythm, or level of consciousness.
3. Assess the site after the procedure.	Monitors for signs and symptoms of complications.	• Bleeding, hematoma, and infection

Documentation

Documentation should include the following:

- Patient and family education
- Informed consent
- Date and time of the procedure
- Indication for the procedure
- Preparation for the procedure
- Any complications that occurred

- Any medications used
- Specimens obtained
- Additional interventions
- For patients receiving conscious sedation, institution-approved discharge criteria that have been met

Additional Readings

Aboul-Nasr, R., et al. (1999). Comparison of touch imprints with aspirate smears for evaluating bone marrow specimens. *Am J Clin Pathol*, (6)III, 753-8.

Bain, B.J. (2001). Bone marrow trephine biopsy. *J Clin Pathol*, Oct, 54, 737-42.

DeVita, V.T., et al. (2001). *Cancer Principles and Practice*. 3rd ed. Philadelphia: Lippincott Williams & Wilkins.

Huyn, B.H., Stevenson, A.J., and Hanua, C.A. (1994). Fundamentals of bone marrow examination. *Hematology/ Oncology Clinics of North America*, 8, 651-63.

Lawson, S., et al. (1999). Trained nurses can obtain satisfactory bone marrow aspirates and trephine biopsies. *J Clin Pathol*, Feb, 52, 154-6.

Lin, E.M. (2001). *Advanced Practice in Oncology Nursing: Case Studies and Review*. Philadelphia: W.B. Saunders.

Litwack, K. (1999). *Core Curriculum for Perianesthesia Nursing*. 4th ed. Philadelphia: W.B. Saunders.

Quinn, D.M.D., and Schick, L. (2004). *Perianesthesia Nursing Core Curriculum: Preoperative, Phase I and Phase II PACU Nursing*. Philadelphia: W.B. Saunders.

Ryan, D.H., and Cohen, H.J. (2000). *Bone Marrow Aspiration and Morphology, Hematology Basic Principles and Practice*. 3rd ed. New York: Churchill Livingstone.

Trewhitt, K.G. (2001). Bone marrow aspirate and biopsy collection and interpretation. *Oncology Nursing Forum*, 28, 1409-15.

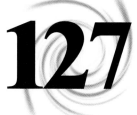
PROCEDURE **127**

Bone Marrow Biopsy and Aspiration (Assist)

P U R P O S E :   Bone marrow aspiration and biopsy are used to diagnose and classify various hematopoietic diseases, identify metastatic disease, monitor clinical response to treatment, and assess engraftment after stem cell transplant.

M.J. Heffernan

PREREQUISITE NURSING KNOWLEDGE

- Anatomy of the posterior and anterior iliac crest should be understood.
- Clinical and technical competence in performing a bone marrow aspirate and biopsy is necessary.
- Knowledge of sterile technique is essential.
- Institutional policies and procedures for administration of intravenous (IV) pharmacologic agents, including conscious sedation (if indicated).
- Procedural care of the patient receiving conscious sedation (if indicated).
- Bone marrow aspirate is used to identify normal and abnormal hematopoietic elements. The aspirate is also used to identify malignant clones by flow cytometry, to identify chromosomal abnormalities that occur in hematologic malignancies, to perform molecular diagnostic studies of gene rearrangements and translocations, and to perform chimerism studies in patients after allogenic transplant.
- A bone marrow biopsy is used for morphologic analysis of hematopoietic cells and for assessing the architecture of the bone marrow that may be abnormal in certain disease states.
- Indications for bone marrow aspiration and biopsy include the following:
  - To diagnose a hematologic abnormality
  - To monitor a hematologic disease state after therapy
  - To rule out bone marrow metastasis before stem cell collection and for staging of various malignant states
  - In all patients after bone marrow transplant, assess to the status of engraftment
  - In patients after allogenic transplant, to assess for chimerism and immune reconstitution
  - To evaluate of immunodeficiency syndromes or to confirm an infectious disease process in the marrow
- Contraindications to bone marrow biopsy and aspirate include *severe* bleeding dyscrasias such as hemophilia. The use of anticoagulant medications such as warfarin or Lovenox may pose serious bleeding risk; therefore coagulation studies should be obtained in these patients. Thrombocytopenia alone is not a contraindication to bone marrow examination.

EQUIPMENT

- Bone marrow aspiration and biopsy kit, which includes the following:
  - Povidone-iodine or chlorhexidine-alcohol antiseptic preparation
  - Sterile fenestrated drape
  - 1 vial of lidocaine (1% or 2%)
  - 5-ml syringe for drawing up lidocaine
  - Needles of appropriate lengths to anesthetize both skin and periosteum
  - Sterile 4 × 4 gauze pads
  - Small scalpel blade
  - Bone marrow aspirate needle
  - Jamshidi bone biopsy needle
  - 20-ml syringe for bone marrow aspirate
  - Two 10-ml syringes with needles
  - Adhesive bandage
- Sterile gloves
- Required tubes for specimen processing: two EDTA (lavender top) and two sodium heparin (green top) tubes
- Glass slides
- 2½- to 3½-inch spinal needle (may be required for anesthetizing periosteum in the obese patient)

- Container for bone biopsy specimen, including appropriate fixative (10% formalin)
- 1 vial of 1000 unit/ml heparin
- 1 additional vial of lidocaine (1% or 2%)

Additional equipment for patients receiving conscious sedation:

- Pulse oximeter
- Automated blood pressure monitor
- Oxygen
- Suction
- Ambu bag
- IV pharmacologic agents (i.e., midazolam 2-4 mg, fentanyl 25-50 mcg, lorazepam 1-2 mg)
- IV opiate and benzodiazepine antagonist agents (i.e., naloxone and flumazenil)

PATIENT AND FAMILY EDUCATION

- Assess patient and family understanding of the bone marrow aspiration and biopsy procedure and the reason for it. ➥*Rationale:* Clarification of the procedure and reinforcement of information are expressed patient and family needs in times of stress and anxiety.
- Inform the patient and family that the results will be shared with them as soon as they are available. ➥*Rationale:* The patient and family are usually anxious about the results.
- Explain the actual procedure to the patient and family. ➥*Rationale:* Prepares the patient and family for what to expect and may decrease anxiety.
- Review safety requirements for patients who will receive pharmacologic agents for sedation (i.e., must have transportation and escort home and may not drive until the following day). ➥*Rationale:* Ensures patient safety and health care provider's accountability for patients receiving sedation.
- Encourage the patient to verbalize any pain experienced during the procedure. ➥*Rationale:* Additional lidocaine, pain medication, or sedation medication can be administered.
- Instruct patient and family to keep pressure dressing clean, dry, and in place for 24 hours after the procedure. ➥*Rationale:* Reduces chance of bleeding, minimizes chance of infection at the site.

PATIENT ASSESSMENT AND PREPARATION

Patient Assessment

- Assess the need for antianxiety, analgesic medication, or conscious sedation. ➥*Rationale:* If the patient is very anxious before the procedure or has experienced severe pain with previous bone marrow procedures, small doses of analgesia or sedation will promote patient comfort.
- Assess coagulation studies in patients who are taking anticoagulant medications. ➥*Rationale:* Identifies patients at risk for bleeding complications.

- Assess the ability of the patient to lie on his or her stomach or side, with the head of the bed at no greater than a 25-degree elevation. ➥*Rationale:* Access to, and control of, the posterior iliac crest is best obtained with the patient lying flat, or with the head of the bed only slightly raised, in a side-lying or prone position.
- Assess vital signs and oxygenation status. ➥*Rationale:* Provides baseline data. Ensures that the blood pressure and oxygenation status can be maintained if the patient is placed on his or her side or prone.
- Assess the posterior iliac crest by palpation. In select cases, the anterior iliac crest may be used because of positioning limitations or excessive tissue surrounding the posterior iliac crest. The sternum is used for aspiration only in very select cases because of potential fatal complications with this procedure; therefore, this procedure should be performed only by physicians. ➥*Rationale:* Identifies the most suitable area for obtaining optimal samples with a minimum of risk or discomfort for the patient.
- Assess for recent bone marrow aspiration and biopsy sites. ➥*Rationale:* It may be painful for the patient if an additional biopsy is performed at a site that has not yet healed from a previous procedure.

Patient Preparation

- Ensure that the patient and family understand preprocedural teaching and discharge instructions. Answer questions as they arise and reinforce information as needed. ➥*Rationale:* Evaluates and reinforces understanding of previously taught information. Ensures that patient and family understand postprocedure care.
- Obtain informed consent for bone marrow aspiration and biopsy and, if indicated, conscious sedation. ➥*Rationale:* Protects the rights of the patient.
- Prescribe analgesia or sedation, if needed. ➥*Rationale:* Patient may need analgesia or sedation to ensure adequate cooperation and minimize discomfort during the procedure.
- Per individual institutional policy, prepare necessary equipment and personnel for care of the patient receiving conscious sedation. ➥*Rationale:* Ensures that appropriate emergency equipment and medical staff are available.
- Obtain IV access for patients receiving conscious sedation. ➥*Rationale:* A secure patent IV is necessary for administration of IV pharmacologic agents and, if necessary, emergency antagonist agents.
- Obtain a complete blood count and differential. ➥*Rationale:* Many pathologists prefer to review a peripheral blood sample in conjunction with the marrow in order to make a complete and accurate diagnostic evaluation.
- Confirm availability of personnel who will assist with the procedure. ➥*Rationale:* Slide preparation, specimen processing, and obtaining additional supplies require an appropriately trained assistant for the procedure.
- Assist the patient to a side-lying or prone position depending on the patient's comfort and the practitioner's preference. ➥*Rationale:* Ensures good visualization and control of the posterior iliac crest.

Procedure for Assisting With Bone Marrow Biopsy and Aspiration

Steps	Rationale	Special Considerations
1. Wash hands.	Reduces transmission of microorganisms; standard precautions.	
2. Ensure that the patient is positioned appropriately.	Prepares patient for the procedure.	
3. Assist the physician or advanced practice nurse with obtaining necessary supplies.	Prepares supplies.	
4. Don gloves and protective eyewear.	Standard precautions.	
5. Assist the physician or advanced practice nurse with syringe preparation.	Ensures adequate preparation for the procedure. Reduces distraction once procedure is started.	
6. Divide 1 ml of 1000 unit/ml heparin into two 10-ml syringes.	Heparinized aspirate is used for flow cytometry, chromosome analysis, and chimerism studies.	
7. Follow institutional procedure for administering prescribed IV pharmacologic agents, including conscious sedation.		
8. Assist with processing the aspirate obtained in the nonheparinized syringe first.	Nonheparinized bone marrow aspirate can clot if it is not placed in the appropriate tubes soon after it is obtained.	If there are no spicules visible in the aspirate syringe, there will be no hematopoietic elements for morphologic analysis.
A. The aspirate in the 20-ml nonheparinized syringe should be placed in a purple-top tube for slide preparation, clot analysis, and PCR studies.		
B. The aspirate in the heparinized syringes should be placed into green-top sodium heparin tubes.		
9. Assist as needed with performing touch prep with the bone biopsy core sample and place sample in 10% formalin fixative.	A touch prep can be very useful for a complete pathology analysis.	
10. Assist with placing a dressing over the site as needed.	Prevents infection.	
11. Follow institutional postprocedural recovery plan for patients who have received conscious sedation.	Ensures recovery parameters have been met.	
12. Label and send samples for laboratory analysis.	Ensures accuracy of results and timeliness of laboratory analyses.	
13. Discard supplies and wash hands.	Reduces transmission of microorganisms; standard precautions.	
14. Document in patient record.		

Expected Outcomes

- Adequate bone marrow aspirate and core biopsy specimens obtained
- Minimal bleeding and discomfort (patient may feel a dull ache for a few days after the procedure)
- Spicules in the aspirate (unless the patient is aplastic); aspirate not clotted

Unexpected Outcomes

- Inability to obtain specimens
- Unrelieved pain

Patient Monitoring and Care

Steps	Rationale	Reportable Conditions
		These conditions should be reported if they persist despite nursing interventions. • Unrelieved discomfort
1. Administer analgesia or sedatives as needed before and during the procedure.	Promotes patient comfort.	
2. Monitor vital signs, level of consciousness, oxygenation, and electrocardiogram rhythm during the procedure.	Determines the patient response to positioning and the procedure.	• Changes in vital signs or level of consciousness • Decreased SaO_2 • Cardiac dysrhythmias
3. Assess the site after the procedure.	Monitors for signs and symptoms of complications.	• Bleeding • Hematoma • Infection

Documentation

Documentation should include the following:

- Patient and family education
- Informed consent
- Indication for the procedure
- Date and time of the procedure
- Any complications that occurred

- Any medications used
- Specimens obtained
- Additional interventions
- For patients receiving conscious sedation, institution-approved discharge criteria that have been met

Additional Readings

Aboul-Nasr, R., et al. (1999). Comparison of touch imprints with aspirate smears for evaluating bone marrow specimens. *Am J Clin Pathol,* (6)III, 753-8.

Bain, B.J. (2001). Bone marrow trephine biopsy. *J Clin Pathol,* Oct, 54, 737-42.

DeVita, V.T., et al. (2001). *Cancer Principles and Practice.* 3rd ed. Philadelphia: Lippincott Williams & Wilkins.

Huyn, B.H., Stevenson, A.J., and Hanua, C.A. (1994). Fundamentals of bone marrow examination. *Hematology/Oncology Clinics of North America,* 8, 651-63.

Lawson, S., et al. (1999). Trained nurses can obtain satisfactory bone marrow aspirates and trephine biopsies. *J Clin Pathol,* Feb, 52, 154-6.

Lin, E.M. (2001). *Advanced Practice in Oncology Nursing: Case Studies and Review.* Philadelphia: W.B. Saunders.

Litwack, K. (1999). *Core Curriculum for Perianesthesia Nursing.* 4th ed. Philadelphia: W.B. Saunders.

Quinn, D.M.D., and Schick, L. (2004). *Perianesthesia Nursing Core Curriculum: Preoperative, Phase I and Phase II PACU Nursing.* Philadelphia: W.B. Saunders.

Ryan, D.H., and Cohen, H.J. (2000). *Bone Marrow Aspiration and Morphology, Hematology Basic Principles and Practice.* 3rd ed. New York: Churchill Livingstone.

Trewhitt, K.G. (2001). Bone marrow aspirate and biopsy collection and interpretation. *Oncology Nursing Forum,* 28, 1409-15.

P R O C E D U R E

128

Determination of Microhematocrit via Centrifuge

P U R P O S E : Determining the microhematocrit via centrifuge is a point-of-care test usually performed within a critical care unit. A capillary tube of blood is used to obtain the hematocrit value.

Maribeth Wooldridge-King

PREREQUISITE NURSING KNOWLEDGE

- The hematocrit measures the percentage of the total volume of red blood cells within a given blood sample. It is the ratio of the volume of red blood cells to that of whole blood expressed as a percentage.
- The hematocrit provides a relative indication of the degree of anemia or hemorrhage; the hemoglobin level is more accurate for measuring the red blood cell count.
- A microhematocrit is determined by centrifuging an anticoagulated specimen of blood under standardized conditions.
- A patient's hematocrit is useful in evaluating fluid status, in evaluating volume status after fluid resuscitation, and in classifying various types of anemia.

EQUIPMENT

- Two heparinized capillary tubes (75 × 1.55 mm internal diameter) or self-sealing capillary tubes
- Standardized high-speed centrifuge
- Sealing clay
- Hematocrit linear scale for direct reading (Fig. 128-1)
- Nonsterile gloves
  Additional equipment, as needed, includes the following:
- One 3-ml syringe and one 5-ml syringe and or needleless connector (for sample from arterial line)
- Lancet device (for fingerstick)
- Tourniquet (for venipuncture if necessary)

PATIENT AND FAMILY EDUCATION

- Explain why the microhematocrit is being performed. **➤➤Rationale:** Promotes patient and family understanding of the treatment plan and encourages the patient and family to ask questions.
- Explain how the procedure is done and discomfort the patient may experience. **➤➤Rationale:** Elicits patient cooperation, although anxiety may be heightened by knowledge that the patient may need a fingerstick or venipuncture if an arterial line sample is not available.

PATIENT ASSESSMENT AND PREPARATION

Patient Assessment

- Assess for signs and symptoms of fluid volume deficit, including dry mucous membranes, decreased skin turgor, lethargy, hyperventilation, decreased pulmonary artery pressures, increased urine specific gravity, and hypotension. **➤➤Rationale:** The hematocrit is increased with dehydration.
- Assess for signs and symptoms of fluid volume excess, including edema, dyspnea, crackles, jugular vein distention, hypertension, decreased urine specific gravity, and elevated pulmonary artery pressures. **➤➤Rationale:** The hematocrit is decreased in the presence of fluid volume excess.
- Assess for signs and symptoms of anemia or a decreased circulating volume caused by hemorrhage or

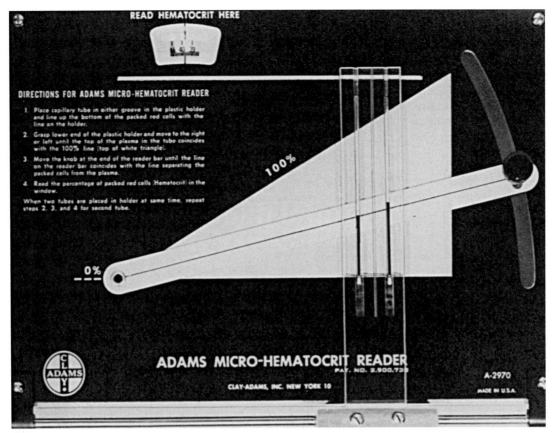

FIGURE 128-1 Adams Micro-Hematocrit Reader. *(From Simmons, A. [1989].* Hematology: A Combined Theoretical and Technical Approach. *Philadelphia: W.B. Saunders.)*

"third-spacing" of fluid from the intravascular compartment to the extravascular compartment. These symptoms include restlessness, dizziness, syncope, severe headaches, disorientation, pallor, diaphoresis, rapid thready pulse, hypotension, and rapid, deep respirations progressing to shallow respirations. ➤➤*Rationale:* The hematocrit provides a relative indication of the degree of anemia and should be compared with the patient's previous hematocrit.

- Assess for evidence of increased intravascular volume caused by congestive heart failure, an overinfusion of intravenous fluids, or the return of "third-spaced" fluids to the intravascular compartment. ➤➤*Rationale:* These clinical states commonly have a dilutional effect on the hematocrit and should be considered when evaluating the patient's fluid and electrolyte status or effects of transfusion therapy.

- Note past medical history of massive hemolysis. ➤➤*Rationale:* Massive red blood cell hemolysis increases the hematocrit.

Patient Preparation

- Ensure that the patient and family understand preprocedural teaching. Answer questions as they arise and reinforce information as needed. ➤➤*Rationale:* Evaluates and reinforces understanding of previously taught information.
- If performing a fingerstick, either wash the patient's hands or have the patient wash his or her hands with soap and water. ➤➤*Rationale:* Reduces risk for infection. Warm water dilates peripheral vessels and facilitates the process of obtaining a specimen.
- Help the patient hold his or her arm in a dependent position for at least 30 seconds. ➤➤*Rationale:* Encourages increased blood flow into fingertips.

Procedure **for Determination of Microhematocrit via Centrifuge**

Steps	Rationale	Special Considerations
1. Wash hands and don gloves.	Reduces transmission of microorganisms; standard precautions.	
2. Obtain blood sample. If patient does not have an arterial line, perform venipuncture (see Procedure 85) or fingerstick.	Provides blood for analysis.	The 1.4 mm lancet is used for most adult patients. The 1.9 mm lancet is used for adults with thick or callused skin or when an inadequate amount of blood is obtained using the smaller lancet.
3. Keeping the index finger of your dominant hand over one end of the capillary tube, place the other end to the hub of the syringe or the puncture site of the fingerstick to fill with blood. Remove your index finger and reposition it; repeat until the capillary tube is filled to within 5 to 10 mm of the end of the tube.	Placing your finger over the small diameter of the capillary tube creates a pressure gradient, which causes the tube to fill.	
4. Fill the second capillary tube in the same fashion.	Two tubes are necessary to balance within the centrifuge.	
5. Place one end of each capillary tube into the special sealing clay.	Capillary tubes must be sealed before they are centrifuged.	Make sure the sealing clay forms a straight edge across the interior of the tube.
6. Place one capillary tube on the centrifuge head with the sealed end directed outward; place the second tube directly opposite the first tube.	Avoids spillage of blood and balances the tubes within the machine.	
7. Place the cover on the centrifuge and set the automatic timer to 5 minutes at 10,000 to 15,000 × gravity. Then turn the machine on.	Separates red blood cells from plasma so that the hematocrit can be determined.	
8. When the machine stops, remove the capillary tubes from the centrifuge and obtain the graphic reader (see Fig. 128-1).	The graphic reader is used to read hematocrit.	
9. Place a capillary tube in the holder on the graphic reader.	Correct placement of the tube is necessary to obtain an accurate reading.	
10. Align the bottom of the red blood cells with the line on the holder (Fig. 128-2; also see Fig. 128-1).	The tube is now adjusted for the amount of blood in this specific tube.	
11. Take the plastic capillary tube holder and move it until the top of the plasma (not the red blood cells) coincides with the 100% line that is at the top of the white triangle (see Figs. 128-1 and 128-2).	Prepares tube so that hematocrit can be read.	

Procedure continues on the following page

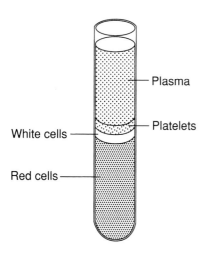

Plasma

Platelets

White cells

Red cells

FIGURE 128-2 Cell layers in centrifuged whole blood.

Procedure for Determination of Microhematocrit via Centrifuge—*Continued*

Steps	Rationale	Special Considerations
12. Turn the knob to the right of the reader and move it until the line coincides with the line where the plasma and red blood cells separate (see Figs. 128-1 and 128-2).	Identifies the microhematocrit.	
13. Read the microhematocrit in the window.	This is the microhematocrit measurement that is to be documented.	
14. Validate the microhematocrit obtained with the second capillary tube.	Duplicate results should agree to within ±1%.	
15. Remove and discard gloves and wash hands.	Reduces transmission of microorganisms; standard precautions.	

Expected Outcome

- Accurate identification of hematocrit

Unexpected Outcomes

- Inability to identify hematocrit level
- Continued bleeding from fingerstick site
- Hemolyzed microhematocrit

Patient Monitoring and Care

Steps	Rationale	Reportable Conditions
		These conditions should be reported if they persist despite nursing interventions.
1. Monitor the microhematocrit as prescribed and as needed.	Provides data for future interventions.	• Abnormal hematocrit
2. Assess hematocrit levels in relation to blood loss and previous hematocrit and microhematocrit levels.	Contributes to decision making with regard to blood or blood component transfusion requirements.	• Signs and symptoms correlating with hematocrit level

Patient Monitoring and Care—*Continued*

Steps	Rationale	Reportable Conditions
3. If a fingerstick was performed, examine the puncture site to determine whether the bleeding has stopped. If the site continues to bleed, apply continuous pressure and elevate the extremity until bleeding has stopped.	Establishes that hemostasis has occurred.	• Unresolved bleeding

Documentation

Documentation should include the following:

- Patient and family education
- Date and time the procedure was performed
- Microhematocrit obtained by centrifuge
- Pertinent assessment findings that correlate with microhematocrit
- Unexpected outcomes
- Interventions taken based on the assessed findings and patient's response

Additional Readings

Dirk, J.L. (1996). Diagnostic blood analysis using point of care technology. *AACN Clin Iss,* 7, 249-59.

Lamb, L.S., et al. (1995). Current nursing practice of point of care laboratory diagnostic testing in critical care units. *Am J Crit Care,* 4, 429-34.

Simmons, A. (1989). *Hematology: A Combined Theoretical and Technical Approach.* Philadelphia: W.B. Saunders.

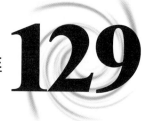
UNIT VII
Integumentary System

SECTION TWENTY-ONE

Burn Wound Management

Across the United States, there is diversity among burn units concerning policy, practice, and procedure in the care of the thermally injured population. This in no way intimates that the diversity in practice corresponds with diversity in quality. The burn care community, consisting of 135 burn units, regularly benchmarks among themselves, both formally and informally. This is done to compare outcomes and update practice to ensure that patients receive the quality of care they deserve. As is true with any specialty, the effects of research and the trial of new techniques and products will always be part of the search for best practice.

PROCEDURE **129**

Donor Site Care

PURPOSE: Care of the donor site is performed to promote wound healing and maintain function. Pain control is a priority during donor site care.

Elizabeth I. Helvig

PREREQUISITE NURSING KNOWLEDGE

* A partial-thickness wound is surgically created when a donor site (Fig. 129-1) is harvested to obtain skin for a full-thickness defect. The more dermis moved with the skin graft, the less the graft will shrink upon healing. Therefore deeper donor sites may be created to obtain skin for cosmetically significant areas such as the face or hands.[9] Depending on the percentage of dermis moved with the graft, donor sites created may be superficial or deep partial thickness wounds that heal in 10-20 days[12] (typically 10-14 days) (Fig. 129-2).
* Factors that can disrupt or prolong healing include infection, desiccation, changing adherent dressings, poor nutrition, and a variety of preexisting medical conditions.[2]
* The longer it takes for a partial-thickness wound to heal, the more significant the scarring; therefore donor sites can produce minimal or hypertrophic scars.[6,9,12]
* Donor sites retain deep epidermal appendages, so they are generally capable of sweating and bearing hair after they heal. The donor site may be reharvested once healing is complete, but skin from the first harvest of a donor site is always of higher quality than that of repeat harvesting.

* Because the dermis is richly supplied with capillaries and nerve endings, donor sites are at risk for bleeding in the first 24 hours and are exquisitely tender to touch. They produce large volumes of serous exudate.
* Donor site treatment goals include minimizing bleeding, supporting reepithelialization, managing exudate, preventing infection, controlling pain, and minimizing scarring.[12]
* Epinephrine-soaked dressings or fibrin sealant may be applied in the operating room to attain stasis.[4,5,10,11]

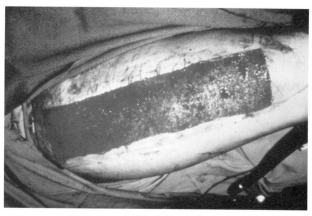

FIGURE 129-1 Fresh donor site.

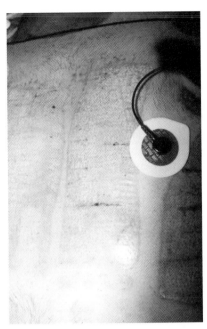

FIGURE 129-2 Donor sites in various stages of healing.

A compression dressing is usually used for the first 12 to 24 hours to ensure stasis.[11] After this initial period compression may be applied for comfort.

- Wounds epithelialize most rapidly in a moist environment. If donor sites are small enough, use of a thin-film or hydrocolloid dressing have been shown to promote rapid healing while providing comfort through dressing flexibility and occlusive coverage of nerve endings.[7,12]
- Occlusive dressings (sealed on all sides) can be difficult to maintain on larger donor sites because of the substantial volume of exudate.[8] A small drain (attached to a vacutainer tube) can be used to remove excess drainage from under a thin-film dressing. Calcium alginates have also been used successfully under occlusive dressings.[3,8]
- Multilayer occlusive dressings may also be used, with a nonstick dressing (e.g., greasy gauze, meshed silicone) applied next to the donor site and a bulky absorbent outer layer to maintain a moist environment and wick away excess drainage.[6,8] The outer dressing may be changed periodically, leaving the inner dressing intact until the wound heals beneath it.
- One of the oldest methods for treating donor sites was to apply a mesh gauze, wrap with an outer wrap for 12-24 hours, then remove the outer wrap and allow the inner dressing to remain exposed and dry until the wound heals beneath. This has been done with fine mesh gauze, scarlet red, and xeroform/xeroflo. The technique is only effective if the dressing dries well and becomes impermeable to bacteria, essentially acting as a scab.[8] Positioning the patient for maximum exposure of the donor sites, preventing prolonged donor site contact with sheets and clothing, and increasing air flow across the wound are important for making this technique work. If the donor site is large, this procedure creates a rather stiff and uncomfortable protective layer.

- Biobrane, a biosynthetic product, produces a more flexible donor site dressing. When exposed to air at 24 hours post-harvesting, it dries to form a fibrous bond with the collagen in the wound.[2] This dressing provides improved pain control, exudate management, and rate of healing when compared with a fine-mesh gauze dressing.[8,9]
- Antimicrobial creams or ointments have also been used on donor sites, essentially treating the wounds in the same way as partial-thickness burns. The disadvantage to this approach is that it requires daily washing of the wound and reapplication of cream and dressings.[8]
- Slow-release silver dressings are gaining popularity for donor site use. These dressings are moistened twice daily with sterile water to release the silver. In highly exudating wounds, the wound moisture may be adequate to promote silver release without exogenously applied moisture. These dressings release silver for 3 or more days; ideally, they are placed on the donor site in the operating room and the wound is allowed to heal beneath with infrequent or no dressing changes.[7,8]
- Donor sites need to be assessed daily for signs of infection, including periwound warmth and erythema, increased pain, or purulent drainage. Bacteria can delay healing and increase scarring or convert a partial-thickness donor site to a full-thickness wound. Erythema should be outlined to monitor progression, with consideration of either removing the donor site dressing or applying a topical antimicrobial to penetrate the donor site dressing. Reopening or "melting" of epithelium in previously healed donor sites is often the result of colonization with gram-positive organisms and may require antibacterial intervention.[6]
- Heavy hair-bearing donor sites such as the scalp provide special challenges. Heavy hair growth can lead to matting of hair in the exudate, leading to accumulation of protein, proliferation of bacteria and ingrowth of hair, a condition referred to as chronic folliculitis,[1] or "concrete scalp." This problem can lead to chronic, nonhealing, inflamed wounds or conversion of partial-thickness donor sites to full-thickness wounds. Dressings that prevent drying and wick away the exudate work well. The donor site will require gentle shaving about every 3 days to control hair growth, as well as possible topical antimicrobial therapy.[1]
- Donor sites are often very painful, with the amount of pain being variable depending on the dressing technique used. Patients with donor sites usually require scheduled round-the-clock pain medication.[6]
- The donor site should not be exposed to the sun for a year after the burn. Skin discoloration can be present for up to a year.[6]

EQUIPMENT

- Personal protective equipment
- Examination gloves
- Scissors
- Replacement dressing as needed

PATIENT AND FAMILY EDUCATION

• Teach the patient and family that donor sites generally heal in 10-12 days with variable scarring. Provide realistic expectations about healing and scarring.

• Provide donor site care instructions,[11] and review them with the patient and family. Demonstrate how to assess and manage the donor site dressing and have the patient and family return the demonstration. Encourage the patient and family to ask questions. Provide positive feedback. Arrange for home care or clinic visits to follow up on dressings and wound care. ➥*Rationale:* Validates the patient's and family's understanding and ability to perform wound care.

• Patients should be encouraged to avoid smoking. ➥*Rationale:* Smoking causes vasoconstriction, inhibits epithelialization, and decreases tissue oxygenation, all of which delay healing.[2]

• Explain to the patient about the pain and itching sensations associated with donor site healing.[2] ➥*Rationale:* Patients need to know that donor site pain and itching, although unpleasant, are normal and not cause for concern.

• Teach the patient and family about appropriate use of medications to manage pain and itching. Encourage application of a topical moisturizer after healing.[11] ➥*Rationale:* Enhances comfort.

• Teach the patient and family about signs and symptoms of infection and the importance of reporting these in a timely manner.[11] ➥*Rationale:* Ensures that patient and family will recognize problems early so that appropriate measures can be instituted by the health care professional.

• Provide the patient and family with follow-up appointments and a contact to call if there is a problem. ➥*Rationale:* Provides necessary information for further care and follow-up.

• Assess the family's ability to provide care at home at each follow-up visit. ➥*Rationale:* Continued care of the wound will be required after discharge.

• Stress the importance of wearing pressure garments if they are indicated. ➥*Rationale:* Reduces scarring.[6]

• Inform the patient and family that the donor site should not be exposed to the sun for a year after the burn and that discoloration can be present for up to a year.[6,11] Patients should wear clothing that covers wounds and/or a sunscreen containing SPF higher than 15. ➥*Rationale:* Prepares the patient and family for changes that will occur after healing.

PATIENT ASSESSMENT AND PREPARATION

Patient Assessment

• Evaluate for signs of healing, as follows:
  ❖ Decreased pain
  ❖ Decreased edema
  ❖ Dressing separation at wound edges with reepithelialization beneath it

• Compare degree of healing with expected rate of healing based on number of days since skin harvested. ➥*Rationale:* Healing should occur within 10 to 12[11] days unless there are complications.

• Evaluate for signs and symptoms of infection, as follows:
  ❖ Foul odor
  ❖ Purulent drainage
  ❖ Increased pain
  ❖ Increasing edema
  ❖ Cellulitis
  ❖ Fever or increasing WBC[11]
  ➥*Rationale:* Donor site infection may require antimicrobial intervention.[6]

• Evaluate the adequacy of the pain control by asking the patient to rate the pain on a scale of 0 to 10, both before and during wound care. ➥*Rationale:* An individualized plan for pain control should be in place for background and procedural pain.[6]

• Evaluate the patient's range of motion in the vicinity of the donor site. Physical and occupational therapists may be consulted to assist the patient in maintaining ROM and for scar management. ➥*Rationale:* Wounds contract during healing; pain and tightness can decrease range of motion. The patient should be encouraged to continue normal movement and range-of-motion exercises.

Patient Preparation

• Ensure that the patient understands preprocedural teaching. Answer questions and reinforce information as needed. ➥*Rationale:* Evaluates and reinforces understanding of previously taught information.

• Premedicate the patient for pain and anxiety, as needed. Wait until the medication has had time to work. ➥*Rationale:* Allows time for medication to take effect and promotes optimal comfort for the patient. Reduces pain and anxiety. Encourages patient trust and compliance with procedure.

Procedure for Care of Donor Sites

Steps	Rationale	Special Considerations
1. Prepare all necessary equipment and supplies.	Preparation facilitates efficient wound care and prevents needless delays.	
2. Wash hands well and don examination gloves as needed.	Reduces transmission of microorganisms to the patient; standard precautions.	

Procedure for Care of Donor Sites—*Continued*

Steps	Rationale	Special Considerations
3. Remove gauze roll and any padding covering inner dressing.	Inner dressing is left in place until the wound heals unless there is a problem with infection.	Gauze roll or outer dressing is usually removed after 24 hours if goal is for inner dressing layer to be exposed to air and dry.
4. Assess the donor site for signs of healing and complications; assess whether the inner dressing needs to be changed. Proceed to step 8 if inner donor dressing needs to be changed.	Validates the healing process and identifies complications.	If inner dressing was stapled in place, staples will need to be removed when inner dressing is fully adherent (generally between postop days 4-7).
5. Remove and discard gloves; don a pair of clean gloves.	Handling the burn dressing contaminates examination gloves, and clean gloves are needed for wound care.	
6. Gently wash exudate from wound edges with warm tap water and pat dry.	Clears exudate that can harbor microorganisms from area of donor site.	
7. Use scissors to trim loose edges of donor site dressing. If inner dressing does not need to be changed, proceed to step 14 to complete donor site care.	Because dry inner dressing is not covered, loose edges of dressing can snag and displace inner dressing.	Assess need for outer dressing and apply as needed.
Inner Dressing Change		
8. Remove inner dressing and discard it.		If dressing is adherent, soak with warm tap water to loosen.
9. Remove and discard gloves; don a pair of clean gloves.	Handling the burn dressing contaminates examination gloves, and clean gloves are needed for wound care.	
10. Gently wash wound with mild solution, rinse with warm tap water, and pat dry.	Cleanses donor site.	Cleanse beyond donor site to reduce microbial count on surrounding tissue. Patients may do better if allowed to cleanse their own wounds.
11. Assess the donor site for progression of healing and complications; outline any inflammation with a marking pen.	Validates the healing process and identifies complications.	Notify health care providers from other disciplines who need to observe the wound ahead of time so that they can be present while the wound is uncovered.
12. Remove and discard gloves. Don a pair of sterile or clean gloves.	Clean gloves are applied after washing a wound.	Sterile gloves may be used when applying dressings to large burn wounds.
13. Cut dressing to the size of donor site with sterile scissors, apply, and secure in place.	Ensures correct fit and adherence.	Dressing may be secured with tubular netting or cloth tape applied to the dressing margins.
14. Remove and discard gloves. Wash hands.	Reduces transmission of microorganisms.	
15. Reapply bulky outer dressing if indicated.	Donor sites may be covered with bulky dressing to maintain moisture barrier, maintain a moist wound surface, or apply a topical antimicrobial soak.	Gauze roll or outer supportive dressing may be ordered over inner dressing until wound has healed.

Expected Outcomes

- Donor site heals within 2 weeks without complications.
- Patient maintains a self-identified, acceptable level of pain relief.
- Patient maintains comfort from measures taken for anxiety and itching.
- Patient and family verbalize knowledge of patient condition and plan of care.
- An optimal level of function is maintained or attained.
- Patient and family response and interactions demonstrate adaptation to injury.
- Patient and family collaborate in management of care.
- At the time of discharge, patient and family verbalize and demonstrate an understanding of posthospital care.

Unexpected Outcomes

- Bleeding
- Infection
- Conversion of donor site to deep partial-thickness or full-thickness wound

Patient Monitoring and Care

Steps	Rationale	Reportable Conditions
		These conditions should be reported if they persist despite nursing interventions.
1. Evaluate and treat the patient's pain. Have the patient rate pain on a validated pain scale; check pain medication orders; review patient's previous response to pain medication and assess the need to increase the dose. Incorporate nonpharmacologic pain relief techniques (e.g., relaxation techniques, massage therapy, music, visual imaging).	The donor site pain will be minimized by an intact dressing that does not require a dressing change; the patient will have increased pain medication requirements if the dressing needs to be changed; attention to the patient's pain will foster the patient's trust in health care personnel.	- Increased heart rate - Increased or decreased blood pressure - Increased respiratory rate - Verbalization of pain - Nonverbal indications of pain (e.g., restlessness, grimacing, teeth clenching) - Inability to cooperate with wound care
2. Obtain baseline vital signs before procedure, monitor them throughout procedure, and check them for 30 minutes after procedure is complete.	Changes in vital signs can be a sign that the patient is experiencing pain or anxiety. Decreasing blood pressure, heart rate, and respiratory rate can be complications of pain medication (especially after dressing change is complete and stimulation has stopped).	- Increased or decreased heart rate - Increased or decreased blood pressure - Increased or decreased respiratory rate - High peak pressures on ventilator
3. Assess the donor site for appearance (e.g., dressing wet or dry, dressing adherent, presence of drainage or bleeding, redness at edges) and progression toward healing (e.g., reepithelialization at wound edges).	Observe for usual progression of wound healing versus complications of infection, progression of donor site to deeper wound, and bleeding.	- Foul odor - Purulent or increased amounts of drainage - Cellulitis or edema - Healing tissue developing eschar - Discoloration of wound - Bleeding
4. Encourage exercise and activities of daily living; place patient in position of optimal function and assess need for pain medication to facilitate movement. Physical therapy may be necessary to maintain range of motion.	Donor site wounds contract during the healing phase. Pain also inhibits movement.	

Documentation

Documentation should include the following:

- Patient and family education
- Date and time of wound care
- Appearance (e.g., dressing wet or dry, dressing adherent, presence of drainage or bleeding, redness at edges)
- Progression toward healing (e.g., reepithelialization at wound edges)

- Assessment of pain before, during, and after procedure
- Medications given for pain and sedation
- Other comfort measures used
- Patient's tolerance of the procedure
- Unexpected outcomes
- Nursing interventions

References

1. Barret, J.P., et al. (1999). Outcome of scalp donor sites in 450 consecutive pediatric burn patients. *Plastic & Reconstruct Surg,* 103, 1139-42.
2. Cho, C.Y., and Lo, J.S. (1998). Excision and repair: Dressing the part. *Dermatologic Clinics,* 16, 25-47.
3. Disa, J.J., et al. (2001). Evaluation of a combined calcium sodium alginate and bio-occlusive membrane dressing in the management of split-thickness skin graft donor sites. *Annals Plastic Surg,* 46, 405-8.
4. Gomez, M., Logsetty, S., and Fish, J.S. (2001). Reduced blood loss during burn surgery. *J Burn Care & Rehab,* 22, 111-7.
5. Greenhalgh, D.G., et al. (1999). Multicenter trial to evaluate safety and potential efficacy of pooled human fibrin sealant for the treatment of burn wounds. *J Trauma,* 46, 433-40.
6. Helvig, E.I. (2002). Managing thermal injuries within WOCN practice. *J Wound Ostomy Continence Nurs,* 29, 76-82.
7. Innes, M.E., et al. (2001). The use of silver coated dressings on donor site wounds: A prospective, controlled matched pair study. *Burns,* 27, 621-7.
8. Lionelli, G.T., and Lawrence, W.T. (2003). Wound dressings. *Surgical Clinics North Am,* 83, 617-38.
9. Mann, R., et al. (2001). Prospective trial of thick vs standard split-thickness skin grafts in burns of the hand. *J Burn Care & Rehab,* 22, 390-2.
10. Nervi, C., et al. (2001). A multicenter clinical trial to evaluate the topical hemostatic efficacy of fibrin sealant in burn patients. *J Burn Care & Rehab,* 22, 99-103.
11. University of Iowa Hospitals. (1998). *Split-Thickness Skin Graft Donor Site Care.* Available at: www.guideline.gov.
12. Valencia, I.C., Falabella, A.F., and Eaglstein, W.H. (2000). Skin grafting. *Dermatologic Clinics,* 18, 521-32.

Additional Readings

Arpey, C.J., and Whitaker, D.C. (2001). Postsurgical wound management. *Dermatologic Clinics,* 19, 787-97.
Cenetoglu, S. (2000). Topical lignocaine gel for split-thickness skin graft donor-site pain management. *Plastic & Reconstruct Surg,* 105, 2633.
Chuenkongkaew, T. (2003). Modification of split-thickness skin graft: Cosmetic donor site and better recipient site. *Annals Plastic Surg,* 50, 212-4.
Davey, R.B., Sparnon, A.L., and Byard, R.W. (2000). Unusual donor site reactions to calcium alginate dressings. *Burns,* 26, 393-8.
Fang, P., et al. (2002). Dermatome setting for autografts to cover INTEGRA.® *J Burn Care & Rehab,* 23, 327-32.
Flynn, M.B., ed. (2004). Burn and wound care. *Crit Care Nurs Clinics North Am,* 16.
Hallock, G.G. (1999). The cosmetic split-thickness skin graft donor site. *Plastic & Reconstruct Surg,* 104, 2286-8.
Kilinc, H., et al. (2001). Which dressing for split-thickness skin graft donor sites? *Annals Plastic Surg,* 46, 409-14.
Long, T.D., et al. (2001). Morphine-infused silver sulfadiazine (MISS) cream for burn analgesia: A pilot study. *J Burn Care & Rehab,* 22, 118-23.
Pierre, E.J., et al. (1998). Effects of insulin on wound healing. *J Trauma,* 44, 342-5.
Summer, G.J., et al. (1999). The Unna "cap" as a scalp donor site dressing. *J Burn Care & Rehab,* 20, 183-8.

PROCEDURE **130**

Burn Wound Care

PURPOSE: Burn wound care is performed to promote healing, maintain function, and prevent infection and burn wound sepsis. A major focus must be on pain control.

Elizabeth I. Helvig

PREREQUISITE NURSING KNOWLEDGE

- Burns destroy the structural integrity of the skin, disrupting its normal functions of regulating temperature, maintaining fluid status, protecting against infection, covering nerve endings, and establishing identity.[18]
- The skin is composed of two layers, the epidermis and the dermis supported by a subcutaneous layer that is rich in blood vessels (Fig. 130-1).

- ❖ The epidermis is the outermost layer. It is capable of rapid regeneration through division of cells closest to the dermis; older epidermal cells are pushed outward as the epidermis is regenerated.[30] The epidermis provides a barrier to the environment, containing melanocytes (protection from the sun) and Langerhans cells (protection against foreign organisms).
- ❖ The dermis contains blood vessels, sensory fibers (for pain, touch, pressure, and temperature), collagen, sebaceous glands, and sweat glands. Epidermal cells line

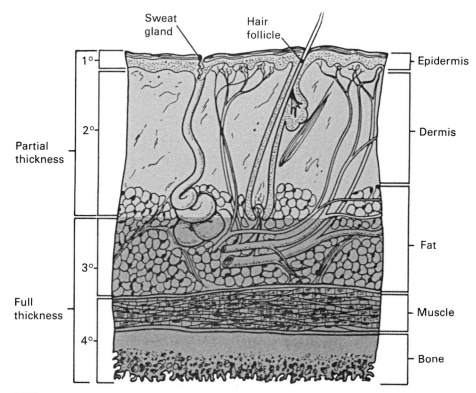

FIGURE 130-1 Cross-section of skin with areas affected by partial- and full-thickness burns. *(From Lewis, S.M., and Cox, I.C. [1987]. Medical-Surgical Nursing: Assessment and Management of Clinical Problems. 2nd ed. New York: McGraw-Hill.)*

deep dermal structures (hair follicles and sweat glands); these epidermal elements provide the ability for the skin to regenerate (the more epidermal cells remaining in the wound bed, the faster the healing).

- The depth of burns has historically been classified as first-degree (into epidermis), second-degree (into dermis) or third-degree (through skin into subcutaneous tissue) (Table 130-1).[2,11,18,26]

  ❖ First-degree burns extend only partially through the epidermis, thereby maintaining the barrier function of the skin. These burns are not included when estimating the percentage of total body surface area burned (% TBSA) because they do not result in an open wound.

  ❖ Second-degree burns extend into the dermis and can be superficial (loss of the epidermis and part of the dermis) or deep (destruction of most of the dermis). They are also referred to as "partial-thickness" burns because they are partially through the skin (Fig. 130-2). These wounds heal by epithelialization from epidermal cells remaining in the dermis. Shallower wounds are associated with rapid healing and less scarring. Deeper wounds may result in slow-healing (more than 21 days) and fragile-healed wounds that are prone to hypertrophic scarring. For that reason, it may be preferable to surgically convert deep partial-thickness wounds to full-thickness wounds and apply skin grafts.

  ❖ A third-degree, or full-thickness, burn involves complete destruction of the dermis. Because the skin is unable to regenerate, the dead tissue is removed and the wound is grafted with skin from another part of the patient's own body (autograft).[18] The grafted wound loses epidermal appendages and is unable to sweat after healing (Fig. 130-3).[26]

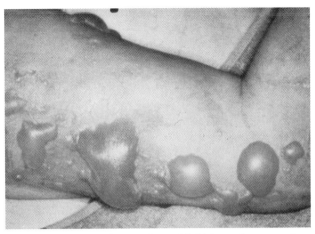

FIGURE 130-2 Blisters of a partial-thickness burn wound on the arm.

- The depth of a burn wound is directly related to the temperature intensity and the duration of contact with the burning agent. The burning agent can be thermal (i.e., flame, contact, or scald), chemical, or electrical. An inhalation injury should always be suspected if the patient was in an enclosed space with a fire, because the mortality rate is increased when burns are compounded by smoke inhalation.

- The burn injury produces three zones of injury: the zone of coagulation (cellular death), zone of stasis (vascular impairment, potentially reversible tissue injury), and zone of hyperemia (increased blood flow and inflammatory response). Decreased perfusion of the burn wound can cause the zone of stasis to deteriorate, deepening the initial wound. This progressive destruction can be minimized by providing adequate oxygenation and fluid resuscitation, alleviating pressure on the injured tissue,

TABLE 130-1	Depth Characteristics of Burn Wounds	
Type	**Physical Characteristics**	**Healing**
Superficial burn (first-degree): Destruction of epidermis, usually caused by overexposure to sun or brief exposure to hot liquid. This type of injury is not included when calculating burn size.	Red; hypersensitive; no blisters.	Injured layers peel away from totally healed skin at 5-7 days without residual scarring.
Superficial partial-thickness burn (superficial second-degree): Destruction of epidermis and upper dermis. Usually results from scalding or brief contact with hot objects.	Blistered; very moist; red or pink in color; exquisitely painful; capillary refill intact.	Reepithelializes from epidermal appendages in 7 to 14 days. Usually has minimal scarring but variable repigmentation.
Deep partial-thickness burn (deep second-degree): Destruction of epidermis through to lower dermis. May result from grease or longer contact with hot objects.	Mottled pink to white; drier than superficial burns; less sensitive to pinprick; does not blanch to pressure; hair follicles and sweat glands intact.	Slower regeneration from epidermal elements: 14-21+ days in absence of grafting. Prone to hypertrophic scars and contracture formation. May require grafting to reduce healing time and complications.
Full-thickness burn (third-degree): Destruction of epidermis and all of dermis. Results from exposure to flames, chemicals that are not immediately washed, electrical injury, or prolonged contact with heat source.	Dry; leathery and firm to touch; pearly white, brown or charred in appearance; no blanching to pressure; no pain, may see thrombosed vessels.	Incapable of self-regeneration. Preferred treatment is early excision and autografting.

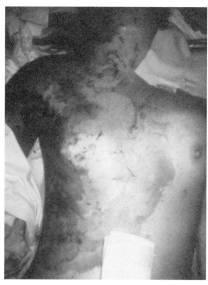

FIGURE 130-3 A fresh burn that is partial-thickness toward the patient's left side and progresses to full-thickness on the patient's right side.

maintaining local and systemic warmth, and decreasing edema by elevating the burned area.[2]

- Assess for areas where full-thickness eschar wraps circumferentially. Because of the inelastic nature of eschar, it may act like a tourniquet as edema develops, requiring surgical release (escharotomy) to prevent circulatory or respiratory compromise (Fig. 130-4).
- Monitor pulses, capillary refill, and sensation distal to circumferential eschar. Signs and symptoms indicating a need for escharotomy include cyanosis of distal unburned skin, unrelenting deep tissue pain, progressive paresthesias, and progressive decrease or absence of pulse.[2]
- Adequacy of respiratory excursion must be assessed because circumferential eschar of the trunk can lead to decreased tidal volume and agitation (Fig. 130-5).[2]
- Escharotomy is performed at the bedside by a physician, using a scalpel or electrocautery to cut the eschar longitudinally. Bleeding should be minimal since only dead tissue is cut; any bleeding can be controlled with sutures,

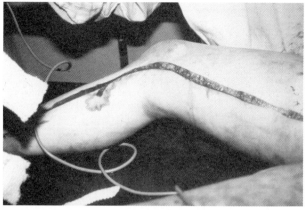

FIGURE 130-4 Escharotomy of the leg to improve circulation.

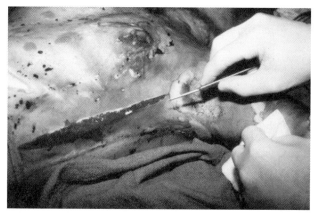

FIGURE 130-5 Full-thickness burn with chest escharotomy to improve chest expansion.

silver nitrate sticks, collagen packing, or electrocautery. Pain is usually managed with small intravenous doses of opiates.
- Burn size may be determined by several methods.[29]
  - ❖ The rule of nines may be used to quickly calculate burn size. In an adult, the head and neck and each upper extremity represent 9% of the patient's body surface area. The anterior trunk, posterior trunk, and each leg represent 18% of the patient's body surface area. This rule only applies to adults; infants and young children have much larger heads in proportion to their body size.
  - ❖ The Lund and Browder chart (Fig. 130-6) breaks the body into smaller areas and takes into consideration the proportional differences of persons of different ages.[22]
  - ❖ The rule of the palm notes that the patient's hand may be used as a template to represent roughly 1% of the total body surface area.
- The inflammatory response causes a massive fluid shift to the interstitial space during the first 24 hours, with mobilization of fluid starting after 72 hours. Fluid resuscitation with a balanced salt solution is based on the patient's weight and burn size.[18] Large wounds are prone to huge evaporative water losses, requiring close monitoring of volume status.
- Burns of specific anatomic areas need special consideration. Assess eyes for injury and treat chemical exposure with normal saline irrigation; treat burned ears with a topical antimicrobial cream and protect from pressure by eliminating use of pillows or dressings about the head; elevate burned extremities; consider the need for a Foley catheter in the patient with perineal burns; shave hair growing through the burn wounds. Two burned surfaces that contact each other require dressings between them to prevent fusing as they heal (e.g., between toes, skinfolds).
- Emergency treatment of thermal injuries includes initially cooling the burned skin with tepid water (never with ice) while recognizing the importance of preventing hypothermia.[3] In preparation for transfer, airway should be assessed and 100% oxygen administered, IV access should be established and fluid resuscitation started, patients should

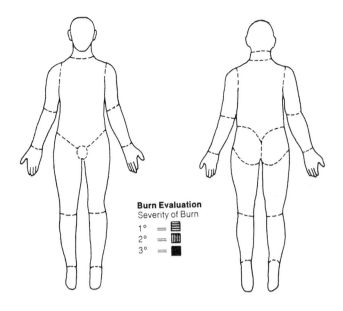

Burn Evaluation
Severity of Burn
1° =
2° =
3° =

Lund and Browder chart

AREA	AGE—YEARS					% 2°	% 3°	% TOTAL
	0–1	1–4	5–9	10–15	ADULT			
Head	19	17	13	10	7			
Neck	2	2	2	2	2			
Ant. Trunk	13	17	13	13	13			
Post. Trunk	13	13	13	13	13			
R. Buttock	2½	2½	2½	2½	2½			
L. Buttock	2½	2½	2½	2½	2½			
Genitalia	1	1	1	1	1			
R.U. Arm	4	4	4	4	4			
L. U. Arm	4	4	4	4	4			
R.L. Arm	3	3	3	3	3			
L.L. Arm	3	3	3	3	3			
R. Hand	2½	2½	2½	2½	2½			
L. Hand	2½	2½	2½	2½	2½			
R. Thigh	5½	6½	8½	8½	9½			
L. Thigh	5½	6½	8½	8½	9½			
R. Leg	5	5	5½	6	7			
L. Leg	5	5	5 ½	6	7			
R. Foot	3½	3½	3½	3½	3½			
L. Foot	3½	3½	3½	3½	3½			
					Total			

FIGURE 130-6 The Lund and Browder chart is used to assess and graphically document size and depth of the burn wound.

be NPO, wounds should be wrapped with a clean dry sheet and possibly blanket, pain medication should be given in small intravenous doses while recognizing that coexisting injury or medical conditions will exacerbate the effects of opiates, tetanus prophylaxis should be administered, and all initial treatment should be documented.[2,29]

- Initial treatment of chemical burns includes removing saturated clothing, brushing off any powdered chemical, and continuously irrigating involved skin with copious amounts of water for 20-30 minutes. Neutralizing chemical burns with another chemical is contraindicated because the procedure generates heat. Burned eyes must be irrigated with large volumes of normal saline followed by an eye examination.[2] Some chemicals are absorbed systemically through burn wounds; contact the local poison control center to determine whether further treatment is indicated.[29]

- Tar can be removed using mineral oil, a petrolatum-based ointment, or solvent.[18,23]

- Electrical injuries (Fig. 130-7) result when the body becomes part of the pathway for the electrical current. Deep burns may occur secondary to tissue resistance where the patient contacted the electrical source and where he or she was grounded. Initially of greater concern than the burns is the high incidence of cardiac dysrhythmias, myoglobinuria resulting in acute tubular necrosis, and neurologic sequelae. Monitoring ECG, increasing urine output to 100 ml/hr in the presence of dark port-colored urine, assessing for associated trauma, and establishing baseline neurologic status are vital in the patient who has been electrocuted.[2,20]

- Criteria for transferring patients to a specialized burn care facility have been adopted by the American Burn Association and the American College of Surgeons. These criteria are listed in Table 130-2.

- Care of the burn wound and associated healing are determined by the extent and depth of the injury and the overall condition of the patient.

- Most burn centers use clean technique for dressing removal and wound cleansing, using sterile technique for sterile dressing application only.[23]

- Wound care should be done in a warm area. Many burn units have replaced traditional hydrotherapy tanks with shower tables for large wound care procedures to allow water run-off, thus decreasing leaching of electrolytes and minimizing wound exposure to perineal-contaminated water. Emergency equipment must always be immediately available during hydrotherapy procedures. As wounds decrease in size and patients approach discharge, bathtubs and showers offer reasonable options for wound cleansing.

- Topical antimicrobial agents limit bacterial proliferation and fungal colonization in burn wounds. The three most commonly used agents are silver sulfadiazine (Silvadene), mafenide acetate (Sulfamylon), and 0.5%

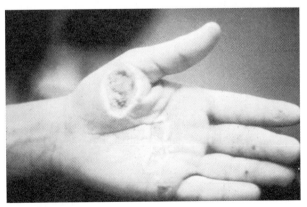

FIGURE 130-7 Entry site of an electrical burn.

TABLE 130-2	Criteria for Patient Transfer to a Specialized Burn Care Facility

Partial-thickness burns on more than 10% total body surface area (TBSA)
Burns that involve the face, hands, feet, genitalia, perineum, or major joints
Third-degree burns in any age group
Electrical burns, including lightening injury
Chemical burns
Inhalation injury
Burn injury in patients with preexisting medical disorders that could complicate management, prolong recovery, or affect mortality
Any patient with burns and concomitant trauma (such as fractures) in which the burn injury poses the greatest risk for morbidity or mortality
Burned children in hospitals without qualified personnel or equipment to care for children
Burn injury in patients who will require special social, emotional or long-term rehabilitative intervention

From American Burn Association. (1994). *Advanced Burn Life Support Course.* Chicago: American Burn Association.

silver nitrate solution (Table 130-3).[19,21,29] Antibiotics are not routinely administered to burn patients because of the high risk for developing antibiotic resistance.[8]

- Eschar is a leathery layer of devitalized tissue that covers full-thickness burns. Bacterial action will cause eschar to separate from the wound bed. However, the use of topical antimicrobial agents and early excision has minimized the nurses' involvement in eschar removal.
- Survival rates for burn patients are markedly improved with early excision and grafting.[4] The most important predictors of mortality are the patient age and the extent of the burn, with the presence of inhalation injury and comorbidity being crucial factors. Even though the burn wound has the most obvious potential for infection, the lower respiratory tract is the most common site of infection and carries the highest incidence of sepsis and death.

- An autograft (skin graft taken from the same person) is the only treatment that can heal a full-thickness burn wound.[32] Wounds with higher than 10^5 organisms per gram of tissue will impede graft adherence, so expedient grafting is desireable.[4,8]
- A debrided full-thickness wound may be protected from infection and drying through the use of biologic dressings when donor sites are not available for autografting. Allograft, or homograft, refers to the use of "nonself" human skin grafts; such a graft becomes vascularized by the patient and risks rejection if it stays in place too long. Xenograft, or heterograft, is nonhuman skin obtained from commercial pigskin (porcine) processing companies; it forms a collagen bond with the wound and protects it for a period of time until donor sites are available for autografting. Porcine xenograft may be placed over

TABLE 130-3	Topical Antimicrobial Agents		
Agent	**Activity**	**Advantages**	**Disadvantages**
Silver sulfadiazine 1% cream (Silvadine, Flamazine, Thermazine)	Bactericidal effect on cell membrane and wall; excellent against *P. aeruginosa, S. aureus,* other burn flora, and yeast	Broad spectrum antimicrobial coverage; low toxicity; no discomfort on application; easy to remove, rare hypersensitivity to sulfa component; may increase neovascularization	Poor eschar penetration; infrequent hypersensitivity; macerates surrounding tissues; contraindicated in pregnant women and newborns (risk for kernicterus); early transient neutropenia when applied to large burns
Mafenide acetate 0.5% cream (Sulfamylon)	Broad-spectrum against gram-positive and gram-negative organisms; not effective against yeast; diffuses through devascularized areas; is absorbed, metabolized, and excreted by kidneys	Highly soluble and penetrates eschar well. Persistent activity against *Pseudomonas*	Pain on application of cream; systemically absorbed; may cause metabolic acidosis (through carbonic anhydrase inhibition); cutaneous hypersensitivity reactions occur; may see yeast overgrowth
Mafenide acetate (Sulfamylon) solution 5.0%	Broad-spectrum against gram-positive and gram-negative organisms; not effective against yeast	Moist dressings may be used over wounds, such as a new graft, when a liquid soak antibiotic is desired	Expensive; wet dressings often uncomfortable and may result in hypothermia
Silver nitrate, 0.5% in water (if dressing allowed to dry, concentration of silver nitrate increases and becomes caustic at 2.0%)[16]	Bacteriostatic against many organisms; doesn't penetrate drainage or debris	Painless application; few organisms resistant to silver	Must be kept wet; poor penetration of eschar; stains unburned tissue and environment brown-black; hypotonicity of dressing may lead to hyponatremia and hypochloremia; requires thick dressings and resoaking every 4 hrs to prevent drying
Acticoat (a nonadherent nanocrystalline silver-coated dressing with sustained silver release for several days)	Lower minimum inhibitory concentration; a lower minimum bactericidal concentration; faster bacterial killing than other topicals	Decreases dressing changes by being left in place 3 days	Decreases ability to visualize wound

clean partial-thickness wounds to protect the wound while it heals beneath the xenograft.[23]

- Integra is an acellular matrix composite graft that may be placed on debrided full-thickness burns. Capillaries and collagen grow into this matrix over about 3 weeks, forming a neodermis, which is then grafted with the patient's own epidermal cells. The matrix is slowly biodegradable and cannot be detected by wound biopsy after complete healing.[32] This allows for better wound coverage and use of thinner donor sites but requires two surgeries.[17] Thinner autografts allow more rapid healing of donor sites and produce less hypertrophic donor site scarring.[6]

- Biosynthetic dressings such as Biobrane have been used to cover clean partial-thickness wounds to facilitate healing.[6] Biobrane is a two-layer, semisynthetic dressing composed of knitted-elastic nylon fabric that is mechanically bonded to a thin, silastic, semipermeable membrane and coated with collagen polypeptides.[7] As the wound heals beneath, the dressing can be peeled away.[17] Interest in impregnating biosynthetic dressings with neonatal foreskin fibroblasts is based on topically applied human growth factors to stimulate healing.

- The burn patient is hypermetabolic until burn wounds are closed and healing is complete. Splanchnic hemodynamics are thought to benefit from early enteral nutrition, with reduction of paralytic ileus postinjury.[10,29] Increased caloric and protein requirements for wound healing are usually met through nasogastric or nasojejunal tube-feeding to maintain mucosal integrity. Zinc and vitamin C have also been shown to be important in wound healing. Current research is evaluating the role of arginine and fish oil in decreasing infections,[1] glutamine's role in maintaining mucosal integrity, and insulin's ability to preserve muscle mass.[28] It is important to keep the patient warm during wound care because heat lost through the wound, along with shivering, increases the metabolic rate.

- An individualized plan for pain control should be in place for both background pain (pain that is continuously present) and procedural pain (intermittent pain related to procedures). Unrelieved pain can lead to stress-related immunosuppression, an increased potential for infection, delayed wound healing, and depression. Subcutaneous and intramuscular injections should be avoided because absorption will be poor and unreliable as a result of edema. Intravenous administration of medication is preferred in critically ill patients; oral medication is preferred in noncritical patients with a functioning gastrointestinal system.[12] As the wound heals, the patient will experience more discomfort from itchiness and less discomfort from pain.[23] A water-based lotion will prevent drying and reduce pruritus. Nonpharmacologic techniques can be learned to assist with the management of pain and itch.[5]

- Burn wounds contract during the healing phase. Self-care and range-of-motion exercises are encouraged. Stretching exercises and proper positioning are vital to prevent contractures and loss of function.[29] Static splinting is sometimes added to maintain sustained stretch.[23] Hypertrophic scar formation is countered through the use of topical silicone gel sheeting[23,24,28] and/or pressure garments worn 24 hours a day until the scars mature and soften (6-18 months).[27] Keloids, if they form, may require surgery, steroid injections, and pressure treatment.[14]

- The burn wound should not be exposed to the sun for a year because new scars burn easily and tend to permanently hyperpigment when exposed to light.[13] Patients should be instructed to select clothing that blocks sun and use sunscreen on exposed skin.

EQUIPMENT

- Personal protective equipment
- Examination gloves
- Sterile gloves
- Warm tap water
- Mild liquid soap, as ordered
- Normal saline (NS)
- Basins
- Washcloths
- Towels
- Scissors and forceps (clean and sterile)
- Topical agents, as ordered
- Tongue depressors
- Sterile dressings as needed (e.g., gauze, Exu-dry)
- Rolled dressing, gentle tape, or netting to secure dressings
- Pillows to elevate extremities
- Pain and sedation medication (as prescribed)

PATIENT AND FAMILY EDUCATION

- Provide detailed wound care instructions in writing or on videotape or DVD. Demonstrate wound care and have patient and family return the demonstration before the planned discharge. Continue to involve patient and family in wound care for the remainder of the admission and encourage them to ask questions. Provide positive feedback. Arrange for home care or clinic visits to follow up on wound care. ➤**Rationale:** Validates patient and family understanding and ability to perform wound care and allows time for them to develop a level of comfort. Provides the opportunity to reinforce important points.

- Explore resources patient will have for doing wound care at home (e.g., availability of running water, tub versus shower). ➤**Rationale:** Ensures that patient is knowledgeable about care based on what adjustments will need to be made at home.

- Simplify wound care and assess the family's ability to provide care at home. ➤**Rationale:** Continued care of the wound may be required after discharge.

- Teach patient and family about signs and symptoms of infection and the importance of reporting these in a timely manner. ➤**Rationale:** Ensures that patient and family will recognize problems early so that appropriate measures can be instituted by the health care professional.

- Teach patient and family about pain control; assess the patient's personal acceptable level of pain. ➤*Rationale:* Decreases concerns about pain, facilitates individualized pain relief plan, and fosters cooperation with care.
- Teach patient and family about pain management, including types of medications to take, timing of medications in relation to wound care, and nonpharmacologic pain strategies.[9] ➤*Rationale:* Supports comfort at home.
- Teach the patient and family about the normal changes seen in the wound, including epithelial islands, healing margins, dryness upon epithelialization, epidermal fragility upon shearing, hypervascularization of the healed wound, venous congestion in the dependent wound. ➤*Rationale:* Reduces anxiety about appearance.
- Teach patient and family about care of healed burns, including medications to reduce itching,[23] use of nonperfumed moisturizers, protection from shear, and protection from sun exposure for a minimum of a year. ➤*Rationale:* Reduces complications and promotes patient satisfaction.
- Teach patient and family about the wearing and care of pressure garments. ➤*Rationale:* Pressure garments need to fit properly to reduce scar formation, and they can be difficult to apply.[27,31]
- Discuss the importance of mobility and proper positioning (e.g., splinting) on function. Self-care (activities of daily living) and range-of-motion exercises should be encouraged during the healing phase. ➤*Rationale:* Prevents contractures associated with healing skin, improper positioning, and immobility.
- Inform patient and family that nightmares, alterations in body image, and psychologic disturbances are experienced by many burned patients.[15,29] Provide resources, including someone to follow up with, if desired. ➤*Rationale:* Increases awareness of these problems and reassures patient and family that these experiences, although unpleasant, are not abnormal.
- Provide patient and family with follow-up appointments and someone to call if there is a problem. ➤*Rationale:* Provides necessary information for further care and follow-up.

PATIENT ASSESSMENT AND PREPARATION

Patient Assessment

- Assess vital signs, including temperature. ➤*Rationale:* Baseline vital signs will allow for comparison during and following the procedure to evaluate patient tolerance and need for pain medication.
- Evaluate for signs of healing, including the following:
  - ❖ Decreased pain
  - ❖ Reepithelialization from epithelial islands within wound
  - ❖ Decreasing wound size
  - ❖ Decreased edema
- Compare patient's level of healing with expected level of healing for number of days postburn. ➤*Rationale:* Healing should occur within a predictable time-frame

determined by the depth of burns, unless there are complications.

- Evaluate for the following signs and symptoms of infection[25]:
  - ❖ Foul odor
  - ❖ Purulent drainage
  - ❖ Increased pain
  - ❖ Increasing edema
  - ❖ Cellulitis
  - ❖ Fever
  - ❖ Development of eschar or early eschar separation
  - ❖ Increase in burn size or depth
  - ❖ Blurring of wound edges
  ➤*Rationale:* Infection can result in delayed wound healing, prolonged hospitalization, or death.
- Monitor for distal circulation (pulses, pain, color, sensation, movement, and capillary refill) to areas with circumferential burns and increased edema. ➤*Rationale:* Edema and circumferential burns impede distal circulation and cause worsening tissue perfusion and cell death.
- Determine patient's understanding of pain management strategies. Assess patient's pain level on a standardized pain scale (such as the 0-10 scale) before, during, and after the procedure. Explore discrepancies between the patient's level of pain and desired level of pain. ➤*Rationale:* An individualized plan for pain control should be in place for background and procedural pain. In addition to the traditional use of pain and anxiety medications, alternative therapies should be included (e.g., relaxation techniques, massage therapy, music therapy). The patient's needs will change based on changes in the wound (e.g., healing, debridement, conversion to deeper wound).
- Evaluate patient's general level of function, particularly in burned areas. ➤*Rationale:* An individualized plan for range-of-motion exercises, positioning, and splinting should be made to optimize the patient's level of function. Burns contract during the healing phase, and immobility enhances loss of function.

Patient Preparation

- Ensure that patient understands procedural teaching. Answer questions as they arise and reinforce information as needed. ➤*Rationale:* Evaluates and reinforces understanding of previously taught information.
- Notify other appropriate health care professionals who need to assess the burn wound (e.g., physician) or perform a task (e.g., quantitative wound biopsies, range-of-motion exercises by physical therapist) of time of dressing change. ➤*Rationale:* Organization of care allows important assessment and intervention to take place without causing extra pain and stress to the patient.
- After checking what was previously needed for patient comfort during the dressing change, premedicate the patient with pain medication and any sedation that is ordered an appropriate amount of time before starting wound care. ➤*Rationale:* Allows time for medication to take effect and promotes optimal comfort for the patient.

Procedure for Care of Burn Wounds

Steps	Rationale	Special Considerations
1. Prepare all necessary equipment and supplies. The treatment area should be warmed.	Preparation facilitates efficient wound care and prevents needless delays. Warming the room decreases risk for hypothermia.	
2. Wash hands well and don examination gloves.	Reduces transmission of microorganisms to the patient and staff; standard isolation precautions.	
3. Remove old dressings and discard them in infectious waste container. Place towel or pad under exposed extremity.	Old dressings can contain large amounts of body secretions and blood. A clean field under the extremity will allow the patient a place to rest the extremity during care.	Remove dressings only from areas that can be redressed within 20 to 30 min at one time. Finish wound care to these areas before moving to new areas (decreases heat loss and pain related to nerve endings being exposed to air).
4. Remove and discard gloves; don a pair of clean gloves.	Used gloves are contaminated by handling of the burn dressing. Clean gloves are needed for wound care.	
5. Wash wound with mild soap solution or wound cleanser, rinse with warm tap water, and pat dry.	Cleanses wound of debris by mechanical debridement and reduces microorganisms.	Cleanse beyond wound to reduce microbial count on surrounding tissue. Patients may do better if allowed to cleanse their own wounds.
6. Use scissors and forceps to remove loose necrotic tissue and to remove any broken blister tissue.	Bacteria proliferate in necrotic tissue.	Typically, physicians perform this function in hospitals that do not specialize in burn wound care.
7. Assess the burn wound for color, size, odor, depth, drainage, bleeding, edema, cellulitis, epithelial budding, eschar separation, sensation, movement, peripheral pulses, and any signs of pressure areas from splints. For wet dressings, proceed to step 10.	Validates the healing process and identifies complications.	Other health care professionals that need to observe the wound should be notified ahead of time so that they can be present while the wound is uncovered.
8. Remove and discard gloves. Apply sterile gloves.	Gloves are contaminated from burn wound care. Sterile gloves should be used for application of the sterile dressing.	
9. Use sterile tongue depressor to remove required amount of topical agent from container. Place on sterile surface before applying $\frac{1}{4}$-in layer directly to burn wound and covering with burn dressing, or apply $\frac{1}{4}$-in layer on burn dressing and cover wound. Proceed to step 13 to continue wound care.	Using sterile tongue depressor and removing only what is needed from container prevent contamination of topical agent.	If the area to be covered has folds and crevices, or if the wound consists of scattered areas, topical agents should be placed directly on the wound, rather than on the burn dressing (ensures good coverage without applying unnecessary amounts of an absorbable topical agent to uninjured areas).
10. Pour prescribed solution into sterile bowl, and drop in sterile gauze pads.		Wet dressings must be moistened every 4 hours. If dressing is adherent to epithelial buds or granulation tissue, wet the dressing with sterile NS to loosen.

Procedure continues on the following page

Procedure **for Care of Burn Wounds**—*Continued*

Steps	Rationale	Special Considerations
11. Remove and discard gloves. Apply sterile gloves.	Gloves are contaminated from burn wound care. Sterile gloves should be used for application of the sterile dressing.	
12. Squeeze excess solution from gauze, and place dressing on wound.		
13. Loosely wrap extremities with gauze rolls.	Holds dressings in place.	Wrap extremities from distal to proximal. Check pulses and capillary refill after wrapping to ensure circulation is not compromised.
14. Assess need for more pain medication before continuing. *(Level II: Theory-based; no research data to support recommendations; recommendations from expert consensus group may exist.)*	Patients have a right to good pain control. The success or failure of pain control for the current dressing change will affect the way the patient responds to future dressing changes.	
15. Repeat steps, starting at step 3, until all burn wounds have been cared for.	Isolating areas for dressing changes prevents unnecessary temperature loss, pain from increased nerve ending exposure to air movement, and cross-contamination of wounds.	The size of the team doing the dressing and the amount of debridement time required will determine how much of the wound should reasonably be exposed at any given time.
16. Apply splints as needed and elevate burned extremities with pillows or elastic net sling or both; elevate head of bed. *(Level II: Theory-based; no research data to support recommendations; recommendations from expert consensus group may exist.)*	Maintains position of function, prevents contractures, and reduces edema and pain.	Do not "gatch" knees if popliteal space is burned. Do not put pillow under head if neck or ears are burned. Do not inhibit movement with splints if patient is awake and able to use involved extremity.
17. Remove and discard gloves. Wash hands.	Reduces transmission of microorganisms.	

Expected Outcomes

- Wounds heals without infectious complications.
- Patient maintains a self-identified acceptable level of pain relief.
- Patient attains comfort from measures taken for anxiety and itching.
- Patient and family verbalize knowledge of patient condition and plan of care.
- An optimal level of function is maintained or attained.
- Patient and family response and interactions demonstrate adaptation to injury.
- Patient and family collaborate in management of care.
- At the time of discharge, patient and family verbalize and demonstrate an understanding of posthospital care.

Unexpected Outcomes

- Wound converts to deeper injury.
- Wound sepsis occurs.
- Wound heals with unnecessary loss of function.

Patient Monitoring and Care

Steps	Rationale	Reportable Conditions
		These conditions should be reported if they persist despite nursing interventions.
1. Evaluate and treat the patient for pain. Ask the patient to rate pain on a scale of 0 to 10; check the orders for pain and sedation for dressing changes; check to see what the patient's medication requirements were with previous dressing changes and have that amount of medication available in the room before starting the dressing; assess the need for more medication throughout the dressing change. Incorporate alternative pain relief techniques (e.g., relaxation techniques, massage therapy, music, visual imaging).	The burn patient will have baseline pain requiring pain medication and increased pain medication requirements and possibly sedation requirements for the pain involved in dressing changes. Attention to the patient's pain will foster the patient's trust in health care personnel to control pain and will promote cooperation with future burn wound care.	• Increased heart rate • Increased or decreased blood pressure • Increased respiratory rate • Verbalization of pain • Nonverbal indications of pain (restlessness, grimacing, teeth clenching) • Inability to cooperate with dressing change
2. Obtain baseline vital signs before procedure, monitor throughout procedure, and check for 30 min after procedure is complete.	Changes in vital signs can be an indication that the patient is experiencing pain or anxiety. Decreasing blood pressure, heart rate, and respiratory rate can be complications of pain medication (especially after dressing change is complete and stimulation has stopped).	• Increased or decreased heart rate • Increased or decreased blood pressure • Increased or decreased respiratory rate • High peak pressures on ventilator
3. Check patient's temperature before dressing change. Make sure patient environment is warm; cover the portions of patient's body that are not involved in dressing change. Check temperature at end of dressing change.	Heat is lost through burn wounds.	• Hypothermia
4. Monitor peripheral pulses and circulation in burned extremity during the dressing change, within 1 hr after applying dressing, and every 2 hr thereafter. Keep extremities elevated and assess for increased edema.	Circumferential burns can decrease or prevent blood flow to involved extremity. The dressing can be too tight, especially if edema increases.	• Increased peripheral edema • Decreased or absent pulses • Pain or numbness in extremity • Prolonged or absent capillary refill in extremity • Conversion to deeper burn wound
5. Assess the burn wound for color, size, odor, depth, drainage, bleeding, pain, early eschar separation, healing, and cellulitis in the surrounding tissue. Obtain wound cultures as needed for suspected infection.	Observes for usual progression of wound healing versus complications of infection, progression of burn to deeper wound, and bleeding.	• Foul odor • Purulent or increased amounts of drainage • Patient spiking temperatures • Cellulitis • Healthy granulation tissue developing eschar • Increasing necrosis • Blurring of burn wound edges • Discoloration of wound • Early eschar separation • Bleeding

Procedure continues on the following page

Patient Monitoring and Care—*Continued*

Steps	Rationale	Reportable Conditions
6. Encourage exercise and activities of daily living; perform range-of-motion exercises during dressing changes; place patient in position of optimal function, using splints as needed to maintain. Use pain medication as needed to facilitate mobility.	Burns contract during the healing phase if not correctly splinted and exercised; loss of function is a complication of immobility. Pain inhibits patients from moving.	• Contractures • Loss of function
7. Monitor patient's tolerance of tube feedings or patient's ingestion of a high-calorie and high-protein diet with supplements; encourage nutritious diet and discourage empty calories. Limit free water intake.	Nutrition is necessary for wound healing; burn patients are hypermetabolic. Protein-rich fluids promote healing; free water decreases intake of nutritional supplements and can lead to hyponatremia.	• Refusal to eat or inability to ingest adequate amount of nutrition • Poor wound healing

Documentation

Documentation should include the following:

- Patient and family education
- Date and time of wound care
- Areas of burn, other wounds, and pressure ulcers; weekly diagrams (or digital photos) of unhealed wounds done to monitor healing and wound changes
- Appearance of the wound (color, size, odor, depth, drainage, bleeding)
- Assessment of wound areas for level of pain (appropriate for depth and level of healing)
- Progression toward healing (e.g., presence of epithelial budding)
- Evidence of cellulitis around the wound (red, warm, tender)

- Assessment of peripheral pulses; color, movement, sensation, and capillary refill distal to a circumferential wound or an extremity wrapped in dressings
- Assessment of pain before, during, and after procedure
- Medications given for pain and sedation
- Other comfort measures used
- Dressings and topical agents applied
- Patient's tolerance of the procedure
- Unexpected outcomes
- Nursing interventions

References

1. Alexander, J.W. (2002). Nutritional pharmacology in surgical patients. *Am J Surgery*, 183, 349-52.
2. American Burn Association. (1994). *Advanced Burn Life Support Course.* Chicago: Author.
3. American Burn Association. (2001). Practice guidelines for burn care: outpatient management of burn patients. *J Burn Care & Rehab*, 10S-3S.
4. Barret, J.P., and Herndon, D.N. (2003). Effects of burn wound excision on bacterial colonization and invasion. *Plastic & Reconstruct Surgery*, 111, 744-50.
5. Barrows, K.A., and Jacobs, B.P. (2002). Mind-body medicine: an introduction and review of the literature. *Med Clinics North Am*, 86, 11-31.
6. Bello, Y.M., and Falabella, A.F. (2001). Use of skin substitutes in dermatology. *Dermatologic Clinics*, 19, 555-61.
7. Chung, J.Y., and Herbert, M.E. (2001). Myth: silver sulfadiazine is the best treatment for minor burns. *Western J Med*, 175, 205-6.
8. Edwards-Jones, V., and Greenwood, J.E. (2001). What's new in burn microbiology: James Laing Memorial Prize Essay 2000. *Burns*, 29, 15-24.
9. Fauerbach, J.A., et al. (2002). Coping with the stress of a painful medical procedure. *Behav Res Ther*, 40, 1003-15.
10. Gottschlich, M.M., et al. (2002). An evaluation of the safety of early vs delayed enteral support and effects on clinical, nutritional, and endocrine outcomes after severe burns. *J Burn Care & Rehab*, 23, 401-15.
11. Helvig, E.I. (2002). Managing thermal injuries within WOCN practice. *J Wound Ostomy & Continence Nurs*, 29, 76-82.
12. Henry, D.B., and Foster, R.L. (2000). Burn pain management in children. *Pediatr Clin North Am*, 47, 681-699.
13. Ho, W.S., et al. (2003). Prospective study on the treatment of postburn hyperpigmentation by intense pulsed light. *Lasers Surgery & Med*, 32, 42-5.
14. Horswell, B.B. (1998). Scar modification. Techniques for revision and camouflage. *Atlas Oral Maxillofac Surg Clin North Am*, 6, 55-72.
15. Ilechukwu, S.T. (2002). Psychiatry of the medically ill in the burn unit. *Psychiatr Clin North Am*, 25, 129-47.
16. Innes, M.E., et al. (2001). The use of silver coated dressings on donor site wounds: a prospective, controlled matched pair study. *Burns*, 27, 621-7.
17. Jones, I., Currie, L., and Martin, R. (2002). A guide to biologic skin substitutes. *Brit J Plastic Surgery*, 55, 185-93.
18. Kagan, R.J., and Smith, S.C. (2000). Evaluation and treatment of thermal injuries. *Dermatol Nurs*, 12, 334-50.
19. Kaye, E.T. (2000). Topical antibacterial agents. *Infectious Dis Clin North Am*, 14, 321-39.
20. Koumbourlis, A.C. (2002). Electrical injuries. *Crit Care Med*, 30, 424-30.
21. Lionelli, G.T., and Lawrence, W.T. (2003). Wound dressings. *Surg Clin North Am*, 83, 617-38.
22. Lund, C.C., and Browder, N.C. (1944). The estimate of areas of burns. *Surgery, Gynecology & Obstetrics*, 79, 352-8.
23. Morgan, E.D. (2000). Ambulatory management of burns. *American Family Physician*, 62, 2015-26, 2029-30, 2032.

24. Musgrave, M.A., et al. (2002). The effect of silicone gel sheets on perfusion of hypertrophic burn scars. *J Burn Care & Rehab,* 223, 208-14.
25. Osborn, K. (2003). Nursing burn injuries. *Nurs Manage,* 34, 49-56.
26. Purdue, G.F., Hunt, J.L., and Burris, A.M. (2002). Pediatric burn care. *Clin Pediatr Emerg Med,* 3, 76-82.
27. Roques, C. (2002). Pressure therapy to treat burn scars. *Wound Repair & Regeneration,* 10, 122-5.
28. Saffle, J.R. (2003). What's new in general surgery: burns and metabolism. *J American College Surgery,* 196, 267-89.
29. Sheridan, R.L. (2002). Burns. *Crit Care Med,* 30(11 Suppl), S500-14.
30. Singer, A.J., and McClain, S.A. (2002). Persistent wound infection delays epidermal maturation and increases scarring in thermal burns. *Wound Repair & Regeneration,* 10, 372-7.
31. Staley, M.J., and Richard, R.L. (1997). Use of pressure to treat hypertrophic burn scars. *Advances Wound Care,* 10, 44-6.
32. Valencia, I.C., Falabella, A.F., and Eaglstein, W.H. (2000). Skin grafting. *Dermatologic Clinics,* 18, 521-32.

Additional Reading

Flynn, M.B., ed. (2004). Burn and wound care. *Crit Care Nurs Clinics North Am,* 16.

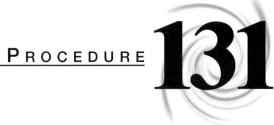

PROCEDURE **131**

Skin Graft Care

P U R P O S E : Skin-graft care is performed to promote graft take, to prevent infection, and to maximize function.

Jeanne R. Lowe

PREREQUISITE NURSING KNOWLEDGE

- An autograft is a skin graft taken from one area of a patient's body and transplanted to a different area of the same patient's body to cover a full-thickness wound. It involves the surgical removal of a section of the epidermis (and sometimes superficial dermis), thus creating a new, partial-thickness wound called a donor site.[3] The graft, a split-thickness skin graft (STSG), is applied over a clean, surgically excised wound that has been debrided of all nonviable tissue.

- An autograft is the only permanent treatment that can heal a large, full-thickness wound. Autografts are also frequently used over deep partial-thickness burn wounds after surgically converting the wound to full thickness. This reduces healing time and thus the risk for complications such as infection, contractures, and hypertrophic scarring.[3]

- The autograft is harvested from an appropriate donor site on the patient's body using a dermatome, a surgical instrument that resembles a cheese slicer. It is common to mesh the STSG (Fig. 131-1) so that it can be stretched to cover approximately 1.5 to 9 times more surface area than the original donor site. The ability to stretch the donor graft is important when there is a limited availability of suitable donor sites or when the burn is extensive. The goals following a meshed graft placement are to protect the wound bed from infection and desiccation and to ensure that there is no movement of the graft while it is becoming vascularized. Neovascularization begins within the first 24 hours of surgery as capillaries grow up into the graft, securing the graft permanently to its new site within 5 to 7 days. Either a barrier dressing (e.g., Biobrane, allograft) protects the wound (with or without a bulky

dressing added), or a minimal nonadherent dressing (e.g., Xeroform) is used with a bulky dressing acting as the barrier to infection and drying. The spaces created by meshing (the interstices) fill in as the epithelial cells from the graft migrate across the meshed spaces, much like a lawn seeding itself. Because of cosmetic and functional concerns related to appearance and increased shrinkage, meshed grafts are not used on the face and are avoided over joints.

- If the STSG is not meshed, it is called a sheet graft. A sheet graft covers the same amount of surface area as the donor site and is used for cosmetic or functional reasons. Pockets of serous fluid or blood tend to accumulate under these grafts (the interstices of meshed grafts allow the fluid to escape), separating the graft from the wound bed that is vital for blood supply. It is imperative to evacuate this fluid. Sheet grafts on the face, neck, and hands are generally inspected within the first 12 to 24 hours to look for

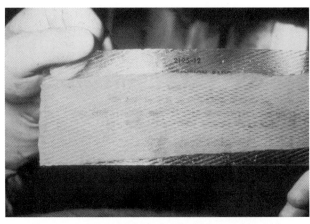

FIGURE 131-1 Meshed split-thickness skin graft.

fluid collections or graft dislodgement. If the sheet graft has been in place for less than 48 hours and the fluid is near the edge of sheet graft, the fluid can be rolled to the edge and out (Fig. 131-2).[2] However, doing this after vascularization begins can disrupt the attachment and endanger graft take. Therefore, practice should be to make a small nick in the sheet graft directly over the area of fluid accumulation and gently express the fluid through the hole.[2] In either case, the fluid should be gently dabbed away with gauze dampened with sterile normal saline or sterile water. Seromas and hematomas tend to redevelop in the same areas, so careful charting should reflect location of any blebs. Close monitoring of these areas should occur at least every 8 hours until bleb formation is no longer noted.

- Cultured epidermal autografts are commercially available and are an option when the patient does not have enough unburned tissue for donor sites to cover the burn in a reasonable period of time.[1] Cultured epidermal autografts are grown from a sample of the patient's own epidermal cells in a laboratory. However, the cost is prohibitive, the grafts are extremely fragile, and successful take of the graft is much more likely if the burn team has experience with this treatment.[3,8]

- The use of artificial skin and other options for wound coverage has expanded in recent years. Currently, the use of these wound coverings is limited to providing temporary wound coverage or allowing for dermal regeneration while waiting for suitable donor sites for definitive wound closure by autografting. Table 131-1 lists a few of the skin substitutes available.[1]

- Within the last decade, the use of Integra® Dermal Regeneration Template (Ethicon Endo-Surgery, Inc., Cincinnati, OH) has been shown to decrease LOS in severely injured burned adults.[9] Integra® is a commercial bilayer dermal regeneration template system that is now being widely used in burn centers worldwide to treat severely burned patients. Early surgical excision of eschar, with immediate coverage of the excised wounds with Integra® leads to decreased wound infections, reduced fluid loss and pain, and diminished catabolism. Integra® is composed of two layers. The first layer is made from cross-linked bovine collagen and chondroitin 6-sulfate (glycosaminoglycan) from shark collagen, which is a permanent dermal template providing a scaffolding for the patient's own dermis to grow into. The second layer, the outer layer, is a temporary Silastic covering that acts

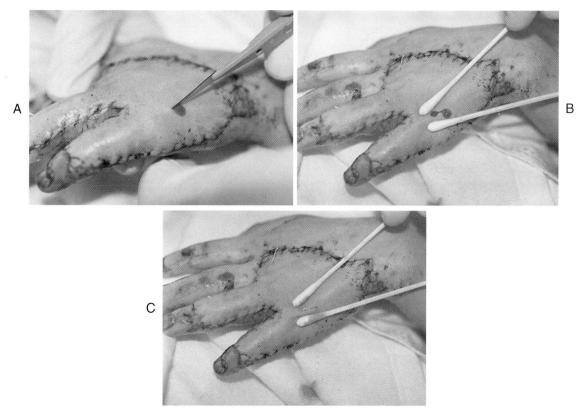

FIGURE 131-2 **A,** A No. 11 surgical blade and cotton-tipped applicator are used to blade a new sheet graft. Note that the blade is held so that the tip of the cutting surface comes into contact with only the graft. **B,** Cotton-tipped applicators are rolled gently over the graft toward the slit in order to express fluid that has collected between the graft and the wound bed surface. When deblebbing thick grafts, it is important to make adequate-sized slits to avoid recurring buildup of fluid, which may jeopardize graft survivability and result in scarring. **C,** Blebs tend to recur in the same place. It is advisable to be vigilant about deblebbing at least once every 8 hours until bleb formation ceases. Documentation of bleb formation and location ensures that the next caregiver will be aware of graft sites in need of close monitoring. *(From Carrougher, G.J. [1998].* Burn Care and Therapy. *St. Louis: Mosby.)*

TABLE 131-1	Types of Skin Substitutes Used as Wound Coverings
Skin Substitutes	**Description**
Permanent Wound Coverings	
Sheet autograft	Thin, intact layer of skin (epidermis and dermis) used for small or cosmetic areas including portion of dermis.
Meshed autograft	Thin layer of skin with small holes that allow for expansion in order to cover more area, including portion of dermis.
Cultured epithelial autograft	Patient's own keratinocytes laboratory grown into sheets of cells. Used when patient's own skin is limited; lacks dermis (fragile).
Temporary Wound Coverings	
Allograft/homograft	Human cadaver skin donated and harvested after death; becomes vascularized but rejected.
Heterograft/xenograft	Porcine skin harvested after slaughter; cryopreserved or lyophilized for storage; develops collagen bond; not vascularized.
Biologicals	
Integra	Permanent dermal replacement bovine; hide collagen and chondroitin 6-sulfate obtained from shark collagen; neodermis; degrades and grafted with epidermal cells.
DermoGraft	Permanent dermal replacement made from fibroblasts of neonatal foreskin.
Apligraft	Cultured skin equivalent containing kerationcytes and fibroblasts (derived from neonatal foreskin).

From Bryant, R.A. (2000). *Acute and Chronic Wounds,* ed. 2. St. Louis: Mosby, p. 210.

as an artificial epidermis until the patient is ready for autografting, usually 2 to 3 weeks after the Integra® is placed. Because of enhanced dermal regeneration, the graft bed requires only a very thin meshed donor graft from the patient to heal the wound. This allows quicker healing of donor sites and the ability to reharvest from the same donor site multiple times, if necessary, in a very short time period. Clinical trials have demonstrated that the epidermal autograft over Integra® usually heals without the formation of the meshed appearance typical of meshed autografts, thereby resulting in a better cosmetic outcome for the patient.[5]

- Postoperative care of Integra® should be similar to treatment of sheet or meshed autografts. The outer dressing should be changed every 3 to 5 days, with or without the use of topical antimicrobial solutions. The patient should be monitored closely for signs of systemic infection. Graft sites should be monitored for fluid formation and infection. Staples or sutures securing the Silastic covering should remain in place until the patient is taken to the operating room for epidermal autografting.
- In the operating room, all nonviable tissue is surgically excised to create a wound bed able to support a skin graft (Fig. 131-3). Therefore the grafted area should be observed for bleeding for the first 24 hours.
- The graft is usually stapled or sutured in place or secured with Steri-Strips or Hypafix, covered with a nonadherent

dressing, and padded with a bulky bolster dressing to prevent mechanical dislodgement of the graft. Fibrin glue, a surgical hemostatic agent derived from human plasma, is often applied topically to the wound bed to decrease blood loss and promote graft adherence.[7]

- Postoperatively, the patient is immobilized for 3 to 5 days to prevent graft shearing or dislodgement of the graft from the wound bed. The first dressing change is usually done after 3 to 5 days. Most burn centers use clean technique for dressing removal and donor-site cleansing and use sterile technique for dressing application only.[4]
- If a patient is allowed to mobilize after surgery, leg grafts must be supported with Ace wraps or other compressive dressings when the patient's legs are dependent for the first 3 to 5 days after surgery to prevent capillary engorgement and hematoma formation beneath the graft. Grafted extremities should be elevated when the patient is supine.
- Initial healing of the grafted area should occur in 7 to 10 days, with vascularization occurring in the first 4 to 5 days. The graft area is immobilized for 4 to 5 days to prevent dislocation and shearing. Splints and immobilizers are used during this time to prevent disruption of grafts and to provide therapeutic positioning of extremities.
- Signs of successful graft take include vascularization of the graft, reepithelialization of the interstices, decreased pain, and adherence of the graft. Signs of complications include graft necrosis, graft loss, cellulitis, purulent drainage, and fever.
- Skin grafts contract during the healing and remodeling phases.[11] Continuing mobility and proper positioning are vital to prevent contractures and loss of function. Self-care and range-of-motion exercises should be encouraged as soon as the graft is adherent. Once the wounds heal, pressure garments may be ordered to be worn at all times, except during bathing, to reduce hypertrophic scar formation.[8]
- An individualized plan for pain control should be in place for both background pain (pain that is continuously present) and procedural pain (intermittent pain related to procedures and routine care). Unrelieved pain can lead to

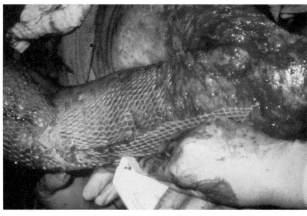

FIGURE 131-3 Meshed split-thickness skin graft covering the arm, with the remainder of the wound bed ready to be grafted.

stress-related immunosuppression, increased potential for infection, delayed wound healing, and depression.[10] Subcutaneous and intramuscular injections should be avoided when edema is present because absorption will be poor and unreliable. Intravenous administration of medication is preferred in critically ill patients; oral medication is preferred in noncritical patients with a functioning gastrointestinal system. As the wound heals, the patient will experience more discomfort from itchiness and less discomfort from pain. A water-based lotion will prevent drying and reduce urticaria.

- The burn patient is hypermetabolic until burn wounds are closed and healing is complete.[3] This is important to note because the patient's baseline body temperature will be higher than normal by 1°F to 2°F[1] (observe for temperature spikes rather than an absolute number), and the patient will be catabolic (resting energy expenditure can increase by as much as 100%),[3] requiring an increased caloric and protein intake for wound healing. It is important to keep the patient warm during wound care because a large amount of heat is lost from the wound, further increasing the metabolic rate.[6]

- Exposure of the healed skin graft to the sun should be avoided. The newly healed area is extremely sensitive to sunlight, and permanent discoloration can occur. To prevent discoloration, the patient should protect grafted areas with clothing or sunscreen. Over the first year, as the patient's graft matures, the risk for skin discoloration slowly decreases.

EQUIPMENT

- Personal protective equipment
- Examination gloves
- Sterile gloves
- Scissors and forceps
- Warm tap water (sometimes sterile water or sterile NS are used for first dressing change)
- Basin
- Clean washcloths
- Staple remover
- Nonadherent gauze (e.g., Adaptic, Xeroform)
- Bulky or thin dressings, as needed
- Pain and antianxiolytic medication (as prescribed)
  Additional equipment, as needed, includes the following:
- Splints (to be secured with gauze roll, Velcro, or Ace wraps or Coban self-adherent wrap)
- Towels or waterproof pads

PATIENT AND FAMILY EDUCATION

- Explain the procedure for skin graft care to patient and family. ➤➤*Rationale:* Diminishes fear of the unknown; ensures that patient and family are knowledgeable about graft care.
- Inform patient and family that the grafted area needs to be immobilized for 5 to 7 days to encourage graft take and reduce the risk for mechanical trauma to graft site.

➤➤*Rationale:* Increases patient's and family's assistance in maintaining immobilization.

- Inform patient and family that the skin graft should not be exposed to the sun for 1 year after the burn, that sunscreen and protective clothing should be used thereafter, and that there will be some scarring and discoloration, which will improve over the first year. Explain that grafted area will never grow hair or be able to sweat, because of permanent loss of these dermal appendages. ➤➤*Rationale:* Prepares patient and family for changes that will be present after hospital discharge and addresses anxieties about body image.

- Discuss the importance of proper positioning. Explain the need for continuing mobility through self-care and range-of-motion exercises as soon as the graft is adherent and throughout the healing phase. ➤➤*Rationale:* Prevents contractures and loss of function associated with healing skin grafts.[8,11]

- Assess family's ability to provide care at home. ➤➤*Rationale:* Continued care of the wound will be required after discharge.

- As appropriate, provide detailed wound care instructions in writing and review with patient and family. Demonstrate exactly what to do and have patient and family return demonstrations before the planned discharge. Continue to involve patient and family in the wound care for the remainder of the admission and encourage them to ask questions. Provide positive feedback. Arrange for home care or clinic visits to follow up on dressings and wound care. ➤➤*Rationale:* Validates patient and family understanding and ability to perform wound care independently and allows time for them to develop a level of comfort. Provides the opportunity to reinforce important points.

- Teach patient and family about pain and pruritus medications as needed. Provide the name of a water-based lotion to apply to healed areas. ➤➤*Rationale:* Supports comfort at home.

- Teach patient and family about signs and symptoms of infection and the importance of reporting these in a timely manner. ➤➤*Rationale:* Ensures that patient and family will recognize problems early so that appropriate measures can be instituted by the health care team.

- Emphasize the importance of wearing pressure garments and splints. ➤➤*Rationale:* Reduces scar formation and contractures.[6,8]

- Schedule follow-up appointments and provide the name of someone to call if there is a problem. ➤➤*Rationale:* Provides necessary information for further care and follow-up.

- Work with vocational rehabilitation counselor to formulate plan for patient's return to work. ➤➤*Rationale:* Depending on the severity of the patient's injuries, the patient may be physically unable to return to former employment or may need assistance with job modifications and accommodations. Developing a back-to-work plan based on any new limitations increases the patient's chance of successfully returning to work.

PATIENT ASSESSMENT AND PREPARATION

Patient Assessment

- Assess vital signs, including temperature. **➤Rationale:** Baseline vital signs allow for comparison during and following the procedure to evaluate patient tolerance and need for pain medication.
- Evaluate for success of graft take:
  - ❖ Vascularization of the graft
  - ❖ Reepithelialization of the interstices
  - ❖ Decreased pain
  - ❖ Adherence of the graft
- Monitor for signs of complications:
  - ❖ Graft necrosis
  - ❖ Graft loss
  - ❖ Cellulitis
  - ❖ Purulent drainage
  - ❖ Fever
- Compare patient's level of healing to expected level of healing for number of days after skin graft. **➤Rationale:** Initial healing of grafted area should occur in 7 to 10 days.
- Determine adequacy of the pain control regimen by asking the patient to rate the pain on a scale of 0 to 10, both before wound care (background) and during the dressing change.[10] **➤Rationale:** An individualized plan for pain control should be in place for background and procedural pain. In addition to the traditional use of pain and anxiety medications, alternative therapies should be included (e.g., relaxation techniques, distraction, massage therapy, music therapy). The patient's medication requirements should decrease as the grafted area heals.
- Assess patient's level of function in the grafted area. **➤Rationale:** Skin grafts contract during the healing phase, and immobility enhances loss of function. The patient should be encouraged to continue normal movement and range-of-motion exercises after graft take has been established.[8]

Patient Preparation

- Ensure that patient understands preprocedural teaching. Answer questions as they arise, and reinforce information as needed. **➤Rationale:** Evaluates and reinforces understanding of previously taught information.
- Make sure that other appropriate health care professionals who need to assess the graft (e.g., physician) or perform a task (e.g., range-of-motion exercises by physical therapist) are notified of the time of dressing change. **➤Rationale:** Organization of care allows important assessment and intervention to take place without causing extra pain and stress to the patient.
- After checking what was previously needed for patient comfort during the dressing change, premedicate the patient with pain medication and any sedation that is ordered. Allow an appropriate amount of time before starting wound care.[10] **➤Rationale:** Allows time for medication to take effect and promotes optimal comfort for the patient. Reduces pain and anxiety. Encourages patient trust and compliance with procedure.

Procedure for Care of Skin Grafts

Steps	Rationale	Special Considerations
1. Prepare all necessary equipment and supplies.	Preparation facilitates efficient wound care and prevents needless delays.	
2. Wash hands and don cap, mask, gown, and examination gloves (this applies to every health care person involved in the procedure).	Reduces transmission of microorganisms to the patient; standard precautions.	If family is doing dressing change at home, mask, cap, and gown are not used.
3. Remove bulky, outer dressings and discard. Place towel or pad under exposed extremity.	Old dressings can contain large amounts of body secretions and blood. Towel allows a place for patient to rest extremity during care.	Initial dressing is commonly left in place for 3 to 5 days; or bulky, outer dressings are changed while leaving nonadherent gauze in place (check orders).
4. Remove and discard gloves; and don a pair of clean gloves.	Examination gloves are contaminated by handling the burn dressing; clean gloves are needed for wound care.	

Procedure for Care of Skin Grafts—*Continued*

Steps	Rationale	Special Considerations
5. If ordered, gently lift nonadherent gauze from grafted site, anchoring graft in place as needed. Note: surgeon may staple on dressing that is to remain in place until skin graft heals (e.g., Biobrane).	Grafts are not firmly attached to the wound bed and can be pulled loose for up to 5 days after grafting.	Warm tap water may be used to loosen dressings stuck to graft area.
6. Gently rinse graft site and surrounding tissue with warm tap water and gauze or wash cloths.	Cleanses wound of exudate and reduces microorganisms.[11]	Special care is necessary not to displace skin graft.
7. Use scissors and forceps to remove loose necrotic tissue.[6] If it is a sheet graft, check for and remove any pockets of fluid under the graft.	Clears debris that can harbor microorganisms.[11] Pockets of fluid will separate the graft from the wound bed, which is vital for blood supply, causing graft loss in that area.	Remove pockets of fluid. If the sheet graft has been in place for less than 48 hours and the fluid is near the edge of sheet graft, roll the fluid to the edge and out; otherwise, make a small nick in the sheet graft directly over the area of fluid accumulation and gently express the fluid through the hole.[6] Gently remove exudate with gauze dampened with sterile NS or sterile water.
8. Remove staples that are no longer needed to hold graft or dressing in place.	Prevents embedding of staples, local irritation, and infection,[6] and scarring.	Staples can be removed starting 5 to 7 days after grafting. A large number of staples may require an anesthesia assisted procedure.
9. Assess graft for progression of healing and for complications.	Validates the healing process and identifies complications.	Notify other disciplines that need to observe the wound ahead of time so that they can be present while the wound is uncovered.
10. Apply nonadherent dressing (if interstices are open), cover with bulky dressings, and secure; or apply moisturizer to healed adherent graft areas where interstices are closed and cover with thin dressings to promote mobility.	Protects graft while healing.	A water-based lotion is used to prevent drying and reduce itching when interstices are closed.
11. Apply splints and elevate hands with pillows or elastic net sling; elevate head of bed.	Maintains position of function,[2] prevents contractures, and reduces edema[6] and pain.	If possible, prevent patient from lying on grafted areas. Consider use of pressure reduction mattress for grafts or donor sites on posterior surfaces. After the initial period of immobilization, splints are used only when the patient is unable to participate in range-of-motion exercises or self-care.
12. Remove and discard gloves. Wash hands.	Reduces transmission of microorganisms.	
13. Continue to monitor patient vital signs.	Patient may be hypothermic following wound care.	Removal of painful stimuli may result in over sedation following wound care.

Expected Outcomes

- Graft take of greater than 90% is attained.
- Patient maintains a self-identified acceptable level of pain relief.
- Patient attains comfort from measures taken for anxiety and itching.
- Patient and family verbalize knowledge of patient condition and plan of care.
- An optimal level of function is maintained or attained.
- Patient and family response and interactions demonstrate adaptation to injury.
- Patient and family collaborate in management of care.
- At the time of discharge, patient and family verbalize and demonstrate an understanding of posthospital care.

Unexpected Outcomes

- Bleeding
- Infection
- Graft loss

Patient Monitoring and Care

Steps	Rationale	Reportable Conditions
		These conditions should be reported if they persist despite nursing interventions.
1. Evaluate and treat the patient for pain. Ask the patient to rate his or her pain on a scale of 0 to 10; check the orders for pain and sedation for dressing changes; check to see what the patient's medication requirements were with previous dressing changes and have that amount of medication available in the room before starting the dressing; assess the need for more medication throughout the dressing change. Incorporate alternative pain relief techniques (e.g., relaxation techniques, distraction, massage therapy, music therapy, visual imaging). *(Level II: Theory-based, no research data to support recommendations; recommendations from expert consensus group may exist.)*	The patient with new skin grafts will have some baseline pain that requires pain medication and increased pain medication requirements and possibly sedation requirements for the procedural pain involved in graft care.[10] Attention to the patient's pain fosters the patient's trust in health care personnel to control pain and promotes cooperation with future graft care.	- Increased heart rate - Increased or decreased blood pressure - Increased respiratory rate - Verbalization of pain - Nonverbal indications of pain (restlessness, grimacing, teeth clenching) - Inability to cooperate with dressing change
2. Obtain baseline vital signs (including pulse oximetry, if using narcotics) before graft care, monitor throughout procedure, and check for 30 minutes after procedure is complete.	Changes in vital signs can be an indication that the patient is experiencing pain or anxiety. Decreasing blood pressure, heart rate, and respiratory rate can be complications of pain medication (especially after dressing change is complete and stimulation has stopped).	- Increased or decreased heart rate - Increased or decreased blood pressure - Increased or decreased respiratory rate - High peak pressures on ventilator
3. Assess graft site for appearance (e.g., color, drainage, bleeding, graft necrosis, graft loss, cellulitis) and progression toward healing (e.g., vascularization of the graft, reepithelialization of the interstices, decreased pain, adherence of the graft).	Observe for usual progression of wound healing versus complications.	- Foul odor - Purulent or increased amounts of drainage - Cellulitis - Hematoma or fluid collection under sheet grafts - Graft necrosis - Sloughing - Bleeding

Patient Monitoring and Care—*Continued*

Steps	Rationale	Reportable Conditions
4. Place patient in position of optimal function during initial period of immobilization of newly grafted areas, using splints to maintain. After the first 5 days, encourage exercise, activities of daily living, and range-of-motion exercises during dressing changes. Use pain medication as needed to facilitate mobility.	Grafted skin contracts during the healing phase if not correctly splinted and exercised.[8,11] Loss of function is a complication of immobility. Pain inhibits patients from moving.[10]	• Contractures • Loss of function
5. Monitor patient's tolerance of tube feedings or ingestion of a high-calorie, high-protein diet with supplements; encourage nutritious diet and discourage empty calories. Limit free water.	Nutrition is necessary for wound healing.[8] Burn patients are hypermetabolic.	• Poor wound healing • Graft loss

Documentation

Documentation should include the following:

- Patient and family education
- Date and time of graft care
- Appearance of graft site (e.g., color, drainage, bleeding, graft necrosis, sloughing, cellulitis)
- Progression toward healing (e.g., adherence and vascularization of the graft, reepithelialization of the interstices, decreased pain)
- Dressings and topicals applied
- Assessment of pain before, during, and after procedure
- Medications given for pain and sedation
- Other comfort measures used
- Patient's tolerance of the procedure
- Unexpected outcomes
- Nursing interventions

References

1. Bryant, R.A. (2000). *Acute & Chronic Wounds.* 2nd ed. St. Louis: Mosby.
2. Carrougher, G.J. (1998). *Burn Care and Therapy.* 1st ed. St. Louis: Mosby.
3. Greenfield, E. (1998). Integumentary disorders. In: Kinney, M.R., et al., eds. *AACN's Clinical Reference for Critical Care Nursing.* 4th ed. St. Louis: Mosby, 1065-87.
4. Herndon, D.N., ed. (2001). *Total Burn Care.* 2nd ed. London: W.B. Saunders Company Ltd., 548.
5. Heimbach, D., et al. (1988). Artificial dermis for major burns: A multi-center randomized clinical trial. *Ann Surg,* Sep, 208, 313-20.
6. Jordan, B.S., and Harrington, D.T. (1997). Management of the burn wound. *Nurs Clin North Am,* 32, 251-73.
7. Mankad, P.S., and Codispoti, M. (2001). The role of fibrin sealants in hemostasis. *Am J Surg,* 182(2 Suppl), 21S-8S (Review).
8. Rose, J.K., et al. (1996). Advances in burn care. *Adv Surg,* 30, 71-95.
9. Ryan, C.M., et al. (2002). Use of Integra artificial skin is associated with decreased length of stay for severely injured adult burn survivors. *J Burn Care Rehab,* Sep/Oct, 23, 311-7.
10. Ulmer, J.F. (1998). Burn pain management: A guideline-based approach. *J Burn Care Rehab,* 19, 151-9.
11. Ward, R.S., and Saffle, J.R. (1995). Topical agents in burn and wound care. *Phys Ther,* 75, 526-38.

Additional Readings

Barret, J.P., and Herndon, D.N. (2003). Effects of burn wound excision on bacterial colonization and invasion. *Plast Reconstruct Surg,* Feb, 111, 744-50.
Blackburn, J.H., II, et al. (1998). Negative pressure dressings as a bolster for skin grafts. *Ann Plast Surg,* 40, 453-7.
Flynn, M.B., ed. (2004). Burn and wound care. *Crit Care Nurs Clinics North Am,* 16.
Heimbach, D.M., et al. (2003). Multicenter postapproval clinical trial of Integra Dermal Regeneration Template for burn treatment. *J Burn Care Rehab,* 24, 42-8.
Jones, I., Currie, L., and Martin, R. (2002). A guide to biological skin substitutes. *Br J Plast Surg,* 55, 185-93 (Review).
Lorenz, C., et al. (1997). Early wound closure and early reconstruction. Experience with a dermal substitute in a child with 60 percent surface area burn. *Burns,* Sep, 23, 505-8.
McCain, D., and Sutherland, S. (1998). Nursing essentials: Skin grafts for patients with burns. *Am J Nurs,* 98, 34-8.
Ward, C.G. (1998). Burns. *J Am Coll Surg,* 186, 123-6.
Valencia, I.C., Falabella, A.F., and Eaglstein, W.H. (2000). Skin grafting. *Dermatol Clin,* 18, 521-32 (Review).
Young, T., and Fowler, A. (1998). Nursing management of skin grafts and donor sites. *Br J Nurs,* 7, 324-6, 328, 330.

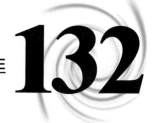

SECTION TWENTY-TWO

Special Integumentary
Procedures

P R O C E D U R E **132**

Intracompartmental Pressure Monitoring

P U R P O S E :   Compartment syndrome results from increased pressure within a limited anatomic space. Compartment syndrome can affect any confined anatomic space where there is an increase in pressure. Most commonly, the upper and lower extremities are involved. Intracompartmental pressure monitoring detects pressure within the muscle compartments.

John J. Gallagher

PREREQUISITE NURSING KNOWLEDGE

- Anatomy of the involved limb compartments (Fig. 132-1) should be understood.
- Knowledge of aseptic technique is essential.
- Two general factors may contribute to the development of compartment syndrome. First, there may be an increase in the contents of the compartment in excess of compartment size secondary to tissue edema or hemorrhage. Second, there may be restriction applied to the compartment from bandages, casts, or pneumatic antishock garment (PASG), reducing tissue expandability and thereby increasing compartment pressure.[1-7,9,10-11]
- The elevation of tissue pressure within the compartment causes compression or occlusion of arteriole flow resulting in ischemia and eventual necrosis of the tissues in the compartment.
- Tissue edema may be worsened as venous outflow is compromised and additional tissue edema results. Interventions to relieve the pressure within the compartment, such as fasciotomy, should be initiated within 4 to 6 hours to prevent ischemia or severe complications.[10]
- Patients at risk for the development of limb compartment syndrome include those who have sustained vascular, soft-tissue, or orthopedic trauma; patients with burns; patients with shock; and those who have undergone massive fluid resuscitation (Table 132-1).
- In general, initial symptoms of compartment syndrome may be observed within 2 hours of the initial trauma or

insult. Ischemia may result in 4 to 6 hours, with ischemic contractures and nerve injury resulting in permanent functional loss in 12 to 24 hours.[10]
- Intracompartmental pressures are monitored in patients who are at risk for the development of compartment syndrome.[5,10] If left untreated, compartment syndrome results in tissue ischemia and necrosis, permanent nerve damage, limb contractures, and possibly, loss of the involved limb. The degree of tissue injury and functional loss depends on the severity and duration of compartment pressure elevation.
- Intracompartmental pressures are obtained from the muscle compartments in the upper and lower extremities using a variety of invasive measuring devices.[5,12]
- Compartment pressure monitoring of the extremities is performed using a pressure monitoring device attached to a needle, wick, or slit catheter (Figs. 132-2 and 132-3).[5,8,11]
- Normal limb compartment pressure is 0 mm Hg. Compartment pressures that are within 10 to 30 mm Hg of the diastolic blood pressure may indicate the presence of compartment syndrome (e.g., a compartment pressure increase to 40 to 45 mm Hg in a person with a diastolic blood pressure of 70 mm Hg may indicate compartment syndrome).[10]
- Compartment syndrome in the extremities is heralded by the five "Ps": pain, paresthesia, pallor, pulselessness, and paralysis[3-4,10-11]:
  ❖ *Pain* is the earliest symptom of compartment syndrome; however, it may not be distinguishable from the pain related to injuries to the extremity. The pain is

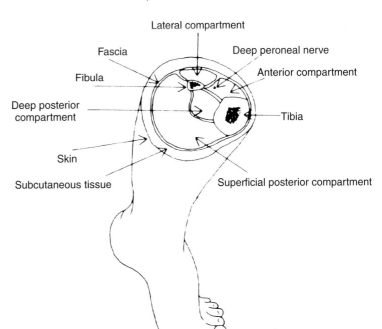

FIGURE 132-1 Muscle compartments of the lower extremity. *(From Ross, D. [1991]. Acute compartment syndrome.* Orthop Nurs, *10[2], 33-8. Reprinted with permission of the National Association of Orthopaedic Nurses.)*

generally unremitting and is not responsive to therapeutic measures such as fracture stabilization or the administration of analgesic agents. Pain is generally exacerbated by passive flexion and extension of the hand or foot in the affected extremity.

TABLE 132-1	Etiology of Compartment Syndrome

Trauma
- Fractures
- Surgery of the extremity
- Hematomas
- Postischemic swelling
- Crush injuries
- Electric injuries
- Vascular injuries

Factors Precipitating Edema Formation
- Prolonged use of tourniquets in surgery
- Vascular obstruction (arterial and venous)
- Replantation surgery
- Nephrotic syndrome
- Thermal injury (frostbite or burns)
- Excessive use (athletic injury)

Coagulopathies
- Anticoagulant therapy
- Hemophilia

Other
- Constrictive dressings, splints, or casts
- Premature or "tight" closure of a fascial defect
- Pneumatic antishock garment
- Hyperthermia or hypothermia
- Infiltration of intravenous infusions
- Intraarterial injections
- Snake bite
- Legionnaire's disease
- Rocky Mountain spotted fever
- *Clostridium perfringens* infection
- Excessive pressure from prolonged immobility in one position

Adapted from Ross, D. (2001). Compartment syndrome. In: Swearingen, P.L., and Keen, J.H., eds. *Manual of Critical Care Nursing: Nursing Interventions and Collaborative Management.* 4th ed. St. Louis: Mosby, 161-6.

❖ *Paresthesia* is one of the earliest signs of impending, yet reversible, compartment syndrome. Paresthesia generally precedes motor dysfunction. Hypothesia of the nerves traversing the affected compartment may also occur (Fig. 132-4).

❖ *Pallor* may be seen in the affected limb, which could also be mottled or cyanotic.

❖ *Pulselessness* is an extremely late finding. Compromised arteriole flow may result in compartment syndrome while palpable pulses are still present.

❖ *Paralysis* is a late sign and signals advanced compartment syndrome.

EQUIPMENT

- Introducer needle (angiocath), 16 G or larger
- Slit or wick catheter
- Electronic pressure monitoring device (bedside pressure monitor or a handheld monitoring device)
- Transducer and pressure tubing setup
- 30-ml syringe
- 50-ml sterile normal saline (NS)
- Sterile gloves

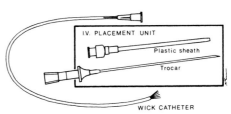

FIGURE 132-2 A wick catheter for intracompartmental pressure monitoring. *(From Mubarak, S.J., and Hargens, A.R. [1981].* Compartment Syndromes and Volkmann's Contracture. *Philadelphia: W.B. Saunders.)*

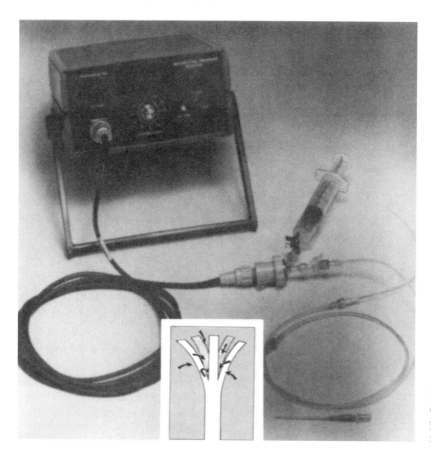

FIGURE 132-3 Slit catheter setup. Slit tip on catheter consists of five petals that allow a patent fluid path and prevent occlusion with material or tissue. *(Courtesy Howmedica, Inc.)*

- Povidone pads, swab-sticks, or solution
- Sterile dressing
- One roll of hypoallergenic tape
- 1% lidocaine without epinephrine

Additional equipment to have available, as needed, includes the following:

- Scissors

PATIENT AND FAMILY EDUCATION

- Explain the indication for compartment pressure monitoring to the patient and family. ➤*Rationale:* Improves patient and family understanding of why the procedure is needed.
- Explain the procedure to the patient and family. ➤*Rationale:* Explaining the procedure may decrease patient and family anxiety and assist in patient cooperation.

PATIENT ASSESSMENT AND PREPARATION

Patient Assessment

- Review the patient's health history for conditions predisposing the patient to compartment syndrome (see Table 132-1).

➤*Rationale:* Patients with certain pathologies and injuries are at increased risk for compartment syndrome.

- Assess the patient's involved extremity for signs and symptoms that may indicate the onset of compartment syndrome. These include pain, paresthesia, changes in skin color and temperature, limitations in movement, change in the strength of distal pulses, tenseness of the tissue, and increase in the girth of the extremity.[10-11] ➤*Rationale:* These symptoms alone indicate the onset of compartment syndrome and the need for intracompartmental pressure measurement and therapeutic intervention.

Patient Preparation

- Ensure that the patient and family understand preprocedural teaching. Answer questions as they arise and reinforce information as needed. ➤*Rationale:* Evaluates and reinforces understanding of previously taught information.
- Remove constricting dressings and bandages. Assist with the removal and modification of splints, casts, PSAGs, or other devices on the affected extremity.[5,10,11] ➤*Rationale:* Reduces external pressure on the tissue of the affected extremity.
- Assist the patient to the supine position. ➤*Rationale:* Provides access to the affected compartment.

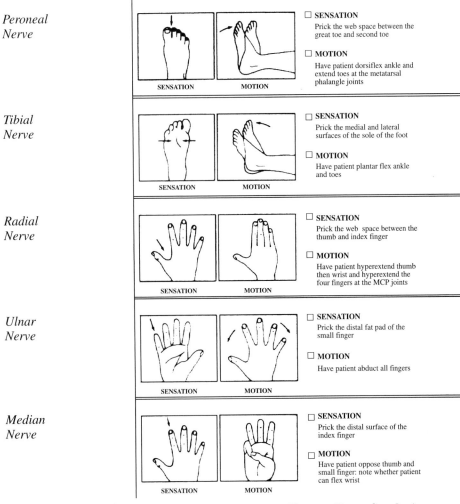

FIGURE 132-4 Neurovascular assessment. *(Courtesy Howmedica, Inc.)*

Procedure | for Intracompartmental Pressure Monitoring

Steps	Rationale	Special Considerations
1. Wash hands.	Reduces transmission of microorganisms; standard precautions.	
2. Assemble the pressure transducer and tubing system (Fig. 132-5).	Prepares the monitoring system.	
3. Fill the 30-ml syringe with normal saline and flush the tubing.	Ensures that there is no air in the system.	
4. Turn on the electronic monitoring device.	Establishes power to the monitoring system.	A portable bedside electronic monitoring device (see Fig. 132-5) designed for the purpose of monitoring compartment pressures can be used or a standard cardiac monitoring system with an available invasive pressure monitoring channel can be used.

Procedure continues on the following page

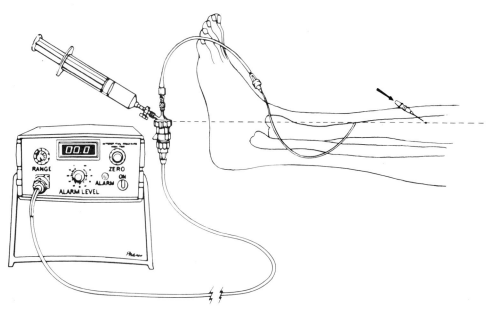

FIGURE 132-5 The open part of the venting stopcock is placed at the level of the tip of the intracompartmental catheter *(arrow)*. Dashes show this level.

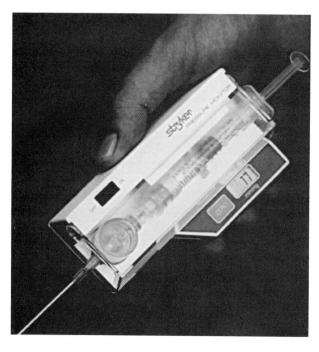

FIGURE 132-6 Stryker intracompartmental pressure monitor. *(Courtesy Stryker Instruments.)*

Procedure for Intracompartmental Pressure Monitoring—*Continued*

Steps	Rationale	Special Considerations
		In addition, a handheld unit such as the Stryker Intracompartmental Pressure Monitor (Fig. 132-6) may be used.
5. Select the appropriate pressure scale on the monitor.	The 30 or 60 mm Hg scale will be sufficient to measure the majority of pressure ranges.	
6. Connect the transducer system to the monitoring device.	Prepares the monitoring system.	

Procedure for Intracompartmental Pressure Monitoring—*Continued*

Steps	Rationale	Special Considerations
7. Wash hands and don clean gloves.	Reduces the transmission of microorganisms; standard precautions.	
8. Assist the physician with preparation of the intended site: A. Clip hairs in the area if necessary. B. Cleanse with povidone-iodine in a circular motion. C. Repeat the povidone-iodine cleansing.	Reduces the potential for infection.	
9. Remove gloves and wash hands.	Reduces the transmission of microorganisms; standard precautions.	
10. Prepare the local anesthetic agent according to physician request or institutional protocol.	Local anesthetic agents may be used before insertion of the introducer needle for patient analgesia.	Other concomitant analgesic or antianxiety agents may be indicated depending on patient need.
11. Level the air-fluid interface (zeroing stopcock) with the planned insertion site of the catheter (see Fig. 132-5).	The intended insertion site of the catheter is the reference point.	
12. Set the system to zero.	Negates the effect of atmospheric system. Ensures accuracy of the system with the established reference point.	
13. Attach the sterile wick or slit catheter to the end of the pressure tubing (see Fig. 132-5).	Connects the monitoring system to the catheter.	
14. Check the responsiveness of the wick or slit catheter to changes in pressure by holding the catheter level with the air-fluid interface (monitor should read "zero"). Raise the catheter to eye level (monitor pressure should rise to 30 to 50 mm Hg).	Ensures the system is able to read changes in pressure.	Failure of the pressure to increase when the catheter is elevated or an increase in pressure with a rapid drop in pressure may indicate a system leak. A slow increase in pressure with elevation of the catheter may indicate air in the system.
15. Assist the physician as needed with insertion of the introducer needle and the wick or slit catheter (Figs. 132-7 and 132-8).	The introducer catheter is inserted first; then the wick or slit catheter is inserted through the introducer needle.	If only a single reading is being obtained, the pressure tubing may be attached directly to the introducer needle after insertion. A handheld device (see Fig. 132-6) equipped with a needle may be a better choice for single measurement use.

Procedure continues on the following page

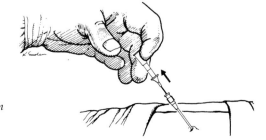

FIGURE 132-7 Jelco catheter used for insertion of wick catheter. (*From Mubarak, S.J., and Hargens, A.R. [1981].* Compartment Syndromes and Volkmann's Contracture. *Philadelphia: W.B. Saunders.)*

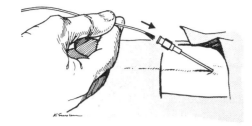

FIGURE 132-8 Threading wick catheter through Jelco catheter and into compartment to be measured. *(From Mubarak, S.J., and Hargens, A.R. [1981]. Compartment Syndromes and Volkmann's Contracture. Philadelphia: W.B. Saunders.)*

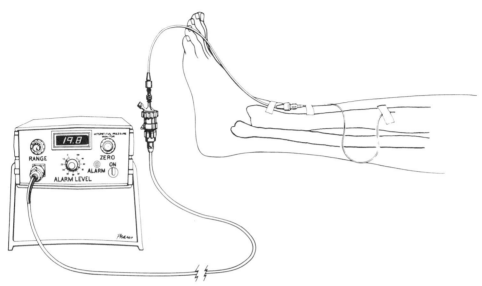

FIGURE 132-9 Tape and sutures are used to secure the catheter.

Procedure for Intracompartmental Pressure Monitoring—*Continued*

Steps	Rationale	Special Considerations
16. Measure the intracompartmental pressure.	Determines presence or absence of pressure.	If measuring lower extremity pressure the extremity can be resting on the bed, but the heel should be elevated to suspend the lower leg above the bed. This is important when the posterior compartments are measured because increased pressure is applied to the compartments resting on the bed.
17. Secure the wick or slit catheter to the patient (Fig. 132-9).	Prevents the catheter from becoming dislodged.	
18. Apply an occlusive sterile dressing to the catheter insertion site.	Reduces the risk for infection.	
19. Check the accuracy of the monitoring system by palpating the area over the catheter tip or by having the patient flex and extend the appropriate distal joint (Fig. 132-10).	Fluctuations in pressure should be noted with patient movement or palpation over the catheter tip. A rapid increase in pressure will be noted with applied pressure or contraction of the muscle.	Patients with normal compartment physiology will demonstrate a rapid rise in pressure during palpation or contraction of the muscle with a rapid return to baseline pressure. Patients with compartment syndrome will have a slow return to baseline pressure after relaxation of the muscle.

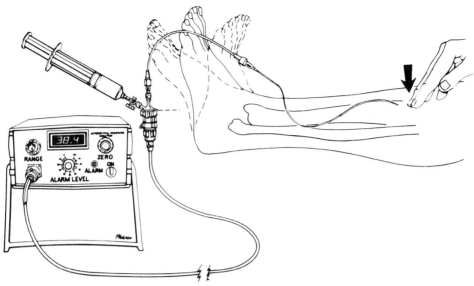

FIGURE 132-10 The system's response can be checked either by palpating the area over the catheter tip *(arrow)* or by having the patient flex-extend the appropriate distal joint; observe the scope for small, temporary elevations in the pressure pattern.

Procedure for Intracompartmental Pressure Monitoring—*Continued*

Steps	Rationale	Special Considerations
20. Assist with removal of the wick or slit catheter when monitoring is complete.	The catheter should not be left in place longer than 48 hours because there is an increased risk for infection.	
21. After removal, apply a dry sterile dressing secured with tape.	Protects the insertion site and assists in control of bleeding.	Do not apply dressing snugly, because this may further impede blood flow and raise compartment pressure.
22. Discard used supplies and wash hands.	Reduces transmission of microorganisms; standard precautions.	
23. Document in patient record.		

Expected Outcomes

- Insertion of the monitoring device completed without complications and with minimal patient discomfort
- Compartment pressure within normal limits
- If physical signs and symptoms of compartment syndrome are identified and compartment pressures are elevated, compartment syndrome is diagnosed and therapeutic interventions are initiated
- Patient tolerates the procedure

Unexpected Outcomes

- Inaccurate pressure readings obtained
- Excessive bleeding from the catheter insertion site
- Signs and symptoms of procedure-related infection

Patient Monitoring and Care

Steps	Rationale	Reportable Conditions
		These conditions should be reported if they persist despite nursing interventions.
1. Complete a neurovascular assessment of the affected extremity every hour and more often as needed.	Detects the onset of signs and symptoms associated with compartment syndrome.	• Onset of *pain* or worsening of pain despite administration of analgesic agents • *Paresthesia* or hypothesia of the affected extremity

Procedure continues on the following page

Patient Monitoring and Care—*Continued*

Steps	Rationale	Reportable Conditions
		• Changes in extremity skin color (mottling, cyanosis, pallor) and skin temperature • Decrease or loss of peripheral pulses • Paralysis of the affected extremity • Increase in circumference and tenseness of the extremity
2. Assess the insertion site for signs and symptoms of infection.	The catheter insertion site may be a source of infection because of the presence of an invasive catheter.	• Erythema, swelling, or drainage around the insertion site • Increase in skin warmth surrounding the insertion site • Increased pain and tenderness at the insertion site • Increase in white blood cell (WBC) count on complete blood count • Fever
3. Measure compartment pressure every hour and more often if needed.	Assessment of compartment pressures along with physical assessment findings is necessary to detect the development of compartment syndrome.	• Elevations and changes in compartment pressure

Documentation

Documentation should include the following:

- Patient and family education
- Extremity assessment findings before compartment pressure measurement
- Identification of the compartments to be assessed
- Medications administered
- The compartment pressure measured

- The condition of the insertion site with the wick or slit catheter in place and after removal of the catheter or needle
- Postprocedure assessment of the limb
- Elevations in compartment pressure or physical assessment findings that are indicative of compartment syndrome onset
- Unexpected outcomes
- Additional interventions

References

1. Chan, P.S., et al. (1998). The significance of the three volar spaces in forearm compartment syndrome: A clinical and cadaver correlation. *J Hand Surg, 23,* 1077-81.
2. Childs, S.A. (1994). Musculoskeletal trauma: Implications for critical care nursing practice. *Crit Care Nurs Clin North Am, 6,* 483-90.
3. Csongradi, J.J., and Nagel, D.A. (1994). Complications of surgery on muscles, fasciae, tendons, tendon sheaths, ligaments and bursae. In: Epps, C.H., ed. *Complications in Orthopaedic Surgery.* 3rd ed, vol II. Philadelphia: J.B. Lippincott, 1123.
4. Fecht-Gramley, M.E. (1994). Emergency: Recognizing compartment syndrome. *Am J Nurs, 94,* 41.
5. Good, L.P. (1992). Compartment syndrome: A closer look at etiology, treatment. *AORN, 56,* 904-11.
6. Johansen, K., and Watson, J. (1998). Compartment syndrome: New insights. *Semin Vasc Surg, 11,* 294-301.
7. Kracun, M.D., and Wooten, C.L. (1998). Crush injuries: A case of entrapment. *Crit Care Nurs Q, 21,* 81-6.
8. Mubarak, S.J. (1981). Laboratory diagnosis of compartment syndromes. In: Mubarak, S.J., Hargens, A.R., and Akeson, W.H., eds. *Compartment Syndrome and Volkmann's Contractures.* Philadelphia: W.B. Saunders.
9. Peck, S.A. (1990). Crush syndrome: Pathophysiology and management. *Orthop Nurs, 9,* 33-40.
10. Pelligrini, V.D., Reid, J.S., and McCollister, E. (1996). Complications. In: Bucholz, R.W., et al., eds. *Rockwood and Green's Fractures in Adults.* 4th ed, vol 1. Philadelphia: Lippincott-Raven, 487.
11. Ross, D. (1991). Acute compartment syndrome. *Orthop Nurs, 10(2),* 33-8.
12. Wilson, S.C., Vrahas, M.S., and Paul, E.M. (1997). A simple method to measure compartment pressures using an intravenous catheter. *Orthopedics, 20,* 403.

PROCEDURE **133**

Pressure-Reducing Devices: Lateral Rotation Therapy

P U R P O S E : The purpose of lateral rotation therapy is to provide dynamic pressure reduction to assist in preventing and treating complications of immobility, especially for patients who would benefit from chest percussion or continuous turning.

Nancy L. Tomaselli
Margaret T. Goldberg
Sandi Wind

PREREQUISITE NURSING KNOWLEDGE

- Principles of preventing pressure-induced injury should be understood.
- Understanding of the pathophysiology of tissue ischemia is needed.
- Knowledge is needed of the effects of immobility on the body systems, including factors contributing to impaired circulation[1] such as venous stasis and thrombosis, pulmonary stasis, urinary stasis, pressure ulcers,[2,6] and friction and shear.[2]
- Principles of wound healing should be understood.
- Understanding of the principles of lateral rotation therapy is needed.[8]
- Indications for lateral rotation therapy include the following:
  - ❖ Coma
  - ❖ Trauma rehabilitation
  - ❖ Chronic neurologic disorders
  - ❖ Stroke
  - ❖ Pulmonary conditions[3,4,5,7]
  - ❖ Spinal cord injury
  - ❖ Cervical traction
  - ❖ Skeletal traction
- Technical and clinical competence in caring for patients receiving lateral rotation therapy is essential.
- The surface below the patient and the positioning packs consist of pressure-reducing foam and a pad of nonliquid polymer gel with a low-friction, low-shear Gore-Tex fabric cover that does not absorb body fluids or odors.
- The gel pads prevent the patient from bottoming out and transfer body heat evenly; they are x-ray transparent.
- The bed provides continuous, slow, side-to-side turning of the patient by rotating the bed frame.
- The bed can turn more than 62 degrees on each side, either intermittently or constantly, providing either unilateral or bilateral rotation.
- The amount of time the patient is held at the rotation limit before rotating in the opposite direction can be adjusted from 7 seconds to 30 minutes.
- Head and shoulder packs provide cervical stability but should not be used as the primary means of stabilizing cervical spine fractures. Cervical traction, halo, and vest or internal fixation may be required. Lateral arm and leg hatches facilitate range of motion.
- Hatches underneath the bed (located in the cervical, thoracic, and rectal areas) provide access for skin care, catheter maintenance, and bladder and bowel management. Do not open thoracic and sacral hatches at the same time.
- The bed has a built-in scale with a maximum patient weight of 300 lb.
- An optional vibrator pack is available to provide chest physiotherapy to further mobilize pulmonary secretions.
- Patients should be placed on a lateral rotation bed as soon as possible to prevent effects of immobility.

EQUIPMENT

- Lateral rotation therapy table (Fig. 133-1).

PATIENT AND FAMILY EDUCATION

- Explain to patient and family the effects of tissue compression. ➤*Rationale:* Encourages understanding and enables patient and family to ask questions.
- Explain how therapy achieves pressure relief. ➤*Rationale:* Increases understanding and cooperation.
- Evaluate the patient's need for long-term pressure reduction (e.g., acute or chronic health problems remaining uncontrolled or chronic pressure ulcers or both). ➤*Rationale:* Allows the nurse to anticipate the need for patient discharge with pressure-reducing device.

PATIENT ASSESSMENT AND PREPARATION

Patient Assessment

- Assess the patient's skin for evidence of pressure ulcer formation. ➤*Rationale:* Provides baseline data.
- Assess the patient's wounds: location, size, stage of ulcer, type of tissue in wound bed, type and amount of drainage, surrounding skin for maceration and inflammation, and any pain on palpation of surrounding skin. ➤*Rationale:* Provides baseline data. Relief of external pressure facilitates wound healing.
- Assess the patient's vascular system: edema in lower extremities, DVT. ➤*Rationale:* Provides baseline data. Lateral movement minimizes venous stasis.
- Assess the patient's pulmonary status: adventitious breath sounds, rate and depth of respirations, cough, cyanosis, dyspnea, nasal flaring, arterial blood gases, chest x-ray, decreased mental acuity, and restlessness. ➤*Rationale:* Provides baseline data. Lateral movement provides postural drainage and mobilizes secretions.
- Assess the patient's bladder: distended bladder, feeling of incomplete bladder emptying, or urinary infrequency. ➤*Rationale:* Provides baseline data. Lateral movement decreases urinary stasis and decreases the incidence of urinary tract infections.

Patient Preparation

- Ensure that the patient and family understand preprocedural teaching. Answer questions as they arise and reinforce information as needed. ➤*Rationale:* Evaluates and reinforces understanding of previously taught information.
- Assist the patient to the supine position with the head of the bed flat or slightly elevated. ➤*Rationale:* Eases transfer of the patient from one bed to another.

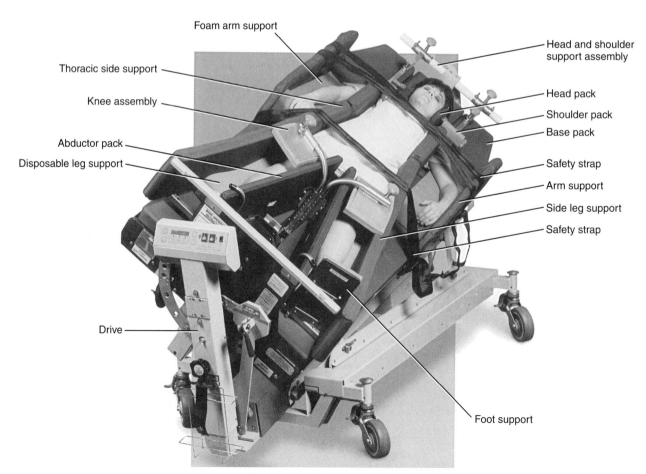

FIGURE 133-1 KCI RotoRest® Delta Kinetic Therapy™ Bed. *(Courtesy KCI, San Antonio, TX.)*

Procedure for Lateral Rotation Therapy

Steps	Rationale	Special Considerations
Placing a Patient on a Lateral Rotation Therapy Table		
	Rental beds require an MD order	FDA-regulated
1. Wash hands.	Reduces transmission of microorganisms; standard precautions.	
2. Ensure that bed is locked in horizontal position and that the drive is disengaged.	Ensures patient safety.	The holes in the frame in which the side supports fit are near the surface of the base packs.
3. Check all hatches to be certain they are properly latched; be sure castors are locked.	Prevents unplanned movement of bed.	
4. Using a drawsheet, move the patient gently to the center of the bed while maintaining body alignment. *(Level I: Manufacturer's recommendations only.)*	Bouncing of patient can result in skin abrasions.	Pillar bars can be covered with a towel or folded paper sheet to avoid possibility of abrasion.
Positioning a Patient on a Lateral Rotation Therapy Table		
1. Center the patient on the bed by aligning the nose, umbilicus, and pubis with the center posts. *(Level I: Manufacturer's recommendations only.)*	Facilitates proper balance. Rotating to one side indicates that the patient is not centered.	To initiate cardiopulmonary resuscitation (CPR), return the bed to the horizontal position and lock in place.
2. Place thoracic side supports in appropriate holes provided in the frame and ensure that they are tightened securely.	These are the main supporting apparatus.	Packs and supports are labeled for patient's right and left sides. Maintain 1-in clearance between the end of the pack and the axilla.
3. Adjust the knee assembly to a position slightly above the patient's knee.	Provides support.	
4. Place the disposable leg support in a position under the thigh and calf so that it fits under the ankle and knee but not beneath the heel.	Decreases external pressure on the heels.	Leg supports should be changed when soiled.
5. Place the foot supports in the foot bracket assembly. The assembly should be positioned so that the footrest is in anatomic position. Tighten the foot assembly. *(Level I: Manufacturer's recommendations only.)*	Maintains each foot in proper anatomic position.	The foot supports should not be left in place for longer than 2 hours at a time. A schedule of 2 hours on and 2 hours off should be maintained continuously. Side-to-side motion does not relieve pressure on the soles of the feet.
6. Install the abductor packs into the preset metal brackets.	Provides support.	
7. Place the side leg supports snugly against the patient's hips; tighten securely.	Provides support.	
8. Install the knee pads in a position so that your hand just fits between the knee and the pack. *(Level II: Theory-based, no research data to support recommendations: recommendations from expert consensus group may exist.)*	Prevents pressure on the knee.	Knee packs can be adjusted to allow for variation in abduction and flexion of the patient's legs. They maintain proper posture of the lower limbs in the patient with spasticity, discouraging contracture formation.

Procedure continues on the following page

Procedure for Lateral Rotation Therapy—*Continued*

Steps	Rationale	Special Considerations
9. Adjust the head and shoulder support assembly.	Provides further support.	
10. Place a hand on the patient's shoulder and adjust the shoulder pack to lightly touch your hand. *(Level II: Theory-based, no research data to support recommendations: recommendations from expert consensus group may exist.)*	Prevents pressure ulcers.	There should always be a 1-in (2.54-cm) clearance between the patient's shoulders and the shoulder packs. If cervical traction causes the patient to slide up on the bed during rotation, place the patient in the reverse Trendelenburg position.
11. Adjust the head pack so that it does not touch the patient's ears or come in contact with the tongs of cervical traction. Tighten head and shoulder assemblies securely.	Provides support.	To remove the head and shoulder packs, loosen the handle of the shoulder pack and slide to the side or lift the entire assembly.
12. Tighten the clamps on the crossbar to secure the assemblies in correct lateral position.	Provides support.	
13. Install the disposable foam arm supports. *(Level I: Manufacturer's recommendations only.)*	Ensures that the patient's hands are in a position of function and that the ulnar nerve and elbows are protected.	
14. Secure the arm supports in the holes provided on the frame.	Provides support.	
15. **Safety straps are to be in place at all times**. One safety strap is used to hold down the shoulder assembly. Place the other strap in proper position.	Prevents falls and patient injury.	
16. Wash hands.	Reduces transmission of microorganisms; standard precautions.	
17. Document in patient record.		

Expected Outcomes

- Intact skin integrity
- Wound healing
- Absence of friction, shearing, and moisture on skin
- Improved peripheral circulation
- Improved urinary elimination
- Maximum pulmonary function achieved

Unexpected Outcomes

- Friction, shearing, motion sickness, agitation, disorientation, and falls due to lateral movement of table if patient is not strapped in properly
- Pressure ulcer formation or further deterioration of existing pressure ulcers
- Desaturation or hemodynamic instability with rotation
- Dislodged invasive lines or tubes
- Development of urinary tract infection
- Development of worsening pulmonary status

Patient Monitoring and Care

Steps	Rationale	Reportable Conditions
		These conditions should be reported if they persist despite nursing interventions.
1. To initiate cardiopulmonary resuscitation (CPR), return the bed to the horizontal position by disengaging the clutch and lock in place with locking pin.	A flat, firm surface is required for CPR.	
2. Evaluate the patient's skin (particularly areas over bony prominences) for evidence of pressure necrosis every 4 to 8 hours.	Relief of external pressure prevents pressure ulcers.	• Development of pressure ulcers
3. Evaluate the patient's existing pressure ulcers, wounds, flaps, and grafts for evidence of healing at least every 8 hours.	Relief of external pressure facilitates healing.	• Deterioration or failure to heal
4. Evaluate the skin for evidence of pressure (especially on the occiput), friction, shearing, or moisture.	These factors contribute to pressure ulcer formation.	• Development of skin breakdown
5. Evaluate the patient's peripheral vascular circulation.	Lateral movement discourages venous stasis.	• Edema, decreased or absent pulses, discoloration, pain
6. Evaluate the patient's pulmonary function.	Lateral movement provides continuous postural drainage and mobilization of secretions.	• Adventitious breath sounds • Decreased respiratory rate and depth • Cough • Cyanosis • Dyspnea • Nasal flaring • Decreased oxygen saturation • Abnormal blood gases • Decreased mental acuity • Restlessness • Abnormal chest x-ray
7. Evaluate the patient for urinary retention.	Lateral movement decreases urinary stasis.	• Decreased urine output • Bladder distention
8. Evaluate the patient's acceptance of and adaptation to the device (motion sickness, agitation, disorientation).	Increases cooperation and decreases anxiety.	• Intolerance to device
9. Maintain bed in motion for 18 hours of every 24-hour period.	Target rotation is 62 degrees. Provides proper rotation and adequate mobility.	• Inability to rotate as per schedule
10. Maintain safety straps at all times.	Prevents falls and patient injury.	• Falls or injury
11. Maintain schedule for foot supports—2 hours on and 2 hours off continuously.	Side-to-side movement does not relieve pressure on soles of feet.	• Breakdown on soles of feet
12. Determine when therapy should be discontinued. Reassess need every 5 days.	Lateral rotation therapy is no longer required.	

Documentation

Documentation should include the following:

- Patient and family education
- Date and time therapy is instituted
- Rationale for use of lateral rotation therapy table
- Number of hours patient is in rotation mode
- Serial skin assessments

- Status of wound healing, if applicable
- Patient's response to therapy
- Any unexpected outcomes and interventions taken
- Phone number and name of company representative

References

1. Brennan, C. (1999). Proper positioning vital for the critically ill patient. *Advance for Nurses, Greater Philadelphia*, 28-30.
2. Bryant, R.A. (2000). Skin pathology and types of damage. In: Bryant, R.A., ed. *Acute and Chronic Wounds: Nursing Management*. 2nd ed. St. Louis: Mosby, 125-56.
3. Fisher, J.A. (2000). How to promote pulmonary healing with Kinetic Therapy. *Nurs Manage, 31*, 38-40.
4. McKay, C. (1999). Best practices: Reducing nosocomial pneumonia. *RN Supplement*, 1-12.
5. Raoof, S., et al. (1999). Effect of combined kinetic therapy and percussion therapy on the resolution of atelectasis in critically ill patients. *Chest, 115*, 1658-66.
6. Russell, T., and Logsdon, A. (2003). Pressure ulcers and lateral rotation beds: A case study. *J Wound, Ostomy & Continence Nurs, 30*, 143-5.
7. Staudinger, T., et al. (2001). Comparison of prone positioning and continuous rotation of patients with adult respiratory distress syndrome: Results of a pilot study. *Crit Care Med, 29*, 51-6.
8. Tomaselli, N. (2004). Special mattresses and beds. In: Elkin, M.K., Perry, A.G., and Potter, P.A., eds. *Nursing Interventions and Clinical Skills*. 3rd ed. Mosby, 611-28.

Additional Readings

Agency for Health Care Policy and Research (AHCPR). (1992). *Pressure Ulcers in Adults: Prediction and Prevention*. Rockville, MD: U.S. Department of Health and Human Services, AHCPR Publication 92-0047.

Agency for Health Care Policy and Research (AHCPR). (1994). *Treatment of Pressure Ulcers*. Rockville, MD: U.S. Department of Health and Human Services, AHCPR Publication 95-0652.

Kinetic Concepts, Inc. Roto-Rest Delta. (1995). *Operations and Maintenance Manual*. San Antonio: Kinetic Concepts.

Kuhrik, M., and Kuhrik, N.S. (2004). Support surfaces and specialty beds. In: Perry, A.G., and Potter, P.A., eds. *Clinical Nursing Skills and Techniques*. 5th ed. St. Louis: Mosby, 916-20.

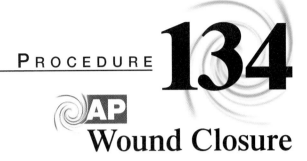
PROCEDURE **134**

⊚AP
Wound Closure

P U R P O S E : Wound closure is the process of holding body tissues together to promote wound healing. It is used to achieve hemostasis, approximate tissues separated by a surgical or accidental trauma, expedite healing with minimal scarring and without infection, provide strength until the natural tensile strength of the healing wound is sufficient to maintain closure, and maintain appropriate positioning of tubes or drains.

Peggy Kirkwood

PREREQUISITE NURSING KNOWLEDGE

- The skin is the largest organ of the body and has two major tissue layers. The outermost layer, the epidermis, is made of stratified, squamous cells with keratin and melanin. This layer protects against environmental exposure, restricts water loss, and gives color. The inner layer, the dermis, is made of fibroelastic connective tissue with capillaries, lymphatics, and nerve endings, providing nourishment and strength. The layer beneath the dermis is the subcutaneous tissue, composed of areolar and fatty connective tissue to provide insulation, shock absorption, and calorie reserve.
- The natural components of wound healing include the following:
  - Inflammation—Vascular and cellular responses are designed to protect the body against alien substances. Blood loss is limited by immediate vasoconstriction of the small vessels that lasts 5 to 10 minutes, the initiation of the coagulation cascade, the tendency for leukocytes to "stick" to the endothelium, and the stimulation of red blood cell (RBC) adherence to each other to plug the cut ends of capillaries. Hemostasis with fibrin formation creates a protective wound scab.

Kinins and prostaglandins produce local vasodilation and increase permeability of the vasculature, thereby promoting development of inflammatory exudate. Inflammation brings chemical stimuli for wound repair. Wounds left open for 3 hours show a dramatic increase in vascular permeability, which results in thick inflammatory exudate and limits the therapeutic value of antibiotics.[4]
  - Epitheliazation—After an incision, the divided parts of the epithelium are closed by cellular migration and mitosis, forming an epithelial bridge that protects the wound against bacteria. When the skin edges are slightly everted with suturing, epithelial bridging occurs within 18 to 24 hours. Wounds that have approximated skin edges may take 36 hours to epithelialize. If the edges are inverted, it may take up to 72 hours to completely epithelialize.[4]
- The goals of primary wound closure are to stop bleeding, prevent infection, preserve function, and restore appearance.
- Principles of proper wound closure include the following:
  - Elimination of dead space where serum and blood can accumulate, thus decreasing the risk for infection
  - Accurate approximation of deep tissue layers to each other with minimal tension on the surrounding tissues
  - Avoidance of tissue ischemia and strangulation from tying sutures too tightly
  - Decreased risk for infection by closing clean wounds within 3 to 8 hours of injury and using aseptic technique in all aspects of wound management

- Risk factors for surgical site infections include intrinsic factors (such as age, active skin condition, smoking status, body mass index, and comorbidities) and extrinsic factors (e.g., pre-, peri- and postoperative patient care practices such as preoperative skin preparation and postoperative dressings).[13] Risk factors for infection in a traumatic laceration include increasing patient age, history of diabetes mellitus, jagged wound edges, stellate shape, visible contamination, injury deeper than the subcutaneous tissue, and presence of a foreign body.[8,21]
- Depending on the clinical setting, referral to an appropriate specialist (e.g., vascular, orthopedic, plastic, or general surgeon) may be warranted for wounds with damage to the blood supply, nerves, or joint; wounds on the face; or wounds with extensive tissue damage or infection.
- Wounds contaminated or infected with saliva, feces, or purulent exudate or that have been open longer than 8 hours may benefit from delayed closure on or after the fourth day to decrease the risk for infection.[12,18,21]
- Wounds may be closed using several techniques: sutures, staples, Steri-Strips, or skin adhesives.
    - Staples provide the strongest closure, skin adhesives and sutures are next strongest, and Steri-Strips are the weakest.[2,7]
    - Stapling is faster, less expensive, and more cosmetically acceptable than suturing in the repair of many types of traumatic lacerations.[7-9,12,15] Staples are useful for lacerations to the scalp, trunk and extremities. They are slightly more painful to remove.[10]
    - Steri-Strips and skin adhesives are found to be equal in cosmetic outcomes and acceptability.[14] They are best used on wounds that are not under tension.
    - Skin adhesives such as 2-octyl cyanoacrylate (Dermabond) have been shown to be equivalent to sutures in repair of simple, clean wounds on children. Adhesives should not be used over joints; on hands, feet, lips, or mucosa; on infected, puncture or stellate wounds; or in patients with poor circulation or a propensity to form keloids.[6,20,23] They are best suited for lacerations that are short (less than 6-8 cm), low-tension, clean-edged, straight to curvilinear wounds that do not cross joints or creases.[12]
- When considering suturing:
    - Curved needles are either tapered or cutting. Needles used for skin closure have an angle of 135 degrees.
    - Tapered needles are used in soft tissues (intestine, blood vessels, muscle, and fascia) and produce minimal tissue damage.
    - Cutting needles are used to approximate tougher tissue, such as skin. Reverse cutting needles have a cutting edge on the outside of the curve and provide a wall of tissue, rather than an incision, for the suture to rest against. This resists suture cut-through and is therefore preferred.
    - Most needles are swaged, or molded, around the suture, providing convenience, safety, and speed in placing sutures.
    - Needles should be handled only with needle holders to prevent needle damage to surrounding tissue and to the user.
    - Suture material is characterized by tissue reactivity, flexibility, knot-holding ability, wick action, and tensile strength. Suture size is indicated by "0." The higher the number that precedes "0," the smaller the suture (e.g., 4-0 is smaller than 3-0).
    - Sutures are absorbable or nonabsorbable, braided or monofilament.
        - Absorbable suture (i.e., natural gut, synthetic polymers) is used for layered closures. Gut suture is broken down by phagocytosis and induces a moderate inflammatory reaction. Chromic gut suture has increased strength and lasts longer in tissue, but it is not used on the skin because it can cause a severe tissue reaction. Synthetic absorbable sutures are favored over gut because of decreased infection rates and increased strength and longevity.[3]
        - Nonabsorbable sutures are either natural fibers (i.e., silk, cotton, linen) or synthetic (i.e., nylon, Dacron, polyethylene) and are best for superficial lacerations because they are supple and easily handled and they facilitate knot construction.
        - Braided sutures are stronger, but the small spaces between the braids may harbor infection.
        - Monofilament is best suited for skin closure because it produces less inflammatory response; however, the knots are less dependable.
        - Nonabsorbable synthetic monofilament sutures (i.e., 4-0 or 5-0 nylon) are preferred for skin closure. Synthetic braided absorbable sutures provide the best closure for interrupted dermal sutures and ligating bleeding vessels.
    - Preferred knotting technique involves a square knot or double loop followed by a square knot tie.
    - Injured tissue will become edematous, and the suture will tighten automatically within 12 to 24 hours. Therefore, the practitioner must avoid tying the suture too tightly, which could produce tissue necrosis.
    - The number of sutures required is the minimum needed to hold the wound edges exactly opposed without crimping. Tension should be minimized but not eliminated on the wound edges. The more tension on a wound, the closer the sutures should be placed.
    - Lacerations are approximated using a variety of suturing techniques:[4]
        - Simple interrupted dermal suture (Fig. 134-1) is used when the skin margins are level or slightly everted. The needle should enter and exit the skin surface at a right angle. The stitch should be as wide as the suture is deep and no closer than 2 mm apart. The knot should be tied using an instrument tie and repeated four or five times. The first suture is placed in the midportion of the wound. Additional sutures are placed in bisected portions of the wound until it is appropriately closed.

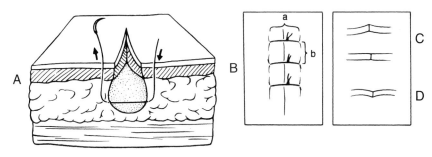

FIGURE 134-1 Interrupted dermal suture. **A,** Proper depth. **B,** Proper spacing (a = b). **C,** Proper final appearance. **D,** Improper final appearance. *(From Pfenninger, J.L., and Fowler, G.C., eds. [2003]. Pfenninger and Fowler's Procedures for Primary Care. 2nd ed. St. Louis: Mosby.)*

○ Subcutaneous suture with inverted knot or buried stitch (Fig. 134-2) is used for deeper wounds or wounds under tension. Absorbable sutures are used with the knot inverted below the skin margin. Begin at the bottom of the wound, come up and go straight across the incision to the base again, and tie. Deep, buried subcutaneous sutures are used to reduce the tension on skin sutures, close dead space beneath a wound, and allow for early suture removal.[17,24]

○ Vertical mattress suture (Fig. 134-3) promotes eversion of the skin, which promotes less prominent scarring.[24] Mattress sutures are used when skin tension is present or where the skin is very thick (palms and soles of feet). Identical to a simple suture, but an additional suture is taken very close to the edge of each side of the wound.

○ Three-point or half-buried mattress suture (Fig. 134-4) is used to close an acute corner of a laceration without impairing blood flow to the tip. The needle is inserted into the skin on the nonflap portion of the wound, passed transversely through the tip, and returned on the opposite side of the wound, paralleling the point of entrance. The suture is then tied, drawing the tip snugly in place.[24]

○ Subcuticular running suture (Fig. 134-5) is used for linear wounds under little or no tension and allows

for edema formation. Wound approximation may not be as meticulous as with an interrupted dermal suture. An anchor suture is placed at one end of the wound; then continuous sutures are placed at right angles to the wound less than 3 mm apart. The wound is pulled together and the other end secured with either another square knot or tape under slight tension.

❖ Sutures must be completely removed in a timely fashion to avoid further tissue inflammation and possible infection. Sutures on extremities and the trunk should be removed in 8 to 14 days; those on the face should be removed in 3 to 5 days; and those on the palms, soles, back, and skin over mobile joints should be removed in 10 to 14 days.[4,19]

EQUIPMENT

- Local anesthetic (with or without epinephrine)
- Chlorhexidine soap[3,16] and sterile normal saline (NS)
- Eight to ten 4 × 4 gauze sponges
- Sterile metal prep basin
- 30-ml or 60-ml syringe and 18-G needle
- Sterile drape
- Fenestrated drape
- Sterile gloves, mask, eye protection
- Electric clippers, if needed

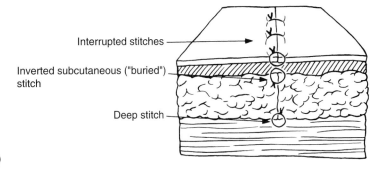

Interrupted stitches

Inverted subcutaneous ("buried") stitch

Deep stitch

FIGURE 134-2 Inverted subcutaneous suture. Also shown is layered closure. *(From Pfenninger, J.L., and Fowler, G.C., eds. [2003]. Pfenninger and Fowler's Procedures for Primary Care. 2nd ed. St. Louis: Mosby.)*

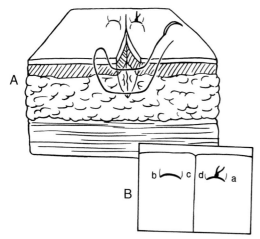

FIGURE 134-3 Vertical mattress suture. **A,** Cross-section. **B,** Overhead view. Begin at *a*, and go under skin to *b*. Come out, go in at *c*, and exit at *d*. *(From Pfenninger, J.L., and Fowler, G.C., eds. [2003]. Pfenninger and Fowler's Procedures for Primary Care. 2nd ed. St. Louis: Mosby.)*

For suturing:
- 6-inch needle holder
- Suture material and needle
- Curved dissecting scissors
- Two mosquito hemostats—one curved, one straight
- Suture scissors
- Tissue forceps
- Scalpel handle and No. 15 knife blade
- Skin hooks (for atraumatic tissue handling)
  For other wound closures:
- Staple gun
- Steri-Strips
- Skin adhesive

PATIENT AND FAMILY EDUCATION

- Explain the procedure and risks and reassure the patient and family. ➤*Rationale:* Decreases patient anxiety and

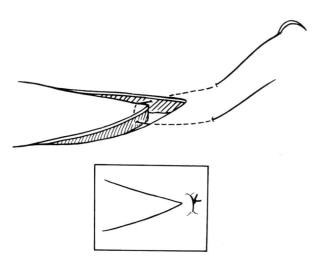

FIGURE 134-4 Three-point or half-buried mattress. *(From Pfenninger, J.L., and Fowler, G.C., eds. [2003]. Pfenninger and Fowler's Procedures for Primary Care. 2nd ed. St. Louis: Mosby.)*

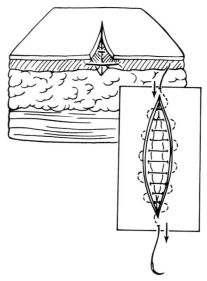

FIGURE 134-5 Subcuticular running suture. *(From Pfenninger, J.L., and Fowler, G.C., eds. [2003]. Pfenninger and Fowler's Procedures for Primary Care. 2nd ed. St. Louis: Mosby.)*

encourages patient and family cooperation and understanding of procedure.
- As appropriate, instruct the patient and family on aftercare: pain medication, wound care, observation for signs and symptoms of infection and when to have wound closure material removed. ➤*Rationale:* Facilitates patient comfort, decreases risk for infection, and encourages prompt intervention to treat possible infection.

PATIENT ASSESSMENT AND PREPARATION

Patient Assessment

- History of present injury and past medical history. ➤*Rationale:* This allows a better understanding of the nature of the injury and any complicating factors to wound healing.
- Damage to peripheral nerve, blood supply, or motor function; x-rays may be needed to assess for bone injury. ➤*Rationale:* Determines the need for referral to a specialist.

Patient Preparation

- Ensure that patient understands preprocedural teaching. Answer questions as they arise and reinforce information as needed. ➤*Rationale:* Evaluates and reinforces understanding of previously taught information.
- Administer pain medication as necessary. Consider conscious sedation for laceration repair in children.[12] ➤*Rationale:* Reduces activity significantly during suturing to provide a stable field.
- Administer tetanus prophylaxis, if necessary (Table 134-1). ➤*Rationale:* Prevents possibility of tetanus from unclean wound.

TABLE 134-1	Summary Guide to Tetanus Prophylaxis in Routine Wound Management			
	Clean, Minor Wounds		All Other Wounds[a]	
History of absorbed tetanus toxoid (doses)	dT[b]	TIG[c]	dT[b]	TIG[c]
Unknown or less than three doses	Yes	No	Yes	Yes
Three or more doses[d]	No[e]	No	No[f]	No

[a]Such as, but not limited to, wounds contaminated with dirt, feces, soil, and saliva; puncture wounds; avulsions; and wounds resulting from missiles, crushing, burns, and frostbite.
[b]For children younger than 7 years old, diphtheria and tetanus toxoids and acellular pertussis vaccine (DtaP) is recommended; if pertussis vaccine is contraindicated, DT is given. For children 7 years of age or older, dT is recommended. *dT,* indicates adult-type diphtheria and tetanus toxoids; *TIG,* tetanus immune globulin (human).
[c]Equine tetanus antitoxin should be used when TIG is not available.
[d]If only three doses of *fluid* toxoid have been received, a fourth dose of toxoid, preferably an absorbed toxoid, should be given. Although licensed, fluid tetanus toxoid is rarely used.
[e]Yes, if older than 10 years since last dose.
[f]Yes, if older than 5 years since last dose. More frequent boosters are not needed and can accentuate side effects.
Data from Centers for Disease Control and Prevention. (2002). *VPD Surveillance Manual.* 3rd ed, Atlanta, GA: CDC.

Procedure for Wound Closure

Steps	Rationale	Special Considerations
1. Wash hands and don personal protective equipment.	Reduces transmission of microorganisms and body secretions; standard precautions.	
2. Anesthetize the wound. Use local anesthetic with or without epinephrine and a 27- to 30-gauge needle to infiltrate the area.[1] *(Level IV: Limited clinical studies to support recommendations.)*	Provides for maximum patient comfort and cooperation during suturing.	Immobilization of site also aids in decreasing pain. Generally, lidocaine without epinephrine should be used in areas with limited vascular supply (fingers, toes, ears, penis, and nose) because of possible vasoconstriction resulting in compromised tissue.[1,23]
3. Examine wound thoroughly for foreign bodies, deep tissue layer damage, joint involvement, and injury to nerve, vessel, or tendon.	Prevents further damage. Assess need for referral.	Use aseptic technique to decrease contamination of wound.
4. Clean the wound.	Removes foreign substances and bacteria and reduces risk for infection.	
A. Mechanical—wiping, brushing, and irrigating with copious amounts of high-pressure saline using a 30-ml or 60-ml syringe with 18-gauge needle.		Mechanical cleaning is important for prevention of infection. Wound must be properly scrubbed and irrigated with high pressure. Care must be taken to avoid damage to the tissues.
B. Chemical—antiseptic soaps. Apply in concentric circles, moving toward the periphery.[13] *(Level V: Clinical studies in more than one patient population and situation.)*	Chlorhexidine reduces bacterial colony counts.[3,13]	Use a soap that is nontoxic to tissues.
C. Only if necessary, remove any hair in the area with an electric clipper. *(Level V: Clinical studies in more than one patient population and situation.)*	Do not remove hair at or around the suture site unless it will interfere with the procedure.[4,10,22] Electric clippers (rather than razors) have been associated with significantly fewer infections.[5,11]	

Procedure continues on the following page

Procedure for Wound Closure—*Continued*

Steps	Rationale	Special Considerations
5. Remove protective gloves used for cleaning wound; don sterile gloves.		
6. Apply sterile drapes over and under the area as necessary.	Creates a sterile field. Reduces risk for infection.	
7. Examine the wound again for devitalized tissue that needs removal or debridement (see Procedure 137). Use a scalpel or sharp tissue scissors, if necessary.	Debridement may convert a jagged, contaminated wound into a clean surgical one and allow better approximation of tissues.	Debridement should be conservative and limited to removal of devitalized tissue that could act as a medium promoting bacterial growth.[23]
8. If needed, loosen the wound from the subcutaneous tissue beneath the dermis using scissors or scalpel. **Note: For wound closure methods other than suturing, skip to step 20.**	Allows the skin to glide together easily and aids approximation of skin edges.	
9. Select the appropriate needle and suture material according to type of wound.	Provides maximum support with the least amount of further tissue trauma.	
10. Arm the needle between the jaws of the needle holder (Fig. 134-6).	Prevents needle bending and provides for guided insertion.	The needle holder should be perpendicular to the needle and should grasp the needle 3 mm beyond the swag hole. The handle of the needle holder should be closed to first or second ratchet.
11. Grasp the needle holder (Fig. 134-7).	Correct grasp ensures smooth entry of needle and proper stitch placement with minimal manipulation.	

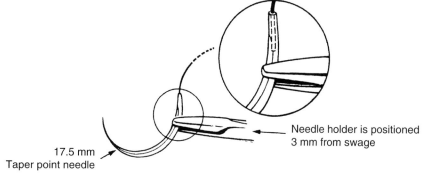

17.5 mm
Taper point needle

Needle holder is positioned 3 mm from swage

FIGURE 134-6 Because the laser-drilled hole is 15 mm long, this needle can be grasped by the needle holder 3 mm from the swage *(insert)*. Needle holder grasps the needle 3 mm from its swage. *(From United States Surgical Corporation. [1996]. Scientific Basis of Wound Closure Techniques, 48. Copyright© 1996, 1999, United States Surgical Corporation. All rights reserved. Reprinted with the permission of the United States Surgical Corporation.)*

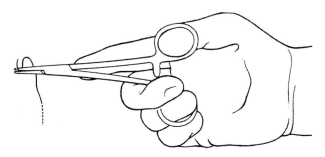

FIGURE 134-7 Thumb-ring finger grip of needle holder. *(From United States Surgical Corporation. [1996]. Scientific Basis of Wound Closure Techniques, 48. Copyright© 1996, 1999, United States Surgical Corporation. All rights reserved. Reprinted with the permission of the United States Surgical Corporation.)*

Procedure for Wound Closure—*Continued*

Steps	Rationale	Special Considerations
12. Position the free end of the suture away from operator.	Allows optimum visualization of the free end of the suture and ensures that it does not become entangled during knot construction.	
13. Pass the needle through the tissue until the needle point is visualized.		Hand should start prone; supination of the wrist will pass needle in a direction toward person suturing and in the direction of the curvature of the needle.
14. Using tissue forceps to grasp the needle point, unclamp the needle holder jaws.	Stabilizes the needle to maintain its position in the tissue.	
15. Regrasp the needle between the needle holder jaws and pull the desired length of suture through the wound.	Prepares for tying knot.	Keep wrist in prone position.
16. Tie the suture knot. Edges should be slightly everted.		Secure the precise approximation of the wound edges without strangulating the tissue. The suture should be tied snugly, but gently.
A. Form suture loop—wrap fixed suture end over and around needle holder twice.	Double-wrap provides increased strength.	Keep length of free suture end less than 2 cm.
B. Pass free end of suture through the loop to create a throw.		Will have a figure-8 shape.
C. Advance the throw to the wound surface by applying tension perpendicular to the wound.		
D. Repeat four or five times.		With each throw, your hands must reverse positions and apply equal and opposing tension to the suture ends in the same plane.
17. Cut suture by holding scissors blades perpendicular to the suture, keeping knot in view between the blades, allowing 3-mm ears to remain.	All knots slip to some degree. The ears of the knot must compensate for enlarged suture loop and prevent the knot from untying.	
18. Reposition knot away from wound edges.	Facilitates suture line care.	
19. Repeat steps 9 through 17 until wound is appropriately closed. Dress wound appropriately. Go to step 22.		
20. **Other wound closure techniques:** Select wound closure technique to be used.		

Procedure continues on the following page

Procedure for Wound Closure—*Continued*

Steps	Rationale	Special Considerations
A. **Staples:** Use fingers or forceps to approximate the edges. Apply firm pressure with stapler and dispense staples as directed. Place staples 0.5 to 1 cm apart. An assistant can help evert the wound edges while the primary operator uses the stapler.		
B. **Steri-Strips:** Ensure that skin is not oily or hairy and wound has minimal drainage. Benzoin may be applied to the area to increase adhesion. The strips should overlap the wound about 2-3 cm on each side of the wound. Start at the midpoint of the wound to approximate the sides and work out to the ends of the wound. Strips should be placed about 2-3 cm apart. Additional strips can be placed over the cross tapes to prevent the ends from coming loose.[2]	**Steri-Strips:** Skin that is not oily or hairy enhances proper adherence of Steri-Strips to skin.	**Steri-Strips:** Should not be used for large wounds or on patients who may remove them (confused, uncooperative, very young patients).
C. **Skin adhesive:** Apply to dry, well-opposed wound edges. Use fingers or forceps to approximate wound edges. Open the product, saturate the porous applicator tip, and paint the edges of the wound using short brush strokes in a multilayering process. Allow 15 sec between layers. Usually four layers are applied. Hold edges together for 30-60 sec.		**Skin adhesive:** Obtaining an even, controlled flow of adhesive is critical to minimize drips and prevent complications. Do not place adhesive *in* the wound. It is ineffective and will impair healing and increase potential for foreign-body reaction.[12]
21. **Staples and Steri-Strips:** Cover wound with nonadherent dressing for the first 24-48 hr. Depending on institutional protocol, topical triple antibiotic ointment may be added prior to dressing application. Staples are removed using sterile technique and appropriate device. *(Level IV: Limited clinical studies to support recommendations.)* **Skin adhesive**: Dressing is unnecessary, but a dry gauze pad may be used. Do not use ointments, creams, or tape strips. Do not soak, scrub, or expose to prolonged wetness. May shower or gently bathe.[2,7]	Protects the wound from further injury; prevents microorganisms from colonizing[2]; minimizes bleeding, edema; and potential dead space; provides physiologic environment that is conducive to epithelial migration and scab formation; takes tension off the wound edges; cushions the wound from extraneous trauma; restricts motion, which decreases lymphatic flow and minimizes the spread of wound microflora.[4,17,19]	For continued oozing, apply a pressure dressing.

Procedure for Wound Closure—*Continued*

Steps	Rationale	Special Considerations
22. Dispose of equipment in appropriate receptacle.	Standard precautions.	
23. Wash hands.	Decreases transmission of microorganisms.	
24. Document in patient record.		

Expected Outcomes

- Bleeding is stopped.
- Wound remains infection free.
- Function is preserved.
- Appearance is restored.

Unexpected Outcomes

- Continued bleeding from the wound site or hematoma
- Wound infection and possible sepsis
- Skin necrosis
- Loss of function
- Abnormal appearance
- Wound dehiscence

Patient Monitoring and Care

Steps	Rationale	Reportable Conditions
1. Monitor for evidence of infection.	Allows for early treatment and prevents systemic infection.	*These conditions should be reported if they persist despite nursing interventions.* • Wound that is red, swollen, tender, or warm • Wound that drains or festers • Red streaks around the wound • Tender lumps in the groin or under the arm • Chills or fever
2. Administer prophylactic antibiotics if: A. Contamination of trauma site is suspected. B. Animal or human bite wounds exist. C. Preexisting medical conditions subject the patient to increased risk for infection (e.g., valvular heart disease, diabetes).	Prevents wound infection.	
3. Administer analgesic medication (agent and dose is determined by the extent of the trauma, the pain threshold of the patient, and the concerns of the patient and family).	Promotes patient comfort and cooperation.	• Excessive pain not relieved with analgesics
4. Splint wounds under considerable tension, as needed.	Decreases lymphatic flow, thereby decreasing the spread of wound bacteria. Provides support and limitation of movement to allow for proper wound healing and patient comfort.	

Procedure continues on the following page

Patient Monitoring and Care—*Continued*

Steps	Rationale	Reportable Conditions
5. Keep wound and dressing clean and dry. If dressing gets wet, use sterile technique to remove it, blot dry with gauze pad, and reapply a clean, dry dressing.[13]	Decreases opportunity for infection due to wicking action of a wet dressing.	
6. Keep dressed for 24-48 hours. If needed, clean with half-strength hydrogen peroxide, blot dry, apply triple antibiotic ointment, and reapply a sterile, nonadherent dressing. *(Level V: Clinical studies in more than one or two different patient populations and situations to support recommendations.)*	Decreases risk for wound contamination and infection. Beyond 48 hours, it is unclear whether an incision must be covered by a dressing or whether showering or bathing is detrimental to healing.[13]	
7. Remove sutures (see Procedure 135): A. Facial wounds—3 to 5 days B. Scalp and extremity wounds—7 to 14 days C. Palms, soles, back, and skin over mobile joints—10 to 14 days	Prevents infection, enhances proper healing, and facilitates desirable cosmetic effects.	
8. Provide detailed patient and family education, including wound care, medications, signs and symptoms of infection, and follow-up appointments.	Facilitates patient and family cooperation.	

Documentation

Documentation should include the following:

- Patient and family education
- Location and appearance of wound
- Time since injury
- Procedure used to clean wound
- Procedure and technique used to close wound
- How patient tolerated the procedure

- Care of wound after closure
- Instructions given to patient and family
- Pain medication or antibiotics given
- Tetanus status, if given
- Unexpected outcomes
- Nursing intervention

References

1. Andrades, P.R., Olguin, F.A., and Calderon, W. (2003). Digital blocks with or without epinephrine. *Plast Reconstr Surg,* 111, 1769-70.
2. Autio, L., and Olson, K.K. (2002). The four S's of wound management: Staples, sutures, Steri-Strips, and sticky stuff. *Holist Nurs Pract,* 16, 80-8.
3. Chaiyakunapruk, N., et al. (2002). Chlorhexidine compared with povidone-iodine solution for vascular catheter-site care: A meta-analysis. *Ann Intern Med,* 136, 792-801.
4. Edlich, R.F., Woods, J.A., and Drake, D.B. (1996). *Scientific Basis of Wound Closure Techniques.* Norwalk, CT: Auto Suture Company.
5. Edlich, R.F., et al. (2000). A scientific basis for choosing the technique of hair removal used prior to wound closure. *J Emerg Nurs,* 26, 134-9.
6. Farion, K.J., et al. (2003). Tissue adhesives for traumatic lacerations: A systematic review of randomized controlled trials. *Acad Emerg Med,* 10, 110-8.
7. Hollander, J.E., and Singer, A.J. (1999). Laceration management. *Ann Emerg Med,* 34, 356-67.
8. Hollander, J.E., et al. (2001). Risk factors for infection in patients with traumatic lacerations. *Acad Emerg Med,* 8, 716-20.
9. Kanegaye, J.T., et al. (1999). Comparison of skin stapling devices and standard sutures for pediatric scalp lacerations: A randomized study of cost and time benefits. *J Pediatr,* 130, 808-13.
10. Khan, A.N., et al. (2002). Cosmetic outcome of scalp wound closure with staples in the pediatric emergency department: A prospective, randomized trial. *Pediatr Emerg Care,* 18, 171-3.
11. Kjonniksen, I., et al. (2002). Preoperative hair removal—a systematic literature review. *AORN J,* 75, 928-38.
12. Knapp, J.F. (1999). Updates in wound management for the pediatrician. *Pediatr Clin North Am,* 46, 1201-13.
13. Mangram, A.J., et al. (1999). Guideline for prevention of surgical site infection, 1999. *Infection Control and Hospital Epidemiology,* 20, 247-78.
14. Mattick, A., et al. (2002). A randomized, controlled trial comparing a tissue adhesive with adhesive strips for paediatric laceration repair. *Emerg Med J,* 19, 405-7.
15. Mayrose, J., et al. (1999). Comparison of staples versus sutures in the repair of penetrating cardiac wounds. *J Trauma,* 46, 441-3.
16. Mimoz, O., et al. (1999). Chlorhexidine compared with povidone-iodine as skin preparation before blood culture. A randomized, controlled trial. *Ann Intern Med,* 131, 834-7.

17. Phillips, S.J. (2000). Physiology of wound healing and surgical wound care. *ASAIO J,* 46, S2-5.
18. Quirinia, A., and Viidik, A. (1996). Effect of delayed primary closure on the healing of ischemic wounds. *J Trauma,* 41, 1018-22.
19. Reilly, J. (2002). Evidence-based surgical wound care on surgical wound infection. *Br J Nurs,* 11(16 Suppl), S4, S6, S8, S10, S12.
20. Shapiro, A.J., Dinsmore, R.C., and North, J.H., Jr. (2001). Tensile strength of wound closure with cyanoacraylate glue. *Am Surg,* 67, 1113-5.
21. Stierman, K.L., et al. (2003). Treatment and outcome of human bites in the head and neck. *Otolaryngol Head Neck Surg,* 128, 795-801.
22. Tang, K., Yeh, J.S., and Sgouros, S. (2001). The influence of hair shave on the infection rate in neurosurgery. A prospective study. *Pediatr Neurosurg,* 35, 13-7.
23. Wilson, J.L., Kocurek, K., and Doty, B.J. (2000). A systematic approach to laceration repair. Tricks to ensure the desired cosmetic result. *Postgrad Med,* 107, 77-83, 87-8.
24. Zuber, T.J. (2002). The mattress sutures: Vertical, horizontal, and corner stitch. *Am Fam Physician,* 66, 2231-6.

Additional Readings

Bower, M.G. (2001). Managing dog, cat, and human bite wounds. *Nurse Pract,* 26, 36-8, 41-2, 45-7.
Chen, E., Harnig, S., and Shepherd, S. (2000). Primary closure of mammalian bites. *Acad Emerg Med,* 7, 157-61.
Snell, G. (2003). Laceration repair. In: Pfenninger, J.L., and Fowler, G.C., eds. *Pfenninger and Fowler's Procedures for Primary Care.* 2nd ed. St. Louis: Mosby, 12-9.
Zuber, T.J. (1998). Skin biopsy, excision, and repair techniques. In: *Soft Tissue Surgery for the Family Physician* (illustrated manuals, videotapes, and CD-ROMs of soft tissue surgery techniques). Kansas City, MO: American Academy of Family Physicians, 100-6.

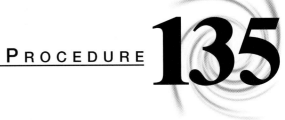
PROCEDURE **135**

Suture Removal

P U R P O S E :   Sutures are placed to approximate tissues that have been separated. When wound healing is sufficient to maintain closure, sutures are removed.

Peggy Kirkwood

PREREQUISITE NURSING KNOWLEDGE

- Wound healing is a nonspecific response to injury. It involves the biologic processes of inflammation, collagen metabolism, and contraction in an overlapping, integrated continuum. Wound healing is divided into three phases—an inflammatory, a fibroblastic, and a remodeling phase. The condition of the tissues and the mechanism of wound closure determine the relative duration of these phases and the end-result of the healing process.
- Sutures must be completely removed to avoid further tissue inflammation and possible infection.
- Timing of suture removal depends on the following:
  - ❖ Shape, size and location of the incision
  - ❖ Absence of inflammation, drainage, and infection
  - ❖ Patient's general condition
- Timing of suture removal is as follows:
  - ❖ Sutures on extremities, scalp, and trunk should be removed in 7 to 14 days.
  - ❖ Sutures on the face should be removed in 3 to 5 days.
  - ❖ Sutures on the palms, soles, back, and skin over mobile joints should be removed in 10 to 14 days.
- Timing of suture removal may be prolonged in the following cases:
  - ❖ Steroid use
  - ❖ Irradiation
  - ❖ Cytotoxics
  - ❖ Diabetes
  - ❖ Rheumatoid arthritis
  - ❖ Trace element imbalance
  - ❖ Elderly patient

EQUIPMENT

- Sterile gloves and mask
- Sterile towel or drape
- Sterile swab with antiseptic cleaning solution according to your facility's policy (iodophor or chlorhexidine)
- 4 × 4 gauze pads
- Suture removal kit with scissors and forceps
  or
- Sterile forceps
- Sterile suture scissors
- Skin tape or Steri-Strips of appropriate width
- Skin adherent, if desired

PATIENT AND FAMILY EDUCATION

- Explain the procedure and risks and reassure the patient and family. Explain that the patient may feel a tickling or pulling sensation as the stitches come out. Assure the patient that the wound is healing properly and removing the stitches won't weaken the incision. ➡ *Rationale:* Decreases patient anxiety and encourages patient and family cooperation and understanding of procedure.
- Instruct the patient and family on aftercare: pain medication, wound care and observation for signs and symptoms of infections. ➡ *Rationale:* Facilitates patient comfort, decreases risk for infection, and encourages prompt intervention to treat possible infection.

PATIENT ASSESSMENT AND PREPARATION

Patient Assessment

- History of present injury and past medical history. ➤*Rationale:* Allows a better understanding of the nature of the injury and any complicating factors to suture removal.
- Patient allergies, especially to adhesive tape and povidone-iodine or other topical solutions or medications. ➤*Rationale:* To prevent further tissue damage.
- Observe wound for signs of gaping, drainage, inflammation, signs of infection, or embedded sutures. ➤*Rationale:* May need to delay suture removal.

Patient Preparation

- Ensure that patient understands preprocedural teaching. Answer questions as they arise and reinforce information as needed. ➤*Rationale:* Evaluates and reinforces understanding of previously taught information.
- Administer pain medication as necessary. ➤*Rationale:* Reduces activity during suture removal to provide a stable field.
- Provide privacy and position the patient for comfort without undue tension on the suture line. Adjust the light to shine directly on the suture line. ➤*Rationale:* To provide ease of removal and patient comfort.
- Prepare sterile field. ➤*Rationale:* To prevent contamination.

Procedure for Suture Removal

Steps	Rationale	Special Considerations
1. Check physician's order to confirm exact timing and other relevant information.	Ensures appropriate treatment.	Physician may want to leave some sutures in place for an additional day or two to support the suture line.
2. Wash hands and don personal protective equipment.	Reduces transmission of microorganisms and body secretions; standard precautions.	
3. Apply sterile drapes or towels over or under the area as needed.		
4. Test the wound line before removal to be sure the wound does not separate. If there is any doubt, apply a skin adherent and skin strips between sutures before removing them.	Ensures that wound is healed sufficiently prior to removal of sutures.	If patient has both retention and regular sutures in place, retention sutures may remain inplace for 14-21 days.
5. Clean the suture line with antiseptic skin cleanser. The wound is considered clean, so when cleaning it, wipe from clean to dirty, inner to outer.	Decreases the number of microorganisms and reduces the risk for infection.	Be particularly careful to clean the suture line before removing mattress sutures, especially if the visible, contaminated part of the stitch is too small to cut twice for sterile removal.
6. Use sterile technique to remove suture[1] (Fig. 135-1): A. Use sterile forceps to grasp the knot and gently raise off the skin. B. Use rounded tip of sterile suture scissors to cut suture at the skin edge on one side of the visible part.	Visible part of suture is exposed to skin bacteria and is considered contaminated.	

Procedure continues on the following page

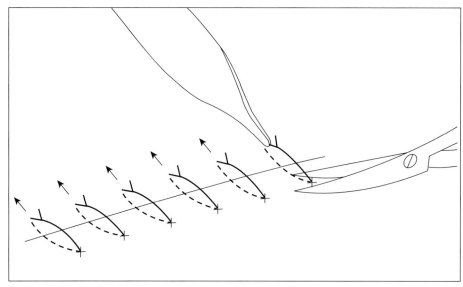

FᴵGUʀᴇ 135-1 Removing plain interrupted sutures with sterile forceps and scissors.

Procedure for Suture Removal—*Continued*

Steps	Rationale	Special Considerations
C. Remove the suture by lifting the visible end off the skin to avoid drawing contaminated portion through subcutaneous tissue.	To prevent pulling it though and contaminating subcutaneous tissue.	
7. To remove mattress sutures[2] (Fig. 135-2): A. Remove the small visible portion of the suture opposite the knot by cutting it at each visible end and lifting the small piece away from the skin. B. Remove the rest of the suture by pulling it out in the direction of the knot. C. If the visible portion is too small to cut twice, cut once and pull the entire suture out in the opposite direction.		
8. If the wound dehisces, apply butterfly adhesive strips or paper tape to support and approximate the edges and call the physician.		

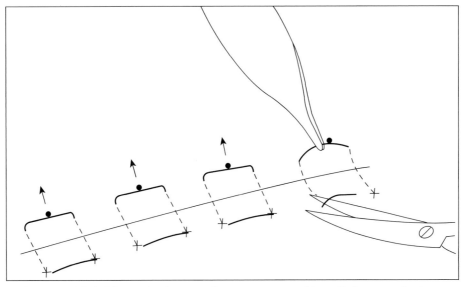

FIGURE 135-2 Removing interrupted mattress sutures with sterile forceps and scissors.

Procedure for Suture Removal—*Continued*

Steps	Rationale	Special Considerations
9. Wipe incision line gently with gauze sponges soaked in antiseptic skin cleanser or prepackaged swab.	Removes serous or bloody drainage from the suture line.	
10. Apply adhesive skin strips or paper tape and a light, sterile gauze dressing, if desired. Leave strips in place for 3-5 days or as ordered.	Holds incision edges together, decreases transmission of microorganisms, and decreased irritation from clothing.	
11. Dispose of gloves and equipment in appropriate receptacle.		
12. Wash hands.		
13. Document in patient record.		

Expected Outcomes

- Wound remains infection free.
- Function is preserved.
- Appearance is restored.

Unexpected Outcomes

- Wound infection and possible sepsis
- Loss of function
- Abnormal appearance
- Wound dehiscence

Patient Monitoring and Care

Steps	Rationale	Reportable Conditions
		These conditions should be reported if they persist despite nursing interventions.
1. Retest range of motion and sensory perception after suture removal.	To ensure no further damage was imposed.	
2. Observe for wound discharge or other abnormal change.	Allows for early treatment and prevents systemic infection.	• Wound that is red, swollen, tender, or warm • Wound that begins to drain or fester • Red streaks around the wound • Tender lumps in the groin or under the arm • Chills or fever • Redness that surrounds the incision and does not gradually disappear or show only a thin line after a few weeks[1]
3. Provide detailed patient and family education, including wound care, medications, signs and symptoms of infection, when the patient can get the incision wet, and follow-up.	Facilitates patient and family cooperation.	

Documentation

Documentation should include the following:

- Patient and family education and aftercare instructions
- Time since suturing
- Care of the wound after suture removal
- Location and appearance of wound
- Range of motion and sensory perception

References

1. Hrouda, B.S. (2000). How to remove surgical sutures and staples. *Nursing 2000,* Feb, 30, 54-5.
2. McConnell, E.A., and DuFour, J.L. (2002). Wound care. In: *Illustrated Manual of Nursing Practice.* 3rd ed. Springhouse, PA: Lippincott Williams & Wilkins, 159-67.

Additional Readings

Berk, W.A., Welck, R.D., and Bock, B.F. (1992). Controversial issues in clinical management of the simple wound. *Ann Emerg Med,* 21, 72.

Edlich, R.F., and Sutton, S.T. (1995). Postrepair wound care revisited. *Acad Emerg Med,* 2, 2.
Lanros, N.E. (1983). Surface trauma and wound management. In: *Assessment and Intervention in Emergency Nursing.* 2nd ed. Bowie, MD: Robert J. Brady Co., 391-415.
Yaremchuk, M.J., and Gallico, G.G. (2000). Principles and practice of plastic surgery. In: Morris, P.J., and Wood, W.C., eds. *Oxford Textbook of Surgery.* 2nd ed. New York: Oxford University Press, Inc., 3533-7.

P R O C E D U R E **136**

Cleaning, Irrigating, Culturing, and Dressing an Open Wound

P U R P O S E : Cleaning, irrigating, culturing, and dressing open wounds is performed to optimize healing. Wound culturing may be necessary to isolate and allow for treatment of organisms.

Mary Beth Flynn Makic

PREREQUISITE NURSING KNOWLEDGE

- Goals of wound care must be clearly outlined so that proper wound care products are used. Wound care products have multiple properties, and technology is rapidly providing advanced products. Wound care products must be matched to the patient and wound conditions.
- Dressings may be categorized as semiocclusive or occlusive. Semiocclusive dressings are semipermeable to gases (oxygen, carbon dioxide, moisture) and impermeable to liquids. Occlusive dressings lack permeability to gases and liquids. Semiocclusive dressings provide moist wound healing environments that optimize wound healing.
- Coarse gauze, used in a wet-to-dry dressing, nonselectively debrides the wound bed mechanically and absorbs wound fluid; absorptive wound dressings such as calcium alginates, foams, and hydrofibers enhance wound absorption; hydrogels provide moisture to nondraining wounds; hydrocolloids provide wound moisture with minimal absorption; transparent films provide moist wound environment without absorption.
- Wounds heal by either primary or secondary intention (Fig. 136-1).
  - ❖ Most clean or clean/contaminated surgical wounds heal by primary intention. Suturing each layer of tissue approximates the wound edges. These wounds typically heal quickly and require minimal wound care. Contaminated surgical or traumatic wounds (open wounds) heal by secondary intention.
  - ❖ Wounds healing by secondary intention granulate from the base of the wound to the skin surfaces; care must

be taken to allow for uniform granulation and prevention of open pockets/tunneling.
- Open wounds must be clean and moist to promote effective and efficient wound healing. To that end, open wound care strives to maintain a clean, moist wound bed that allows for effective wound healing under the support of a dressing.
- Openly granulating wounds heal more slowly, must remain moist to enhance tissue granulation, and may be more painful for the patient.
- Open wounds may have excessive wound drainage, requiring application of absorptive dressings, protection of periwound skin, and more frequent dressing changes to facilitate healing.
- Wound cleaning should be accomplished with minimal chemical or mechanical trauma. Cytotoxic cleaning agents should be avoided because they may delay healing and increase the risk for infection. Normal saline (NS) is the cleaning agent of choice for clinicians; however, tap water is safe and effective for cleaning of most acute and chronic wounds.[1-2,7]
- Wound contamination is the presence of bacteria on the wound surface that are not actively multiplying. Signs of infection are not present, and healing is not impaired.[6]
- Colonization is the presence of bacteria in the wound that are actively multiplying or forming colonies. Wound colonization may not elicit signs of local or systemic infection but may delay healing.
- Wound infection is present if organisms are present at 10^5 colony-forming units per ml in conjunction with local and systemic clinical findings such as erythema, edema, pain, purulence, fever, and leukocytosis.

FIRST INTENTION (Primary union)   SECOND INTENTION (Granulation)   THIRD INTENTION (Secondary suture)

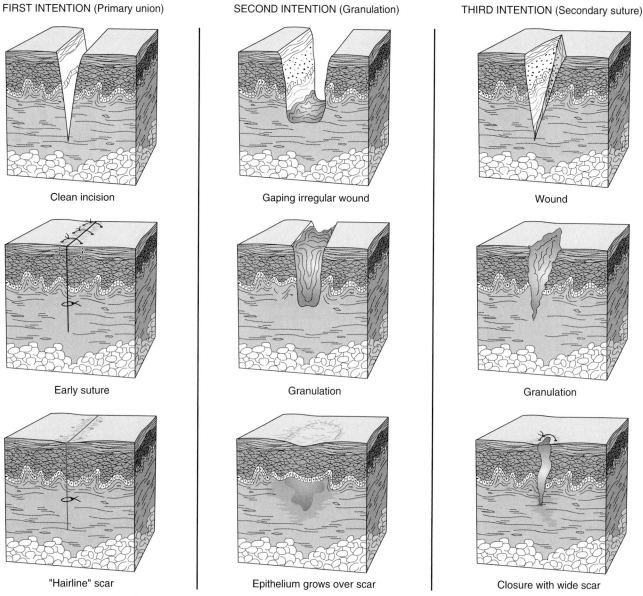

Clean incision   Gaping irregular wound   Wound

Early suture   Granulation   Granulation

"Hairline" scar   Epithelium grows over scar   Closure with wide scar

FIGURE 136-1 Wound healing by primary, secondary, and tertiary intention.

- Bacterial invasion of wounds is best managed with wound cleaning, debridement (see Procedure 137), and antibiotic therapy (local, systemic or combination therapy) dependent on the type and amount of bacteria in the wound.
- Wound cleaning must deliver solution to the wound surface with enough force to physically loosen foreign materials and bacteria with minimal injury to the tissue. Pressure of a stream of solution on a surface is measured in pounds per square inch (psi). Research suggests effective wound cleaning is best achieved when solution is delivered 8-13 psi. Pressures greater than 15 psi may actually force bacteria and debris deeper into the wound bed.[6]
- The use of a 35-ml syringe attached to a 19-gauge angiocatheter tip delivers a stream of fluid at 8 psi. A 12-ml syringe attached to a 22-gauge angiocatheter tip delivers fluid at 13 psi. Increasing the syringe size will decrease the pressure of the stream and increasing the bore of the catheter tip will increase the pressure.[6-7]
- Wound infections may delay wound healing; sterile wound cultures or tissue biopsy may be obtained to isolate organisms and differentiate between colonization and active infection within a wound bed.

EQUIPMENT

- Nonsterile and sterile gloves (two pairs); sterile field (depending on type and age of wound)
- Gowns and face protection
- Sterile gauze (4 × 4)
- Normal saline (NS)

- Sterile basin
- Waterproof barrier
- Sterile 35-ml slip-tip syringe and 19-G needle for irrigation (if necessary)
- Sterile gauze (4 × 4); possibly, ABD dressings (if the wound has excessive drainage, an absorptive dressing may be necessary or if the wound has minimal drainage, a moisture-enhancing dressing may be needed)
- Hypoallergenic tape; one set of Montgomery straps
- Liquid skin barrier for applying Montgomery straps; hydrocolloid wafer

Additional equipment to have available, if needed, includes the following:
- Swab culture: two sterile serum-tipped swabs
- Tissue biopsy: scalpel, sterile forceps, and container
- Needle aspiration: 10-ml syringe and 22-G needle

PATIENT AND FAMILY EDUCATION

- Explain the procedure, rationale, and patient's role in wound cleaning, irrigation, culture, and dressing management. ➤*Rationale:* Decreases patient anxiety and discomfort.
- Discuss patient's role in wound cleaning, irrigation, culturing, and dressing management. ➤*Rationale:* Elicits patient cooperation; prepares patient for wound management on discharge (as appropriate).
- Explain the procedure and reason for obtaining a wound culture. ➤*Rationale:* Decreases patient anxiety and discomfort.
- Discuss signs and symptoms of local and systemic wound infection (erythema, pain, increased wound drainage, odor, fever) and inform patient that they should consult their health care provider. ➤*Rationale:* Prepares the patient for wound management on discharge.

PATIENT ASSESSMENT AND PREPARATION

Patient Assessment

- Assess for the following:
  - ❖ Wound drainage (amount and color)
  - ❖ Foul drainage or odor
  - ❖ Appearance of wound bed (color, debris—i.e., darkened areas on tissue bed, pale red, green, or yellow tissue bed)
  - ❖ Erythema
  - ❖ Pain or tenderness
  - ❖ Change in wound drainage amount or color
  - ❖ Elevated temperature
  - ❖ Elevated white blood cell count
  - ❖ Presence and depth of pocket/tunnel
  - ➤*Rationale:* Assessment of the wound bed provides information about the healing process and assists in early identification of wound infection. True wound bed assessment cannot be completed until after the wound bed has been cleansed.

Patient Preparation

- Ensure that patient understands preprocedural teaching. Answer questions as they arise and reinforce information as needed. ➤*Rationale:* Evaluates and reinforces understanding of previously taught information.
- Place patient in position of optimal comfort and visualization for wound care procedures. ➤*Rationale:* Provides for effective wound visualization and enhances patient tolerance of procedure.
- Optimize lighting in room and provide privacy for patient. ➤*Rationale:* Allows for optimal wound assessment and patient comfort.
- Premedicate patient with prescribed analgesic, if indicated. ➤*Rationale:* Decreases patient anxiety and increases comfort.

Procedure for Cleaning, Irrigating, Culturing, and Dressing an Open Wound

Steps	Rationale	Special Considerations
Cleaning and Irrigating Wounds		
1. Wash hands; position patient to facilitate drainage and cleaning of wound.	Decreases contamination; uses gravity to direct flow of solution away from wound bed.	
2. Position waterproof barrier to collect drainage.	Controls flow of cleansing solution and wound drainage; minimizes solution contact with intact skin.	
3. Position wound cleaning materials and soiled contamination container within reach of practitioner and patient; conform to principles of aseptic technique.	Decrease cross-contamination during wound cleaning process; enhances body mechanics for practitioner.	

Procedure continues on the following page

Procedure for Cleaning, Irrigating, Culturing, and Dressing an Open Wound—*Continued*

Steps	Rationale	Special Considerations
4. Wash hands and don personal protective equipment.	Reduces transmission of microorganisms; standard precautions.	
5. Remove soiled dressing and discard in appropriate container. Assess wound bed. Remove soiled gloves.	Assess wound upon dressing removal for type, odor, and amount of drainage.	True wound bed assessment cannot be completed until after the wound bed has been cleansed.
6. Establish sterile field; open sterile gauze; place sterile water or NS cleaning solution in sterile container. *(Level VI: Clinical studies in a variety of patient populations and situations.)*	Decreases cross-contamination during the wound cleaning process. Cleansing solution should not be cytotoxic.[1-2,7]	There is no evidence to support use of sterile technique when changing dressings on chronic wounds.
7. If irrigation (Fig. 136-2) is necessary, attach 19-G needle to syringe for irrigation. A. Draw up solution into syringe. B. Don sterile gloves. C. Maintain needle 1 to 3 cm from wound surface. D. Direct solution onto wound bed from area of least contamination to greatest.	Irrigation removes excess debris to enhance healing. A 35-ml syringe with a 19-G needle provides approximately 8 psi, which is sufficient force to remove debris without creating wound bed damage. The smaller the syringe, the greater the psi.[1,6-7] Too great a force during irrigation can create tissue damage, reinitiating the inflammatory process and delaying wound healing.	Not all open wound beds need irrigation with a needle. Gentle irrigation using a slip-tip 35-ml syringe is indicated for open wounds that are granulating well.[1,6-7]

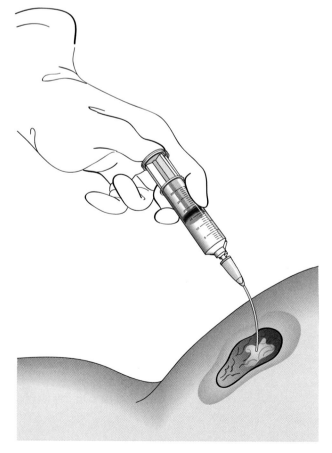

FIGURE 136-2 Irrigating a wound.

Procedure for Cleaning, Irrigating, Culturing, and Dressing an Open Wound—*Continued*

Steps	Rationale	Special Considerations
E. Continue with irrigation until return solution is clear. *(Level VI: Clinical studies in a variety of patient populations and situations to support recommendations.)*		
8. Cleaning a closed wound: A. Using moistened gauze, cleanse from top of wound to base (or center of wound to edges). B. Discard gauze C. Clean from area of least contamination to greatest (Fig. 136-3).	Prevents wound contamination during the cleaning process.	If cleaning around a drain, clean from drain site outward in a circular motion; discard gauze with each circle.
9. Dry intact skin surrounding wound with gauze.	Limits maceration of healthy skin surrounding the wound.	
Culturing Wounds *Swab Culture* 1. Don clean gloves and remove swab from culturette tube; maintain sterile technique. *(Level V: Clinical studies in more than one patient population and situation.)*	Must clean wound before obtaining culture to ensure that debris contamination is not cultured.[3-4,8] Wound culturing is a sterile procedure.	
2. Swab firmly across the surface of the wound in a zigzag manner, simultaneously rotating the swab between finger and thumb. *(Level IV: Limited clinical studies to support recommendations.)*	Ensures collection of an adequate specimen.[3-4,8]	

Procedure continues on the following page

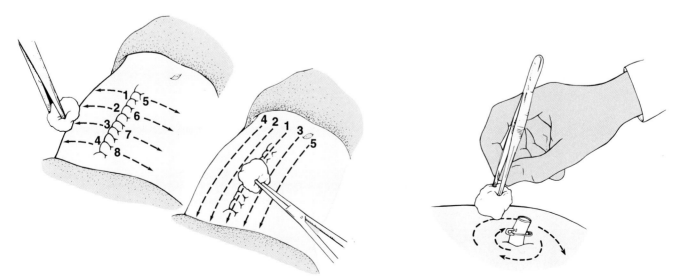

FIGURE 136-3 Cleaning a wound. *(From Potter, P.A., and Perry, A. [2003]. Basic Nursing: Essentials for Practice. 5th ed. St. Louis: Mosby.)*

Procedure for Cleaning, Irrigating, Culturing, and Dressing an Open Wound—*Continued*

Steps	Rationale	Special Considerations
3. Carefully place swab into culturette tube without touching swab or inside of container.	Prevents contamination.	Swab center of wound and not wound edges. Culturing of wound edges may result in contamination from skin flora and wound debris.
4. Crush ampule of medium in culturette and close securely; observe that culture medium surrounds swab.	Keeps specimen from drying and provides growth-supporting medium for culture.	If collecting an anaerobic culture, ensure tube is maintained upright to prevent carbon dioxide from escaping.
5. Label specimen with patient name, date, wound site; transport to laboratory as soon as possible.		

Tissue Biopsy

Steps	Rationale	Special Considerations
1. Don sterile gloves; using sterile scalpel and forceps, obtain a tissue sample approximately 1 to 2 cm in size (width and depth); apply pressure with sterile gauze to tissue sampling site. (*Level IV: Limited clinical studies to support recommendations.*)	Ensures good sample size; provides for homeostasis of tissue bed.[1,3-4,8]	Caution must be exercised in obtaining a tissue biopsy; assess for excessive bleeding and damage to underlying and surrounding structures. Advanced training is encouraged for practitioners performing this skill.
2. Place tissue sample in sterile container and close tightly; sample may be placed on agar plate, if indicated.	Prevents contamination of sample.	
3. Label specimen with patient name, date, wound site; transport to laboratory as soon as possible. Proceed to "Dressing Open Wounds."		

Needle Aspiration

Steps	Rationale	Special Considerations
1. Don clean gloves; insert sterile needle into drainage; aspirate approximately 5 to 10 ml of drainage into sterile syringe. (*Level IV: Limited clinical studies to support recommendations.*)	Ensures good specimen collection. Use syringe method only when large amounts of drainage are present or for collecting specimens from deep wounds.[1,7]	
2. Express excess air out of syringe.		
3. Remove needle and replace with a needleless blunt end cap; maintain sterile technique.	Maintains standard precautions; prevents contamination.	
4. Label specimen with patient name, date, wound site; transport to laboratory as soon as possible.		

Dressing Open Wounds

Steps	Rationale	Special Considerations
1. Open sterile gauze 4 × 4 pads and saturate with normal saline; don sterile gloves; wring out excessive moisture; apply 4 × 4s loosely over wound bed; gently pack gauze to wound edge but do not exceed wound edge. (*Level V: Clinical studies in more than one patient population and situation.*)	Open, moist gauze protects wound bed and allows for placement of dressing without creating open areas or pockets; dressing must be moist but not wet to allow for absorption.[1,5]	Moist dressing must stay within parameters of wound bed to prevent surrounding skin maceration. Dressings packed too firmly into wound will compromise perfusion and wound healing. Wound care dressing products that absorb drainage or provide moisture may also be used.

Procedure for Cleaning, Irrigating, Culturing, and Dressing an Open Wound—*Continued*		
Steps	**Rationale**	**Special Considerations**
2. Place dry gauze 4 × 4s and ABDs over moist dressing.	Provides protection and absorption.	
3. Secure dressing with tape or Montgomery straps. A. Tape: Apply tape across the wound dressing, extending approximately 2 in beyond dressing onto skin.	Hypoallergenic tape is less traumatic to noninjured skin; secures dressing in place.	
B. Montgomery straps (Fig. 136-4): (1) Apply a liquid or hydrocolloid barrier to surround skin where Montgomery straps will be applied.	Assists with providing a protective skin barrier and more effective anchoring of Montgomery straps.	
(2) Peel paper backing off Montgomery straps and apply to skin surface using gentle, even pressure.	Secures Montgomery straps to skin.	

Procedure continues on the following page

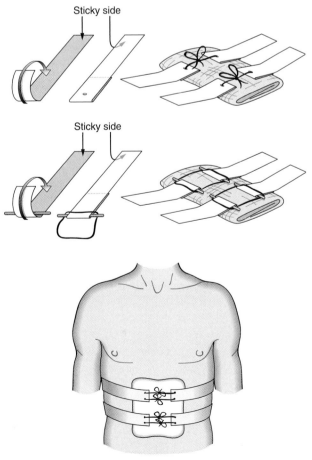

FIGURE 136-4 Montgomery straps.

Procedure	for Cleaning, Irrigating, Culturing, and Dressing an Open Wound—*Continued*		
Steps	**Rationale**	**Special Considerations**	
(3) Lace the cotton type (twill tape, umbilical tape, tracheotomy tape, large rubber bands) through holes in the Montgomery straps in a criss-cross fashion.	Secures dressing in place beneath Montgomery strap.	

Expected Outcomes

- Wound bed will be clean.
- Wound culture specimen obtained will confirm and identify causative organism of infection.
- Wound will heal uniformly without tunneling or tracking or infection.
- Surrounding skin is free of maceration and erosion.
- Wound is free of signs of infection or compromised perfusion.

Unexpected Outcomes

- Cross-contamination of wound
- Damage to wound bed (hemorrhage, dehiscence) from excessive force during irrigation
- Maceration or inflammation of surrounding skin
- Hemorrhage from tissue biopsy culture technique
- Signs of infection; changes in amount and character of wound drainage
- Wound healing (granulation and contraction) not noticeably progressing on a weekly basis
- Development of wound tunneling or tracking

Patient Monitoring and Care

Steps	**Rationale**	**Reportable Conditions**
		These conditions should be reported if they persist despite nursing interventions.
1. Assess patient, wound bed, and skin surrounding wound. *(Level VI: Clinical studies in a variety of patient populations and situation.)*	Continued assessment for wound infection is essential; wounds must be free of infection to heal. Wound colonization is the presence of bacteria in a wound in quantities that do not interfere with wound healing.[1,6] Infection is the presence of bacteria in a wound that elicits an inflammatory response and interferes with wound healing.[1,3-4,6,8] Healthy granulation tissue will be red in color. Discoloration may indicate infection, necrotic tissue, and poor perfusion or hypoxemia at the wound bed site.	- Foul drainage or odor - Darkened areas on tissue bed; pale red, green, or yellow tissue bed - Erythema - Pain - Change in wound drainage (amount, color, odor) - Elevated temperature - Elevated white blood cell count - Hyperglycemia in a diabetic patient
2. Monitor wound dressing site for bleeding.	Capillary bed of a healing wound is very fragile. Excessive stimulation created during the collection of a culture by tissue biopsy or needle aspiration may disrupt the capillary integrity, creating excessive bleeding.	- Bleeding that does not stop with mild pressure to wound bed - Excessive bleeding

Patient Monitoring and Care—*Continued*

Steps	Rationale	Reportable Conditions
3. Assess wound bed and edges for pockets or tunnels.	Wounds healing by secondary intention are at increased risk for developing pockets or tunnels.	• Presence and depth of pocket or tunnel

Documentation

Documentation should include the following:

- Patient and family education
- Premedication given, patient tolerance of procedure, and response to pain medication
- Wound cleaning and irrigation procedure completed; date; time
- Description of wound bed before and after cleaning or irritation; drainage and odors if appropriate; presence of necrotic and granulation tissue
- Description of surrounding skin (color, moisture, integrity)
- Size of wound (measure or trace wound area and depth when appropriate)

- Progression of difficult-to-heal or complex wounds (consider use of digital photography to document)
- Wound culture completed, date, time; type of culture obtained (swab, aerobic, anaerobic, needle aspiration, tissue biopsy)
- Description of approximate site where wound culture was obtained
- Description of wound drains, surrounding skin, and characteristics of wound drainage
- Type of dressing applied after wound care
- Unexpected outcomes
- Nursing interventions

References

1. Agency for Health Care Policy and Research. (1994). *Clinical Practice Guideline: Treatment of Pressure Ulcers.* Rockville, MD: U.S. Department of Health and Human Services.
2. Fernandez, R., Griffiths, R., and Ussic, C. (2002). Water for wound cleansing. *The Cochrane Database of Systematic Review,* Vol. 1, September.
3. McGuckin, M., et al. (2003). The clinical relevance of microbiology in acute and chronic wounds. *Advances Skin & Wound Care,* 16, 12-23.
4. Neil, J.A., and Munro, C.L. (1997). A comparison of two culturing methods for chronic wounds. *Ostomy/Wound Manage,* 43, 20-30.
5. Ovington, L.G. (2001). Wound care products: How to choose. *Home Healthcare Nurse,* 19, 224-31.
6. Ovington, L.G. (2001). Battling bacteria in wound care. *Home Healthcare Nurse,* 19, 622-30.
7. The Joanna Briggs Institute. (2003). Solutions, techniques and pressure for wound cleansing. *Best Practice,* 7, 1-6.
8. Wysocki, A.B. (2002). Evaluating and managing open skin wounds: colonization versus infection. *AACN Clin Iss,* 13, 382-97.

Additional Readings

Bates-Jensen, B.M. (2001). Management of exudates and infection. In: Sussman, C., and Bates-Jensen, B.M., eds. *Wound Care.* 2nd ed. Gaithersburg, MD: Aspen Publication, 216-32.

Bello, Y., and Phillips, T. (2000). Recent advances in wound healing. *JAMA,* 283, 716-8.

Boynton, P.R., and Paustian, C. (1996). Wound assessment and decision making options. *Crit Care Nurs Clin North Am,* 8, 125-39.

Harding, K.G., Morris, H.L., and Patel, G.K. (2002). Healing chronic wounds. *BMJ,* 324, 160-3.

Maklebust, J. (1996). Using wound care products to promote a healing environment. *Crit Care Nurs Clin North Am,* 8, 141-58.

Ovington, L.G. (2002). Dealing with drainage: The what, why, and how of wound exudates. *Home Healthcare Nurse,* 20, 368-72.

Rijswijk, L.V. (1996). The fundamentals of wound assessment. *Ostomy/Wound Management,* 42, 40-52.

Rook, J.L. (1996). Wound care pain management. *Adv Wound Care,* 9, 24-31.

Sussman, C. (2001). Assessment of the skin and wound. In: Sussman, C., and Bates-Jensen, B.M., eds. *Wound Care.* 2nd ed. Gaithersburg, MD: Aspen Publication, 85-118.

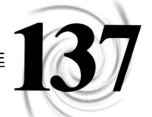

PROCEDURE **137**

Debridement: Pressure Ulcers, Burns, and Wounds

P U R P O S E : Wound debridement is the removal of necrotic nonviable tissue to promote wound healing.

Mary Beth Flynn Makic

PREREQUISITE NURSING KNOWLEDGE

- Prior to wound debridement, the patient and wound should be assessed for underlying causes, patient's physical condition, nutritional status, and current health care treatment plan, including medications.[2-3,9,11]
- Normal wound healing progresses through an orderly sequence of three overlapping phases: inflammation, proliferation, and reepithelization and remodeling.
- The presence of necrotic tissue or debris will interrupt the normal sequence of wound healing; retards healing processes and provides a medium that promotes bacterial growth.[2-3,6,9,11,13]
- Acute wounds may be classified as either partial-thickness or full-thickness. Partial-thickness wounds penetrate the epidermis and part of the dermis; partial-thickness wounds can be further described as superficial or deep partial-thickness wounds. Full-thickness wounds extend to all skin layers, the epidermis and dermis, and may penetrate subcutaneous tissues.[2]
- Pressure ulcers are defined as localized areas of tissue necrosis that develop when soft tissue is compressed between a bony prominence and an external surface for a prolonged period of time.[5] The National Pressure Ulcer Advisory Panel (NPUAP) staging system is used to describe pressure ulcers.[1,5]
  - ❖ Stage I: Pressure ulcer is an observable pressure-related alteration of intact skin whose indicators, when compared to an adjacent or opposite area on the body, may include changes in one or more of the following: skin temperature (warmth or coolness), tissue consistency (firm or boggy feel), and/or sensation (pain, itching). The ulcer appears as a defined area of persistent redness in lightly pigmented skin, whereas in darker skin tones, the ulcer may appear with persistent red, blue, or purple hues.
  - ❖ Stage II: Partial-thickness skin loss involving epidermis, dermis, or both. The ulcer is superficial and presents clinically as an abrasion, blister, or shallow crater.
  - ❖ Stage III: Full-thickness skin loss involving damage to or necrosis of subcutaneous tissue that may extend down to, but not through, underlying fascia. The ulcer presents clinically as a deep crater with or without undermining of adjacent tissue.
  - ❖ Stage IV: Full-thickness skin loss with extensive destruction, tissue necrosis, or damage to muscle, bone, or supporting structures (e.g., tendon, joint). Undermining and sinus tracts also may be associated with Stage IV pressure ulcers.[1,5]
- Necrotic tissue is nonviable tissue and may range in color from whitish gray, tan, yellow, and finally progressing to black.[2]
- Debridement provides a mechanism of removing necrotic tissue and reestablishes normal phases of wound healing.
- Debridement may be achieved by several methods:[1,4,6,9,10]
  - ❖ *Surgical debridement:* Fast and effective means of removing devitalized tissue. Requires local anesthesia, use of sterile instruments, and conditions and availability of a qualified clinician.[2,9,10]
  - ❖ *Sharp debridement:* Similar to surgical debridement but instruments may be clean and local anesthesia may or may not be administered. A qualified clinician performs procedure.[2,9,10]
  - ❖ *Chemical (enzymatic) debridement:* Highly selective method of removing necrotic tissue. Relies on naturally

occurring enzymes that are exogenously applied to the wound surface to degrade tissue. This is a slower process that requires a moist wound bed with adequate secondary dressing to absorb wound exudates.

❖ *Mechanical debridement:* Method of physically removing debris from the wound. Methods range from wet to dry gauze dressings, irrigation, pulsatile lavage, and whirlpool therapy; debridement is nonselective, and healthy tissue as well as necrotic tissue and debris may be removed in the process.

❖ *Autolytic debridement:* Employs the properties of moisture-interactive dressings to facilitate digestion of devitalized tissue by the body's own enzymes. Typically, if tissue autolysis does not begin to appear in the wound in 24-72 hours, another method of debridement should be considered.[9]

• Vascular evaluation is essential prior to wound debridement. Inadequate perfusion may result in the wound extending into a deeper dermal or full-thickness wound after debridement.[2-3,8,10,11]

• Pressure ulcers, burns, and chronic wounds may develop necrotic tissue that requires debridement for wound healing to progress.

• Surgical debridement should be performed by physicians. Sharp debridement may be performed by physicians, registered nurses, and physical therapists with documented educational course completion and validation of knowledge and skill. It is wise to check with state regulatory agencies prior to performing sharp wound debridement.[2,12]

• A key to successful safe sharp debridement is knowledge of anatomy and assessment.[2]

• All wound care procedures should adhere to principles of aseptic technique. Clinical judgment should be used in determining whether clean or sterile technique is indicated in the wound dressing procedure. Generally speaking, acute wounds may be cared for using sterile technique and chronic wounds may be cared for with clean technique.[1] The clinician must assess the patient, type or stage of wound, and type of procedure in deciding which technique should be used in providing wound care.

EQUIPMENT

• Sharp debridement
  ❖ Sterile gloves and field
  ❖ Normal saline
  ❖ Gauze 4 × 4 pads
  ❖ Instrument set (scissors, forceps, No. 10 scalpel)
  ❖ Wound dressing
  ❖ Tape
• Chemical debridement
  ❖ Normal saline or water to clean wound
  ❖ Clean gloves and/or sterile gloves (depending on type and age of wound)

❖ Enzymatic preparation or solution (prescribed)
❖ Tongue blade
❖ Filler dressing if needed; secondary absorptive dressing
❖ No. 10 scalpel for crosshatching (optional)
❖ Tape
• Mechanical debridement (wet to dry gauze dressing)
  ❖ Clean or sterile gloves (depending on type and age of wound)
  ❖ Normal saline
  ❖ Gauze (rolled or 4 × 4 pads)
  ❖ Secondary absorptive dressing
  ❖ Tape
• Autolytic debridement
  ❖ Clean gloves
  ❖ Normal saline or water to clean wound
  ❖ Moisture-retentive dressing (transparent film, hydrocolloid dressing, hydrogels)
  ❖ Secondary absorptive dressing as indicated
  ❖ Tape

PATIENT AND FAMILY EDUCATION

• Explain procedure and reason for wound debridement; educate regarding potential complications such as bleeding if sharp debridement is the prescribed procedure. ➤*Rationale:* Decreases patient anxiety and comfort; informs patient.

PATIENT ASSESSMENT AND PREPARATION

Patient Assessment

• Vascular assessment should be completed prior to debridement. ➤*Rationale:* Poor perfusion may result in the extension of the wound after debridement.

• Assess for signs and symptoms of local and systemic infection. ➤*Rationale:* Debridement may seed bacteria into systemic circulation; appropriate antibiotics should be considered prior to debridement in at-risk patient populations.[8] Sharp debridement, the most aggressive type of debridement, is the method of choice when signs of severe cellulitis or sepsis are present.[1]

• Ensure that coagulation parameters are within normal limits. ➤*Rationale:* Coagulation abnormalities may result in unwanted bleeding complications due to debridement process.

Patient Preparation

• Ensure that patient understands preprocedural teaching. Answer questions as they arise and reinforce information as needed. ➤*Rationale:* Evaluates and reinforces understanding of previously taught information.

• Premedicate patient with prescribed analgesic, if needed. ➤*Rationale:* Decreases patient anxiety and discomfort.

• Place patient in position of optimal comfort and visualization for dressing the wound. ➤*Rationale:* Provides for effective wound visualization and enhances patient tolerance of procedure.

• Optimize lighting in room and provide privacy for patient. ➤*Rationale:* Allows for optimal wound assessment and patient comfort.

Procedure for Debridement: Pressure Ulcers, Burns, and Wounds

Steps	Rationale	Special Considerations
Sharp Debridement		
1. Premedicate patient for pain.	Systemic analgesic may be administered prior to procedure for patient tolerance and compliance.	Assess patient response to analgesic.
2. Position patient to allow for optimal lighting and view of wound.	Maintains aseptic technique.	Sharp debridement may be difficult on hard, dry wounds; consider enzymatic debridement as first option.[2,10]
3. Don clean gloves and clean wound.	Reduces transmission of microorganisms; standard precautions.	
4. Prepare sterile field of instruments, NS, gauze, and secondary dressing.	Maintains aseptic technique.	Gauze may be needed to provide hemostasis during procedure.
5. Don sterile gloves.		
6. Using forceps, lift eschar and gently cut with scalpel or scissors. Debride tissue to line of demarcation of healthy tissue.	Goal of sharp debridement is removal of devitalized tissue without damage to healthy wound bed.	Pain and bleeding are signs of healthy tissue. Stop procedure if bleeding is excessive or if there is impending bone, tendon, or proximity to fascial plane.[2]
7. Clean wound bed with normal saline.	Allows for removal of loose devitalized tissue and debris.	Reassess wound bed postprocedure.
8. Apply moist wound dressing of choice.	Promotes wound healing of newly exposed tissues.	Assess for hemostasis prior to application of dressing.
Chemical Debridement	Selective debridement technique.	Requires prescription for desired enzyme preparation.
1. Don clean gloves and clean wound.	Maintains aseptic technique.	
2. Discard dirty gloves and don clean gloves.	Maintains clean technique.	
3. If wound eschar is hard and dry, No. 10 scalpel may be used to cross hatch necrotic tissue. (*Level IV: Limited clinical studies to support recommendation.*)	Cross-hatching technique may allow better penetration of enzymatic agent and enhance enzyme activity.[2]	
4. Establish sterile field: enzymatic agent, NS, and secondary moist healing dressing.	Maintains aseptic technique.	
5. Apply enzymatic agent with tongue blade to eschar in the wound bed.	Assists with even application of enzymatic agent over necrotic wound tissue.	Concentrate enzymatic agent over nonviable tissue.
6. Place moisture-retentive dressing (typically, gauze moistened with NS) over wound.	Most enzymatic agents require a moist dressing medium to be applied over agent for effective action.	Other dressings that promote moist wound healing may be used.
7. Secure secondary dressing in place.	Secondary dressing is needed to absorb wound exudates.[2-3,10]	Assess periwound for irritation and breakdown from moisture. Consider applying liquid skin barrier to periwound edge.

Procedure for Debridement: Pressure Ulcers, Burns, and Wounds—*Continued*

Steps	Rationale	Special Considerations
Mechanical Debridement—Wet-to-Dry-Gauze Dressing	Nonselective debridement technique.	Nonviable and viable tissue may be lost with this method of debridement.
1. Wash hands and don clean gloves.	Maintains clean technique.	
2. Establish sterile field: gauze dressing moistened with normal saline.	Maintains aseptic technique.	
3. Clean wound.	Wound cleansing is a means of mechanical debridement; also removes nonadherent bacteria.	
4. Don gloves.	Maintains aseptic technique.	
5. Place moistened gauze loosely into wound bed.	Excessive packing of gauze into wound bed may compromise perfusion.[7]	If more than one gauze dressing is used, place ends of two dressings close to each other for easy removal.
6. Cover wound with secondary absorptive dressing and secure.	Protects wound from external contamination and absorbs exudates.	Consider changing dressing if 75% or greater strikethrough is present on secondary dressing.[6,7] Assess periwound area for maceration; consider use of liquid skin barrier or hydrocolloid to protect periwound skin.
7. After prescribed time interval, don clean gloves and remove dressing to create mechanical debridement action.	Drying action of gauze adheres it to necrotic tissue, which will be detached with dressing removal.	If dressing is dry and adherent to viable tissue, lightly moisten gauze to prevent excessive debridement of viable tissue and minimize pain.[7]
Autolytic Debridement	Selective debridement technique that utilizes the body's natural enzymes to destroy necrotic tissue.	May not be effective for large wound surfaces.
1. Don clean gloves	Maintains aseptic technique.	
2. Clean wound bed with NS or water.		
3. Apply moisture-retentive dressing.	Provides moist wound healing environment that enhances autolytic debridement process.	Assess dressing for absorptive properties; dressing should be changed with 75% saturation or presence of drainage strikethrough to prevent bacterial contamination into the wound.[6,7]
4. Apply secondary dressing as indicated.	Autolyic debridement will result in production of wound exudates that should be absorbed into a secondary dressing away from wound bed to prevent bacterial adherence to tissues.	

Procedure continues on the following page

Expected Outcomes

- Wound bed will be free of necrotic tissue and debris.
- Inflammatory stage of wound healing is reestablished and wound healing progresses along normal trajectory.
- Wound is free of infection or signs of compromised perfusion.
- Wound hemostasis is established after sharp debridement.

Unexpected Outcomes

- Depth of wound extends, and necrotic tissue is reestablished.
- Normal wound healing process is not reestablished by removal of devitalized tissue and wound healing fails to progress.[1-3]
- Bacterial infection is present; signs of local or systemic infection are present.
- Excessive bleeding from lack of wound hemostasis.

Patient Monitoring and Care

Steps	Rationale	Reportable Conditions
		These conditions should be reported if they persist despite nursing interventions.
1. Assess patient, wound bed, and surrounding skin for signs of infection. (*Level V: Clinical studies in more than one patient population.*)	Wound debridement may not effectively remove all bacteria; continued assessment for wound infection is essential for healing.[2-3,5,6,9,11]	• Erythema and warmth at wound site • Pain and tenderness • Edema • Change in wound drainage amount, color, odor • Fever • Elevated white blood cell count
2. Monitor dressing for signs of bleeding.	Wound debridement may disturb newly formed, fragile blood vessels, as well as established blood vessels, and cause bleeding.	• Bleeding that does not stop with mild pressure to wound bed • Excessive bleeding
3. Assess wound for signs of healing after debridement. (*Level V: Clinical studies in more than one patient population.*)	Goal of necrotic tissue debridement is to establish would healing in the form of granulation tissue and wound contracture.[2-3,9]	• Discoloration of wound bed noted • Development of necrotic tissue in wound bed • Changed, diminished, or absent pulses distal to wound bed

Documentation

Documentation should include the following:

- Patient and family education
- Description of wound bed prior to debridement and after debridement
- Description of periwound skin assessment (color, moisture, integrity)
- Size of wound after wound debridement procedure
- Description of dressing applied to wound bed (primary and secondary dressings as appropriate)

- Premedication given, patient tolerance of procedure, and response to pain medication
- Description of wound debridement process and any unexpected complications
- Vascular assessment
- Description of established wound hemostasis obtain at completion of procedure
- Digital photography is recommended to document progression of wound healing[1]

References

1. Agency for Health Care Policy and Research. (1994). *Treatment of Pressure Ulcers*. Rockville, MD: U.S. Department of Health and Human Services, AHCPR Publication No. 95-0652.
2. Bates-Jensen, B.M. (2001). Management of necrotic tissues. In: Sussman, C., and Bates-Jensen, B.M., eds. *Wound Care*. 2nd ed. Gaithersburg, MD: Aspen Publications, 197-215.
3. Chalk, L. (1999). Wound prevention and healing: Everyone's problem. *Surg Services Manage*, 5, 35-8.
4. McGuckin, M., et al. (2003). The clinical relevance of microbiology in acute and chronic wounds. *Advances Skin & Wound Care*, 16, 12-23.

5. NPUAP Staging Report. Available at: *www.npuap.org*. Accessed Jan. 5, 2005.
6. Ovington, L.G. (2001). Battling bacteria in wound care. *Home Healthcare Nurse*, 19, 622-30.
7. Ovington, L.G. (2002). Hanging wet-to-dry dressings out to dry. *Advances Skin & Wound Care*, 15, 79-89.
8. Patterson, G.K. (2001). Vascular evaluation. In: Sussman, C., and Bates-Jensen, B.M., eds. *Wound Care*. 2nd ed. Gaithersburg, MD: Aspen Publications, 177-92.
9. Sibbald, R.G., et al. (2000). Preparing the wound bed: Debridement, bacterial balance, and moisture balance. *Ostomy Wound Manage*, 46, 14-34.

10. Rodeheaver, G.T. (1999). Pressure ulcer debridement and cleansing: A review of current literature. *Ostomy Wound Manage,* 45, 80-6.

11. Rudolph, D. (2002). Why won't this wound heal? *Am J Nurs,* 102, 24DD-24HH.

12. Thomaselli, N. (1995). WOCN position statement: Conservative sharp wound debridement for registered nurses. *J Wound Ostomy Continence Nurses,* 22, 32A.

13. Wysocki, A.B. (2002). Evaluating and managing open skin wounds: Colonization versus infection. *AACN Clin Issues,* 13, 382-97.

Harding, K.G., Morris, H.L., and Patel, G.K. (2002). Healing chronic wounds. *BMJ,* 324, 160-3.

Martin, S.J., Corrado, O.J., and Day, E.A. (1996). Enzymatic debridement for necrotic wounds. *J Wound Care,* 5, 310-1.

Rose, J.K., and Herndon, D.N. (1997). Advances in the treatment of burn patients. *Burns,* 23(Suppl 1), S19-26.

Sussman, C., Fowler, E., and Wethe, J. (1995). *Sharp Debridement of Wounds* (video series). Torrance, CA: Sussman Physical Therapy, Inc.

Additional Readings

Bello, Y., and Phillips, T. (2000). Recent advances in wound healing. *JAMA,* 283, 716-8.

PROCEDURE

138

Dressing Wounds With Drains

P U R P O S E :   Dressing wounds with drains is performed to manage wound drainage and protect surrounding skin.

Mary Beth Flynn Makic

PREREQUISITE NURSING KNOWLEDGE

- Wound healing is best achieved through adequate cleansing, debridement, and dressing of the wound bed based on patient and wound characteristics.
- Goals of wound care must be clearly outlined so that proper wound care products are used. Coarse gauze nonselectively debrides the wound bed mechanically and absorbs wound fluid; calcium alginates, foams, and hydrofiber dressings enhance drainage absorption; hydrogels provide moisture to nondraining wounds; hydrocolloids provide wound moisture with moderate absorption; film dressings are for nonexudating wounds.[3,7-8]
- Drains are placed in wounds to facilitate healing by providing an exit for excessive fluid accumulating in or near the wound bed.
- Excessive wound fluid may create pressure in the wound bed and compromise perfusion. Continually assess the patient for adequate blood supply distal to the wound bed.
- Assessment of wound exudate should include the quantity, color, consistency, and odor of drainage.
- Assess the patient's nutritional needs, specifically for protein, with exudating wounds. Excessive wound exudates production may result in the loss of up to 100 g of protein daily in wound exudates.[7]
- Excessive wound fluid may provide a source for proliferation of microorganisms.
- Wound drains may be ports of microorganism entry[3,6,7-8]; aseptic techniques must be strictly observed.
- Most wound drains are surgically placed; drains may or may not be sutured in place.[3,6]

- Topical negative pressure, or vacuum-assisted closure (V.A.C)® (see Procedure 141), provides negative pressure to a wound bed that stimulates cell growth and wound healing. The closed system also provides active withdrawal of excessive wound fluid. All nonviable tissue should be removed prior to application of a V.A.C® dressing.
- V.A.C® dressings are usually changed every 48 hours.[1-2,4-5] Infected wound beds may require more frequent dressing changes (every 12 hours), and V.A.C® dressings over grafts may be changed less frequently (every 3-5 days).[1,2,4-5]

EQUIPMENT

- Nonsterile and/or sterile gloves; sterile field (depending on type and age of wound)
- Gowns and face protection
- Sterile gauze (4 × 4 pads); ABD or other absorptive dressings may be needed
- Sterile water or normal saline (NS) for cleansing
- Hypoallergenic tape; one set of Montgomery straps
- Liquid skin barrier to protect periwound skin and for applying Montgomery straps; hydrocolloid wafer

PATIENT AND FAMILY EDUCATION

- Explain the procedure and the reason for changing wound dressing. ➤*Rationale:* Decreases patient anxiety and discomfort.
- Discuss patient's role in dressing change procedure and maintenance of wound drains or VAC. ➤*Rationale:* Elicits patient cooperation; prepares patient for wound management on discharge.

PATIENT ASSESSMENT AND PREPARATION

Patient Assessment

- Monitor for signs and symptoms of wound infection, including the following:
  ❖ Erythema at drainage site
  ❖ Heat
  ❖ Edema
  ❖ Pain
  ❖ Elevated temperature and white blood cell count
  ❖ Wound drainage becoming cloudy and foul-smelling
  ❖ Increase in amount of wound exudate
  ➤➤*Rationale:* Drains assist with removal of excessive fluid but also provide a portal of entry for microorganisms.

- Assess patency of wound drainage system. ➤➤*Rationale:* Drains are frequently soft and pliable and thus can easily become kinked or blocked if wound drainage is fibrous in composition.

Patient Preparation

- Premedicate patient with prescribed analgesic if needed. ➤➤*Rationale:* Decreases patient anxiety and discomfort.
- Place patient in position of optimal comfort and visualization for dressing the wound. ➤➤*Rationale:* Provides for effective wound visualization and enhances patient tolerance of procedure.
- Optimize lighting in room and provide privacy for patient. ➤➤*Rationale:* Allows for optimal wound assessment and patient comfort.

Procedure | for Dressing Wounds With Drains

Steps	Rationale	Special Considerations
Dressing Wounds With Drains		
1. Wash hands, don gloves, and remove old dressing.	Maintains clean technique.	Use caution with dressing removal to ensure that drains are not dislodged.
2. Remove gloves and wash hands.		
3. Establish sterile field.	Maintains aseptic technique.	There is no evidence to support use of sterile technique when changing dressings on chronic wounds.
4. Don personal protective equipment.	Standard precautions.	
5. Clean and irrigate wound (see Procedure 136) as indicated.	Removes contaminated drainage and debris from wound.	Irrigation of wound drains should be performed only if indicated and only by physician or advanced practice nurse.[3,7-8]
6. Change gloves; apply liquid skin barrier to periwound area allow to dry; open 4 × 4 gauze pad and apply on top of wound and around drains (Fig. 138-1). Avoid wrapping gauze around drain site.	Gauze absorbs drainage to keep underlying skin dry; wrapping gauze around drain may result in inadvertent drain removal with future dressing changes.	Drains are placed to remove excessive wound fluid. Care must be taken to provide a dressing capable of absorbing wound drainage and preventing moisture accumulation on surrounding healthy skin.[7-8]

Procedure continues on the following page

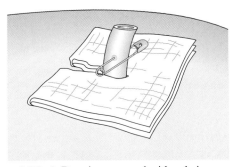

FIGURE 138-1 Dressing a wound with a drain.

Procedure for Dressing Wounds With Drains—*Continued*

Steps	Rationale	Special Considerations
7. Apply gauze dressings from area of least contamination to area of greatest contamination.	Prevents cross-contamination of wound bed.	
8. If necessary, apply ABD or other absorptive dressing over 4 × 4 gauze pads.	Gauze 4 × 4 pads enhance removal of drainage away from skin; secondary dressing prevents contamination and protects clothing from drainage.	Wound exudate that leaks from edges or outer layer of dressing (strikethrough) creates a portal for bacteria to enter the wound. Dressings should be changed when they are 75% saturated or when strikethrough is present.[7]
9. Apply tape or Montgomery straps to secure dressing. Hydrocolloid wafers may be placed on skin, creating a protective barrier for application of tape or Montgomery straps.	When tape is used to secure dressings, frequent dressing changes may result in skin irritation or disruption from the adhesive tape. Hypoallergenic tape, Montgomery straps, and skin barriers help decrease mechanical irritation caused by frequent tape removal.	Assess periwound edge for chemical and moisture irritation or skin breakdown from wound exudate.
A. Tape: Apply hypoallergenic tape across the wound dressing extending approximately 2 in beyond dressing onto skin.	Hypoallergenic tape is less traumatic to noninjured skin; it is necessary to extend tape beyond dressing edges to anchor and secure dressing well.	
B. Montgomery straps (see Fig. 136-4): (1) Apply a liquid or hydrocolloid barrier to surrounding skin when Montgomery straps are used.	Assists with providing protective skin barrier and more effective anchoring of Montgomery strap.	
(2) Peel paper backing off Montgomery straps and apply to skin surface using gentle, even pressure.	Secures Montgomery straps to skin.	
(3) Lace cotton tape (twill tape, umbilical tape, tracheostomy ties) through holes in the Montgomery straps in a criss-cross fashion.	Secures dressing in place beneath Montgomery strap.	

Expected Outcomes

- Drains remain intact and patent and effectively remove excessive wound fluid.
- Surrounding skin is dry and free of excessive wound drainage moisture (maceration).
- Wound drainage exit sites are clean and dry, without signs of infection or irritation.
- Wound healing is enhanced because of effective wound drainage removal.
- Wound drainage decreases in volume (over time) and is absent of foul odor or undesirable color.

Unexpected Outcomes

- Wound drain becomes dislodged, blocked, or kinked.
- Skin erosion or maceration occurs around wound drainage sites or skin sites or both.

Patient Monitoring and Care

Steps	Rationale	Reportable Conditions
1. Observe for signs of wound infection.	Drains assist with removal of excessive fluid but also provide a portal of entry of microorganisms.[3,7-8]	*These conditions should be reported if they persist despite nursing interventions.* • Erythema at drainage site • Heat • Edema • Pain • Elevated temperature and white blood cell count • Wound drainage becoming cloudy and foul-smelling • Wound drainage amount increases
2. Assess for patency of wound drainage system.	Drains are frequently soft and pliable and thus can easily become kinked or blocked if wound drainage is fibrous in composition. V.A.C® system may become disconnected, seal may be lost from outer drape, or system becomes unplugged from energy source.	• Wound drainage suddenly decreasing in amount or stopping
3. Monitor amount of wound drainage relative to patient intake and output.	If a wound produces excessive fluid, the patient may experience a fluid imbalance requiring intravenous or oral fluid replacements. Nutritional consult to replace protein loss from wound exudates may be indicated.	• Tachycardia • Hypotension • Oliguria • Increasing amounts of drainage • Laboratory analysis suggestive of hypoalbuminemia[7]

Documentation

Documentation should include the following:

- Patient and family education
- Premedication given, patient tolerance of procedure, and response to pain medication
- Wound cleansing and dressing change completed/date, time
- Description of wound bed, drains (suction if applied), surrounding skin, and characteristics of wound drainage

- Dressing applied after wound care
- Amount of drainage
- Unexpected outcomes
- Nursing interventions

References

1. Argenta, L.C., and Morykwas, M.J. (1997). Vacuum-assisted closure: A new method for wound control and treatment. *Annals Plastic Surgery,* 38, 563-77.
2. Bates-Jensen, B.M., et al. (2001). Management of the wound environment with advanced therapies. In: Sussman, C., and Bates-Jensen, B.M., eds. *Wound Care.* 2nd ed. Gaithersburg, MD: Aspen Publication, 272-92.
3. Bates-Jensen, B.M., and Wethe, J.D. (2001). Acute surgical wound management. In: Sussman, C., and Bates-Jensen, B.M., eds. *Wound Care.* 2nd ed. Gaithersburg, MD: Aspen Publication, 310-20.
4. Chua-Patel, C.T., et al. (2000). Vacuum-assisted wound closure. *Am J Nurs,* 100, 45-8.
5. Evans, D., and Land, L. (2001). Topical negative pressure for treating chronic wounds. *The Cochrane Database of Systematic Reviews,* Vol. 1, November.
6. Hochberg, J., and Murray, G. (2004). Principles of operative surgery: Antisepsis, technique, sutures, and drains. In: Townsend, C.M., et al., eds. *Sabiston Textbook of Surgery.* 17th ed. Philadelphia: W.B. Saunders, 253-80.
7. Ovington, L.G. (2002). Dealing with drainage: The what, why, and how of wound exudates. *Home Healthcare Nurse,* 20, 368-74.
8. Sibbald, R.G., et al. (2000). Preparing the wound bed: Debridement, bacterial balance, and moisture balance. *Ostomy Wound Manage,* 46, 14-35.

Additional Reading

Armstrong, D.G., et al. (2002). Outcomes of subatmospheric pressure dressing therapy on wounds of the diabetic foot. *Ostomy Wound Manage,* 48, 64-7.

Collier, M. (1997). Know how: Vacuum-assisted closure. *Nurs Times,* 137-8.

Maklebust, J. (1996). Using wound care products to promote a healing environment. *Crit Care Nurs Clin North Am,* 8,141-58.

McCallon, S.K., et al. (2000). Vacuum-assisted closure versus saline-moistened gauze in the healing of postoperative diabetic foot wounds. *Ostomy Wound Manage,* 46, 28-34.

Mendez-Eastman, S. (1998). When wounds won't heal. *RN,* 61, 20-3.

Ovington, L.G. (2001). Wound care products: How to choose. *Home Healthcare Nurse,* 19, 224-31.

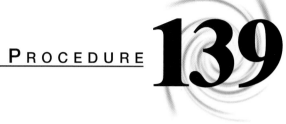

Drain Removal

PURPOSE: Drain removal is performed when the drain is longer needed for drainage management.

Mary Beth Flynn Makic

PREREQUISITE NURSING KNOWLEDGE

- Goals of wound care must be clearly outlined so that proper wound care products are used after drain removal. The wound care products selected will be based on the size and location of the wound, as well as the amount and nature of any remaining drainage.
- Coarse gauze nonselectively debrides the wound bed mechanically and absorbs wound fluid; calcium alginates, foams, and hydrofiber dressings enhance wound absorption; hydrogels provide moisture to nondraining wounds; hydrocolloids provide wound moisture with minimal absorption; film dressings are for nonexudating wounds.[1,3-4]
- Drains are placed in wounds to facilitate healing by providing an exit for excessive fluid accumulating in or near the wound bed. Drains may be removed when drainage is considered to be minimal.[2-4]
- Type of drain, location, and how the drain is secured must be known before drain removal. Competence should be demonstrated by the clinician performing drain removal, because significant tissue injury may result from an improperly removed drain.[1]

EQUIPMENT

- Nonsterile gloves
- Gowns and face protection
- Sterile gauze (4 × 4 pads)
- Suture removal kit or sterile scissors
- Hypoallergenic tape

PATIENT AND FAMILY EDUCATION

- Explain the procedure and reason for drain removal. ➤*Rationale:* Decreases patient anxiety and discomfort.

- Discuss patient's role in drain removal. ➤*Rationale:* Elicits patient cooperation; prepares patient for wound management on discharge.

PATIENT ASSESSMENT AND PREPARATION

Patient Assessment

- Signs of wound infection at drain site include the following:
  - ❖ Change in the amount, odor, or characteristics of the wound drainage
  - ❖ Erythema
  - ❖ Pain
  - ❖ Edema
  - ❖ Elevated temperature
  - ❖ White blood cell count
  - ❖ Foul drainage from exit site
  - ❖ Pressure or tenderness at exit site.

  ➤*Rationale:* Although drains are placed to remove excessive wound fluid and decrease the risk for infection, early detection of infection facilitates prompt, appropriate intervention.

Patient Preparation

- Ensure that patient understands preprocedural teaching. Answer questions as they arise and reinforce information as needed. ➤*Rationale:* Evaluates and reinforces understanding of previously taught information.
- Premedicate patient with prescribed analgesic, if needed. ➤*Rationale:* Although many patients do not require premedication for drain removal, all patients should be assessed for the need prior to the procedure and treated appropriately.

Procedure for Drain Removal

Steps	Rationale	Special Considerations
1. Don gloves and personal protective equipment.	Maintain aseptic technique; standard precautions.	
2. Open sterile scissors; cut any sutures, if present.	Releases drain from tissue suture anchors.	
3. Open gauze 4 × 4; place gauze close to drain skin exit site; instruct patient to take a deep, easy breath; withdraw drain swiftly and evenly. *(Level IV: Limited clinical studies to support recommendations.)*	Gauze is used to capture body fluids as you remove the drain. Deep breathing may decrease the pain the patient feels with drain removal.[4]	Do not force removal of drain. If resistance is felt, stop.
4. Place sterile dressing over drain exit site and secure with tape.	Provides protection of open wound site; prevents entrance of microorganisms.	

Expected Outcomes

- Intact drain is removed without resistance.
- Wound drainage is minimal from exit site.
- Drain exit site is free of signs of fluid accumulation, inflammation, or infection.
- Wound healing continues to progress without presence of excessive wound fluid.

Unexpected Outcomes

- Resistance is felt on drain removal, creating tissue trauma beneath skin surface.
- Wound fluid accumulates beneath skin at drain exit site.[1,4]
- Infection or inflammation occurs at drain exit site.
- Poor approximation of skin edges occurs at drain exit site, requiring wound healing by secondary intention.
- A portion of the drain remains in the wound tract.

Patient Monitoring and Care

Steps	Rationale	Reportable Conditions
		These conditions should be reported if they persist despite nursing interventions.
1. Assess for presence of drainage from drain exit site.	Drainage should be minimal and potentially cease within 24 hours. Continued drainage from drain exit site may indicate accumulation of wound fluid beneath the skin that needs to be evacuated.	• Continued drainage • Edema or pain at exit site
2. Monitor for signs of infection.	Drains are placed to remove excessive wound fluid and to decrease risk for infection.	• Erythema • Pain • Edema • Elevated temperature and white blood cell count • Foul-smelling drainage from exit site • Pressure or tenderness at exit site

Documentation

Documentation should include the following:

- Patient and family education
- Type of drain removed, placement, date, time
- Amount of wound drainage documented in the last 24 hours prior to drain removal
- Premedication given, patient tolerance of procedure, and response to pain medication
- Dressing applied after drain removal
- Appearance of exit site
- Unexpected outcomes
- Nursing interventions

References

1. Bates-Jensen, B.M., and Wethe, J.D. (2001). Acute surgical wound management. In: Sussman, C., and Bates-Jensen, B.M., eds. *Wound Care*. 2nd ed. Gaithersburg, MD: Aspen Publication, 310-20.
2. Hochberg, J., and Murray, G. (2004). Principles of operative surgery: Antisepsis, technique, sutures, and drains. In: Townsend, C.M., et al., eds. *Sabiston Textbook of Surgery*. 17th ed. Philadelphia: W.B. Saunders, 253-80.
3. Ovington, L.G. (2002). Dealing with drainage: The what, why, and how of wound exudates. *Home Healthcare Nurse,* 20, 368-74.
4. Sibbald, R.G., et al. (2000). Preparing the wound bed: Debridement, bacterial balance, and moisture balance. *Ostomy Wound Manage,* 46, 14-35.

Additional Readings

Bello, Y., and Phillips, T. (2000). Recent advances in wound healing. *JAMA,* 283, 716-8.
Harding, K.G., Morris, H.L., and Patel, G.K. (2002). Healing chronic wounds. *BMJ,* 324, 160-3.
Maklebust, J. (1996). Using wound care products to promote a healing environment. *Crit Care Nurs Clin North Am,* 8, 141-58.
Mendez-Eastman, S. (1998). When wounds won't heal. *RN,* 61, 20-3.
Ovington, L.G. (2001). Wound care products: How to choose. *Home Healthcare Nurse,* 19, 224-31.
Rudolph, D.M. (2002). Why won't this wound heal? *AJN,* 102, 24DD-24HH.

PROCEDURE **140**

Pouching a Wound

PURPOSE: Pouching a draining wound is performed to provide a method for containing excessive drainage or accurately measuring drainage output.

Mary Beth Flynn Makic

PREREQUISITE NURSING KNOWLEDGE

- Goals for wound pouching must be clearly outlined; wound pouching is an effective means of collecting fistula drainage.[2-3]
- Wound drainage systems that are applied to suction or collection chamber must have wound care goals and prescribed amount of suction outlined by the health care team.
- Excessive wound drainage is removed to allow for wound healing to occur without tissue congestion, microorganism proliferation, and skin maceration.[1]
- Excessive wound drainage may need to be calculated into the assessment of a patient's daily intake and output.
- Assess the patient's nutritional needs, specifically for protein, with exudating wounds. Excessive wound exudates production may result in the loss of up to 100 g of protein daily in wound exudates.[3-4]
- Vacuum-assisted Wound Closure (VAC)™ (see Procedure 141) may also be used with exudating wounds.

EQUIPMENT

- Nonsterile and/or sterile gloves; sterile field
- Gowns and face protection
- Sterile gauze (4 × 4 pads)
- Normal saline (NS) or water for cleansing wound
- Drainage bag or pouch: ostomy type appliance
- Liquid skin barrier, hydrocolloid dressing, or skin barrier wafers; paste; powder and sealant, if appropriate
- Clean scissors; forceps, if appropriate
- Tape

PATIENT AND FAMILY EDUCATION

- Explain the procedure and reason for changing wound dressing or pouch; educate regarding potential odor during procedure. ➡*Rationale:* Decreases patient anxiety and discomfort.
- Discuss patient's role in dressing/pouch change procedure and maintenance of wound drains/stomas. ➡*Rationale:* Elicits patient cooperation; prepares patient for wound management on discharge.

PATIENT ASSESSMENT AND PREPARATION

Patient Assessment

- Assess for signs and symptoms of local and systemic wound infection, including the following:
  - ❖ Erythema
  - ❖ Pain
  - ❖ Edema
  - ❖ Elevated temperature and white blood cell count
  - ❖ Wound drainage changes in color, odor, or amount
  - ❖ Pressure or tenderness at wound site

  ➡*Rationale:* Early detection of infection facilitates prompt, appropriate intervention.

Patient Preparation

- Ensure that patient understands preprocedural teaching. Answer questions as they arise and reinforce information as needed. ➡*Rationale:* Evaluates and reinforces understanding of previously taught information.

- Premedicate patient with prescribed analgesic if needed. ➤*Rationale:* Decreases patient anxiety and discomfort.
- Place patient in position of optimal comfort and visualization for dressing the wound. ➤*Rationale:* Provides for effective wound visualization and enhances patient tolerance of procedure.
- Optimize lighting in room and provide privacy for patient. ➤*Rationale:* Allows for optimal wound assessment and patient comfort.

Procedure for Pouching a Wound

Steps	Rationale	Special Considerations
1. Wash hands; don clean gloves and personal protective equipment.	Reduces transmission of microorganisms; standard precautions.	
2. If current drainage pouch has external opening, drain and measure content volume and discard.	Reduces transmission of microorganisms during dressing change; provides documentation of wound or fistula drainage.	Ensure that you have all needed supplies before removing old pouching system.
3. Gently remove old drainage pouch; support underlying skin with fingertips while drainage pouch is being removed; dispose of pouch.	Prevents tissue trauma to underlying skin.	A moist cloth may be applied to loosen edges of drainage pouch and assist with the removal process.
4. Using wet gauze 4 × 4s, gently clean wound site from area of least contamination to greatest (see Procedure 136); clean and dry surrounding intact skin.	Maintains clean wound environment; surrounding skin should be free of moisture.	
5. If ordered, irrigate wound/fistula (see Procedure 136) with NS or water until drainage is clear.	Cleans wound bed; decreases microorganism count.	
6. Using wrapper from wound drainage pouch or wafer, draw (measure) wound or fistula edge onto wrapper; cut out the center of the pattern on the wound skin barrier and drainage pouch (cut the pattern *slightly* larger than the tracing).	Irregular shapes and sizes of draining wounds are difficult to estimate; tracing wound onto wrapper will allow for a better fit, with less potential for leaking on intact surrounding skin.	
7. Apply skin barrier (wafer, liquid, paste, sealant).	Assists in providing a good seal for the drainage pouch.	A good seal is important to prevent moisture/wound exudate undermining the dressing and creating skin maceration.
8. Remove adhesive paper from drainage pouch; apply drainage pouch over wound and, using gentle, even pressure, secure pouch edges to skin barrier. *(Level IV: Limited clinical studies to support recommendations.)*	Gentle, even pressure helps ensure a better seal from the drainage pouch to skin barrier; care must be taken to avoid wrinkles from developing during pouch application; wrinkles in pouch barrier create a leak, and fluid will not be contained within drainage pouch.[2-3]	If wrinkles are present, sealant paste may be added to drainage pouch edges to fill spaces created by wrinkles. However, fluid may still track in the wrinkles, despite paste.
9. Close drainage pouch; wound drainage may be allowed to collect in pouch, or suction may be attached to end of pouch to pull fluid away from wound into a more distant collection container. *(Level IV: Limited clinical studies to support recommendations.)*	The type and amount of drainage coming from a wound determines whether or not suction is added to the drainage pouch.[2-3,5]	If suction is not used, care should be taken to empty the appliance regularly. Excessive drainage weight can cause loosening of the appliance.

Expected Outcomes

- Skin surrounding a draining wound remains intact.
- Wound drainage is effectively collected.
- Wound healing is enhanced because of removal of wound drainage into collection device.
- Risk for wound infection is minimized because of effective removal of wound drainage.

Unexpected Outcomes

- Wound drainage is not effectively collected, and surrounding skin is macerated.
- Wound drain (if present) is dislodged during dressing or pouching procedure.
- Wound is not healing efficiently because management of wound drainage is not effective.
- Wound infection is suspected because of inadequate removal of wound drainage that allowed for bacterial growth.

Patient Monitoring and Care

Steps	Rationale	Reportable Conditions
		These conditions should be reported if they persist despite nursing interventions.
1. Observe for signs of wound infection.	Wounds with unmanaged excessive drainage are at higher risk for infection. Wound drainage should slowly decrease as the wound is healing.	• Erythema • Pain • Elevated temperature and white blood cell count • Wound drainage changes in color, odor, or amount
2. Monitor amount of wound drainage relative to patient intake and output.	Excessive wound drainage may cause a fluid imbalance, requiring intravenous or oral fluid replacements.	• Tachycardia • Hypotension • Oliguria • Decreased filling pressures
3. Monitor caloric and protein intake in the presence of heavily draining wounds. Initiate a nutritional consult as needed.	Excessive wound drainage may result in the loss of 100 g of protein a day. Adequate protein will need to be replaced for wound healing.[3-4]	• Hypoalbuminemia
4. Assess for continued adherence of drainage pouch (seal).	Leaking of the pouch may lead to maceration and skin breakdown in the area surrounding the wound.	• Leaking of drainage • Skin breakdown

Documentation

Documentation should include the following:

- Patient and family education
- Wound cleansing, irrigation (if performed), date and time dressing or pouch change was completed
- Description of wound, drainage, odors, presence of drains, suction, and surrounding skin
- Premedication given, patient tolerance of procedure, response to pain medication
- Type of dressing or pouch applied and sealant used
- Unexpected outcomes
- Nursing interventions

References

1. Bates-Jensen, B.M. (2001). Management of exudates and infection. In: Sussman, C., and Bates-Jensen, B.M., eds. *Wound Care*. 2nd ed. Gaithersburg, MD: Aspen Publication, 216-32.
2. Bates-Jensen, B.M., and Seaman, S. (2001). Management of malignant wounds and fistulas. In: Sussman, C., and Bates-Jensen, B.M., eds. *Wound Care*. 2nd ed. Gaithersburg, MD: Aspen Publication, 465-83.
3. Ovington, L.G. (2002). Dealing with drainage: The what, why, and how of wound exudates. *Home Healthcare Nurse*, 20, 368-74.
4. Posthauer, M.E. (2001). Nutritional assessment and treatment. In: Sussman, C., and Bates-Jensen, B.M., eds. *Wound Care*. 2nd ed. Gaithersburg, MD: Aspen Publication, 52-84.
5. Sibbald, R.G., et al. (2000). Preparing the wound bed: Debridement, bacterial balance, and moisture balance. *Ostomy Wound Manage*, 46, 14-35.

Additional Readings

Ovington, L.G. (2001). Wound care products: How to choose. *Home Healthcare Nurse*, 19, 224-31.
Ovington, L.G. (1998). The well-dressed wound: An overview of dressing types. *Wounds*, 10(Suppl A), 1A-11A.

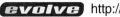

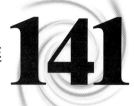
P R O C E D U R E **141**

Vacuum-Assisted Closure™ (V.A.C.)® System for Wounds

P U R P O S E :   To apply subatmospheric (negative) pressure to the wound bed to stimulate granulation and reduce edema, thus enhancing wound healing.

Eleanor R. Fitzpatrick
Mary Beth Flynn Makic

PREREQUISITE NURSING KNOWLEDGE

- Negative-pressure wound therapy, or Vacuum-Assisted Closure™ (V.A.C.®) therapy (V.A.C.® Kinetic Concepts Inc., San Antonio, TX) (Fig. 141-1), is an exclusive system for wound closure that applies subatmospheric (negative) pressure evenly over a wound bed (Fig. 141-2). This mechanical stress creates a noncompressive force on the wound bed that dilates the arterioles, increasing the effectiveness of local circulation and enhancing the proliferation of granulation tissue.[1] The system also enhances lymphatic flow and removal of excessive fluid, decreasing wound edema and bacterial load at the wound site, further aiding wound healing[1] (Fig. 141-3A and B).
- Wound healing is best achieved through adequate cleansing, debridement, and dressing of the wound bed based on patient and wound characteristics.
- Wounds heal by either primary or secondary intention (see Fig. 136-1). Most clean or clean/contaminated surgical wounds heal by primary intention. Suturing each layer of tissue approximates the wound edges. These wounds typically heal quickly and require minimal wound care. Contaminated surgical or traumatic wounds (open wounds) heal by secondary intention.
- Wounds healing by secondary intention granulate from the base of the wound to the skin surfaces; care must be taken to allow for uniform granulation and prevention of open pockets/tunneling.

- Open wounds must be clean and moist to promote effective and efficient wound healing. To that end, open wound care strives to maintain a clean, moist wound bed that allows for effective wound healing under the support of a dressing.
- Openly granulating wounds heal more slowly, must remain moist to enhance tissue granulation, and may be more painful for the patient.
- Open wounds may have excessive wound drainage, requiring application of absorptive dressings, protection of periwound skin, and more frequent dressing changes to facilitate healing.
- The V.A.C.® system is indicated for wounds in which subatmospheric pressure may promote wound healing—for example, chronic, acute, traumatic, subacute, and dehisced wounds, diabetic ulcers, pressure ulcers, flaps, and grafts). The V.A.C.® will draw wound edges together and create a less edematous, clean, vascularized wound bed. The wound may fully heal, or improved adherence of the flap or graft closure can be achieved.
- The V.A.C.® has been approved by the Food and Drug Administration (FDA) for clinical use in the treatment of these wounds. A newer system called the Mini VAC® is portable and battery-powered and can be carried by the patient, allowing for increased mobility. The V.A.C.® device requires an electrical outlet for therapy; however, some units have limited battery reserve. Optimal therapy is achieved by delivering uninterrupted therapy at least 22 out of 24 hours (battery power is maintained).

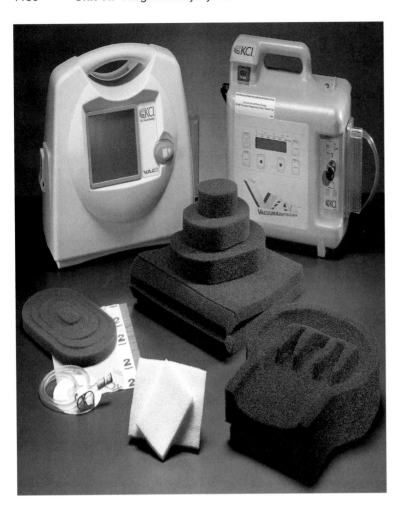

FIGURE 141-1 Components of the Vacuum-Assisted Closure™ System. *(Kinetic Concepts, Inc., San Antonio, TX.)*

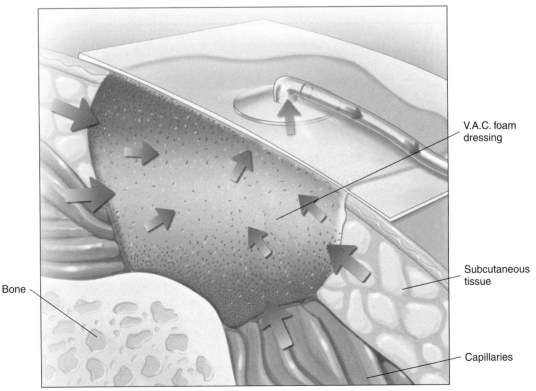

V.A.C. foam dressing

Subcutaneous tissue

Bone

Capillaries

FIGURE 141-2 V.A.C.® Therapy. Fluid, exudate, and debris removed from wound bed. *(Courtesy: Kinetic Concepts, Inc., San Antonio, TX.)*

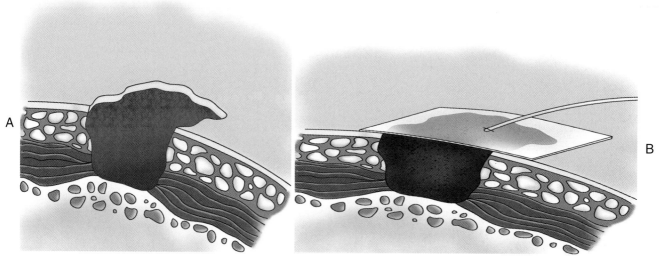

FIGURE 141-3 **A,** Wound defect. **B,** Wound defect with V.A.C.® therapy applied. *(Courtesy: Kinetic Concepts, Inc., San Antonio, TX.)*

- Contraindications to use of the V.A.C.® system include malignancy in the wound margins, untreated osteomyelitis, fistulas to organs or body cavities, necrotic tissue with eschar present, exposed arteries or veins in the wound. Precautions should be used for wounds with active bleeding, difficult wound hemostasis, or patients taking anticoagulants.[25]
- Negative therapy may be applied to the wound by selecting continuous or cycling pressure (intervals of 5 min on/2 min off). After this period the dressing is removed and the wound is cleansed, assessed, and prepared for V.A.C.® therapy to continue if needed.
- V.A.C.® dressings are usually changed every 48 hours.[3,5,7,13] However, infected wound beds may require more frequent dressing changes (every 12 hours); V.A.C.® dressings over grafts may be changed less frequently (every 3-5 days).[3,5,7,13]
- The wound bed should be free of necrotic tissue and debris prior to applying the V.A.C.® In highly exudating wounds, draining from the wound bed may be significant in the first 24-48 hours of therapy, requiring monitoring of urine output and hemodynamic stability. Studies have not suggested fluid replacements have been necessary to ensure hemostasis in highly exudating wounds.[1,13]
- Nutritional requirements for wound healing are great. These needs must be assessed, met, and monitored frequently as fluids and some proteins are removed via V.A.C.® therapy.
- Inflammatory cytokines and protein-degrading enzymes impair wound healing and can be removed with negative-pressure systems such as the V.A.C.®

EQUIPMENT

- Personal protective equipment (gown, goggles)
- Nonsterile and sterile gloves; sterile field
- Sterile water or normal saline (NS) for cleansing
- Liquid skin barrier to protect periwound skin and/or hydrocolloid wafer

- V.A.C.® collection chamber and suction pump (commercially available)
- Sterile foam dressing
- Sterile adhesive drape
- Noncollapsible evacuation tube
- Adhesive drape
- Sterile scissors

Additional equipment to have available, as needed, includes the following:

- Razor

PATIENT AND FAMILY EDUCATION

- Assess patient and family readiness to learn and any factors that may affect learning. It is also important to identify how best the patient learns. ➤*Rationale:* Allows the nurse to develop the most appropriate teaching strategy for each patient.
- Provide information about the V.A.C.® system, the procedure, and the equipment. ➤*Rationale:* May decrease or alleviate anxiety by assisting patient and family to understand the procedure, why it is needed, and the preferred outcomes.
- Explain the procedure and the reason for changing wound dressing. ➤*Rationale:* Decreases patient anxiety and discomfort.
- Discuss patient's role in dressing change procedure and maintenance of V.A.C.® ➤*Rationale:* Elicits patient cooperation; prepares patient for wound management on discharge.

PATIENT ASSESSMENT AND PREPARATION

Patient Assessment

- Fully assess wound to determine its characteristics and appropriateness for the procedure. ➤*Rationale:* Insures that there is no contraindication to use of the V.A.C.®

system. Provides data that can be used for comparison at successive dressing changes.

- Monitor for signs and symptoms of wound infection, including the following:
  - ❖ Erythema at drainage site
  - ❖ Heat
  - ❖ Edema
  - ❖ Pain
  - ❖ Elevated temperature and white blood cell count
  - ❖ Wound drainage becoming cloudy and foul-smelling
  - ❖ Increasing in amount of wound exudate

  ➤*Rationale:* Although negative-pressure wound therapy assists with removal of excessive fluid, thus reducing the presence of bacteria in the wound bed, assessment for signs and symptoms of wound infection is necessary, especially in compromised patients.
- Determine baseline pain assessment of the patient. ➤*Rationale:* Provides data that can be used for comparison with past procedure assessment data. Allows the nurse to plan for pre- and intraprocedure analgesia.
- Determine baseline nutritional status and fluid volume status. ➤*Rationale:* Fluids and protein may be lost during V.A.C.® therapy.
- Assess past medical history, especially related to problems with bleeding, fistula formation, or malignancy. ➤*Rationale:* The use of the V.A.C.® may be contraindicated in these conditions.
- Assess current medications specifically related to anticoagulant use. ➤*Rationale:* Identify possible areas of caution which should be monitored with V.A.C.® use.

- Assess current laboratory values especially coagulation studies and protein levels. ➤*Rationale:* Identifies abnormalities possibly associated with risks or areas to monitor related to V.A.C.® use.

Patient Preparation

- Ensure patient and family understanding of preprocedural teaching. Reinforce teaching points as needed. ➤*Rationale:* Evaluates understanding of previously taught information and provides a conduit for questions.
- Validate presence of patent intravenous access. ➤*Rationale:* Access may be needed for administration of analgesic medications.
- If debridement or other invasive intervention is to be performed in conjunction with the V.A.C.® procedure, ensure that informed consent has been obtained. ➤*Rationale:* Allows patient to make decision with appropriate information and health care providers can document this.
- Position the patient in a manner which will facilitate dressing application and patient comfort. ➤*Rationale:* Prepares patient to undergo procedure.
- Sedate the patient or administer prescribed analgesics if needed. ➤*Rationale:* Improve comfort level and tolerance of the procedure. Decreases patient anxiety and discomfort. Typically pain medication is not required for V.A.C.® therapy; however, if the patient required analgesia for previous dressing therapy, pain medications may be required for V.A.C.® therapy.[1,5]

Procedure for Vacuum-Assisted Closure™ (V.A.C.)® System for Wounds

Steps	Rationale	Special Considerations
1. Wash hands and don gloves.	Reduces possibility of transmission of microorganisms.	
2. Establish a sterile field with all cleansing supplies and materials for appropriately sized V.A.C.® dressing.	The V.A.C.® dressing size should be chosen so that it will fill the entire wound cavity.	
3. Position the patient to facilitate cleansing and dressing application.	Provides for patient comfort and allows for visualization and access to the wound.	
4. Cleanse the wound according to orders (see Procedure 136) and/or institution protocol. *(Level VI: Clinical studies in a variety of patient populations and situations to support recommendations.)*	Exudate and debris are removed prior to dressing application. This process facilitates healing and decreases bacterial burden.[4,21-22]	
5. Physician or advanced practice nurse may debride (see Procedure 137) necrotic tissue or eschar if applicable. *(Level VI: Clinical studies in a variety of patient populations and situations to support recommendations.)*	Healthy, vascularized tissue is reached, and with a clean wound bed there is enhanced granulation tissue development.[4,6,15,21-23]	If extensive debridement is necessary, it may require an operative suite.

Procedure for Vacuum-Assisted Closure™ (V.A.C.)® System for Wounds—*Continued*

Steps	Rationale	Special Considerations
6. Shave hair on the border around the wound (if needed) and thoroughly cleanse skin surrounding wound. *(Level I: Manufacturer's recommendations only.)*	Improves dressing adherence.	
7. Dry and prepare the periwound tissue as appropriate. Skin degreasing/medical cleansing agents may be necessary to apply to periwound tissue. *(Level I: Manufacturer's recommendations only.)*	Moisture from perspiration, oil, or body fluids may cause difficulty in achieving an air-tight seal with V.A.C.® dressing.	
8. Choose V.A.C.® soft foam (white), a hydrophilic (water-attracting) material or the black foam (polyurethane), a hydrophobic (water-repelling) dressing (Table 141-1). *(Level I: Manufacturer's recommendations only.)*	White, polyvinyl alcohol foam is denser with smaller pores, which restricts granulation tissue growth into the foam and may be used in cases in which black foam cannot be tolerated due to pain. Larger pores in black foam are considered to be most effective in stimulating granulation tissue and wound contraction.	The white V.A.C.® dressing holds moisture but also allows exudate to be removed through it. It is nonadherent and can be used in tunnels and shallow undermining due to its higher tensile strength. The black V.A.C.® dressing does not hold moisture and allows exudates to be removed. Its design results in rapid growth of new granulation.
9. Remove gloves. Wash hands. Apply sterile gloves.		
10. Open the V.A.C.® dressing onto sterile, dry surface; inspect it for any defects.	Faulty dressings should be replaced.	
11. Cut the V.A.C.® foam with sterile scissors in a location away from the wound (Fig. 141-4A). *(Level IV: Limited clinical studies to support recommendations.)*	This prevents small particles from the dressing falling into the wound. The dressing should be cut to fit the size and shape of the wound, including tunnels and undermined areas (Fig. 141-4B). Tunneling can result in a cyst or abscess when the main body of a wound heals	Any exposed tendons, nerves, or blood vessels should be protected by moving muscle or fascia over exposed structures or by placing a layer of nonadherent dressing over them.

Procedure continues on the following page

TABLE 141-1 Recommended Guidelines for Foam Use	V.A.C.® Polyurethane (Black Foam)	V.A.C.® Soft Foam	Both	Either
Deep, acute wounds with moderate granulation tissue growth	X			
Deep wounds with extremely rapid growth in granulation tissue			X	
Deep pressure ulcers	X			
Superficial wounds		X		
Shallow chronic ulcers		X		
Postgraft therapy				X
Compromised flaps	X			
Fresh flaps	X			
Tunneling/sinus tracks/undermining		X		
Diabetic ulcers				X
Dry wounds	X			
Deep trauma wounds			X	
Superficial trauma wounds				X

Responsible physician or advanced practice nurse should be consulted for individual patient conditions. Consult device user manual and manufacturer's recommended guidelines before use.
Courtesy Kinetic Concepts, Inc., San Antonio, TX.

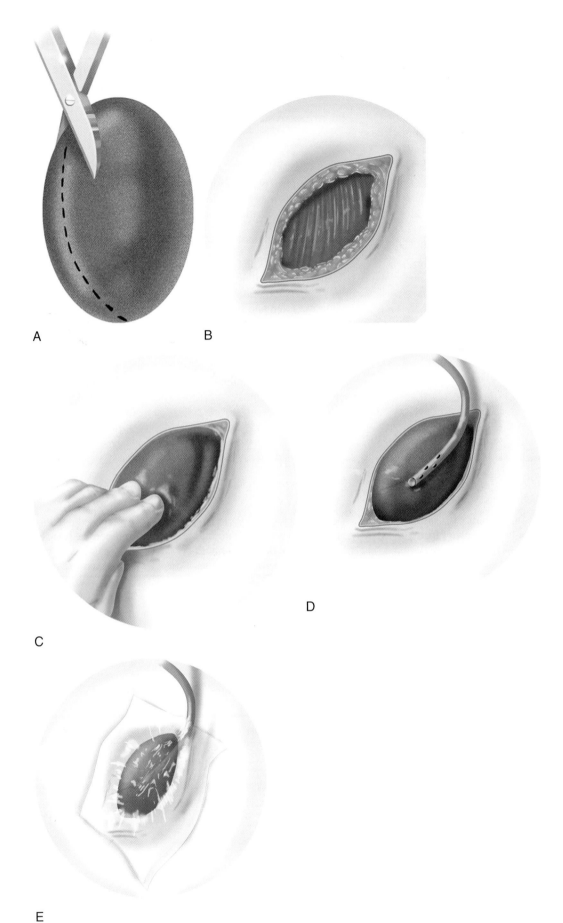

A

B

C

D

E

FIGURE 141-4 **A** and **B,** Cut the V.A.C.® foam to appropriate size to fill the wound defect. **C,** Apply V.A.C.® foam into wound bed. **D,** Apply V.A.C.® tubing to foam in the wound. **E,** Cover foam and 3 to 5 cm of surrounding healthy tissue with transparent dressing drape to ensure an occlusive seal. *(Courtesy Medical Media Department, Thomas Jefferson University Hospital, Philadelphia, PA.)*

Procedure for Vacuum-Assisted Closure™ (V.A.C.)® System for Wounds—*Continued*		
Steps	**Rationale**	**Special Considerations**
	and closes the entrance to the tunnel. Bacterial invasion and impaired healing results from unfilled dead space.[4,24]	
12. Size and trim the dressing drape to cover the foam plus a 3-5 cm border of intact skin. Do not discard excess drape.	Excess drape may be needed later as a patch.	Drape can be placed over prepared skin or the barrier.
13. Gently place the foam into the wound cavity covering the entire wound base and sides as well as areas of tunneling and undermining (Fig. 141-4C). *(Level IV: Limited clinical studies to support recommendations.)*	Capillaries could be compressed if packed too tightly, and pressure on newly formed granulation tissue may prevent or delay healing.[4,24] If periwound skin is fragile, use a skin preparation (Matisol®, No-Sting®) prior to drape application or frame the wound with a skin barrier or hydrocolloid dressing. This affords protection for periwound skin.	More than one dressing may be needed for larger wounds. More than one piece of foam may be used to fill the wound bed. Foam pieces should be in contact but not overlapping each other to allow equalization of negative pressure applied to the wound bed by the suction device.[1,3,5,7,13]
14. Apply tubing to foam in the wound. Tubing can be laid on top of the foam or inside the foam dressing. The tubing should be positioned away from bony prominences (Fig. 141-4D). *(Level I: Manufacturer's recommendations only.)*	This will prevent the development of pressure.	For deeper wounds the tubing should be repositioned regularly to minimize pressure on wound edges. Cushion skin under tubing with excess foam.
15. Cover foam and 3 to 5 cm of surrounding healthy tissue with drape to ensure an occlusive seal (Fig. 141-4E). *(Level IV: Limited clinical studies to support recommendations.)*	The vacuum will not function without an occlusive seal. The drape may also help maintain a moist wound environment.[2]	The drape is vapor-permeable and allows for gas exchange. It also protects the wound from external contamination. Foam will contract into wound bed if seal is obtained. If foam does not contract, reassess outer dressing for possible leaks in the system or dressing seal.[1,3,5,7,13]
16. Lift the tubing and pinch 1 to 3 cm of drape together under the tubing to help hold the tubing away from the skin and pad underneath the tubing.	This will reduce pressure on the skin from the tubing.	
17. Avoid stretching the drape and compressing the foam into the wound with transparent occlusive drape. Simply cover and seal around the foam. *(Level I: Manufacturer's recommendations only.)*	Avoids tension and shearing forces on wound and surrounding tissue. Allows distribution of pressure throughout all wounds with the use of one pump.	More than one wound of similar pathology in close proximity can be managed with one negative-pressure pump. Such wounds can be bridged by placing the V.A.C.® drape on intact skin and a strip of foam from one wound bed to the other. All edges of the foam should be in contact and the tubing placed in a central location.

Procedure continues on the following page

Procedure **for Vacuum-Assisted Closure™ (V.A.C.)® System for Wounds**—*Continued*

Steps	Rationale	Special Considerations
18. Secure tubing with an additional piece of drape or tape (pad underneath tubing) several centimeters away from the dressing. *(Level I: Manufacturer's recommendations only.)*	Prevents pull on the primary dressing area, which can cause leaks.	
19. Use excess drape to patch leaks and secure borders as needed.	Leaks prevent activation of the V.A.C.® system.	
Applying the V.A.C.® Device		
1. Remove canister from the sterile packaging and push it into the V.A.C.® unit until it clicks.	If the canister is not engaged properly, it will not function and an alarm will sound.	
2. Connect the dressing tubing to the canister tubing, making sure both clamps are open.	Closed clamps prevent activation of the negative pressure.	
3. Place the V.A.C.® unit on a level surface or hang from the footboard. *(Level I: Manufacturer's recommendations only.)*	The V.A.C.® unit will alarm and deactivate therapy if the unit is tilted beyond 45 degrees.	
4. Press the green-lit power button.	Activates subatmospheric pressure therapy.	In less than 1 min of operation, the V.A.C.® dressing will collapse unless leaks are present.
5. Adjust the V.A.C.® unit settings based on individual patient's needs. Variable negative-pressure settings can be chosen, as well as a continuous or intermittent mode (Table 141-2). *(Level IV: Limited clinical studies to support recommendations.)*	Continuous vacuum mode removes cellular edema and debris, enhancing perfusion through vessels previously compressed.[1,10,12,14,17,18] Healing inhibitory factors present in this fluid are also removed.[20,26] After edema has been sufficiently withdrawn, the intermittent mode promotes granulation tissue formation and prevents wound dehydration.[1,8,16,17] Negative pressures ranging from 50 to 175 mm Hg can be chosen, depending on the amount of exudate and granulation tissue within the wound and the type of foam used (see Table 141-2).	Premedicate patient if necessary. Application of negative-pressure systems may cause mild discomfort for the patient during initial activation of the V.A.C.® system.[1,11] Blood flow may be inhibited by application of higher negative pressures. If you suspect a leak (small leaks may create a whistling noise), gently press around the tubing to better seal the drape. Excess drape can also be used to patch over leaks. Air leaks most often occur around tubing.
6. Slowly increase negative pressure on suction device to desired setting of 125 mm Hg. *(Level I: Manufacturer's recommendations only.)*	Negative pressure may be initiated at 75 mm Hg and gradually increased to 125 mm Hg. Maintain therapy continuously. Subatmospheric pressure therapy should not be off for more than 2 hr per day. Treatment is discontinued when goals for V.A.C.® therapy are achieved or after 1 to 2 weeks without improvement in the condition of the wound.	Physician or advanced practice nurse will order desired negative-pressure settings. Lower pressure settings may be ordered for special wound beds (meshed grafts); higher pressure settings (125-175 mm Hg) may be ordered for high-effluent wounds.[1,3,5,7,13] V.A.C.® therapy is delivered for 48 hr. After this period the dressing is removed and the wound cleansed, assessed, and prepared for V.A.C.® therapy to

TABLE 141-2	Recommended Guidelines for Treating Wound Types with V.A.C.® System				
Wound Type	Initial Cycle	Subsequent Cycles	Target Pressure for Black Polyurethane Dressing	Target Pressure Polyvinylalcohol Soft Foam	Dressing Change Interval
Acute/traumatic wound	Continuous for first 48 hr	Intermittent (5 min on/2 min off) for rest of therapy	125 mm Hg	125-175 mm Hg	Every 48 hr (every 12 hr with infection)
Surgical wound dehiscence	Continuous for first 48 hr	Intermittent (5 min on/2 min off) for rest of therapy	125 mm Hg	125-175 mm Hg (titrated up for increased drainage)	Every 48 hr (every 12 hr with infection)
Meshed graft	Continuous	Continuous	75-125 mm Hg	125 mm Hg; (titrated up for increased drainage)	None; remove dressing after 4-5 days when using either foam
Pressure ulcer	Continuous for first 48 hr	Intermittent (5 min on/2 min off) for rest of therapy	125 mm Hg	125-175 mm Hg (titrated up for increased drainage)	Every 48 hr (every 12 hr with infection)
Chronic ulcer	Continuous	Continuous	50-125 mm Hg	125-175 mm Hg (titrated up for increased drainage)	Every 48 hr (every 12 hr with infection)
Fresh flap	Continuous	Continuous	125-150 mm Hg	125-175 mm Hg (titrated up for increased drainage)	Every 72 hr (every 12 hr with infection)
Compromised flap	Continuous	Continuous	125 mm Hg	125-175 mm Hg (titrated up for increased drainage)	Every 48 hr (every 12 hr with infection)

Responsible physician or advanced practice nurse should be consulted for individual patient conditions. Consult device user manual and manufacturer's recommended guidelines before use.
Courtesy Kinetic Concepts, Inc., San Antonio, TX.

Procedure for Vacuum-Assisted Closure™ (V.A.C.)® System for Wounds—Continued

Steps	Rationale	Special Considerations
		continue if needed. If infection is present, the dressing change interval should be every 12 to 24 hr. Negative pressure may enhance bacterial clearance from the wound.[9,11,19]
Dressing Removal		
1. To remove the dressing, raise the tubing connector above the level of the pump unit.	Drains fluid from tubing into canister.	
2. Tighten clamps on the dressing tube.	Prevents leakage.	
3. Separate canister tube and dressing tube by disconnecting the connector.	Allows canister to be emptied and/or discarded.	
4. Allow the pump unit to pull the exudate in the canister tubing into the canister; then tighten clamps on the canister tube.	Removes any remaining fluid from the dressing.	
5. Press Therapy button Off.	Deactivates pump.	
6. Gently stretch drape horizontally and slowly pull up from skin. Do not peel. Gently remove.	Decreases patient discomfort and potential for skin and wound trauma.	
7. Discard disposables according to institution policy.	Reduces transmission of microorganisms; universal precautions.	
8. Document procedure in patient record.		

Expected Outcomes

- Wound healing/granulation enhanced by consistent negative-pressure therapy; early signs of contraction of wound margins
- Decreased volume of wound exudate (over time) and absence of foul odor or color
- Enhanced wound healing because of effective wound fluid/edema removal
- Decrease in size of wound with ability for surgical closure with flap/graft or skin graft; complete healing of wound
- Decreased time to satisfactory healing (may decrease hospital length of stay and cost)

Unexpected Outcomes

- Infection
- Bleeding
- Fistula formation
- Disruption of underlying tissue/structures
- Pain
- Misplacement over exposed vessel, ligaments, other structures
- Lack of improvement in wound after 1 to 2 weeks of therapy
- Tissue loss
- Ischemia and necrosis
- Skin erosion or maceration around wound sites, or pressure breakdown at dressing tubing site, or both

Patient Monitoring and Care

Steps	Rationale	Reportable Conditions
		These conditions should be reported if they persist despite nursing interventions.
1. Assess location of wound and placement of V.A.C.® evacuation tube to avoid excessive pressure on surround tissue/structures.	Excessive pressure may result in tissue breakdown at evacuation tube site.	• Tissue breakdown
2. Assess patency of V.A.C.® system.	The V.A.C.® dressing should be collapsed when seal is maintained and negative pressure is being delivered in a consistent manner. Alarms on the device indicate loss of seal; raised foam dressing indicates loss of negative-pressure therapy.	• Loss of seal • Raised foam dressing • Wound drainage suddenly decreasing in amount or stopping
3. Monitor condition of wound bed and periwound skin with dressing changes; observe for signs of wound infection.	Identifies any evidence of wound healing or of any changes or abnormalities indicative of complications.	• Erythema at drainage site • Heat, edema, pain • Elevated temperature and white blood cell count • Cloudy or foul-smelling wound drainage • Increased wound drainage • Excess bleeding • Discolored tissue in wound bed • Macerated periwound skin • New tunneling or undermining
4. Change the dressing every 48 hr. If infection is present, increase the frequency of dressing change to every 12 to 24 hr. *(Level II: Theory-based, no research data to support recommendations: recommendations from expert consensus group may exist.)*	Removes infectious material from a healing wound bed. If dressing adheres to the wound base, consider imposing a single layer of nonadherent porous material (e.g. wide-meshed Vaseline-impregnated gauze) between the dressing and the wound when reapplying the dressing. The nonadherent material must have wide enough pores to allow unrestricted passage of air and fluid. Because tissue growth into the V.A.C.® dressing may cause adherence, also consider more frequent dressing changes.	• Signs or symptoms of infection (erythema, heat, discolored or purulent drainage, fever)

Patient Monitoring and Care—*Continued*

Steps	Rationale	Reportable Conditions
	If previous dressings were difficult to remove, make sure the dressing tubing is unclamped; introduce 10 to 30 ml of NS solution into the tubing to soak underneath the foam for 15 to 30 min. NS can be injected directly into the foam while low vacuum (50 mm Hg) is applied to the dressing. Clamp the tube when the NS starts to flow into the dressing tube. Wait 15 to 30 min; then gently remove dressing. If the patient experiences pain during dressing change, 1% lidocaine solution may be ordered by the physician or advanced practice nurse. This can be introduced down the tubing or injected into the foam with the pump turned on at a lower pressure (50 mm Hg). After instilling the lidocaine, clamp the tube and wait 15 to 20 min before gently removing the dressing.	
5. Monitor the mode (continuous or intermittent) and level of suction (50-175 mm Hg). *(Level IV: Limited clinical studies to support recommendations.)*	Removal of edema and debris alleviates compressive forces, thus improving perfusion. Suctioning fluid from within the wound may remove factors that inhibit healing.[25] Negative-pressure wound therapy decreases the bacterial load of deliberately infected wounds.[1] Application and release of force on tissue stimulates cell proliferation and protein synthesis. Mechanical stretch on the tissue by the negative pressure draws the wound toward the center closing the defect.[16] Once edema of the wound has resolved (typically after 48 hr of continuous therapy) the intermittent mode allows a more aggressive stimulus for granulation tissue formation, possibly due to rhythmic perfusion or increased cell mitosis stimulated by a rest and stimulation cycle.[1,8,17]	• Patient discomfort • Excess granulation tissue overgrowth into the dressing when removed • Continued edema within wound bed
6. Maintain an air tight seal. *(Level I: Manufacturer's recommendation only.)*	Loss of an air-tight seal can result in a decreased amount of drainage removal and in desiccation of the wound.	
7. Use sterile technique with new dressing application.	Prevents bacterial contamination of system.	
8. Label dressing with date and time of application.	Identifies when system should be changed.	
9. Keep canister position level.	Prevents malfunction of suction apparatus and an inoperative status.	

Procedure continues on the following page

Patient Monitoring and Care—*Continued*

Steps	Rationale	Reportable Conditions
10. The V.A.C.® canister should be changed when full (unit will alarm) or at least weekly. Label with date and time of change.	Controls odor.	• Wound drainage becoming foul-smelling and cloudy
11. Monitor amount of wound drainage. *(Level II: Theory-based; no research data to support recommendations: recommendations from expert consensus group may exist.)*	If a wound produces excessive fluid, the patient may experience a fluid imbalance, requiring intravenous or oral fluid replacements. Excess drainage may also result in some protein loss. Nutritional consult to replace protein loss from wound exudates may be indicated.	• Increasing amounts of drainage • Tachycardia • Hypotension • Oliguria • Decreasing serum protein levels
12. Encourage patient hygiene, shower, or bath during V.A.C.® dressing changes.		

Documentation

Documentation should include the following:

- Patient and family education
- Patient tolerance of the procedure
- Condition of the wound bed and periwound skin description
- Characteristics of wound drainage
- Degree of suction (mm Hg) and continuous or intermittent mode
- Nursing interventions
- Premedication given and patient's response to the pain medication

- Wound debridement procedure (if applicable), wound cleansing procedure completed, dated, and timed
- Size of the wound measured by length, width, and depth (consider obtaining a photograph of the wound, depending on institution policy)
- Size and type of V.A.C.® foam dressing applied and total number placed in the wound
- Unexpected outcomes, reportable conditions

References

1. Argenta, L.C., and Morykwas, M.J. (1997). Vacuum-assisted closure: A new method for wound control and treatment: clinical experience. *Ann Plastic Surg,* 38, 563-76.
2. Banwell, P.E. (1999). Topical negative pressure therapy in wound care. *J Wound Care,* 8, 79-84.
3. Bates-Jensen, B.M., et al. (2001). Management of the wound environment with advanced therapies. In: Sussman, C., and Bates-Jensen, B.M., eds. *Wound Care.* 2nd ed. Gaithersburg, MD: Aspen Publication, 272-92.
4. Bergstrom, N., et al. (1994). Treatment of pressure ulcers. *Clinical Practice Guideline, No. 15.* Rockville, MD: U.S. Department of Health and Human Services, Public Health Service, Agency for Healthcare Policy and Research, AHCPR Publication No. 95-0652.
5. Chua-Patel, C.T., et al. (2000). Vacuum-assisted wound closure. *Am J Nurs,* 100, 45-8.
6. d'Udekem, Y., et al. (1998). Radical debridement and omental transposition for post-sternotomy mediastinitis. *Cardiovasc Surg,* 6, 415-8.
7. Evans, D., and Land, L. (2001). Topical negative pressure for treating chronic wounds. *The Cochrane Database of Systematic Reviews,* 4:CD001898.
8. Fabian, T.S., et al. (2000). The evaluation of subatmospheric pressure and hyperbaric oxygen in ischemic, full-thickness wound healing. *Am Surg,* 66, 1136-43.
9. Ford, C.N., et al. (2001). Interim analysis of a prospective, randomized trial of a vacuum-assisted closure versus the healthpoint system in the management of pressure ulcers. *Ann Plast Surg,* 49, 55-61.
10. Genecov, D.G., et al. (1998). A controlled subatmospheric pressure dressing increases the rate of skin graft donor site re-epithelialization. *Ann Plast Surg,* 40, 219-25.
11. Hersh, R.E., et al. (2001). The vacuum-assisted closure device as a bridge to sternal closure. *Ann Plast Surg,* 46, 250-4.
12. Joseph, E., et al. (2000). A prospective randomized trial of vacuum-assisted closure versus standard therapy of chronic, nonhealing wounds. *Wounds,* 12, 60-7.
13. Kirby, J.P., et al. (2002). Novel uses of a negative pressure wound care system. *J Trauma,* 53, 117-21.
14. McCallon, S.K., et al. (2000). The effectiveness of vacuum-assisted closure vs. saline moistened gauze in the healing of post-operative diabetic foot wounds. *Ostomy/Wound Manage,* 46, 28-35.
15. Meara, J.G., et al. (1999). Vacuum-assisted closure in the treatment of degloving injuries. *Ann Plast Surg,* 42, 589-94.
16. Morykwas, M.J., and Argenta, L.C. (1997). Nonsurgical modalities to enhance healing and care of soft tissue wounds. *J South Ortho Assoc,* 6, 279-88.
17. Morykwas, M.J., et al. (1997). Vacuum-assisted closure: a new method for wound control and treatment: Animal studies and basic foundation. *Ann Plast Surg,* 38, 553-62.
18. Mullner, T., et al. (1997). The use of negative pressure to promote the healing of tissue defects: A clinical trial using the vacuum seal technique. *Br J Plast Surg,* 50, 194-9.

19. Obdeijn, M.C., et al. (1999). Vacuum-assisted closure in the treatment of poststernotomy mediastinitis, *Ann Thorac Surg,* 68, 2358-60.
20. Philbeck, T.E., et al. (1999). The clinical and cost effectiveness of externally applied negative pressure wound therapy in the treatment of wounds in home healthcare Medicare patients. *Ostomy/Wound Manage,* 45, 41-50.
21. Rodeheaver, G., et al. (1994). Wound healing and wound management: Focus on debridement. *Adv Wound Care,* 7, 22-4, 26-9, 32-6.
22. Sibbald, R.G., et al. (2000). Preparing the wound bed-debridement, bacterial balance and moisture balance. *Ostomy/Wound Manage,* 46, 14-35.
23. Steed, D.L., et al. (1996). Effect of extensive debridement and treatment on the healing of diabetic foot ulcers. Diabetic Ulcer Study Group. *J Am Coll Surg,* 183, 61-4.
24. Stotts, N. (1997). Co-factors in impaired wound healing. In: Krasner, D., and Kane, D., eds. *Chronic Wound Care: A Clinical Source Book for Healthcare Professionals.* 2nd ed. Wayne, PA: Health Management Publications, Inc.
25. Wysocki, A.B. (1996). Wound fluids and the pathogenesis of chronic wounds. *J WOCN,* 23, 283-90.
26. *www.kci1.com/clinicalevidence/indexVAC.* Accessed May 17, 2004.

Additional Readings

Barker, D.E., et al. (2000). Vacuum pack technique of temporary abdominal closure: A 7-year experience with 112 patients. *J Trauma,* 48, 201-7.

Casey, G. (2003). Nutritional support in wound healing. *Nurs Stand,* 17, 55-6, 58.
Dolynchuk, K. (2000). Best practices for the prevention and treatment of pressure ulcers. *Ostomy/Wound Manage,* 46, 38-52.
Erdman, D., et al. (2001). Abdominal wall defect and entero-cutaneous fistula treatment with the vacuum-assisted (V.A.C.) system. *Plast Reconstr Surg,* 108, 2066-8.
Falanga, V., ed. (2000). *Text Atlas of Wound Management.* London: Martin Dunitz Ltd.
Falanga, V., ed. (2001). *Cutaneous Wound Healing.* London: Martin Dunitz Ltd.
Irion, G. (2002). *Comprehensive Wound Management.* Thorofare, NJ: Slack Incorporated.
Kinetic Concepts, Inc. (2001). *V.A.C. Physician and Caregiver Reference Manual.* San Antonio: Kinetic Concepts, Inc.
Kloth, L.C., and McCulloch, J.M., eds. (2002). *Wound Healing: Alternatives in Management.* 3rd ed. Philadelphia: F.A. Davis Company.
Krasner, D.L., et al. (1999). Nursing management of chronic wounds. *Nurs Clin N Am,* 34, 933-949.
Krasner, D.L. (2002). Managing wound pain in patients with vacuum-assisted closure devices. *Ostomy/Wound Manage,* 48, 38-43.
Mendez-Eastman, S. (2001). Guidelines for using negative pressure wound therapy. *Adv Skin & Wound Care,* 14, 314-22.
Mendez-Eastman, S. (1999). Use of hyperbaric oxygen and negative pressure therapy in the multidisciplinary care of a patient with nonhealing wounds. *J Wound Ostomy Continence Nurs,* 26, 67-76.

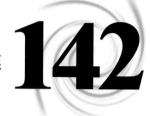
UNIT **VIII**
Nutrition

PROCEDURE **142**

Enteral Nutrition

P U R P O S E : Enteral tube nutrition is provided to achieve nutrition requirements, recommended daily allowance of vitamins and minerals, and administration of free water in patients who cannot consume nutrients orally. The use of enteral feedings also maintains gastrointestinal (GI) function and integrity.

Deborah C. Stamps

PREREQUISITE NURSING KNOWLEDGE

- The first principle in providing nutrition for critically ill patients is to use the GI tract whenever possible. The absence of bowel sounds and stool or flatus does not preclude the use of the GI tract for feeding, particularly when feedings are administered distal to the pylorus. Increasing abdominal distention or severe GI disease may be reasons to administer parenteral nutrition (see Procedure 143).
- The goals of nutrition support include the provision of nutritional support consistent with the patient's available route of administration, nutritional status, and medical condition. They also include the prevention or treatment of macro- and micronutrient deficiencies, prevention of complications related to the technique of nutrition delivery, the improvement of patient outcomes, and enhanced recovery from illness.
- Use of the algorithm in Fig. 142-1 can assist the nutritional support team in choosing the appropriate type of nutrition to best meet the patient's needs.
- Prior to administering enteral tube feedings, an individualized nutrition plan should be developed in collaboration with the multidisciplinary team. This would include a review of past medical history, current clinical status, laboratory values, and calculation of calorie and protein needs.
- The nurse should understand insertion, flushing, and confirmation of feeding tube placement (see Procedure 145).

EQUIPMENT

- Enteral feeding bag and administration set
- One 60-ml irrigation tip syringe
- One clean cup
- Prescribed enteral formula
- One enteral feeding pump
- 1-in roll of paper tape

PATIENT AND FAMILY EDUCATION

- Explain procedure for enteral nutrition to both patient and family. ➤➤*Rationale:* Decreases anxiety and promotes understanding of treatment regimen and possible length of therapy.
- If possible, teach patient to report signs and symptoms of nausea, abdominal cramping, and abdominal fullness. ➤➤*Rationale:* These symptoms indicate a potential intolerance to rate of infusion or type of formula and decrease the patient's comfort.
- Discuss patient's need for long-term enteral nutritional support. ➤➤*Rationale:* Allows for planning for long-term access, if needed.

PATIENT ASSESSMENT AND PREPARATION

Patient Assessment
- Fluid balance assessment includes the following:
  ❖ Patient's baseline weight
  ❖ Edema (pedal, sacral, generalized)
  ❖ Breath sounds
  ❖ Jugular venous distention
  ❖ Intake and output
  ➤➤*Rationale:* Baseline weight and fluid balance assessment will promote evidence of the effectiveness of enteral nutrition support after it has begun.

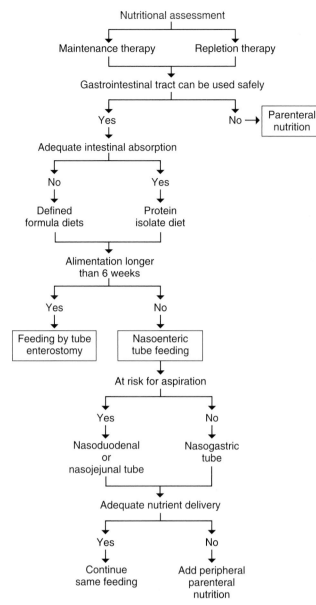

FIGURE 142-1 Patient selection for enteral feeding. *(From Rolandelli, M.D., et al. [2004]. Clinical Nutrition: Enteral and Tube Feeding. 4th ed. Philadelphia: W.B. Saunders.)*

- Protein-calorie malnutrition assessment includes the following:
  ❖ Weight loss
  ❖ Muscle atrophy
  ❖ Edema
  ❖ Weakness or lethargy
  ❖ Failure to wean from ventilator support
  ➥*Rationale:* Physical signs and symptoms provide an indication of the severity of malnutrition and baseline for later evaluation.
- Medical history for presence of chronic cardiac, hepatic, renal, or pulmonary disease. ➥*Rationale:* Chronic illness may dictate restrictions in volume of fluid or type of enteral formula administered.
- Serum proteins indicative of nutritional deficits include the following:
  ❖ Albumin less than 3.5 g/dl

- ❖ Total protein less than 7.0 mg/dl
- ❖ Serum transferrin less than 150 g/dl
- ❖ Prealbumin less than 200 g/dl
  ➥*Rationale:* Depressed levels indicate a patient with nutritional deficits or liver dysfunction.
- Past and current medication profile for use of catabolic steroids (e.g., prednisone, dexamethasone). ➥*Rationale:* Catabolic steroids increase protein requirements.
- Medications. ➥*Rationale:* Note potential food and drug interactions and collaborate with the physician, advanced practice nurse, or pharmacist, as needed.
- GI tract function assessment includes the following:
  ❖ Presence of bowel sounds
  ❖ Abdomen soft and nondistended
  ❖ Flatus or stool present
  ➥*Rationale:* Enteral feeding tolerance is improved when administered via a functioning GI tract.
- Baseline blood glucose, sodium, potassium, calcium, phosphate, magnesium, renal function, and liver function studies (Table 142-1). ➥*Rationale:* Baseline laboratory values provide data for decision making about the type and amount of enteral feedings, as well as the need for any supplementation or deletion of electrolytes.
- Skin integrity. ➥*Rationale:* Pressure wounds or large wounds require increased protein needs.

Patient Preparation

- Ensure that patient understands preprocedural teaching. Answer questions as they arise and reinforce information as needed. ➥*Rationale:* Evaluates and reinforces understanding of previously taught information.
- Assist the patient to a semi-Fowler's or high Fowler's position. The head of the bed should be at least 30-45 degrees during infusion of enteral feedings (in patients requiring prepyloric feedings). ➥*Rationale:* Decreases the risk for aspiration of gastric contents. Patients who must remain supine (e.g., unstable neck fracture) must be monitored closely for aspiration during infusion of enteral feedings.
- Aspirate gastric or intestinal contents using a 60-ml syringe and assess pH. Be sure to consider the impact of certain drugs on pH (e.g., H_2 blockers) (see Procedure 111). ➥*Rationale:* Verifies correct placement of feeding tube.

TABLE 142-1	Suggested Laboratory Monitoring	
Baseline Tests	**Until on Stable Rate**	**When on Goal***
Body weight	Twice weekly	Weekly
Fluid intake/output	Daily	Daily
Glucose		
Nondiabetic	Daily	2-3 times/wk
Diabetic	Daily	Daily
Electrolytes	Daily	1-3 times/wk
Renal function	Daily	1-3 times/wk
Phosphorus	2-3 times/wk	Weekly
Liver function	1-2 times/wk	Weekly
Calcium/magnesium	2-3 times/wk	Weekly
Prealbumin	2 times/wk	Weekly
Albumin	Weekly	Monthly

*In the hospitalized patient. Patients at home or at long-term care facilities may require less frequent monitoring.
From Gottschlich, M.M., ed. (2001). *The Science and Practice of Nutrition Support: A Case-Based Core Curriculum.* Silver Spring, MD: ASPEN.

Procedure for Enteral Nutrition

Steps	Rationale	Special Considerations
1. Assemble all equipment and supplies at the bedside.	This ensures that enteral feedings will be initiated quickly and efficiently.	
2. Wash hands and don gloves. *(Level IV: Limited clinical studies to support recommendations.)*	Decreases the transmission of microorganisms; standard precautions.[2,10]	
3. Check placement of feeding tube (see Procedure 145).	Prevents delivery of feeding tube into the lungs.[2]	
4. Verify order for enteral feedings.	Prescriber's order should include type of formula, volume to be delivered, and rate or length of infusion. Decreases the risk for error.[10]	
5. Elevate the head of the bed at least 30-45 degrees for patients receiving prepyloric feedings. *(Level IV: Limited clinical studies to support recommendations.)*	Decrease risk for aspiration of gastric contents during administration of feeding.[2,3,5,7]	If patient must be supine (e.g., because of a neck fracture), extreme caution must be exercised to monitor for aspiration.
6. For continuous feeding: close the clamp on the enteral feeding bag and pour up to 8 hours' worth of formula into the bag; or hang prepackaged closed system container of prescribed formula. For intermittent feeding: hang 100 to 480 ml of formula in the bag at a time. *(Level IV: Limited clinical studies to support recommendations.)*	Hang no more than 8 hours' worth of feeding to prevent bacterial overgrowth in formula. With the high-carbohydrate concentration and frequent exposure of formula to multiple personnel, bacterial growth can occur rapidly, leading to gastritis, nausea, vomiting, and diarrhea. Limit hang time or use a closed delivery system to reduce risk for contamination.[1,7,10]	
7. Hang bag on IV pole and prime tubing. For continuous enteral feeding, load administration set into enteral feeding pump. *(Level IV: Limited clinical studies to support recommendations.)*	Priming tubing will purge the system of air.[2,6,7,9-10]	
8. Evaluate for residual tube feeding every 4 hours. Attach a 60-ml syringe to the feeding tube. A. Nasogastric, nasoenteric, or gastrostomy tube: aspirate intestinal contents if greater than 60 ml, place returns in a clean cup at the bedside.	Determines patient's tolerance to feeding. If gastric residual is more than 200 ml with continuous feedings or greater than 50% of bolus volume for intermittent feedings, the feeding should be delayed 1 hour.[5,11]	Gastric residual may be elevated because of formula intolerance, delayed gastric emptying, sepsis, or GI disease. Residual is also dependent on infusion rate and gastric emptying time. Notify the physician or nurse practitioner if the residual is greater than 150 ml after 2 hours.
B. Jejunostomy tube: unable to assess intestinal residual.	If unable to withdraw residual from small-bore feeding tube, some manufacturers recommend first instilling 30 to 60 ml of air through the tube. This helps to move the tube away from the gastric or intestinal wall and clear it of any residual water, formula, or medications.[1,7]	

Procedure for Enteral Nutrition—*Continued*

Steps	Rationale	Special Considerations
9. After determining the volume of residual, complete guaiac test. If guaiac is negative, return up to 125 ml of gastric aspirate to stomach using the same syringe. *(Level V: Clinical studies in more than one patient population and situation.)*	If guaiac is positive, do not reinstill contents. Gastric aspirate contains enzymes and secretions essential for digestion of the nutrients administered. Returning more than 150 ml of gastric aspirate may overfill the stomach when enteral feeding is started.[1,2,6,9,10,12,13]	
10. Flush feeding tube with 30 to 50 ml of water. *(Level V: Clinical studies in more than one patient population and situation.)*	Prevents clogging of tube and provides additional free water to patient.[1,2,9,10]	Patients on fluid restrictions (e.g., renal failure, congestive heart failure) should have 10 to 20 ml of flush to clean the tube.
11. Connect feeding bag administration set to distal end of feeding tube with safety tape connection. *(Level II: Theory-based, no research data to support recommendations: recommendations from expert consensus group may exist.)*	Decreases risk for accidental disconnection.	
12. Remove gloves and wash hands.	Decreases the transmission of microorganisms; standard precautions.	
13. Begin infusion. A. Feeding pump: set prescribed infusion flow rate for continuous feeding; begin infusion via pump. B. Gravity feeding: adjust roller clamp to infuse formula via gravity over 30 to 60 minutes for intermittent feeding. C. Syringe method: Remove the plunger from a 60-ml syringe. Pour the enteral formula to be administered slowly, trying not to introduce air into the GI system. Allow formula to flow in by gravity. *(Level IV: Limited clinical studies to support recommendations.)*	Initiates administration of feeding.[1,2,9,10]	For intermittent feeding, infuse 100 to 480 ml of formula every 4 to 6 hours (depending on total volume prescribed).
14. Label enteral feeding bag and administration set with date and time hung and type and amount of formula. Change bag and administration set every 24 hours. *(Level IV: Limited clinical studies to support recommendations.)*	Changing enteral administration set every 24 hours prevents bacterial overgrowth in set.[1,2,6,9,12,13]	
15. Administer water boluses as prescribed. *(Level IV: Limited clinical studies to support recommendations.)*	Enteral formulas do not contain sufficient water to meet some patient's needs. High-osmolality formulas could lead to dehydration.[1,2,6,9,12,13]	Adults require 25 to 35 ml/kg of water each day (i.e., for a 70-kg patient receiving 2000 ml of an isotonic formula, 600 ml of additional water will need to be

Procedure continues on the following page

Procedure for Enteral Nutrition—*Continued*

Steps	Rationale	Special Considerations
		administered). Water boluses can be given with a syringe into feeding tube in 100-ml increments every 4 hours. The formula also could be diluted with necessary water and the infusion rate increased. The greater the formula's osmolarity, the less free water in the formula.
16. Remove gloves and wash hands.	Decreases the transmission of microorganisms; standard precautions.	
17. Medication administration: prior to administration of medications via feeding tube, determine drug-nutrient incompatibilities (Table 142-2). *(Level IV: Limited clinical studies to support recommendations.)*	Medications and enteral formulas may interact, reducing the effectiveness of the medication or causing enteral feeding side effects.[1,4,6,8,12]	
18. To administer medications: stop feeding infusion. Flush feeding tube with 20 to 30 ml of water. Liquid medications are preferred for administration via feeding tube. If tablets need to be crushed, do so with the use of a commercial tablet crusher. Administer crushed tablets or liquid medications. Flush with 20 to 30 ml of water. Resume feeding. *(Level IV: Limited clinical studies to support recommendations.)*	Prevents clogging of tube and decreases GI upset.[1,6,8]	

Declogging the Tube

1. Attach a 60-ml syringe to the end of the enteral tube and aspirate as much fluid as possible.	The key to maintaining a patent feeding tube is to flush frequently with water.	
2. Fill the syringe with 5 ml of warm water. Instill using manual pressure for 1 minute; use a back-and-forth motion with the plunger.		

TABLE 142-2	Drug and Nutrient Interactions*	
Drug	**Interaction**	**Nursing Intervention**
Phenytoin[4,8]	Enteral feedings affect the absorption of phenytoin.	Phenytoin suspension is recommended. Shake the suspension well before measuring the dose from the bottle. Stop the tube feeding for 1 hour before and 2 hours after each dose. The rate of feeding administration may need to be adjusted to accommodate these changes and still meet the nutrition goals.
Warfarin[3]	Enteral feedings containing vitamin K may inhibit anticoagulation, decreasing the effectiveness of warfarin therapy.	Select feedings with minimal or no vitamin K. If an enteral feeding with vitamin K is being used in a patient on warfarin therapy, close monitoring of the INR should be done if changes are made to the feeding formula, feeding rate, or warfarin dose.
Ciprofloxacin[3,15]	Enteral feeding formulas will decrease ciprofloxacin absorption, resulting in treatment failure.	Alternate medication delivery times with intermittent feeding doses. Obtain order from physician or advanced practice nurse to change from enteral route of administration to parenteral route, if possible.

*The three medications most commonly associated with drug and nutrient interactions are phenytoin, warfarin, and ciprofloxacin.
INR, International Normalized Ratio.

Procedure for Enteral Nutrition—*Continued*

Steps	Rationale	Special Considerations
3. Clamp the tube for 5 to 15 minutes.		
4. Try to aspirate or flush the tube.		
5. If tube remains clogged, use the following solution: 1 crushed Viokase tablet or 1 teaspoon Viokase powder mixed with 1 tablet baking soda or ½ teaspoon of baking soda (NaHCO$_3$) in 5 ml of water.		Papin, combinations of activated pancreatic enzymes (Viokase) and sodium bicarbonate mixed with water,[1,14] may also be used.

Expected Outcomes

- Maintenance of baseline weight or weight gain of 0.5 to 1 pound every week
- Maintenance or elevation of serum visceral proteins, improved wound healing, maintenance of muscle mass, and positive nitrogen balance
- Fluid balance stable
- Patent feeding tube

Unexpected Outcomes

- Intolerance of enteral feeding formula
- Aspiration
- Dehydration
- Hyperosmolar hyperglycemic nonketotic dehydration or coma
- Persistent elevated glucose level
- Diarrhea
- Drug/nutrient interactions

Patient Monitoring and Care

Steps	Rationale	Reportable Conditions
		These conditions should be reported if they persist despite nursing interventions.
1. Monitor serum glucose levels daily (commonly by fingerstick).	High carbohydrate concentration of formula may exceed endogenous insulin production.	- Glucose higher than 200 mg/dl
2. Weigh patient daily; compare with baseline weight. Document trends of weight gain or loss.	Evaluates patient's response to enteral feeding. Additionally, dehydration can occur as a result of hyperosmolar formulas, patient fluid losses, and inadequate water intake. Overhydration can occur in a patient with hepatic, cardiac, and renal failure. Fluid needs increase when a patient has an elevated temperature.	- Weight gain or loss - Poor skin turgor - Dry mucous membrane - Hypernatremia - Oliguria - Elevated blood urea nitrogen levels
3. Monitor intake and output every shift. Quantify diarrheal stool as output. Observe for a change in urine output.	Diarrhea can occur as a result of the use of hyperosmolar enteral formulas, lactose intolerance, prolonged use of antibiotics, bacterial contamination of formulas, or severe hypoalbuminemia (less than 2 mg/dl).	- Intake greater than output for more than 24 hours - More than three loose or liquid stools in 24 hours
4. If persistent diarrhea occurs, send a stool culture to rule out *Clostridium difficile* and other pathogens.	*C. difficile* can be a cause of diarrhea.	

Procedure continues on the following page

Patient Monitoring and Care—*Continued*

Steps	Rationale	Reportable Conditions
5. Assess patient's medications for A. Potential cause or relationship to persistent diarrhea B. Drug and nutrient interactions	Osmolarity of medications may cause diarrhea. Antibiotics cause bacterial overgrowth in GI tract, resulting in diarrhea. Elixir forms of medications may contain large amounts of sorbitol. Actions of medications alter GI tolerance of enteral feedings and may necessitate a change in administration regimen.	
6. Administer antidiarrheal medications as indicated (if *C. difficile* is negative).	Narcotic antidiarrheal medications are an effective and appropriate treatment for many patients. Control of diarrhea prevents dehydration and improves absorption of nutrients. Banana flakes have been shown to be a successful natural way to firm up stool consistency.[6]	• More than three loose or liquid stools in 24 hours
7. Auscultate bowel sounds every 8 hours to assess for GI mobility.	GI function will affect patient's tolerance to enteral feedings.	• Decreased or absent bowel sounds
8. Aspirate intestinal residuals before every feeding or at least every 8 hours.	Residuals greater than 200 ml indicate decreased gastric mobility or emptying. Continued feeds with high residuals increase the risk for vomiting and aspiration. Residuals may be increased because of intolerance to enteral formulas, indicating a need for reevaluation of the formula.[1,5]	• Residual greater than 125 ml for more than 2 hours
9. Hold enteral feeding for 30 to 60 minutes before patient requires supine position (e.g., transport, procedures).	Decreases the risk for aspiration.	
10. Administer mouth care every 2 hours, including brushing teeth or dentures at least daily. Moisten mouth with water-soaked sponge or gauze. Apply petroleum-based ointment to lips.	Decreases bacterial flora in the oral cavity, therefore reducing the risk for aspiration. Prevents drying and cracking of oral mucosa.	
11. Assess patency of feeding tube.	Feeding tubes that are not patent prevent the administration of nutrients, medications, and water.	• Inability to aspirate or flush feeding tube
12. Monitor laboratory values (see Table 142-1).	Baseline and ongoing laboratory values provide data for decision making about the type and amount of enteral feedings, as well as the need for any supplementation of electrolytes.	• Hyper- or hypoglycemia • Hyper- or hyponatremia • Hyper- or hypokalemia • Hyper- or hypocalcemia • Hyper- or hypophosphatemia • Hyper- or hypomagnesemia • Abnormal renal function or liver function studies

Documentation

Documentation should include the following:

- Patient and family teaching
- GI assessment
- Fluid balance (daily weight, intake and output, number of stools)
- Date and time enteral feeding was initiated
- Strength and type of enteral feeding
- Volumes of residuals
- Infusion rate

- Tolerance to feedings
- Total volume delivered
- Condition of oral cavity and mouth care completed
- Laboratory values
- Unexpected outcomes
- Nursing interventions

References

1. ASPEN Board of Directors. (2002). Guidelines for the use of parenteral and enteral in adult and pediatric patients. *Nutr Clin Pract,* 26, 1SA-44SA.
2. Bowers, S. (1996). Tubes: A nurse's guide to enteral feeding devices. *Medsurg Nurs,* 5, 313-24.
3. Davis, A.E., et al. (1995). Preventing feeding-associated aspiration. *Medsurg Nurs,* 4, 111-9.
4. Doak, K.K., et al. (1998). Bioavailability of phenytoin acid and phenytoin sodium with enteral feedings. *Pharmacotherapy,* 18, 637-45.
5. Edwards, S.J., and Metheny, N.A. (2000). Measurement of gastric residual volume: State of the science. *Medsurg Nurs,* 9, 125-8.
6. Emery, E.A., et al. (1997). Banana flakes control diarrhea in enterally fed patients. *Nutr Clin Prac,* 12, 72-5.
7. Fellows, L.S., et al. (2000). Evidence-based practice for enteral feedings: Aspiration prevention strategies, bedside detection, and practice change. *Medsurg Nurs,* 9, 27-31.
8. Gilbar, P.J. (1999). A guide to enteral drug administration in palliative care. *J Pain & Symptom Manage,* 17, 197-207.
9. Goff, K.L. (1997). The nuts and bolts of enteral infusion pumps. *Medsurg Nurs,* 6, 9-15.
10. Guenter, P., Jones, S., and Ericson, M. (1997). Enteral nutrition therapy. *Nurs Clin North Am,* 32, 651-67.
11. Ideno, K.T. (1996). Enteral nutrition formulas: An overview. *Medsurg Nurs,* 5, 264-8.
12. Lord, L.M. (1997). Enteral access devices. *Nurs Clin North Am,* 32, 685-703.
13. Lord, L.M., and Lipp, J.S. (1996). Adult tube feeding formulas. *Medsurg Nurs,* 5, 407-19.
14. Marcuard, P., and Stegall, K.S. (1990). Unclogging feeding tubes with pancreatic enzyme. *J Parenteral & Enteral Nutrition,* 2, 198-200.
15. Nyffeler, M.S. (1999). Ciprofloxacin use in the enterally fed patient. *Nutr Clin Prac,* 14, 73-7.

Additional Readings

Bellini, L.M. (2002). Fundamentals of nutritional support in the critically ill. *Up to Date.* Available at: www.uptodate.com.

Guenter, P., and Silkraski, M. (2001). *Tube Feeding: Practical Guidelines and Nursing Protocols.* Silver Springs, MD: Aspen Publishers.

Marian, M.J., and Allen, P. (1998). Nutrition support in long-term acute care and subacute care facilities. *AACN Clinical Issues: Adv Pract Acute & Crit Care,* 9, 427-40.

Metheny, N., et al. (1998). Testing tube placement: Auscultation vs. pH method. *Am J Nurs,* 98, 37-42.

Penrod, L.E., Allen, J.B., and Cabacungan, L.R. (2001). Warfarin resistance and enteral feedings: 2 case reports and a supporting in vitro study. *Arch Phys Med Rehabil,* 82, 1270-3.

Shikora, S.A., Martindale, R.G., and Schwaitzberg, S.D. (2002). *Nutritional Considerations in the Intensive Care Unit.* Dubuque, IA: Kendall-Hunt Publishing.

PROCEDURE **143**

Parenteral Nutrition

PURPOSE: Parenteral nutrition (PN) is an important adjunctive therapy that provides macro- and micronutrients to patients who are unable to be adequately nourished via their gastrointestinal (GI) tracts.

Deborah C. Stamps

PREREQUISITE NURSING KNOWLEDGE

- Principles of fluid and electrolyte balance should be understood.
- The goals of nutritional support include the provision of nutritional support consistent with the patient's available route of administration, nutritional status, and medical condition. They also include the prevention or treatment of macro- and micronutrient deficiencies, prevention of complications related to the technique of nutrition delivery, the improvement of patient outcomes, and enhanced recovery from illness.
- Use of the algorithm in Fig. 142-1 can assist the nutritional support team in choosing the appropriate type of nutrition to best meet the patient's needs.
- Before administering PN, an individualized nutrition plan should be developed in collaboration with the multidisciplinary team. This would include a review of past medical history, current clinical status, laboratory values, and calculation of calorie and protein needs.
- There are two types of PN. Total parenteral nutrition (TPN) consists of a complex formulation of hyperosmolar dextrose, amino acids, lipids, minerals, vitamins, trace elements, and water. It is administered via a large-bore central catheter by an electronic infusion device. TPN formulations can meet the patient's complete or total nutritional needs. Peripheral parenteral nutrition (PPN) has a final concentration of dextrose of 10% or less. It is administered via a peripheral catheter. PPN does not provide enough carbohydrates to meet patient's daily nutritional needs. Instead, PPN is intended to supplement dietary

intake or provide minimal support to uncompromised patients.

- The first principle in providing nutrition for critically ill patients is to use the GI tract whenever possible. The absence of bowel sounds and stool or flatus does not preclude the use of the GI tract for feeding, particularly when feedings are administered distal to the pylorus. Increasing abdominal distention or severe GI disease states may be reasons to administer PN.
- The indications for PN should be evaluated daily. The patient should receive oral or enteral nutrition once GI function returns. Clinical studies demonstrate that the use of the GI tract and enteral feedings are associated with preservation of GI tract integrity and immune function and a reduction in infections and complications.
- Prevention of the metabolic and infectious complications associated with the use of PN is accomplished by close monitoring and strict adherence to aseptic technique.
- Indications for PN include the following:
  ❖ Patient whose GI tract is not functioning
  ❖ Patient whose GI tract cannot be accessed
  ❖ Patient who cannot be adequately nourished by oral or enteral diets

EQUIPMENT

- Prescribed PN solution
- IV administration set for electronic infusion device
- In-line IV filter (i.e., 0.22 micron for PN solutions without lipids; 1.2 micron for PN solution containing lipids)
- Nonsterile gloves
- Syringes and needleless injection cannula

- Normal saline (NS) for injection
- Heparin (100 units/ml)
- Electronic infusion device
- Central venous catheter (CVC) placed in the superior vena cava, *or*
- Peripheral venous catheter

PATIENT AND FAMILY EDUCATION

- Assess patient and family understanding of PN therapy and the reason for its use. ➤*Rationale:* Clarification or reinforcement of information is an expressed family need during times of stress and anxiety.
- Explain standard care to the patient and family, including catheter site care and dressings, physical assessment and laboratory monitoring, infusion device function and alarms, and parameters for change in route of nutritional administration. ➤*Rationale:* Encourages patient and family to ask questions and voice concerns about PN therapy and patient's nutrition.
- Explain the procedure. ➤*Rationale:* Teaching provides information and may decrease anxiety and fear.

PATIENT ASSESSMENT AND PREPARATION

Patient Assessment

- Preadmission nutritional status (including history of weight loss), current nutritional status, including patient weight and lean body mass, if available. ➤*Rationale:* An individualized nutritional plan should be created to

TABLE 143-1	Suggested Weekly Laboratory Monitoring for PN Patients

Electrolytes (sodium, potassium, chloride, CO_2)*
Renal function tests (blood urea nitrogen, serum creatinine)*
Glucose, phosphate, magnesium*
Liver function tests (SGOT, alkaline phosphatase, total bilirubin)
Ionized and total calcium
Prealbumin/albumin
CBC

*These laboratory values should be done at initiation, then daily for 5 days, and then weekly.
CBC, Complete blood count; *SGOT,* serum glutamic-oxalo-acetic transaminase.

meet the patient's needs based on individual assessment. An evaluation by a nutrition support team member or dietitian may be very helpful in patients with sepsis, significant trauma, burns, multiple organ failure, and other conditions that require complex nutritional requirement evaluation.

- Current laboratory profile (Table 143-1). ➤*Rationale:* An individualized nutritional plan and nutritional formulas should be created to meet the patient's needs based on individual assessment.
- Patency of venous access. *Rationale:* TPN is administered via a central venous line; PPN via a peripheral venous line.

Patient Preparation

- Ensure that patient understands preprocedural teaching. Answer questions as they arise and reinforce information as needed. ➤*Rationale:* Evaluates and reinforces understanding of previously taught information.

Procedure	**for Parenteral Nutrition**		
Steps	Rationale		Special Considerations
1. Verify orders with pharmacy label on PN bag. Remove PN bag from refrigeration 1 hour before initiation of infusion.	Reduces risk for error. The solution can be warmed to room temperature before infusion, increasing the patient's comfort.		Order should indicate volume to be infused, rate of delivery, and the number of hours of the PN infusion. If the rate is to be gradually increased or tapered, the length of time at each rate should be indicated. Note the expiration time and date of the PN solution.
2. Wash hands.	Reduces transmission of microorganisms; standard precautions.		
3. Compare patient's identification band with label on PN bag.	Prevents administration of PN to wrong patient.		
4. Aseptically spike PN bag with administration set for electronic infusion device.	Reduces transmission of microorganisms.		Volume-controlled electronic devices are preferred for PN solutions.

Procedure continues on the following page

Procedure for Parenteral Nutrition—*Continued*

Steps	Rationale	Special Considerations
5. Add appropriate in-line filter, fill the drip chamber to the appropriate level, prime tubing so that it is free of bubbles, and clamp tubing. *(Level IV: Limited clinical studies to support recommendations.)*	Traps particulate matter, bacteria, and endotoxins and vents air from intravenous tubing.[1,3-5,7]	If using PN solution that contains lipids (three-in-one solutions), use a 1.2-micron filter to prevent clogging.
6. Don nonsterile gloves.	Reduces exposure to blood and body fluids.	
7. Clamp catheter port.	Prevents air embolism and blood backup.	
8. Cleanse catheter port or hub with povidone-iodine prep pad. If lipids are to be administered separately, that injection port also must be cleaned with povidone-iodine, 70% isopropyl alcohol, 2% chlorhexadine solution). *(Level IV: Limited clinical studies to support recommendations.)*	Reduces microorganisms at catheter hub connection.[1-6]	PN should be administered in a dedicated line or lumen. If the lumen has been previously used, the line should be changed over a guide wire before initiation of PN. Use of the catheter lumen for other IV fluids or medications increases the risk for contamination. Subsequent infusion of PN via the lumen may promote growth of microorganisms in the presence of high concentrations of dextrose.
9. Remove cap or IV tubing from catheter hub and attach PN administration set using needleless connection. *(Level IV: Limited clinical studies to support recommendations.)*	Needleless connections decrease the risk for accidental needle sticks.[2,3,5]	Use of a needle or needleless injection cannula through an injection cap is not recommended. There is an increased risk for accidental disconnection, resulting in blood loss, air embolism, or hypoglycemia.
10. Place IV tubing into electronic infusion device. *(Level 1: Manufacturer's recommendation only.)*	Use of an infusion device ensures accurate, consistent delivery of PN.	
11. Set prescribed rate of infusion and other parameters on infusion device.	Consistent delivery of PN decreases the risk for metabolic complications[1,3-6] (Table 143-2).	If PN needs to be suddenly interrupted, notify physician or nurse practitioner. $D_{10}W$ should be infused at the same rate as the PN to prevent hypoglycemia.
12. Open clamps on IV set and catheter; start pump.		
13. Assess patency of catheter or venous access device.		
14. Label PN bag and IV set with date and time and other required information.		Change set and filter every 24 hours to reduce risk for infection.

TABLE 143-2	Metabolic Complications of Parenteral Nutrition (PN)		
Complication	**Etiology**	**Symptoms**	**Treatment**
Carbohydrate Metabolism			
Hyperglycemia	Too-rapid administration of PN, diabetes mellitus, sepsis, stress, steroids	Elevated blood glucose levels, glycosuria, diuresis, thirst	Decrease PN infusion rate Add insulin to PN solution
Hypoglycemia	Abrupt decrease or discontinuance of PN infusion, too much insulin	Blood glucose lower than 80 mg/dl, lethargy, diaphoresis, headache, pallor	Administer glucose by IV bolus or orally, depending on patient condition
Hyperglycemic hyperosmolar nonketotic (HHNK) dehydration/coma	Uncontrolled hyperglycemia	Blood glucose higher than 500 mg/dl, increased BUN, increased serum osmolality/ sodium levels, increased urine output, lethargy, coma	Decrease or stop PN, administer insulin to correct hyperglycemia, administer isotonic saline to rehydrate, administer potassium to correct hypokalemia
Respiratory compromise from excessive CO_2 production/retention	Overfeeding, excess calories, and total carbohydrate load	Respiratory quotient higher than 1.0	Decrease total calorie load; decrease carbohydrates and fat
Protein Metabolism			
Azotemia	Excessive protein administration, impaired renal or liver function	Increased serum BUN	Decrease protein amounts in PN solution; current recommendation, 0.8 to 1.5 g/kg/day
Fat Metabolism			
Essential fatty acid deficiency	Lack of adequate fat intake or supplement	Dry, flaky skin; hair loss; coarse hair; impaired wound healing	Administer 10% to 20% lipid emulsion IV at a minimal rate of 4% of required daily calories per week
Hyperlipidemia	Overinfusion of lipid emulsions	Increased serum cholesterol, triglyceride, and phospholipid levels	Decrease amount or concentration of lipid emulsion administration
		Exacerbation of arteriosclerotic cardiovascular disease	Discontinue lipid infusions and monitor serum lipid levels
Volume Administration			
Hypovolemia	Inadequate free water administration or excessive glucose administration	Increased serum BUN and sodium levels, decreased urine output, dehydration, thirst	Increase free water in PN solution; administer additional free water IV; decrease glucose calories
Hypervolemia	Fluid volume overload in renal, cardiovascular, pulmonary, or hepatic disease	Jugular venous distention, dyspnea, pedal and sacral edema, increased right atrium/central venous pressures	Concentrate fluids in PN; decrease or concentrate other IV solutions; consider renal replacement in patients with renal impairment
Electrolyte Metabolism			
Hypokalemia	Inadequate administration or increased losses of potassium	Cardiac dysrhythmias, muscle weakness	Increase potassium in PN formula
Hyperkalemia	Excess administration or inadequate excretion of potassium, as in renal impairment	Cardiac dysrhythmias	Discontinue current PN infusion and decrease potassium amounts in subsequent formulas
Hypocalcemia	Inadequate calcium administration or excessive phosphorus administration	Paresthesias, positive Chvostek's sign	Increase calcium in PN
Hypomagnesemia	Inadequate magnesium administration	Tingling around the mouth, dizziness, paresthesias	Increase magnesium in PN
Hypophosphatemia	Inadequate phosphate administration	Lethargy, paresthesias, respiratory distress, coma	Add phosphates as potassium or sodium salts to PN
Anemia, iron deficiency	Excessive blood loss, inadequate iron, copper, B_{12}, folate replacement	Pallor, fatigue, exertional dyspnea	Addition of iron to PN; blood transfusion as indicated
Trace element deficiencies	Inadequate trace element administration, excessive losses	Dependent on specific element deficiency, impaired wound healing, glucose intolerance, hair loss	Appropriate replacement of trace elements Routine monitoring not helpful Measure individual element level when deficiency is clinically suspected
Acid-Base Metabolism			
Metabolic acidosis	Too rapid administration of PN, diabetes mellitus, sepsis	Arterial pH less than 7.35	Correct hyperglycemia, treat sepsis

BUN, Blood urea nitrogen; *HHNK*, hyperglycemic hyperosmolar nonketotic; *IV*, intravenous.

Procedure for Parenteral Nutrition—*Continued*

Steps	Rationale	Special Considerations
Separate Lipid Emulsion Infusion 1. If lipids are to be piggy-backed into PN line via injection site on the tubing, repeat steps 1 through 14 above. When spiking lipids bottle, remove metal cap from the top. Spike with administration set. Cleanse the rubber cap per institutional policy.	In-line filter used for lipids is 1.2 micron.	Lipid emulsions are available in 10% and 20% concentrations in 250-ml and 500-ml bottles. 1.2-micron filters are used on lipids to prevent clogging. If lipids are not filtered, introduce the line below the level of the PN filter. Lipids should be infused over 16 to 24 hours. Lipid administration sets are changed with each new bottle.
Cycled PN 1. Infuse PN at prescribed rate. Physician or nurse practitioner may order rate to be increased over 1 to 2 hours or to begin at full rate. *(Level II: Theory-based, no research data to support recommendations: recommendations from expert consensus group may exist.)*	Gradual increase in PN may improve patient tolerance to glucose.[1,3-4,6]	Cycled PN is infused over 10 to 14 hours. This may help to stimulate patient's appetite and supplement oral intake. Patients with hepatobiliary dysfunction may be able to clear excess glycogen during hours when PN is off.
2. Decrease rate of PN infusion as prescribed, typically decreasing in half 1 to 2 hours before end of cycle. *(Level II: Theory-based, no research data to support recommendations: recommendations from expert consensus group may exist.)*	Decreases glucose load, thus decreasing insulin secretion, to prevent rebound hypoglycemia.[1,3,4,6]	
3. At the end of PN infusion, turn off infusion device; disconnect PN from catheter.		
4. Flush catheter with NS or heparin per institutional standard (see Procedure 65).		

Expected Outcomes

- Maintenance of baseline body weight or weight gain of 1 to 2 pounds per week in patients with weight loss
- Maintenance or repletion of serum proteins
- Normal or improved wound healing
- Positive nitrogen balance
- Maintenance of muscle mass
- Fluid balance slightly positive (greater than or equal to 500 ml/24 hr)
- Laboratory values within normal limits

Unexpected Outcomes

- Fluid overload
- Dehydration
- Hyperglycemic hyperosmolar nonketotic (HHNK) coma
- Azotemia
- Hyperlipidemia
- Metabolic acidosis
- Refeeding syndrome
- Catheter site infection
- Systemic infection
- Venous access disruption or nonpatency of catheter/port

Patient Monitoring and Care

Steps	Rationale	Reportable Conditions
		These conditions should be reported if they persist despite nursing interventions.
1. Obtain serum glucose measurements; assess patient's insulin requirements every 6 hours.	High carbohydrate intake in PN solution may lead to glucose intolerance. Early treatment of hyperglycemia may prevent HHNK coma. Glycosuria may occur as a later symptom of hyperglycemia. Sudden increases in insulin requirements and glucose intolerance are early indicators of sepsis. Use of a bedside glucose monitor will facilitate measurement of patient's serum glucose level.	• Serum blood glucose higher than 220 mg/dl • Glycosuria • Unexplained lethargy or coma

2. Evaluate patient's fluid status on a daily basis.
    A. Daily weights
    B. Skin turgor
    C. Breath sounds
    D. Jugular venous distention
    E. Peripheral edema
    F. Dyspnea
	Weight changes occurring within 24-hour periods are indicative of fluid imbalance. Dehydration may occur as a result of fluid loss and inadequate fluid intake. Fluid excess may occur, especially in patients with cardiac, hepatic, or renal compromise.	• Weight gain of 1 to 2 pounds in 24 hours
		• Changes in baseline breath sounds
		• Dyspnea
		• Peripheral edema
		• Jugular venous distention
		• Change in skin turgor

3. Monitor intake and output.	Intake and output is another indication of overall fluid balance. Trends over several days may indicate a positive or negative fluid balance, indicating need for adjustment in PN formula or volume.	• Positive or negative fluid balance of 1 to 2 L/24 hours
4. Monitor electrolytes, glucose, and renal function tests daily for first 5 days of PN therapy; weekly thereafter.	PN may alter electrolyte values if PN formulas are not adjusted to serum levels. Protein metabolism may elevate blood urea nitrogen (BUN), especially in patients with renal compromise.	• BUN higher than 50 mg/dl, elevated serum creatinine • Hyper- or hypoglycemia • Hyper- or hypophosphatemia • Hyper- or hypomagnesemia • Hyper- or hypokalemia • Hyper- or hyponatremia
5. Monitor liver function studies, albumin, and prealbumin at initiation of PN and weekly thereafter.	Infusion of PN may elevate liver function tests as a result of metabolism of amino acids, carbohydrates, or lipids.	• Total bilirubin higher than 1 mg/dl • Alkaline phosphatase higher than 130 milliunit/ml • Serum glutamic-oxalo-acetic transaminase (SGOT) higher than 40 milliunit/ml • Albumin lower than 3 g/dl • Prealbumin lower than 20 mg/dl
6. Monitor complete blood count (CBC) weekly and iron, ferritin, vitamin B_{12}, and folate levels as necessary.	Excess blood loss and inadequate administration of iron, copper, and vitamins result in anemia and iron and vitamin deficiencies.	• Iron level lower than 45 mcg/dl • Hematocrit (Hct) lower than 35% • Decreased vitamin B_{12} • Ferritin lower than 10 mcg/ml

Procedure continues on the following page

Patient Monitoring and Care—*Continued*

Steps	Rationale	Reportable Conditions
7. Assess patient for signs of trace mineral deficiencies.	Deficiencies in trace minerals (e.g., copper, zinc, chromium) may cause abnormalities in metabolism and impairment in skin integrity. Trace elements should be added to PN daily to prevent these deficiencies.	• Impaired wound healing • Glucose intolerance without signs of sepsis • Hair loss • Acne lesions • Anemia • Clotting abnormalities
8. Assess for hyperlipidemia.	Administration of lipids may cause increased serum lipid levels.	• Elevated total cholesterol, triglycerides, or phospholipids
9. Evaluate patient for evidence of refeeding syndrome.	Patients at risk include those with severely or moderately depleted nutritional states, in which efforts to provide nutritional support are too aggressive.	• Rapid decreases in serum phosphorus, potassium, and magnesium levels • Altered glucose metabolism • Altered cardiac function • Fluid shifts
10. Monitor temperature and vital signs every 4 hours. Monitor white blood cell count every 3 days.	Elevated temperature and white cell count may indicate the development of systemic infection. PN should be considered the cause of such infection until ruled out.	• Leukocytosis • Fever • Chills • Positive blood cultures
11. Monitor catheter insertion site daily or per institutional standard.	Local infection can progress to systemic infection if left untreated.	• Erythema • Pain/tenderness • Warmth • Purulent drainage

Documentation

Documentation should include the following:

- Patient and family education
- Laboratory assessment result
- Fluid balance assessment
- Temperature, vital signs, weights

- Observation of patient response to PN
- Unexpected outcomes
- Nursing interventions

References

1. ASPEN Board of Directors. (2002). Guidelines for the use of parenteral and enteral nutrition in adult and pediatric patients. *Nutr Clin Pract,* 260, 1SA-44SA.
2. Attar, A., and Messing, B. (2001). Evidence-based prevention of catheter infection during parenteral nutrition. *Curr Opin Clin Nutr Care,* 4, 211-18.
3. Collier, D., and Duggan, C. (2001). Overview of parenteral and enteral nutrition. *Up to Date.* Available at: www.uptodate.com.
4. Goff, K. (1997). Metabolic monitoring in nutrition support. *Nurs Clin North Am,* 32, 741-53.
5. Schwartz, D.B. (1996). Enhanced enteral and parenteral nutritional practice and outcomes in an intensive care unit with a hospital-wide performance improvement process. *J Am Diet Assoc,* 5, 484-9.
6. Skipper, A. (1995). *Nutrition Support Policies, Forms, and Formulas.* Gaithersburg, MD: Aspen Publishers.

7. Worthington, P., et al. (2000). Parenteral nutrition for the acutely ill. *AACN Clinical Issues,* 11, 559-79, 634-6.

Additional Readings

Alverdy, J.C., and Burke, D. (1992). Total parenteral nutrition: Iatrogenic immunosuppression. *Nutrition,* 8, 359-65.
Cerra, F.B., et al. (1997). Applied nutrition in ICU patients: A consensus statement of the American College of Chest Physicians. *Chest,* 111, 769-78.
Dark, D.S., Pingleton, S.K., and Kerby, G.R. (1995). Hypercapnia during weaning: A complication of nutritional support. *Chest,* 88, 141-3.
Gallica, L.A. (1997). Parenteral nutrition. *Nurs Clin North Am,* 32, 704-17.
Pearson, M.L., et al. (1995). Guidelines for prevention of intravascular device-related infection.

Percutaneous Endoscopic Gastrostomy (PEG), Gastrostomy, or Jejunostomy Tube Care

P U R P O S E : Gastrostomy, percutaneous endoscopic gastrostomy (PEG), and jejunostomy tubes provide long-term access to the gastrointestinal (GI) tract for nutrition.

Margaret M. Ecklund

PREREQUISITE NURSING KNOWLEDGE

- Anatomy and physiology of the upper and lower GI system is necessary.
- Patients who cannot have enteral tubes passed orally or nasally secondary to anatomy or surgery and those who require supplemental enteral nutrition support for longer than 4 weeks should be considered as candidates for long-term enteral access.
- The most commonly used long-term enteral access is the PEG tube. The PEG tube is inserted without general anesthesia. The use of a local anesthetic (i.e., 1% lidocaine injection) is used at the abdominal puncture site. A guide wire is threaded via endoscope through the oropharynx, esophagus, and stomach and brought out through the abdominal wall. The tube is then threaded over the guide wire and passed into the stomach. The tapered end of the tube is brought through a stab wound in the abdominal wall until the mushroomed end of the tube is set against the stomach wall. An adapter for infusion is attached to the end of the tube, and a disk on the tube is moved up to the abdominal wall to stabilize the tube in place.
- PEG tubes are large-bore catheters ranging from 18 French to 22 French, having a mushroom-shaped curved end in the stomach and a two-port distal end to instill enteral

nutrition, medications, and fluid. PEG tubes have disks, perpendicular to the tube, to hold the device close to the skin and lessen shift of tube in and out of the skin (Fig. 144-1).

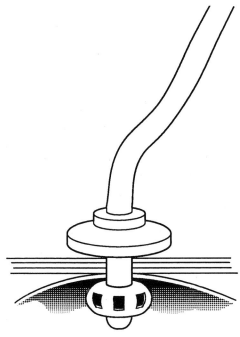

FIGURE 144-1 Percutaneous endoscopic gastrostomy.

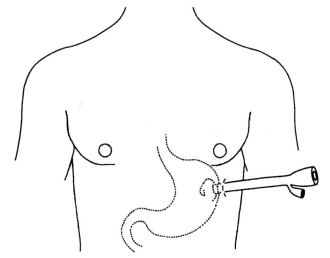

FIGURE 144-2 Gastrostomy tube.

- Contraindications for PEG placement include the following:
  - Previous gastric resection
  - Tumors blocking the passage of the endoscope
  - Ascites
  - Morbid obesity
  - Esophageal or gastric varices
- Gastrostomy tubes usually have a balloon in the intestinal lumen to prevent dislocation, which is inflated with sterile water. The distal end has an infusion port and a port for the balloon instillation (Fig. 144-2). A jejunostomy tube, which does not have a balloon, is indicated in those patients at risk for aspiration or who are unable to tolerate enteral feedings into the stomach, and are routinely sutured in place for stability (Fig. 144-3).
- If the tubes are removed, reinsertion of the tubes is a routine procedure after the tunnel and stoma are healed (approximately 2-6 weeks after insertion).
- Because these tubes all enter through the abdominal wall, skin care at the site of insertion is important for skin integrity and prevention of infection.
- Consult with the multidisciplinary team to individualize nutrition goals. The nutrition plan is developed based on the collaborative assessment of the nurse, dietitian, and physician or nurse practitioner.

EQUIPMENT

- Nonsterile gloves
- 4 × 4 gauze pads
- Cotton-tipped swabs
- 4 × 4 gauze pads—drain cut
- Protective skin barrier (e.g., vitamin A and D ointment)
- Silk tape (or paper tape if patient has a sensitivity to silk tape)

Additional equipment to have available, as needed includes the following:

- Hydrogen peroxide
- Abdominal binder

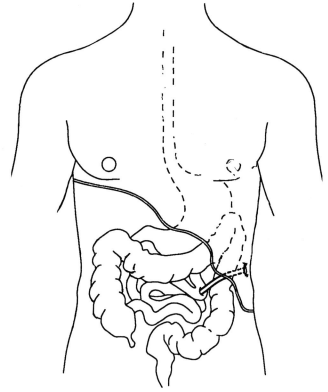

FIGURE 144-3 Jejunostomy tube placement.

PATIENT AND FAMILY EDUCATION

- Explain the purpose for the tube. ➤*Rationale:* Knowledge decreases anxiety and fear of the unknown.
- Explain reason for skin care assessment and maintenance. ➤*Rationale:* Knowledge decreases anxiety and fear of the unknown.
- Stress the importance of not pulling at the tube. ➤*Rationale:* Avoids unnecessary pain and skin irritation.
- Oral nutrition is possible with the long-term enteral access catheter. ➤*Rationale:* Knowledge decreases anxiety and fear of the unknown.
- Long-term enteral access catheters can be removed when oral intake meets the needs of the individual. ➤*Rationale:* Knowledge decreases anxiety and fear of the unknown. This also may be a goal for the patient to consume more via the oral route.

PATIENT ASSESSMENT AND PREPARATION

Patient Assessment

- Gastrointestinal assessment. ➤*Rationale:* A patient needs a functional gut to receive enteral nutrition.
- Skin condition at the feeding tube stoma; signs and symptoms of infection include the following:
  - Site redness/edema
  - Warmth
  - Purulent drainage
  - Pain or tenderness
  - Fever

➤➤*Rationale:* Intact skin integrity is a defense against infection. Early assessment of signs of infection promotes early, appropriate intervention.

Patient Preparation

* Ensure that patient understands preprocedural teaching. Answer questions as they arise and reinforce information as needed. ➤➤*Rationale:* Evaluates and reinforces understanding of previously taught information.
* Assist patient to position of comfort. ➤➤*Rationale:* Stoma of tube is easily accessible.

Procedure	**for Percutaneous Endoscopic Gastrostomy (PEG), Gastrostomy, or Jejunostomy Tube Care**		
Steps	**Rationale**	**Special Considerations**	
1. Wash hands and don nonsterile gloves.	Prevents transmission of microorganisms; standard precautions.		
2. Use soap and warm water to moisten gauze pads and two cotton-tipped applicators. *(Level II: Theory-based, no research data to support recommendations: recommendations from expert consensus group may exist.)*	Soap and water will clean the skin surface at the stoma.	Hydrogen peroxide, diluted to half strength with water, should be reserved for use for situations in which wound cleansing is a goal. Hydrogen peroxide will dry skin at the stoma.[1,5]	
3. Wipe the area closest to the tube (stoma) with the cotton-tipped applicators and proximal skin with the moistened gauze. Rinse with water. *(Level II: Theory-based, no research data to support recommendations: recommendations from expert consensus group may exist.)*			
4. Dry skin and stoma thoroughly with a dry gauze pad.	Prevents chafing and skin maceration.		
5. Using cotton-tipped applicator, apply protective skin barrier (e.g., vitamin A and D ointment or other commercial topical moisture barrier products) in a circular motion around stoma. *(Level II: Theory-based, no research data to support recommendations: recommendations from expert consensus group may exist.)*	Protective barrier ointment provides a moisture barrier for skin and assists wound healing. If purulent drainage is persistent, collaborate with physician or nurse practitioner for an antimicrobial ointment after skin cleansing.[1,4,5]		
6. Apply a 4 × 4 split gauze sponge around tube and secure with tape along edges. Change gauze every 12 hours or when soiled or moist. *(Level II: Theory-based, no research data to support recommendations: recommendations from expert consensus group may exist.)*	If no drainage is evident, gauze pad may be left off.[1,5]		

Procedure continues on the following page

Procedure for Percutaneous Endoscopic Gastrostomy (PEG), Gastrostomy, or Jejunostomy Tube Care—*Continued*

Steps	Rationale	Special Considerations
7. Anchor tube to skin at adjacent spot on abdomen. Site should be rotated to avoid skin damage from repeated taping. *(Level II: Theory-based, no research data to support recommendations: recommendations from expert consensus group may exist.)*	Reduces tension on the tube.	

Expected Outcomes

- Intact skin at stoma of long-term enteral access device
- Patent long-term enteral access for enteral feeding and fluid

Unexpected Outcomes

- Infection at stoma
- Tube removal by patient or accidental dislodgment with patient movement
- Migration of tube into intestinal lumen
- Peritonitis
- Aspiration

Patient Monitoring and Care

Steps	Rationale	Reportable Conditions
		These conditions should be reported if they persist despite nursing interventions.
1. Assess skin integrity and quality of drainage from stoma.	Intact skin is the first line of prevention against infection.	• Erosion of stoma • Change in drainage • Increased volume of foul-smelling, purulent drainage from around stoma • Redness or pain at stoma
2. Ensure that PEG tube has disk aligned next to skin without pressure into skin.	Disk helps prevent excess movement of tube in and out of skin. If the disk pushes with excess pressure, tissue injury may occur.[3]	• Pressure injury adjacent to stoma • Removal of tube by the patient • Clogging of the device
3. Ensure that the patient does not remove long-term enteral access device. A loosely applied abdominal binder is helpful to deter a confused patient from pulling at the tube.	A tube removed before the tract is established is a surgical emergency and requires immediate return to the operating room for repair and replacement.[2] Consult with the physician or nurse practitioner to determine the urgency of replacement follow-up. Tubes with established tracts can be replaced by the nurse at the bedside with a tube of comparable size and length.	
4. Note distance of tube from adapter to entrance into skin. Label tube with insertion date and measurement at entrance to skin.	Evaluates whether tube has migrated inward or pulled outward. Emesis or nausea may indicate pyloric obstruction.	• Length has deviated significantly • Emesis or nausea
5. Evaluate wearing of tube with ongoing use.	No routine change is indicated. Change of tube is indicated with device failure.[2]	• Tube wearing

Documentation

Documentation should include the following:

- Patient and family education
- Condition of stoma
- Any treatment rendered related to site complications
- Tube patency

- Type of tube and distance of tube from adapter to entrance into skin
- Unexpected outcomes
- Nursing interventions

References

1. Broscious, S.K. (1995). Preventing complications of PEG tubes. *DCCN,* 14, 37-41.
2. Graham, S., et al. (1996). Percutaneous feeding tube changes in long-term care facility patients. *Infect Control Hosp Epidemiol,* 17, 732-6.
3. Haslam, N., Hughes, S., and Harrison, R.F. (1996). Peritoneal leakage of gastric contents, a rare complication of percutaneous endoscopic gastrostomy. *JPEN,* 20, 433-4.
4. Holmes, S. (1996). Percutaneous endoscopic gastrostomy: A review. *Nursing Times,* 92, 34-5.
5. Lord, L.M. (1997). Enteral access devices. *Nurs Clin North Am,* 32, 685-702.

Additional Readings

Bowers, S. (1996). Tubes: A nurse's guide to enteral feeding devices. *Medsurg Nurs,* 5, 313-24.
Guenter, P., and Silkroski, M. (2001). *Tube Feeding: Practical Guidelines and Nursing Protocols.* Silver Springs, MD: Aspen Publishing.
Heiser, M., and Malaty, H. (2001). Ballon type versus nonballoon type replacement percutaneous endoscopic gastrostomy: Which is better? *Gastroenterol Nurs,* 24, 58-63.
Kelley, E., and Gokhali, C. (1998). Replacing displaced PEG tubes with a Foley catheter. *Gastroenterol Nurs,* 21, 254-5.
McMeekin, K. (2000). Replacing PEG tubes. *Nurs Times,* 96, 9-10.

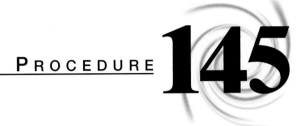
PROCEDURE **145**

Small-Bore Feeding Tube Insertion and Care

PURPOSE: A small-bore feeding tube is inserted to provide access to the gastrointestinal (GI) tract for the patient who is unable to consume adequate calories orally. The tube can be used for administration of nutrients, fluid, and medications.

Margaret M. Ecklund

PREREQUISITE NURSING KNOWLEDGE

- Anatomy and physiology of the upper and lower GI tract is needed.
- The GI tract should be functioning (bowel sounds audible and active peristalsis) for gastric feedings to be digested and absorbed.
- Small-bore feeding tubes are preferable over larger-bore nasogastric tubes during the course of critical illness, because the risk for tissue necrosis at the nares and sinusitis is lower.
- The small diameter of the tube allows simultaneous oral intake if the patient is able to consume orally without aspiration.
- Both weighted (tubes with an enlarged tip, filled with tungsten) and unweighted (bolus tip) small-bore nasogastric tubes are available. They typically are packaged with guide wires already in the lumen to assist passage of the tube. After successful placement, the guide wire is removed and discarded. The size of tubes range from 7 to 12 French.
- Unweighted tipped tubes migrate postpylorically into the duodenum more often than tubes with weighted tips. Weighted-tip tubes are harder for the compromised patient to swallow; ultimately, the unweighted tube may be a more comfortable choice for the patient.
- Absolute contraindications for insertion of a nasogastric feeding tube are basilar skull fracture, trans-sphenoidal surgical approaches, and esophageal varices. Oral insertions are usually appropriate in these situations. Esophageal varices are a contraindication for any tube that transgresses the esophagus.

- Small-bore feeding tubes are not designed for drainage of gastric contents. If gastric decompression is desired, the small-bore nasogastric tube should be replaced with a large-bore tube (Procedure 111).
- It is important to review institutional standards regarding insertion of small-bore feeding tubes. Some institutions restrict insertion to physicians and advanced practice nurses.

EQUIPMENT

- Small-bore feeding tube
- Small glass of tap water
- 60-ml Luer-Lok tip, or catheter-tip syringe, appropriate for feeding tube
- Skin preparation agent
- Plastic adhesive or clear tape
- Nonsterile gloves
- Water-soluble lubricant (if tube is not prelubricated)

PATIENT AND FAMILY EDUCATION

- Explain reason for insertion of tube and need for support of enteral nutrition. ➤*Rationale:* Knowledge decreases anxiety and fear of the unknown.
- Explain how patient can assist with passage of the tube, by positioning (e.g., sitting upright, head tipped forward and swallowing) when cued. ➤*Rationale:* Tube passes easier with patient cooperation.
- Explain the risk for the gag reflex being stimulated during insertion. ➤*Rationale:* Knowledge decreases anxiety and fear of the unknown.
- Explain the reason for the x-ray after insertion. ➤*Rationale:* Knowledge decreases anxiety and fear of the unknown.

- Discuss reasons for not pulling at tube once it has been placed and secured. ➤➤*Rationale:* Leaving the tube in place avoids the need for reinsertion and another x-ray for verification. Reinsertion increases risk for trauma to nasopharyngeal passages.

PATIENT ASSESSMENT AND PREPARATION

Patient Assessment

- Medical history of head and neck cancer and surgery, basilar skull fracture, esophageal cancer, decreased pharyngeal reflexes, trans-sphenoidal pituitary resection. ➤➤*Rationale:* These conditions prohibit safe passage of a tube nasally through pharynx. Inadvertent intracranial placement of the small bore feeding tube is possible with a basilar skull fracture.[5]
- Patency of the nares for potential obstructions to feeding tube passage. ➤➤*Rationale:* A tube cannot pass through occlusion.
- Gastrointestinal function. ➤➤*Rationale:* A functional gut is needed to administer enteral feedings.

Patient Preparation

- Ensure that patient understands preprocedural teaching. Answer questions as they arise and reinforce information as needed. ➤➤*Rationale:* Evaluates and reinforces understanding of previously taught information.
- If the patient has a large-bore nasogastric tube, it needs to be removed prior to placement of the small-bore nasogastric tube. ➤➤*Rationale:* Attempting to pass a small-bore tube will be extremely difficult with an oral or nasal tube already in place. Removal of the large-bore tube after placement of the small-bore tube, will likely cause displacement of the newly placed small tube.

Procedure for Small-Bore Feeding Tube Insertion and Care

Steps	Rationale	Special Considerations
1. Wash hands.	Reduces transmission of microorganisms.	
2. Don nonsterile gloves.	Standard precautions.	
3. Sit patient upright and tip head forward. *(Level IV: Limited clinical studies to support recommendations.)*	Facilitates passage of tube into esophagus. If patient cannot tolerate upright positioning, position laterally to the right side to insert tube.[4,6]	
4. Estimate depth of tube insertion by measuring tube from tip of nose to ear, then inferior to stomach (see Fig. 111-3). *(Level IV: Limited clinical studies to support recommendations.)*	Approximates length of tube to insert. If postpyloric placement is desired, add 10 to 15 cm to length of tube measured.[4]	
5. Lubricate tip of tube with water. *(Level I: Manufacturer's recommendations only.)*	Water activates a lubricant on the surface of tube to facilitate passage through nares.	If tube does not have self-lubrication, a water-soluble lubricant can be applied to the tube.
6. Insert tip of tube into either nare; advance to posterior pharynx until resistance is met. *(Level IV: Limited clinical studies to support recommendations.)*	Once tube is advanced through the nares, the oropharynx is reached, and the tube will stop.[3,6]	
7. At this point, ask patient to swallow. If the patient is able to cooperate, give sips of water to trigger swallow reflex and ease tube passage. *(Level IV: Limited clinical studies to support recommendations.)*	Swallowing immediately assists passage of the tube into the esophagus.[1-3] If the patient is unable to cooperate with swallowing, neck positioning may facilitate passage.	If coughing begins immediately with advancing tube, immediately pull back to nares.

Procedure continues on the following page

Procedure for Small-Bore Feeding Tube Insertion and Care—*Continued*

Steps	Rationale	Special Considerations
8. As patient swallows, advance tube to desired marking. Remove guide wire with one hand, while holding the tube securely at the nares.	The initial swallow gets the tube into the esophagus, and the nurse can advance it to desired position without repeated swallowing. Removing the guide wire without holding the tube can cause the tube to pull out with the guide wire.	If the patient is unconscious or unable to cooperate, do not attempt to use water orally to pass tube.
9. Apply skin preparation to nose and securing surface of the face; allow to dry.	Prepares surface of skin to help with the tape adhering.	
10. Tape tube securely to nose, using one half of a 3-cm strip. The lower portion of the tape is then split up to the tip of the nose and wrapped around the tube (see Fig. 111-4). *(Level IV: Limited clinical studies to support recommendations.)*	The tape needs to hold the tube to prevent slipping it out. Pink plastic tape has shown an ability to stay secure for a greater length of time compared with other methods.[1]	Tape the tube so that it does not press against the skin. Excess pressure can cause breakdown.
11. Remove gloves and wash hands.		
12. Obtain chest x-ray (lower chest view) to verify placement. *(Level IV: Limited clinical studies to support recommendations.)*	Chest x-ray verification is the safest way to ensure correct placement. A lower chest view will ensure the tip is in stomach or intestine.[2-4,6]	
13. If postpyloric placement is desired, tape additional length with coil in stomach. *(Level IV: Limited clinical studies to support recommendations.)*	The extra length can allow the migration of tube past the pyloric valve.[4]	
14. Position patient on right side.	This assists with peristalsis. If tube is in stomach, peristalsis should move it beyond the sphincter.	
15. Obtain abdominal x-ray.	Abdominal x-ray verification is the standard of care to ensure correct placement.	Postpyloric placement is verified with abdominal film to ensure tip is visualized.
16. If tube has not migrated postpylorically, continue to position patient on right side and recheck x-ray. *(Level IV: Limited clinical studies to support recommendations.)*	Right-side positioning potentially helps pass the tube postpyloric with the aid of peristalsis. The best location is at the beginning of the jejunum, or the fourth portion of the duodenum.[3,6]	
17. If tube remains in stomach, consult with physician or nurse practitioner to administer metoclopramide IV and repeat x-ray. *(Level IV: Limited clinical studies to support recommendations.)*	Promotility agents have shown benefit in moving tube through pyloric valve.[4]	

Expected Outcomes

- Distal tip of tube is placed in either stomach or small bowel.
- Patent tube accepts enteral feedings, medications, and fluid.
- Patient is able to swallow oral foods and fluids while small-bore feeding tube is in place, if allowed.

Unexpected Outcomes

- Coughing or dyspnea, indicating potential bronchial placement
- Pneumothorax from inadvertent pleural placement
- Tube coiled in esophagus or posterior pharynx
- Esophageal tear from trauma of tube passing
- Tube dislodging during therapy, necessitating removal and new tube placement
- Aspiration of stomach contents despite appropriate placement
- Clogging of enteral tube with medication fragments or enteral formula
- Skin irritation at nose

Patient Monitoring and Care

Steps	Rationale	Reportable Conditions
		These conditions should be reported if they persist despite nursing interventions.
1. Monitor tolerance to tube placement.	Agitation may inhibit successful placement	• Self-extubation • Agitation and inability to cooperate with tube placement • Recurrent vomiting • Continued coughing and dyspnea
2. Assess oral cavity and perform oral care every 2-4 hours and prn.	Patients with orogastric or NG tubes in place tend to mouth-breathe, thus drying their mouths and increasing the risk for mucosal breakdown and ulceration. Tube presence also may predispose a patient to sinusitis or oral infections.	• Ulceration, drainage, foul odor
3. Monitor insertion site of tube for redness, swelling, drainage, bleeding, or skin breakdown. Use only water-soluble lubricants at site.	Many critically ill patients have fragile skin and have associated conditions that predispose them to skin breakdown. Frequent monitoring and subsequent repositioning of the tube can prevent serious damage.	• Redness • Swelling • Drainage • Bleeding • Skin breakdown at insertion site
4. Reposition and retape tube every 24 hours or when tape is soiled.	Decreases risk for tissue damage to mouth or nares.	

Documentation

Documentation should include the following:

- Patient and family education
- Size and type of tube placed
- Patient response to insertion
- Length of tube external to patient, from nose to end of tube
- X-ray interpretation
- Unexpected outcomes
- Nursing intervention

References

1. Burns, S.M., et al. (1995). Comparison of nasogastric tube securing methods and tube types in medical intensive care patients. *AJCC*, 4, 198-203.
2. Fater, K.H. (1995). Determining nasoenteral feeding tube placement. *Medsurg Nurs*, 4, 27-32.
3. Lord, L.M. (1997). Enteral access devices. *Nurs Clin North Am*, 32, 685-702.
4. Lord, L.M., et al. (1993). Comparison of weighted vs unweighted enteral feeding tubes for efficacy of transpyloric intubation. *JPEN*, 17, 271-3.
5. Metheny, N.A. (2002). Inadvertent intracranial nasogastric tube placement. *AJN*, 102, 25-7.
6. Welch, S.K. (1996). Certification of staff nurses to insert enteral feeding tubes using a research-based procedure. *Nutr Clin Prac*, 11, 21-7.

Additional Readings

Bowers, S. (1996). Tubes: A nurse's guide to enteral feeding devices. *Medsurg Nurs*, 5, 313-24.

Davies, A.R., et al. (2002). Randomized comparison of nasojejunal and nasogastric feeding in critically ill patients. *Crit Care Med*, 30, 586-90.

Fitch, L., et al. (1999). Oral care in the adult intensive care unit. *Am J Crit Care*, 8, 314-8.

Guenter, P., and Silkroski, M. (2001). *Tube Feeding: Practical Guidelines and Nursing Protocols.* Silver Springs, MD: Aspen Publishers.

Metheny, N. (2002). Assessing placement of feeding tubes. *AJN*, 101, 36-45.

Powers, J., et al. (2003). Bedside placement of small bowel feeding tubes in the intensive care unit. *Crit Care Nurse*, 23, 16-24.

Zaloga, G.P. (1991). Bedside method for placing small bowel feeding tubes in critically ill patients. *Chest*, 100, 1643-6.

PROCEDURE **146**

Advance Directives

PURPOSE: Advance directives are designed to document patients' treatment choices in the event that they are unable to actively participate in the decision-making process, as well as to inform members of the health care team of those decisions.

Barbara B. Ott

PREREQUISITE NURSING KNOWLEDGE

- Documentation of an individual's wishes for future health care is called an *advance directive* and may include a living will and/or a health care proxy (Fig. 146-1).
- A living will is a document that expresses a person's wishes for medical treatments when that person is terminally ill or in a persistent vegetative state or a coma and unable to make his or her own decisions.[12] Using a living will, a patient can choose to accept or refuse specific life-sustaining medical treatments (e.g., mechanical ventilation, cardiopulmonary resuscitation, tube feedings, blood products, dialysis, antibiotics).
- A health care proxy (also referred to as a *durable power of attorney for health care*) is a document that identifies a person who can make medical decisions for an individual if he or she becomes unable to make decisions in the future.[12] The patient's designated decision maker is called a *surrogate* or *proxy decision maker.*[14]
- Patients have the right to make treatment decisions.[16] The development of an advance directive encourages understanding, reflection, and discussion of treatment options by the patient, surrogate, family, and health care team.
- Treatment decisions differ from patient to patient because decisions are based on individual values.[5,9]
- Living wills and health care proxies are easy to prepare, and both documents can be changed or revoked at any time. A patient can change or revoke a living will by telling the physician or nurse that he or she wishes to change or revoke it.
- The Patient Self-Determination Act[3,13] is a federal law requiring hospitals to do the following:
  - ❖ Ask patients whether they have an advance directive

  - ❖ Give patients and families information about advance directives
  - ❖ Tell patients what state law says about advance directives
  - ❖ Tell patients what hospital policies say about advance directives
- The Joint Commission on Accreditation of Healthcare Organizations (JCAHO) requires hospitals to have clear standards on advance directives[9]; these standards may differ from institution to institution and state to state. Universally, patients are not required to have an advance directive, nor are institutions allowed to discriminate against patients based on whether or not they have an advance directive.
- Under most circumstances, the hospital is required to honor the patient's wishes when they are communicated to the hospital staff. A hospital's policy will explain any specific information or procedures.
- Most hospitals will not guarantee that a health care provider will follow advance directives in every circumstance. The physician should tell the patient or family if the physician cannot, in good conscience, honor the patient's wishes as stated in the advance directive.
- Although not necessary in most states, specific forms may be available to make the preparation of an advance directive easier. Additionally, some states require an advance directive to be signed by two witnesses or notarized by a notary public. Hospitals have state-specific forms for both living wills and health care proxies. Typically, there are hospital employees (social workers, chaplains, patient services representatives) available to help patients prepare an advance directive. Focusing on the outcomes of treatment rather than specific treatments helps with decision making.[10] It is best if advance directive documents are prepared before a health care crisis occurs.

DECLARATION

I, _____ , being of sound mind,

willfully and voluntarily make this declaration to be followed if I become incompetent.

This declaration reflects my firm and settled commitment to refuse life-sustaining

treatment under the circumstances indicated below.

I direct my attending physician to withhold or withdraw life-sustaining

treatment that serves only to prolong the process of my dying, if I should be in

a terminal condition or in a state of permanent unconsciousness.

I direct that treatment be limited to measures to keep me comfortable

and to relieve pain, including any pain that might occur by withholding or withdrawing

life-sustaining treatment.

In addition, if I am in the condition described above, I feel especially

strongly about the following forms of treatment:

I ( ) do ( ) do not want cardiac resuscitation.

I ( ) do ( ) do not want mechanical respiration.

I ( ) do ( ) do not want tube feeding or any other artificial

or invasive form of nutrition (food) or hydration (water).

I ( ) do ( ) do not want blood or blood products.

I ( ) do ( ) do not want any form of surgery or invasive

diagnostic tests.

I ( ) do ( ) do not want kidney dialysis.

I ( ) do ( ) do not want antibiotics.

I realize that if I do not specifically indicate my preference regarding any of

the forms of treatment listed above, I may receive that form of treatment.

FIGURE 146-1 Pennsylvania Declaration Form.

Other instructions:

I ( ) do ( ) do not want to designate another person as my surrogate to make medical treatment decisions for me if I should be incompetent and in a terminal condition or in a state of permanent unconsciousness.

Name and address of surrogate (if applicable):

Name and address of substitute surrogate (if surrogate designated above is unable to serve):

I made this declaration on ————————————————— , 20 ——.

Declarant s signature: ————————————————————

Declarant s address: ————————————————————

————————————————————

The declarant knowingly and voluntarily signed this writing by signature or mark in my presence.

———————————————————
Signature of Witness

———————————————————
Address of Witness

———————————————————
Signature of Witness

———————————————————
Address of Witness

FIGURE 146-1—*Cont'd.*

Good communication between the patient, family and health care team can help prevent ethical emergencies.[6]

- Physicians, nurses, and other health care professionals can recommend various treatment options; the patient can choose among the various options or refuse all recommended treatments.[2] Communication is very important.[1]

Terminology used in advanced care planning must be clear to the patient, family, and health care team.[8]

- Patients make decisions regarding medical care with advice from their physician, nurse, and others.[17] Religious, cultural, and personal values can influence these decisions.[11]

- If a person becomes too ill to make decisions about health care, a previously prepared advance directive can be used to help with those decisions.
- If a patient who does not have an advance directive becomes ill and is unable to make medical decisions, the physician asks a relative or close friend for guidance regarding what treatments the patient would want.[7]
- The hospital ethics committee may be consulted when concerns about patient care and medical decision making for patients are present.[4] The ethics committee also is available to provide additional information, answer questions, or address concerns about advance directives and the care of patients requiring end-of-life care.[4,9,16]
- It is best to keep a copy of the patient's living will or health care proxy in the patient's chart so that all individuals involved in patient care are aware of the patient's choices. It can be problematic if the only copy of the advance directive is locked in a safe deposit box or stored in a place without easy access.

EQUIPMENT

- State-specific advance directive forms (if required)
- Notary or witness (if required by the state).

PATIENT AND FAMILY EDUCATION

- Give the patient and family the hospital's information about advance directives. ➤*Rationale:* Although patients are not required to have an advance directive, institutions have an obligation to inform patients about advance directives. This information should be provided in a manner that is not too difficult to read.[13]
- Answer any questions about advance directives. ➤*Rationale:* Advance directives are best prepared by well-informed patients.
- Encourage patients to think carefully about these important medical decisions with a focus on the goals of treatment. Discussions with loved ones are essential. ➤*Rationale:* Discussions can help clarify values and desired treatments. An advance directive document should reflect an individual's values and beliefs.

PATIENT ASSESSMENT AND PREPARATION

Patient Assessment

- On admission, determine the existence of or interest in developing an advance directive. ➤*Rationale:* The Patient Self-Determination Act[6] requires that all patients are asked, on admission, if they have an advance directive. Admission to a health care facility provides an opportunity for health care providers to open discussion with patients about their personal wishes for their health care.
- Confirm accuracy of the advance directive (if present). ➤*Rationale:* Verifies the accuracy of the document and its usefulness during the patient's stay.
- Assess the patient's decision-making capacity. ➤*Rationale:* Usually, the physician or advanced practice nurse determines the patient's decisional capacity with input from other sources, such as nursing assessments, patient history, patient examination including mental status examination, conference with family, friends, or psychiatric consultation.[14] Decision-making capacity usually consists of three attributes:
  - ❖ Understanding: Can the patient understand information about his or her diagnosis and prognosis and information about the particular decision(s) to be made (treatment options, risks, benefits, burdens)?
  - ❖ Evaluation: Can the patient determine how this information relates to his or her values, beliefs, and goals of treatment?
  - ❖ Reasoning: Can the patient analyze how health care decisions will affect him or her personally? This includes a basic understanding of probability and percentages.[11]

  Reassessment is appropriate. The patient may be only temporarily unable to make decisions. Document this process following institutional policies.
- Determine whether the patient is 18 years of age or older. ➤*Rationale:* Persons over the age of 18 are assumed to be legally competent unless a court has determined otherwise. In the clinical setting, some legally competent individuals may have diminished capacity to make health care decisions.
- Assess whether the family knows about a patient's advance directive. ➤*Rationale:* It is possible that the patient did not discuss the advance directive choices with the family.

Patient Preparation

- Ensure that the patient and family understand preprocedural teaching. Answer questions as they arise and reinforce information as needed. ➤*Rationale:* Evaluates and reinforces understanding of previously taught information.
- If the patient wishes to develop an advance directive, arrange for a time and place for the patient, family, and health care provider to talk about advance directives. ➤*Rationale:* A quiet place, with comfortable seating away from the noises of the critical care unit, would be ideal for these important discussions to take place.

Procedure for Advance Directives

Steps	Rationale	Special Considerations
1. Ask the patient whether he or she has an advance directive (a living will and/or health care proxy).	The Patient Self-Determination Act requires that hospitals ask whether patients have an advance directive.[6]	If the patient is unconscious or too ill to respond to the question, ask family members or friends if they know whether the patient has an advance directive.
2. Document the patient's response (Yes or No; the patient has or does not have an advance directive).	It is important to know whether the patient has already prepared an advance directive.	It may be necessary to ask more than one family member or friend whether the patient has an advance directive.
3. If the patient has an advance directive, place a copy of it on the current medical record (see Fig. 146-1).	Advance directive choices must be communicated to the health care team.	Some hospitals have special procedures for documenting the presence of an advance directive (e.g., special sticker for the chart, designated placement in the medical record, special checklist). Advance directives can be changed or revoked by the patient verbally or in writing. The presence of an advance directive on the chart does not mean the patient has an order for Do Not Resuscitate.[15]
4. If the patient has an advance directive, but does not have a copy of it with him or her, make arrangements with a family member or friend to bring it to the hospital for incorporation into the medical record.	Copies of advance directives often are kept with other important papers in secure places (e.g., bank safety deposit boxes and household safes). It is essential that the patient's advance directive is reviewed and is a part of the patient's chart.	Copies of advance directives can sometimes be found in medical records from the physician's office or from an old hospital record.
5. Assess that choices recorded on the advance directive document are accurate and up to date.	It is important to ensure that previously prepared documents reflect the patient's current choices.	
6. Confirm that medical treatments and nursing care are consistent with the patient's advance directive choices.	Patients may change their minds regarding treatment choices. These changes must be communicated to the staff.	
Developing an Advance Directive		
1. Assist the physician or advanced practice nurse with assessment of the patient's decision-making capacity.	Illness can cause a patient to have difficulty understanding information, relating the information to personal values, or communicating choices to the health care team.	
2. Provide the patient with information about advance directives and answer any questions about advance directives.	Federal law requires hospitals to give patients information about advance directives.[6]	
3. Provide the patient with appropriate resources (i.e., hospital personnel who can assist with more information about advance directives) and with preparation of an advance directive document, if desired.	Provides assistance with the development of an advance directive.	

Procedure continues on the following page

Procedure **for Advance Directives**—*Continued*

Steps	Rationale	Special Considerations
4. Encourage the patient to discuss medical treatment decisions with his or her physician, surrogate, and family.	Providing information and encouraging discussion is important, so that the patient's treatment wishes are known.	Patients should not be pressured to sign an advance directive. Encourage discussion of all options.
5. Have a follow-up discussion with the patient about his or her advance directive.	Upon admission, patients and family members may be quite stressed and overloaded with information. Patients and family members may need time to reflect on treatment wishes.	

Expected Outcomes

- Patient treatment wishes are known.
- Patient treatment wishes are honored.

Unexpected Outcomes

- Patient treatment wishes are unknown.
- Patient treatment wishes are not honored.

Patient Monitoring and Care

Steps	Rationale	Reportable Conditions
		These conditions should be reported if they persist despite nursing interventions.
1. The patient should be asked whether he or she has a current advance directive and if it is accurate.	Advance directives can be prepared many months or years before a patient becomes sick. It is advisable to ask the patient if the choices in his or her advance directives are still current. Sometimes, as a patient's physical condition changes through the course of an illness, the patient may want to modify decisions previously stated in the advance directive. A patient with decision-making capacity can revoke or change his or her advance directive at any time.	- The patient wishes to modify his or her advance directive
2. Ensure that the advance directive is communicated with members of the health care team and family.	It is possible that decisions made by a patient and reflected in an advance directive may not have been communicated to the patient's family or friends or the health care provider.	- Misunderstanding by health care professionals or family about the patient's choices for health care
3. Consult the hospital ethics committee as needed.	The patient, family, or health care providers may need to consult the ethics committee if there are misunderstandings or disagreements about what treatment options should be pursued.	- Advance directive not honored or treatment not in accordance with the patient's advance directive - Involvement of the ethics committee

Documentation

Documentation should include the following:

- Patient and family education
- Existence of an advance directive
- Location of the advance directive document, if the patient has one
- Name and phone number of the individual who brought a copy of the advance directive to the hospital
- A copy of the living will or health care proxy in the front of the chart or in a location in the chart where it is easy to find

- Discussions with patient, surrogate, and family members regarding the advance directive
- Misunderstandings the patient or family may have about the law, institutional policy, or content of an advance directive
- Unexpected outcomes
- Additional nursing interventions

References

1. American Association of Critical-Care Nurses. (1985). *Clarification of Resuscitation Status in Critical Care Settings: Position Statement.* Aliso Viejo, CA: Author.
2. American Association of Critical-Care Nurses. (1990). *Withholding and/or Withdrawing Life-Sustaining Treatment: Position Statement.* Aliso Viejo, CA: Author.
3. American Nurses Association. (1992). *Position Statement on Nursing and the Patient Self-Determination Act.* Kansas City, MO: Author.
4. American Society for Bioethics and Humanities Task Force on Standards for Bioethics Consultation. (1998). *Core Competencies for Health Care Ethics Consultation. Monograph.* Available at: www.asbh.org/resources/publications/index.html.
5. Beauchamp, T.L., and Childress, J.F. (2001). *Principles of Biomedical Ethics.* New York: Oxford University Press.
6. Benner, P. (2003). Avoiding ethical emergencies. *Am J Crit Care,* 12, 71-2.
7. Buchanan, A.E., and Brock, D.W. (1989). *Deciding for Others.* New York: Cambridge University Press.
8. Calvin, A.O., and Clark, A.P. (2002). How are you facilitating advance directives in your clinical nurse specialist practice? *Clin Nurse Specialist,* 16, 293-4.
9. Davis, A.J., et al. (1997). *Ethical Dilemmas and Nursing Practice.* Stamford, CT: Appleton & Lange.
10. Fried, T.R., et al. (2002). Understanding the treatment preferences of seriously ill patients. *N Engl J Med,* 346, 1061-6.
11. Kundhal, K.K., and Kundhal, P.S. (2003). Cultural diversity: An evolving challenge to physician-patient communication. *JAMA,* 289-94.
12. Monagler, J.F., and Thomasma, D.C. (1998). *Health Care Ethics.* Gaithersburg, MD: Aspen Publications.
13. Omnibus Budget Reconciliation Act of 1990. (1990). *Patient Self-Determination Act. Pub L10-508.* Washington, DC: Government Printing Office.
14. Ott, B.B. (1999). Advance directives: The emerging body of research. *Am J Crit Care,* 8, 514-9.
15. Ott, B.B., and Hardie, T.L. (1997). Readability of advance directive documents. *Image,* 29, 53-7.
16. President's Commission for the Study of Ethical Problems in Medicine and Biomedical and Behavioral Research. (1982). *Making Health Care Decisions.* Washington, DC: Government Printing Office.
17. SUPPORT. (1995). A controlled trial to improve care for seriously ill hospitalized patients. *JAMA,* 274, 1591-8.

Additional Readings

American Association of Critical-Care Nurses. (1997). *Discovering Your Beliefs About Healthcare Choices.* Aliso Viejo, CA: Author.

Prendergast, T.J., and Puntillo, K.A. (2002). Withdrawal of life support: Intensive caring at the end of life. *JAMA,* 288, 2732-40.

Wallace, S.K., et al. (2001). Influence of an advance directive on the initiation of life support technology in critically ill cancer patients. *Crit Care Med,* 29, 2294-8.

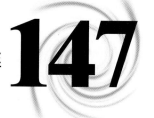
PROCEDURE **147**

AP
Determination of Death

PURPOSE: This procedure will describe how death is determined. Institutional policies and legislation governing declaration of death may vary across practice settings and states. However, standardized evidence-based criteria provide guidelines for practices involving determination of cardiopulmonary and brain death.

Jacqueline Sullivan
Liza Severance-Lossin

PREREQUISITE NURSING KNOWLEDGE

- Death is determined when there is either (1) irreversible cessation of circulatory and respiratory functions or (2) irreversible cessation of all functions of the entire brain, including the brain stem.
- In cases of either cardiopulmonary or brain death, diagnosis of death requires both cessation of function and irreversibility.
- In cardiopulmonary death cessation of function is determined by clinical examination.
- In cardiopulmonary death irreversibility is confirmed by persistent cessation of functions during a period of observation.
- In brain death cessation of function is determined when clinical evaluation discloses absence of both cerebral and brain stem function.
- In brain death irreversibility is determined when (1) the etiology of coma sufficient to account for loss of brain functions is established, (2) the possibility of recovery of brain function is excluded, and (3) the cessation of all brain functions persists for a period of observation or therapy.
- Previously, death had been described as the cessation of circulation and respiration (cardiopulmonary death). The advent of mechanical ventilation and cardiovascular support, however, presented new challenges for determining

death in patients with catastrophic cerebral insults whose cardiopulmonary function could be preserved using complex technology.[4,5]

- Initial efforts to define death in an age of technologic advancement included the development of the Harvard criteria, which described determination of a condition known as "irreversible coma," "cerebral death," or "brain death."[2]
- Since the initial introduction of the Harvard criteria, the Uniform Determination of Death Act (UDDA) was published in 1980 and recommended by the President's Commission for the Study of Ethical Problems in Medicine and Biomedical and Biobehavioral Research as a model statute for state legislation defining death.[4]
- UDDA asserts that "an individual who has sustained either (1) irreversible cessation of circulatory and respiratory functions, or (2) irreversible cessation of all functions of the entire brain, including the brain stem, is dead. A determination of death must be made in accordance with accepted medical standards."[4]
- The concept of brain death continues to be a topic of international debate among clinicians, anthropologists, philosophers, and ethicists. This ongoing dialogue concerning determination of death is a process of developing multidisciplinary consensus responsive to continually changing technology.[7,14,16,19]
- Although conceptualization of death continues to evolve, experts have generated clinical practice parameters for brain death diagnosis that are grounded in empirical knowledge, supported by sufficiently rigorous research, and substantiated by moderate to high degrees of clinical certainty.[26]
- Neuroscience experts continue to define brain death as irreversible cessation of all functions of the entire brain,

including the brain stem. This definition remains consistent with the definition of brain death initially presented by the President's Commission for the Study of Ethical Problems in Medicine and Biomedical and Biobehavioral Research.[4,26]

- Cardinal findings in brain death include coma or unresponsiveness, apnea, absence of cerebral motor responses to pain in all extremities, and absence of brain stem reflexes including pupillary signs, ocular movements, facial sensory and motor responses, pharyngeal and tracheal reflexes.

- Legal responsibility for assessment and declaration of death varies by state. Many states permit advanced practice nurses to determine death. Other states allow registered nurses to do so under certain circumstances. Often these circumstances include written authorization from a physician in cases where a death is anticipated due to illness, infirmity, or disease.

EQUIPMENT

- For cardiopulmonary death determination
  - Stethoscope
  - Electrocardiogram (ECG) monitor
  - ECG leads
  - ECG electrodes
- For brain death determination
  - Flashlight
  - Laboratory testing supplies
  - Iced saline or water solution
  - 60-ml Luer-Lok syringe and 18- or 20-G angiocatheter with needle removed (*or* 60-ml syringe)
  - Small basin
  - Towels and protective bedding
  - Nonsterile gloves
  - Oxygen delivery via endotracheal airway using nasal cannula or straight tubing for oxygen delivery
  - Arterial blood gas kit supplies

PATIENT AND FAMILY EDUCATION

- Assess family understanding of the death determination procedure and its purpose. ➥*Rationale:* Clarification and repeat explanation may assist in allaying some stress and anxiety for grief-stricken family members.
- Explain potential outcomes of the death determination procedure. ➥*Rationale:* Awareness of the duration and expectations of death determination procedures may allay some stress and anxiety in grief-stricken family members.
- If testing for brain death, assess family understanding of the concept of being "brain-dead." Give clear definition of brain death and death as synonymous and reinforce repeatedly with the family. ➥*Rationale:* The concept of

brain death may be confusing to family members, because the term "brain-dead" may imply that only the brain is dead and the rest of the body is alive. Brain death must be described as death.

- If a patient has conclusively been declared brain-dead, facilitate the discussion of organ donation by appropriate members of the health care team. ➥*Rationale:* Patients who are brain-dead are potential candidates for organ donation. Experts recommend separating the interaction involving declaration of death to the family from the interaction requesting consideration for organ donation (a process otherwise known as "decoupling"). Request for organ donation is the responsibility of representatives from the organ procurement organization (OPO) or a specially trained designated hospital requester (see Procedure 150).

PATIENT ASSESSMENT AND PREPARATION

Patient Assessment

- Assess the patient's baseline cardiopulmonary and neurologic status in preparation for determination of death. ➥*Rationale:* In cardiopulmonary death, clinical examination discloses absence of responsiveness, heartbeat, and respiratory effort. In brain death, clinical examination reveals an absence of both cerebral and brain stem function.
- For brain death determination, the following prerequisites must also be met:
  - Acquire clinical or neuroimaging evidence of an acute catastrophic cerebral event consistent with the clinical diagnosis of brain death
  - Exclude conditions that may confound the clinical assessment of brain death, such as acute metabolic or endocrine derangements or neuromuscular blockade
  - Confirm the absence of drug intoxication or poisoning
  - Maintain the patient's core body temperature greater than or equal to 32°C
  ➥*Rationale:* The brain death determination procedure must confirm both cessation and irreversibility of all brain function (including both cerebral and brain stem function). The above four criteria are required for the confirmation of irreversible cessation of brain function.

Patient Preparation

- Ensure that the family understands preprocedural teaching. Answer questions as they arise and reinforce information as needed. ➥*Rationale:* Evaluates and reinforces understanding of previously taught information.
- Place the patient in a supine position. ➥*Rationale:* Facilitates patient assessment, oculovestibular testing, and arterial puncture.

Procedure for Determination of Death

Steps	Rationale	Special Considerations
Determination of Cardiopulmonary Death		
1. Wash hands.	Reduces the transmission of microorganisms; standard precautions.	

2. Conduct a clinical examination:
  A. Assess level of consciousness.
  B. Assess airway. Assess breathing. Assess circulation.
	The clinical examination in cardiopulmonary death reveals absence of responsiveness, heartbeat, and respiratory effort.	

3. Perform an ECG if available (see Procedures 54 and 57).	A confirmatory test such as ECG monitoring or 12-lead ECG may be performed to rule out reversible nonperfusing dysrhythmias.	
4. Confirm the irreversibility of the cessation of cardiopulmonary function.	Irreversibility is confirmed by persistent cessation of functions, including pulselessness, apnea, and loss of consciousness.	In clinical situations, where death is expected and where the course has been gradual, the period of observation following cessation may be limited to the time required to complete the examination. If ventricular fibrillation and cardiac standstill develop in a monitored patient and resuscitation is not undertaken or is unsuccessful, the required period of observation may be limited to the time required to complete the examination. When a possible death is unobserved, unexpected, or sudden, the duration of the examination should be commensurate with continued resuscitative efforts. Declaration of death in patients who are first observed with rigor mortis may require only the period of observation necessary to establish that condition.
Determination of Brain Death		
1. Wash hands.	Reduces the transmission of microorganisms; standard precautions.	
2. Ensure that the patient's core body temperature is at least 32°C at the time of the clinical examination for brain death determination.	Hypothermia may artificially alter the results of the neurologic examination, leading to confounding results regarding irreversible cessation of brain function.[7,16,26]	
3. Perform the necessary endocrine screenings as required for the individual patient to rule out reversible conditions such as diabetic ketoacidosis.	Endocrine screening may exclude conditions that could confound the clinical assessment of brain death.[26]	
4. Perform the necessary toxicology screenings as required for the individual patient.	In cases where the possibility of excessive sedation is present, toxicology screening for all likely drugs should be considered.[26]	If exogenous intoxication of drugs is determined to exist, death should not be declared until the intoxicant is metabolized or until

Procedure **for Determination of Death**—*Continued*

Steps	Rationale	Special Considerations
		confirmatory testing for cessation of intracranial circulation is considered.
5. Establish evidence of coma or unresponsiveness.	In brain death, intense stimulation evokes no verbal or voluntary motor responses.	Spontaneous voluntary motor activity, shivering, or seizure activity are absent in brain death.
6. Assess the patient's cerebral motor responses to pain using noxious stimulation such as a sternal rub or pinching the trapezius (Fig. 147-1).	Absence of cerebral motor responses to pain is a cardinal finding consistent with brain death.[7,14,16] Peripheral stimuli such as nailbed pressure may evoke a reflex arc as opposed to a true brain stem response.	Motor responses may occur spontaneously during apnea testing with the occurrence of hypoxia or hypotension and are considered to be of spinal reflex origin. Respiratory acidosis and brisk neck flexion also may generate spinal cord reflexes. Spinal reflex responses occur more frequently in young adults and include rapid spontaneous flexion and muscle stretch reflexes in the arms and legs, with resulting grasplike walking-like movements. Spinal reflex movements are not cerebrally modulated. Spinal reflex movements may occur in the presence of brain death. Involuntary posturing movements are absent in brain death.
7. In the presence of neuromuscular blockade use, assessment with a peripheral nerve stimulator is required before testing for cerebrally modulated motor responses (see Procedure 104).	Clinical brain death determination procedures cannot be undertaken in the presence of neuromuscular blockade. Neuromuscular blockade may confound motor testing in brain death due to pharmacologically induced motor weakness.[26]	In cases where neuromuscular blocking agents may have been previously used, testing with a peripheral nerve stimulator may determine whether adequate neuromuscular function is present for valid clinical brain death determination.

Procedure continues on the following page

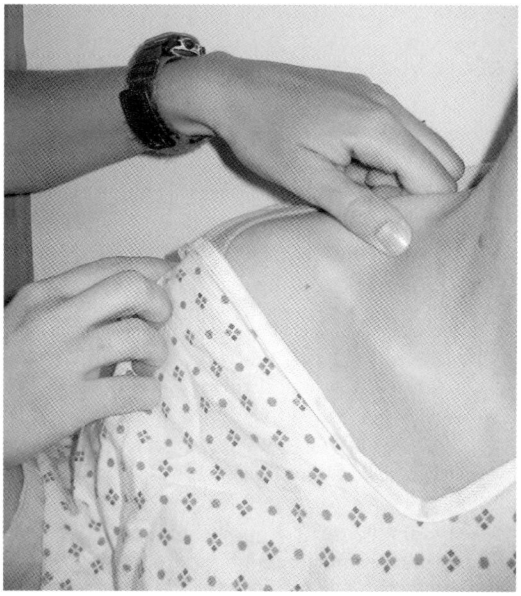

FIGURE 147-1 The trapezius pinch.

Procedure for Determination of Death—*Continued*

Steps	Rationale	Special Considerations
8. Assess the patient's pupillary size and response to light bilaterally.	Round, oval, or irregularly shaped pupils are compatible with brain death.[7,16,26] Pupillary light reflex must be absent in brain death. Absence of pupillary light reflexes, as a component of brain stem reflexes, is a cardinal finding consistent with brain death. Most pupils are midposition size (4 to 6 mm) in brain death.	Dilated pupils may occur even in the presence of brain death because sympathetic cervical pathways connected to the pupillary dilator muscle may still be intact. Standard doses of atropine administered intravenously do not markedly affect pupillary response. Neuromuscular blocking agents do not significantly influence pupil size. Topical administration of medications and ocular trauma may influence pupillary size and reactivity. Preexisting ocular anatomic abnormalities may also confound pupillary assessment in brain death.
9. Assess the patient's oculocephalic (doll's eye) reflexes: A. Oculocephalic reflexes are elicited by rapidly and vigorously turning the head 90 degrees laterally on both sides. B. If the oculocephalic reflexes are intact, the patient's eyes will deviate from the direction in which the patient's nose points. C. In brain death, oculocephalic reflexes are absent, with no eye movements occurring in response to head movements.	Absence of oculocephalic reflexes, as a component of brain stem reflexes, is a cardinal finding consistent with brain death.[7,16,26]	Contraindications to performance of oculocephalic reflex testing include suspicion of cervical spine fracture or instability.
10. Assess the patient's oculovestibular (caloric) reflexes (see Procedure 96). A. Elevate the head of the bed to 30 degrees B. Instill 50 ml of iced water or saline into the ear over 30 seconds—3 minutes. C. Observe the patient's eyes for 1 minute. D. After 5 minutes, perform the same procedure to the patient's other ear. E. In brain death the oculovestibular reflexes are absent, with no deviation of the eyes in response to ear irrigation.	Absence of oculovestibular reflexes, as a component of brain stem reflexes, is a cardinal finding consistent with brain death.	Contraindications to testing of oculovestibular reflexes include impaired integrity of the tympanic membranes. Several medications may diminish oculovestibular reflexes, such as sedatives, aminoglycosides, tricyclic antidepressants, anticholinergics, antiseizure agents, and neuromuscular blocking agents. Preexisting vestibular disease, preexisting cranial nerve disorders, and facial trauma involving the auditory canal and petrous bone also may inhibit oculovestibular reflex responses.
11. Assess the patient's corneal and jaw reflexes. Corneal reflexes should be tested with a cotton-tipped swab. Jaw reflexes are described as grimacing to pain and may be tested by application of deep pressure on the nailbeds, the supraorbital ridge, or the temporomandibular joint.	Absence of facial and motor responses, as a component of brain stem reflexes, is a cardinal finding consistent with brain death.[26] Corneal and jaw reflexes are absent in brain death.	Severe facial trauma may inhibit interpretation of facial brain stem reflexes.

Procedure for Determination of Death—*Continued*

Steps	Rationale	Special Considerations
12. Assess the patient's gag and cough reflexes. The gag reflex may be elicited by stimulating the posterior pharynx with a tongue blade. The cough reflex may be tested by bronchial suctioning.	The absence of pharyngeal and tracheal reflexes, as a component of brainstem reflexes, is a cardinal finding consistent with brain death.[7,16,26] Gag and cough reflexes are absent in brain death.	Gag reflex may be difficult to evaluate in orally intubated patients.
13. Prepare for the performance of an apnea test.	A cardinal finding and essential component in the clinical determination of brain death is the demonstration of apnea. Loss of brainstem function definitively results in loss of centrally controlled breathing function, with resultant apnea.	
14. Achieve conditions necessary for apnea test precautions.[1,6,8,11,15,25,26] A. Maintain core body temperature greater than or equal to 36.5°C. B. Maintain systolic blood pressure greater than or equal to 90 mm Hg. C. Achieve euvolemia. D. Achieve eucapnea (arterial $Paco_2$ of greater than or equal to 40 mm Hg). E. Maintain/achieve normoxemia (arterial Pao_2 of greater than or equal to 200 mm Hg).	Apnea test precautions will minimize cardiac dysrhythmias and systemic hypotension, which may occur during the apnea test.	Cardiac dysrhythmias and systemic hypotension may occur during apnea testing. Cardiac dysrhythmias usually result from hypercarbia and respiratory acidosis and occur most frequently in patients with hypoxia. Severe hypotension may occur in well-oxygenated patients whose arterial $Paco_2$ rises to high levels with acidosis. Hemodynamic disturbances may be avoided during apnea testing when respiratory acidosis is limited to a pH of 7.17 ($\pm$0.02) with an arterial $Paco_2$ of 60 to 80 mm Hg.[8] Pretest hyperoxygenation and procedural administration of oxygen also have resulted in avoidance of significant hypoxemia in apnea testing.
15. Perform an apnea test: A. Obtain a baseline arterial blood gas (ABG). B. Disconnect the ventilator. C. Deliver 100% oxygen, 6 L/min. May place oxygen cannula at the level of carina. D. Observe closely for respiratory movements that produce adequate tidal volumes. E. Obtain an ABG after approximately 8 minutes. F. Reconnect the ventilator.	Determines respiratory status.	In many institutions a physician must be present during performance of apnea testing. The exact level of arterial $Paco_2$ necessary to maximally stimulate the chemoreceptors of central respiratory centers remains unknown in conditions consistent with hyperoxygenation and brain stem destruction. Advisory guidelines for determination of death based on clinical and research data recommend achieving $Paco_2$ levels of greater than 60 mm Hg for maximal stimulation of brain stem respiratory centers.[4] Target $Paco_2$ levels for apnea tests in brain death determination may be higher in patients with chronic hypercapnia.

Procedure continues on the following page

Procedure for Determination of Death—*Continued*

Steps	Rationale	Special Considerations
		Hypocarbia may also occur in patients with acute catastrophic cerebral insults and may result from therapeutic hyperventilation or hypothermia. Although correction of hypocarbia should precede apnea testing, use of carbon dioxide admixtures should probably be avoided because of associated consequences, including severe hypercarbia and respiratory acidosis.
16. Interpret the apnea test results (Table 147-1).	Aids in determination of brain death.[1,6,8,11,15,25,26]	Apnea test results may be interpreted in the following four ways: (1) positive, (2) negative, (3) occurrence of cardiovascular/pulmonary instability, and (4) inconclusive.
17. Facilitate compliance with institutional recommendations regarding persistent observation in brain death determination.	Persistent observation further confirms irreversibility in the clinical determination of brain death.[26] A repeat clinical evalution of cardinal findings in brain death is recommended.	Most experts recommend an arbitrary interval of 6 hours between initial and repeat observations for the clinical determination of brain death in adults; however, a firm recommendation based on scientific literature cannot be given.[26] All clinical tests of cardinal findings are equally essential in declaring brain death.
18. Assist in obtaining confirmatory tests for brain death determination as indicated (Table 147-2).	Confirmatory testing may aid diagnosis.[3,9,10,12,13,17,18,20-24] Although confirmatory tests are not mandatory in most situations, diagnostic testing may be necessary for declaring brain death with patients in whom specific components of clinical testing cannot be reliably evaluated.[26] Clinical experience with confirmatory tests mostly involves use of conventional angiography, electroencephalogram (EEG), transcranial Doppler ultrasonography (TCD), and cerebral blood flow studies.	
19. Discard used supplies and wash hands.	Reduces the transmission of microorganisms; standard precautions.	

TABLE 147-1   Apnea Test Results

Positive apnea test	Respiratory movements are absent.
	Posttest arterial Pa_{CO_2} is greater than or equal to 60 mm Hg.
	Supports clinical determination of brain death.
Negative apnea test	Respiratory movements are observed regardless of arterial Pa_{CO_2} level.
	Does *not* support clinical determination of brain death; apnea test may be repeated.
Apnea test resulting in cardiovascular or pulmonary instability	Systolic blood pressure falls below 90 mm Hg.
	Arterial oxygen desaturation below therapeutic levels occurs.
	Cardiac dysrhythmia occurs.
	Immediately draw an arterial blood gas sample and reconnect the ventilator.
	Confirmatory test to finalize clinical determination of brain death may be performed at the discretion of the physician.
Inconclusive apnea test	No respiratory movements are observed.
	Posttest arterial Pa_{CO_2} is less than 60 mm Hg without significant cardiovascular instability.
	Apnea test may be repeated with 10 minutes of apnea.

TABLE 147-2	Confirmatory Brain Death Test Results
Cerebral angiography	No intracerebral filling at the level of the carotid bifurcation or circle of Willis External carotid circulation patent
Electroencephalogram (EEG)	No electrical activity during a period of at least 30 minutes of recording
Transcranial Doppler ultrasonography	Absent diastolic or reverberating flow Flow only through systole or retrograde diastolic flow Small systolic peaks in early systole
Technetium 99m brain scan (cerebral blood flow scan)	No uptake of isotope in brain parenchyma ("hollow skull phenomenon")

Expected Outcomes

- Clinical or diagnostic determination of death
- Declaration of death and notification of the family

Unexpected Outcome

- Indecisive results regarding determination of death

Patient Monitoring and Care

Steps	Rationale	Reportable Conditions
		These conditions should be reported if they persist despite nursing interventions.
1. Assess family understanding of and response to death determination procedure.	Family understanding of and response to death determination situations may vary based on religious beliefs and cultural practices. Adequate assessment of the family provides the necessary foundation for provision of support.	
2. Solicit family support from spiritual and psychologic counselors (e.g., grief counselors).	Support of spiritual and psychologic counselors may assist the family in the grieving process.	
3. Provide adequate private time for family members to visit with and grieve for the loss of their loved one.	Private visiting time provides family members with the opportunity for grieving and closure.	
4. In cases of brain death, facilitate discussion of organ donation options (see Procedure 150).	The OPO will screen the patient with brain death for possible organ donation.	
5. In cases where brain death has not been confirmed but where quality-of-life issues are being considered, be prepared to facilitate and provide support during discussions regarding possible withdrawal of therapy (Procedure 152).	Indecisive results regarding brain death determination may lead to consideration of other treatment options, including withdrawal of therapy. In cases of devastating neurologic insults without the occurrence of brain death, the health care team, in collaboration with the patient's family, may make decisions regarding continuation or initiation of resuscitation measures, provision of supportive care, and withdrawal of therapy.	

Documentation

Documentation should include the following:

- Family education and support
- Description of the specific procedure(s) performed for death determination, results of such procedures, and the patient's tolerance of procedures
- Clinical examination components consistent with the determination of death and the exact time of the death determination
- Time of brain death (documented as the time of the clinical diagnostic confirmation of complete and irreversible cessation

of all brain function; not listed as the time of removal of mechanical ventilation or the time of organ donation)
- Time of cardiopulmonary death (documented as the time of clinical or diagnostic confirmation of complete and irreversible cessation of circulatory and respiratory function); ECG strips, if obtained, should be interpreted and included in the patient's permanent medical record

References

1. al Jumah, M., et al. (1992). Balk diffusion apnea test in the diagnosis of brain death. *Crit Care Med,* 20, 1564-7.
2. Anonymous. (1968). A definition of irreversible coma. Report of the Ad Hoc Committee of the Harvard Medical School to Examine the Definition of Brain Death. *JAMA,* 205, 337-40.
3. Anonymous. (1994). Guideline three: Minimum technical standards for EEG recording in suspected cerebral death. American Electroencephalographic Society. *J Clin Neurophysiol,* 11, 10-3.
4. Anonymous. (1981). Guidelines for the determination of death. Report of the Medical Consultants on the Diagnosis of Death to the President's Commission for the Study of Ethical Problems in Medicine and Biomedical and Behavioral Research. *JAMA,* 246, 2184-6.
5. Anonymous. (1995). *Practice Parameters for Determining Brain Death in Adults: Summary Statement.* Report of the Quality Standards Subcommittee of the American Academy of Neurology. *Neurology,* 45, 1012-4.
6. Benzel, E.C., et al. (1992). Apnea testing for the determination of brain death: A modified protocol. Technical note. *J Neurosurg,* 76, 1029-31.
7. Calliauw, L. (1990). Brain death. *Acta Neurochir,* 105, 85-6.
8. Ebata, T., et al. (1991). Haemodynamic changes during the apnea test for diagnosis of brain death. *Can J Anesth,* 38, 436-40.
9. Erbengi, A., et al. (1991). Brain death: Determination with brain stem evoked potentials and radionuclide isotope studies. *Acta Neurochir,* 112, 118-25.
10. Goldie, W.D., et al. (1981). Brainstem auditory and short-latency somatosensory evoked responses in brain death. *Neurology,* 31, 248-56.
11. Gutmann, D.H., and Marino, P.L. (1991). An alternative apnea test for the evaluation of brain death. *Ann Neurol,* 30, 852-3.
12. Ishii, K., et al. (1996). Brain death: MR and MR angiography. *Am J Neuroradiol,* 17, 731-5.
13. Jalili, M., Crade, M., and Davis, A.L. (1994). Carotid blood flow velocity changes detected by Doppler ultrasound in determination of brain death in children: A preliminary report. *Clin Pediatr,* 33, 669-74.
14. Kennedy, M., and Kiloh, N. (1996). Drugs and brain death. *Drug Safety,* 14, 171-80.
15. Lang, C.J. (1997). Blood pressure and heart rate changes during apnea testing with or without CO_2 insufflation. *Intens Care Med,* 23, 903-7.

16. Link, J., Schaefer, M., and Lang, M. (1994). Concepts and diagnosis of brain death. *Forensic Sci Int,* 69, 195-203.
17. Machado, C. (1993). Multimodality evoked potentials and electroretinography in a test battery for an early diagnosis of brain death. *J Neurol Sci,* 37, 125-31.
18. Matsumura, A., et al. (1996). Magnetic resonance imaging of brain death. *Neurol Med Chir,* 36, 166-71.
19. Morenski, J.D., et al. (2003). Determination of death by neurologic criteria. *J Intens Care Med,* 18, 211-21.
20. Newell, D.W. (1995). Transcranial Doppler measurements. *New Horiz,* 3, 423-30.
21. Palma, V., and Guadagnino, M. (1992). Evoked potentials in brain death: A critical review. *Acta Neurol,* 14, 363-8.
22. Payen, D.M., et al. (1990). Evaluation of pulsed Doppler common carotid blood flow as a noninvasive method for brain death diagnosis: A prospective study. *Anesthesiology,* 72, 222-9.
23. Petty, G.W., et al. (1990). The role of transcranial Doppler in confirming brain death: Sensitivity, specificity, and suggestions for performance and interpretation. *Neurology,* 40, 300-3.
24. Silverman, D., et al. (1969). Cerebral death and the electroencephalogram. Report of the Ad Hoc Committee of the American Electroencephalographic Society on EEG Criteria for Determination of Cerebral Death. *JAMA,* 209, 1505-10.
25. Visram, A., and Marshall, C. (1997). $PaCO_2$ and apnoea testing for brain stem death. *Anesthesia,* 52, 503.
26. Wijdicks, E.F.M. (1995). Determining brain death in adults. *Neurology,* 45, 1003-11.

Additional Readings

Black, P.M. (1991). Conceptual and practical issues in the declaration of death by brain criteria. *Neurosurg Clin North Am,* 2, 493-501.

Byrne, P.A., and Nilges, R.G. (1993). The brain stem in brain death: A critical review. *Issues Law Med,* 9, 3-21.

Lock, M. (1996). Death in technological time: Locating the end of meaningful life. *Med Anthropol Q,* 10, 575-600.

Nau, R., et al. (1992). Results of four technical investigations in fifty clinically brain dead patients. *Intens Care Med,* 18, 82-8.

Paolin, A., et al. (1995). Reliability in diagnosis of brain death. *Intens Care Med,* 21, 657-62.

Ying, Z., et al. (1992). Motor and somatosensory evoked potentials in coma: Analysis and relation to clinical status and outcome. *J Neurol Neurosurg Psychiatry,* 55, 470-4.

PROCEDURE **148**

Care of the Organ Donor

P U R P O S E :   To preserve organ function until transplantation.

June Hinkle

PREREQUISITE NURSING KNOWLEDGE

- Knowledge of federal rules, state laws, organ procurement organization (OPO) policies, and hospital policies regarding organ donation from patients diagnosed with brain death and from patients who are non-heart-beating donors.
- The only persons who should approach the family about organ donation is the designated hospital requestor or the OPO coordinator. The designated requestor must complete an OPO-approved program.[1] The training is OPO specific but usually includes information on brain death testing, techniques on how to explain brain death to families, grief, cultural differences, and role playing the consent process.
- In brain death, cessation of function is determined when clinical evaluation discloses absence of both cerebral and brain stem function (see Procedure 147).
- Non-heart-beating donors are those who have experienced a cardiopulmonary arrest or are being removed from life support and the family or significant other wishes to donate organs (see Procedure 151).[2]
- The patient remains in the intensive care unit (ICU) until the organ donor matching process is completed.
- Hemodynamic instability may occur because of autonomic nervous system failure. Management goals should focus on maintenance of intravascular volume, normothermia, acid-base balance, and the optimization of oxygenation and perfusion.
- Costs associated with organ recovery are billed to the OPO.
- If organ recovery is occurring from a patient meeting brain death criteria, the donor remains on the ventilator until organ recovery is complete.
- If organ recovery is occurring from a non-heart-beating donor on a ventilator, the ventilator is stopped and death

must be pronounced after the heart stops beating. Recovery of organs must occur quickly after the heart stops beating to ensure the organs are viable. All organs may be recovered from a non-heart-beating donor, but the kidney is the most frequently recovered organ.[2] OPO and hospital policies regarding non-heart-beating donors vary between institutions and states (see Procedure 151).

- If the donor experiences cardiac arrest, cardiopulmonary resuscitation (CPR) and advanced cardiac life support are initiated. If resuscitation is not successful, organ recovery is performed as soon as feasible.
- If the patient was designated as Do Not Resuscitate (DNR) before consent for organ donation, this may be reversed if there is consent for donation. This is discussed with the family as part of the donation discussion.
- Organ donation is a cooperative effort between the family, critical care nurses, physicians, transplant coordinator, designated requestor, OPO coordinator, operating room personnel, and the surgical recovery team.

EQUIPMENT

- Thermometer
- Electrocardiogram (ECG) monitor and electrodes
- Consent form
- Laboratory specimen containers and laboratory forms
- Prescribed intravenous fluids
- Urinary catheter
- Ventilator
- IV equipment and IV pumps
- Arterial blood gas (ABG) kits

Additional equipment to have available, as needed, includes the following:

- Arterial line and monitoring system
- Pulse oximetry
- Medications

PATIENT AND FAMILY EDUCATION

- Evaluate the family's understanding of the organ recovery process. ➺*Rationale:* Allows the critical care nurse to correct misunderstandings, clarify information, evaluate the efficacy of coping strategies, and reduce anxiety related to the care of the patient.
- Reinforce to the family that surgical removal of the organs takes place with respect and careful technique, similar to any operation. ➺*Rationale:* Decreases the family's anxiety about the care of their loved one during organ recovery.

PATIENT ASSESSMENT AND PREPARATION

Patient Assessment

- Assess the patient's oxygenation. ➺*Rationale:* Provides baseline data.
- Assess the patient's vital signs and hemodynamic parameters. ➺*Rationale:* Provides baseline data.
- Assess the patient's current laboratory results (e.g., electrolytes, blood urea nitrogen, creatinine). ➺*Rationale:* Provides baseline data.

Patient Preparation

- Ensure that the family understands preprocedural teaching. Answer questions as they arise and reinforce information as needed. ➺*Rationale:* Evaluates and reinforces understanding of previously taught information.
- An arterial catheter may be inserted, if not already in place. ➺*Rationale:* Facilitates assessment of blood pressure and ease of blood sampling.
- Communicate with the OPO coordinator to determine the timing and logistics of the organ recovery surgery. ➺*Rationale:* The OPO coordinator has the responsibility of organ placement and the coordination of the arriving surgical recovery teams.
- Determine a plan for communicating with the family during the organ recovery process. This should be developed with the critical care nurse, OPO coordinator, and the family. ➺*Rationale:* Each family has unique needs during the organ recovery process. Some families wish to leave the hospital as soon as the consent for donation is signed; others wish to see their deceased loved one after organ recovery has occurred.

Procedure for Care of the Organ Donor

Steps	Rationale	Special Considerations
1. Ensure that brain death criteria have been met and proper documentation is in the chart (see Procedure 147).	This is a necessary criterion for organ donation.	Non-heart-beating donors also may donate organs in some states. Institution guidelines are helpful in guiding this process (see Procedure 151).
2. Ensure that the consent form for organ donation has been completed.	This is a necessary criterion for organ donation.	
3. Obtain blood samples for laboratory analysis as prescribed by the OPO coordinator.	Multiple laboratory analyses are needed before final placement of the patient's organs.	Common tests include: complete blood count, liver and kidney function tests, electrolytes, hepatitis panels, and HIV testing.
4. Administer intravenous fluids and medications (including vasoactive agents) as prescribed by the OPO coordinator or medical team.	Therapies may be necessary to optimize organ function before recovery.	
5. If the family is present, allow the family visitation with the patient.	Promotes family togetherness; prepares for family goodbyes and grieving.	
6. Transfer the patient to the operating room as directed by the OPO coordinator.	Prepares the patient for the donation process.	
7. Provide family support.	Aids family coping.	
8. Provide a method for the family to obtain information about the organ recovery process.	Keeps the family informed of the recovered organs.	

Expected Outcomes

- Organ recovery completed
- Recovered organs viable

Unexpected Outcomes

- Determination that the potential donor is medically unsuitable for organ donation
- Inability to recover viable organs for transplantation

Patient Monitoring and Care

Steps	Rationale	Reportable Conditions
		These conditions should be reported if they persist despite nursing interventions.
1. Monitor the patient's cardiac and hemodynamic status continuously.	If the donor is unstable, it may compromise organ viability.	• Systolic blood pressure less than 90 mm Hg • Changes in heart rate or other parameters set by the OPO coordinator • Dysrhythmias
2. Monitor the patient's oxygenation status via continuous pulse oximetry and arterial blood gases.	Determines the presence of hypoxemia.	• Pao_2 less than 100 mm Hg • Sao_2 less than or equal to 96% or other parameters as set by the OPO coordinator
3. Monitor the patient's body temperature and intervene as necessary to achieve normothermia.	Hypothermia or hyperthermia may lead to coagulopathies.[2]	• Temperature less than 96°F • Temperature greater than 99°F • Other parameters set by OPO coordinator
4. Monitor the patient's urine output hourly.	Determines renal perfusion.	• Urine output less than 0.5 ml/kg/h
5. Monitor laboratory studies as determined by the OPO coordinator (e.g., electrolytes, renal and liver function tests).	Determines organ function.	• Abnormal laboratory results
6. Provide family support. Incorporate the grief counselor, social worker, and pastoral care.	Offers family resources during grieving.	• Ineffective family coping

Documentation

Documentation should include the following:

- Family education
- Determination of brain death or cessation of respirations and cardiac activity
- Completed consent form for organ donation and recovery
- Complete donor record, including vital signs, assessments, treatment, and the clinical status of the donor
- Communication with the family, including summary of information provided and response of the family
- Preoperative checklist
- Unexpected outcomes
- Additional interventions

References

1. Health Care Financing Administration. (1998). Medicare and Medicaid programs: Hospital condition of participation; Identification of potential organ, tissue and eye donors. Title 42, Vol 3, *Federal Register.*
2. Herdman, R., and Potts, J.T. (1997). *Non-Heart-Beating Organ Transplantation: Medical and Ethical Issues in Procurement.* Washington, DC: National Academy Press.
3. Power, D.J., and Reich, H.S. (2000). Regulation of coagulation abnormalities and temperature in organ donors. *Progress Transplantation,* 10, 146-53.

Additional Readings

Church, E.J. (2002). Organ donation and transplantation. *Radiologic Technology,* 73, 537-72.
Coleman-Musser, L. (1997). The physician's perspective: A survey of attitudes toward organ donor management. *J Trans Coor,* 7, 55-8.
Day, L. (2001). How nurses shift from care of a brain-injuries patient to maintenance of a brain-dead organ donor. *AJCC,* 10, 306-12.
DeVita, M.A. (2001). The death watch: Certifying death using cardiac criteria. *Progress Transplantation,* 11, 58-66.

Duckworth, R.M., et al. (1998). Acute bereavement services as a mechanism to increase donation. *J Trans Coor,* 8, 16-8.

Holmquist, M. (1996). Organ donor care map: A multidisciplinary approach. *J Trans Nurs,* 6, 101-4.

Jordan, M.L., et al. (1999). High-risk donors: Expanding donor criteria. *Transplant Proc,* 31, 1401-3.

McCoy, J., and Argue, P.C. (1999). The role of the critical care nurse in the donation process: A case study. *Crit Care Nurs,* 19, 48-52.

Novitzky, D. (1997). Donor management: State of the art. *Transplant Proc,* 28, 3773-5.

Novitsky, D. (1997). Detrimental effects of brain death on the potential organ donor. *Transplant Proc,* 29, 3770-2.

Park, K.M., et al. (1996). Proper donor management and multiorgan procurement: Practical ways to cope with the organ shortage. *Transplant Proc,* 28, 1869-70.

Ptacek, J.T., and Eberhardt, T.L. (1996). Breaking bad news. *JAMA,* 276, 496-502.

Rosendale, J.D., et al. (2003). Hormonal resuscitation yields more transplanted hearts with improved early function. *UNOS Update,* May/June, 8.

Verbal, M., and Worth, J. (1997). Reservations and preferences among procurement professionals concerning the donation of specific organs and tissues. *J Trans Coor,* 7, 111-5.

Wood, R.F. (1996). Donor management: Multiorgan procurement and renal preservation. *J R Med,* 89, 23-4.

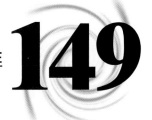

Identification of Potential Organ Donors

PURPOSE: Potential organ donors are cared for in the critical care environment. They are ventilator-dependent and usually require vasoactive agents for blood pressure support. The early identification of potential donors maximizes the availability of organs for transplantation.

June Hinkle

PREREQUISITE NURSING KNOWLEDGE

- Knowledge of federal rules, state laws, organ procurement organization (OPO) policies, and hospital policies regarding organ donation from patients diagnosed with brain death and from patients who are non-heart-beating donors.
- Organ recovery takes place either from patients who have been declared brain-dead or from non-heart-beating donors. The medical suitability of the patient must be determined before any discussion about donation.
- OPOs are nonprofit agencies that determine the medical suitability of potential donors. OPO coordinators do the following:
  - ❖ Approach families for consent to donate
  - ❖ Explain to the family that the patient is an organ donor due to registration in a donation registry
  - ❖ Coordinate the recovery of organs
- In brain death, cessation of function is determined when clinical evaluation discloses absence of both cerebral and brain stem function (see Procedure 147).
- Non-heart-beating donors are those who have experienced a cardiopulmonary arrest or are being removed from life support and the family or significant other wishes to donate organs.[6] OPO and hospital policies regarding non-heart-beating donors vary between institutions and states (see Procedure 151).
- As of August 1998, every death or imminent death in a United States hospital must be reported to an organ procurement agency to meet the federal rules of the U.S. Department of Health and Human Services.[4]

- The only persons who should approach the family about organ donation is the designated hospital requestor or the OPO coordinator.[4] If the hospital has identified designated requestors, they are trained by the OPO to explain donation options and obtain consent if indicated.
- Before caring for potential organ donors and their families, critical care nurses should explore his or her own personal values and beliefs about life, death, and ethical issues surrounding transplantation.[2,5]
- Organ transplantation is a viable therapeutic modality for patients with end-stage organ disease. Thousands of patients currently are waiting for the availability of an organ for their end-stage disease.
- The Joint Commission on Accreditation of Healthcare Organizations (JCAHO) has established standards for accreditation related to organ donation. These standards are updated as federal regulations and rules change. They can be found under Standard RI.2.[1]
- A patient's driver's license may indicate the desire to be an organ donor or may be consent for donation.
- Depending on the laws of the state, organ donor information on a driver license may be consent for donation regardless of family wishes, or it may be helpful for the family when they make a decision about donation.
- It is important not to offer the family the option of donation. The designated hospital requestor or OPO coordinator will know the laws of your state, the implications of a donation registry in your state, and the patient's driver license designation, if appropriate. A donation registry allows a patient to designate whether he or she wishes to be a donor after death and allows for first-person consent. The registry may supercede the family desires regarding donation.

EQUIPMENT

- Flashlight
- Neurologic checklist
- Tongue blade
- Cotton-tipped applicator
- Ventilator
- Arterial line or automatic blood pressure cuff
- Urinary catheter
- Electrocardiogram (ECG) monitor and electrodes
- Two blood gas kits
- Nonsterile gloves

Additional equipment to have available, as needed, includes the following:

- Cotton ball
- Suction catheter

PATIENT AND FAMILY EDUCATION

- Explain the medical and nursing care provided to the patient. ➸***Rationale:*** Ensures that the family has some level of understanding about the therapies used to treat or support the patient. Also assures family members that the appropriate therapies are being employed and that the patient is not experiencing increased discomfort because of these therapies.
- Inform the family of the patient's current condition. ➸***Rationale:*** Keeps family informed and prepares the family for realistic expectations of the patient's outcome.

PATIENT ASSESSMENT AND PREPARATION

Patient Assessment

- Obtain a thorough medical and social history from the family about the patient that includes current age, injuries, chronic diseases, surgical history, familial history, and social habits. Of particular interest is a history of renal disease, hypertension, diabetes mellitus, malignant disease, hepatitis, and human immunodeficiency virus (HIV). ➸***Rationale:*** Allows the OPO transplant coordinator to assess the medical suitability of the patient for organ donation.
- Perform a physical assessment, with emphasis on the following: old surgical scars, needle track marks, tattoos, body piercing, congenital anomalies, and injuries. ➸***Rationale:*** Provides indicators of physical conditions or social behaviors that may influence organ suitability for transplantation. Patients with recent tattoos and body piercings or fresh needle tracks are considered high risk and may not be accepted as a donor by the transplant team.
- Assess the patient's neurologic status, including response to pain, eye opening, communication attempts, pupillary response, gag reflex, cough reflex, corneal reflex, and observation of attempts to breathe spontaneously at a rate greater than that set on the ventilator. ➸***Rationale:*** Identifies changes in the neurologic status; implement treatment as appropriate.
- Assess the patient's Glasgow Coma Scale (GCS) score and whether the patient is receiving any sedating medications that may alter the GCS. ➸***Rationale:*** Provides baseline neurologic data.
- Monitor pertinent data, including urine output, liver function studies, renal function studies, electrolytes, serum osmolality, coagulation panel, urine studies including specific gravity, and culture results. ➸***Rationale:*** Provides data that may influence organ suitability for transplantation.
- Determine an accurate measurement of height and weight. ➸***Rationale:*** Provides information for matching organs to a recipient of a corresponding body size.

Patient Preparation

- Ensure that the family understands preprocedural teaching. Answer questions as they arise and reinforce information as needed. ➸***Rationale:*** Evaluates and reinforces understanding of previously taught information.
- Any patient with a significant and potentially life-threatening injury to the head, whether caused by trauma, an intracerebral hemorrhage, or an anoxic event, should be referred to the OPO as early as possible for evaluation as a potential organ donor.[3] ➸***Rationale:*** This allows the OPO coordinator to evaluate the patient and provides the critical care nurse with information about the patient's potential as an organ donor.
- When neurologic testing to determine clinical brain death begins, ensure that the patient is normothermic and that no sedating medications have been given (see Procedure 147). ➸***Rationale:*** Hypothermia and sedating medications will interfere with brain death testing by clinical criteria.

Procedure for Identification of Potential Organ Donors

Steps	Rationale	Special Considerations
1. Discuss the patient's prognosis with the health care team.	Ensures that all members of the health care team have the same understanding of the patient's prognosis.	
2. Contact the OPO coordinator if the patient has a life-threatening illness.	Early referral provides information about the potential for organ donation.	

Procedure for Identification of Potential Organ Donors—*Continued*

Steps	Rationale	Special Considerations
3. Wash hands and don nonsterile gloves.	Reduces the transmission of microorganisms; standard precautions.	
4. Obtain laboratory samples as prescribed (e.g., complete blood count, liver and renal function tests, electrolyte levels, hepatitis and HIV testing).	Provides data to assess organ function.	
5. Monitor vital signs.	Determines the presence of hemodynamic stability or instability. Decreased perfusion to the organs may alter organ donor potential.	
6. Monitor fluid status.	Determines kidney perfusion or hypoperfusion. Decreased urine output may alter organ donor potential.	
7. Assist with brain death determination (see Procedure 147).	Facilitates the process and assesses whether the patient may be a possible organ donor.	
8. Assist the physician when he or she informs the family of the results of the brain death determination.	Facilitates the process and offers support.	This meeting is best done in a quiet, private setting. Do not discuss donation.
9. Contact the OPO when the patient is declared brain-dead.	OPO coordinators will discuss possible organ donation with the family.	

Expected Outcomes

- Timely determination of brain death occurs.
- A representative of the OPO is notified of a patient determined to be brain-dead.
- If the patient meets the criteria of brain death and is medically suitable to be a donor, the OPO coordinator is notified. The OPO coordinator, along with members of the health care team, approaches the family with the option of organ donation.
- The family comprehends the patient's status and prognosis.

Unexpected Outcomes

- The recognition and documentation of brain death does not occur.
- The OPO is not notified before the pronouncement of brain death or the discussion of organ donation.
- The OPO is not notified when life support is removed from a patient who meets brain death criteria (institution-and state-specific).
- The family fails to comprehend the patient's status and prognosis.

Patient Monitoring and Care

Steps	Rationale	Reportable Conditions
		These conditions should be reported if they persist despite nursing interventions.
1. Monitor the patient's neurologic status and monitor intracranial pressure (if available) every hour and more frequently, as needed.	Determines changes in neurologic status so that treatment can be initiated.	• Changes in neurologic function • Sudden, sustained increase in intracranial pressure
2. Monitor vital signs every hour and more frequently, as needed.	Determines cardiovascular status and needed treatment.	• Changes in vital signs
3. Continuously monitor cardiac rhythm.	Assesses cardiac status.	• Dysrhythmias

Procedure continues on the following page

Patient Monitoring and Care—*Continued*

Steps	Rationale	Reportable Conditions
4. Continuously monitor pulse oximetry and intermittent blood gases.	Determines oxygenation status.	• Changes in pulse oximetry • Abnormal ABG results
5. Monitor urinary output every hour.	Determines perfusion to the kidneys; may affect organ donation.	• Changes in urinary output; urinary output less than 0.5 ml/kg/h
6. Obtain laboratory samples for liver function tests, renal function tests, coagulation values, urine specific gravity, hemoglobin, white blood cell count, electrolytes, osmolality, hepatitis screen, HIV screening, and cultures. Frequency and prescriptions vary depending on the organs being recovered and the patient's health status.	Determines organ function; may affect organ donation.	• Abnormal laboratory results

Documentation

Documentation should include the following:

- Family education
- Patient history and physical findings
- Vital signs, neurologic findings, and if applicable, intracranial pressures
- Intake and output

- Communication with the physician about changes in the patient's physiologic status
- Communications with the OPO coordinators
- Unexpected outcomes
- Additional interventions

References

1. CAMH 2003. (2003). *Automated Hospitals, Patient Rights and Organization Ethics,* Joint Commission on Accreditation of Healthcare Organizations.
2. Davies, M., et al. (2002). The impact of health professionals' attitudes about being registered donors on the availability of organs. *Nurs Times, 1,* 36-9.
3. Ehrle, R.N., Shafer, T.J., and Nelson, K.R. (1999). Determination and referral of potential organ donors and consent for organ donation: Best practices—a blueprint for success. *Crit Care Nurs, 19,* 21-36.
4. Health Care Financing Administration. (1998). Medicare and Medicaid programs: Hospital condition of participation; identification of potential organ, tissue and eye donors. Title 42, Vol 3, *Federal Register.*
5. Heitman, L.K. (1987). Organ donation in community hospitals: A nursing perspective. *Curr Concepts Nurs, 1,* 2-5.
6. Herdman, R., and Potts, J.T. (1997). *Non-Heart-Beating Organ Transplantation: Medical and Ethical Issues in Procurement.* Washington, DC: National Academy Press.

Additional Readings

Alleman, K., et al. (1996). Public perceptions of an appropriate donor card/brochure. *J Trans Nurs, 6,* 105-8.
American Academy of Neurology. (1995). Summary statement: Practice parameters for determining brain death in adults. *Neurology, 45,* 1012-14.

Day, L. (2001). How nurses shift from care of a brain-injured patient to maintenance of a brain-dead organ donor. *AJCC,* 10, 306-12.
Flick, C., and Metules, T. (2002). Organ donation: A delicate balance. *RN, 65,* 43-7.
Holmquist, M. (1996). Organ donor care map: A multidisciplinary approach. *J Trans Nurs, 6,* 101-5.
Ingram, J.E., Buckner, E.B., and Rayburn, A.B. (2002). Critical care nurses' attitudes and knowledge related to organ donation. *DCCN, 21,* 249-55.
Lewis, D.D., and Valerius, W. (1999). Non-heart-beating organ donation: An answer to the organ shortage. *Crit Care Nurs,* 19, 70-5.
McConnell, E.A. (2001). Myths & facts...about organ donation. *Nurs, 31,* 76.
Molzahn, A.E., Starzomski, R., and McCormick, J. (2003). The supply of organs for transplantation: Issues and challenges. *Neph Nurs J, 30,* 17-28.
Morgan, S.E., and Miller, J.K. (2002). Beyond the organ donor card: The effect of knowledge, attitudes, and values on willingness to communicate about organ donation to family members. *Health Comm, 14,* 121-34.
Olson, L., et al. (1996). Twelve years' experience with non-heart-beating donors. *J Trans Nurs, 6,* 196-9.
Winsett, R.P. (2002). Attitudes about organ transplantation reflected different conceptions of the body. *Evidence-Based Nurs, 5,* 31.

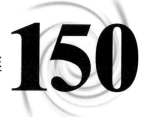

PROCEDURE **150**

Request for Organ Donation

P U R P O S E :   To facilitate a discussion about organ donation. The focus of the discussion may be informing family of the patient's prior consent to be a donor or asking the family to make a decision to donate. If the family makes the decision, the focus of the discussion should be the best decision for the family—and that decision may not be organ donation.

June Hinkle

PREREQUISITE NURSING KNOWLEDGE

- Knowledge of federal, state, organ procurement organization (OPO), and hospital policies regarding organ donation from patients diagnosed with brain death and from patients who are non-heart-beating donors.
- Every death or imminent death in a United States hospital must be reported to an OPO to meet the federal rules of the U.S. Department of Health and Human Services.[2]
- The only person who should approach the family about organ donation is the designated hospital requestor or the OPO coordinator. The designated requestor must complete an OPO-approved program.[2] The training is OPO specific but usually includes information on brain death testing, explaining brain death to families, dealing with grief, understanding cultural differences, and role playing the consent process.
- Consent rates for organ donation increase when families are given time to accept their relative's death, when the request for donation is made by a member of the OPO with the hospital designated requestor, and when the request is made in a quiet, private setting.[1]
- According to a survey conducted in 1993, only 52% of people wishing to be organ donors have told their families of their desire and only 28% have signed a donor card or designated their wishes on their driver's license.[3]
- Most states use some form of designation for organ donation on the driver's license. The designation may be legal consent for donation despite family wishes, or it may serve as an indication of the patient's desire. If the family does not know the patient's desire related to organ donation, it is sometimes helpful to locate the patient's driver's license.
- Knowledge about state donation registries, advance directives and laws related to organ donation is essential. Donation registries are usually associated with the driver license and may indicate an individual's desire to be a donor or actual consent for donation. The health care proxy may be the decision maker for organ donation or the decision related to organ donation may revert to the nearest next-of-kin.

EQUIPMENT

- Brain death information materials for the family
- Donor information materials for the family
- Forms needed for consent for organ donation

PATIENT AND FAMILY EDUCATION

- Assess the family's understanding of brain death. ➡️*Rationale:* The diagnosis may be difficult for the family to understand and frequently requires multiple explanations before the diagnosis is understood.
- Allow a designated, trained requestor to provide information to the family regarding organ donation. This may be an OPO coordinator or a hospital-based designated requestor.[2] ➡️*Rationale:* Meets the federal mandate and provides the family with accurate, complete information about the organ donation process.

PATIENT ASSESSMENT AND PREPARATION

Patient Assessment

- Determine whether the patient is a potential organ donor. ➤*Rationale:* The coordinator from the OPO determines the appropriateness of potential organ donors. Donation should not be offered to family members as an option unless the OPO has determined that the patient is a potential donor.
- Assess the family's ability to verbalize and understand brain death. ➤*Rationale:* The family is more likely to donate organs if they accept the diagnosis of brain death.[2]

Patient Preparation

- Ensure that the family understands teaching related to brain death. Answer questions as they arise and reinforce information as needed. ➤*Rationale:* Evaluates and reinforces understanding of previously taught information.
- Consult the designated requestor and OPO coordinator to determine when and how they will approach the family about organ donation. ➤*Rationale:* Coordinates the request process.

Procedure for Request for Organ Donation

Steps	Rationale	Special Considerations
1. Assist with the determination of brain death (see Procedure 147).	Facilitates the process and assesses whether the patient may be a possible organ donor.	
2. Consult the OPO when brain death testing begins.	Early assessment by the OPO coordinator determines whether the family is offered the option of donation.	
3. Ensure that the patient's brain death has been declared.	Family can be approached for an organ donation discussion after brain death criteria have been met.	
4. Coordinate a meeting between the family, designated requestor, and/or OPO coordinator.	Facilitates the process.	This meeting is best done in a quiet, private setting.
5. The designated requestor or the OPO coordinator will determine whether the patient had an advance directive about organ donation or is listed in a donor registry.	If a family discussion about organ donation had occurred, the family is more likely to donate organs.	According to a survey, 93% of family members would donate organs if their loved one had requested it, whereas only 47% of family members would donate organs if no discussion had taken place.[3]
6. The designated requestor or OPO coordinator will explain the process of recovery if the patient has an advance directive requesting organ donation.	Keeps the family informed of the process that will take place.	
7. If there is no advance directive, the designated requestor or the OPO coordinator determines whether the family will consent to organ donation.	Determines family willingness to consider organ donation.	
8. If the family decides to donate or there is an advance directive for organ donation, the OPO will coordinate the donation process of the brain-dead patient. If there is conflict among family members or disagreement about the prior consent, the OPO will work with the family to understand and resolve issues.	The OPO coordinator becomes responsible for prescribing care for the patient until organ recovery occurs.	All laboratory values and changes in patient condition should be reported to the OPO coordinator.

Procedure **for Request for Organ Donation**—*Continued*

Steps	Rationale	Special Considerations
9. If the patient is having life support withdrawn and the family has consented to non-heart-beating donation, the OPO works with the medical and nursing team to coordinate the donation (see Procedure 151).	The patient's care is the responsibility of the medical team until death is pronounced. This may be in the ICU or operating room.	All laboratory values and changes in patient condition should be reported to the medical staff and the OPO coordinator.
10. If the patient is brain-dead and the family decides not to donate, discuss with the physician, family, and health care team when and how to discontinue therapy.	Coordinates end-of-life care.	Ensure that the family understands what will happen when therapy is withdrawn.
11. Provide the emotional support the family needs to cope with the death of their loved one.	Supports the grieving family.	
12. Involve pastoral care, social workers, and/or grief counselors.	Provides additional support to the grieving family.	

Expected Outcomes

- The family receives accurate, timely information about organ donation provided by a hospital designated requestor and/or the OPO coordinator.
- Patient wishes related to organ donation are honored.
- The family makes a decision about organ donation based on the prior expressed desires of the patient, cultural and religious beliefs, and the information provided about the organ donation process.
- The family understands the organ donation recovery process.

Unexpected Outcomes

- The family is approached about organ donation before the determination of brain death.
- An untrained staff member approaches the family about organ donation.
- The family members are not kept informed as to the care of their loved one.

Patient Monitoring and Care

Steps	Rationale	Reportable Conditions
		These conditions should be reported if they persist despite nursing interventions.
1. Encourage the family to be at the bedside and to be involved as much as possible with patient care.	Promotes patient and family time together.	• Changes in family preferences for care
2. The OPO will coordinate the care of a brain-dead patient if the family decides to donate organs.	Facilitates patient management and the donation process.	• Changes in patient condition
3. If the family of a patient who is brain-dead decides not to donate, coordinate a plan for removal of therapy (see Procedure 152).	Facilitates the removal of therapy.	• Family's wishes for removal of therapy
4. Support the family decision, whether the family decides for or against organ donation.	Organ donation is a personal decision for each patient and family. The family members needs to make the decision they feel is right for their loved one and their family.	
5. Encourage family involvement in end-of-life care.	Promotes family involvement, family presence, family control, and family time together.	

Documentation

Documentation should include the following:

- Family education
- Date and time of brain death determination or when respirations and cardiac activity cease
- Notification of the OPO
- Presentation of organ donation options to the family, including the date, time, and location; name of requestor; summary of information provided; and response of family

- If family requests organ donation, completion of appropriate donation consent forms
- Unexpected outcomes
- Additional interventions

References

1. Beasley, C.L., et al. (1997). The impact of a comprehensive, hospital-focused intervention to increase organ donation. *J Trans Coor,* 7, 6-13.
2. Health Care Financing Administration. (1998). Medicare and Medicaid programs: Hospital condition of participation; identification of potential organ, tissue and eye donors. Title 42, Vol 3, *Federal Register.*
3. The Gallup Organization. (1993). *The American Public's Attitudes Toward Organ Donation and Transplantation.* The Partnership for Organ Donation.

Additional Readings

DeJong, W., and Franz, H.G. (1998). Requesting organ donation: An interview study of donor and nondonor families. *Am J Crit Care,* 7, 13-23.

Duckworth, R.M., et al. (1998). Acute bereavement services and routine referral as a mechanism to increase donation. *J Trans Coor,* 8, 16-8.

Ehrle, R.N., Shafer, T.J., and Nelson, K.R. (1999). Referral, request, and consent for organ donation: Best practice: a blueprint for success. *Crit Care Nurs,* 19, 21-33.

Frants, H.G., et al. (1997). Explaining brain death: A critical feature of the donation process. *J Trans Coor,* 7, 14-21.

Gortmaker, S.L., Beasley, C.L., and Sheehy, E. (1998). Improving the request process to increase family consent for organ donation. *J Trans Coor,* 8, 210-7.

Holmquist, M., et al. (1999). A critical pathway: Guiding care for organ donors. *Crit Care Nurs,* 19, 84-98.

Latour, T. (1998). Should we be more aggressive in honoring a donor's wishes? *Nephrol News Issues,* 12, 41-3.

Riley, L.P., and Collican, M.B. (1999). Needs of families of organ donors: Facing death and life. *Crit Care Nurs,* 19, 53-9.

Rocheleau, C.A. (2001). Increasing family consent for organ donation: Findings and challenges. *Prog in Transpl,* 11, 194-200.

Schaefdfer, M.J., Johnson, E., and Suddaby, E.C. (1998). Analysis of donor versus non-donor demographics. *J Trans Coor,* 8, 9-15.

Siminoff, L.A., and Lawrence, R.H. (2002). Knowing patients' preferences about organ donation: Does it make a difference? *J of Trauma,* 53, 754-60.

Siminoff, L.A., Lawrence, R.H., and Arnold, R.M. (2003). Comparison of black and white families' experiences and perceptions regarding organ donation requests. *Crit Care Med,* 31, 146-51.

Siminoff, L.A., Lawrence, R.H., and Zhang, A. (2002). Decoupling: What is it and does it really help increase consent to organ donation? *Progress in Transp,* 12, 52-60.

Sullivan, H., Blakely, D., and Davis, K. (1998). An in-house coordinator program to increase organ donation in public teaching hospitals. *J Trans Coor,* 8, 40-2.

U.S. Department of Health and Human Services. (2002). *Annual Report Transplant Data 1992-2001.* Department of Health and Human Services.

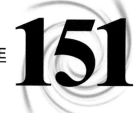

PROCEDURE **151**

Non-Heart-Beating Organ Donation (Donation After Cardiac Death)

PURPOSE: Typically, organ donation follows death determined by neurologic criteria. Organ donation can also occur when a person has suffered an unexpected cardiac arrest and resuscitation has not been achieved or when a person's life is sustained by technologies and for whom life support will be withdrawn.

Margaret M. Mahon

PREREQUISITE NURSING KNOWLEDGE

- Knowledge of federal rules, state laws, organ procurement organization (OPO) policies, and hospital policies regarding organ donation from patients considered as potential non-heart-beating donors.[1-5]
- For non-heart-beating organ donation to occur, patient death is determined by cessation of cardiac and respiratory function, rather than by absence of cerebral and brain stem function.
- The Institute of Medicine has issued several reports on donation after cardiac death,[2,3] one of which includes recommendations for policy development related to procurement of organs from non-heart-beating organ donors.[2] These recommendations have come to shape programs and practice related to donation after cardiac death, including the following:
  - ❖ Written, locally approved non-heart-beating donor protocols
  - ❖ Public openness of non-heart-beating donor protocols
  - ❖ Case-by-case decisions about the premortem administration of medication
  - ❖ Family consent for premortem cannulation
  - ❖ Conflict-of-interest safeguards
  - ❖ Determination of death (in controlled non-heart-beating donations) by cessation of cardiopulmonary function for at least 5 minutes by electrocardiographic and arterial pressure monitoring

- ❖ Family options (e.g., attendance at life support withdrawal) and financial protection
- Donor criteria for non-heart-beating organ donation includes:
  - ❖ A ventilator-dependent patient who has sustained a neurologic injury from which recovery is not possible, but who does not meet brain death criteria
  - ❖ A severely ill patient receiving life-sustaining therapy
  - ❖ A patient who has had an unexpected cardiac arrest and for whom resuscitation has not been achieved
- Families of patients being considered for donation after cardiac death are dealing only secondarily with the request for organ donation. First and foremost, these families are dealing with the usually sudden and severe injury or illness of the patient. They must integrate the fact of the illness, and then the likelihood or inevitability of death. It is only after those facts are presented that the possibility of donation can be broached.
- Many myths and misunderstandings are common in families confronted with the request for donation. For instance, some people still believe that a donor's life is shortened to ensure adequate organ supply. This belief must be considered when explaining the process of donation after cardiac death. The standard for death is not brain death, but rather cardiac death. The patient is still dead, but understanding that different criteria are applied to "diagnose" death can be difficult for families.
- Families should never be told, "We've tried everything. There is nothing else we can do." This often engenders

feelings or fear of abandonment of the patient by the health care team. Until death is declared, there is an aggressive focus on symptom management. Decisions about what symptoms to manage and how to manage them should be based on the standard of care for a specific type of injury (e.g., multiple internal and orthopedic injuries following a motor vehicle accident) or illness (surgery that necessitated opening a patient's chest or abdomen).

- More appropriate language would be, for example, "When your brother was admitted, our goal was to heal him, and we did many procedures to try to achieve that. We have been unable to cure him. We have to shift the focus of our interventions from cure to comfort." Rather than going from "everything" to "nothing," a *goals of care* framework is used. When it becomes evident that the patient may or will die, language should be specific: "I'm sorry, but we believe that your brother will die from his injuries." Avoiding the use of the words "die," "dying," or "death" can result in some family members being unsure about what the message really is. The shock and tension can interfere with integration of reality.

- Determination of "Do Not Resuscitate" (DNR) or "Do Not Attempt Resuscitation" (DNAR) status and the decision to discontinue life-prolonging therapies must occur before the discussion about donation after cardiac death can occur. Documentation of the process and the decisions must be put in the medical record. Most institutions have specific guidelines about DNR/DNAR status. The health care team that has cared for the patient donor *must* be a separate team from the team that participates in the organ recovery.

EQUIPMENT

- Consent forms
- Prepared operating room

PATIENT AND FAMILY EDUCATION

- Inform the family of the patient's current condition. ➤*Rationale:* Keeps the family informed and prepares the family for realistic expectations of the patient's outcome.
- Explain the medical and nursing care provided to the patient. ➤*Rationale:* Ensures that the family understands therapies provided to treat and support the patient.

PATIENT ASSESSMENT AND PREPARATION

Patient Assessment

- Obtain a thorough medical and social history from the family about the patient, including current age, injuries, chronic diseases, surgical history, familial history, and social habits. Of particular interest is a history of renal disease, hypertension, diabetes mellitus, malignant disease, hepatitis, and human immunodeficiency virus (HIV). ➤*Rationale:* Allows the OPO transplant coordinator to assess the medical suitability of the patient for organ donation.
- Perform a physical assessment, with emphasis on old surgical scars, needle track marks, tattoos, body piercing, congenital anomalies, and injuries. ➤*Rationale:* These are indicators of physical conditions or social behaviors that may influence organ suitability for transplantation. Patients with recent tattoos and body piercings or fresh needle tracks are considered high risk and may not be accepted as a donor by the transplant team.
- Monitor pertinent patient data, including urine output, liver function studies, renal function studies, electrolytes, serum osmolality, coagulation panel, and urine studies, including specific gravity and culture results. ➤*Rationale:* Provides data that may influence organ suitability for transplantation.
- Determine an accurate measurement of the patient's height and weight. ➤*Rationale:* Provides information for matching organs to a recipient of a corresponding body size.

Patient Preparation

- Ensure that the family understands preprocedural teaching. Answer questions as they arise and reinforce information as needed. ➤*Rationale:* Evaluates and reinforces understanding of previously taught information.
- Refer patients with a potentially life-threatening illness or injury to the OPO as early as possible for evaluation as a potential organ donor. ➤*Rationale:* This allows the OPO coordinator to evaluate the patient and provides the critical care nurse with information about the patient's potential as an organ donor.

Procedure	**for Non-Heart-Beating Organ Donation (Donation After Cardiac Death)**	
Steps	**Rationale**	**Special Considerations**
1. Discuss the patient's prognosis with the health care team and identify whether the patient has a grave prognosis.	Early implementation of the process ensures that all involved can take the time needed for adequate decision making.	

Procedure **for Non-Heart-Beating Organ Donation (Donation After Cardiac Death)**—*Continued*

Steps	Rationale	Special Considerations
2. Collaborate with the physician when he or she discusses the patient's prognosis with the family.	Prepares the family for the expected patient outcome and provides an opportunity to offer family support.	No mention of organ donation should be made in this meeting. The decoupling of prognosis and the discussion of possible organ donation is essential.
3. Contact the OPO coordinator to determine whether the patient is eligible for organ donation.	The OPO does an independent evaluation to determine eligibility for donation.	If the patient is deemed ineligible for donation, the process ceases here.
4. If it is determined that the patient is not a suitable candidate for organ donation, complete and place the OPO referral form on the patient's chart.	Documents the referral and that the patient is not eligible for organ donation.	
5. If, after initial consultation between the OPO coordinator and the health care team, it is determined that the patient might be an appropriate donor, the donation process will commence.	Ongoing collaboration is necessary for an optimal outcome.	
6. If the patient is a possible candidate for donation, coordinate a meeting between the family, designated requestor and/or OPO coordinator.	Family consent for organ donation is greatest when the OPO and the hospital staff collaborate in the consent process.[1] Contact with the family by the OPO coordinator must not be made until a decision has been made to forgo life-prolonging therapies and the likelihood of medical suitability has been determined by the OPO representative.	Many states have legislated guidelines as to who can consent for organ donation. Know the next-of-kin order for consent in your jurisdiction. The Uniform Anatomical Gift Act also has a designated hierarchy for contact.
7. If there is an appropriate designation by the patient indicating a desire not to be an organ donor, or the same stated in a valid advance directive or by an appropriate surrogate decision maker, further approaches for donation should not be made.	The patient is his or her own decision maker, even when the patient is no longer able to communicate. A patient's wishes as appropriately communicated though an advance directive or an informed surrogate optimizes respect for patient autonomy.	
8. The OPO coordinator discusses the option of organ donation with the patient's family.	Determines patient desires and family willingness to consider organ donation.	
9. If the decision is made by the family to consider organ donation, the OPO coordinator coordinates the process with the health care team.	OPO involvement increases the likelihood of successful procurement. In addition, they can provide guidance and support during the process.	If the patient's death is likely to be a coroner or medical examiner case, consent should be obtained from the medical examiner or the coroner prior to tissue or organ recovery. The OPO representative coordinates this consent process.
10. Allow the family to spend as much time as they desire with the patient prior to discontinuation of life-sustaining therapy.	This is an important opportunity in the family's process of saying good-bye and beginning the grieving process.	

Procedure continues on the following page

Procedure for Non-Heart-Beating Organ Donation (Donation After Cardiac Death)—*Continued*

Steps	Rationale	Special Considerations
11. Administer medications as needed to promote patient comfort (e.g., manage pain, dyspnea, and anxiety).	Symptoms known to be associated with dying should be aggressively managed.	
12. Determine the approximate time that the patient will be taken to the operating room.	Allows the family and the health care team to know what to expect.	
13. Determine the roles of various personnel when the patient is taken to the OR: A. OPO coordinator B. Anesthesiologist C. Critical care nurse D. Operating room nurse E. Physician F. Respiratory therapist G. Family support (e.g., clergy, grief counselor)	Determines who will be in the operating room setting and defines health care provider responsibilities.	
14. Determine in advance who will withdraw life-sustaining therapy.	Facilitates the withdrawal of life-sustaining therapy process.	Some health care providers, including anesthesiologists, may not want to be a part of this process.[4]
15. Determine family preference for being physically present or absent during the process of withdrawing life-sustaining therapy (e.g., mechanical ventilation).	Care of the dying patient and family is of primary importance through the time of death. Families should be given the option of being present until the patient dies.	Patients who will be donors after cardiac death are often taken to the OR prior to withdrawal. Accommodations for family presence in the OR must be made. Since family members are almost never allowed in the OR, this may require time-consuming and skilled negotiation with the OR staff. Follow institutional policy regarding family presence and support during this process.
16. Transport the patient to the OR.	Prepares for the organ donation process.	Prior to transporting the patient, the process and timeline should be explained to the OR, and the family should again be given the opportunity to be present prior to and at the time of withdrawal.
17. When the patient arrives in the OR, the patient may be prepped and draped by the organ recovery team. This team then leaves the room. In some cases, the draping is done after death has been declared.	It is essential to keep separate the health care team members who will provide for the patient until death and those who will harvest the organs.	The family has consented to donation, and draping and preparing the patient is non-invasive and non-burdensome. If the withdrawal did not occur in the OR, the donor will immediately be transported to the OR. The withdrawal may occur in the PACU, outside the OR, or even in a patient room if the OR is nearby.
18. When the entire health care team and family are ready, life-sustaining therapy will be withdrawn.	Coordinates the end-of-life process.	
19. If ventilatory and hemodynamic support have been discontinued, there must be an interval of at least	Organ donation can occur only after cardiopulmonary death is confirmed.	

Procedure	for Non-Heart-Beating Organ Donation (Donation After Cardiac Death)—*Continued*	
Steps	**Rationale**	**Special Considerations**
5 minutes of cessation of circulatory function (evidenced by ECG and blood pressure monitoring via an arterial catheter) before death is pronounced and the organ removal process begins.		
20. After discontinuation of life-sustaining therapy, but prior to the 5-minute interval, a femoral cannula may be inserted if prior consent has been obtained from the individual consenting for organ donation.	Cannulation is an invasive procedure that does not benefit the patient; therefore, a separate consent is necessary for this procedure.[4]	In some cases, cannulation is done prior to discontinuation from life-sustaining therapy. This should be done only (1) after a decision to withdraw therapies has been made, (2) with local anesthesia if needed, and (3) with specific and distinct consent. Some institutions initiate a surgical approach for recovery using an abdominal aortic approach, and do not use a femoral cannula.
21. If the patient continues to breath or has a pulse and blood pressure for more than 30 minutes after the discontinuation of ventilatory and hemodynamic support, the donation is canceled; assist in transfer of the patient back to the original room.	Family must be informed of the time limit to the donation process ahead of time.	Ensure that the family is aware of possible outcomes, as well as of bereavement resources.
22. The patient's attending physician should be present and should pronounce death when it occurs.	One patient's life cannot be shortened to ascertain organs for another; the donor must have died before organ and tissue recovery can begin.	While attending physicians are not always present for deaths, especially when the time of death cannot be predicted, their presence conveys a message of respect for the patient, the family, and the act of donation.
23. Provide family support.	Supports the grieving family.	

Expected Outcomes

- The patient's wishes regarding donation are respected.
- The patient dies immediately or within a few minutes of discontinuation of life-sustaining therapy.

Unexpected Outcomes

- The family does not agree with patient preferences.
- Dying is prolonged.

Patient Monitoring and Care

Steps	**Rationale**	**Reportable Conditions**
		These conditions should be reported if they persist despite nursing interventions.
1. Monitor the patient's temperature and intervene as necessary to achieve normothermia.	Minimizes coagulopathies.	- Temperature less than 96°F
2. Monitor the patient's cardiac and hemodynamic status continuously.	Determines hemodynamic stability.	- Systolic BP less than 90 mm Hg - Changes in heart rate or other parameters set by the OPO coordinator

Procedure continues on the following page

Patient Monitoring and Care—*Continued*

Steps	Rationale	Reportable Conditions
3. Monitor the patient's oxygenation status via continuous pulse oximetry and arterial blood gases.	Determines the presence of hypoxemia.	• Pao_2 less than 100 mm Hg • Sao_2 less than or equal to 96% or other parameters as set by the OPO coordinator
4. Monitor the patient's urine output.	Determines renal function.	• Urine output less than 0.5 ml/kg/hr
5. Monitor laboratory studies as determined by the OPO coordinator (e.g., electrolytes, renal and live function tests).	Determines organ function.	• Abnormal laboratory results
6. Provide family support. Incorporate the grief counselor and pastoral care.	Offers family resources during grieving.	• Ineffective family coping

Documentation

Documentation should include the following:

- Family education
- Prognosis and family discussion
- Knowledge of patient preferences
- Completed consent form for organ donation and recovery
- Complete donor record, including vital signs, assessments, treatment, and the clinical status of the donor
- Plan for withdrawal
- Time of withdrawal of life-sustaining therapy

- Plan and implementation of symptom management
- Communication with the family, including summary of information provided and response of the family
- Time of transportation to the OR
- Determination of cessation of respirations and cardiac activity
- Unexpected outcomes
- Family coping
- Additional interventions

References

1. Gortmaker, E.T. (1998). Improving the request process to increase family consent for organ donation. *J Transplant Coord,* Dec.
2. Institute of Medicine, Potts, J., Principal Investigator. (1997). *Non-Heart-Beating Organ Transplantation: Medical and Ethics Issues in Procurement.* Washington, DC: National Academy Press.
3. Institute of Medicine. (2000). *Non-Heart-Beating Organ Transplantation. Practice and Protocols.* Washington, DC: National Academy Press.
4. Van Norman, G.A. (2003). Another matter of life and death. What every anesthesiologist should know about the ethical, legal, and policy implications of the non-heart-beating cadaver organ donor. *Anesthesiology,* 98, 763-73.

Additional Readings

American College of Critical Care Medicine, Society of Critical Care Medicine. (2001). Recommendations for non-heart-beating organ donation. A position paper by the ethics committee. *Crit Care Med,* 29, 1826-31.

Arnold, R.M., and Youngner, S.J. (1995). Time is of the essence: The pressing need for comprehensive non-heart-beating cadaveric donation policies. *Transplant Proceedings,* 27, 2913-21.

D'Alessandro, A.M., Hoffman, R.M., and Belzer, F.O. (1995). Non-heart-beating donors: One response to the organ shortage. *Transplantation Reviews,* 9, 168-76.

Edwards, J.M., Hasz, R.D., and Robertson, A.M. (1999). Non-heart-beating organ donation: Process and review. *AACN Clinical Issues in Critical Care,* 10, 293-300.

Frader, J. (1993). Non-heart-beating organ donation: Personal and institutional conflicts of interest. *Kennedy Institute of Ethics Journal,* 3, 189-98. JHU Press.

Koogler, T., and Costarino, A.T. (1998). The potential benefits of the pediatric non-heart-beating organ donor. *Pediatrics,* 101, 1049-52.

Younger, S.J., and Arnold, R.M. (1993). Ethical, psychosocial, and public policy implications of procuring organs from non-heart-beating cadaver donors. *JAMA,* 269, 2769-74.

P R O C E D U R E **152**

Withholding and Withdrawing Life-Sustaining Therapy

P U R P O S E :   To assist patients and family members with the process of withholding or withdrawing life-sustaining therapy. Life-sustaining therapy may include nutrition, hydration, antibiotics, dialysis, ventilatory therapy, vasoactive therapy, and additional therapies.

Debra Lynn-McHale Wiegand
Margaret M. Mahon

PREREQUISITE NURSING KNOWLEDGE

- Withholding and withdrawing life-sustaining therapy involve end-of-life decisions that commonly result in the death of the patient.
- It is essential to know the state regulations, as well as hospital policies or procedures, regarding end-of-life decision making.
- Hospitals should have policies that direct the process to withhold and withdraw life-sustaining therapy.[1]
- As much information as possible should be obtained from the patient and the patient's family regarding the patient's desired wishes regarding life-sustaining therapy. This information may be ascertained from an advance directive or from verbal conversations with family, friends, or health care providers.
- Advance directives (see Procedure 146) may exist in the form of a living will or a health care proxy.
  - ❖ A living will is a document that identifies treatments a patient would or would not want under specific end-of-life situations. (Most are specific to terminal illness or a permanent state of unconsciousness.)
  - ❖ A health care proxy or a durable power of attorney for health care is a document that identifies a predetermined person who has been given the authority to represent the patient's preferences in health care decision making if the patient is unable to make decisions (e.g., comatose state).
- Patients have a moral and legal right and responsibility to make decisions about their health care and the use of life-sustaining therapy.[1]

- Decision-making capacity is determined by an individual's ability to[3]:
  - ❖ Understand relevant information
  - ❖ Make a judgment about the information in light of his or her values
  - ❖ Intend a certain outcome
  - ❖ Communicate his or her decision to health care providers
- If a patient no longer has decision-making capability, the patient's preferences should be represented by the patient's health care proxy. That is decisions made by the health care proxy should be based on the patient's previously stated wishes or presumed preferences based on lifestyle and prior choices.
- Usually the patient's family is very involved in the process of withholding and withdrawing life-sustaining therapy. On occasion, the patient prefers that the family not be involved. If the patient does not want the family to be involved, the health care team should work with the patient to identify another person who can serve as his or her health care proxy in the event that the patient loses decision-making capacity.
- Dialogue regarding end-of-life care should be comprehensive. Discussions should include what treatments are going to be withheld or withdrawn. Discussions should focus on patient wishes and goals of care. If the goal of care is a peaceful death, then all therapies that do not contribute toward this goal should be considered for discontinuation, including cessation of vasoactive agents, intravenous fluids, nutrition, laboratory studies, x-rays, extubation, etc. Therapies that support the goal of a peaceful death should

be continued, such as pain management, use of anxiolytics to decrease anxiety, frequent skin and mouth care, family presence, etc.

- Health care providers are responsible for knowing how their personal beliefs affect interactions and decisions about withholding and withdrawing of life-sustaining therapy.
- Patients, families, and health care providers often have different values.
- Patients and their families should be actively involved in all health care decisions, including end-of-life decisions (unless the patient requests that family members not be involved; see above).
- Family members involved in end-of-life decision making should be guided by their knowledge of what the patient wants or would want.
- If a critical care nurse cannot support the patient and family in the process of withholding or withdrawing life-sustaining therapy, the critical care nurse should proceed through the appropriate channels to transfer care to another critical care nurse.[1]
- Paralyzing agents must be discontinued and cleared from the patient's body before withdrawal of life-sustaining therapy.
- Maintaining patient dignity and comfort is essential at all times, and especially at the end of life.
- Medications given to relieve pain often have sedative or respiratory depressant side effects; yet this should not be an overriding consideration in their use for dying patients, as long as such use is consistent with the patient's wishes.[2]
- Pain medication titrated to achieve adequate symptom control is ethically justified, even at the expense of maintaining life or hastening death secondarily.[2]
- Family meetings can be very helpful in aiding patients, families, and health care providers in planning end-of-life care.
- Hospital ethics committees can be very helpful in aiding patients, families, and health care providers when conflicts arise with decision making or during the process of withholding or withdrawing life-sustaining therapy discussions.

PATIENT AND FAMILY EDUCATION

- In collaboration with the physician, inform the patient or family of the patient's current condition and prognosis. ➤*Rationale:* Informs and prepares the patient or family of anticipated outcomes.
- Explain resources available to aid with end-of-life decision making (e.g., nurses, physicians, social workers, pastoral care, grief counselors, palliative care team, ethics consultation, ethics committee). ➤*Rationale:* Offers additional resources and support to assist the patient or family with end-of-life decisions.
- Describe how the patient is likely to respond to withholding or withdrawing of therapies, including expected outcomes and unexpected outcomes. ➤*Rationale:* Prepares the patient and the family for the process. If death is anticipated, the dying process may progress quickly or slowly (e.g., occurring within minutes or lasting days). Although rare, death may not ensue after life-sustaining therapy is withheld or withdrawn.
- Explain that analgesia or sedatives will be administered to relieve discomfort that may be experienced during withholding or withdrawing life-sustaining therapy. ➤*Rationale:* Decreases patient and family anxiety to know that patient comfort will be promoted.

PATIENT ASSESSMENT AND PREPARATION

Patient Assessment

- Assist the physician or advanced practice nurse to assess the patient's decision-making capacity (see Procedure 146). ➤*Rationale:* Patients with decision-making capacity should make their own therapy decisions.
- If patients do not have decision-making capacity, determine whether the patient has a designated health care proxy. ➤*Rationale:* The patient's health care proxy should make decisions for the patient if he or she no longer has decision-making capacity.
- If patients do not have decision-making capacity or a health care proxy, identify key individuals who can best represent patient preferences and who will be active participants in therapy decisions. ➤*Rationale:* It is essential that family members are able to communicate patient wishes for end-of-life care or are able to determine to the best of their knowledge what therapies the patient would or would not want. The patient may also have communicated therapy wishes to primary care providers and friends.

Patient Preparation

- Ensure that the patient or family understands preprocedural teaching. Answer questions as they arise and reinforce information as needed. ➤*Rationale:* Evaluates and reinforces understanding of previously taught information.
- Plan the day and time that life-sustaining therapy will be withheld or withdrawn. ➤*Rationale:* Allows family and friends to spend time with the patient and to arrive from out of town. Allows the health care team time to plan availability to be present during therapy changes.
- Identify family or friends whom the patient or family would like present during the withholding or withdrawal process. ➤*Rationale:* Involves the patient or family in planning of the withholding or withdrawal of therapy.
- In addition to nursing, medicine, and possibly respiratory therapy, identify additional members of the health care team whom the patient or family would like present during the withholding or withdrawal process (e.g., clergy, social worker, grief counselor). ➤*Rationale:* Provides

control to the patient or family as they determine essential members of the health care team who should be involved with the withholding or withdrawing of therapy process.

- Encourage the patient and family to personalize the environment by bringing in music or other items that will make the room as the patient would want it to be. ➤➤*Rationale:* Promotes a peaceful, caring environment.

- Establish a patent intravenous access. ➤➤*Rationale:* Necessary for administration of analgesia and anxiolytics.

Procedure | for Withholding and Withdrawing Life-Sustaining Therapy

Steps	Rationale	Special Considerations
1. With the patient, family, and health care team, coordinate a comprehensive plan for the process of withholding and/or withdrawing life-sustaining therapy.	Ensures that key individuals are aware of the plan of end-of-life care. Addresses what aspects of therapy will be withheld and what aspects of therapy will be withdrawn.	The patient, family, and health care providers need to work together to facilitate the process. Thorough preplanning facilitates the process of end-of-life care.
2. Ensure that the patient, health care proxy, and/or family understand and agree to the process of withholding and/or withdrawing life-sustaining therapy.	Ensures the understanding of what will be withheld or withdrawn, when it will be withheld or withdrawn, and in what order (or all at once).	Consult the ethics committee if conflicts arise.
3. Ensure that the patient, health care proxy, or family understand the probable outcome of withholding and/or withdrawing life-sustaining therapy.	Ensures that there are no misperceptions regarding what will happen after therapy is withheld or withdrawn.	
4. Allow the patient and family time to complete family affairs, communicate with each other, spend time together, and say goodbyes.	Facilitates family functioning and the grief process.	
5. Ensure that key members of the health care team are actively involved in the process of withholding and/or withdrawing life-sustaining therapy.	Presents a team approach to support the patient, family, and each other.	Predetermine who will withdraw therapy (e.g., endotracheal tube, pacing wires, central lines).
6. In collaboration with the physician, determine the type, route of administration, dosage, and time that analgesia and other medications such as anxiolytics will be initiated.	Allows time to ensure intravenous access and to obtain and prepare the medication.	Continuous intravenous infusion of pain medication (e.g., morphine sulfate) facilitates constant administration and ease of dosage adjustment.
7. In collaboration with the physician, determine how medications for pain and other symptoms will be titrated to signs of patient discomfort.	Provides a pain management plan to promote patient comfort.	Pain medication should be titrated to increasing dosages only if signs of patient discomfort are present. Signs of discomfort might include verbalization of pain, moaning, grimacing, increase in heart rate, increase in blood pressure, or labored respirations.
8. Assist or place the patient in a preferred position of comfort.	Promotes comfort.	Supine position with the head of bed elevated may facilitate comfort and ease of respirations.
9. Lower the side rails if family and/or friends are present.	Allows the family access to be close to the patient, hold his or her hand, or sit on the bed.	Side rails may need to be raised if the patient is moving, experiencing a seizure, etc.

Procedure continues on the following page

Procedure for Withholding and Withdrawing Life-Sustaining Therapy—*Continued*

Steps	Rationale	Special Considerations
10. Turn off all monitors.	Eliminates focus on the monitor.	Pulse can be checked by palpation. Blood pressure can be checked manually, if necessary, to assess whether additional pain medication is necessary.
11. Ensure that the family is present.	Ensures that significant family members are there to support the patient and each other.	Some family members may choose to be close by but not in the room when life-sustaining therapy is withheld or withdrawn.
12. Ensure that the environment is as the patient or family wants it.	Promotes patient and family involvement.	
13. Ensure that key members of the health care team are present (e.g., critical care nurse, attending physician, respiratory therapy, pastor).	Presents a team approach to support the patient, family, and each other.	There may be health care providers who the patient or family specifically wish to be present.
14. Initiate pain medication as prescribed (e.g., low dose of pain medication; less than 5 mg/hr of morphine).	Promotes comfort.	If the patient was already receiving pain medication at a constant infusion, the same rate of infusion would continue.
15. Withhold or withdraw therapy.	Discontinues unwanted therapy.	
16. Titrate intravenous pain medication to signs of patient distress.	Minimizes distress and promotes comfort.	Bolus doses of pain medication should be administered, and the infusion rate should be titrated until comfort is promoted.
17. Support the patient and the family.	Aids comfort.	
18. Provide time for the patient and the family to be alone, if so desired.	Aids the grief process.	
19. Assist the family with the grief process.	Aids family coping.	

Expected Outcomes

- Patient wishes regarding end-of-life care are honored.
- Therapies that are not wanted by the patient or family or both are withheld or withdrawn.
- Patient dignity and comfort are achieved.
- Family is actively involved in end-of-life care.
- Patient and family receive needed support.
- Patient death occurs (time frame may vary from minutes to hours to days).

Unexpected Outcomes

- The patient receives unwanted therapies.
- The patient has discomfort.
- Family members are not involved in end-of-life care.
- Family conflicts arise regarding end-of-life therapy decisions.
- Patient survives withholding or withdrawing of life support, necessitating consideration of a new plan of care and the possibility of long-term care.

Patient Monitoring and Care

Steps	Rationale	Reportable Conditions
		These conditions should be reported if they persist despite nursing interventions.

1. Assess the patient for discomfort:
  A. Verbalization of pain
  B. Moaning
  C. Grimacing
	Signs of discomfort indicate ineffective management of comfort.	• Discomfort

Patient Monitoring and Care—*Continued*

Steps	Rationale	Reportable Conditions
D. Increase in heart rate E. Increase in blood pressure F. Labored respirations G. Restlessness H. Delirium		
2. Titrate analgesia or anxiolytics to comfort.	Promotes patient dignity and comfort.	• Unrelieved pain • Dyspnea • Anxiety
3. Assess vital signs before withholding or withdrawing life-sustaining therapy, then only as necessary to ensure that the patient is not experiencing pain.	Promotes patient dignity and comfort. Minimizes unnecessary data.	• Decreasing values of vital signs are normal and expected as life-sustaining therapy is being withheld or withdrawn; thus these should be reported only as needed to keep the health team informed. • Increasing values of vital signs may indicate that pain medication is insufficient.
4. Support the patient and the family through the entire process.	Provides additional emotional support, promotes family functioning, aids in the grief process.	• Ineffective family functioning or need for additional support services

Documentation

Documentation should include the following:

- Patient and family education
- Patient, health care proxy, or family wishes regarding end-of-life care
- Coordination of the end-of-life process
- Patient, health care proxy, or family understanding of the withholding or withdrawing process and the anticipated outcome
- Involved family and health care team members
- When and how life-sustaining therapy was withheld or withdrawn

- Patient level of comfort
- How comfort was promoted
- Medication administered
- Time of patient death
- Unexpected outcomes
- Additional interventions

References

1. American Association of Critical-Care Nurses. (1990). *Withholding and/or Withdrawing Life-Sustaining Therapy.* Laguna Niguel, CA: Author.
2. American Nurses Association. (1991). *Position Statement on Promotion of Comfort and Relief in Dying Patients.* Kansas City, MO: Author.
3. Beauchamp, T.L., and Childress, J.F. (1994). *Principles of Biomedical Ethics.* 4th ed. New York: Oxford University Press.

Additional Readings

American Nurses Association. (1992). *Position Statement on Nursing Care and Do-Not-Resuscitate Decisions.* Washington, DC: Author.

American Nurses Association. (1992). *Position Statement on Foregoing Artificial Nutrition and Hydration.* Washington, DC: Author.
American Nurses Association. (1991). *Position Statement on Nursing and the Patient Self-Determination Act.* Kansas City, MO: Author.
Campbell, M.L. (1998). *Forgoing Life-Sustaining Therapy.* Laguna Niguel, CA: AACN.
President's Commission for the Study of Ethical Problems in Medicine and Biomedical and Behavioral Research. (1983). Washington, DC: Government Printing Office.
The Hastings Center. (1987). *Guidelines on the Termination of Life-Sustaining Therapy and the Care of the Dying.* Briarcliff Manor, NY: Author.

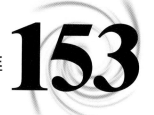

P R O C E D U R E **153**

Calculating Doses, Flow Rates, and Administration of Continuous Intravenous Infusions

P U R P O S E : Calculation of dosages and flow rates for continuous intravenous (IV) infusions is done to ensure delivery of the correct amount of medication. Many of the medications delivered by continuous IV infusion have potent effects and narrow margins of safety; therefore, accuracy in calculating and administering these agents is imperative.

Barbara A. Brown

PREREQUISITE NURSING KNOWLEDGE

- Knowledge of aseptic technique is important.
- Many different types of medications are delivered as continuous IV infusions in acute and critical care. These medications include, but are not limited to, vasoactive, inotropic, antidysrhythmic, sedative, and analgesic agents. Nurses must possess knowledge about the actions, indications, desired patient response, dosage, and adverse effects of the medication being administered.
- Hemodynamic assessment and electrocardiographic (ECG) monitoring are frequently necessary to evaluate the patient response to the infusion. The nurse must be familiar with monitoring equipment such as noninvasive blood pressure cuffs, cardiac monitors, arterial lines, and pulmonary artery catheters.
- Titration is adjustment of the dose, either increasing or decreasing, to attain the desired patient response. Weaning is a gradual decrease of the dose when the medication is being discontinued.
- Volume-controlled infusion devices are required to precisely deliver and titrate continuous infusions. Alterations or interruptions of the flow rate can significantly affect the dose of medication being delivered and adversely affect the patient.

- "Smart technologies" are electronic devices such as computers, bedside monitors, or infusion pumps, which will perform calculations of doses and flow rates after information is entered and programmed by the user. Although these devices are not universally available, their use may help to reduce medication errors.[1]
- There are three factors involved in the calculations for continuous IV infusions:
  - ❖ The concentration is the amount of medication diluted in a given volume of IV solution (e.g., 400 mg dopamine diluted in 250 ml normal saline (NS), or 2 g lidocaine diluted in 500 ml 5% dextrose in water [D_5W]).
  - ❖ The dose of the medication is the amount of medication to be administered over a certain length of time (e.g., dopamine 5 mcg/kg/min, or lidocaine 2 mg/min). The units of measure for the dose will differ for various medications. The length of time is 1 minute or 1 hour. If the medication is weight-based, the dose of the medication is per kilogram of patient weight.
  - ❖ The flow rate is the rate of delivery of the IV fluid solution (e.g., 20 ml/hr). The units of measure of the flow rate are always ml/hr.
- All units of measure in the formula must be the same. It frequently is necessary to perform some conversions on the concentration prior to entering it into the formula. The units of measure of the concentration must be

converted to the same units of measure of the dose (e.g., the concentration of dopamine is measured in mg, but the dose of dopamine is measured in mcg). Additionally, the mathematical calculations are simplified if the concentration is expressed per milliliter of fluid, rather than the total volume of the IV container.

- The mathematical formula for continuous IV infusions contains the three factors involved in continuous infusions (Table 153-1). When two factors are known, the third can be calculated by using the basic formula. Therefore, when the concentration of the solution and the prescribed dose are known, the flow rate can be determined. When the concentration of the solution and the flow rate are known, the dose can be determined. The two known factors are entered into the formula, and the mathematical computations are solved to determine the third factor. Variations on the basic formula are used to allow for medications delivered per hour or per minute and for medications that are weight-based (Tables 153-2 and 153-3).

- Calculations for weight-based medications include the patient's weight in the formula. The choice of which weight to use can be challenging. There is much disagreement

---

TABLE 153-1 **Basic Formulae***

1. To determine an unknown flow rate

$$\frac{\text{Dose (mg/hr or mcg/hr)}}{\text{Concentration (mg/ml or mcg/ml)}} = \text{Flow rate (ml/hr)}$$

2. To determine an unknown dose

$$\text{Flow rate (ml/hr)} \times \text{Concentration (mg/ml or mcg/ml)} = \text{Dose (mg/hr or mcg/hr)}$$

3. To determine the concentration of drug in 1 ml of fluid

$$\frac{\text{Total amount of drug (mg or mcg)}}{\text{Total volume of fluid (ml)}} = \text{Concentration} \frac{\text{(mg or mcg)}}{\text{(ml)}}$$

Example: when flow rate is unknown: diltiazem 125 mg/125 ml D$_5$W to be administered at 10 mg/hr.

A. Calculate concentration of drug in 1 ml of fluid

$$\frac{125 \text{ mg}}{125 \text{ ml}} = \frac{1 \text{ mg}}{\text{ml}}$$

B. Enter known factors into the formula and solve

Flow rate (ml/hr) × Concentration (mg or mcg/ml) = Dose (mg or mcg/ml)

$$\frac{10 \text{ ml/hr}}{1 \text{ mg/ml}} = 10 \text{ ml/hr}$$

Example: when dose is unknown: diltiazem 125 mg/125 ml D$_5$W is infusing at 15 ml/hr.

A. Calculate concentration of drug in 1 ml of fluid

$$\frac{125 \text{ mg}}{125 \text{ ml}} = \frac{1 \text{ mg}}{1 \text{ ml}}$$

B. Enter known factors into the formula and solve

15 ml/hr × 1 mg/ml = 15 mg/hr

---

*Since there are units on the top of the equation and units on the bottom of the equation, to ensure that the final units are correct, the units on the bottom of the equation must be inverted and multiplied by the units of the top of the equation. Example:

$$\frac{1800 \text{ mcg/hr}}{200 \text{ mcg/ml}} = \frac{9 \times \text{ml}}{\text{hr}} = 9 \text{ ml/hr}$$

TABLE 153-2 **Variation for Medication Doses Measured per Minute (mg/min or mcg/min)***

To determine unknown flow rate

$$\frac{\text{Dose (mg/min or mcg/min} \times 60 \text{ min/hr)}}{\text{Concentration (mg/ml or mcg/ml)}} = \text{Flow rate (ml/hr)}$$

To determine unknown dose

$$\frac{\text{Flow rate (ml/hr)} \times \text{Concentration (mg/ml or mcg/ml)}}{60 \text{ min/hr}}$$

$$= \text{Dose (mg/min or mcg/min)}$$

Example: when flow rate is unknown: nitroglycerin 50 mg/250 ml D$_5$W to be administered at 30 mcg/min.

A. Convert the concentration to like units of measure

$$\frac{50 \text{ mg}}{250 \text{ ml}} \times \frac{1000 \text{ mcg}}{1 \text{ mg}} = \frac{50,000 \text{ mcg}}{250 \text{ ml}}$$

B. Calculate concentration of drug in 1 ml of fluid

$$\frac{50,000 \text{ mcg}}{250 \text{ ml}} = \frac{200 \text{ mcg}}{1 \text{ ml}}$$

C. Enter known factors into the formula and solve

$$\frac{30 \text{ mcg/min} \times 60 \text{ min/hr}}{200 \text{ mcg/ml}} = 9 \text{ ml/hr}$$

Example: when dose is unknown: lidocaine 2 g/500 ml D$_5$W is infusing at 30 ml/hr.

A. Convert the concentration to like units of measure

$$\frac{2 \text{ g}}{500 \text{ ml}} \times \frac{1000 \text{ mg}}{1 \text{ g}} = \frac{2000 \text{ mg}}{500 \text{ ml}}$$

B. Calculate concentration of drug in 1 ml of fluid

$$\frac{2000 \text{ mg}}{500 \text{ ml}} = \frac{4 \text{ mg}}{\text{ml}}$$

C. Enter known factors into formula and solve

$$\frac{30 \text{ ml/hr} \times 4 \text{ mg/ml}}{60 \text{ min/hr}} = 2 \text{ mg/min}$$

---

*The time factor of 60 min/hr must be added to the basic formula.

---

and inconsistency in the literature as to which weight to use, ideal body weight, actual body weight, or dry body weight.[2,3] Distribution of specific medications across fat and fluid body compartments varies, thus affecting the therapeutic level. Since most medications will be titrated to patient response and a desired clinical end-point, a consistent approach is to use the patient's admission weight for initial dose calculations. The clinical pharmacist then should be consulted for obese patients and for medications that have potentially dangerous toxicities.

- Central IV access should be utilized for vasoconstrictive medications and for medications that can cause tissue damage when extravasated.[4] Mechanisms and agents that may cause tissue damage include osmotic damage secondary to hyperosmolar solutions, ischemic necrosis caused by vasoconstrictors and certain cation solutions, direct cellular toxicity caused by antineoplastic agents, direct tissue damage from pH strong acids and bases, and direct irritation.[5]

TABLE 153-3	**Variation for Weight-Based Medication Doses Measured per Minute (mcg/kg/min)***

To determine unknown flow rate

$$\frac{\text{Dose (mcg/kg/min)} \times 60 \text{ min/hr} \times \text{Patient weight (kg)}}{\text{Concentration (mcg/ml)}}$$

$$= \text{Flow rate (ml/hr)}$$

To determine unknown dose

$$\frac{\text{Flow rate (ml/hr)} \times \text{Concentration (mcg/ml)}}{60 \text{ min/hr} \times \text{Patient weight (kg)}} = \text{Dose (mcg/kg/min)}$$

Example: when flow rate is unknown: dopamine 400 mg/250 ml D$_5$W to infuse at 5 mcg/kg/min. Patient weighs 100 kg.

A. Convert the concentration to like units of measure

$$\frac{400 \text{ mg}}{250 \text{ ml}} \times \frac{1000 \text{ mcg}}{1 \text{ mg}} = \frac{400,000 \text{ mcg}}{250 \text{ ml}}$$

B. Calculate concentration of drug in 1 ml of fluid

$$\frac{400,000 \text{ mcg}}{250 \text{ ml}} = \frac{1600 \text{ mcg}}{1 \text{ ml}}$$

C. Enter known factors into the formula and solve

$$\frac{5 \text{ mcg/kg/min} \times 60 \text{ min/hr} \times 100 \text{ kg}}{1600 \text{ mcg/ml}} = 18.75 \text{ ml/hr}$$

Example: when dose is unknown: dobutamine 500 mg/250 ml D$_5$W is infusing at 15 ml/hr. Patient weighs 70 kg.

A. Convert the concentration to like units of measure

$$\frac{500 \text{ mg}}{250 \text{ ml}} \times \frac{1000 \text{ mcg}}{\text{mg}} = \frac{50,000 \text{ mcg}}{250 \text{ ml}}$$

B. Calculate concentration of drug in 1 ml of fluid

$$\frac{50,000 \text{ mcg}}{250 \text{ ml}} = \frac{2000 \text{ mcg}}{\text{ml}}$$

C. Enter known factors into the formula and solve

$$\frac{15 \text{ ml/hr} \times 2000 \text{ mcg/ml}}{60 \text{ min/hr} \times 70 \text{ kg}} = 7.14 \text{ mcg/kg/min}$$

*The patient's weight in kilograms and the time factor of 60 min/hr must be added to the basic formula.

EQUIPMENT

- Prepared IV solution with medication to be administered
- IV tubing
- IV infusion device
- Nonsterile gloves
- Alcohol pads
- Calculator (optional)

PATIENT AND FAMILY EDUCATION

- Explain the indications and expected response to the pharmacologic therapy. ➤*Rationale:* Patients and families need explanations of the plan of care and interventions.
- Instruct the patient to report adverse symptoms, as indicated. Reportable symptoms include, but are not limited to pain, burning, itching, or swelling at the IV site; dizziness; shortness of breath; palpitations; and chest pain. ➤*Rationale:* Assists the nurse to evaluate response to the pharmacologic therapy and to identify adverse reactions.

PATIENT ASSESSMENT AND PREPARATION

Patient Assessment

- Assess medication allergies. ➤*Rationale:* Identification and prevention of allergic reactions.
- Obtain vital signs and hemodynamic parameters. ➤*Rationale:* Establishes the need for vasoactive agents and provides baseline data to evaluate response to therapy.
- Assess the ECG. ➤*Rationale:* Establishes the need for antidysrhythmic therapy and provides baseline data.
- Obtain other assessments relevant to the medication being administered, e.g., sedation scale for continuous IV sedatives.

Patient Preparation

- Ensure that the patient and family understand preprocedural teaching. Answer questions as they arise and reinforce information as needed. ➤*Rationale:* Evaluates and reinforces understanding of previously taught information.
- Weigh the patient, if the medication is weight-based. ➤*Rationale:* Permits calculation of the correct dose based on patient weight. Use of dry weight is preferable.
- Verify patency or obtain patent, appropriate IV access. ➤*Rationale:* Ensures delivery of the medication into the IV space. Some continuous infusion medications require central line access to prevent irritation or damage to smaller peripheral veins and to reduce the risk for extravasation.

Procedure	**for Calculating Doses, Flow Rates, and Administration of Continuous Intravenous Infusions**	
Steps	**Rationale**	**Special Considerations**
1. Verify the prescription ordered by the physician or the advanced practice nurse.	Prevents errors in medication administration.	The prescription should include the medication, dose, and the prescribed parameters for titration of the dose. The concentration of the solution and the diluent should be indicated in the order or determined by institutional policy.

Procedure	for Calculating Doses, Flow Rates, and Administration of Continuous Intravenous Infusions—*Continued*		
Steps	**Rationale**	**Special Considerations**	
2. Wash hands and don gloves.	Reduces transmission of microorganisms; standard precautions.		
3. Connect and flush the IV solution (with prescribed medication) through the tubing system.	Prepares the infusion system.		
4. Place the IV infusion in the infusion device. *There are two methods to perform the next step; choose either step 5 or step 6, or both as a double-check.*			
5. Determine the correct flow rate using manual mathematical calculation method. A. Convert the concentration of the solution to the same units of measure as the dose. B. Calculate the concentration of the medication per ml of fluid. C. Enter the concentration and the dose into the formula and solve for the flow rate.	The infusion device controls the consistent and accurate delivery of the flow rate. All units of measure must be the same to perform the mathematical functions. Necessary for medication calculation. Necessary for medication calculation. Entering information into the device is required for the device to perform the calculations.	Infusion devices are electrical equipment and may malfunction. Monitor the infusion for accuracy in flow rate. Use alternate formulas if medication dose is a per-minute or weight-based dose (Tables 153-1, 153-2 and 153-3).	
6. Determine correct flow rate using electronic devices. A. Enter necessary information into the device, including—but not limited to—patient weight, drug name, concentration of solution, dose ordered. B. Program device to electronically calculate the flow rate.	Prevents errors in medication administration. Ensures patient safety. Prevents mathematical errors or data entry and programming errors.		
7. Verify the five rights of medication administration: right patient, right drug, right dose, right time, right route.			
8. Double-check flow rate calculations or programming with another qualified individual.			
9. Connect the infusion system to the intended IV line or catheter.	Prepares the infusion.	Alcohol is used to cleanse the IV port before connecting the infusion, or the infusion system may be connected into a stopcock port.	
10. Discard used supplies and wash hands.	Reduces transmission of microorganisms; standard precautions.		
11. Set the flow rate on the infusion pump; initiate the infusion.	Initiates therapy.		
12. Document in patient record.			

Expected Outcomes

- Desired patient response is achieved.
- Correct dose of medication is administered.
- Dose is titrated to achieve/maintain desired patient response.

Unexpected Outcomes

- Adverse reactions to the medication occur.
- Incorrect dose of medication is administered.
- Desired patient response is not achieved/maintained.
- Infiltration or extravasation of medication occurs.

Patient Monitoring and Care

Steps	Rationale	Reportable Conditions
		These conditions should be reported if they persist despite nursing interventions. • Adverse reactions • Hemodynamic instability • Cardiac dysrhythmias • Excessive sedation • Respiratory depression
1. Evaluate patient response by monitoring the indicated parameters for the medication being infused.	Medications given as continuous infusions often have potent effects and potentially serious adverse effects. Most medications given as continuous infusions have a quick onset of action. Frequent monitoring of parameters is necessary during initiation of the infusion.	
2. If the patient response is inadequate, titrate the infusion as prescribed until the prescribed parameters are met.	The patient's response to many continuous infusions is dose-dependent. To achieve the desired response, titration of the dose is necessary.	• Desired response not achieved within an acceptable dosage
3. Assess IV access for catheter placement, catheter patency, and signs of infiltration or extravasation every 1 to 4 hours and as needed.	Ensures delivery of the medication into the venous system. Prevents interruptions in delivery of the medication. Provides early recognition of complications.	• Extravasation of any medication

Documentation

Documentation should include the following:

- Patient and family education
- Name of the medication and the type of solution in which medication is diluted; concentration of the solution; dose; flow rate; and administration times
- Assessment of the IV access and site
- Parameters monitored and patient response
- Adverse reactions and interventions to treat the reaction
- Titration

References

1. Institute for Safe Medication Practices (ISMP) Medication Safety Alert. (2002). *Smart Infusion Pumps Join CPOE and Bar Coding as Important Ways to Prevent Medications Errors.* Feb. 7, 2002. Huntington Valley, PA: Institute for Safe Medication Practices.
2. Varon, J., and Marik, P. (2001). Management of the obese critically ill patient. *Critical Care Clinics,* 17, 187-200.
3. Deglin, J.H., and Vallerand, A.H. (2003). *Davis's Drug Guide for Nurses.* 8th ed. Philadelphia: F.A. Davis Co.
4. Nursing. (2001). *IV Drug Handbook.* 7th ed. Springhouse, PA: Springhouse.
5. Upton, J., Mulliken, J.B., and Murray, J.E. (1979). Major intravenous extravasation injuries. *Am J Surg,* 137, 497-506.

Additional Readings

Guiliano, K., et al. (1993). A new strategy for calculating medication infusion rates. *Crit Care Nurs,* 13, 77-82.
Hadaway, L.C. (2001). How to safeguard delivery of high-alert IV drugs. *Nursing,* 31, 36-42.
McMillen, P. (2000). Calculating medication dosages. *Crit Care Nurs,* 20, 17-9.
Springhouse's Dosage Calculations Made Incredibly Easy. (2002). 2nd ed. Springhouse, PA: Springhouse.

Index